# SCIENCE

NEW SERIES. VOLUME LXXVII

JANUARY-JUNE, 1933

NEW YORK
THE SCIENCE PRESS
1933

THE SCIENCE PRESS PRINTING COMPANY
LANCASTER, PENNSYLVANIA

3 77

# CONTENTS AND INDEX

## NEW SERIES. VOL. LXXVII—JANUARY TO JUNE, 1933

THE NAMES OF CONTRIBUTORS ARE PRINTED IN SMALL CAPITALS


Absorption of Carbon Dioxide by Leaves, A. J. HEINICKE and M. B. HOFFMAN, 55

Academy, of Arts and Sciences, Amer., 485; of Natural Sciences, Philadelphia, 512; of Science, Texas, H. B. PARKS, 54, 565; of Oklahoma, H. J. HARPER, 55; of Tennessee, J. T. MCGILL, 192; Colorado-Wyoming, R. J. GILMORE, 329; Alabama, E. B. CARMICHAEL, 329; of Minnesota, 405; of Ohio, W. H. ALEXANDER, 539; of Illinois, H. R. WANLESS, 540; of Tennessee, F. G. SLACK, 541; of Virginia, E. C. L. MILLER, 541; of Iowa, J. C. GILMAN, 563; of Kansas, G. E. JOHNSON, 564; of Sciences, Washington, 83; of California, 383; National, 422, 454, 494, 517; Medals, 514; W. W. CAMPBELL, 549

Adrenal Cortical Hormone, N. E. FREEMAN, 211; W. W. SWINGLE and OTHERS, 58; S. W. BRITTON and H. SILVETTE, 366; J. MCK. CATTELL, 428

Aerated Water, H. B. SIFTON, 431

Agricultural Exper. Sta., C. G. WILLIAMS, 155

Agriculture and Research, H. A. WALLACE, 475

ALEXANDER, J., Bacterial Filtrability, 449; Food Products, 489

ALEXANDER, W. H., Ohio Acad. of Science, 539

Alkali Treatment of Soils, G. T. SHAW and R. R. MCKIBBIN, 411

ALLEN, E., D. B. CALVIN and M. D. OVERHOLSER, Harry Hayward Charlton, 598

American Association for the Advancement of Science, Pacific Div., 44, Salt Lake City Meeting, 460; Atlantic City Meeting, B. E. LIVINGSTON, 123; Officers for 1933, 15, General, 126; Membership and Financial Reports, 126; Secretaries' Conference, 128; Academy Conference, 128; Press Service, 129; Science Exhibition, 129; Association Prize, 130; President Elect, 132; Newly Elected Permanent Secretary, 133; General Sessions, 134; Scientific Sessions: A—135; B—137; C—139; D—139, 375; E—140; F—140; G—142; Programs Related to both F and G, 145; H—147, 29; I—147, 578; K—148; L—149; M—150, Address, 1; N—150; O—152, 155; Q—153; Organizations related to the Association as a Whole, 154; Southwestern Division, New Mexico Meeting, 278; Meeting of Executive Committee, H. B. WARD, 452; Chicago Meeting, Geology and Geography at, 345; Hotel Headquarters, 453; Preliminary Program, H. B. WARD, 461, 467; Evening Meetings, 462, Entertainment for Ladies, 464; Century of Progress Exposition, 464; Points of Interest and Excursions, 465; Press Service, 465; Membership, 466; Business Sessions, 466; Hotel Headquarters and Transportation, 466; Scientific Sections and Societies, 467; Mathematics, 554; Chemistry, 555; Medical Sciences, 556; 622

Amoeba, The Spelling of, M. F. GUYER, 307

Anatomical Preparations, Mounting, H. W. SCHOENBORN and C. P. HICKMAN, 287

ANDERSON, C. D., Free Positive Electrons, 432

Anemia, Nutritional, in Rats, R. E. REMINGTON, 115

Anesthesia, Electric, F. PETERSON, 326

Anthrax, Active Immunization, G. E. ROCKWELL, 612

Antiprothrombin and Globulins, I. P. EARLE and P. E. HOWE, 213

Ants, Swarming and Mating of, C. C. GUTHRIE, 627

Aquarium Aerator, E. C. DRIVER, 565

Arboretum, Morris, 184, 404, 503

ASCHAM, L., Vitamin A in Pimiento Pepper, 351

Asphyxiation, Deaths from, 442

Atomic Weight of Lead from Pitchblende, G. P. BAXTER and C. M. ALTER, 431

Australia, Central, J. B. CLELAND, 260

Australian Fossils for Harvard Museum, 232

AVINOFF, A., William Jacob Holland, 204

Bacteria and Ultra-violet Light, F. L. GATES, 350; Growth of, J. M. SHERMAN and G. M. CAMERON, 537

Bacterial Gall Disease of Douglas Fir, H. N. HANSEN and R. E. SMITH, 628

BALCH, W. B., Respirometer, 116

Bancroft, Wilder D., Award of Nichols Medal, 164

Banting Research Foundation, V. E. HENDERSON and D. T. FRASER, 192

BARRON, D. H., Albino Rats and Amytal, 372

BARROWS, A. L., National Research Council, 356

BATEMAN, J. B., Medusae, 451

BAUDISCH, O., Active Iron, 317

Bausch, Edward, Dinner in Honor of, 110

BAXTER, G. P., and C. M. ALTER, Atomic Weight of Lead from Pitchblende, 431

Beds, Red, Hamilton, G. H. CHADWICK, 86

Belling, John, C. B. DAVENPORT, 250

BELLING, J., Univalent Chromosomes, 260

BENGTSON, I. A., Bacterium Granulosis and Trachoma, 218

BERKSON, J., Coefficient of Correlation, 259

BERRY, J. A., Lactobacilli in Peas, 350

BEVANS, C. A., Illuminator, 116

Biological, Laboratory, Cold Spring Harbor, Conferences, 530; Sciences, National Research Fellowships in, 577; Literature, D. REDDICK, 625

BISHOPP, F. C., Mosquitoes and Live Stock, 115

BLAKE, C. H., Nomenclatorial Notes on Gastrotricha, 606

BLAKESLEE, A. F., Genetics, E. W. Sinnott and L. C. Dunn, 284; F. W. Sansome and J. Philp, 284

Blood Cells, R. C. PARKER, 544

Bloodsucking Insects, A. DAMPF, 20

BLUMENTHAL, L. M., "A Correlation Curiosity," 88

Bog, Sphagnum, G. B. RIGG, 535

BOGERT, M. T., Mechanism of the Ionene Synthesis, 197; Phenanthrene and Derivatives, 289

BONAR, R., F. BONAR and E. C. H. DAVIES, Cellophane Roll Films, 217

BOND, W. R., Artificial Respiration, 515

BORING, E. G., Law of Effect, 307

Borreliotoses, E. W. GOODPASTURE, 119

BORSOOK, H., and G. KEIGHLEY, Urea Synthesis, 114

BOSS, L. F., Current for Potentiometers, 331

Botanical Garden, New York, 82

Boulder, Dam Project Area, 233; Canyon Lake, 276

BOWIE, W., Gravity Apparatus, 308

Bragg, Sir William, and Royal Institution, 484

BRAND, E., and M. M. HARRIS, Protein Metabolism, 589

BRASCH, F. E., Rufus Lot Green, 11

British, East African Expedition, 404; Entomological Society, 421; Association for Advancement of Science, 484; Academic Assistance Council, 620, 629

BRITTON, S. W., and H. SILVETTE, Cortico-adrenal Function, 366

Brooklyn Botanic Garden, 362

Brooks, Fred E., C. R. CUTRIGHT, 527

BROOKS, S. C., Species Differences, 221

BROWN, F. M., Meteor Crater, 239

BROWNE, C. A., Spontaneous Heating and Ignition, 223

BRUCE, W. F., Disintegrator for Yeast Cells, 543

BRYANT, E. C., The Pinhole Image, 428

Bulbs from Holland, F. P. MCWHORTER, 21

BURKE, J. J., Eocene Lagomorpha, 191

BUSH, V., In Honor of Elihu Thomson, 418

California Academy of Sciences, 383
CAMPBELL, W. W., National Academy of Sciences, 549
Cancer Research, C. C. LITTLE, 214
Caribbean Region, 109
CARMAN, A. P., Ether Structure, 114
CARMICHAEL, E. B., Alabama Academy of Science, 329
Carty, John Joseph, F. B. JEWETT, 41
CATTELL, J. MCK., American Men of Science in 1932, 264; The Adrenal Glands, 428; Opportunity for Exceptional Ability, 491
Cellophane for Lantern Slides, B. H. WALDEN, 91; F. F. YONKMAN, 218; Roll Films, R. BONAR, F. BONAR and E. C. H. DAVIES, 217
Century of Progress Exposition, 164
CHADWICK, G. H., Hamilton Red Beds, 86
Charlton, Harry Hayward, E. ALLEN, D. B. CALVIN and M. D. OVERHOLSER, 598
Chemical, Education, *Journal* of, 110; Analysis, J. F. MCCLENDON, 189; Soc., Amer., Meeting, 234
Chemistry, Council for, 300
Chicago Museum of Science, Danish Exhibit, 206
Chicks, a "Scurvy-like" Disease in, W. F. HOLST and E. R. HALBROOK, 354
CHILD, G. P., and R. B. HOWLAND, Developmental Processes in Egg of Drosophila, 396
Chromosomes, Univalent, J. BELLING, 260
Cirriped, Cretaceous, H. A. PILSBRY, 283
Citrus Fruits, E. K. NELSON and G. L. KEENAN, 561
Clamp, Stop-cock, A. F. ROE, 566
CLARK, E. P., Rotenone, 311
CLAYTON, H. H., Solar Variations and Atmospheric Pressure, 568
CLELAND, J. B., Expedition to Central Australia, 260
COCKERELL, T. D. A., Creative Evolution, C. C. Hurst, 89
COE, W. R., Destruction of Mooring Ropes, 447
COFFMAN, F. A., Heterosis, 114
COFMAN, V., Mendeleev Congress, 286
Colleges, Land Grant, Reduction in Aid for, 599
Collier, John, Commissioner of Indian Affairs, 384
Color Blindness, T. R. GARTH, 333
COLTON, H. S., Earliest Dated Dwelling, 240
COMPTON, A. H., Cosmic Rays, 480
COMPTON, K. T., Greeting to Professor Einstein, 271; Professor Thomson's Work in Electrical Engineering, 415
Conjunctivitis, Experimental Granular, P. K. OLITSKY, J. T. SYVERTON and J. R. TYLER, 25
Conservation, V. E. SHELFORD, 535
COOPER, G. A., Preparation of Fossils, 394
COPISAROW, M., Twisted Trees, 581
Cornell University, Heckscher Grants, 207
"Correlation, Curiosity, A," L. M. BLUMENTHAL, 88; Coefficient of, J. BERKSON, 259
Cortin and Traumatic Shock, N. E. FREEMAN, 212
Cosmic, Parade, H. SHAPLEY, 272; Rays, A. H. COMPTON, 480
Councilman, William Thomas, H. CUSHING, 613
Criticisms, C. D. PERRINE, 20
Culture Methods, J. G. NEEDHAM, 427
CUNNINGHAM, E. R., German Periodicals, 409
Curme, George Oliver, Chandler Medal, 83
CURTIS, M. R., W. F. DUNNING and F. D. BULLOCK, Malignancy, 175
Curve, Normal, Anniversary of, C. J. MARSH, 583
CUSHING, H., William Thomas Councilman, 613
CUTRIGHT, C. R., Fred E. Brooks, 527
Cytology, Vicious Circle in, E. C. JEFFREY, 49

DALE, H. H., Therapeutics, 521
DALY, C. A., Air Supply of Micro Burners, 413
DALY, R. A., The Depths of the Earth, 95
DAMPF, A., Bloodsucking Insects, 20
Danish Exhibit at Chicago Museum of Science, 206
DARROW, G. M., and G. F. WALDO, Photoperiodism, 353
DARROW, K. K., Electricity Released from Matter, 591
Darwinism, Revivals of, H. F. OSBORN, 199
DAVENPORT, C. B., John Belling, 250
DAVIS, R. O. E. and W. SCHOLL, Ammoniation of Peat, 330
DELLENBAUGH, F. S., Naming the Grand Canyon, 349
DE TERRA, H., Yale North India Expedition, 497
Diabetes, J. F. REGAN and B. O. BARNES, 214
DICKSON, L. E., Eliakim Hastings Moore, 79
Dilatometer, Universal, R. HOLCOMB, 261
DOYLE, W. L., Microdetermination of Carbon, 173
DRIVER, E. C., Aquarium Aerator, 565
Drosophila, Developmental Processes in Egg of, G. P. CHILD and R. B. HOWLAND, 396
DUSSER DE BARENNE, J. G., Nerve Cells of the Cerebral Cortex, 546
Dwelling, Earliest, Dated, H. S. COLTON, 240

EARLE, I. P., and P. E. HOWE, Antiprothrombin and Globulins, 213
Earth, the Depths of, R. A. DALY, 95
Earthquakes, B. WILLIS, 351
Ectocarpus siliculosus Dillw., G. F. PAPENFUSS, 390
Effect, Law of, E. L. THORNDIKE, 173; E. G. BORING, 307
EGGLESTON, W. W., Timothy E. Wilcox, 300
Eggs, Stored, "Pink White" in, F. W. LORENZ, H. J. ALMQUIST and G. W. HENDRY, 606
Einstein, Professor, K. T. COMPTON, 271, H. SHAPLEY, 272; and Prussian Academy, 346, 444
EINSTEIN, A., Address, 274
Electrical Units, International, Revision, 251
Electricity Released from Matter, K. K. DARROW, 591
Electrons, Free Positive, C. D. ANDERSON, 432
Electroscope, B. A. WOOTEN and W. T. HARRIS, 630
Embedding Mixture, Paraffin, R. T. HANCE, 353
EMERSON, J. L., and A. C. HILDRETH, Transpiration of Evergreens, 433
Encephalomyelitis, Equine, Virus, A. P. KRUEGER, B. HOWITT and V. ZEILOR, 288
Engineering, Studies, 14; Week, 164
Entomological Society, British, 421
Eocene Lagomorpha, J. J. BURKE, 191
ESSIG, E. O., Nomenclature of Vegetable Weevil, 605
Ether Structure, A. P. CARMAN, 114
Everest, Mount, Natural History of, 43
Evolution, Vertebrate, W. K. GREGORY, 29
Evolutionist, Forgotten, S. J. HOLMES, 48
Exposition, Yale North India, 301; H. DE TERRA, 497
Eye Color in Drosophila melanogaster, J. W. GOWEN and E. H. GAY, 312
Eyes, Blue for Brown, V. STEFANSSON, 191
EYRING, H., Quantum Mechanics and Chemistry, 158

Faraday's Diary, W. F. MAGIE, 52, 308
Fellowships, National, at Johns Hopkins Univ., 109; of Mellon Institute, 503
FENTON, C. L., and M. A. FENTON, Hail Prints of Proterozoic Age, 491
Ferns, Eusporangiate, Tapetum of the W. N. STEIL, 606
FIELD, A. M., B. H. ALEXANDER and E. B. SYLVANUS, Soy-bean Paste, 91
Field Museum of Natural History, 13, 420
Films, Roll, Cellophane, R. BONAR, F. BONAR and E. C. H. DAVIES, 217
Filtrability, Bacterial, J. ALEXANDER, 449
Filtrable Cycle of Bacteria, C. V. SEASTONE and M. B. LAWRENCE, 259
FINCH, F. H., Sibling Resemblance, 373
Fisk, Harlan Wilbur, J. A. FLEMING, 80
Fixing Fluids, A. PETRUNKEVITCH, 117
FLEMING, J. A., Harlan Wilbur Fisk, 80; Nuclear Physics, 298; American Geophysical Union, 607
FLEXNER, A., University Patents, 325
FLEXNER, S., Poliomyelitis, 7, 413
Food Products, J. ALEXANDER, 489
FORBES, E. B., Normal Nutritive Value, 306
Forestry Program for Southeastern States, 43

Fossils, Vertebrate, E. W. SHULER, 368; Preparation of, G. A. COOPER, 394
FOX, W. J., A Rare Publication, 351
Franklin Institute, Honors, 538
FREEMAN, N. E., Cortin and Traumatic Shock, 211
Fungi and Termites, E. C. HENDEE, 212
Fungus, Root-rot, in Texas, H. C. McNAMARA, R. E. WESTER and K. C. GUNN, 510
Fusarium Disease of Peas, W. C. SNYDER, 327

G., F. P., Leonard Wood Memorial for the Eradication of Leprosy, 562
GAEHR, P. F., A Two-field Stroboscope, 412
Galactose Feeding of Dogs, J. H. ROE and R. F. CAHOON, 331
GALTSOFF, P. S., and L. E. CABLE, Current Rotor, 242
GARTH, T. R., Color Blindness, 333
Gases, Permeability of, A. L. ROMANOFF, 393
Gastrotricha, Nomenclatorial, C. H. BLAKE, 606
GATES, F. L., Bacteria and Ultra-violet Light, 350
Genetics, and Embryology, C. ZELENY, 177; of Fish, A. B. HOWELL, 389
Geological, Congress, International, 252; Classification, F. LEVERETT, 560
Geology and Boys and Girls, K. VER STEEG, 169
Geophysical Union, Amer., J. A. FLEMING, 607
GERICKE, W. F., Bread Wheat, 229
German Periodicals, E. R. CUNNINGHAM, 409
Germany, Situation in, 528
Gestalt Doctrines, E. L. THORNDIKE, 368
GIESE, A. C., and P. A. LEIGHTON, Fluorescence of Cells in the Ultra-violet, 509
GILMAN, J. C., Iowa Academy of Science, 563
GILMORE, R. J., Colorado-Wyoming Academy of Science, 329
Glacial Age in Wisconsin, M. M. LEIGHTON, 168
GODFREY, G. H., Greenhouse Plants, 583
Goiter Prevention, K. G. ZWICK, 627
GOODPASTURE, E. W., Borreliotoses, 119
Gorham, Frederic Poole, H. E. WALTER, 597
GORTNER, R. A., Medusae, 282
GOULD, C. N., Mesquite on the Great Plains, 511
GOWEN, J. W., and E. H. GAY, Eye Color in Drosophila melanogaster, 312
GRAHAM, C. F., Telephonic Drop Counter, 542
Grains, Clastic, C. K. WENTWORTH, 633
Grand Canyon, Naming, F. S. DELLENBAUGH, 349
Grapes, Seedless, A. B. STOUT, 310
Gravity Apparatus, W. BOWIE, 308
Green, Rufus Lot, F. E. BRASCH, 11
GREGG, A., University Patents, 257
GREGORY, W. K., Vertebrate Evolution, the New Anthropogeny, 29
GRODINSKY, M., M. BEBER and C. P. BAKER, Novocaine in Nervous Tissue, 450
Growth Retardation, F. S. HAMMETT, 190
GUTHRIE, C. C., Swarming of Ants, 627
GUYER, M. F., Spelling of Amoeba, 307

HAHN, O., Ponderable and Imponderable, 397
Hail Prints of Proterozoic Age, C. L. FENTON and M. A. FENTON, 491
HAMMETT, F. S., Growth Retardation, 190; Questions, 584
HANCE, R. T., Staining Action of Iron Haematoxylin, 287; Paraffin Embedding Mixture, 353
HANSEN, H. N., and R. E. SMITH, Bacterial Gall Disease of Douglas Fir, 628
Harding, Everhart Percy, S. C. LIND, 12
HARPER, H. J., Oklahoma Academy of Science, 55
HARRINGTON, E. L., ''Rotette'' for Liquids, 21
Harrison, Professor, as Croonian Lecturer, 530
Harvard Museum, Australian Fossils for, 232
HARVEY, E. N., Centrifuge-Microscope, 430
HASKINS, C. P., and C. N. MOORE, Twisting Habit, 283
Heart, Mammalian, Perfusion of, J. W. WILSON and J. M. DARLINGTON, 370
Heckscher Grants at Cornell University, 207
HEDRICK, E. R., Logic of Mathematics, 335
HEIDELBERGER, M., and A. E. O. MENZEL, Tubercle Bacillus, 24
HEINICKE, A. J., Photosynthesis, 516; and M. B. HOFFMAN, Absorption of Carbon Dioxide by Leaves, 55
HENDEE, E. C., Termites and Fungi, 212
HENDERSON, V. E., and D. T. FRASER, The Banting Research Foundation, 192
HENDERSON, Y., Patents are Ethical, 324; Public Service, 584
Henry, William Arnon, F. B. MORRISON, 160
Herbarium of W. W. Ashe, 206
HERRICK, G. W., and G. H. GRISWOLD, Webbing Clothes Moth, 391
Heterosis, F. A. COFFMAN, 114
Hicks, John F. G., R. W. HUFFERD, 108
HOLCOMB, R., Universal Dilatometer, 261
Holland, William Jacob, A. AVINOFF, 204
Hollick, Arthur, E. C. JEFFREY, 440
Holm, Herman Theodor, A. F. WOODS, 183
HOLMAN, R. M., Microscope Lamp, 610
HOLMES, S. J., A Forgotten Evolutionist, 48
Holmes, William Henry, W. HOUGH, 482
HOLST, W. F., and E. R. HALBROOK, ''Scurvy-like'' Disease in Chicks, 354
Hookworm Disease, C. W. STILES, 237
Hormone, Adrenal Cortical, W. W. SWINGLE, 58; N. E. FREEMAN, 211; S. W. BRITTON and H. SILVETTE, 366; J. McK. CATTELL, 428; Ovarian Follicular, 344
Hormone-like Substance, Extraction from Urine, D. PERLA and J. MARMORSTON, 432
HOUGH, W., William Henry Holmes, 482
Howard Method, J. D. WILDMAN, 263
HOWELL, A. B., Genetics of Fish, 389
HOWELL, W. H., Grants of National Research Council, 214; History of, 355
HRUBY, K., Double Staining, 352
HUFFERD, R. W., John F. G. Hicks, 108
Human Necrobacillosis, F. W. SHAW, 392
HUNGATE, J. W., Northwest Scientific Assoc., 193
HUNTINGTON, E. V., Attraction of a Sphere, 489
Hurst, C. C., Evolution, T. D. A. COCKERELL, 89

Ignition and Spontaneous Heating, C. A. BROWNE, 223
Illinois Academy of Science, H. R. WANLESS, 540
Illuminator, C. A. BEVANS, 116
Indian Affairs, New Commissioner, 384
Ionene Synthesis, M. T. BOGERT, 197
Ions, Adsorbed, Utilization by Plants, H. JENNY and E. W. COWAN, 394
Iowa Academy of Science, J. C. GILMAN, 563
Iron, Active, O. BAUDISCH, 317

JACKSON, D. C., National Research Council, 500
JAMES, E. S., Slide Technique, 369
JEFFREY, E. C., Vicious Circle in Cytology, 49; Maturation Divisions, 325; Arthur Hollick, 440
JENNY, H. and E. W. COWAN, Utilization of Adsorbed Ions by Plants, 394
JEWETT, F. B., John Joseph Carty, 41; Transmission and Reproduction of Music, 435
Jewish Scientific Men in Germany, 492, 620, 629
Johns Hopkins Univ., National Fellowships, 109; Conference on Chemistry, 320; Conference of Donors, 504
JOHNSON, D., Scientific Investigation, 569
JOHNSON, G. E., Kansas Academy of Science, 564
Joule, Pronunciation of Name, J. O. THOMPSON, 88

Kansas Academy of Science, G. E. JOHNSON, 564
Kentucky, Univ. of, Museums, 277
KEYES, D. B., Organic Reactions, 202
de Khotinsky, Achilles, P. E. KLOPSTEG, 382
KIMBALL, D. S., Mass Production, 1
KLOPSTEG, P. E., Achilles de Khotinsky, 382

KNIGHT, J. B., Zoological Nomenclature, 389
KRAATZ, W. C., Medusae, 87, 308
KRAUS, C. A., National Research Council, 552
KRUEGER, A. P., B. HOWITT and V. ZEILOR, Equine Encephalomyelitis, 288
Kymograph Recording, F. F. YONKMAN, 172

Laboratory Unit for Lighting, S. E. POND and O. MEIER, JR., 585
Lactobacilli in Peas, J. A. BERRY, 350
Lake San Augustin, N. M., W. E. POWERS, 51
Lammert, Olive M., M. L. SAGUE, 275
LANGFELD, H. S., Response Psychology, 243
LEIGHTON, M. M., Wisconsin Glacial Age, 168
Leonard, Arthur Gray, H. E. SIMPSON, 108
LEVERETT, F., Geological Classification, 560
LIND, S. C., Everhart Percy Harding, 12
LITTLE, C. C., Variability and Individuality, 195; Cancer Research, 214
LIVINGSTON, B. E., Atlantic City Meeting of the American Association for the Advancement of Science, 123
Longevity and Optimum Growth, C. M. MCCAY, 410
LORENZ, F. W., H. J. ALMQUIST and G. W. HENDRY, "Pink White" in Stored Eggs, 606
Loubat, Prizes, Award of, to C. O. Paullin, J. K. Wright and W. P. Webb, 421
Louse and Its Host, F. H. WILSON, 490

MCCAY, C. M., Longevity and Optimum Growth, 410
MCCLENDON, J. F., Chemical Analysis, 189
MACFARLAND, F. M., Edwin Chapin Starks, 182
MCGILL, J. T., Tennessee Acad. of Science, 192
MCNAMARA, H. C., R. E. WESTER and K. C. GUNN, Root-rot Fungus in Texas, 510
MCWHORTER, F. P., Bulbs from Holland, 21
MAGIE, W. F., Faraday's Diary, 52, 308
Malignancy, M. R. CURTIS, W. F. DUNNING and F. D. BULLOCK, 175
MARSH, C. J., Anniversary of the Normal Curve, 583
Massachusetts Institute of Technology, Spectroscopy at, 162, 577; George Eastman Laboratories, 405, 443
Mathematics, Logic of, E. R. HEDRICK, 335; Native, G. A. MILLER, 366
Mather, Stephen Tyng, 529
Maturation Divisions, E. C. JEFFREY, 325
MAUGHAN, G. H., and E. MAUGHAN, Vitamin D, 198
Medal, Perkin, George Oenslager, 14; Chandler, George Oliver Curme, 83; Nichols, Wilder D. Bancroft, 164; Lamme, Edward Weston, 302; Inst. of Chemists, H. C. Sherman, 346; Willard Gibbs, Dr. Willstaetter, 385
Medical, Care, C.-E. A. WINSLOW, 102; Students, 277; Patents, 451
Medicine, School of, of Rosario, 232; of Paris, 251
Medusae, Fresh-water, W. C. KRAATZ, 87, Ohio, 308; R. A. GORTNER, 282; J. B. BATEMAN, 451
Mellon Inst., Fellowships of, 503
Mendeleev Congress, V. COFMAN, 286
MERA, H. P., "Mescal Pits," 168
Mercury, Perihelion of, T. MERRIMAN, 371
MERRIMAN, T., The Perihelion of Mercury, 371
"Mescal Pits," H. P. MERA, 168
Mesquite on the Great Plains, C. N. GOULD, 511
Metabolism, Protein, E. BRAND and M. M. HARRIS, 589
Metallic Conduction, J. C. SLATER, 595
Meteor Crater, F. M. BROWN, 239
Meteorite, No, R. W. STONE, 87
Mice, Demonstration Jar for, C. REYNOLDS, 195; Measuring, A. SVIHLA, 331; Infection in, P. K. OLITSKY, H. R. COX and J. T. SYVERTON, 611; Spontaneous Tumors of, J. B. MURPHY and E. STURM, 631
Michigan, Univ. of, Greenland Expedition, 163; Symposium in Theoretical Physics, 320
Micro Burners, C. A. DALY, 413
Microdetermination of Carbon, W. L. DOYLE, 173
Micro-organisms, Slime-producing, J. R. SANBORN, 290
Microscope, Centrifuge, E. N. HARVEY, 430; Lamp, R. M. HOLMAN, 610
MILLER, D. C., Absolute Motion of the Solar System and the Orbital Motion of the Earth, 587
MILLER, E. C. L., Virginia Acad. of Science, 541
MILLER, G. A., Native Mathematics, 366
Minnesota Academy of Science, 405
Mirror Demonstration Apparatus, W. B. UNGER, 23
MITCHELL, S. A., Ormond Stone, 107
MOBERG, E. G., and M. W. HARDING, Boron Content of Sea Water, 510
MOORE, E. J., Staining Fungi on Culture Media, 23
Moore, Eliakim Hastings, L. E. DICKSON, 79
MOORE, J. H., Solar Eclipse Problems, 375
Morris Arboretum, 184, 404, 503
MORRISON, F. B., William Arnon Henry, 160
Mosquitoes and Live Stock, F. C. BISHOPP, 115
Moth, Webbing Clothes, G. W. HERRICK and G. H. GRISWOLD, 391
Mount, Specimen, for Insects, H. OSBORN, 587
Munroe, Charles E., in Honor of, 384
MURPHY, J. B. and E. STURM, Spontaneous Tumors of Mice, 631
Muscle Contraction, and Action-Current, R. H. STETSON and H. D. BOUMAN, 219
Museums, at Univ. Ky., 277; Century of Progress, 442; International Conference of, 599
Music, Transmission and Reproduction of, F. B. JEWETT, 435
MYERS, E. H., Mouth Pipette and Containers, 609

National, Research Council, Grants, W. H. HOWELL, 214, 355; A. L. BARROWS, 356; F. K. RICHTMYER, 358; D. C. JACKSON, 500; C. A. KRAUS, 552; W. H. TWENHOFEL, 618; Acad. of Sciences, 422, 454, 494, 512, 517; Medals, 514; W. W. CAMPBELL, 549
Natural Sciences, Acad. of, of Philadelphia, 512
Nature Sanctuaries, V. E. SHELFORD, 281
NEEDHAM, C. E., Sponge Spicules, 450
NEEDHAM, J. G., Culture Methods, 427
NELSON, E. K. and G. L. KEENAN, Citrus Fruits, 561
Nerve, Areas, Cutaneous, I. M. THOMPSON and V. T. INMAN, 216; Cells of the Cerebral Cortex, J. G. DUSSER DE BARENNE, 546
New York, Botanical Garden, 82; State Geological Assoc., Field Conference, 530
Nomenclature, Stratigraphic, F. X. SCHAFFER, 368; Zoological, J. B. KNIGHT, 389
Northwest Scientific Assoc., J. W. HUNGATE, 193
Novocaine in Nervous Tissue, M. GRODINSKY, M. BEBER and C. P. BAKER, 450
Nuclei, Physics of, 505
Nutritional Organs in Embryos of Top Minnows, C. L. TURNER, 93
Nutritive Value, Normal, E. B. FORBES, 306

Observatory, McDonald, 483
Oenslager, George, Award of Perkin Medal, 14
OGDEN, R. M., Thorndike on Law of Effect, 240
Ohio Academy of Science, W. H. ALEXANDER, 539
Oklahoma Academy of Science, H. J. HARPER, 55
OLITSKY, P. K., J. T. SYVERTON and J. R. TYLER, Experimental Granular Conjunctivitis, 25; H. R. COX and J. T. SYVERTON, Infection in Mice, 611.
Opportunity for Exceptional Ability, J. MCK. CATTELL, 491
Organic Reactions, D. B. KEYES, 202
OSBORN, H., Specimen Mount for Insects, 587
OSBORN, H. F., Revivals of Darwinism, 199
Oxygen Tension and Protein Synthesis, C. VOEGTLIN, M. E. MAVER and J. M. JOHNSON, 92

Pacific Science Congress, 163
Pack, Charles Lathrop, Forest Fellowships, 363
PAPENFUSS, G. F., Ectocarpus siliculosus Dillw., 390

Parasites, Prehistoric, G. E. WILSON, 560
Park, National, Everglades, 185
PARKER, R. C., Blood Cells, 544
Parks, Buildings and Reservations, 620
PARKS, H. B., Texas Acad. of Science, 54, 565
Patents, University, A. GREGG, 257; A. FLEXNER, 325; Ethical, Y. HENDERSON, 324
Paullin, C. O., Award of Loubat Prize, 421
PAYNE, F., Edward Bruce Williamson, 344
PEARSE, A. S., Zoological Text-books, 169
Peat, Ammoniation of, for Fertilizers, R. O. E. DAVIS and W. SCHOLL, 330
Pennsylvania, Univ. of, Morris Arboretum, 184, 404, 503
PERLA, D. and J. MARMORSTON, Suprarenal Cortical-Hormone-like Substance Extracted from Urine, 432
PERRINE, C. D., Two Criticisms, 20
PETERSON, F., Electric Anesthesia, 326
PETRUNKEVITCH, A., Fixing Fluids, 117
Pharmacology and Experimental Therapeutics, Amer. Soc. and *Journal*, 557
Phenanthrene and Derivatives, M. T. BOGERT, 289
Philadelphia College of Pharmacy and Science, 301
Phosphorescence of Solid Nitrogen, L. VEGARD, 588
Photoperiodism, G. M. DARROW and G. F. WALDO, 353
Photosynthesis, A. J. HEINICKE, 516
*Physical Review*, Format of, 109
Physics, Nuclear, J. A. FLEMING, 298; International Symposium on, 345
PILSBRY, H. A., Cretaceous Cirriped, 283
Pinhole Image, E. C. BRYANT, 428
Pipette, Mouth, and Containers, E. H. MYERS, 609
Planetarium for Amer. Museum Natural History, 361
Plants, Greenhouse, G. H. GODFREY, 583
Plotz, Ella Sachs, Foundation, 328
Poliomyelitis, S. FLEXNER, 7, 413
POND, S. E. and O. MEIER, JR., Laboratory Unit for Lighting, 585
Ponderable and Imponderable, O. HAHN, 397
Potentiometers, Current for, L. F. BOSS, 331
POWERS, W. E., Lake San Augustin, N. M., 51
Priestley Lectures at Pa. State College, 252
Production, Mass, D. S. KIMBALL, 1
Psychology, Response, H. S. LANGFELD, 243; at Chicago, 578
Psychrometer, J. F. TOWNSEND, 241
Public Service, Y. HENDERSON, 584
Publication, N. E. STEVENS, 239; W. J. FOX, 351
Pyrometer, W. C. STADIE and S. L. WRIGHT, JR., 172

Quantum Mechanics and Chemistry, H. EYRING, 158
Questions, F. S. HAMMETT, 584

Radiation and Plant Life, 554
Radio Research Facilities in Great Britain, 576
Radio-mat, F. L. WELLS, 91
Rats, Albino, and Amytal, D. H. BARRON, 372
Reactions in Biological Systems, H. F. SCHOTT and H. BORSOOK, 589
REDDICK, D., Biological Literature, 625
REGAN, J. F. and B. O. BARNES, Experimental Diabetes, 214
REMINGTON, R. E., Nutritional Anemia in Rats, 115
Research, Laboratories, Industrial, 420; Scientific, S. TSCHACHOTIN, 426
Respiration, Artificial, W. R. BOND, 515
Respirometer, W. B. BALCH, 116
''Reticulo-endothelial'' Cells, P. ROUS and J. W. BEARD, 92
REYNOLDS, C., Demonstration Jar for Mice, 195
RICHTMYER, F. K., National Research Council, 358
RIGG, G. B., A Sphagnum Bog, 535
RILEY, H. P., Self-sterility in Nemesia, 326
ROCKWELL, G. E., Immunization to Anthrax, 612
ROE, A. F., Stop-cock Clamp, 566
ROE, J. H. and R. F. CAHOON, Galactose Feeding of Dogs, 331
ROMANOFF, A. L., Permeability of Gases, 393
Ropes, Mooring, W. R. COE, 447
Rotenone, E. P. CLARK, 311
''Rotette'' for Liquids, E. L. HARRINGTON, 21
Rotor, Current, P. S. GALTSOFF and L. E. CABLE, 242
ROUS, P. and J. W. BEARD, ''Reticulo-endothelial'' Cells, 92
Royal, Society, 302; Institution, 576
RUSSELL, H. N., Constitution of the Stars, 65; Attraction of Spheres, 412

SAGUE, M. L., Olive M. Lammert, 275
SANBORN, J. R., Slime-producing Micro-organisms, 290
Sansome, F. W. and J. Philp, Genetics, A. F. BLAKESLEE, 284
SCHAEFFER, A. B. and M. D. FULTON, Staining Endospores, 194
SCHAFFER, F. X., Stratigraphic Nomenclature, 368
SCHOENBORN, H. W. and C. P. HICKMAN, Mounting Anatomical Preparations, 287
SCHOTT, H. F. and H. BORSOOK, Reactions in Biological Systems, 589
Science, Amer. Journal of, 207; American Men of, J. McK. CATTELL, 264; Junior Clubs, 319; Service Conference, 505
Scientific, Investigation, Analysis in, D. JOHNSON, 569; Work under Government, 600
Sea Water, Photochemical Nitrification in, C. E. ZOBELL, 27; Boron Content of, E. G. MOBERG and M. W. HARDING, 510; Lithium in, B. D. THOMAS and T. G. THOMPSON, 547
SEASTONE, C. V. and M. B. LAWRENCE, Filtrable Cycle of Bacteria, 259
Sedimentation and Sedimentology, H. WADELL, 536
SEIFRIZ, W., Twisted Trees, 50
Self-sterility in Nemesia, H. P. RILEY, 326
Serapias Helleborine in New York, V. A. YOUNG, 560
SHAPLEY, H., The Cosmic Parade, 272
SHAW, F. W., Human Necrobacillosis, 392
SHAW, G. T. and R. R. MCKIBBIN, Alkali Treatment of Soils, 411
SHELFORD, V. E., Nature Sanctuaries, 281; Conservation, 535
Sherman, H. C., Award of Medal of Inst. Chemists, 346
SHERMAN, J. M. and G. M. CAMERON, Growth of Bacteria, 537
SHULER, E. W., Vertebrate Fossils, 368
Sibling Resemblance, F. H. FINCH, 373
SIFTON, H. B., Agitation of Material in Aerated Water, 431
SIMPSON, H. E., Arthur Gray Leonard, 108
Sinnott, E. W. and L. C. Dunn, Genetics, A. F. BLAKESLEE, 284
SKILLING, H., Vowel Production, 604
SLACK, F. G., Tennessee Acad. of Science, 541
SLATER, J. C., Metallic Conduction, 595
SLEGGS, G. F., Sub-surface Thermometer, 586
Slide Technique, E. S. JAMES, 369
SNYDER, W. C., Fusarium Disease of Peas, 327
Solar, Light Visible during Submarine Measurements, C. L. UTTERBACK, 118; Eclipse Problems, J. H. MOORE, 375; Variations and Atmospheric Pressure, H. H. CLAYTON, 568; System, Absolute Motion of, and Orbital Motion of Earth, D. C. MILLER, 587
Soy-bean Paste, A. M. FIELD, B. H. ALEXANDER and E. B. SYLVANUS, 91
Species Differences, S. C. BROOKS, 221
Spectroscopy, at Mass. Inst. Tech., 162, 577
Sphere, Attraction of, E. V. HUNTINGTON, 489; H. N. RUSSELL, 412
Sponge Spicules, C. E. NEEDHAM, 450
STADIE, W. C. and S. L. WRIGHT, JR., Pyrometer, 172
Staining, Fungi on Culture Media, E. J. MOORE, 23; Endospores, A. B. SCHAEFFER and M. D. FULTON, 194; Action of Iron Haematoxylin, R. T. HANCE, 287; Double, K. HRUBY, 352

Starks, Edwin Chapin, F. M. MACFARLAND, 182
Stars, Constitution of, H. N. RUSSELL, 65
STEFANSSON, V., Blue Eyes for Brown, 191
STEIL, W. N., Tapetum of Eusporangiate Ferns, 606
STETSON, R. H. and H. D. BOUMAN, Action-Current and Muscle Contraction, 219
STEVENS, N. E., Publication, 239
STILES, C. W., Hookworm Disease, 237
Stone, Ormond, S. A. MITCHELL, 107
STONE, R. W., No Meteorite, 87
STOUT, A. B., Seedless Grapes, 310
Stroboscope, Two-Field, P. F. GAEHR, 412
SVIHLA, A., Measuring Mice, 331
SWANBACK, T. R. and H. G. M. JACOBSON, Brown Root-rot of Tobacco, 169
SWINGLE, W. W., Adrenal Cortical Hormone, 58

TAKAHASHI, W. N. and T. E. RAWLINS, Rod-shaped Particles in Tobacco Mosaic Virus, 26; Stream Double Refraction, 284
Technocracy, Amer. Engineering Council on, 81
Telephonic Drop Counter, C. F. GRAHAM, 542
Tennessee Acad. of Science, J. T. MCGILL, 192; F. G. SLACK, 541
Testing Materials, American Society for, 81
Texas Acad. of Science, H. B. PARKS, 54, 565
Therapeutics, H. H. DALE, 521
Thermodynamics and Relativity, R. C. TOLMAN, 291, 313
Thermometer, Sub-surface, G. F. SLEGGS, 586
THOMAS, B. D., and T. G. THOMPSON, Lithium in Sea Water, 547
THOMPSON, I. M. and V. T. INMAN, Cutaneous Nerve Areas, 216
THOMPSON, J. O., How Did Joule Pronounce Name? 88
Thomson, Elihu, 185; 321; Work in Electrical Engineering, K. T. COMPTON, 415; in Honor of, V. BUSH, 418
THORNDIKE, E. L., Law of Effect, 173; "Spread" or "Scatter" in Relation to Gestalt Doctrines, 368
Thorndike on Law of Effect, R. M. OGDEN, 240
Tissues, Hydrogen-ion Concentration of, C. VOEGTLIN, H. KAHLER and R. H. FITCH, 567
Tobacco, Mosaic Virus, W. N. TAKAHASHI and T. E. RAWLINS, 26; Brown Root-rot of, T. R. SWANBACK and H. G. M. JACOBSON, 169; Plants, W. N. TAKAHASHI and T. E. RAWLINS, 284
TOLMAN, R. C., Thermodynamics and Relativity, 291, 313
TOWNSEND, J. F., Psychrometer, 241
Trachoma and Bacterium Granulosis, I. A. BENGTSON, 218
Transpiration of Evergreens, J. L. EMERSON and A. C. HILDRETH, 433
TRAVIS, L. E. and A. R. BUCHANAN, Vowel Theory, 121
TSCHACHOTIN, S., Scientific Research, 426
Tubercle Bacillus, M. HEIDELBERGER and A. E. O. MENZEL, 24
TURNER, C. L., Nutritional Organs in the Embryos of the Top Minnows, 93
TWENHOFEL, W. H., National Research Council, 618
Twisted Trees, W. SEIFRIZ, 50; M. COPISAROW, 581
Twisting Habit, C. P. HASKINS and C. N. MOORE, 283

Ultra-violet, Fluorescence of Cells in, A. C. GIESE and P. A. LEIGHTON, 509
UNGER, W. B., Mirror Demonstration Apparatus, 23
Urea Synthesis, H. BORSOOK and G. KEIGHLEY, 114
UTTERBACK, C. L., Variations in Visible Solar Light during Submarine Measurements, 118

Variability and Individuality, C. C. LITTLE, 195
VEGARD, L., Solid Nitrogen, 588
VER STEEG, K., Geology and Boys and Girls, 169
Virginia Acad. of Science, E. C. L. MILLER, 541
Vitamin, D, T. F. ZUCKER, 19; G. H. MAUGHAN and E. MAUGHAN, 198; Standards, 184; Advisory Board, 233; A in Pimiento Pepper, L. ASCHAM, 351
VOEGTLIN, C., M. E. MAVER and J. M. JOHNSON, Protein Synthesis, 92; H. KAHLER and R. H. FITCH, Hydrogen-ion Concentration of Tissues, 567
Vowel, Theory, L. E. TRAVIS and A. R. BUCHANAN, 121; Production, H. SKILLING, 604

WADELL, H., Sedimentation and Sedimentology, 536
WALDEN, B. H., Cellophane for Lantern Slides, 91
WALLACE, H. A., Research and Agriculture, 475
WALTER, H. E., Frederic Poole Gorham, 597
WANLESS, H. R., Illinois Acad. of Science, 540
WARD, H. B., American Association for the Advancement of Science, 452, 461, 467
Washington Academy of Sciences, 83
Wawona Road Tunnel in Yosemite Nat. Park, 599
Weather Station on Mt. Wachusett, 362
Webb, W. P., Award of Loubat Prize, 421
Weevil, Vegetable, Nomenclature, E. O. ESSIG, 605
WELLS, F. L., Radio-mat, 91
WENTWORTH, C. K., Sizes of Clastic Grains, 633
Weston, Edward, Lamme Medal, 302
Wheat, Bread, W. F. GERICKE, 229
Wilcox, Timothy E., W. W. EGGLESTON, 300
WILDMAN, J. D., Howard Method, 263
WILLARD, B., Field Conference of Geologists, 629
WILLIAMS, C. G., Agricultural Exper. Sta., 155
Williamson, Edward Bruce, F. PAYNE, 344
WILLIS, B., Earthquakes, 351
Willstaetter, Dr., Willard Gibbs Medal, 385
WILSON, F. H., A Louse and Its Host, 490
WILSON, G. E., Prehistoric Parasites, 560
WILSON, J. W. and J. M. DARLINGTON, Perfusion of the Mammalian Heart, 370
WINSLOW, C.-E. A., Medical Care for U. S., 102
Wisconsin Alumni Research Foundation, 44
Wood, Leonard, Memorial, F. P. G., 562
WOODS, A. F., Herman Theodor Holm, 183
WOOTEN, B. A. and W. T. HARRIS, Electroscope, 630
Wright, J. K., Loubat Prize, 421

Yale, North India Expedition, 301; H. DE TERRA, 497; Univ., Honorary Degrees, 621
Yeast Cells, Disintegrator for, W. F. BRUCE, 543
YONKMAN, F. F., Kymograph Recording, 172; Cellophane for Lantern Slides, 218
YOUNG, V. A., Serapias Helleborine in N. Y., 560

ZELENY, C., Genetics and Embryology, 177
ZOBELL, C. E., Nitrification in Sea Water, 27
Zoological Text-books, A. S. PEARSE, 169
ZUCKER, T. F., Vitamin D in Milk and Bread, 19
ZWICK, K. G., Goiter Prevention, 627

# SCIENCE

VOL. 77 FRIDAY, JANUARY 6, 1933 No. 1984

*The American Association for the Advancement of Science:*
*The Social Effects of Mass Production:* DR. DEXTER S. KIMBALL 1
*Prevention of Poliomyelitis:* DR. SIMON FLEXNER 7
*Obituary:*
*Rufus Lot Green:* FREDERICK E. BRASCH; *Everhart Percy Harding:* DR. S. C. LIND; *Recent Deaths; Memorials* 11
*Scientific Events:*
*The Year at the Field Museum of Natural History; Advanced Studies in Engineering and Business for Disengaged Engineers; Award of the Perkin Medal to Mr. Oenslager; Officers of the American Association for the Advancement of Science* 13
*Scientific Notes and News* 16
*Discussion:*
*The Use of Vitamin D from Cod-liver Oil in Milk and Bread:* DR. THEODORE F. ZUCKER. *Two Criticisms:* PROFESSOR C. D. PERRINE. *Concentration of Microfilariae by the Salivary Secretions of Bloodsucking Insects:* DR. ALFONS DAMPF. *Bulbs from Holland:* PROFESSOR FRANK P. MCWHORTER 19
*Scientific Apparatus and Laboratory Methods:*
*The "Rotette" or an Apparatus for Handling Small Quantities of Liquids with Rapidity and Precision:* PROFESSOR E. L. HARRINGTON. *Mirror Demonstration Apparatus:* DR. W. BYERS UNGER. *The Use of Phenosafranin for Staining Fungi on Culture Media or in Host Tissue:* ELIZABETH JANE MOORE 21
*Special Articles:*
*Protein Fractions of the H 37 (Human) Strain of Tubercle Bacillus:* DR. MICHAEL HEIDELBERGER and DR. ARTHUR E. O. MENZEL. *Induction of Experimental Granular Conjunctivitis by Direct Inoculation of Trachomatous Tissue:* DR. PETER K. OLITSKY, DR. JEROME T. SYVERTON and JOSEPH R. TYLER. *Rod-shaped Particles in Tobacco Mosaic Virus Demonstrated by Stream Double Refraction:* WILLIAM N. TAKAHASHI and DR. T. E. RAWLINS. *Photochemical Nitrification in Sea Water:* DR. C. E. ZOBELL 24
*Index to Volume 76* i
*Science News* 8

SCIENCE: A Weekly Journal devoted to the Advancement of Science, edited by J. MCKEEN CATTELL and published every Friday by

THE SCIENCE PRESS

New York City: Grand Central Terminal
Lancaster, Pa. Garrison, N. Y.
Annual Subscription, $6.00 Single Copies, 15 Cts.

SCIENCE is the official organ of the American Association for the Advancement of Science. Information regarding membership in the Association may be secured from the office of the permanent secretary, in the Smithsonian Institution Building, Washington, D. C.

## THE SOCIAL EFFECTS OF MASS PRODUCTION[1]

By Dr. DEXTER S. KIMBALL

DEAN OF THE COLLEGE OF ENGINEERING, CORNELL UNIVERSITY

IN the center of the theater district on Broadway, New York City, behind large plate glass windows there stood a short time since a modern cigarette-making plant. One machine, fed constantly with pulverized tobacco leaf and wrapping paper, ejects continuously a cigarette bar which is cut into standard lengths as it issues from the machine at the rate of 500 cigarettes a minute. A neighboring machine takes the cigarettes and automatically places them in packages, closes them and delivers the finished marketable product. The degree of skill required to operate the machine is small, though, of course, some one must fully understand the mechanism and be competent to make adjustments. At the other extreme of size, consider the automatic factory of the A. O. Smith Company of Milwaukee. This great machine literally takes in steel plates at one end and ejects finished automobile frames at the other at the rate of 8,000 daily. The machine, for such it virtually is, cost $10,000,000 and requires only 200 men to operate it. Probably 5,000 men would be required to produce the same result with ordinary processes. Here again, of course, there must be a certain number of skilled engineers who can adjust the machine, but the labor cost of actual operation is comparatively insignificant.

A survey of any progressive industry will reveal similar developments and constant progress toward the mechanization of its processes. Everywhere one finds the handicraftsman displaced by the machine and the semi-skilled operators, backed by the most lavish use of power the world has ever witnessed. In many instances the product is equal to or better than the

[1] Address of the vice-president and chairman of Section M—Engineering, American Association for the Advancement of Science, Atlantic City, December, 1932.

work of the artisan and in all cases the volume of product per worker is vastly greater than can be achieved by handicraft. Of course, there is nothing new *in principle* in these developments, which began with the first stone axe and culminated in the industrial revolution. Until that event the tool had always been an adjunct to the skill of the worker; but the developments of the industrial revolution made the worker an adjunct to the machine.

Since 1900 the mechanization of industry has proceeded at a rapid and apparently at an accelerated pace. As long as industry was prosperous and displaced workers, in some measure, could find work elsewhere, little attention was given to this tendency, though thoughtful writers have from time to time called attention to the problem. But the present depression has aroused more interest in the basic reasons for unemployment than any other in modern times, and for the first time technological unemployment, as this displacement of labor is called, appears as a vital issue and as a possible factor, in a large way, in the general problem of unemployment.

The most natural reaction on first observing productive processes such as have been described is one of concern for the skilled workers who may have been displaced by the new invention and a consequent belief that such advanced methods can not be conducive to the welfare of the workers. If, however, the observer should voice such fears probably he would be reminded of the great economic gains made by this country since modern manufacturing methods came into use and his attention would be directed to the high scale of living that the workers in this country enjoy, the inference being that modern methods of production can not in the long run be anything but helpful for all. While much can be said in support of both of these somewhat antipodal assertions, neither of them reveal the trials and tribulations through which many men have passed in building up our present level of existence, they throw no light upon the complex forces operating in the industrial field, nor do they even in a remote manner advise us as to whether the net trend is for good or evil.

Whenever an advanced process, such as those referred to in the foregoing, is set in motion, several economic changes at once become operative. The first is an increase in the capital investment and a further separation of the worker from the ownership of the tools of industry. This tendency is not connected directly with this present discussion, except that it has progressively closed certain avenues of escape open formerly to the worker under simpler industrial conditions. As industrial equipment has grown more complex and more expensive, the worker's industrial independence has decreased until to-day he is no longer an economic self-sufficient unit, but dependent largely upon capitalistic management for an opportunity to earn his daily bread. Consequently, the need of protective measures in his behalf increases daily.

The greatest and most immediate menace to the worker because of industrial progress is this displacement in favor of more highly developed machines in the hands of less skilled workers or "degradation of labor," as it has been called. In the early days of the industrial revolution in England the ruthless application of improved methods in the textile industries and the displacement of handicraft workers by machinery operated by children of tender years forms one of the darkest pictures in modern industrial history. Such direful conditions never prevailed in this country, even from the earliest days. Industry itself was in the making, the frontier was always accessible and a change from one calling to another not so difficult as at present. Even during the rapid expansion and development of industry in the latter half of the last century, technological unemployment was never a serious issue, though it had begun to raise its head. This is not to deny, of course, that at times and places much distress has occurred because of such displacement. Industrial progress is necessarily accompanied by change and apparently such change is necessarily accompanied by suffering on the part of some one. Progress, change and distress for some persons appear to be concomitant. The U. S. Census Report of 1900 mentions this tendency specifically as a menace to the wage-earner and predicts a doleful future for the wage-earning class in the following words:

> A factor that has a real tendency to lower the actual earnings of the wage earner in many industries is the displacement of the skilled operator by machinery which permits the substitution of a comparatively unskilled machine hand. This tendency is noticeable in many lines of industry. Its effects are twofold; to reduce the number of employees producing the same or an increased quantity of product and hence to lower the total wages of the group; and to reduce the average rate of wages because of the lower degree of skill required. The effect of the introduction and improvement of machinery upon the condition of the skilled artisan is an economic question of the greatest importance.

Here is analysis and prophecy, the accuracy of which will be discussed subsequently, after an examination of some other phases of the problem.

If this displacement of labor, as described in the foregoing, were the only effect of modern productive methods we should have found ourselves long ago in great difficulties. But improved machinery, while frequently displacing labor of a certain degree of skill, provides employment for workers of a lesser degree of skill, and thereby "extends" the field of industry to workers who otherwise could take no part in modern manufacturing. Hence in the older callings that have been mechanized, shoes are no longer made by shoemakers, watches by watchmakers, or knives, forks and spoons by skilled cutlers and silversmiths, but by semi-skilled workers operating highly developed machines. More important still, these new methods and processes have made possible the building up of new enterprises of vast proportions, such as the sewing machine, the automobile, telephone, radio, refrigeration and other new industries, and which, but for modern methods, must have remained small in size with their products classed as luxuries. And these new mechanized industries in turn have given rise to supporting industries of great importance. Thus it is estimated that the automotive industry when busy gives direct employment to 800,000 workers and indirectly to 4,000,000 workers who supply equipment, raw materials, accessory parts, gasoline, etc. The plants of the Western Electric Company, which is the manufacturing arm of the American Telephone and Telegraph Company, have a normal capacity of over 50,000 workmen and the supporting industries must employ many thousands of workers. One wonders what this army of men would be doing if these new developments had not appeared.

The history of the development of these new factors in our existence should be noted, for it gives a clue to the character of the inventions which may be needed to hold the pace that has been set. The story of one is the story of all. First, there appears the period of invention and incredulity on the part of the public. It is only a few years ago that the electric motor was looked upon as an interesting toy, and the same was true of the telephone. A very few years ago the drivers of "horseless carriages" were viewed with mild amusement. Then comes the period when it is a luxury to possess one of the new devices. In the year 1880, for instance, it cost as high as $280 to have a private telephone. Finally, when the new device has proven its usefulness, mass production reduces the cost, and it becomes an economic necessity, the number in use depending sometimes, as in the case of the watch, almost solely upon the population. The sewing machine, the telephone, the automobile and other modern products have all justified their existence economically. It should also be noted that the driving power back of these modern methods is increased production and decreased costs. And it is a peculiar characteristic of these methods that as the quantity to be manufactured is increased, the unit costs can be decreased, which stimulates consumption, and this in turn reacts upon production, thus creating an ever-widening cycle of increasing production and decreasing costs until some limiting factor checks the movement. The results of this cycle are too well known to merit discussion, but it may be noted that in all probability the greatest value ever offered the public for every hour of labor expended is to be found in some of the moderate priced automobiles. How cheaply they may be produced time, only, will tell. The net result of modern methods, therefore, has been a vast increase in the quantity of manufactured goods and a remarkable decrease in the cost of them. It should be remembered that these methods have also been reflected in the basic industry, agriculture, and it would appear that the problem of production is fairly well solved, since at this moment we are producing more goods and more food than we can conveniently use, or rather more than we can intelligently distribute.

In résumé, therefore, as industry advances, some classes of workers are displaced, while at the same time other workers of lower degree of skill are given employment in callings hitherto closed to them. The displaced workers may find employment at the same economic level elsewhere, or they may be compelled to drop to the level of the new semi-skilled group. If the displaced workers are skilled in the machine building trades, they are usually absorbed by these callings, and the movement in general has been of advantage to the so-called "mechanic arts" group through the great development of the machine-construction industries. Other classes of workers have not been so fortunate, for it should be remembered that it is very difficult for a mature man of limited education to change his calling, to say nothing of the restrictions now imposed by trade unionism upon such changes. The statement so often made that displaced workers "find work elsewhere" is not always true, and if they do so it may be at an economic sacrifice. In time, of course, the displaced workers pass out of the picture so far as their old vocation is concerned, and the calling appears in a greatly modified form.

For the new groups that have been recruited, the conditions are usually the reverse. Given a small amount of training, they can be made more highly productive than formerly, they can render a greater service to society, and their remuneration in general is increased. That is, they may be, and generally are, elevated economically and as a natural result socially. The absorption of immigrant people and their descendants by the industries of New England and their economic and social elevation is too well known to need discussion, and the process still continues, not only there, but in every manufacturing center of this country.

Until quite recently, our industrial progress was viewed with considerable satisfaction. Our per capita wealth has risen from $383 in 1850 to about $3,500 at the present time. Our national wealth has reached the unprecedented total of about $400,000,000,000 and our national income approximated $90,000,000,000, a most remarkable amount. Our scale of living exceeded anything in history, and despite the present depression, other nations, notably Germany and Russia, are eagerly studying our methods and adopting those that may help them to emulate our success. It appeared to many of us that we had really entered a new era and that we had in some measure solved the problem of living through high wages and a constant increase in the manufacturing cycle that has been described. The depression, therefore, came as a very painful reaction to many.

Economists in times past have usually looked for the causes of depression in the law of supply and demand, a change in the supply of gold or in some disturbance in international trade, all of which would be adjusted with time. But now for the first time a new and sharp question is raised concerning our manufacturing methods and equipment, and the fear is expressed that our industrial equipment is so efficient that permanent overproduction, for the markets available, has occurred and that consequently technological unemployment has become a permanent factor unless remedial efforts are put in force. Other critics contend that our methods of distributing the products and profits of industry are hopelessly antiquated, and that overproduction can not occur as long as there is poverty, want and ignorance. It is indeed a paradox to see storerooms filled with raw material, shoe factories equipped with the most efficient machinery man had ever produced, and workmen, anxious and willing to work, walking the streets almost without shoes for themselves or their families. It is not the province of this article to discuss this last contention, but it must be admitted that our present methods of distribution are hopelessly behind our powers of production in scientific background and direction. And without doubt we shall not achieve any marked relief from some of our industrial troubles until the same methods of analysis are applied to distribution, including tariff-making, that have produced our magnificent machinery of production.

Many economists believe that permanent technological unemployment is unlikely or even impossible. Briefly, they argue that, as has been stated, technological progress increases the quantity and reduces the cost of production. This in turn creates a greater demand and hence enlarges the opportunities for labor. Or, if the demand is inelastic, even at reduced costs, the savings, either to the consumer or the producer, are eventually invested through banks in the production of other products, and thus the field of industry is indirectly expanded. Unfortunately, we have little quantitative knowledge concerning these complex relations. There are some facts concerning some individual industries, however, that are illuminating.

The census of 1900 lists the number of workers in the shoemaking industry, both handicraft and factory, as 153,600 and gives their earnings as $63,304,344, or about $415 per person. This industry has been very fully mechanized, yet in 1914 the number employed was 191,555, with average earnings of about $522 per person. In 1925 there were 206,992 workers in the industry, with total earnings of $225,787,981, or about $1,090 per person. The purchasing power of the dollar of 1925 was about 66 per cent. of that of 1914 and 53 per cent. of that of 1900, but even with these allowances there has been a gain in real wages since 1900. Furthermore, in 1900 there were 4,849 children under 16 years of age employed in the industry, with yearly earnings of about $177 per year per child. No such conditions are tolerated to-day in progressive states.

Again, in the printing industry, which also has been highly mechanized, the census of 1900 gives the number of workers as 162,992 with yearly earnings of $84,249,963, or about $517 per person. The census of 1925 lists 251,276 persons as employed in this calling with total annual earnings of $438,832,974, or about $1,746 per person. Here again, allowing for the difference in the value of the dollar, there has been a decided gain in earnings. Furthermore, such statistics do not take into account the increased employment due to the production of machinery for these industries. In 1925 the value of the printing machinery produced in the United States was $69,216,683, and the corresponding value of shoemaking machinery was $11,769,137, and each of these machine industries in turn has many ramifications, the money value of which would be difficult to compute. No doubt an analysis of other industries over this period of rapid mechanization would show similar results and it would appear that so far as some individual callings are concerned, the recorded experience does not bear out in any way the gloomy predictions of the editor of the Census of 1900 quoted in a preceding paragraph. And it is fair to assume that under present circumstances any calling that is transformed by mechanization will stabilize "in the long run," as economists say, on a higher level so far as those workers who survive the change are concerned. We need not be troubled apparently at the *final* results of such metamorphoses. It is the *immediate* results of such changes that are now engaging the attention of thoughtful men.

It is usually assumed by ardent advocates of industrial progress that the workers who are displaced by reason of advanced technological methods, whether mechanical or administrative, will find work elsewhere. This is not so easy to do. In former days, when industry was simpler, less specialized and less highly organized, such a transfer was not so difficult without great loss of time or economic standing: but conditions are vastly changed. The displaced worker is, in general, debarred from engaging in his wonted calling on his own responsibility, both for lack of funds and administrative experience. It is this lack, indeed, that makes cooperative production so difficult, if not impossible, under modern conditions. Again, the displaced worker can not, in general, engage in some other calling, at the same economic level, since his knowledge, skill and experience are not transmutable. If he does find employment in some other calling it is usually at a lower salary, that is, he suffers degradation of labor, so called. The few statistical studies that have been made of this problem indicate clearly that many displaced workers find employment elsewhere only after a considerable period of idleness and often at a lower wage scale. These difficulties are, of course, greatly increased where the decline in employment is such as to require the worker and perhaps his family to migrate to some distant point, a procedure that he faces with greatest reluctance. The most startling index of these new and changed conditions is the growing group of men over forty years of age that are finding it very difficult to get a foothold in industry once they are displaced for any cause. In this sense it may be that permanent technological unemployment already exists to a certain extent. It is, therefore, the immediate and not the ultimate results of technological progress that are of greatest concern and it is an open question as to how far we should permit the good of the majority to be advanced at the cost of suffering and poverty on the part of the minority. We are sadly lacking in accurate data as to the quantitative results of modern methods as affecting permanent unemployment. Perhaps nothing but a careful study of these phenomena or a pragmatic return to normal production can reveal to us with surety just what the true trends are, but in the meantime there are indications enough to put us on our guard as industry becomes increasingly scientific in its background and practices.

If an understanding of past progress and present conditions be important, some estimate of what the future may hold is even more so. The last thirty years has witnessed an unprecedented improvement in the science and art of production. Not only has this reshaped many of the old callings, but in some cases new and unheard-of industries based upon scientific processes have placed products on the market that have threatened or even obliterated old industries. In addition, the entire philosophy of industrial management has been rebuilt and made much more efficient. In its effect modern management is analogous to improved mechanical methods in that it aims to produce more per worker and hence tends to technological unemployment. There has also been a vastly greater use of power, particularly in heavy construction. Dean W. B. Donham, of the Harvard Graduate School of Business Administration, in his excellent and thought-provoking book, "Business Adrift," voices the opinion that "technological progress in the direction of better processes and methods will continue and accelerate during the generation ahead of us." He makes a similar prediction concerning the progress of efficient management. This may or may not be a true prediction, but if it be true, there are certain features of our economic life that must be studied carefully if our present system is to endure and if we are to keep up the present level of existence and escape extreme technological unemployment.

First, our home markets must be developed extensively. Foreign trade must, of course, be cultivated as heretofore, for the United States is far from being self-sufficient in the materials needed in modern industry, and it would appear that progressive nations are increasingly interdependent. But the field of foreign trade promises to be a very crowded place in the near future, and one in which our high tariff will not be a welcome passport. This means also the full evaluation of such economic theories as high wages and consequent high purchasing power. Our own people now purchase 90 per cent. of our products, it is said. Can this ratio be maintained if new methods greatly increase production? New inventions of economic value must be found, which, like the automobile, the radio, etc., will absorb the surplus labor and the increase in population. No such inventions are at present on the horizon, but no one knows what the day may bring forth. Industry individually and collectively must plan a program years in advance and thus endeavor to reduce the periods of feverish activity and corresponding periods of depression. Much thought is even now being given to this problem by forward-looking industrialists and economists in the hope that the business cycle can be controlled. Manufacturing must be freed from the incubus of speculation. Its inherent troubles are great enough without being thrown out of balance periodically by spasms in the stock market. It is inevitable, I believe, that we shall come to a shorter working week. There is nothing new or startling in this idea. Not many years ago the working day in most factories was twelve hours long for six days in the week, or 72 hours for the week. This working period has fallen steadily to approximately 44 hours a week of eight working hours a day. How much shorter the working week may be, time and technical developments alone will determine. And, lastly, management must provide a greater degree of security for the worker against unemployment and indigence in old age, the two calamities most dreaded by the worker. In such a program the effect of new technological processes in effecting unemployment must be studied in advance of their application. It may well be that we shall see legislation making it obligatory upon the part of ownership to provide some means of escape for displaced workers, though a happier solution would be a humanitarian interest in this problem on the part of the employing class that will minimize this difficulty by allowing longer period of readjustment and such provision for the transfer of displaced workers as may be possible. Unless some such program as this can be put into effect, an acceleration of our industrial machinery will make life unbearable for a large part of our population.

Personally, I am not convinced that the rate of progress during the next thirty years will be as rapid as during the last thirty. Scientific progress we shall surely see, and this is sure to be reflected in our industrial methods. But there are reasons, also, for believing that retarding factors are already at work. The most important of these is the old law of diminishing returns that so far has never failed to put in an appearance where economic progress has been active. Only a few of the more easily recognized indications of the working of this principle can be given here.

Consider first the transmission of intelligence by the telegraph and the telephone, which probably have accelerated the pace of modern industry as much as or more than any other factors. It is not conceivable that this quickening effect can be greatly increased. The solution of this problem is practically perfected. Since 1880 the time required to cross the continent by rail has been reduced from eight days to less than four. It is not conceivable that the next fifty years will witness anything like a proportionate reduction in rail time, and flying is still to be fully developed. Again in 1880 steamships were crossing the Atlantic in about eight days. The new giant liners now under construction are expected to make the passage in four days. Again it is not conceivable that this time will be reduced to two days in the next fifty years. The new methods of industrial management have accelerated industry and much more can be done in that field, but its limitations have already been evaluated by thoughtful observers. It is a well-known fact that in all engineering it is becoming progressively difficult to increase the efficiency of operation of power plants and machinery, in general.

Lastly, and most important of all, there are good reasons for believing that there are economic limitations to the growth in the size of manufacturing enterprises and consequently to the efficiency of mass production itself. Indeed, if the facts were known, it probably would be found that many modern industrial enterprises have already passed the point of greatest efficiency and greatest economic returns. The value of the industrial product per worker in this country in 1900 was about $1,600, while in 1919 (the last census in which such data are available) this ratio had risen to $7,500. Making due allowance for the changed value of the dollar, this is a great gain in production per worker. But *the ratio of the value of products to the capital invested has decreased* steadily for a number of years. In 1850 this ratio was close to 2, but it has fallen progressively until in 1919 it was only 1.39. This would appear to indicate that even if the number of workers were materially reduced in favor of more refined machinery the cost of production will eventually rise with increased complexity of mechanisms. This is already foreshadowed in some industries where the fully automatic machine as yet is not so economical. as the semi-automatic operated by a skilled worker. Barring some new and eruptive change like the industrial revolution there is little likelihood of startling changes in the immediate future.

Finally, whether industrial progress be slow or rapid, these new methods are here to stay and their deeper significance should not be forgotten. Through them there is held out a hope that as we have achieved political and religious freedom, so we may also achieve economic freedom, freedom from physical drudgery and an opportunity for all men to live like men and not like beasts of the field, as the majority of our ancestors have done. But this will be no easy task, for it involves many changes in our ideas of economics and government. It involves the discarding of some economic ideas and taboos of Adam Smith and others who viewed industry as handicraft and the worker as a self-sufficient economic unit. And it also involves a realization on the part of ownership that it can no longer absolve itself from the responsibility of either controlling the business cycle or making the effort to provide continuous dividends to industry as it now does to insure continuous returns to capital. We can not continue with the present uncertain methods faced with even moderate technological progress.

Make no mistake in this matter. If we shall achieve a semblance of economic freedom for all men, a high standard of life, security and delight in work, and leisure, it will be through much trouble and opposition, such as men have always encountered in winning political and religious freedom. There is an opportunity to attain this economic freedom in the United States by peaceful means, and this problem offers a challenge to business men, economists and engineers such as no similar group has ever had. Will they have the vision, courage and intelligent statesmanship to accept this challenge?

# PREVENTION OF POLIOMYELITIS[1]

By Dr. SIMON FLEXNER

DIRECTOR OF THE ROCKEFELLER INSTITUTE FOR MEDICAL RESEARCH, NEW YORK

THE evidence presented on the mode of infection in poliomyelitis has established two important facts: First, that the disease is a particular form of infection of the upper respiratory tract; and second, that in harmony with other epidemic diseases of respiratory origin, the cases arising during an epidemic cover a wide latitude in degree of symptoms and pathological effects. There is consensus of opinion among clinicians that the number of children suffering some degree of infection, the slight cases expressing themselves as minor illnesses only, is very large, being in comparison with the number that are frankly paralyzed many times as great. The wide occurrence of the slighter forms of infection can be taken as a means, favorable in character, of delimiting the prevalence of the severer affection, since early experimental observations showed Lewis and myself[2] that any degree of actual infection, irrespective of whether muscular paralysis arose or not, protected the inoculated monkeys from the effects of a second administration of the virus.

Hence the investigation of the immunological phenomena in poliomyelitis became at once a rewarding field of experiment. The knowledge of the phenomena has become considerable during the twenty-year period of the experimental study of the disease, and the application of this knowledge to the prevention of epidemic poliomyelitis has met with encouraging results in the severe outbreaks occurring in New York State in 1931 and in Pennsylvania in 1932. I shall endeavor to guide you quickly through the main discoveries which have led to the practical achievements to be described. It is, however, necessary at the outset to explain that I have taken the lecturer's privilege of including in this statement certain later results bearing out the earlier ones presented, which were obviously not available when the lecture was delivered. It is sometimes advantageous to defer writing a lecture until the time of publication arrives, especially when, as in this instance, a new method has been under trial. During the intervening period, the method may have been given a wider test, with results sometimes favorable, and of course sometimes unfavorable to its employment. We appear in this instance to be in the happier situation, and while it is still too early to pass final judgment on available means of preventing poliomyelitis in the young during the prevalence of an epidemic, it is desirable that the nature of such means shall become widely known, since epidemic poliomyelitis continues to appear annually in some parts of America and Europe during the summer and autumn season.

The observation of Lewis and myself, already referred to, that monkeys which had recovered from an attack—irrespective of its severity—of experimentally induced poliomyelitis were not subject to reinfection, led quickly to the testing of the blood of recovered monkeys and human beings for immune substances to which the protection might be attributable.[3] Tests made almost simultaneously in France, Germany and the United States disclosed the existence in the blood, after recovery from the disease, of neutralizing, antiviral bodies. A mixture consisting of the virus of poliomyelitis and the serum of the blood was injected into monkeys. No symptoms of disease tended to arise from this injection; while mixtures of virus and normal monkey serum, or the serum of many, but not all persons not known to have had poliomyelitis, proved incapable of protecting the animals against the onset of the symptoms, including paralysis, characteristic of the experimental disease. I shall return a little later to a consideration of the circumstances under which the blood of supposedly normal individuals acts in a measure similar to that of persons known to have had paralytic poliomyelitis, since this action has come to have such pregnant meaning.

Let me repeat, the blood of normal monkeys invariably failed to act upon or neutralize the virus of

1 Abstracted from the John M. Anders Lecture on Poliomyelitis delivered at the College of Physicians, Philadelphia, January 6, 1932.

2 S. Flexner and P. A. Lewis, *Jour. Am. Med. Assn.*, liv, 45, 1910; *Jour. Exp. Med.*, xii, 227, 1910.

3 P. H. Römer and K. Joseph, *Münch. med. Woch.*, lvii, 568, 1910; C. Levaditi and K. Landsteiner, *Compt. rend. Soc. biol.*, lxviii, 311, 1910; S. Flexner and P. A. Lewis, *Jour. Am. Med. Assn.*, liv, 1780, 1910; A. Netter and C. Levaditi, *Presse méd.*, xviii, 268, 1910.

poliomyelitis. The neutralizing property was detectable only when the inoculated monkeys had shown unmistakable signs of infection, although these signs may have been fleeting in character and wholly devoid of a paralyzing effect. Monkeys which receive the virus in the ordinary process of inoculation and resist all infection—either because the virus employed is too weak or too small a quantity is used, or because individual monkeys are exceptionally refractory—remain normal in regard to the antiviral action of the blood and capacity to respond with paralytic symptoms when a more effective inoculation is made.

In the light of the fact that monkeys are not naturally afflicted with poliomyelitis, as is man, it is significant to note not only that normal monkeys do not exhibit the blood antiviral property, but that the blood of recovered monkeys is weaker in antiviral substances than is the blood of recovered persons. For the sake of convenience it is customary to speak of the neutralizing, antiviral blood serum obtained from recovered persons and monkeys as "convalescent serum." Thus, monkey convalescent serum is less potent than human convalescent serum. But the potency of the former can be markedly increased by the additional injection of virus into recovered monkeys, a process which Lewis and I called reinforcement.[4] Reinforced (or hyperimmune) monkey serum equals or even surpasses in neutralizing power the convalescent serum obtained from human beings.

Neutralization of the virus by convalescent serum, monkey and human, was established originally by test tube experiments. As already stated, virus and serum were mixed before the mixture was injected into monkeys. Since under such conditions no infection occurred, the immediate question which arose was whether neutralization could also be effected inside the animal body, that is, when virus and convalescent serum were injected separately. While the test tube, or *in vitro* demonstration, of the presence of antiviral bodies in the blood undoubtedly threw light on immunity in poliomyelitis, it was thought that the determination of neutralization *in vivo* might possibly lead to therapeutic application. The tests carried out by Lewis and myself[5] consisted of the intracerebral inoculation of virus and the intraspinal injection of convalescent serum into monkeys. The intracerebral method is the most effective that is known for inducing the infection; the intrathecal injection is the most certain and efficient procedure for bringing the neutralizing serum into intimate relation with the nervous tissues, including the nerve cells, and hence for the blocking of the cells against the entrance of the virus, the injurious effects of which are responsible for the severe symptoms of the disease. While it is true that under physiological conditions the flow of the cerebrospinal fluid, into which the serum is introduced, is away from the nerve tissues, the small rise in pressure produced by the injection suffices to reverse the current, bringing the serum into intimate contact with all the constituents of the tissues, including the nerve cells.[6]

The results of the *in vivo* experiments can be stated briefly. When the virus is injected not longer than from 18 to 24 hours before the serum, and the amount of virus introduced into the brain does not exceed a fixed quantity, neutralization *in vivo* can be accomplished. Neutralization may be complete, when no symptoms whatever arise; or it may be partial, in which instance mild symptoms appear after a longer incubation period. Ordinarily the experimentally produced paralytic disease in the monkey is severer than the paralytic disease in man. While the mortality of the human affection is 20 per cent. or less, that of the frankly paralyzed monkey is 60 per cent. or more. When monkeys recover at all, they have as a rule merely passed through a mild attack of the experimental disease, such as is produced with weak virus strains or after partial neutralization of the virus. The *in vivo* experiments showed, therefore, that the action of the virus already present in the animal body could, under certain conditions, be suppressed. Suppression is, however, possible only when the immune serum is injected before symptoms of infection arise; once signs of infection are present, the serum is incapable of preventing the ordinary course of the disease from supervening.

The test by intracerebral inoculation is the most drastic one that can be devised. It exceeds in severity the conditions of infection occurring in man. In the human being, the virus is believed both to enter and to leave the nervous system by way of the nasal mucous membrane; we[7] early found that the virus implanted in the brain escapes into the nasal mucosa. This observation was quickly followed by the induction of the experimental paralytic disease through the instillation of the virus into the nares,[8] which finding in turn soon gave rise to the discovery that the intrathecal injection of serum prevents the development of infection by way of the nasal membrane.[9] It has,

[4] S. Flexner and P. A. Lewis, *Jour. Am. Med. Assn.*, liv, 1780, 1910; lv, 662.

[5] S. Flexner and P. A. Lewis, *Jour. Am. Med. Assn.*, liv, 1780, 1910.

[6] L. H. Weed and P. S. McKibben, *Am. Jour. Physiol.*, xlviii, 512, 1919.

[7] S. Flexner and P. A. Lewis, *Jour. Am. Med. Assn.*, liv, 535, 1910.

[8] S. Flexner and P. A. Lewis, *Jour. Am. Med. Assn.*, liv, 1140, 1910; S. Flexner, *Jour. Am. Med. Assn.*, lv, 1105, 1910.

[9] S. Flexner and P. A. Lewis, *Jour. Am. Med. Assn.*,

indeed, proven easier to prevent infection by the nasal than by the cerebral route of inoculation.[10] An important consideration is that the time interval between the nasal instillation of virus and the intrameningeal injection of serum may be lengthened with security beyond the period of safety that has been determined when the virus is inoculated into the brain. Moreover, convalescent serum injected into the meninges is equally capable of preventing infection by virus introduced into the blood;[11] and the immune serum is also protective, under certain circumstances, when the injection is made into the blood stream instead of into the membranes surrounding the brain and spinal cord.[12]

Professor Netter, of Paris, in 1911,[13] seized upon these experimental results and introduced into practice the convalescent serum treatment of poliomyelitis which has since been the subject of so much discussion. It soon became apparent that, once paralysis had appeared in human beings, the serum was quite powerless to influence the disease. As means of diagnosis became more accurate and instances of preparalytic poliomyelitis could be diagnosed with greater certainty, the use of the convalescent serum was increasingly restricted to these early cases. Medical opinion is still divided as to whether the serum is effective even under these circumstances. The matter has indeed become largely a statistical one, and hence it is not likely that a definite decision will be made immediately.[14] Epidemic poliomyelitis is a protean disease, symptomatically considered, and its effects are so varied that the outcome of individual preparalytic cases can not be predicted with certainty. Even the comparison of alternate cases in which serum is given with those from which it is withheld, is at best but a rough measure of effectiveness, since so much may depend on the way in which the choice of cases is made. I have attempted to formulate my own views on this debated subject[15] which I venture to restate here:

> My own experience has been chiefly with the experimental disease in monkeys. There the use of immune serum does make a difference. As between human beings and monkeys, the conditions are not identical; but the advantage is in part with human beings. Among them we find far more of the mild or preparalytic cases. In man there is, therefore, an inherently effective agency at work in aborting poliomyelitis. This agency is far less effective in monkeys in which the experimental disease tends to be severe and fatal. The severe form of the experimental disease in monkeys can be prevented or mitigated by means of immune serum. Since the practice of medicine is applied to individual cases of disease and does not, except statistically, deal with disease in mass, the question may fairly be asked whether the preexisting mechanisms in man tending to confine and abort the virus infection, can not in some instances be supplemented and fortified by convalescent serum. It is generally agreed that the use of the serum does no harm. Since it can not be affirmed that in individual cases it does no good, and a body of medical opinion exists in its favor, the question arises of whether its use should be withheld. This question is to be answered not by the pathologist, but by the physician. If a better, more calculable method of preventing paralysis were known, that is, a surer way of supplementing the normal mechanism tending to restrain the action of the virus before it causes functional injury to the nerve cells, this question would not arise. But there is no better or more calculable method known. The choice is, therefore, between no therapeutic intervention at all and a kind of intervention believed to be harmless and not known actually not to be sometimes useful in cases of this tragic disease.

Up to this point we have dealt with the restraint of the virus when it is mixed with immune serum in the test tube, or when the virus introduced into the animal body is followed by the injection of serum before symptoms of infection have arisen. The next problem to be considered related to the possibility of restraint of the virus when the serum is injected several days in advance of the virus. The answer to this question received from experimental work promises to bear on a possible preventive measure—passive serum protection—against epidemic poliomyelitis.

Stewart and I on addressing ourselves to the solution of this problem found that serum prevention is not only experimentally possible, but that the blocking effect against the entrance of the virus into the nerve cells endures for several days after an intraspinal injection, and occurs even after an intravenous injection of convalescent serum. Having in mind the practical implications of these observations, we proposed "that in the event of severe outbreaks of epidemic poliomyelitis, convalescent human serum be employed to afford passive protection to persons—children especially—menaced by the disease."[16]

The experimental results having been successful, we regarded it desirable to apply the method of protection to children and young adults exposed to epidemic

liv, 1780, 1910; S. Flexner, *Tr. Assn. Am. Physn.*, xxvi, 67, 1911.

[10] S. Flexner and H. L. Amoss, *Jour. Exp. Med.*, xxxi, 123, 1920.

[11] S. Flexner and H. L. Amoss, *Jour. Exp. Med.*, xxv, 525, 1917.

[12] S. Flexner and F. W. Stewart, *Jour. Am. Med. Assn.*, xci, 383, 1928; *New England Jour. Med.*, cxcix, 213, 1928.

[13] A. Netter, A. Gendron and Touraine, *Compt. rend. Soc. biol.*, lxx, 625, 1911.

[14] S. D. Kramer, W. L. Aycock, C. I. Solomon and C. L. Thenebe, *New England Jour. Med.*, ccvi, 432, 1932; W. H. Park, *Tr. Assn. Am. Physn.*, xlvii, 123, 1932.

[15] S. Flexner, *Jour. Am. Med. Assn.*, xcix, 70, 1932.

[16] S. Flexner and F. W. Stewart, *Jour. Am. Med. Assn.*, xci, 383, 1928; *New England Jour. Med.*, cxcix, 213, 1928.

poliomyelitis. During the next two or three years, of a number of such persons injected with convalescent serum, none developed the disease; but the number was too small to permit decisive conclusions. An opportunity came, however, with the overwhelming New York City epidemic of 1931, at which time we recommended the protective injection of convalescent serum or its near equivalent, blood from normal adults, parents by preference.[17] The amounts of convalescent serum available are too limited to serve for mass immunization. Several thousand children were treated in this manner, and among them the incidence of poliomyelitis was believed to be lower than in the uninjected population. The procedure employed was to withdraw from parents blood taken under sterile conditions and to inject 30 cubic centimeters or more of the uncoagulated blood intramuscularly into the children.

Allusion has been made to the fact that the blood of normal adults offers a substitute for the convalescent serum. The history of the discovery of the virus neutralizing property possessed by the blood serum of normal adults on the virus of poliomyelitis is instructive. In the year 1911, Anderson and Frost[18] investigated the so-called "abortive cases" of poliomyelitis to which Wickman's attention has been forcibly directed in the Swedish epidemic of 1905–1906.[19] The American investigators paid particular attention to the blood neutralizing reaction which had been described a short time before[20] by the employment of which they endeavored to establish the poliomyelitic nature of certain indefinite cases of illness which accompanied those of frank paralysis arising in the epidemic of poliomyelitis at Mason City, Iowa. In the course of their studies they made two observations, since confirmed, which are of special significance: first, that the blood of adults who had shown no signs of illness may possess considerable antiviral properties; and second, that the blood of young children, even when they have had an attack of the disease, may not develop promptly neutralizing power against poliomyelitis, or may develop it in a lesser degree than adults. Similar observations were made by Peabody, Draper and Dochez,[21] who studied the New York City epidemic of 1911. But it was Aycock and his associates[22] who studied the phenomenon more widely and concluded that a process of unperceived—subclinical—immunization of the adult population is taking place extensively to-day, thus explaining the antiviral activities now so generally found in the blood of normal persons. Aycock relates this subtle process to the similar one long known to be occurring in widely prevalent infectious diseases such as diphtheria and scarlet fever. Normal adult blood not only tends to contain the neutralizing substances in appreciable amounts, but in rare instances in quantities surpassing those present in the blood of persons who have recovered from undoubted attacks of poliomyelitis.[23]

However, it was not until the epidemic of 1932 in Philadelphia and other places in Pennsylvania that the method of passive immunization by the use of normal adult blood received not only wide, but more measured application. The analysis of these tests is being awaited with great interest. Certain favorable results have already been reported. But the completion of final results, and especially their interpretation, will require time and critical judgment. It is obvious, of course, that comparison should be made, where practicable, between large groups of children, injected and uninjected, both groups being similarly circumstanced as to age, environment and exposure. But it is also desirable to take into account the fact that certain adults are known not to possess the antiviral blood property; hence a standardized protective material can not be generally employed in the effort to produce passive immunization.

Finally, it must be remembered that tests on monkeys have disclosed two modes of intra-vitam action of the convalescent serum. In one, the virus is completely suppressed and no symptoms of infection arise; in the other, the action of the virus is mitigated, the incubation period before the appearance of symptoms being prolonged, and the symptoms themselves are milder. It is probable, therefore, that among the passively immunized children many will escape all signs of disease, and others—depending on all the circumstances stated—will fail to be protected, or will develop milder symptoms, taking into account the number receiving the adult blood in comparison with a corresponding number not so treated. We must await future events before attempting any general prediction on this important subject; but enough would appear to have been achieved already to warrant a further and wider trial of this safe and readily available means of preventing epidemic paliomyelitis which continues to be a serious menace on a world-wide scale.

One aspect of the subject of immunity in polio-

[17] S. Flexner, SCIENCE, lxxiv, 251, 1931.

[18] J. F. Anderson and W. H. Frost, *Jour. Am. Med. Assn.*, lvi, 663, 1911.

[19] I. Wickman, Beiträge zur Kenntnis der Heine-Medinischen Krankheit (Poliomyelitis acuta und verwandter Erkrankungen), Berlin, S. Karger, 1907.

[20] P. H. Römer and K. Joseph, etc., *loc. cit.*

[21] F. W. Peabody, G. Draper and A. R. Dochez, Monographs of The Rockefeller Institute No. 4, 1912.

[22] W. L. Aycock and S. D. Kramer, *Jour. Prevent. Med.*, iv, 189, 1930.

[23] H. J. Shaughnessy, P. H. Harmon and F. B. Gordon, *Jour. Prevent. Med.*, iv, 463, 1930; M. Brodie, *Jour. Exp. Med.*, lvi, 507, 1932.

myelitis remains to be considered. We have long known that monkeys may be rendered actively immune by successive small injections, or one large injection, of poliomyelitis virus made beneath the skin[24] or by successive inoculations made into the skin.[25] Both these methods of securing immunity suffer from the disadvantage that occasionally monkeys develop paralysis instead of immunity. It appears that monkeys, in common with human beings, exhibit varying degrees of susceptibility to the presence of the virus in the body. An effort is being made to improve and perfect this means of active immunization in order to avoid the rare onset of disease. The combined use of immune serum and virus offers greater security. That active immunity can be obtained by the injection of mixtures of the serum and virus has been shown by Rhoads.[26] Recently we have carried out experiments on a larger scale, in which virus and serum have been injected separately into the body of monkeys. These animals developed active immunity and, up to the present, without the appearance of symptoms of infection in any case. Moreover, evidence is accumulating that as the original, human virus is passed from monkey to monkey, it undergoes modification, and while retaining its immunizing properties, changes its infective power. Whether or not use may be made of this transformation in securing active immunization of human beings when menaced by epidemic poliomyelitis, future study alone can determine.[27]

# OBITUARY

## RUFUS LOT GREEN

PROFESSOR RUFUS LOT GREEN, professor emeritus of mathematics at Stanford University, died in Palo Alto, California, on November 19 at the age of 71. With the death of Professor Green, Stanford University loses one of its most faithful servants, teachers, counselors and friends, and the community one of its most serviceable citizens.

It does not fall to the lot of every man in academic work to stand out as a teacher par excellence, a counselor with wise judgment, a citizen with a high sense of public duty and a friend with understanding mind and heart. So did this man, best known, however, only to his colleagues, students and friends. The name of Professor Green does not stand out in the annals of science, nor will historians of science record any great achievements of his in mathematical research or published monographs—but in the hearts of his students are indelibly impressed the sterling and modest qualities of a quiet and unassuming teacher, endowed with high ideals of true scholarship. For a period of over 40 years, teaching mathematics was his one great task.

Professor Green was born in Rush County, Indiana, on March 3, 1862, the son of Samuel and Elizabeth Anne (McKee) Green. He showed early aptitude for both mathematics and natural history. His first two years in college were spent at the University of Indiana from 1879 to 1881 under Daniel Kirkwood in mathematics and David Starr Jordan in natural history. From 1881 to 1883 he attended Cornell University, after which he returned to Indiana University, where he graduated in 1885 with a B.S. degree, and immediately became an instructor in mathematics at his alma mater. During this time he prepared for his master's degree, which he received in 1888. His long teaching career was interrupted only once when he spent one year as a graduate student and fellow by courtesy at Johns Hopkins University in 1887–88 under Sylvester. Professor Green's advancement was rapid; he filled successfully the position of associate professor (1886–90) and attained the position of full professor at the age of 28 (1890–93) during the period of David Starr Jordan's presidency of Indiana University (1885–91). Two years after the new university Leland Stanford first opened its doors in 1891 with Dr. Jordan as president, Professor Green received a call to become associate professor of mathematics, and in 1894 he was promoted to full professorship. He was just a year too late to be classified with the "Old Guards," an affectionate term for the pioneer professors who came with Dr. Jordan. (It was three years later that the writer became a student of his and formed a friendship which endured until Professor Green's death.) He became executive head of the department of mathematics in 1925, from which position he retired in 1927.

In the councils of affairs of the university he assumed more than his full responsibility on various committees. He was best known, however, as chairman of the students' affairs committee. His fairness and justice in administering student disciplinary cases won him great respect and esteem. The students recognized in Professor Green a man of high principles and this made him a favorite among them.

The work in his classroom was unusually interesting

[24] S. Flexner and P. A. Lewis, *Jour. Am. Med. Assn.*, lv, 662, 1910; C. P. Rhoads, *Jour. Exp. Med.*, li, 1, 1930.

[25] W. L. Aycock and J. R. Kagan, *Jour. Immunol.*, xiv, 85, 1927; F. W. Stewart and C. P. Rhoads, *Jour. Exp. Med.*, xlix, 959, 1929.

[26] C. P. Rhoads, *Jour. Exp. Med.*, liii, 115, 1931.

[27] S. Flexner, *Jour. Am. Med. Assn.*, xcix, 1244, 1932.

in that he presented the subject-matter with a feeling of freshness and clarity. For mathematics was to Professor Green a live and growing science; he constantly emphasized the theoretical and practical phases, showing their parallel with the philosophical aspect. One of his favorite and constant admonitions to students on giving an examination was that the purpose of a test was to see what we could do "under pressure." He introduced a number of new courses to Stanford, one of which particularly interested him, namely, statistical mathematics.

His broad and catholic interest in life and its problems manifested itself in his interest in economic, social and political problems. So well was he posted on various issues that during political periods he was constantly sought by his colleagues and by organizations for advice and elucidation of the problems. His was the habit of clear thinking. Although he was never robust in health, he loved outdoor life and during his early days at Stanford, like David Starr Jordan, he was a leader in mountain walking with his students. For many years during the summer period he directed a camp in the Yosemite Valley, later becoming director of the Yosemite Park and Curry Company.

Professor Green was a fellow of the American Association for the Advancement of Science, member of the American Mathematical Society, Mathematical Association of America, American Economic League, Academy of Political and Social Science, American Political Science Association, California Academy of Science, American Museum of Natural History, and American Association of University Professors.

Thus closed an active and full life, devoted to state, church and university.

On August 11, 1886, he had married Miss Emma Edwards, of Knightstown, Indiana, who in addition to two daughters and one son survives him.

FREDERICK E. BRASCH

## EVERHART PERCY HARDING

ON October 10, 1932, Professor Harding died at his home in Minneapolis after an illness of more than two years. Before his retirement, owing to ill health, in September, 1931, he was the only remaining member of the staff of chemistry of the University of Minnesota whose service antedated the foundation in 1904 of the school of chemistry as an independent faculty. His connection with the university as a student and as a staff member extended over more than forty years.

Professor Harding was born on August 15, 1870, at Waseca, Minnesota, where he had his early education. He entered the University of Minnesota in 1890 and maintained a high record of scholarship during his entire career, achieving election to Phi Beta Kappa and later to Sigma Xi. At the same time, he set an all-time record for athletic prowess, especially in football. Participation in intercollegiate athletics was at that time not limited to three years, so that his career as an athlete was continued through the entire period of his undergraduate and graduate years. He took the bachelor's degree in 1894 and was awarded a scholarship, which enabled him to take the M.S. degree in 1895.

After serving as instructor in chemistry from 1896 to 1899, he pursued further studies in chemistry under Professor Curtius at the University of Heidelberg, where he was granted the Ph.D. degree in 1901. From 1905 until his retirement, he was successively assistant professor and associate professor of chemistry. He also took a prominent and responsible part in the management and supervision of intercollegiate athletics.

During the decade prior to his death, Professor Harding was in charge of technological chemistry, a division of the school of chemistry which comprised instruction and research in chemical technology, particularly of foods and fuels. It was in these fields that most of his researches were made, although some of his earlier work was devoted to pure organic chemistry. His interest in fuels led him to investigate extensively the presence and distribution of sulfur in oil shales for the determination of which he developed methods of unusual accuracy.

Professor Harding was frequently called on for public service and acted as consultant for industries of the state, particularly in connection with city gas supplies. Early in his career, he rendered valuable aid in the introduction of the sugar beet industry into Minnesota.

In all his relations, Professor Harding was characterized by his spirit of loyalty and by the strictest conscientiousness in the performance of all duties. He was equally devoted to his students and to research, which he carried on until his health failed. He was a member of Phi Beta Kappa, Sigma Xi, Phi Lambda Upsilon honor societies, of Alpha Chi Sigma and Phi Delta Theta fraternities and of numerous professional and scientific societies.

He is survived by his widow and three children.

S. C. LIND

## RECENT DEATHS

DR. ELIAKIM HASTINGS MOORE, professor emeritus of mathematics at the University of Chicago, died on December 30. He was seventy years old.

DR. JOHN J. CARTY, vice-president and chief engineer of the American Telephone and Telegraph Company, retired, died on December 27 at the age of seventy-one years.

DR. EDWIN CHAPIN STARKS, who recently retired as associate professor of zoology at Stanford University, died on December 30 at the age of sixty-five years.

DR. THEODOR HOLM, known for his work on Arctic botany and on plant anatomy, died in Washington, D. C., on December 26 at the age of seventy-eight years.

DR. GEORGE FETTEROLF, professor of otolaryngology at the University of Pennsylvania, died on December 29 at the age of sixty-three years.

LEON R. STREETER, chief in research, in charge of the chemical work on fungicides and insecticides of the division of chemistry, New York State Agricultural Experiment Station, died on December 26, aged thirty-eight years.

DR. WILLIAM A. LAFIELD, professor of radiology at Yale University, committed suicide on December 26. He was fifty-two years old.

DR. ERNEST HOWE, consulting mining geologist, an editor of the *American Journal of Science,* died on December 18. Dr. Howe was fifty-seven years old.

FRANK W. SKINNER, consulting engineer of New York City, died on December 26 at the age of seventy-four years.

DR. ALLAN DOUGLAS RISTEEN, director of technical research and editor of safety publications for the Travelers Insurance Company of Hartford, Connecticut, died on December 30 at the age os sixty-six years.

JOHN H. STEVENS, chemical expert for the Celluloid Corporation of Newark, New Jersey, died on December 4. He was seventy-nine years old.

W. H. FRY, of the Division of Soils of the U. S. Department of Agriculture, died suddenly at the age of forty-four years on December 28.

SIMON WILLIAM DYKSHORN, assistant at the experimental laboratories of the Carnegie Institution of Washington at Cold Spring Harbor, while hunting for scientific purposes, shot himself fatally on December 25. He was twenty-seven years old.

DR. GEORGES HARET, head of the radiology department at Lariboisière Hospital, Paris, died on December 20, as a result of x-ray burns incurred in the course of his work. He was fifty-eight years old.

### MEMORIALS

THE centenary of the birth of Julius von Sachs, the German botanist who founded plant physiology as a modern experimental science, was celebrated during the Atlantic City meeting of the American Association for the Advancement of Science. The memorial program on December 28 was led by Professor D. H. Campbell, of Stanford University, representing the Botanical Society of America; Professor Rodney H. True, of the University of Pennsylvania, representing the American Society of Plant Physiologists, and Professor C. E. Allen, of the University of Wisconsin, representing the botanical section of the American Association for the Advancement of Science.

THE Johns Hopkins University Institute of the History of Medicine commemorated on December 20 the three hundredth anniversary of the birth of Antony Van Leeuwenhoek, 1632–1723. Dr. William H. Welch, formerly director of the institute, gave an illustrated lecture on Van Leeuwenhoek and his work. A film, made especially in Holland to commemorate the tercentenary, was shown. There was also an exhibit of illustrative books, documents and instruments.

To commemorate the bicentenary of the birth of Sir Richard Arkwright, inventor of the yarn spinning frame, the Newcomen Society arranged a public lecture which was delivered on December 14 by Mr. Frank Nasmith.

THE University of Manchester has received from Mrs. R. W. Williamson a portrait in oils of her father-in-law, the late Professor W. C. Williamson, who was in charge of the teaching of zoology, botany and geology in Owens College from 1851 until 1892.

# SCIENTIFIC EVENTS

## THE YEAR AT THE FIELD MUSEUM OF NATURAL HISTORY

DESPITE enforced economies, due to reduction of its income from endowment and other sources because of the depression, Stephen C. Simms, director of the Field Museum of Natural History, reports that the museum maintained full service to the public during 1932, and its educational benefits were extended to a greater number of persons than in any previous year of its history.

While extra-mural activities such as scientific expeditions were curtailed, the museum carried on a full program of installing new exhibits and making general improvements, presenting free courses of illustrated lectures on science and travel for the general public, maintaining manifold educational activities for school children both at the museum and by extension work in the schools of Chicago, and issuing scientific publications.

A total of more than 1,800,000 persons have visited

the museum during the year. This is the largest attendance of any year, and represents an increase of nearly 300,000 or about 20 per cent. over the 1931 total of 1,515,540 visitors. The year 1932 was the sixth in which attendance has exceeded 1,000,000; and the total for the past five years has been more than 6,840,000, or approximately 1,000,000 more than the 5,839,579 visitors received in the entire twenty-five years during which the museum has occupied its first building in Jackson Park.

The outstanding new exhibit completed during the year is a reproduction of an African water-hole, a group with twenty-three mounted mammals, including giraffes, rhinoceroses, elands, gazelles, zebras and an oryx. This is the largest exhibit in the museum, and is one of the largest animal groups in any museum, possibly exceeding all others in size. Other groups of animals with reproductions of their natural habitats which were completed during 1932 include Alaskan caribou, Asiatic water buffalo, and the mountain lion of states west of the Rockies. In addition to such groups, many other new zoological exhibits were installed, while each of the other departments—anthropology, botany and geology—made notable additions and improvements among their exhibits, especially in the divisions of Chinese archeology, paleontology or historical geology, and in the Hall of Plant Life.

More than 265,000 persons attended the lecture courses and lecture tours provided by the museum for adults, and the series of motion picture programs, extension lectures, and other activities for school children given by the James Nelson and Anna Louise Raymond Foundation for Public School and Children's Lectures (the foundation is a unit of the museum organization with special endowment). Likewise, the more than 1,300 traveling exhibits of the N. W. Harris Public School Extension Department, another specially endowed unit, were circulated continually throughout the school year among public and private schools of Chicago with a total enrolment of about 500,000 children. A large public was served also by the library of the museum and the study collections of specimens maintained in each department.

## ADVANCED STUDIES IN ENGINEERING AND BUSINESS FOR DISENGAGED ENGINEERS

LEADERS in industry, engineering and education are sponsoring "Advanced Studies in Engineering and Business for Disengaged Engineers" to be given during the winter and spring under the auspices of the Engineering Foundation, according to an announcement made by H. Hobart Porter, chairman of the foundation. The courses will be conducted by unemployed or volunteer teachers under the supervision of members of the faculties of Columbia University, New York University, Stevens Institute of Technology and the Polytechnic Institute of Brooklyn. The business courses will be directed by members of the faculty of the School of Commerce of New York University.

The curriculum embraces six courses. Sessions are to be held in the forenoon beginning on January 9 and will continue for twenty weeks to the end of May. The opportunity is open to unemployed engineers who have the requisite education for pursuing the work.

These are free and deal with business finance, sales engineering, power plant engineering, structures and mechanical equipment of buildings, industrial applications of electricity and industrial management. Rooms for class use will be made available in the Engineering Societies Building and the Engineering Societies Library will place text and reference books at the disposal of class members. Requests for application blanks should be addressed to P. H. Littlefield, manager, in care of the Engineering Foundation, 29 West 39th Street, New York City. The movement is sponsored by the following:

Robert P. Lamont, president, American Iron and Steel Institute; A. G. Pratt, president, Babcock and Wilcox Company; Robert Ridgway, consulting engineer, Board of Transportation of New York City; Alfred P. Sloan, president, General Motors Corporation; Morse A. Cartwright, director, Association for Adult Education; Dean J. W. Barker, Engineering School, Columbia University; Dean Collins P. Bliss, Engineering School, New York University; Dean John T. Madden, School of Commerce, New York University; Dr. Harvey N. Davis, president of Stevens Institute of Technology, Hoboken, New Jersey; Dean E. J. Streubel, Polytechnic Institute of Brooklyn; H. A. Kidder, president, United Engineering Trustees, Inc.; H. Hobart Porter, chairman, Engineering Foundation; Admiral F. R. Harris, general chairman, Professional Engineers' Committee on Unemployment; George T. Seabury, secretary, American Society of Civil Engineers; A. B. Parsons, secretary, American Institute of Mining and Metallurgical Engineers; Calvin W. Rice, secretary, American Society of Mechanical Engineers, and H. H. Henline, acting national secretary, American Institute of Electrical Engineers.

## AWARD OF THE PERKIN MEDAL TO MR. OENSLAGER

GEORGE OENSLAGER, of Akron, Ohio, whose researches are said to have revolutionized the rubber industry, will be presented with the 1933 Perkin Medal of the Society of Chemical Industry at a national gathering of the chemical societies on the evening of January 6 at the Electrical Institute Auditorium, Grand Central Palace, New York City.

The award goes to Mr. Oenslager as "the American scientist who has most distinguished himself by his services in applied chemistry." Other organizations participating are the American Chemical Society, the American Electrochemical Society, the American Institute of Chemical Engineers and the American Section of the Société de Chimie industrielle.

Alfred P. Jones, of the Houston Properties Corporation, will detail the accomplishments of Mr. Oenslager which led to the award. Professor Marston T. Bogert, of Columbia University, past president of the American Chemical Society and of the Society of Chemical Industry, will make the presentation. Mr. Oenslager will deliver an address describing the development of organic accelerators for rubber vulcanization. Dr. A. E. Marshall, of New York, chairman of the award committee, will preside.

"Five major achievements mark the change in rubber technology during the past thirty years," according to the announcement of the award committee. "These are reclaimed rubber, the cord tire, the carbon black tread, the nitrogenous organic accelerator and antioxidants. Mr. Oenslager may be credited with two of these—the carbon black tread and the nitrogenous organic accelerator. As a direct result of his efforts the rubber industry has been revolutionized and from it have come economies of manufacture, increase in service and savings to consumers which run into the hundreds of millions of dollars annually."

Mr. Oenslager began his researches in 1906, setting out with the definite object of finding substances to be used in rubber mixtures which would decrease the rate of cure and increase the physical qualities of low grades of crude rubber. He found that the best organic accelerators contained nitrogen and his discovery has been put to wide use.

His experiments also laid the foundation for the most widely accepted theory of vulcanization—that zinc oxide is necessary to vulcanization with most of the nitrogen accelerators. He also viewed rubber as a colloid which needed uniformity of dispersion and toward this end he introduced what is known as the master batch.

In 1911, Mr. Oenslager developed the carbon black tread for automobile tires which was adopted for large scale production the following year.

"Were we to remove these two main features from tires to-day," the award committee points out, "the mileage figures would drop to one half the present values. If the modern tire can show savings to consumers over those of twenty-five years ago of $800,000,000 a year, then appraise the accelerator and the carbon black at a $400,000,000 annual saving and it will not be far out of line."

Mr. Oenslager was born in Harrisburg, Pennsylvania, in 1873. After attending schools in that city he prepared for college at Phillips Exeter Academy, entering Harvard University in 1890. While in college he became greatly interested in chemistry and after his graduation in 1894 he devoted two years of study to that science in the Harvard Graduate School.

In 1896 he became associated with S. D. Warren and Company as a chemist and remained in that post for nine years. In 1905 he was appointed research chemist to the Diamond Rubber Company. This company later was purchased by the B. F. Goodrich Company, with which Mr. Oenslager is now associated.

## OFFICERS OF THE AMERICAN ASSOCIATION FOR THE ADVANCEMENT OF SCIENCE

A FULL account of the Atlantic City meeting of the American Association for the Advancement of Science, and the scientific societies associated with it, edited by the general secretary, Dr. Burton E. Livingston, will be published in the issue of SCIENCE for February 3. Officers of the association were elected on December 30 as follows:

PRESIDENT

Henry Norris Russell, Princeton University.

PERMANENT SECRETARY

Henry B. Ward, University of Illinois.

GENERAL SECRETARY

Burton E. Livingston, the Johns Hopkins University.

TREASURER

John L. Wirt, Carnegie Institution of Washington.

MEMBERS OF THE COUNCIL

George T. Hargitt, Duke University.

Dugald C. Jackson, Massachusetts Institute of Technology.

MEMBERS OF THE EXECUTIVE COMMITTEE OF THE COUNCIL

Edwin B. Wilson, Harvard School of Public Health.

A. F. Woods, U. S. Department of Agriculture.

Philip Fox, Adler Planetarium and Astronomical Museum (to succeed Henry B. Ward)

REPRESENTATIVE ON THE BOARD OF TRUSTEES OF SCIENCE SERVICE

Burton E. Livingston, the Johns Hopkins University.

VICE-PRESIDENTS AND CHAIRMEN OF SECTIONS

A—*Mathematics*. C. N. Moore, University of Cincinnati.

B—*Physics*. C. J. Davisson, Bell Telephone Laboratories.

C—*Chemistry*. Arthur B. Lamb, Harvard University.

D—*Astronomy*. V. M. Slipher, Lowell Observatory.

E—*Geology*. Rollin T. Chamberlin, University of Chicago.

F—*Zoological Sciences*. A. S. Pearse, Duke University.

G—*Botanical Sciences*. K. M. Wiegand, Cornell University.

H—*Anthropology.* T. Wingate Todd, Western Reserve University.

I—*Psychology.* Walter R. Miles, Yale University.

K—*Social and Economic Sciences.* Wesley C. Mitchell, Columbia University.

L—*Historical and Philological Sciences.* Waldo G. Leland, American Council of Learned Societies.

M—*Engineering.* C. F. Kettering, General Motors Corporation.

N—*Medical Sciences.* Charles R. Stockard, Cornell University.

O—*Agriculture.* A. R. Mann, Cornell University.

Q—*Education.* Walter F. Dearborn, Harvard University.

SECRETARIES OF SECTIONS

A—*Mathematics.* E. R. Hedrick, University of California at Los Angeles.

B—*Physics.* H. A. Barton, American Institute of Physics.

C—*Chemistry.* J. H. Simons, Chicago, Ill.

D—*Astronomy.* H. T. Stetson, Ohio Wesleyan University.

E—*Geology.* Kirtley F. Mather, Harvard University.

F—*Zoological Sciences.* George R. La Rue, University of Michigan.

G—*Botanical Sciences.* Sam F. Trelease, Columbia University.

H—*Anthropology.* W. M. Krogman, Northwestern University.

I—*Psychology.* John E. Anderson, University of Minnesota.

K—*Social and Economic Sciences.* James Ford, Harvard University.

L—*Historical and Philological Sciences.* Joseph Mayer, American Association of University Professors.

M—*Engineering.* N. H. Heck, U. S. Coast and Geodetic Survey.

N—*Medical Sciences.* W. M. Simpson, Miami Valley Hospital.

O—*Agriculture.* P. E. Brown, Iowa State College.

Q—*Education.* William S. Gray, University of Chicago.

# SCIENTIFIC NOTES AND NEWS

AT the banquet of the Cambridge meeting of the Geological Society of America the fifth presentation of the Penrose Medal for distinguished achievement was made to Dr. Edward Oscar Ulrich, of Washington, who recently retired after long service with the U. S. Geological Survey. The presentation was made by Dr. W. O. Hotchkiss, president of the Michigan College of Mines. At the same time the society honored the sole survivor of the thirteen men who formed it in 1888, Dr. Herman LeRoy Fairchild, professor emeritus of geology at the University of Rochester, with the presentation of an inscribed copy of "The Geological Society of America," a history which he helped to prepare. Dr. Fairchild is a former president of the society.

AT the close of the recent meeting at Washington of the National Council of Geography Teachers, the first award of the certificate of merit for service in teaching geography was presented to Dr. William Morris Davis, professor emeritus of geology at Harvard University.

DR. HENRY EYRING, research associate in chemistry at the Frick Chemical Laboratory of Princeton University, received the ninth annual $1,000 award of the American Association for the Advancement of Science at the close of the Atlantic City meeting. The prize was given for Dr. Eyring's paper entitled "Quantum Mechanics of Conjugate Double Bonds," presented to the chemical section.

THE annual gold medal award for conspicuous achievement in the medical sciences, given by the Phi Lambda Kappa fraternity, was presented to Dr. Béla Schick, of the Mount Sinai Hospital, New York City, discoverer of the Schick test for diphtheria, at the annual dinner on January 1. The annual gold medal award for the best thesis on a medical subject written by an undergraduate medical student was presented to Myron G. and Maurice M. Rosenbaum, of the University of Buffalo School of Medicine.

THE Rudolf-Virchow Medal of the Berlin Anthropological Society has been awarded to Professor Karl Pearson, director of the Francis Galton Laboratory for National Eugenics, University of London.

*Nature* reports that in commemoration of the seventieth birthday of Sir P. C. Rây, founder, foundation-president and patron of the Indian Chemical Society, a jubilee volume of some 350 pages is being published by the society, containing contributions from many eminent chemists in India and abroad.

DR. MARCHOUX, professor at the Institut Pasteur, Paris, has been nominated a Grand Officer of the Legion of Honor.

DR. CHARLES ZELENY, professor of zoology at the University of Illinois, was elected president of the American Society of Zoologists at the Atlantic City meeting.

AT the Cambridge meeting of the Geological Society of America the following officers were elected: Dr. Charles Kenneth Leith, of the University of Wisconsin, *president;* Professor Rollin T. Chamberlin, University of Chicago; Dr. E. M. Kindle, chief of the Division of Paleontology of the Canadian Geological Survey; Professor E. S. Moore, of the University of

Toronto, and Herbert P. Whitlock, curator of mineralogy at the American Museum of Natural History of New York, *vice-presidents*. Dr. Charles P. Berkey, of Columbia University, continues as secretary for his eleventh term, and Professor Edward B. Mathews, of the Johns Hopkins University, continues as treasurer.

THE Paleontological Society of America elected E. M. Kindle, of Ottawa, *president;* E. B. Branson, University of Missouri, *first vice-president;* J. B. Reeside, Washington, D. C., of the United States Geological Survey, *second vice-president;* M. A. Hanna, Houston, Texas, *third vice-president;* B. F. Howell, Princeton University, *secretary;* C. O. Dunbar, of Yale University, *treasurer,* and Walter Granger, of the American Museum of Natural History, New York City, editor of the *Bulletin.*

OFFICERS elected by the Mineralogical Society of America were Herbert P. Whitlock, curator of mineralogy for the Morgan-Tiffany collection at the American Museum of Natural History, New York City, *president;* Frank R. Van Horn, Case School of Applied Science, Cleveland, Ohio, *secretary,* and Waldemar T. Schaller, of the U. S. Geological Survey, *treasurer.*

As has already been announced, the annual meeting of the British Association will be held next year in Leicester from September 6 to 13, under the presidency of Sir F. Gowland Hopkins, of the University of Cambridge, president of the Royal Society. *Nature* reports that the following sectional presidents have been appointed: Section A—Mathematical and Physical Sciences, Sir Gilbert Walker; B—Chemistry, Professor R. Robinson; C—Geology, Professor W. G. Fearnsides; D—Zoology, Dr. J. Gray; E—Geography, the Right Hon. Lord Meston; F—Economic Science and Statistics, Professor J. H. Jones; G—Engineering, R. W. Allen; H—Anthropology, the Right Hon. Lord Raglan; I—Physiology, Professor E. D. Adrian; J—Psychology, Professor F. Aveling; K—Botany, Professor F. E. Lloyd; L—Educational Science, J. L. Holland; M—Agriculture, Dr. A. Lauder.

THE Royal College of Physicians and Surgeons of Canada has conferred honorary fellowships on Lord Bessborough, and on Dr. John Stewart and Dr. I. H. Cameron, emeritus professors of surgery at Dalhousie and Toronto Universities, respectively.

THE title of emeritus professor has been conferred on Dr. William Savage Boulton, who recently retired from the chair of geology at the University of Birmingham.

PROFESSOR W. M. GARDINER, principal of the Technical College, Bradford, will relinquish the editorship of the *Journal* of the Society of Dyers and Colorists at the end of the present year, after holding it for thirty-four years. Dr. F. M. Rowe, professor of color chemistry at the University of Leeds and foreign editor of the journal, has been appointed in his place as co-editor with Mr. Ellis Clayton, chief lecturer in dyeing and cellulose chemistry at the Technical College, Bradford.

DR. DOUGLAS H. SPRUNT, New York, was recently appointed assistant professor of pathology at Duke University School of Medicine, and Dr. Ernest M. Poate, Southern Pines, professor of psychiatry.

HAROLD P. FAWCETT, instructor in mathematics, Columbia University, has become assistant professor of mathematics in the Ohio State University.

DR. LUDWIG HEKTOEN, professor of pathology at the University of Chicago and director of the John McCormick Institute for Infectious Diseases, has been elected chairman of the Board of Governors of the Chicago Institute of Medicine.

DR. GILBERT E. DOAN, associate professor of metallurgy at Lehigh University, has been granted for 1933 a sum of money sufficient to employ a research fellow in continuation of studies of pure iron for arc welding. The study is foundational to the investigation of quality of steel for arc welding, and is sponsored by the Engineering Foundation.

THE *Journal* of the Washington Academy of Sciences reports that Frank T. Davies, formerly of the Byrd Antarctic Expedition, and now on furlough at the request of the Meteorological Service of Canada, from the Department of Terrestrial Magnetism of the Carnegie Institution of Washington, is in charge of the Polar Year station at Chesterfield Inlet. This station is the nearest point to the North Magnetic Pole at which continuous records will be taken during the Polar Year. W. J. Rooney, of the Department of Terrestrial Magnetism, who was temporarily assigned to the U S. Coast and Geodetic Polar Year Station at College, Alaska, to assist in the installation of the atmospheric-electric and earth-current equipment, has completed his work and returned to Washington. K. L. Sherman will be in charge of the work during the Polar Year.

PROFESSOR H. WEYL, of the University of Göttingen, has accepted the invitation of Swarthmore College to give the William J. Cooper Foundation Lectures for 1932–33. He will reside at Swarthmore from the middle of February until the middle of March. During this period he will give five lectures on the general subject of "Mind and Nature" and will take part in the honors work of the college.

Dr. J. C. Drummond, professor of biochemistry, University College, London, will deliver tne next Lane Lectures early in April at the Stanford University School of Medicine in San Francisco. Professor Drummond expects to arrive in San Francisco about April 1, 1933. There will be five lectures, under the general title of "Recent Advances in the Biochemical Study of Nutritional Disorders." The lectures are to be published later.

Dr. Henry A. Christian, Hersey professor of the theory and practice of physic at Harvard University Medical School, Boston, conducted the third graduate teaching clinic at the Central Maine General Hospital, Lewiston, from November 21 to 22. Dr. Christian gave an address on "Cardiac Disease and Its Treatment."

Dr. Walter B. Cannon, George Higginson professor of physiology at the Harvard Medical School, will give the Beaumont Lectures of the Wayne County Medical Society, on January 30 and 31. The subject tentatively selected is "The Relation of the Autonomic System to the Functions of the Alimentary Canal."

A series of scientific discussions will be offered by the Institute of Arts and Sciences of Columbia University during the next three months. Michael Pupin will discuss the "Future of Science"; Dr. Arthur H. Compton, of the University of Chicago, will speak on "Cosmic Rays and their Significance"; Dr. John Bellamy Taylor, of the General Electric research staff, will speak on "Audible Light"; Albert Edward Wiggam, author of "The New Decalogue of Science," will lecture on "Biology in Human Affairs"; Professor Walter Rautenstrauch, of Columbia University, will analyze technocracy, and Auguste Piccard, of Belgium, will tell of his explorations of the stratosphere.

On behalf of the Geological Society of America, its president, Professor Reginald A. Daly, of Harvard University, has protested the proposed cuts in Congressional appropriations for the U. S. Geological Survey. In a statement to Science Service, Professor Daly said: "Directly and indirectly geological service is a principal aid to American business in locating underground raw materials. If the U. S. Geological Survey is now seriously crippled it will be costly if not impossible to restore personnel and skilled experience. Applied geology and profitable mining depends on research of the survey type and to destroy any of the survey's efficiency would be bad economy from the viewpoint of the American consumer of goods that are made from metallic and non-metallic underground raw materials. The Geological Society of America would regard a serious cut of the survey's budget a major disaster for the producers of wealth in this country."

Support of President Hoover's executive order transferring river and harbor engineering work now directed by army engineers to a new Division of Public Works in the Interior Department is announced by the American Engineering Council, representing 60,000 engineers in this country. The reorganization will remedy the present War Department control that is "exceedingly undemocratic and unfair to the more than 200,000 professional engineers of the United States and particularly so to that faithful and efficient group of civilian engineers" working under the War Department. The council predicted material savings in cost, elimination of waste and increase of efficiency when the reorganization is effective.

A bequest of $150,000 for a professorship of geography at Princeton University and one of $500,000 to the Geographical Society of Philadelphia, are included in the will of Henry Grier Bryant, noted explorer, who died on December 7. The American Philosophical Society will receive $10,000 for its building fund, and $5,000 each is to go to the Museum of the University of Pennsylvania, the Pennsylvania Academy of the Fine Arts, the Children's Country Week Association and the Appalachian Mountain Club of Boston, the interest to be applied "to the maintenance of refuge huts or mountain trails operated by the club."

The twenty-third annual exhibition of scientific instruments and apparatus, arranged by the Physical Society, London, was held from January 3 to 5 at the Imperial College of Science and Technology, South Kensington. If the program given in *Nature* was carried out the leading manufacturers of scientific instruments exhibited their latest products in the Trade Section. The Research and Experimental Section contained contributions from most of the important research laboratories in Great Britain, and there was a special sub-section devoted to experiments of educational interest. In addition, the work submitted for the craftsmanship competition by apprentices and learners was on view. Discourses were delivered each day at 8 p. m. as follows: January 3, Dr. Allan Ferguson: "Surface Tension and its Measurement"; January 4, Mr. R. A. Watson Watt: "Cathode Ray Oscillography"; January 5, Mr. F. Hope-Jones: "Time Measurement: Old and New."

The Morris Foundation that has recently affiliated the Morris Arboretum at Chestnut Hill, Philadelphia, with the University of Pennsylvania, has also provided funds for a number of graduate fellowships for students in botany working for higher degrees. A stipend of $1,250 accompanies each appointment. Since appointments may take effect with the middle of February, applications for consideration should be sent at an early date to the Director of the Morris Arboretum, at the Department of Botany, University of Pennsylvania.

# DISCUSSION

## THE USE OF VITAMIN D FROM COD-LIVER OIL IN MILK AND BREAD

As was pointed out in an editorial which appeared in the *Journal* of the American Medical Association for November 26, 1932, it would be of advantage if antirachitic properties could be imparted in a suitable degree to a few foods (such as milk and bread) that enjoy wide-spread use, particularly in the dietary of childhood, because, in spite of several years of vigorous antirachitic propaganda, rickets remains all too prevalent in many communities.

Work with this specific objective in view has been carried on for some years at Columbia University. During the course of experiments conducted for the purpose of determining what substance in cod-liver oil conferred on this oil its well-known therapeutic value in the treatment of rickets, it was found that the antirachitic factor (to which McCollum gave the name of "vitamin D") could be concentrated in a fraction representing a very small part of the original oil.

The process by which this concentration is effected is briefly as follows: The cod-liver oil is treated with 95 per cent. ethyl alcohol, which dissolves out the antirachtic substance together with some other materials, chiefly fatty acids. The fatty acids are saponified, precipitated as calcium soaps, and treated with acetone which removes the active substance. The acetone solution is concentrated, and then treated with ether. After further purification of the ether solution, the ether is distilled off, leaving a brownish, waxy residue (still a very complex mixture) which can be conveniently handled dissolved in oil.

Rat assays showed this concentrate to be highly antirachitic, and later tests at the Children's Clinic of Bellevue Hospital and other health centers showed that it possessed the same curative effects on rachitic infants known to be produced by cod-liver oil.

In its original form, the concentrate had a restricted usefulness, since it contained much of the bad taste and unpleasant odor of cod-liver oil, but further refinements have made possible the elimination of these disadvantages and have produced a product which can be added to milk without altering its flavor. While we are still dealing with an impure substance, the activity of the more recent concentrates is now approaching that of irradiated ergosterol.

Dr. Barnes, of the Detroit Health Department, has conducted a series of tests with milk so treated on rachitic infants and has found that a quart of milk having 150 units of "vitamin D" (equivalent to 3 teaspoonfuls of cod-liver oil), and also amounts corresponding to about 100 units, give excellent results in the treatment of rickets.

It has also been found practical to add the concentrate to bread, as the vitamin D is not destroyed at baking temperatures. An arbitrary standard of 90 units to a 1-lb. loaf has been temporarily adopted.

An economic advantage of this process lies in the fact that the de-vitaminized cod-liver oil is still suitable for industrial purposes, and can be sold at full price so that the raw material cost of the concentrate is very low.

It was originally taken for granted by those engaged in the development work on the cod-liver oil concentrate that the process would be made freely available to any one who wished to use it, but objections to this plan began to multiply. In the first place, conferences with representatives of drug manufacturers made it clear that no one would undertake the extensive work needed for perfecting production methods and marketing the product unless protected from competitors who could enter the field after the pioneering work was done and secure profits without material outlay. Secondly, it seemed desirable to control the manufacture, application and promotion of the product, so that the public could be protected against improperly treated foods on one hand and false claims on the other.

Finally, the president of Columbia University indicated that he had had in mind for some time the creation within the university of some means of meeting just such situations. At his behest, the Board of Trustees passed a resolution creating a Board of University Patents, which now functions under the name of University Patents, Inc. This board consists of trustees and faculty members and is empowered to accept patent rights and copyrights and administer them for the public good. The vitamin D concentrate process was patented in several countries and the applications were assigned to University Patents, Inc. It was decided that royalties which might accrue were to be used for further research within the university.

License contracts were then entered into between University Patents, Inc., and National Oil Products Company, by which the latter obtained the right to manufacture and sell the concentrate in the United

States, Canada and Newfoundland, while the university undertook strict supervision of all advertising, stipulated control of the quality of the reinforced foods by means of regular assays by independent laboratories, and also maintained certain regulations as to prices to be paid by the public in order to keep these as low as possible. The university's royalty was also kept at a low rate in order to keep the burden on the consumer at a minimum.

Through this arrangement we have hopes of making a useful product available to the public in an efficient manner, at the same time safeguarding the interests of the university. A number of problems have presented themselves, some of which have been successfully met, but new ones are still coming up and await solution. It should be possible to set certain useful precedents.

THEODORE F. ZUCKER
COLLEGE OF PHYSICIANS AND SURGEONS,
COLUMBIA UNIVERSITY

## TWO CRITICISMS

I DESIRE to call attention to two practices which in recent years are occasionally noticed and which are objectionable. One is the use of the *unit* of wave-length, Å, for the wave-length itself, λ. The other is the putting of zeros in the tens columns of catalogues.

With the adoption of the Ångstrom as the official *name* of the unit of wave-length in the spectrum some writers began to use it in place of λ, the wave-length itself. This is neither logical nor advantageous. The use of λ before the number to designate wave-length had become an established practice, a necessity, and entirely satisfactory. It is by no means my feeling or wish to detract from the honor due the great Ångstrom, merely to clarify the use of this honor, which it seems to me is fairly obvious as the intentions of the body bestowing it.

Before the adoption of the Ångstrom as the unit (as well as since) the wave-lengths were given in ten millionths of a millimeter. Sometimes this unit of length was given as μ, but usually it was assumed to be understood. Now the Ångstrom, Å, is merely the *name* of this *unit* of a ten millionth of a millimeter, but obviously not the wave-length itself, which is the *whole number* of these units which go to make up the wave-length λ.

Those who use Å usually omit λ, as, for example, 4,340 Å instead of λ 4,340. While perhaps correct in a sense it is much as if we gave a certain number of inches and failed to say of what they were the measure. The users of Å in the way criticized will probably counter that it is well known that these are wave-lengths, to which I would reply that for a much longer time it has been known what the unit was.

It seems to me that here is where the fundamental conception is wrong—that the old designation λ is correct and that the unit Å applies only *within* the spectrum to specify the distances between lines or an arbitrary number of units. That when we wish to give the wave-length of Hγ we should say λ 4,340, but that if we wish to give the distance between the two calcium lines H and K we should say 35 Ångstroms instead of 35 ten millionths of a millimeter, or sometimes merely "tenth mu" among spectroscopists, as formerly.

The use of zeros in the tens columns in catalogues is not extensive and I have only noticed it in a few cases comparatively recently. The object presumably is to avoid such mistakes as occur occasionally by a number getting wrongly into the tens columns of such data as right ascensions and declinations or omissions thus causing confusion. Such mistakes happen but seldom; rarely indeed if the proofs have been read with sufficient care. In small lists of very miscellaneous data such a practice may find some justification but not in extensive catalogues, where entire pages often have the same tens column.

My objection to this practice is that not only is it in reality unnecessary, but chiefly that it is a bother to those consulting the catalogues—just that many more figures to take mental note of in getting out the data wanted. Unquestionably, the fewer the figures which the user of a catalogue has to even look at, the better.

As to the number of mistakes which would be avoided by filling in the tens columns with zeros, it can safely be said that they would not offset the work caused in preparing MS, typesetting and proofreading as well as in the use of the catalogues.

One hesitates to make any criticism whatever of some of the finest and most useful catalogues of data ever provided the investigator, but that feeling should not deter us from trying to better even them in small but essential practical matters.

I might add the suggestion that it is becoming increasingly useful to have the epochs at which spectroscopic data were obtained given in the catalogues *as far as possible*. This is usually given in original sources, but where possible it is useful to have such data in general catalogues also.

C. D. PERRINE
CORDOBA
OCTOBER 12, 1932

## CONCENTRATION OF MICROFILARIAE BY THE SALIVARY SECRETIONS OF BLOODSUCKING INSECTS

DURING my stay in the Chiapas Mountains, southeast Mexico, in November, 1930, investigating on behalf of the Mexican Public Health Department the biology and distribution of the simulid flies concerned in the transmission of the microfilariae of *Onchocerca caecutiens,* I made the same observation as Strong in Guatemala on the concentration of microfilaria about the point of the bite and suggested also in my report, read before the III Congress of the Pan-American Medical Association, Mexico City, July, 1931, and published on September 10, 1931,[1] the same method for diagnoses of Onchocera infestation in man, in dissecting engorged simulid flies. It is very interesting to know that Professor Chas. F. Craig[2] has made the same observation with respect to the transmission of *Wuchereria bancrofti* by *Culex quinquefasciatus* in the Philippines. It would be an easy task for medical officers stationed in tropical Africa, where microfilaria-infections are frequent, to add more observations to the reported cases.

ALFONS DAMPF

LABORATORIO ENTOMOLOGICO,
OFICINA FEDERAL PARA LA
DEFENSA AGRICOLA,
SAN JACINTO D. F.,
MEXICO

## BULBS FROM HOLLAND

I EXPECT that by now you have learned of the fictitious nature of the "Hollandia's World-Famed Flower Bulbs" advertisement which appeared in SCIENCE in September, and in other American magazines. It was exposed in the Report of the Chicago Better Business Bureau for November 4. According to the report:

A fraud order was issued by the Post Office Department against Bulb Nurseries ''Hollandia'' and Harry Bruhl, its director at Voorhout by Hillegom, Holland, for fraudulent practices in the sale of flower bulbs. A previous fraud order was issued on March 18 against L. H. Straathof and others of Hillegom, Holland, upon evidence showing that under those names a scheme to defraud was being conducted through United States mails.

From an American bulb grower's view-point, this advertisement is of concern because it mentions the "certificate of health" supposed to accompany these bulbs. As a matter of fact, our great American bulb-growing industry has been made possible through the establishment of quarantine regulations necessitated by diseases harbored in foreign grown bulbs. The better Holland growers have tried to control these troubles but with varying success. Plant disease control largely depends on efficient crop rotation. This important measure is exceedingly difficult in a locality where usable land is limited and has given rise to certain rather artificial methods of culture. For example, it is a Holland custom to attain partial crop rotation by deep spading and turning the soil upside down, thus creating a "new" field. From a phytopathological view-point such methods can not compete with those possible in American bulb areas where land for rotation is unlimited and climatological factors more favorable.

Competent observers have pointed out that the success of the Holland bulb growers is not attributable to favorable climatic and edaphic factors but to the industry of the growers who have overcome unfavorable circumstances by what may be considered artificial methods. These methods have produced fine bulbs, but we feel that out of fairness to American growers it should be pointed out that the standard of American grown bulbs on a disease-free basis is equal to or higher than that which obtains abroad.

FRANK P. MCWHORTER

OREGON STATE COLLEGE

# SCIENTIFIC APPARATUS AND LABORATORY METHODS

## THE "ROTETTE" OR AN APPARATUS FOR HANDLING SMALL QUANTITIES OF LIQUIDS WITH RAPIDITY AND PRECISION

IT was found in using the pipette previously described[1] that even higher precision was attained by mounting the pipette in bearings at a convenient angle. In this arrangement it could be used directly as before or it could be connected to another tube, either fixed or movable, by means of a rubber tubing. This greatly extended the usefulness of the device since larger quantities of mercury could be safely handled, though there was still a limitation due to the weight of the mercury and its tendency to surge when large quantities were employed.

The employment of a helical glass tube in place of the two bulbs previously used greatly simplified the problem and extended the practical limits as to quantities for which it might be adaptable. With the helical tube it is no longer necessary to have a volume of mercury equal to the volume of liquid to be handled, since only enough mercury to fill the lower half of one turn of the coil is required. The controlling factors are diameter of tubing and of coils and the number of turns. A proper choice of these makes it possible to control the volume desired. With this form the volume displacement is proportional to

[1] *Medicina, Revista Mexicana:* Vol. xi, Year XII, No. 151, pp. 753–761 (see p. 757).

[2] SCIENCE, 1952, May 27, 1932, pp. 561–2.

[1] E. L. Harrington, SCIENCE, p. 201, Aug. 22, 1930.

the angular rotation and it may be stopped in any position, since it is symmetrical about the axis of the helix.

"Rotettes" of the new form were constructed for hand use, as shown in Fig. 1, and also for mounting

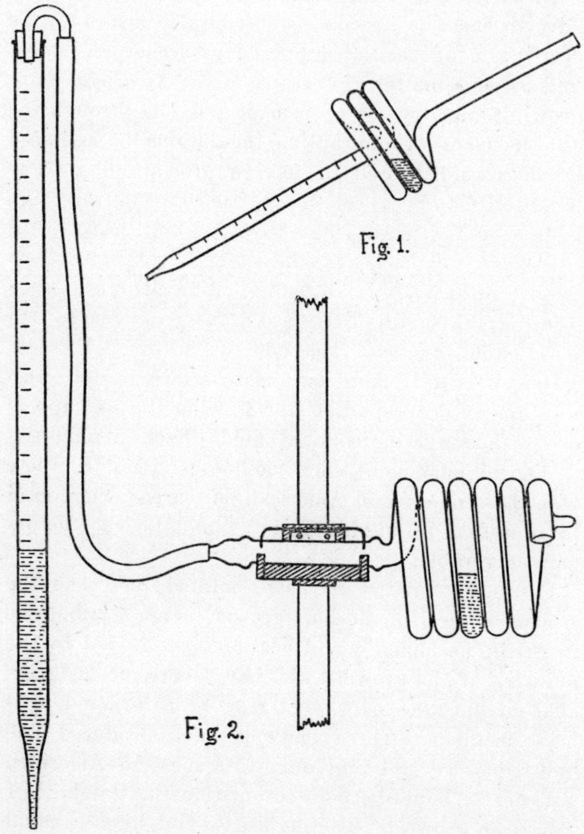


on bearings, as shown in Fig. 2. The advantages of the small form have been discussed.[2] Among these may be mentioned the elimination of the rubber bulb, with all its objections, the necessity of "sucking" directly with the mouth and the difficulty of controlling the outflow of liquid by holding the finger over the upper end of the pipette. In addition may be mentioned the better manual control afforded. It will be observed that the bend leading from the coil to the lower tube is elevated so that the mercury can not run out, even when the pipette is held vertically. In using this form one has merely to hold the rotette at about the angle shown. A rotation in one sense about its axis elevates the liquid, while the reverse rotation ejects it.

When more than a few cubic centimeters are involved, the form shown in Fig. 2 is generally to be preferred. Rotettes with capacities up to 50 cc (but using only 5 or 6 cc of mercury) have been constructed. In this form it has many uses, and a number of advantages over burettes, etc.—among which may be mentioned the following:

(1) It makes for higher precision in operations of the titration type. It is easy to "split" drops without the tedium involved in other methods.

(2) It obviates the use of stop-cocks, pinch-cocks and many other special devices now employed. This is a very important improvement, for leaky cocks, stuck or frozen cocks, contamination by cocks and stop-cock grease, difficulties in cleaning, limitations as to flow, the difficulty of getting "just a drop," are all eliminated.

(3) It eliminates the funnel-bottle method of filling, for the burette is filled directly from the supply container, quickly, and the remnant left after a determination may be returned or ejected just as quickly.

(4) It eliminates the "sucking" of fluids into pipettes, with its dangers to person, and the resulting contaminations by mouth fluids and breath-borne vapors. This makes it possible to put or to hold the rotette in the best position for visibility. The rotating member can be placed in a convenient position, even though the receiving tube has to be introduced into awkward places.

(5) It saves time, since burettes, etc., can be filled to the mark desired without the usual delay or "fiddling." In letting the liquid down, the rate of flow is subject to controlled variation between the full stream of the outlet and a slow dropping. This enables one to "go fast" until he nearly reaches the critical level. It is so easy to restore the liquid to the original level that one need not use long and awkward burettes to avoid having to refill frequently. After practice one learns how much of a turn is required in a certain test. Another great saving in time is gained in the cleansing of the burettes, since the absence of stop-cocks makes cleaning a simple matter. By the same operations cleaning solutions, distilled water, etc., can be introduced without even taking down the burette. When burettes are filled the old way, one has to wait until the liquids have drained down in order to avoid a zero error—with the rotette the surface need not be raised above the zero. With the old method it takes so much time to get the surface just to a mark that students are often tempted to call it "good enough" and to try to carry corrections in the mind. With the rotette a quick adjustment to a line is possible.

(6) It lessens the dangers of contamination. In addition to the points mentioned above it is obvious that stop-cock grease is soluble in many liquids one might want to handle, and in any event one can hardly know when a stop-cock has been really cleaned.

[2] *Loc. cit.*

With stop-cocks, pinch-cocks, rubber tubing, etc., eliminated, one has merely an open tube to clean. The burette is never open at the top to catch contaminating solids or fumes, and no funnels are needed.

(7) It can be used for liquids too viscous to flow readily through a stop-cock, *e.g.,* agar agar—which must often be handled in measured quantities, and handled at a temperature where stop-cock grease would become thin. With the rotette the lower outlet can be made a size suited to the liquid and to the speed employed. The rotette can be used equally well with liquids which attack either stop-cock grease or the ground surface of the glass itself, such as, *e.g.,* KOH or NaOH which so often cause cocks to freeze.

(8) A rotette can not wear out—and while in use it saves the price of a stop-cock on every burette with which it is employed. The burettes without stop-cocks are not only cheaper, but are less fragile—for most of the breakages of burettes are due to stop-cock troubles rather than to accidents. One of these mounted over a stock bottle might facilitate obtaining the definite quantities that may be required in routine tests.

(9) It can be used in places where stop-cocks would be inaccessible, as well as in hot, corrosive or poisonous liquids.

It would appear that the rotette is especially well suited for all types of burette and pipette work, for rapidly measuring out fixed quantities of liquids for routine tests in chemical, biological and clinical laboratories. As the movement is wholly rotational it lends itself to mechanical operation as a rack and pinion arrangement provided with stops would adapt it to the commercial or laboratory filling of vials with definite quantities of liquid. Or, similarly, it could be arranged for foot control in which case both hands would be free for other operations, which would be a very great advantage in many situations.

Suggestion: When connecting the rubber tubing to the burette the mercury should be in the middle coil, as this minimizes the twist that must be given the former in use. The tubing should be one of the smaller commercial sizes, preferably heavy walled to prevent kinking.

E. L. HARRINGTON

UNIVERSITY OF SASKATCHEWAN, CANADA

## MIRROR DEMONSTRATION APPARATUS

IN many lecture rooms the top of the instructor's table is above the line of vision of persons seated in the audience. Demonstrations which must remain flat upon the table are therefore often out of sight of, or at best imperfectly seen by, observers in the lecture room. The difficulty attendant upon demonstrating

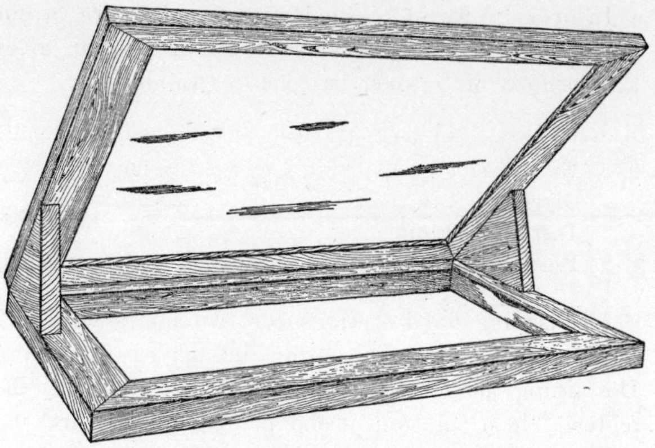

certain materials to large groups of students can be overcome by the device represented in Fig. 1.

A wooden frame holds a mirror at an angle with the table top. The object to be demonstrated is placed inside the base of the frame under the mirror; the reflected image is then visible to students seated in all parts of the room. The angle of the mirror will be determined by the height of the table top above the horizontal line of vision of the audience. In our laboratory, a mirror (size $40 \times 50$ cm) held at a 40° angle gives good results with groups of seventy students. Spot lights may be directed upon the demonstration area from the sides or from above without interfering with the visibility.

The apparatus is particularly useful in demonstrating artificial "amoeboid" action induced by the interaction of various chemicals; in these experiments it is essential that the dishes remain stationary and in a horizontal position. The apparatus is also useful in showing the peculiar movement of waltzing mice; other uses will doubtless suggest themselves to the reader.

The writer is indebted to the department of graphics in Dartmouth College for the perspective drawing in Fig. 1.

W. BYERS UNGER

DARTMOUTH COLLEGE

## THE USE OF PHENOSAFRANIN FOR STAINING FUNGI ON CULTURE MEDIA OR IN HOST TISSUE

THE work of Mangin (1890) first brought out the use of phenosafranin as a differential stain for pectose and lignin. This stain is frequently used in dilute aqueous solution as a desensitizer for panchromatic film. It gives a dark red color in the alkaline condition, which may be removed by means of alcohol or an acid alum solution. This stain has been found useful in mycological studies for both fresh and preserved material and also in the examination of bacterial colonies growing on an agar substratum.

In order to avoid plasmolysis and to restore turgor to the cells the stain was made up in solution after the formula of Satory, as given by Linder:[1]

| | | |
|---|---|---|
| Carbolic acid crystals | 20 | gms. |
| Lactic acid, syrup | 20 | " |
| Glycerine | 40 | " |
| Distilled water | 20 | " |
| Phenosafranin | 0.5 | " or less |

Mordanting fixed sections for two hours with a 2 per cent. iron alum solution intensifies the stain. Destaining may be accomplished by washing the material in a solution of 0.5 per cent. alum and 0.5 per cent. HCl or by means of alcohol. After destaining it is often desirable to set or intensify the stain by applying a 1 per cent. ammonium hydroxide solution. For use in the examination of mycelia in host tissue, the destaining of the parenchymatous tissue is more rapid than that of the parasite, so that by proper control of this process a differential stain may be attained. Sections of Johnson grass leaves infected with a rust stained for twenty minutes in phenosafranin and then destained for ten minutes in acid alum show a differential stain between host and parasite tissue. In the case of mycelia within woody tissue the contrast is not so pronounced, since the lignified walls retain the stain as well as the mycelia.

This stain has proved particularly adaptable in the study of bacterial and fungal colonies growing on an agar substratum. If these colonies be treated with phenosafranin the medium does not absorb the stain as readily as the cells, so that the latter stand out intensely stained against a lighter background, no destaining being necessary.

Phenosafranin is superior to the cotton blue suggested by Linder, because the red is a more intense stain than the blue and also because of the much greater permanence of the phenosafranin color

ELIZABETH JANE MOORE

DEPARTMENT OF BOTANY
AND BACTERIOLOGY,
UNIVERSITY OF TEXAS

# SPECIAL ARTICLES

## PROTEIN FRACTIONS OF THE H 37 (HUMAN) STRAIN OF TUBERCLE BACILLUS[1]

THE method of protein fractionation[2] recently used in the case of the timothy grass bacillus[3] has now been applied to a human strain (H 37) of the tubercle bacillus.

A frozen and dried harvest of the organism[4] (grown on Long's medium) was extracted in the cold with acetone and ether, ground in a ball mill and again extracted, as described previously.[3] The cell residues were stirred for about 6 hours in the cold successively with buffer at pH 4.0 (fraction C), buffer at pH 6.5 (fraction D), water containing enough *N* $NH_4OH$ to keep the pH at 8.3–8.5 (E), water made alkaline to about pH 9 (F), and water made alkaline to about pH 11 (G). The residual material was stirred in turn with 0.1, 0.2 and 0.5 *N* NaOH at room temperature (K, K′, K″). The properties of the fractions obtained by acidifying two lots of the extracts are given in the table. Each fraction was redissolved and reprecipitated twice.

| Fraction | $[\alpha]_D$ degrees | N Per cent. | P Per cent. | Basic ash Per cent. | Precipitin reaction of 1: 2000 solution with anti-human strain serum[4] | Precipitin reaction of 1: 2000 solution with anti-timothy bacillus serum[4] |
|---|---|---|---|---|---|---|
| 701 | | | | | | |
| D | + 9 | 15.7 | 3.4 | 0.7 | ±(±)* | − (+) |
| E | +11 | 15.4 | 2.0 | 0.5 | ±(±) | |
| F | −26 | 15.0 | 1.8 | 1.4 | ±(±) | ±(+) |
| G | −31 | | | | ±(±) | ±(±) |
| K | −61 | 16.2 | 0.4 | 0.4 | ±(±) | +(+±) |
| K′ | −50 | 14.9 | 0.04 | 0.3 | ±(+) | +(+) |
| K″ | −18 | 11.2 | | 1.9 | +++(++++) | +(+±) |
| 702 | | | | | | |
| D | + 9 | 15.6 | 3.7 | 0.8 | ±(±) | +(+±) |
| E | −19 | 15.8 | 2.1 | 0.2 | ±(±) | +(++) |
| G | −28 | 15.7 | 2.1 | 0.2 | ±(±) | +(++) |
| K | −56 | 15.3 | 0.6 | 0.3 | ±(+) | +(+) |
| K′ | −51 | 15.3 | 0.06 | 0.2 | ±(+) | +(+) |
| K″ | −46 | | | | +++(++++) | +(++) |

$[\alpha]_D$, N, P calculated to ash-free basis.
* Values in parentheses obtained after centrifugation.

As in the case of the corresponding fractions of the hemolytic streptococcus,[2] levorotation increases and

[1] David H. Linder, "An Ideal Mounting Medium for Mycologists," SCIENCE, 70: 430, 1929.

[1] From the Department of Medicine, College of Physicians and Surgeons, Columbia University and the Presbyterian Hospital, New York City.

Carried out under a grant from the National Tuberculosis Association and with the aid of the Harkness Research Fund, Presbyterian Hospital, New York City.

[2] M. Heidelberger and F. E. Kendall, *Jour. Exp. Med.*, 54: 513, 1931.

[3] M. Heidelberger and A. E. O. Menzel, *Proc. Soc. Exp. Biol. and Med.*, 29: 512, 1932.

[4] Kindly supplied by the H. K. Mulford Biological Laboratories of Sharp and Dohme, Glenolden, Pa.

phosphorus decreases in general from the D to the K fraction. The percentage of nitrogen, however, remains nearly constant throughout the present series. The exceptional properties of the very small K″ fraction appear due to contamination with specific polysaccharides,[5] especially since the other fractions are practically inactive toward an immune serum known to be rich in polysaccharide antibodies. The products differ in this respect from Johnson's "water soluble" and "alkali-soluble" tubercle bacillus proteins.[6] The relationship of the new fractions to the three proteins indicated by Levene[7] will be investigated.

The somewhat stronger precipitin reactions given by the fractions in an anti-timothy bacillus serum than in the homologous antiserum indicate that all contain group-specific protein. The only additional biological data available at the present preliminary stage of the study are that a proportion of normal rabbits showing a negative skin test to fraction K respond with a "lighting up" of the original test area during a subsequent course of intravenous injections of K, and, as found by Sabin and Smithburn at the Rockefeller Institute for Medical Research, a distinct difference in the type of skin reaction produced by the D and K fractions in tuberculous guinea pigs.

MICHAEL HEIDELBERGER
ARTHUR E. O. MENZEL

## INDUCTION OF EXPERIMENTAL GRANULAR CONJUNCTIVITIS BY DIRECT INOCULATION OF TRACHOMATOUS TISSUE

IN a recent review on the causation of human trachoma Dr. Bengtson[1] writes: "If it can be shown that the condition produced in *Macacus rhesus* monkeys by direct transfer from cases of human trachoma is as definite and as easily transmissible as that induced by inoculation with *Bact. granulosis*, then we would feel more certain of the relationship of *Bact. granulosis* to the human disease."

The observations herein reported demonstrate that direct transfer from such human cases is definitely and easily made and no difference exists between the readiness with which the experimental granular conjunctivitis can be induced by means of human tissue and culture of *Bact. granulosis.*

Through the kind cooperation of Dr. Martin Cohen, of New York, we obtained recently the tarsectomized conjunctival tissue removed for curative purposes from a case of florid trachoma of three years' duration, accompanied by bilateral pannus.

The specimen was employed in two ways: (a) For direct subconjunctival injection of one eye of monkeys having smooth lids, and (b) for bacteriological study. A culture of *Bact. granulosis* was isolated and it also was injected subconjunctivally in one lid of normal *Macacus rhesus* monkeys. Thus human trachomatous tissue, on the one hand, and a culture of *Bact. granulosis,* on the other, both having a common origin, were used to inoculate monkeys.[2]

The first two animals injected with the culture showed within seven days characteristic granular conjunctivitis in the inoculated eye. Within another week, the uninoculated conjunctivae became similarly affected, and after three weeks, the experimental disease, previously described in detail,[3] was fully developed. Conjunctival tissue was removed from one of the affected animals two weeks after inoculation, and employed for subconjunctival injection of two fresh monkeys; they in turn were apparently affected in the same way as the preceding animals. In this manner, monkey to monkey transmission was obtained through seven passages. At this point, when we were convinced that transfer could be carried on indefinitely, the experiment was terminated.

The first two animals inoculated with the suspension of human trachomatous tissue exhibited, within seven days, characteristic granular conjunctivitis, and again the tissue of one of them induced the experimental disease in two fresh animals. The affection was thus transmitted through seven consecutive series, at least, of paired animals. The period of incubation, the conveyance of infection from inoculated to uninoculated eye, the appearance of the early and fully developed lesions of the disease and the histopathological changes were identical with those shown by the animals of the culture series.

The activity of the incitant in both series apparently became "fixed" in the consecutive transmissions, that is, the incubation period and the degree of reaction became constant.

Since transfers were made early in the course of the affection, we were able to study the microscopic changes of beginning conjunctival lesions. These consisted of congestion of blood vessels and marked hypertrophy of their endothelium. The vessels were surrounded by a thick layer containing chiefly monocytes, some lymphocytes, and a few polymorphonuclear cells with acidophilic granules. In later stages, the perivascular agglomerations were coalesced to form the large folliculomata characteristic of trachomatous lesions.

[5] M. Heidelberger and A. E. O. Menzel, *Proc. Soc. Exp. Med. and Biol.,* 29: 631, 1932.
[6] T. B. Johnson, *Am. Rev. Tuberc.,* 14: 169, 1926.
[7] P. A. Levene, *Medical Record,* Dec. 17, 1898.
[1] I. A. Bengston, Public Health Rep., 47: 1914, 1932.
[2] All operative procedures were carried on with the aid of ether anesthesia.
[3] H. Noguchi, *Jour. Exp. Med.,* 48, Suppl. 2, 53 pp. 1928; P. K. Olitsky, R. E. Knutti and J. R. Tyler, *Jour. Exp. Med.,* 53, 753, 1931; 54, 31, 1931.

Finally, cultures of *Bact. granulosis* were isolated from monkeys of the first and second passages of the series of transmissions initiated by inoculation of trachomatous tissue, and from animals of the third and sixth passages of the *Bact. granulosis* series.

In conclusion, we have found that the experimental disease induced by human trachomatous tissue is as definitely transmissible as that produced by cultures of *Bact. granulosis,* and that from different animals of both series the microorganism can be recovered. We also record the fixed character of the incitant in consecutive animal passages and the anatomical changes of early experimental lesions.

PETER K. OLITSKY
JEROME T. SYVERTON
JOSEPH R. TYLER

THE ROCKEFELLER INSTITUTE
FOR MEDICAL RESEARCH,
NEW YORK

## ROD-SHAPED PARTICLES IN TOBACCO MOSAIC VIRUS DEMONSTRATED BY STREAM DOUBLE REFRACTION

FOR some years pathologists have been attempting to obtain evidence regarding the nature of the filterable viruses which cause numerous diseases of man, lower animals and plants. Although much information has been gained regarding the properties of viruses the available evidence is still insufficient to prove whether the virus particles are inanimate colloids or organisms which are too small to be seen through the microscope.

We have recently attempted to obtain evidence regarding the shape of virus particles by the use of polarized light. Methods somewhat similar to those described by Ambronn and Frey[1] and Freundlich[2] for determining the shape of colloid particles have been used in this work. According to these workers minute isotropic rods, disks or leaf-shaped particles contained in a flowing liquid tend to become oriented with their long axis parallel to the direction of flow. Under these conditions a liquid containing rods is doubly refractive when the direction of transmission of the incident light is perpendicular to the direction of flow; a liquid containing disks or leaf-shaped particles is doubly refractive when the incident light is perpendicular to the direction of flow and parallel to the faces of the particles. This so-called form double refraction only occurs when the dispersed phase has a refractive index which differs from that of the continuous phase and when the shortest axis of the particle is small in relation to the wave-length of the light used. Liquids containing anisotropic rods, disks or leaf-shaped particles also show form double refraction under the above conditions, and in addition to this may show an intrinsic double refraction due to the arrangement of atoms in the particles. This intrinsic double refraction occurs when the anisotropic particles are so oriented that their long axis is parallel to the direction of flow, and the direction of transmission of the incident light is not parallel to the optic axis of the particles. Since most of the studies which have been made on virus particles indicate that they are smaller than the wave-lengths of visible light it appears that if virus particles were to have the form of rods, disks or leaves, and the proper refractive index, and were in sufficient concentration, the flowing virus suspension should show double refraction.

In order to test this idea the apparatus shown in Fig. 1 was set up. It consists of an ordinary microscope lamp L and a microscope stand S, from which

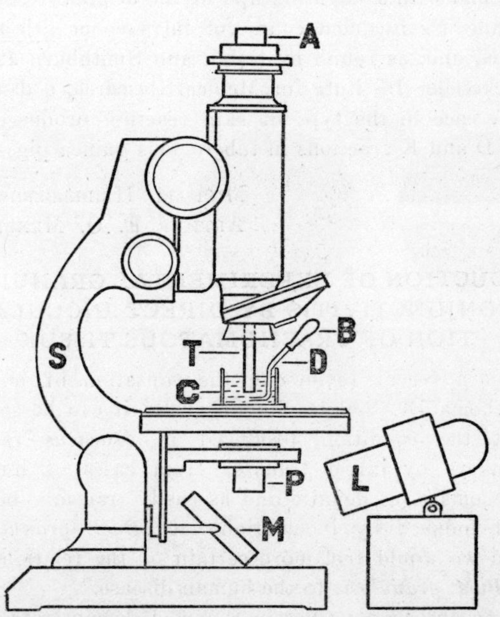


FIG. 1. Apparatus used to detect stream double refraction in virus-containing plant juices and other sols.

the ocular, objectives and condenser have been removed. A polarizer P was placed in the diaphragm carrier and an analyzer A was attached to the microscope tube. A curved glass pipette D, having an inside diameter of 0.5 mm at the orifice, was prepared. This was cemented to the inside of a cylindrical glass chamber C, with its orifice so directed that pressure on the bulb caused a stream to flow across the middle of the chamber. A small round cover glass was cemented to the lower end of the glass tube T, and the upper end of the tube was pushed through a hole in a rubber stopper. The stopper was held in one of the

[1] H. Ambronn and A. Frey, "Das Polarisationsmikroskop." Leipzig. 1926.

[2] H. Freundlich, "Colloid and Capillary Chemistry." E. P. Dutton and Co., New York.

sockets in the nose piece. The glass tube T, the peripheral portion of the cover glass and the lateral surface of the vessel C were painted with black paint so that only light from the polarizer passed up through tube T. The polarizer was turned on its vertical axis until its vibration direction made an angle of 45° with the direction of flow of the liquid expelled from the pipette. The analyzer was then turned until the field was dark as a result of the nicol prisms being crossed.

Leaves of tobacco plants affected with typical mosaic (Johnson's tobacco virus 1) were frozen at 0° F. for 15 hours. The leaves were then thawed at room temperature for about 1 hour and the juice was pressed out of the leaves by means of a screw press. The juice was centrifuged and about 5 cc of the supernatant liquid were poured into the chamber C. A small volume of the liquid was then drawn up into the pipette by means of the rubber bulb B. Upon pressing the bulb while looking through the analyzer the liquid flowing from the pipette was seen to be distinctly doubly refractive, and appeared as a bright streak across the dark field, as seen at A in Fig. 2.

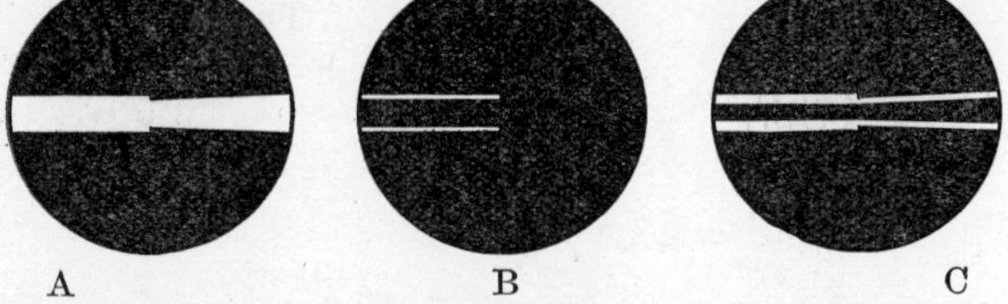


FIG. 2. Showing the appearance of the field when different liquids were expelled from the pipette.

A = Field produced by solutions known to contain rod-shaped particles and by virus-infected plant juice.

B = Field produced by juice from healthy plants.

C = Field produced by ferric oxide sol containing disk-shaped particles.

Juice from healthy leaves prepared in the same way showed no detectable double refraction, the field appearing dark as shown at B in Fig. 2. This experiment was repeated 6 times, with leaves from 6 different healthy and mosaic tobacco plants, once with juice from the roots of a healthy and mosaic tobacco plant, and once with juice from the leaves of a healthy and mosaic tomato plant. In each case double refraction was shown only by juice from the mosaic plants.

Freundlich[2] has reported that sols of vanadium pentoxide, aniline blue and benzopurpurin have rod-shaped particles, while old ferric oxide sols have disk-shaped particles. In order to gain evidence regarding the shape of the particles in the virus-bearing juice which are responsible for the double refraction, sols of vanadium pentoxide, aniline blue, benzopurpurin and ferric oxide were tested in our apparatus. It was found that, like the virus-bearing juice, the sols containing rod-shaped particles produced a stream which showed uniform light intensity throughout the width of the stream as shown at A in Fig. 2. On the other hand, the ferric oxide sol containing disk-shaped particles produced a stream which showed double refraction only along its edges as shown at C in Fig. 2. This behavior is presumably due to the fact that it is only in the edges of the stream that a large proportion of the disk-shaped particles are oriented with their faces parallel to the direction of transmission of the incident light.

It has not been determined whether the double refraction observed in the infective juice is a form double refraction, an intrinsic double refraction or a combination of both types. In any case the occurrence of stream double refraction in the juice of mosaic tobacco plants, its absence in the juice of healthy plants and its similarity to the stream double refraction shown by sols containing rod-shaped particles, indicate that the virus of tobacco mosaic or some substance regularly associated with it, is composed of rod-shaped particles.

WILLIAM N. TAKAHASHI
T. E. RAWLINS
DIVISION OF PLANT PATHOLOGY,
UNIVERSITY OF CALIFORNIA,
BERKELEY

## PHOTOCHEMICAL NITRIFICATION IN SEA WATER

SINCE nitrates frequently are considered to be a limiting factor in the productivity of the sea, phenomena which increase the available nitrogen for plant growth are of great importance. It has been tacitly assumed by many authors that the same biological agencies which are operative in the transfer of nitrogen from one form to another in the soil similarly activate these processes in the sea. However, Lipman,[1] Atkins,[2] Brandt[3] and other investigators have reported their failure to demonstrate nitrifying bacteria in the open seas, although nitrifiers are frequently found near the shore and in bottom muds. Similar observations in the Pacific Ocean off the coast of California in the vicinity of San Diego have been made repeatedly by the writer. Brandt has mentioned the possibility of nitrites being formed from ammonium near the surface, due to the presence of inorganic catalysts in the sea water.

It has been impossible to demonstrate nitrifying bacteria by the conventional soil methods when from 0.1 to 100 cc of sea water was inoculated into Winogradsky's solution and other similar nutrient com-

[1] SCIENCE, 56: 501, 1922.
[2] *Jour. du Conseil,* 1: 197, 1926.
[3] *Wissensch. Meeresuntersuchungen,* 20: 203, 1927.

binations, although controls inoculated with a little garden soil or even sea bottom muds have given positive results. There was no perceptible nitrification in media consisting of raw sea water to which ammonium salts were added in different concentrations. Varying the temperature from 4° to 30° C. by six-degree intervals did not give any evidence of the presence of nitrifiers in the sea water.

On the other hand, soil nitrifiers, *nitrosomonas,* failed to elaborate any nitrites when inoculated into sea water with the addition of magnesium carbonate in excess and ammonium sulfate, although they were still viable after eight weeks at 20° C. In a medium consisting of 50 per cent. sea water and 50 per cent. Winogradsky's solution inoculated with *nitrosomonas,* nitrification occurred, but not as readily as in straight Winogradsky's solution. With 75 per cent. sea water the amount of the reaction was negligible and 90 per cent. sea water stopped it. The addition of 5 to 10 per cent. sea water to Winogradsky's solution accelerated the oxidation of ammonium to nitrites by the biological agents mentioned above. Such evidence seems to warrant the conclusion that if bacterial nitrifiers are in the open seas, they are different from the soil forms, but it does not preclude the possibility of there being bacterial nitrifiers in the sea which require special methods of cultivation. Investigations are now in progress which may help to elucidate this point.

In continuing the inquiry into the mode of origin of nitrates, it was found, contrary to expectation, that sunlight favored nitrification in sea water under certain conditions. When pyrex flasks partly filled with raw sea water plus 0.005 per cent. ammonium sulfate were exposed to light on the top of a building for two weeks there was a measurable increase in nitrites as well as nitrates and a corresponding decrease in the ammonium content. The controls in the dark were unchanged. Examinations revealed that there were fewer viable bacteria in the flasks which had been exposed to sunlight than in the dark controls. The removal of bacteria by filtering the water through a Berkefeld N candle into sterile flasks did not influence the oxidation of ammonium to nitrites when thus irradiated. The reaction was accelerated by the addition of manganese dioxide. No perceptible oxidation of ammonium occurred in distilled water nor in artificial sea water under comparable conditions. Autoclave sterilization (120° C. for 30 minutes) of sea water destroyed its photochemical nitrifying properties. This is attributed to the thermal destruction of certain oxidizing substances or even organic catalysts.

Many of the above experiments were repeated, using ultra-violet light having a maximum intensity in the 2950Å region. Such irradiation of sea water mixtures produced results not unlike those observed under the influence of sunlight, except for the speed of the reaction. Exposure to the mercury arc at thirty inches for two hours caused the oxidation of as much ammonium as the daylight did in two weeks. Again it was found that more ammonium was oxidized to nitrites by irradiation of sea water than distilled water. Ultrafiltration of sea water did not alter it in this respect, but autoclaving it retarded the reaction. Increasing the intensity of the irradiation ten times by bringing the source to within about 9½ inches from the test solutions actually caused the destruction of more ammonium than could be accounted for as nitrites or nitrates.

In view of these observations it appears that at least part of the nitrification which occurs in the sea is photochemically activated. Zolcinski[4] has repeatedly found that chemical nitrification in the soil is activated by sunlight in the exclusion of biological agencies. It is well known that under certain conditions ultra-violet light causes the oxidation of ammonium to nitrites. Due to the slight penetrability of water by these rays, they could play an important rôle only at or a few millimeters from the surface. Inasmuch as no light filters were used in these preliminary tests, many rays other than the ultra-violet may have been the effective ones. The mercury arc did supply visible light of great intensity. As previously stated, the solar rays responsible for the reaction will pass through pyrex glass. The point to be emphasized at this time is not which rays are active, but rather that the irradiation of sea water causes the oxidation of ammonium to nitrites and that sunlight supplies the necessary rays. In a later communication a report of the foregoing experiments will be amplified and additional observations given.

C. E. ZOBELL

SCRIPPS INSTITUTION OF OCEANOGRAPHY
UNIVERSITY OF CALIFORNIA
LA JOLLA, CALIFORNIA

## BOOKS RECEIVED

*Annual Report of the Director of the National Park Service, 1932.* Pp. 100. Illustrated. National Park Service, U. S. Department of the Interior.

JOHNSTONE, JAMES and R. J. DANIEL, Editors. *Report for 1931 on the Lancashire Sea-Fisheries Laboratory, University of Liverpool, and the Annual Report of the Marine Biological Station, Isle of Man.* Pp. 169. Illustrated. University Press of Liverpool. 6s.

*Journal of the Faculty of Science of Hokkaido Imperial University.* Series IV: *Geology and Mineralogy,* Vol. I, Nos. 3–4. Illustrated. The University, Sapporo, Japan.

*Proceedings of the American Council of Learned Societies.* Bulletin No. 18. Pp. 152. The Council, Washington, D. C.

[4] *Int. Rev. Sci. Pract. Agric.,* 2: 838, 1924 (Abstract).

# SCIENCE

VOL. 77 — FRIDAY, JANUARY 13, 1933 — NO. 1985

*The New Anthropogeny—Twenty-five Stages of Vertebrate Evolution, from Silurian Chordate to Man:* DR. WILLIAM K. GREGORY ... 29

*Obituary:*
*John Joseph Carty—an Appreciation:* DR. F. B. JEWETT ... 41

*Scientific Events:*
*The Natural History of Mount Everest; Forestry Program for the Southeastern States; The Wisconsin Alumni Research Foundation; The Pacific Division of the American Association for the Advancement of Science* ... 43

*Scientific Notes and News* ... 45

*Discussion:*
*A Forgotten Evolutionist:* DR. S. J. HOLMES. *A Vicious Circle in Cytology:* PROFESSOR E. C. JEFFREY. *Twisted Trees and the Spiral Habit:* PROFESSOR WILLIAM SEIFRIZ. *The Extinct Lake San Augustin, New Mexico:* PROFESSOR WILLIAM E. POWERS ... 48

*Scientific Books:*
*Faraday's Diary:* PROFESSOR W. F. MAGIE ... 52

*Societies and Meetings:*
*The Texas Academy of Science:* H. B. PARKS. *The Oklahoma Academy of Science:* HORACE J. HARPER ... 54

*Scientific Apparatus and Laboratory Methods:*
*An Apparatus for Determining the Absorption of Carbon Dioxide by Leaves under Natural Conditions:* PROFESSOR A. J. HEINICKE and M. B. HOFFMAN ... 55

*Special Articles:*
*The Function of the Adrenal Cortical Hormone and the Cause of Death from Adrenal Insufficiency:* PROFESSOR W. W. SWINGLE, J. J. PFIFFNER, H. M. VARS, P. A. BOTT and W. M. PARKINS ... 58

*Science News* ... 8

SCIENCE: A Weekly Journal devoted to the Advancement of Science, edited by J. MCKEEN CATTELL and published every Friday by

THE SCIENCE PRESS

New York City: Grand Central Terminal
Lancaster, Pa. — Garrison, N. Y.
Annual Subscription, $6.00 — Single Copies, 15 Cts.

SCIENCE is the official organ of the American Association for the Advancement of Science. Information regarding membership in the Association may be secured from the office of the permanent secretary, in the Smithsonian Institution Building, Washington, D. C.

# THE NEW ANTHROPOGENY: TWENTY-FIVE STAGES OF VERTEBRATE EVOLUTION, FROM SILURIAN CHORDATE TO MAN[1]

By Professor WILLIAM K. GREGORY

COLUMBIA UNIVERSITY AND AMERICAN MUSEUM OF NATURAL HISTORY

THE subject of anthropogeny, as it was developed at the hands of Ernst Haeckel, involved an attempt to read the earlier stages of prehuman evolution largely from the data supplied by human and comparative embryology. Thus its main postulate was the so-called "law of recapitulation." But the attacks of modern zoologists on this "law" seem to have led, in this country at least, to a loss of confidence in Haeckel's chief conclusions. In certain quarters there has sprung up a regular epidemic, which may be named *Haeckelophobia.*

Meanwhile the new anthropogeny has been gradually taking shape. But before speaking of its origins and tentative results to date, it might be well to note that a humble exponent of the new doctrine is liable to experience a slightly guilty feeling if he finds himself obliged to speak in any official gathering of his scientific brethren. For example, the brethren of the orthodox anthropologist sect are always piously busy, wielding their magic measuring wands and ringing the bells on their magic calculators, or thinking machines, while the poor anthropogenist stands idly by and must confess that he is not primarily bent on measuring or counting anything, but only in piecing together the broken story of the "big parade" that nature has staged across the ages.

Another contrast between the anthropogenist and

[1] Address of the vice-president and retiring chairman of Section H—Anthropology, American Association for the Advancement of Science, Atlantic City, December 29, 1932.

the orthodox anthropologist is that the regulars stand happily among the topmost branches of the family tree of man and count all its twigs, while the anthropogenist, like a silly ant, runs up and down the main branches and trunk and gropes blindly around the roots.

Moreover, up to the present time the new anthropogeny is operating to a considerable extent on a borrowed, or perhaps appropriated, capital of facts. And up to date it has found no way to repay the lenders.

For example, from historical geology the new anthropogeny appropriates the standard divisions of geologic time in which the drama of evolution has been played. But until relatively recent times geology could determine only the sequence of terrestrial events, without measuring their duration in years.

To physics, mineralogy and stratigraphy, the new anthropogeny now owes the "radium clock" of geologic time. If the readings of this clock give even a preliminary approach to the truth, as they seem indeed to do, then the events which the new anthropogeny attempts to discover and describe took place during a period of the general order of magnitude of five hundred million years.

From zoology and comparative anatomy the new anthropogeny has received the precious doctrine of the *"Échelle des Êtres,"* or scale of beings, which was elaborated by the French naturalists of the eighteenth century, but which has since been almost abandoned and forgotten. Instead of throwing this doctrine on the junk-heap along with Euclidean geometry, the new anthropogeny finds that after being slightly revamped and fitted with a few new parts, the old apparatus still functions well; for it has led to a fuller recognition of the significance and importance of "living fossils," which have preserved in greater or less degree the successive grades of organization that were characteristic of many past ages. The study of the scale of beings has led also to the realization that if there were no "living fossils," that is, if every phyletic line had evolved at the same equal and constant rate, all the descendants of a common ancestral stock would now be indistinguishable throughout their anatomy. In other words, the very existence of comparative anatomy depends upon the fact that there is a more or less closely graded scale of beings, or rather, many scales of beings, leading not only toward man but toward every other highly specialized animal.

To paleontology, however, we owe the discovery of actual fossil skeletons that correspond more or less closely to the grades of organization inferred from the study of the scale of beings. Thus there is no longer any need of inventing hypothetical stages, as Haeckel did from doubtfully valid extensions of embryological processes, when the paleontological evidence is so unexpectedly adequate if viewed in the light of evidence from several different fields.

If the obligations of the new anthropogeny to all the previously named sciences are great, still greater is its dependence upon the science of vertebrate taxonomy; this branch of science endeavors to identify and follow the large and small branches of the vast tree of the vertebrates. We may be inclined to smile at first at the simplicity of Haeckel's picture of the tree of life, which might now be condemned as "monophyletic" and rejected in favor of a "polyphyletic" diagram with innumerable lines all running back to infinity. However, the cumulative experience of modern paleontologists and zoologists leads to the concept that while the tree of vertebrate life has a fairly large number of minor twigs which run back for long distances in geologic time, the number of major branches is quite limited and can be fairly well grasped during the lifetime of an ordinarily industrious student of fossil and recent vertebrates. But the supreme mistake would be to suppose that the branches have grown at equal rates, that is, that the "chronometer of evolution" runs at the same rate in all lines; it would be another mistake to infer that the branches never did run together because we have not yet located all the junctions. For the progress of vertebrate paleontology constantly leads to the discovery of new forms, yet in most cases the new forms represent branches that lie in between two or more branches already recorded.

Perhaps the most essential of all services rendered to the new anthropogeny by the science of phylogenetic taxonomy is the identification of branches that can be definitely excluded from what we choose to call the main line of ascent to man. Another service is the determination of the probable distance of a given branch from that main line.

Anthropogeny likewise borrows from chemistry, physics and physiology the very basic principle that man, like other organisms, is a sort of solar engine that runs by means of the energy stored up in plant and animal food. It follows that this potential energy forms a hidden prize of great worth, to obtain which all animal life struggles unceasingly. Hence the drama of terrestrial evolution is motivated by the complexly ramifying competition and strife for food and for reproductive mates; this principle operates as strongly in the latest stages of life as it did in the earliest.

We may start then with one of the most firmly grounded landmarks in the new anthropogeny, namely, that man belongs on the vertebrate tree of life, and that, while his present habitus is that of the human biped, his general heritage is that of a quadrupedal vertebrate of the class of mammals and of the order of Primates. These general facts were well known to Huxley, Haeckel, Darwin, Lamarck, and even to a large extent to Linnaeus, but they are always being buried and forgotten under the details about which scientific men love to dispute. What was not known to the older naturalists, however, is the modern wealth of material that supplies us with a paleontological series representing the main successive structural stages in the long ascent from the jawless chordates of the Silurian age up to man.

At present we may distinguish about twenty-five structural stages from and including the oldest known pre-fishes up to modern man. It is not claimed that these stages lie exactly in the direct line of ascent but only that they are more or less near to it after the elimination of more specialized side branches.

Let us attempt to run over these stages very briefly with the lantern slides.

We may consider for a moment the general history of the locomotor apparatus, especially the skeleton. We start with the fact that the larger units of the vertebrate locomotor system are the W-shaped muscle flakes, or myomeres, on the side of the fish; the smaller units are the striped muscle fibers with their far smaller fibrillae, which run into the billions in a human body. The beginnings of all the complex motions of the human body are to be sought in the rhythmic contraction and relaxation of the W-shaped muscle flakes of the fish, and there are already on record many structurally intermediate stages between the simple muscles of the fish and the complex muscles of man. And it is sufficient to mention in passing that the human embryo agrees with that of the fish in that not only its axial muscles but also the segments of the backbone arise from segmentally arranged buds of mesoderm on either side of the embryonic notochord.

*Stage 1. Pre-fishes (Ostracoderms) of Paleozoic times (Ordovician to Devonian).*

For the purpose of this address we must leave out of account the disputed problem of the origin of the vertebrates and begin with a grade of organization that was already far nearer to that of man than to the one-celled starting-point. Thanks to the Danish scientific expeditions to Greenland, Norway and Spitzbergen, we now possess a surprisingly detailed fund of information regarding the general characters of the brain and cranial nerves and blood-vessels of these oldest known Chordates; these have recently been described in the beautiful monographs by Stensiö and Kiaer. Thus we now have a firm foundation of facts to replace conjecture. These pre-fishes, or ostracoderms, were bilaterally symmetrical, with a median axis, or notochord, moving by lateral undulations of the body, by contractions of W-shaped muscle segments. The head was of the complex vertebrate type, including a braincase that contained three pairs of main sense organs, corresponding to the olfactory, optic and otic capsules of higher vertebrates and arranged in a fore-and-aft series.

A continuous endoskeletal tissue, containing bone-cells in one order of ostracoderms, enclosed the three main pairs of sense organs and formed a trough for the brain and tunnels for the cranial nerves and blood-vessels. When these tunnels and this braincase became filled with mud, which subsequently became mineralized, there was left a record of the general anatomy of the nervous system which has endured for perhaps four hundred millions of years, down to our own time.

Beneath the braincase was a greatly expanded chamber containing the mouth cavity, the gill-pouches, the skeletal partitions between the gill-pouches and the ducts leading to and from the gill-openings and the exterior. This arrangement is closely paralleled in the larval stage of the existing lampreys. The same is true of the brain and cranial nerves. The neurologists and students of the classical problem of the vertebrate head-segments had long ago fixed upon the larval stage of the lamprey as standing nearest among existing forms to the archetypal vertebrates. Thanks to the labors of many investigators, we can now affirm that the ostracoderms as a class were the archetypal vertebrates from which were derived, on the one hand, the so-called jawless cyclostomes, or lampreys and hags, and on the other hand, the gnathostomes, or jaw-bearing vertebrates, comprising true fishes, amphibians, reptiles, birds and mammals (including man).

*Stage 2. "Antiarchs" of Devonian age.*

These strange-looking forms had the head and body enclosed in an armor of bony plates and propelled themselves by a pair of jointed appendages that remind us of the walking legs of crabs. They were probably quite far off the direct line leading to higher vertebrates, but the beautiful fossils from Scaumenac Bay, Quebec, described by the late Professor Patten and now by Stensiö, leave little doubt that these antiarchs had recently crossed the line separating the so-called jawless from the true jaw-bearing forms. For they had obviously acquired external jaw plates, homologous with those plates in the true fishes which were destined to give rise ultimately to our own upper and lower jaws; while, according to Stensiö, their external jaw plates could only have been supported internally by cartilaginous bars homologous with the true or inner jaws of adult sharks and of embryonic higher vertebrates.

*Stage 3. "Pre-sharks" of Devonian age.*

The earlier acanthodians may well be called "pre-sharks" because, although shark-like in general characters, they represent an older and more primitive type nearer to the line of ascent to higher vertebrates.

Externally the acanthodians give us a glimpse of an early stage in the evolution of paired limbs. They support the conclusions of Balfour, Dean and others that the paired fins are essentially the same as the median fins and that both arose as folds of skin and projections of the muscular body-wall that served originally as stabilizers and keels. Such fin-folds in the early stages had wide bases and limited mobility.

The pre-sharks had attained an early stage in the evolution of the gnathostomes, or jaw-bearing vertebrates, since they had inner or true jaws, in series with the gill-arches. In another early shark, *Cladoselache,* we see in this view of the under side of the head how closely the upper and lower jaw bars are in series with the gill-arches, from one pair of which the jaws were doubtless derived.

*Stage 4. "Basal ganoid fish" (Palaeoniscoid), Old Red Sandstone (Devonian).*

These earliest known forerunners of the modern bony fishes used to be called "osseous sharks" by the late Professor Bashford Dean, because they combine a generally shark-like body-form with the bony armor over the head and shoulder-girdle of the earlier typical fishes. This bony armor is composed of plates, each one of which has a definite name. Many of these plates, such as the frontals, the parietals and the surface bones of the upper and lower jaws, can be traced forward, as we shall presently see, from these very early fishes up through the amphibians, the earlier reptiles, the mammal-like reptiles, to the earlier mammals and thence through the lower primates to man. Other elements of the fish skull, such as the bones of the opercular series that covered the gill-chamber, disappeared when fish turned into amphibians.

These earlier true fishes also exhibit the fins in successive stages of development. The anal fin is still just like the dorsal fin, with an extended base supported by a regular series of little bony rods. The pelvic fins show an early stage in the crowding of the basal pieces, especially at the front end. The pectoral fin has already attained the stage of a broad paddle with a crowded base.

This sequence is still clearly seen in the fins of the spoon-bill sturgeons, or paddle-fishes, which are the otherwise specialized descendants of the earlier ganoids. Here we see three stages in the evolution of the mobile pectoral paddles, as figured by Dr. Tate Regan, of the British Museum of Natural History.

*Stage 5. "Lobe-finned" fishes, of Upper Devonian and Lower Carboniferous ages.*

The tendency toward the evolution of freely turning paddles, presumably out of fin-folds, reaches a climax among the lobe-finned fishes of late Paleozoic times. In the tassel-finned branch of these forms the paddles grow at the distal end and give rise to a string of joints with slender rods on each side. But in the "fan-finned" branch the paddles spread out like the sticks of a fan, and the bony rods that support them seem destined to give rise to the skeleton of the arm and hand of higher vertebrates. This fan-shaped stage is well illustrated in an Upper Devonian form to which the geologist James Hall in 1843 gave the appropriate name *Sauripterus*—"lizard-fin." We shall see a little later how such a paddle might give rise to the cheiropterygium, or five-rayed hand, of a higher vertebrate.

Before going on to the next higher stage we must pause for a moment in order to rule out the dipnoans, or lung-fishes, from the line of ascent to the higher vertebrates and to expose their true place on a side branch further away from the main line than that which they occupy in the genealogical trees figured by Haeckel and by his modern follower, Professor Naef. The dipnoan lung-fishes are excluded from the main line by three sets of characters: first, they belong in a division with feather-shaped, or leaf-shaped, paddles, in which the many-jointed central axis is predominant; secondly, their dentition is specialized in a very peculiar way, which leads to nothing but that of their modern descendants and is widely different from the dentition of the earliest amphibians. Thirdly, the lung-fishes are excluded from ancestry to the higher forms by the highly peculiar specialization of the extremely massive inner skull, and by the bizarre pattern of the many small plates covering the braincase.

On the other hand, the ancient lobe-finned fishes present nearly ideal conditions, not only of the paddles, but also of the dentition and skull patterns, to favor their claim to be on or near the main line of ascent to the four-footed, air-breathing vertebrates.

The living *Polypterus* of Africa is a justly famous survivor of the most ancient ganoids. From whichever of the two oldest orders of ganoids he may have been derived, he does show us how readily a lobe-finned paddle may be directed downward on either side of the body in a position to assist in wriggling on the mud.

*Stage 6. Basal Amphibian. Upper Devonian and Lower Carboniferous.*

Even the modern amphibians, including the frogs, newts and salamanders, retain so many essentially fish-like characters, especially in their larval stages, and in the general pattern of the cranial and spinal nerves, that zoologists have never had any reason to doubt that amphibians have been derived from ancient air-breathing fishes of some sort.

Thanks to the recent labors of Bryant, Watson, Stensiö and others, on the fossil lobe-finned fishes, and to those of Watson on the Lower Carboniferous amphibians of Great Britain, the gap in our records between fishes and amphibians is being measurably lessened.

Indeed, it may now be said to be highly probable that although no known genus of lobe-finned fish was the immediate ancestor of the amphibians, yet the group as a whole has the characters to be expected in the descendants of an earlier common stock that gave rise, on the left, to the lung-fishes, near the center, to the known lobe-fins, and on the right, to the earliest tetrapods or amphibians.

Since the last sentence was written I have received the latest report of the Danish Geological Survey of Greenland, containing a monograph by G. Säve-Söderbergh entitled "Preliminary Note on Devonian Stegocephalians from East Greenland." These oldest known amphibians, which were discovered in 1931, aroused a great deal of interest in the American press a short time ago under the name of "four-legged fish." The present report fully justifies the expectation that when amphibians of Devonian age became known they would be decidedly nearer to the lobe-finned fishes than were the already known amphibians of the Lower Carboniferous. This now proves to be the case in the patterns of the skull top and palate as figured from beautifully preserved material.

The breathing of atmospheric air had already been acquired by several groups of fishes of the ancient coal swamps, as it has by several unrelated modern fishes. If we may judge from modern conditions, an oxygen-secreting pouch long served to tide the fish over periods of drought, and possibly the stout fan-shaped paddles of the lobe-fins may have assisted them in wriggling from one pool to another.

The greatest advance made by the earliest known amphibians over their fish ancestors is to be seen in their paired limbs. For each limb is now sharply angulated at the elbow and at the wrist, the basal supports of the bony rays have been crowded together so that they converge toward the postaxial arm-bone, while five of the paddle-rays have become modified to serve as fingers and the outer fin-rays have disappeared, leaving only the nails as a trace of their former existence.

As a result of studies in several fields, Gregory, Miner and Noble have attempted to visualize a possible intermediate stage between a fan-shaped lobe-fin of the *Sauripterus* type and the known pattern of the fore limb in a primitive amphibian.

When, however, we compare the skulls and jaws of the lobe-fins with those of the earliest amphibians, we have no difficulty in identifying homologous elements, or in accounting for those which are lacking in the amphibians.

When breathing by the air-sac finally superseded breathing by the gills, in the adult stage, it is not surprising that the opercular bones, which play an important part in branchial respiration, should have failed to ossify, leaving only a dermal flap. The region of the otic notch in Amphibia corresponds closely to that of the opercular flap in fishes.

As in many other stages of vertebrate ascent, we learn much from the highly specialized descendants of to-day, which in this case are the frogs, toads, salamanders, etc. Their skulls represent fenestrated and depauperized derivatives of the ancient amphibian type.

### *Stage 7. The Stem Reptiles (Cotylosaurs), Upper Carboniferous and Permian.*

It used to be supposed that there was a great gap between the Amphibia and the reptiles, the former being classified with the fishes as Ichthyopsida, the latter with the birds and mammals as Amniota. But thanks to the labors of the late Professor Samuel W. Williston and others, we now know certain fossil forms that break down the old distinctions between amphibians and reptiles. It was said by the elder Huxley, for example, that the amphibians had paired condyles at the back of the occiput, while the reptiles had but one median condyle. It is now known that the primitive amphibians had tripartite condyles, from which were evolved, on the one hand, the double condyles of the typical amphibians and, on the other hand, the ball-like median condyle of modern reptiles and birds.

One of these early reptiles, *Seymouria,* is so nearly on the borderline between amphibians and reptiles that one set of his skull characters has been used to classify him as an amphibian, while other skull characters, together with the detailed construction of his vertebral column, justify his claim to be one of the stem reptiles.

In short, the most conspicuous advance among the reptiles was the elimination of the fish-like or aquatic stage of individual development. By enclosing an artificial watery environment within a water-tight egg the reptiles hit upon a "basic patent" which enabled them to invade the uplands and eventually to conquer almost the whole earth.

The earliest reptiles retained generalized 5-rayed hands and feet, and this constitutes one of their many claims to be on or near the "main line" of ascent to man. The opposite course of digital reduction has been followed by most of the descendants of the ancient reptiles. It has invariably carried them away from the "main line" of ascent.

*Stage 8. The Captorhinids, progressive cotylosaurs. Permian.*

In the ancient "lobe-finned" ganoids the entire surface of the head was enclosed in a shiny armor of surface plates with openings only for the paired nostrils, the median pineal eye, the paired eyes. The outer jaws were merely the bony plates covering the inner, or gill-arch, jaws. The upper jaw plates were in series with the bony mask covering the head, the lower jaw plates covered the primary, or gill-arch, jaws. The jaw muscles were hidden under the shining facial mask. All this was equally true of the oldest amphibians and reptiles, except that the shiny surface of the bony skull plates was lost just before the amphibian stage.

In the captorhinids, which were rather progressive stem reptiles, the same conditions obtained, but these enterprising little forms had, so to speak, patented what we may call a "four-way palate brace" and were also using the oldest recorded orthodontic appliance, the "descending pterygoid flange," which kept the lower jaw in vertical alignment. Lack of time forbids further references to these devices except for the statement that they seem to be prerequisites for the development of the peculiar type of palate that appeared in the mammal-like reptiles.

*Stage 9. The Texas Theromorphs, of Permian times.*

As noted above, the jaw muscles of primitive vertebrates were covered externally by a shell or bone, forming the so-called "unperforated temporal roof." While this arrangement may have been advantageous by reason of the protection it afforded to the jaw muscles, it may also have had its inherent disadvantages, such as cramping the free expansion of the jaw muscles. But the Texas theromorphs hit upon the device of "fenestrating" by absorbing the central area of the temporal shell while strengthening its periphery. After this, nothing could or did stop the advance of the jaw muscles until the completely mammalian type of cheek arch had been reached. This was one of the reasons why Professor Cope classified these Texas Permian forms as Theromorpha, or mammal-like reptiles, and regarded them as ancestral to the mammals. The big ones are obviously too specialized in having a chevaux-de-frise of spines on top of the backbone, but the smaller ones, such as Williston's *Mycterosaurus,* avoided these specializations.

*Stage 10. The Earlier Mammal-like Reptiles, of the Permian of South Africa and Russia.*

South Africa is justly famous for its diamond mines, but from the view-point of anthropogeny its extinct mammal-like reptiles are of far greater significance. Even the earlier reptiles of the Karroo series had already progressed far on the long evolutionary road toward the mammalian grade of organization. For, while their own forerunners had been clumsy beasts, crawling with sharply bent elbows and knees, the South African theromorphs had begun to lift the body off the ground by bringing the fore and hind feet under the body. The skeleton, in fact, abounds in indications of progressively heightened activity associated with predatory habits. The skull was beginning to approach the mammalian grade, in the differentiation of the dentition into incisors, canines and cheek teeth, in the presence of a temporal opening and cheek arch of mammalian type, and in other features.

*Stage 11. The Cynodonts or Pro-mammals (Triassic of South Africa and Russia).*

The South African cynodonts advanced so far toward the mammals that they ought to have been called pro-mammals, and they are only technically still within the upper limits of the reptilian class. For instance, the skeleton is now well fitted for running, while the skull abounds in new advanced features directly foreshadowing the mammalian grade. The skull of the smaller cynodonts is strikingly like that of a primitive mammal in general appearance, arrangement of bones of upper jaw and nasal region of cheek bar, fossa for jaw muscles, etc., etc. That these cynodonts stand in between primitive reptiles and typical mammals is shown in almost every feature of their skeletons.

The lower jaw also was very progressive, but their official status as reptiles was validated by the retention of the old "reptilian joint" beneath the new or "mammalian joint."

The secondary palate was approaching that in mammals and stands between the primitive reptilian and the typical mammalian conditions.

The living relatives of the cynodonts are the mammals, including ourselves.

*Stage 12. Ictidosaurians, Upper Triassic of South Africa.*

These highly progressive derivatives of the pro-mammals (recently described by Robert Broom from two skulls) were on the borderline between reptiles and mammals. They practically break down the distinction between reptiles and mammals and show the absurdity of the statement that there are "no links between classes." They possessed the new joint between the mandible and the temporal bone that is characteristic of the mammals, but they also retain the old reptilian joint between the quadrate bone and the articular bone of the mandible.

Possible survivors or relatives of Upper Triassic mammal-like reptiles may be seen in

*Stage 13. The Duckbill Platypus and the Spiny Anteater of Australia.*

Both these forms lay large reptilian eggs, have reptile-like oviducts and many reptilian features in skull and skeleton, also a relatively primitive brain. They represent an early stage in the evolution of mammalian characters, especially those that tend to maintain a higher, more stable body temperature and more sustained activity. These qualities have helped mammals to conquer the world and drive out the reptiles.

*Stage 14. Pretrituberculate, Jurassic mammals.*

There was once a dogma that "no mammals are found in Jurassic rocks," and when one was found there, some denied that it was a mammal, others that the rocks were Jurassic. But Cuvier pronounced it "the jaw of a little opossum," a nearly correct allocation. Three orders, numerous genera and species of Mesozoic mammals have been described from the Jurassic of England and Wyoming, but mostly from broken jaws and teeth.

The teeth represent several stages of evolution toward primitive mammalian types. The skull in general had advanced beyond mammal-like reptiles in the direction of the most primitive marsupials. In the more advanced members the teeth were of primitive tritubercular type, ancestral to those of later mammals, including man.

*Stage 15. Cretaceous Opossum-like Marsupials.*

Huxley, Dollo and later students have emphasized the extremely primitive character of existing American opossums, our oldest and most precious "living fossil."

Unfortunately, most Americans appreciate the opossum more for those qualities which have earned for him the title of "African turkey." It rather pains me to hear of great statesmen taking a holiday down South to hunt these poor animals to eat, when they ought to be securing them for the museums of the future or laboring to establish opossum sanctuaries. The opossum has an American ancestry which would make even the longest known human genealogy look like a last year's birth record from Ellis Island. For Barnum Brown, our curator of Fossil Reptiles, found in rocks of Upper Cretaceous Age in Alberta a fossilized skull of an early member of the opossum family embedded underneath a dinosaur skull. Its estimated age is about eighty to one hundred millions of years.

The opossum skeleton is highly instructive in many ways; *e.g.*, it shows incipient adaptations to tree-living habits, the use of the pectoral limbs as hands and of the hind feet for grasping. While not in the direct line to higher mammals, it preserves many characters which we may confidently look for in the direct ancestors of the Primates.

*Stage 16. Cretaceous Insectivorous Placentals of Mongolia.*

One of the greatest prizes of Dr. Andrews' expedition to Mongolia, discovered by Dr. Granger. Huxley, Osborn and others had predicted that ancestors of the higher or placental mammals would be found to be Mesozoic insectivores. These little forms are judged to be placentals, through the close resemblances of their skulls and teeth to those of existing insectivores. Uniting characters of the earliest insectivores and carnivores, they show an ideally primitive stage in tritubercular upper molars and give long-looked-for paleontological proof that the primitive cusp was not on the inner side, as believed by Cope and Osborn, but was located on the main cusp, homologous with the main tip of the premolars.

The surviving relatives of the Cretaceous insectivores are the Centetid insectivores of Madagascar.

*Stage 17. Primitive Tree-shrews (? Upper Cretaceous to Lower Eocene).*

Somewhere in late Cretaceous times a group of small placental insectivores took to climbing up trees, with momentous consequences. For here they gradually acquired those primary arboreal characters which, as there is much evidence to conclude, were deeply stamped into the anatomy and ways of life of our own remote ancestors.

The tree-shrews, however, took only the initial steps; their skeleton retained much of the generalized mammalian type; but while the hands and feet retained claws, initial stages in the evolution of the nails are seen in late members of the group (from the Tertiary of Mongolia).

The existing tree-shrews suggest ordinary insectivores in their large muzzle, but their skulls and teeth approach those of lemurs in certain important characters. In fact, some authorities want to classify them with the lemurs, but as they were a separate family far back in Eocene times, they may be treated as pre-Primates.

*Stage 18. The earliest true Primates (Eocene).*

There is one fraternal order to which all Americans belong by right of birth, though few are willing to admit it, that is, the Order of Primates. This ancient and honorable order has an antiquity vastly exceeding even the claims of any that hold conventions in the big hotels; the bones of its founders have been discovered in the Bridger formation of Wyoming—their estimated age, about fifty millions of years. This most important skeleton I had the pleasure of naming in honor of the president of the American Museum of Natural History, Henry Fairfield Osborn.

The conspicuous characters are: While retaining five digits, it has grasping hands and feet fitted for climbing; the skull is progressive in its fairly large orbits; the brain is essentially lemur-like but lower and smaller; the dentition is very generalized for a primate; the dental formula is $I\frac{2}{2}C\frac{1}{1}P\frac{4}{4}M\frac{3}{3}$. Thus there were forty teeth in the adult, while in anthropoid apes and man the number has sunk to thirty-two.

Some paleontologists, including Drs. Wortman and Gidley, saw in *Notharctus* an ancestor of the South American monkeys, but to me it is too generalized to be classified with the South American monkeys. It is rather closely related to the Adapidae of Europe, which in turn are probably near the stem of the Madagascar lemuroids. Thus *Notharctus* may not be in direct line of ascent to man, but it is most instructive in showing how deeply arboreal characters had been impressed on the Primates by the Lower Eocene, fifty million years ago. Many lines of evidence support the view that the Primates as an order were fundamentally arboreal and that later semi-terrestrial types, like the baboon, or fully terrestrial types, like man, were all secondary.

*Stage 19. The Tarsioids (Eocene).*

The active arboreal life of the Primates requires a high development of sight. Hence the Primates were primarily big-eyed forms. This tendency early ran to extremes in the tarsioids, which Dr. Wood Jones regards as nearer than any other known forms to remote ancestors of man. But while it is not necessary to accept the tarsioids as *direct* ancestors, they show certain advances in the optical organs which the ancestors of man must have passed through. Excessive specialization, however, even in the Eocene *Anaptomorphus,* has led to extreme squeezing of the interorbital region and extreme diminution of the nasal chamber. The tarsioids were also early overspecialized in the hopping adaptations of their feet; this again rules them out of the direct line. Nevertheless, even in the modern *Tarsius* their brain and soft anatomy are pretty primitive and in many respects they bridge the gap between lemurs and monkeys; not impossibly they stand rather near to the unknown direct line leading to apes and man, though their relationship to man, in the judgment of most students of the subject, is not nearly as close as is the relationship of the apes to man.

*Stage 20. The separation into New World and Old World series.*

The question of the precise degree of relationship between the New World and the Old World monkeys has been considered from many angles, but there is no unanimity of opinion. In spite of certain common characters of the brain, placenta, etc., it seems possible that the New World monkeys were derived from some as yet unknown family other than that which gave rise to the Old World series, as maintained by Stehlin. They are widely separated in space and time and widely differentiated in many anatomical characters; *e.g.,* in details of skull and dentition.

The Old World monkeys are distinguished from the New World series not only by the narrow nostrils ("Catarrhinae") but also by the dental formula, already reduced to the same figures as in man and apes, namely, $I\frac{2}{2}C\frac{1}{1}P\frac{2}{2}M\frac{3}{3}$.

Dr. Wood Jones has referred to certain skull characters in which Old World monkeys appear to be too specialized to give rise to man. The same is true of their molar teeth. Nevertheless, the skeleton as a whole is far nearer the ancient Primate type in that the Old World monkeys are still mostly pronograde, *i.e.,* they do not practice brachiation, or arm-swinging, as much as do the anthropoids. Their hands and feet also are much more primitive, and the same is true of their brains.

*Stage 21. The founding of the Anthropoid dynasty.*

From the Lower Oligocene formation of upper Egypt, Professor Max Schlosser, of Munich, described two priceless little fossil jaws, illustrating two stages of evolution of the Primates. The smaller one, *Parapithecus,* already a living fossil in its own time forty million years ago, was apparently a hold-over from the tarsioids of the Eocene. At least it agreed with them in having a very short jaw, very wide at the back as seen from above, implying a much expanded braincase, and pointed in front. The teeth combine some characters of tarsioids with others of the anthropoid-human series.

The second stage was definitely a small anthropoid ape but of immense antiquity and primitiveness. It was named by its discoverer *Propliopithecus,* as a forerunner of *Pliopithecus,* the ancestor of the gibbon, but much more primitive than the gibbons in jaw and teeth. It has advanced beyond the tarsioid stage in widening of the front end, implying widening of tongue (embryonic jaw moulded by tongue). Dental formula: $I_2C_1P_2M_3$, as in anthropoid apes and man.

Molar teeth of primitive anthropoid type with five main cusps. It has been regarded by an eminent anthropologist (Sergi) as an ideal ancestor of man, but it might be a near ancestor of the entire ape-man series in characters of the lower jaw and dentition.

The modern gibbon, as a descendant of *Propliopithecus,* is a somewhat overspecialized side branch with excessively long arms and legs and saber-like upper canine tusks. Nevertheless, in many ways it represents a transitional stage between monkeys and apes. It retains the last traces of ischial callosities. Several characters of the skull and skeleton, but especially the molar teeth, definitely and surely classify the gibbon as an ape, not a monkey. The Johns Hopkins University school of anatomists concludes that the human line came off far down the anthropoid stem, a little above the level of the origin of the gibbon. I feel that there are too many strong bonds between man and the higher anthropoids to make the pro-gibbon ancestry of man probable, but all are agreed that man has come off from the anthropoid stock either earlier or later.

The gibbon skeleton is thoroughly adapted for brachiating. This is generally defined as "arm-swinging," but if we watch living gibbons we see that the legs play a very important part in leaping. The habit of brachiation has brought the backbone into a vertical position at right angles to its primitive horizontal position, and some authorities believe that brachiation is a prerequisite to human evolution. We may readily concede, however, that the gibbon is now in an advanced overspecialized phase of brachiation which need not be imputed to the early Tertiary anthropoids.

### *Stage 22. The Miocene Anthropoids.*

During the Miocene epoch the anthropoid group was represented by many species found as fossil jaws and teeth in France, Germany, the Vienna basin, Spain, northern Egypt and India; hence there was a broad zone extending across Europe and India with later offshoots in tropical Africa, South Africa, China, and southeastern Asia. This wide-ranging group was highly variable in size and in details of the dentition. They are known to date only from scattered jaws, one humerus and one femur. An eminent mammalogist demands fossil ape skeletons that include well-preserved hands, feet, pelves, etc., before admitting the evidence of fossil apes to his private court of judgment; but fossil apes do not come to us in that form. Nevertheless, these jaws and teeth of fossil apes are of extraordinary value, for they reveal both the wide plasticity and wide geographic distribution of the anthropoid stock. Barnum Brown discovered in India several important jaws shown in composite form in the figure. The jaw is deep and massive; there are thirty-two teeth; the canines are prominent, the opposite tooth rows are parallel as in apes.

The cheek teeth are of great interest because the pattern appears to be archetypal to that of man. The lower molars have three cusps on the outer side, two on the inner side, with elaborate "*Dryopithecus* pattern" of grooves, also a "fovea anterior" and "fovea posterior." Exactly this combination is found in primitive human jaws along with new and distinctly human characters. The characters of the premolars and molars support the view that man is an offshoot from some member of the *Dryopithecus* stock and with closer relationships to the African anthropoids than to the gibbon and the orang. The reduction of the canine in man is quite secondary, as supported by the extensive researches of Remane.

Dr. Gerrit S. Miller, Jr. (as quoted in a recent note in SCIENCE) objects that men and anthropoids are different kinds of giants, as compared with Primates of average size, and that there is no fossil-proved precedent for one kind of giant's turning into a different kind of giant. He therefore classes the derivation of man from a Tertiary anthropoid stock as "an alluring speculation," choosing to ignore the hundreds of anatomical characters that tie man with the anthropoids in a single systematic group. But there are giants and giants. The crown of the third lower molar of *Dryopithecus fontani* measures about 11 by 9.2 millimeters in anteroposterior and transverse diameters, respectively, while that of *Dryopithecus giganteus* measures 19 by 15.3 millimeters.[2] This wide range of variability in size in the older group does not seem to favor Dr. Miller's assumption of unalterable, fixed divergences between the two.

The conclusion that man is closer to the *Dryopithecus* stock than to the gibbons seems also to be opposed by my colleagues in Johns Hopkins University, and although I am prepared to defend it in detail, I do not regard it as essential for the present purpose, which is merely to reaffirm the conclusion that man in much the greater part of his characters is nearer to the anthropoid apes than to the more primitive Primates.

### *Stage 23. The extinct South African Anthropoid (Australopithecus)*

This amazingly well-preserved fossil was described by Professor Raymond Dart, of the University of the Witwatersrand, South Africa, in 1925. It was found in a fissure deposit near Taungs, on the eastern edge of the Kalahari desert. Its geological age is

[2] William K. Gregory and Milo Hellman, Anthropological Papers of the American Museum of Natural History, Vol. xxviii, Part I, 1926, p. 74.

not precisely established but, according to Dr. Robert Broom, two species of fossil baboons and an extinct species of *Hyrax* have been found in the same level. He therefore considers the age of *Australopithecus* to be Pliocene. But whether the age be Pliocene, Pleistocene or Recent, this skull is of exceptional interest. Extremes of judgment about the skull are first, that of Professor Dart, who regards it as the representative of a new family "Homosimiidae" widely removed from the African anthropoids; at the opposite extreme is the conclusion of Dr. Wolfgang Abel, of Vienna, who regards it as closely related to the gorilla and having nothing whatever to do with human ascent. Dr. Milo Hellman and I, who have studied the excellent casts of the upper and lower teeth, conclude that while it is a young anthropoid, related to the existing African genera, yet its deciduous canines and molars and its first permanent molars are, on the whole, unequivocally more man-like than those of the existing young gorilla and chimpanzee; while its permanent molars are definitely not those of *Gorilla* but present beautiful examples of a modified *Dryopithecus* pattern akin to those of the Ehringsdorf and Mousterian fossil human stage. In short, while we do not yet know the form of the adult skull of *Australopithecus,* it is safe to affirm that this child skull is strikingly "prehuman" in the general appearance of its cranium and facial skeleton and that it tends to lessen the phylogenetic gap between man and the existing African anthropoids.

*Stage 24. Man appears.*

With regard to the fossil human remains known as *Pithecanthropus,* found in Java, and *Eoanthropus,* found in England, scientific controversies have raged to such an extent that the eminent mammalogist already cited has urged that these names be, so to speak, wiped off the scientific slate until they are documented by better material. Fortunately, we need not for the moment at least contest this quite arbitrary ruling, for new and unimpeachable material of early man has been discovered near Peking and admirably described by Dr. Davidson Black. One of the Peking skulls was only little more advanced than that of *Pithecanthropus,* while the second was slightly further advanced toward the Neanderthal type. But according to the masterly field investigations of Teilhard de Chardin, the Peking human remains are contemporaneous with an extensive mammalian fauna that retains many elements characteristic of the Pliocene age, along with others indicating Lower Pleistocene age. Moreover, the Peking horizons belong in the Red Earth series, which are older than the thick loess deposits of Pleistocene age. Hence the Peking man, according to Chardin, is far older than the typical Neanderthals of the late Pleistocene of Europe, while its skull-contours, as figured by Black, are all lower and more primitive.

Without entering into controversial questions as to the geological age of the Piltdown and *Pithecanthropus* remains, it seems highly probable that the ancestors of *Sinanthropus* in late Tertiary times would have been properly classifiable as men rather than as apes. Time after time the Pliocene representatives of modern mammalian families have been shown to be almost modern in the appearance of their teeth, skulls and feet.

But here, as always, we must avoid the serious logical error of assuming for man the low average rate of evolution that obtained in non-Primate mammals. Moreover, the Lower Pleistocene *Sinanthropus* stands so far below *Homo sapiens* in cranial capacity that a backward prolongation of the curve at the same rate would presumably bring down the figures to the horizon of the anthropoids at no very distant geological date. Finally, according to the eminent geologist, Professor Schuchert, of Yale University, who has given prolonged consideration to this problem, the duration of the Pliocene epoch is many times greater than that of the Pleistocene. At present I know of no single item of objective evidence for the view that the human family began to diverge from that of the anthropoid apes as far back as Lower Oligocene or Upper Eocene times, forty or fifty million years ago; although in all fairness it should be noted that many other families of mammals did part company with each other at even earlier dates. But upon another occasion I was at some pains to demonstrate that, considering only the molar teeth and the feet, the structural differences between two families, the tapirs and the horses, that are known to have diverged in Lower Eocene times, are now far greater than the differences in the patterns of the molar teeth and of the feet respectively between modern men and modern apes.

But at whatever period, early or late, the human family may have begun to diverge from that of the anthropoid apes, it appears to be virtually proved by hundreds of separate items of evidence that men and apes are the divergent offshoots of a common stock, the existence of which, though not the period, is sufficiently documented by the huge mass of evidence already at hand. But it is not to be expected that this still growing mass of evidence for man's evolution from the lower animals will quiet the loud demands of anti-evolutionists for "objective evidence."

*Stage 25. Homo sapiens, the big-brained devastator.*

The existing anthropoids have a veritable passion for tearing things apart; but in point of destructiveness they are bungling amateurs, compared with their big-brained relative *Homo sapiens*. In him, by a series of conditioned responses, destructiveness within the family and tribal limits was restrained, but when enemies were to be ravaged and pillaged it was given full rein. For untold millions of years the line of vertebrates that led toward man were unblushing thieves and robbers; even now, the human face beneath its smiling mask carries the old mammalian trap set with sharp teeth. Such being the case, it is no wonder that we suffer from grafters, racketeers and gunmen. The wonder is not that so many of us find ourselves in prison but that any of us ever learned to keep out.

However, as soon as apes began to go in families and hordes, the counter principles of more or less unselfish interest in others began to operate; even in the lowest of existing social organizations there seems to be more or less clear proof of the unselfishness of mothers, the devotion of fathers, the generosity and disinterestedness of friends. Such a patchwork of good and evil is *Homo sapiens!*

But it does not seem that the pessimists are necessarily right. As Dr. Clark Wissler has pointed out, particular cultures may disappear, but culture itself goes on. And in view of the nearly world-wide distribution of *Homo sapiens* it would be hard to imagine any purely terrestrial epidemic or insect scourge that could wipe him out over his entire range.

Finally, man, in respect to the high development of his brain and other characters, may well represent an early stage in the differentiation of a virtually new class of vertebrates. The paleontological record shows repeatedly that, in the long past, once a new class gets started it runs for hundreds of millions of years. So that, taking the available evidence into consideration, it seems safe to predict that *Homo sapiens* will eventually muddle through this depression and survive to endure others in the future.

## SUMMARY

The "Anthropogenie" of Ernest Haeckel, a pioneer work of great difficulty, depended to a considerable extent upon the so-called biogenetic law. Since the validity of this law has been attacked by several modern zoologists, public confidence in Haeckel's conclusions seems to have been undermined, at least in certain parts of the country. The "new anthropogeny" has grown chiefly out of the progress of paleontology, comparative anatomy, phylogenetic taxonomy and the comparison of the *échelle des êtres* among recent and fossil series. It seems that we are now in a position to substitute for the more or less hypothetical stages postulated by Haeckel a new and independently discovered series representing groups that depart the least from a continuous ascent. This, of course, involves the exclusion of all other groups which show more than the least observed differences from the more nearly continuous series.

For example, Haeckel relied upon the lung-fishes (Dipnoi) to bridge the gap between earlier fishes and the Amphibia. The Paleozoic Dipnoi are now seen to have been further from the "line of least change" than were their contemporaries, the lobe-finned ganoids (Crossopterygii), which possess in an earlier form a great many of the skeletal characters that were inherited by the Amphibia. It is concluded by Watson and others that the "lobe-fins" were descendants of an earlier group, which also gave rise in one direction to the Dipnoi, in the other to the Amphibia.

The new anthropogeny, as far as developed to date, submits the following series, subject, of course, to correction by further discovery:

(1) *Pre-fish* (*ostracoderm*) of Ordovician, Silurian and Devonian age. Paired sense organs, brain and cranial nerves, all fundamentally identical with those of the larval lamprey. "Gill-arch" jaws not developed.

(2) *Antiarch.* "Gill-arch" jaws incipient, outer jaw bones present. Known forms: *Pterichthys, Bothriolepis,* etc.; probably well off the main line except in characters noted.

(3) *Pre-shark* (*acanthodian*). Devonian. "Gill-arch" jaws (in series with gill-arches) fully developed. Paired fins arising from stabilizing fin-folds.

(4) *Basal ganoid fish.* Devonian. Enamel-covered bony mask over face and gill-chamber. Inner (primary) and outer jaw-parts complete. Anal, pelvic and pectoral fins showing progressive evolution from fin-fold to paddle type. Pectoral girdle complex (surface and deep elements). Near line of ascent to typical true fishes.

(5) *Lobe-finned ganoid.* Devonian and Lower Carboniferous. Paired fins with shortened bases and crowded, fan-like skeleton. Teeth labyrinthodont, primary jaws covered with bony plates. Many bones of skull-roof homologous with those in later vertebrates. Cleithrum predominant in pectoral girdle.

(6) *Basal amphibian.* Lower Carboniferous. Paired limbs with five-rayed digits. Vertebrae cut up, large intercentra. Pectoral girdle at first retained cleithrum from fish stage. Teeth labyrinthodont. Opercular bones absent. Skull patterns archetypal to all later tetrapods. Occipital condyle tripartite. Aquatic (tadpole) mode of development.

(7) *Stem reptile.* Upper Carboniferous. Presumed elimination of tadpole stage. Vertebrae simplified, intercentra small. Occipital condyle tripartite to single and median. Cleithrum reduced. Limbs of crawling type.

(8) *Progressive cotylosaur* (*captorhinid*). Permian. Retaining primitive shell of bone over temporal muscles. "Four-way palate arch" developed from primary upper jaw. Skeleton lizard-like.

(9) *Texas theromorph.* Permian. Temporal roof fenestrated by jaw muscle, leaving zygomatic arch of pre-mammalian type.

(10) *Earlier mammal-like reptile.* Permian of South Africa and Russia. Limbs adapted for running. Dentition carnivorous, with incisors, canines and cheek teeth. Temporal region of pre-mammalian type. Dentary bone of lower jaw with obliquely ascending ramus. Occipital condyle single.

(11) *Cynodont or pro-mammal.* Triassic of South Africa. Skull sub-mammalian in: zygomatic arch, secondary palate, differentiated dentition, double occipital condyle, etc. Lower jaw with increasing ascending ramus finally approaching squamosal bone. Jaw bones behind dentary reduced. Quadrate small. Skeleton of sub-mammalian running type.

(12) *Ictidosaurian, near-mammal.* Upper Triassic, South Africa. Skull almost mammalian. Lower jaw with large, nearly vertical, ascending ramus of dentary and much reduced jaw bones behind dentary.

(13) *Prototherian mammal.* Known chiefly from recent Duckbill (*Ornithorhynchus*) and *Echidna* of Australia. Retaining semi-reptilian type of eggs and oviducts. Primitive skeletal features, especially in girdles and limbs. Incipient stage of milking habit. Lower jaw with new or mammalian type of joint with skull (*i.e.*, between dentary and squamosal bones). Various aberrant specializations in modern representatives.

(14) *Pre-trituberculate mammal.* Jurassic. Lower jaw of primitive mammalian type, crowns of lower cheek teeth with elevated, three-cusped "trigonid" and low, small "talonid" or heel.

(15) *Pre-opossum,* conservative Metatherian. Cretaceous. Not near direct line to placentals but retaining many primitive skeletal features, especially in skull and dentition. Young probably born in very incomplete condition. Brain with only beginning of "neopallium"; corpus callosum not developed.

(16) *Cretaceous insectivorous placental.* Skull of small generalized insectivore type. Small brain with large olfactory lobes. Brain in modern descendants with corpus callosum. Upper cheek teeth with incipiently divided main cusp (paracone) and low inner spur (protocone). A placenta developed in modern relatives.

(17) *Primitive tree-shrew.* Basal Eocene. Incipient adaptations of hands and feet for tree-climbing. Skull essentially as in No. 18, that is, lemur-like but with unreduced olfactory chamber. Skeleton of generalized placental type. Modern tree-shrews retaining many primitive characters.

(18) *Stem Primate.* Lower and Middle Eocene. Adaptations for arboreal habits deeply stamped on hands and feet of grasping type. Dental formula $I\frac{2}{2}C\frac{1}{1}P\frac{4}{4}M\frac{3}{3}$. Eyes large, orbits with postorbital rim.

(19) *Eocene Pre-tarsioid.* Known forms aberrantly specialized; but more generalized stage should be near to main line. Eyes large, protruding forward, interorbital space reduced. Brain very wide, jaw short, wide posteriorly, pointed in front. Extremities grasping (grasping-hopping in known forms). Premolars typically $\frac{3}{3}$. *Parapithecus* possibly belongs here.

(20) *Stem Old World monkey.* Pronograde or essentially quadrupedal, with grasping hands and feet. Dentition $I\frac{2}{2}C\frac{1}{1}P\frac{2}{2}M\frac{3}{3}$. Cheek teeth in recent forms aberrantly specialized; *i.e.*, with well developed cross-crests. Nose catarrhine (V-shaped nostrils). Orbits separated from temporal fossae by bony partition.

(21) *Pre-anthropoid* (*Propliopithecus*). Lower Oligocene. Ancestral gibbons with short, deep lower jaw, more primitive lower canines and premolars. Dentition: $I\frac{2}{2}C\frac{1}{1}P\frac{2}{2}M\frac{3}{3}$. Molars with five cusps. Frugivorous. Recent gibbons overspecialized for upright progression by brachiation, with excessively long arms and legs; nevertheless retain certain monkey characters (*e.g.*, traces of ischial callosities). Brain less advanced than those of the chimpanzee and gorilla.

(22) *Mid-Tertiary anthropoid group.* Ranging from Spain, through France, Germany, Austria, Egypt, East Africa to India and (later) to South Africa. Lower molars with five cusps and "*Dryopithecus* pattern." Limb bones of anthropoid type. Brain capacity of recent great apes ranging from 290 to 610 cc. (Keith).

(23) *Southern Ape* (*Australopithecus*). Pliocene or Pleistocene of South Africa. This "ape-child" skull probably belonged to a race of adults with muzzles more ape-like than its own. Nevertheless, its deciduous teeth and first true molars, while primarily of the "*Dryopithecus*" type, are not very far below the earlier human levels.

(24) *Early Human Stage.* Lower Pleistocene or earlier. Represented at least by *Pithecanthropus* of Java and *Sinanthropus* of China. Vertically low skulls with strongly projecting brow-ridges. Brain of relatively low type; endocranial capacity 900 ± cc. (Dubois). Clear traces of "*Dryopithecus* pattern" in lower molars of Ehringsdorf young.

(25) *Homo sapiens.* Pleistocene and Recent. Braincase typically high, with little or no brow-ridges. Cranial capacity: racial means ranging between 1200 and 1500 cc. (Hooton). Skeleton adapted for upright bipedal posture, but hands and feet retaining many clear traces of generalized ape ancestry. Lower molars often four-cusped, with traces of "*Dryopithecus* pattern" usually on $m_1$. Brain retaining many unmistakable marks of derivation from an anthropoid stage, but with progressive development of centers and areas associated with speech and verbalized thinking.

As to the possible future of mankind, it is pointed out that, to judge from the history of many other new groups (not species), and in consideration of his cosmopolitan distribution, mankind should be a "good risk" for survival for an indefinite period.

# OBITUARY

## JOHN JOSEPH CARTY—AN APPRECIATION

WHEN in the early morning hours of Tuesday, December 27, General John J. Carty died in the Johns Hopkins Hospital, after a valiant but unsuccessful fight to overcome the shock of a major operation, the field of science, the profession of engineering and the community of intellectual life in the United States suffered a great loss. Nor was this loss confined to the nation of which he was a citizen, which he loved with that intellectual fervor which only the great possess, and which throughout his life he had served with such steadfast devotion. In many countries, from those of Europe to far-off Japan, Carty, his works and achievements and his philosophy of life were known and admired.

From every country which has felt during the past half century the stirring of that new force which science and its application has brought into human living, men have at one time or another made the pilgrimage to New York to sit at Carty's feet and to learn and profit from his wisdom. It mattered not what language the pilgrims spoke, all profited from the contact and all returned whence they came not only with a realization of this profit, but also with the realization that they had acquired the lasting friendship of a wise man.

Nor were these contacts one-sided affairs. General Carty had an insatiable desire to enlarge his own fund of information and understanding. All who came in contact with him, from the most wise to the most frivolous and shallow, were subjects for his inquiry. He gave much and willingly of his store of knowledge and wisdom but in return, and frequently in ways unknown to his vis-à-vis, he exacted payment in full measure. At times this payment was in kind; more frequently than not it was in values quite foreign to the main subject-matter of the conversation. At the termination of the contact General Carty had invariably something new added to his already great store of knowledge—a bit of social history or custom, a hitherto unknown item of science, a peculiar slant of political thinking, or any other of the thousand and one things which involve the working of human emotions or the human mind.

His relentless search into the way human beings react and into the motives which guide their thought and action, and whose results he continually marshaled and remarshaled under the guidance of his incisively analytical mind, became a main source of his extraordinary capacity for being always at home in any company. Few men possess the capacity which General Carty had for meeting on a plane of complete understanding men and women of every social and intellectual gradation. It was a capacity which enabled him in every situation to give and receive knowledge and to influence the outcome of events in ways and in a manner which were frequently uncanny.

More than most men, General Carty had at one time or another actually put himself in the position of the other man in the wide variety of situations in which men exercise their powers, their frailties, their hopes and aspirations and their emotions.

For one who attained to such eminence, whose counsel and advice were so sought after in so many fields, and whose opinion always carried such weight, even with those who dissented from his conclusions, the record of General Carty's own writings, even in the field of his profession or that part of it which was his specialized interest—electrical communication—is surprisingly meager. Of course during his long active and creative career he produced a vast volume of letters, memoranda and reports, each bearing the imprint of a master mind but each concerned primarily with some specific question of the moment. At the same time lectures, addresses and articles of the kind which go commonly to build up a reputation for wisdom and which produce a far-reaching and lasting influence were remarkably few in number. Such as do exist are almost without exception just what one would expect from their author.

Why was it that a man who possessed and deserved the reputation which General Carty acquired made so little use of the tool which most men of ability esteem their most powerful weapon? The answer is clear to those in position to know him best. In part it was because he was always too busy seeking to solve the vast array of problems crying for solution, even though he always promised himself and others that he would some time write out something of what he had learned. In part also it was because the act of authorship was for him an incredibly laborious task. Only those of us who have been witness to this labor have any real appreciation of just how difficult and time-consuming it was for him to prepare an important document which would be a permanent record of his thoughts and conclusions and to which he would be willing to sign his name. This labor was not because he in any way failed to have a perfectly definite and clear picture of just what he wished to say, nor because he lacked the full vocabulary in which to express his thoughts. Rather it was because he did have complete clarity of mind and a full vocabulary. To him words and their arrangement were powerful tools which should not be lightly nor thoughtlessly employed. Every word and every sentence in any document of importance must, when finally chosen and arranged, convey to the reader the exact shade of meaning—no more, no less—that he had in mind. This habit and insistence made serious writing far too time-consuming an operation to be indulged in frequently.

Absence of a voluminous printed record does not mean, however, that General Carty left no substantial material evidence of his great creative ability. Modern telephony, whose development owes so much to him, has in the last analysis a very limited number of elements which are prime to its existence. Some, like the telephone itself, or the loading coil or the vacuum tube amplifier, are spectacular and well known. Others of equal or greater importance have become so much the commonplace of telephone engineering that few realize their fundamental character or that their creation was ever looked upon as an outstanding achievement.

The three most important of these foundation stones which are in use wherever telephony is employed are creations of General Carty. His invention of the "common battery" for supplying operating current from a single central office battery to any number of interconnected telephones made practical the commercial development of telephony in metropolitan areas.

His development of the high resistance bridging signal bell for subscribers substations to replace the theretofore universally employed low resistance series bell, tore the hampering shackles from a wide-spread extension in the use of the telephone. Every telephone set now in use employs such a signal.

Equally revolutionary and of a more distinctly scientific character was his discovery that the principal cause of cross interference between telephone circuits was electrostatic and not electromagnetic unbalance. This discovery and the rules which General Carty worked out for the proper construction of adjacent telephone circuits are now universally employed.

A characteristic of each of these achievements is that each came as the direct and logical result of what was one of General Carty's most powerful intellectual weapons—his ability to brush aside non-essentials and grasp the kernel of the problem. Many men had worked on each of the three things just mentioned. They were obvious obstacles to progress. They yielded readily to solution once General Carty had formulated simply and accurately the essentials of the problem and the nature of the answer required.

These things and a host of others similar but less important were personal creations. They belong to his earlier years. The great achievements of his later life and for which he is best known in the field of electrical communication are the achievements of a generalissimo. Long distance telephony over land, transoceanic radio telephony, the coordination of factors which render present-day telephony so marvelously easy bear scarcely a trace of General Carty as a creator of any essential new element. They are, however, almost as surely his creations as any of his earlier work.

He analyzed the problems, picked out the essential elements to be attacked, mobilized just the right forces, provided the supplies by selling confidence in ultimate success to those who must provide the supplies and inspired a sort of fanatic determination in those who looked on him as captain.

Although primarily concerned with scientific, engineering and organization matters in the field of electrical communication and most of all in the well-being and reputation of the Bell System, General Carty looked upon the whole field of science as his hunting ground. Many of his closest friends were men of distinction in fields of science far removed from those of electrical engineering or physics. Denied the privilege of any formal training in science he nevertheless acquired such an understanding in many fields of knowledge and research that masters there sought discussion with him.

Consideration of everything General Carty did shows always the same technique. Painstaking analysis of the problem; exact formulation of the questions to be solved; full consideration of every ascertainable obstacle, human or material, likely to be encountered; assembly of just the right forces and then when all was ready a feverish onslaught quite in contrast with the slow and methodical preparations. But no matter how feverish the attack once all was ready, there was never any lessening of meticulous attention to detail where he thought that detail important. This technique he applied with infinite variations and shades to the material problems of electrical communication; to the delicate political problems involved in the daring attempt to demonstrate transatlantic telephony in the midst of the World War; to the essentially human problems of organization which created the perfect battalions which made the Signal Corps Reserve preeminent; to his part in creating the National Research Council, or to making certain that the solemn ceremonies of the burial of the Unknown Soldier should be broadcast to expectant thousands across the continent unmarred by accident.

Who but General Carty would have realized that the most probable cause of disaster in these august ceremonies would lie in forgetfulness on the part of the great participating personages under the emotional stress of the occasion? Or who but he would have known that insurance of success lay in the little piece of carpet which he himself tacked in exactly the right place where each speaker was to stand?

The lasting record of General Carty's character and

achievements is in the art of communication, of which for nearly fifty years he was an outstanding leader; in the citations by which a large number of great institutions justified their grants to him of honorary degrees or medals of distinction and in the archives of the Departments of State of his own and other nations which conferred upon him high orders in recognition of services rendered in the cause of making this world a better place in which to live.

To General Carty, science and the methods of scientific thought were never narrow things or things apart from the great problems of a fuller life. Nor were the great institutions and academies of science mere machinery for putting the capstones of acknowledged success on recognized achievement. To him their raison d'être was their unique opportunity for service.

It was in this light that he looked upon the National Academy of Sciences, an essentially undemocratic institution in a democratic country. It was knowledge of this feeling which caused his associates to create there the medal which bears his name and of which the academy later made to him its first award. It was for him the most pleasurable and satisfying token of love and esteem which those associates could render since it gave assurance of enhanced opportunity to the academy for lasting service. That he did not live to receive the medal is a source of regret to his friends. To him it mattered little.

F. B. JEWETT

# SCIENTIFIC EVENTS

## THE NATURAL HISTORY OF MOUNT EVEREST

IN view of the forthcoming Everest Expedition, a small selection of the specimens brought back by the expeditions of 1921, 1922 and 1924 has been arranged at the British Museum (Natural History), South Kensington, to illustrate conditions upon the mountain. According to the London *Times,* the general appearance of the upper ranges of Everest is excellently illustrated in a number of enlarged photographs. One of these shows how the high winds, even outside the seasons of the monsoon, give rise to whirling clouds of dry snow. The article in the *Times* continues:

A sectional elevation shows the altitudes up to which various forms of life were found, and objects from every department indicate the peculiarities of the natural history of the mountain. Beetles were found at a height of 16,500 feet, butterflies up to 17,000 feet, moths as far up as 18,000 feet. Each of these specimens had its idiosyncrasies; the butterflies and moths clung with their wings to the mountain side against the high wind; the beetles stiffened out and rolled; and even the ants were remarkably torpid.

The grasshoppers shown from the higher altitudes are all wingless, but are related, save for one endemic group, to winged varieties elsewhere. It is curious to note how much smaller were two specimens, within the same species, which were found at 10,000 feet, than two similar examples from the 7,000-foot level. Spiders were found above the snowline and up to 22,000 feet; they live, apparently, upon diminutive insects which themselves must exist on inconspicuous vegetable life.

Sheep were found up to 20,000 feet on the borders of the lichen-zone, but the highest recorded altitude to be reached by a mammal (20,100 feet) was attained by the Royle's pika or Wollaston's pika (mouse-hare), of which a number are on view.

In general, the fauna below 16,000 feet is of essentially the same type as that of the adjacent areas of Central and Southern Asia, while above 16,000 feet its affinities are predominantly Palearctic. The animals are, however, frequently of smaller size than their lowland relatives. The highest nesting birds were found at 17,000 feet; finches were seen migrating at 21,000 feet, and choughs followed the climbers as high as they went.

The plants found on Everest include willows, primulas, gentians, blue poppies and others known to Western gardeners. The short duration of the growing season (three to four months), the exposure to wind and cold, the brightness of the light, the pressure of snow, the distance of water from surface, the scarcity of insects and the poorness of soil, however, all help to make plant life difficult. The plants on screes and cliffs have a very long, spongy taproot, enabling them to reach down to the moisture and to resist the movement of the loose stony material.

The Himalayan range is comparatively Recent, and reached its present form only in Pliocene times. Fossil ammonites from the 14,000-foot level of the Tibetan plateau show the creatures which formerly lived in the sea, which covered the site of the great range. Examples of Recent rocks were collected up to 27,000 feet.

The exhibition, which has been arranged in the Insect Gallery by Dr. Anna B. Hastings and M. M. Burton, will remain open between six months and a year.

## FORESTRY PROGRAM FOR THE SOUTHEASTERN STATES

A FORESTRY program designed to meet the needs of the eight southeastern states has been adopted by the Southeastern Council according to an announcement made by Colonel J. W. Harrelson, director of the North Carolina State Department of Conservation and Development. This program is given below.

1. Encouragement of teaching forestry in public schools and colleges and the development of an appreciation on the part of the general public of the benefits of forest conservation.

2. Speedy extension of each state's forest fire prevention and control system to include all forest lands needing systematic protection.

3. Promotion of comprehensive economic surveys to provide for land-use zoning to designate areas best suited to agricultural development, private forestry and public forests.

4. Development of a coordinated system of publicly owned forests, national, state and local, to be used for timber production, demonstration of improved timber growing and fire control methods, wild life conservation, public hunting grounds and recreation.

5. Equalization of taxes so that forest property will not carry a greater burden, in proportion to its value, than do other classes of property.

6. State-wide assistance to landowners in the handling of their forestry problems.

7. Encouragement of reforestation of idle and eroding lands by maintaining state forest tree nurseries to provide suitable planting stock.

8. Extension of investigations by federal forest experiment stations and suitable state research agencies upon the various subjects fundamental to economic handling of forest lands.

9. Speedy extension to the entire southeast of a survey inaugurated under the McNary-McSweeney Act to supply information now woefully lacking as to the present quantity and condition of standing timber, its rate of growth and rate of depletion and market demands for the several types of timber.

10. Recognition by the Federal Government of landowners engaged in the practice of forestry as eligible for the same loans, assistance, grants and privileges as are accorded to the producers of other crops that spring from the soil.

## THE WISCONSIN ALUMNI RESEARCH FOUNDATION

A PATENT on another important scientific discovery which will aid in the restoration and protection of health has been assigned to the Wisconsin Alumni Research foundation at the University of Wisconsin, according to an announcement made by Dr. Harry L. Russell, director of the foundation.

A broad basic patent on inorganic compounds of iron and copper for the prevention and treatment of anemia has been granted to Professor Edwin Bret Hart, of the department of agricultural chemistry, University of Wisconsin, and has been assigned to the foundation, becoming one of a number of health-giving discoveries controlled by the foundation in the interests of public welfare. Among the most important of these discoveries is Professor Harry D. Steenbock's process for imparting the health-giving vitamin D properties to food.

The latest patent assigned to the foundation covers various aspects of Professor Hart's discovery of the effect which copper has on unlocking the therapeutic powers of iron in restoring proper hemoglobin content to the blood of anemia patients. Professor Hart made his discovery in 1928 after three years of research and the patent application has been pending since that time.

The foundation has obtained patent control of the discovery, Dr. Russell explained, in order to insure the therapeutic presentation of the compounds in accord with the proper formula. This control is gained through a system of granting licenses for the use of the discovery and other patented articles, and thus the foundation is able to make available these discoveries to the public, while at the same time protecting the public from fraudulent and unchecked exploitation of uncontrolled commercial use.

Professor Hart's experiments showed that iron, long accepted as beneficial in some cases of anemia, required the addition of copper as a catalytic agent, and that "iron" which proved actively useful in treatment of anemias contained traces of copper as a contaminant. The research was narrowed to a study of inorganic materials when vegetable and animal tissues were burned to an ash before being fed and the catalytic properties were found to persist. The blue appearance of such ash led to successful experiments with copper.

Rabbits, chicks and rats developed severe anemia when placed on an exclusive diet of milk, a food naturally deficient in copper, but they evidenced rapid hemoblogin improvement to normal when minute quantities of copper were introduced in their foods.

In application to a hundred cases of secondary anemia in children, it was found in a New York hospital that the administration of copper and iron together increased the hemoglobin content from 64 per cent. to 84 per cent. in four weeks. The red blood cells gained in numbers accordingly. The appetite of the children treated improved materially, and they gained in alertness, weight and color. The copper-iron preparation was mixed with their milk or other foods which it was found neither to discolor nor to alter in taste.

## THE PACIFIC DIVISION OF THE AMERICAN ASSOCIATION FOR THE ADVANCEMENT OF SCIENCE

BY invitation of the University of Utah, the seventeenth annual meeting of the Pacific Division of the American Association for the Advancement of Science and associated societies will be held in Salt Lake City. The period June 12 to 15, 1933, has been approved for the meeting. Up to the present time the following societies have announced their intention to participate:

American Association of Economic Entomologists, Pacific Slope Branch. *Chairman*, Program Committee: G. I. Reeves, University of Utah, Salt Lake City.

American Chemical Society, Pacific Intersectional Division. *Chairman*, Program Committee: C. R. Kinney, University of Utah, Salt Lake City.

American Physical Society. Local Secretary for the Pacific Coast: Leonard B. Loeb, University of California, Berkeley.

American Phytopathological Society, Pacific Division. *Secretary:* B. A. Rudolph, Route 1, Box 232, San Jose.

American Society of Ichthyologists and Herpetologists, Western Division. *Secretary:* L. E. Griffin, Reed College, Portland, Oregon.

Astronomical Society of the Pacific. *Secretary:* C. H. Adams, 506 Merchants Exchange Building, San Francisco.

Botanical Society of the Pacific, Pacific Section. *Secretary:* George R. Hill, American Smelting and Refining Company, Salt Lake City.

California Academy of Sciences. *Secretary:* Susie M. Peers, Golden Gate Park, San Francisco.

San Francisco Aquarium Society. *Secretary:* Mrs. Ethel Seale, Steinhart Aquarium, Golden Gate Park, San Francisco.

Society of American Foresters, California and North Pacific Sections. *Secretary:* H. L. Person, University of California, Berkeley.

Society for Experimental Biology and Medicine. *Secretary:* M. L. Tainter, Stanford Medical School, San Francisco.

Utah Academy of Sciences. *Secretary:* Vasco M. Tanner, Brigham Young University, Provo.

Western Society of Naturalists. *Secretary:* E. G. Moberg, The Scripps Institution, La Jolla, California.

Western Society of Soil Science. *Secretary:* E. E. Thomas, Citrus Experiment Station, Riverside, California.

Members wishing to present papers before any of the scientific sessions are asked to submit the titles of their communications to the secretary or program chairman of the appropriate society. Alternatively, titles may be sent to the office of the Pacific Division. Members of non-participating societies desiring to present papers are cordially invited to do so. A title submitted to any of the above will be placed upon the program of the society most suitable to receive it.

A preliminary announcement containing general information about the meeting will be distributed late in March. The program containing titles of all communications will be mailed about June 1.

# SCIENTIFIC NOTES AND NEWS

DR. H. SPENCER JONES, astronomer at the Cape of Good Hope Observatory, has been appointed astronomer royal at the Royal Observatory, Greenwich, in succession to Sir Frank Dyson, who on reaching the age of sixty-five years will retire from the public service on February 28. Dr. Jones was chief assistant at the Greenwich Observatory from 1913 to 1923.

DR. PAUL D. FOOTE, director of research of the Gulf Oil Companies and lecturer at the University of Pittsburgh, was elected president of the American Physical Society at the recent Atlantic City meeting. He succeeds Dr. W. F. G. Swann, director of the Bartol Research Foundation of the Franklin Institute.

A SOUND film presenting Dr. William H. Welch speaking on "Reminiscences of the Early Days of the Medical School" will be shown at the Rockefeller Institute for Medical Research, New York, at four o'clock on January 18. Admission is by invitation.

DR. EMIL ARTIN, professor at Hamburg, and Dr. Emmy Noether, professor at Göttingen, have been awarded the Ackerman-Teubner Memorial Prize, Leipzig, for research in mathematics.

DR. R. S. BASSLER, head curator of the department of geology of the U. S. National Museum, has been elected an honorary member of the Society of Natural History of Tartu, Esthonia, in recognition of his work on the geology and paleontology of that country published as a museum bulletin some years ago.

*The British Medical Journal* reports that the Dr. Sophie A. Nordhoff-Jung Cancer Prize for the best work in the field of cancer research in recent years has been awarded to Professor Max Askanazy, of the University of Geneva, in recognition of his experimental research work and his critical presentation of larger and general problems in the same field. The commission of award was composed of Professors Borst, Doederlein, von Romberg and Sauerbruch.

WE learn from *Nature* that the Hopkins prize for the period 1924–27 has been awarded by the Cambridge Philosophical Society to Professor G. I. Taylor, Yarrow research professor of the Royal Society, for his researches on hydrodynamics and on the deformation of crystals; and the prize for the period 1927–30 to Professor P. A. M. Dirac, who was recently elected Lucasian professor of mathematics in the University of Cambridge, for his researches on the theory of quantum mechanics.

AT their meeting at Atlantic City on December 27, the trustees of the Mathematical Association of America awarded the Chauvenet Prize of $100 to Professor G. H. Hardy, of the University of Cambridge, England, for his paper entitled "An Introduction to the

Theory of Numbers," which appeared in the *Bulletin* of the American Mathematical Society, Vol. 35 (1929), pages 778–818. This prize is awarded every three years for the best expository paper on a mathematical subject published in English by a member of the Mathematical Association. The award covered the triennium 1929–31.

ON the occasion of the seventieth birthday of Emmanuel de Margerie, the French geologist, thirty-seven American geologists united in sending him a message which included the following: "A few of your American friends and colleagues take this occasion to send you greetings from across the sea. We are mindful of your scholarly acquaintance with the literature of American geology; we appreciate your generous interest in the scientific studies of your American colleagues; and we recall with peculiar pleasure the days when you brought to this country the rich fruits of your ripe experience. And so we gladly join in sending you affectionate greetings, and our cordial wishes for many more years of health in which to enjoy both your own scholarly pursuits and the high honor and esteem in which you are held throughout the world."

DR. CHARLES SINGER, of the University of London, who went to California as Herzstein Lecturer in Medicine in 1930, and who has been professor of the history of science for the past year, has left San Francisco for a trip around the world on his way to England. A farewell luncheon was given to Dr. Singer and Mrs. Singer at the Bohemian Club by the California Medical History Seminar, with Dr. Chauncey D. Leake, professor of pharmacology at the University of California Medical School, presiding.

IN recognition of the work of Dr. Louis E. Wise in the department of forest chemistry at the New York State College of Forestry, Syracuse University, a hand-illumined copy of a resolution by the faculty of the college has been signed by each member and forwarded to him. Dr. Wise, who had been professor of forest chemistry at the college since 1919, resigned on July 1 owing to illness. Through the action of the Board of Trustees, he retains his connection with the college as professor emeritus. His present address is Winter Park, Florida.

DR. COLLIER COBB, since 1893 professor of geology at the University of North Carolina, has retired from active service.

DR. JAMES A. KENNEDY has been appointed director of the division of diagnostic laboratories at the University of Rochester School of Medicine and Dentistry.

DR. EDWARD DELEHANTY has been promoted to the professorship of neurology in the University of Colorado School of Medicine, Denver, succeeding the late Dr. George A. Moleen.

DR. HENRY S. HOUGHTON, dean of the Medical College at the University of Iowa, has been appointed professor and associate dean of the division of the biological sciences at the University of Chicago and director of the south side clinics. Dr. Houghton assumed his post on January 1. As director of the clinics he will succeed Dr. Franklin C. McLean, who has become professor of physiology. Dr. Houghton will be associated with Dr. Frank R. Lillie, dean of the biological sciences, and will supervise the medical work of the various university hospitals and clinics.

DR. REGINALD FITZ, associate professor of medicine at the Harvard Medical School, has been elected a member of the National Board of Medical Examiners.

WE learn from *Museum News* that Arthur C. Parker has resigned as director of the Rochester Museum of Arts and Sciences, effective December 31. The budget cut of the City Council reduced the museum appropriation to about $6,000, making impossible a continuation of the institution as an effective organization. Mr. Parker was recently commissioned by *New York History*, the official organ of the New York State Historical Association, to write "A Manual of Museology for History Museums." A consulting board has also been appointed to participate in the project. Its members include Clark Wissler, Hardinge Scholle, Robert W. Bingham, Alexander J. Wall, Julian P. Boyd and Stephen H. P. Pell.

GOVERNOR A. HARRY MOORE, of the State of New Jersey, has appointed Dr. Robert P. Fischelis, secretary and chief chemist of the Board of Pharmacy of the State of New Jersey, a member of the State Educational Survey Commission. The duties of the commission are to survey the educational system of the state and to propose recommendations for an essential program of modern education and methods of financing it. The commission includes the State Commissioner of Education, a number of school superintendents and principals and a number of prominent laymen, all of whom serve without pay.

AT the annual meeting of the Board of Directors, which followed the annual meeting of the National Committee for Mental Hygiene, the following officers were reelected: *Honorary president,* Dr. William H. Welch, of Baltimore; *President,* Dr. Charles P. Emerson, of Indianapolis; *Vice-Presidents,* President James R. Angell, of Yale University; Dr. William L. Russell, professor of psychiatry at the Cornell University Medical College; Dr. Bernard Sachs, of New York; *General Director,* Dr. C. M. Hincks; *Treasurer,* Frederic W. Allen, and *Secretary,* Clifford W. Beers. Dr.

Arthur H. Ruggles, of Providence, was reelected chairman of the Scientific Administration Committee; Dr. Augustus Knight, of New York, chairman of the Executive Committee, and Mortimer N. Buckner, of New York, chairman of the Finance Committee.

DR. EUGENE LINDSAY OPIE, professor of pathology at Cornell Medical College, and Dr. Louis Israel Dublin, vice-president of the Metropolitan Life Insurance Company, have been appointed Cutter Lecturers on Preventive Medicine at Harvard University for the academic year 1932–33.

DR. FRANCIS R. FRASER, professor of medicine at the University of London, will give the third series of Abraham Flexner Lectures at Vanderbilt University School of Medicine, Nashville, during February and March. Dr. Fraser will lecture on "The Principles of Therapeutics" and will hold clinics under the auspices of the department of medicine. The Abraham Flexner Lectureship, founded at Vanderbilt in 1927 by Mr. Bernard Flexner, New York, is awarded every two years. Previous lecturers have been Dr. Heinrich Poll, director of the Institute of Anatomy, University of Hamburg, Germany, and Sir William Hardy, director of the Low Temperature Research Station, Cambridge, England.

THE REV. JAMES B. MACELWANE, S.J., Dean of the Graduate School and professor of geophysics in St. Louis University, addressed the St. Louis University Sigma Xi Club on December 12 on "Some Results of Recent Studies at the St. Louis University Seismographic Stations."

DR. FREDERIC H. LAHEE recently completed an extensive trip made for the purpose of addressing various groups of members of the American Association of Petroleum Geologists, of which he is president. His itinerary included San Antonio, Los Angeles, San Francisco, Seattle, Calgary, Denver, Wichita, Oklahoma City and Tulsa.

ON the night of December 12, the geologists of Greater Chicago met to dine together and to form the Geological Society of Chicago. After brief organization proceedings an executive committee was elected to direct later meetings. Professors Edson S. Bastin and John R. Ball spoke in honor of the late Professor U. S. Grant, after which a resolution in memory of Dr. Grant was drafted and unanimously approved. The meeting was then addressed by Professor Warren J. Mead, of the University of Wisconsin, on "The Hoover Dam." Some seventy men and women, representing industrial companies, museums and universities of Greater Chicago, attended.

THE American Physical Society and the American Optical Society will meet at Columbia University, New York City, on Friday and Saturday, February 24 and 25.

THE annual general meeting of the American Philosophical Society will be held at Philadelphia on April 20, 21 and 22, beginning at 2 P. M. on Thursday, April 20.

THE new research laboratory of Merck & Company, Rahway, New Jersey, will be dedicated on March 1. The structure, started in 1932, will house in the south wing laboratories for pure research in biochemistry and pharmacology while the north wing will be used for applied research. The central section will be used for offices of the directors of research, Dr. R. T. Major, director of pure research, and Dr. W. H. Engels, director of applied research. Dr. Joseph Rosin, technical director of the company, and his staff will work on the second floor, which will also house a library.

DR. WALTER M. SEWARD, of Brunswick County, Virginia, has left his entire estate, valued at approximately $250,000, to the University of Virginia. Under the terms of his will, the lands and personal property bequeathed to the university will be used for "practical demonstrations in the art of forestry," and "toward the maintenance and upbuilding of the school of forestry at the university."

BY the will of the late William Boyce Thompson the American Museum of Natural History receives Colonel Thompson's jades and crystals, valued at $107,000, and in addition $20,000 to prepare quarters for the collection and $50,000 to maintain it and make additions.

IT is reported from Mexico City that the State of Oaxaca, with the aid of funds from the federal government, will build a museum to house the relics unearthed during the past two years by the Mexican archeological expedition directed by Professor Alfonso Caso.

*Nature* reports that an addition of value has been made to the possessions of the Royal Society for the Protection of Birds in the Eastwood Nature Reserve, Stalybridge. The reserve, originally extending to about eight acres, was bequeathed by the Right Honorable John F. Cheetham, together with £5,000 for its upkeep. To this has been added an adjacent four acres, with £500, by a niece of the donor, Mrs. Wimbush, of Taunton. The reserve is a beautiful ravine within the public park given by Mr. Cheetham to Stalybridge, and his wish that it should be kept in a natural state as regards fauna and flora will insure the continuance of a sample of wild nature in the heart of an industrial area. Already there is abundance of wild plants and unexpected variety of birds.

THE eighth cumulative volume of the Readers' Guide to Periodical Literature, covering the period from

January, 1929, to June, 1932, has been published by the H. W. Wilson Company of New York City. The index is issued monthly, the numbers are cumulated throughout the year and bound volumes are issued annually. These are then superseded by the permanent volumes. The Guide covers the complete contents of the periodicals that it indexes by subjects and authors. 1,047 periodicals are indexed, including SCIENCE, *School and Society* and *The Scientific Monthly*. The first two of these are among nine weekly journals whose contents are selected as most worthy of permanent record and reference.

THE next award of the Alvarenga Prize, amounting to about $300, will be made on July 14, 1933. Essays may be on any subject in medicine and should represent an addition to the knowledge and understanding of the subject based on either original or literary research. The prize was not awarded in 1932. Communications should be addressed to Dr. John H. Girvin, secretary, 19 South Twenty-second Street, Philadelphia.

ACCORDING to the *Journal* of the American Medical Association, the Rumanian Academy of Sciences controls a fund, collected mainly from bequests, the interest of which, according to the wish of the testator, is awarded to the best literary works that have appeared during the year. The committee on awards has just finished reading the contributions for 1931, and out of the many awards the following were given for medical treatises: The Oroveanu prize of 70,000 lei has been awarded to Dr. Mina Minovici, professor of forensic medicine at the University of Budapest, for the second volume of his "Manual of Forensic Medicine." The Riegler 6,000 lei prize was awarded to Professor Peter Tomescu for his "Clinical Experimental Studies," which will be shortly translated into German. The Adamachi prize was given to Dr. Valeriu Bologa for his work "The History of Scientific Medical Work in Rumania," read in part at the recent International Congress on Medical History. The Constantinide prize was divided between Aurel Voina, lecturer at the University of Bucharest, for his treatise "Prostitution and Venereal Disease in Rumania," and Drs. Staicovici and Westfried for their monograph dealing with public health affairs of the city of Bucharest in the post-war years.

A CORRESPONDENT writes: "Cottonwood Cave on the Lincoln National Forest in New Mexico has been used for a goat shed for a great many years, also as a bat loft perhaps for thousands of years; consequently there are great deposits of guano in the bottom of the cave. As it is very rare that any water runs into the upper part of this cave, the deposit has become very dry. Presumably some visitor started a fire in the litter, not knowing that it would continue to burn. Judging from the distance it traveled, the fire had been burning for about three weeks when it was first discovered. At that time, the gas formed by the burning nitrates was so strong that the party could not go down to the fire. However, when it was visited by Supervisor O. Fred Arthur and Mr. Musgrave on September 24, the fumes were not bad except at the entrance to the cave. Fire guards were sent into the cave and put out the fire by packing water from a supply further down in the cave. An interesting phase of the fire was that the gas, evidently nitric acid gas, was so strong that it killed the leaves on oaks and maples at the mouth of the cave and about 200 feet from the fire. At no time during the fire was there enough heat to kill these leaves."

# DISCUSSION

## A FORGOTTEN EVOLUTIONIST

ON looking through the volumes of the short-lived *Archiv für Zoologie und Zootomie* my attention was attracted to an article (Bd. III, p. 167, 1802) entitled "Ueber den ursprünglichen Stamm des Menschengeschlechts," by D. Schelver. Being curious to see what the writer would say upon this topic in the year 1802, I discovered that the article contained a most interesting speculation on the probable original home of the human species and the source from which man was derived. Schelver takes issue with the then prevailing doctrine that man originated somewhere in southwestern Asia, urging that we can not legitimately argue from the origin of culture to the origin of the human race. The natural place in which to seek for the origin of man, he argues, is the region in which the most primitive men are living at the present time. Basing his conclusion on a number of anthropological characteristics, as well as cultural development, Schelver contends that the Negroes are the most primitive members of the human family, and that Africa must, therefore, have been the original cradle of the human race. But whence the Negroes? The Negroes, however, are far from representing the original ancestors of men. They have progressed far, both culturally and structurally, from the original human beings. It is no mere coincidence, according to Schelver, that Africa is the home of both the Negroes and the anthropoid apes. But man can not be derived from any existing species of anthropoids. "I shall not assert," says Schelver, "that the original natural man (Naturmensch) came from any species of ape at present known, because I can not support this by positive proofs; and since we know quite as little of the original source of the apes, as of the human family, the apes may represent a degenerate branch of the original stem of the human species. I am acquainted with no distinguishing characteristic, however, which sharply separates the apes from human beings."

" . . . The bodily nature of the human race must, in its origin, completely integrade with that of animals, and it is not improbable that, for example, we may discover hairy quadrupeds with the capacity for becoming human beings. . . . As to lowly origin, man is clearly worthy of all the more honor the lower the creatures from which he was descended."

Language, says Schelver, is a product of culture. "Der mensch hat sie erfunden, selbst geschaffen." The linguistic shortcomings of the apes, it is suggested, may be associated with the possession of vocal sacs which may, as was suggested by Sömmering, act as an impediment to the imitation of sound. These sacs are lacking in man, who, on the other hand, has another organ in a somewhat similar position, namely, the thyroid gland, which is stated to be absent in the apes. At any rate, the thyroid was not mentioned by Camper, and Schelver remarks that it could scarcely have escaped being noticed by so attentive and accurate an observer. Since the apes have vocal sacs, which man has not, and since man has the thyroid, which Schelver is persuaded is absent in the apes—"aber so viel mir bekannt ist," he cautiously adds—the hypothesis is advanced that the mysterious thyroid, whose function was so long sought for in vain, might represent the degenerate vocal sacs of the anthropoids. This conclusion is supported by certain statements concerning the outlet of the thyroid, which rest upon no better foundation than the alleged absence of this organ in the apes. That Schelver should have been led astray in his attempt at homologizing is quite natural when one considers the facts at his disposal. The point of chief interest is that the attempt was made at all.

What caused the human and anthropoid stems to diverge is a problem for which Schelver has no solution to offer. While his evolutionary concepts have much of the vagueness that characterizes the speculations of the earlier transformists, it is clear that he regards man as having a common origin with the higher apes, and that the higher types of animals are derived from lower ones, as is indicated by his reference to the genealogical table of organic life, "*der Stammtafel der ganzen lebenen Schöpfung, . . . die bis an das erste punctum saliens alles Lebens zurückführet.*"

S. J. HOLMES

UNIVERSITY OF CALIFORNIA

## A VICIOUS CIRCLE IN CYTOLOGY

THE existence of rings and sometimes strings of chromosomes has been known for a number of years and apparently first attracted marked attention in the case of the genus Oenothera. This genus is particularly unfavorable for cytological investigation on account of the extremely small size of its nuclei. It has accordingly been unsuitable for working out the fundamental significance of ring formation. Much more suitable material for such investigations is supplied by the monocotyledonous family Tradescantiae, which have been investigated by various American and European cytologists. The conclusion has been reached that the rings of chromosomes, where they occur, are series of univalents which have more or less become confused with one another and pass over to opposite poles in approximate alternation at the metaphase of the reduction or meiotic division. Unfortunately, this statement is palpably incorrect. Apparently it is due to the study of the material by means of excessively thick sections or by the smear method. Both of these procedures have the fault of obscuring important details. The situation in the case of the Tradescantiae has been studied by means of thin sections appropriately developed by approved methods of staining. It has become clear in this connection that the so-called synaptic mates are actually present in Tradescantia as normally elsewhere and that they present clearly the phenomenon of chiasmotypy, a phenomenon to which, by the way, apparently an entirely disproportionate amount of attention has been given in recent years. The pairs of chromosomes become somewhat indistinct in the pachytene stage which follows the advent of pairs. This is a common phenomenon at pachytene and it is amazing that it has not been noticed in this instance. The whole situation, in fact, suggests a surprising superficiality on the part of certain observers which is in marked contrast to the large claims which they have made on the attention of cytologists in general. It is quite obvious that in *Tradescantia virginiana,* for example, the process of meiosis follows perfectly that which is not uncommon in hybrids. The apparent serially arranged, miscalled univalent chromosomes represent in reality a segmented pachytene in which the synaptic pairs are lined up, back to back. This view of the matter harmonizes further with the observations of Hakansson on hybrid Godetias. Here he noted, while the species showed little or no so-called ring formation, that in contrast this condition was quite often characteristic of the hybrids between species. Muentzing (1932) has more recently called attention to the same tendency in hybrids. There seems to be little excuse for the errors of those who have worked on the cytology of ring formation in the case of Tradescantiae. In the species of Oenothera, however, and in the Onagraceae in general, the formation of pairs in connection with meiosis is very obscure and their separation can in general only be clearly made out at the actual metaphase. The rings and strings in species of Oenothera are also nothing more than persistent pachytenes which become distributed as such to the metaphase plate. It is obvious, if the statements made here are well founded, that the results obtained by Belling, Darlington and Sax in regard to ring formation are without sound foundation in fact.

E. C. JEFFREY

## TWISTED TREES AND THE SPIRAL HABIT

THE behavior of organisms is determined by the physical and chemical nature of their protoplasm and by their environment. The relative importance of hereditary material and environment has long been, and probably ever will be, a controversial subject. This is true because both factors always play a part, sometimes one and sometimes the other having the predominant influence. There is also the very natural tendency of an investigator to attach more significance to the point of view represented by his field of work. A student of protoplasm or of genetics will see in heredity a greater influence, and the ecologist will lay emphasis on environment, though the former must be aware of the fact that protoplasm has come to be what it is primarily because of environmental influences working through the ages. The relationship between hereditary reactions and developmental expressions is presented fully and well by Stockard.[1]

It has occurred to me that a protoplasmic interpretation of the twisting of tree trunks might be a logical view of this interesting behavior concerning which there has been much discussion on the pages of SCIENCE.[2-6] Certain observers[2,4,5], see in the prevailing direction of the wind an explanation of the twisting of tree trunks. Persistent winds might well bring about a twisting of the trunk, in support of which is the fact that trees exposed to the wind often assume an oval shape. There is also the report that twisted trunks rarely occur in the heart of a forest.[4]

Several years ago this subject was again brought to my attention by my friend, Mr. Philip Sawyer, of New York, who told me of the twisted trunks of trees (conifers) along the trail up Mt. Audubon in Boulder County, Colorado. The degree of twist varied considerably, from a very gradual one to a complete twist within a distance equal to twice the diameter of the tree. The clockwise twist was the more usual. The reverse twist was infrequent and occurred among the others. This last remark of Mr. Sawyer's increased my belief that tree trunks twist because of an innate tendency to do so and not because of environmental factors. I was, therefore, very much interested in the recent report by Herrick[6] on twisted trees in the forests of Louisiana. He examined 1,527 trees, of which 364 (23 per cent.) were straight grained, 811 (53 per cent.) showed a right-hand twist, and 352 (24 per cent.) showed left-hand twisting. He observed further the condition of the roots of 57 trees that had been uprooted. Of these, 31 (5 per cent.) showed twisting to the right, 7 (12 per cent.) showed left-hand twisting and 19 (33 per cent.) were straight. He adds that if prevailing winds were the cause it would be expected that the limbs on the one side of a tree would twist in one direction and those on the opposite side would twist in the opposite direction. Actually, however, the limbs of any one tree always twist in the same direction. Herrick, therefore, concludes that as there is both right and left-hand twisting in tree trunks of the same locality, and as the twisting of limbs is in the same direction on all sides of the tree, and as roots also show twisting, winds can not be the cause. Mr. Laurence Moyer adds the old apple tree as another common example of tree trunk twisting.

It is the purpose of the present paper to suggest that the twisting of tree trunks is but one manifestation of a wide-spread tendency in organisms to grow and move spirally, a tendency due to a heritable protoplasmic quality and not to environmental factors.

The formation of spirals is not limited to living things. Crystals show both right-hand and left-hand growth. The precipitation of salts in gels, which goes by the name of the Liesegang phenomenon, is ordinarily rhythmic, resulting in the production of concentric rings, but occasionally a perfect spiral is produced, for which there is no adequate explanation. Organisms, from the lowest to the highest, give various indications of a spiral habit. Schaeffer[7] reports that Amoeba travels in a spiral when moving along a thin glass rod or within a fine capillary tube. The spiral may be to the right or to the left for varying lengths of time, and may alternate frequently, although a species is predominantly to the left or to the right. The shells of mollusks are striking examples of the spiral habit in organisms. Both Mr. Sawyer and my colleague Dr. Zirkle reminded me of this

[1] "The Physical Basis of Personality," 1931.
[2] SCIENCE, February 13, 1931.
[3] *Ibid.*, March 27, 1931.
[4] *Ibid.*, May 22, 1931.
[5] *Ibid.*, January 29, 1932.
[6] *Ibid.*, November 4, 1932.

[7] SCIENCE, July 10, 1931.

fact. The shells of Nautilus and Triton are examples; especially fine are the long, cornucopia-like spiral shells of *Terebra oculata*. Further inquiry brought from Dr. H. E. Crampton the interesting observation that sea snails in the South Pacific show both right- and left-hand twists, the latter being infrequent.

Schaeffer[8] has carried his observations on spiral movement in organisms to man, whom he regards as a spirally twisted right organism. This is true not only of the movements of man but of body structure as well. The gall-duct is the most conspicuously spirally twisted unpaired organ in man, and it is a right spiral. There are numerous other examples of spirally-twisted organs in animals. As for movement, when man is blindfolded he walks in a right spiral. (In this connection there is the old saying that hunters when lost in the woods walk in circles to the right, the circle getting smaller and smaller, *i.e.*, man walks in a spiral. One wonders if the habit which dogs have of turning round and round before finally settling down for a nap, is another manifestation of the spiral tendency in organisms.) Spiral walking in man is also regarded as due simply to the fact that most people are right-legged, as they are right-handed, which results in walking in a curve. But the curve is most often to the right, while right-leggedness should, it would seem, produce a left spiral. However, right-leggedness is a possible cause of spiral walking in man, which, if true, eliminates but one of the many examples of the spiral habit in organisms.

The spiral structure of trees is duplicated in the most delicate of plant cellulose parts, namely, the cotton fiber. Titus and his coworkers[9] report such a structure for the cotton fiber. Denham[10] enumerates four distinct classes of spirals in cotton fibers. The structure does not always proceed in the same direction but suffers more or less regular reversals. Balls[11] has presented a number of papers dealing with the twisting of cotton fibers. He states that reversal from dexter (right) to sinister (left) spirals occur in the same fiber. Causation of the reversals is physiological (*i.e.*, protoplasmic). Ordinary environmental influences do not affect the statistical peculiarities of the reversals. The spiral habit in plants is further illustrated by the tight wrapping of tendrils and of vines. Two vines may twist around each other and give as perfect an example of spiral wrapping as exists in the artificial wound fibers of a rope. It appears, therefore, that the tendency toward spiral growth is as characteristic of the cellulose framework of plants as it is of the parts of animals. The spiral twisting of cotton fibers is convincing evidence that the twisting of tree trunks is an innate heritable property, and not an environmental effect.

The evidence presented here indicates that spiral development among organisms is the expression of a wide-spread tendency which is protoplasmic in origin.

WILLIAM SEIFRIZ
UNIVERSITY OF PENNSYLVANIA

[8] *Jour. Morph. and Physiol.*, p. 294, 1928.
[9] *Jour. Chem.*, 9: 114, 1932.
[10] *Jour. Textile Inst.*, 14: 86T, 1923.
[11] *Proc. Roy. Soc.*, London, 99: 130, 1926.

## THE EXTINCT LAKE SAN AUGUSTIN, NEW MEXICO

A SEMI-ARID basin in western New Mexico, known as the San Augustin Plains, has been described by Bryan as an old lake basin.[1] To this extinct body of water he has given the name Lake San Augustin. Field work by the writer during the summer of 1932 not only supports Bryan's view, but has yielded detailed information on the extent and characteristics of this ancient lake.

The San Augustin basin lies in western Socorro and eastern Catron Counties, and is bordered on the north by the Bear, Gallinas and Datil Mountains; on the west by the Tularosa Mountains; and the south by a mountainous belt, including the O Bar O, Pelona and Tuera Mountains; and on the east by the Magdalena Mountains The basin is 60 miles long from northeast to southwest, and has a maximum width of about 20 miles. During the rainy season (July and August) ephemeral streams make their way from the mountains across broad alluvial slopes to two playas, the larger and westernmost of which is called locally the San Augustin Plains, and contains the lake basin herein described.

Lake San Augustin at its highest stage was about 32 miles long by 11 miles wide, with a surface at about 6,940 feet A. T. The lowest point in the basin is 6,776 feet A. T., and thus the greatest depth of the lake was about 164 feet. The shore lines of this and all the lower stages are strikingly marked by shingle beaches, spits and bay head bars, and by cliffs developed both on rocky mountainsides and on alluvial fans. These shore features form a descending series that indicates many lake stages, the details of which are yet to be worked out from a study of the field notes. At its highest stage Lake San Augustin was connected by a small channel with a basin farther east, as yet unstudied, that probably drained into Lake San Augustin. At all the lower stages Lake San Augustin had no possible outlet, and its waters must have been depleted by evaporation and underground seepage.

The highest beach has a constant altitude on all sides of the playa, and thus gives positive evidence that no differential earth movements have occurred

[1] Kirk Bryan, ''Ground Water Reconnaissance in Socorro County, New Mexico,'' Seventh Biennial Report of the State Engineer, pp. 82–83, 1925–26.

here since the formation of this beach. The beaches can be traced across all the larger alluvial fans surrounding the playa, and thus show that these fans were formed before the lake existed. Subsequent fan development has been feeble. The lake is believed to have existed in the last (Wisconsin) glacial stage.

DEPARTMENT OF GEOLOGY WILLIAM E. POWERS
NORTHWESTERN UNIVERSITY

# SCIENTIFIC BOOKS

*Faraday's Diary.* Vols. I and II. Edited by THOMAS MARTIN, M.Sc., and published by order of the Managers of the Royal Institution of Great Britain, with a Foreword by Sir William H. Bragg, O.M., K.B.E., F.R.S. G. Bell and Sons, Ltd., London.

AFTER Faraday's death the Royal Institution received as a bequest from him a manuscript record containing an account of the experimental work which had been done by him in the years from 1820 to 1862. This record the managers of the Royal Institution decided to publish as a fitting memorial of their most distinguished director. When the publication is complete there will be seven volumes, of which two are now at hand, and the others may be expected within two years. Only 750 copies of the work will be issued, and these will be sold in sets. The price of a set is twelve guineas.

The task of editing this work was undertaken by Thomas Martin, M.Sc., general secretary of the Royal Institution. It has been admirably performed. So far as one can judge without comparison with the original manuscript, the transcription of the text has been carried out with accuracy. The peculiarities of spelling and the abbreviations used by Faraday have been retained, and obvious errors have been noted, with proper reference to the editor. The diagrams and sketches with which the manuscript abounds have been with great judgment and good taste removed from the body of the text and inserted either on the wide exterior margins of the pages or at the bottom below the letterpress. In the latter case the paragraphs to which the diagrams pertain are indicated. The result is that, while the diagrams are immediately available, the text can be read with continuous comfort. An extensive table of contents is prefixed to each volume, and references are made in it to Faraday's published papers in which the matter of the text has been incorporated. An index or synopsis of the whole work is promised for the last volume of the set. The books are beautifully printed, in excellent legible type, on wide pages, with large margins, and are well bound. The publishers, Messrs. G. Bell and Sons, Ltd., should be congratulated on their contribution to the value of the work.

Faraday's first scientific paper was published in 1816, at a time when, as he says of himself, his fear was greater than his confidence, and both far greater than his knowledge; at a time also when he had no thought of ever writing an original paper on science. The favorable reception given to it emboldened him to undertake other researches in the time that was left him after the many duties of his position as assistant in the laboratory had been performed. After a few years he evidently felt that he would be able to carry on research in a sufficiently consecutive way to make regular entries of his experiments advisable, and in September, 1820, he began the notes of his work which ended only with the close of his scientific activity, forty-two years later. They present a complete record of the experiments which he carried out in the laboratory of the Royal Institution. The only important things which he did which do not appear there are his studies of alloys of other metals with iron and steel, carried out by him in collaboration with Mr. Stodart; his researches on the manufacture of glass for optical purposes; and the work which he did for nearly thirty years as scientific adviser of the Trinity House, for the improvement of the lighthouse service.

As was to be expected of an assistant of Sir Humphry Davy, Faraday was first interested in chemistry. With the exception of the invention in 1821 of apparatus to exhibit electromagnetic rotations, most of the entries for the first ten years are concerned with chemical matters. They record the experiments which led to the discovery of two compounds of chlorine with carbon (1820), they describe the liquefaction of chlorine and other gases (1822); and they present the long series of observations which led to the isolation of benzene from coal oil (1825). Many other observations are recorded which led to nothing or to results of minor importance. In 1831 appears the first study —with the exception noted above—of a purely physical subject, the vibrations of plates and the formation of Chladni's figures.

From time to time in these years Faraday had evidently had in mind the possibility of an inductive effect produced by an electric current in a neighboring conductor. On December 28, 1824, he tried the experiment of bringing up a strong magnet to a wire carrying a current, with the expectation that the current would be thereby modified; but no effect was shown on a magnetic needle placed under a distant part of the circuit. On November 28, 1825, he looked for a current in a wire set parallel to another wire carrying a current, but could perceive no action. Again on April 22, 1828, he endeavored to find an effect produced by a magnet pushed through a ring of copper wire, with no result. Why some of these experiments failed it is not easy to determine, unless it was that Faraday was looking for a steady effect, produced so long as the arrangement was maintained, and so either did not look for or did not notice the momentary effects produced while the magnet was moving or when the primary current was closed or broken. That this explanation is the true one may be supported by an entry made on August 29, 1831, the day on which his first successful observations of electromagnetic induction were made: "Hence effect evident but transient; but its recurrence on breaking the connection shews an equilibrium somewhere that must be capable of being rendered more distinct."

The course of Faraday's progress in the discovery of the induced current was entirely different from that of his exposition of the discovery in his "First Series of Researches" read before the Royal Society on November 24, 1831. His first successful observation was made with an iron ring wound with two coils of wire, one of which was joined with a galvanometer, the other to a battery. When the battery circuit was made or broken, a temporary current appeared in the galvanometer. This experiment is the same as that reported by Joseph Henry as made by him before he had any knowledge of Faraday's method. On September 24 Faraday records his obtaining the induced current in a coil wound around an iron bar when the ends of the bar were in contact with the opposite poles of two bar magnets and the other ends of these magnets were brought together or separated. "Here distinct conversion of Magnetism into Electricity."

The first record of an induced current produced in a circuit by making or breaking a current in a neighboring circuit "without the presence of iron" was made on October 1. It was not until October 18 that this effect was confirmed not only with the galvanometer but by using the induced current in a helix to magnetize needles. This observation is the one with which Faraday begins his exposition.

The observation described by him in §18 of the production of the induced current in a circuit made in the shape of a large W, to which another similar circuit carrying a current was moved up or from which it was removed is not recorded in the diary until December 26. This note is evidently misdated, for the observation recorded in it is described in the paper of November 24, and in the following paragraph it is taken as evidence of the existence of an electrotonic state, a hypothesis which Faraday abandoned in his Bakerian Lecture, dated December 21. These two paragraphs belong somewhere in October, if the course of Faraday's thought can serve as a guide.

Volume I closes with this discovery and its elaboration. Faraday evidently felt that he was justified in expecting to succeed in obtaining other important results, for he published this work as his "First Series of Experimental Researches in Electricity" and began numbering the paragraphs consecutively. In the new folio volume of the diary which he opened on August 25, 1832, he also introduced this consecutive numbering of the paragraphs, which is continued until March, 1860.

Volume II opens with the record of many experiments made to show the identity of electricity from different sources. Most of the volume is taken up with the study of electrochemical decomposition, which led to the discovery of the laws of electrolysis. In October, 1835, Faraday left this subject for a while to study the phenomena presented by the induction of a circuit on itself. In this he had been anticipated by Joseph Henry. Before the close of the year he started work on electrostatic induction and the electric discharge, the result of which was his proof of the equality of the positive and negative charges and his discovery of specific inductive capacity. Volume II closes before the account of these researches is complete. He also for a while reverted to chemistry by the examination of the properties of fluorine.

With the work on electrostatic induction closes what Dr. Bence-Jones calls the first period of Faraday's experimental researches. He had for some time been weary and oppressed with giddiness and loss of memory, and shortly after this work was done he was forced to give up his studies altogether and rest. The famous discoveries of the magnetic rotation of the plane of polarized light and of diamagnetism, which were made after he returned to work, together with his speculations and philosophical views on the action of the medium in maintaining and determining the magnetic and electric fields will appear in the later volumes. The two now issued contain a large part of Faraday's experimental achievements.

It is interesting to notice that he tried (May 2, 1833) to obtain an effect on a beam of polarized light by passing it through an electrolyte which was transmitting a current, and also (May 6, 1833) by passing the beam through a piece of his borate of lead glass while it was in a strong electrostatic field (the Kerr effect), but with no positive results. He also (September 19, 1833) observed the same effect as that afterwards applied in the Groves' gas battery, without appreciating its meaning. Probably other hints of future discoveries could be found by a careful study of his records.

On a general view of these volumes one is struck with Faraday's astonishing industry. This is especially noticeable in the earlier years covered by the record. The number of chemical experiments made in one day while he was studying the compounds of chlorine, involving heating the mixtures and measuring the volumes of the gases produced from them, is amazing. Perhaps the most striking example is given by the two days (October 28, November 4, 1831) in which he experimented on electromagnetic induction at Mr. Christie's with the great magnet of the Royal Society. On the first of these days he records no less than 27 separate experiments, and on the second 29, many of which were tried over and over. The number of tests made in one day with the electrolytic cells during his study of electrolysis in 1833 and 1834 is even more astonishing.

The notes exhibit, even better than his published work, the marvelous fertility of Faraday's mind. Every page, nay, nearly every paragraph contains a new thought, often unimportant, occasionally in error, but sometimes, when good fortune and inspiration combine, rising to the highest flights of the scientific imagination. From the best of these he constructed the great scientific poems of his published papers.

It also appears very plainly that a great deal of Faraday's work was done in his mind and is not recorded in his notebooks. To perceive this we need only compare the notes of his discovery of the induced current, with the beautifully ordered presentation of the subject in his first paper and in the Bakerian Lecture, or consider the notes on the phenomena of self-induction before, as Faraday says, he begins to see light. After he saw the light his experiments became more systematic and show how he worked when led by a guiding principle.

This publication constitutes a noble memorial to one of the greatest leaders in experimental science. Its value as a history of the way in which an honest, industrious and powerful mind operates on the facts of nature is inestimable. The thanks of the scientific world should be given to the managers of the Royal Institution and to any others who may have cooperated with them to make it possible.

W. F. MAGIE

PRINCETON UNIVERSITY

# SOCIETIES AND MEETINGS

## THE TEXAS ACADEMY OF SCIENCE

THE Texas Academy of Science held its annual meeting on November 11 and 12 in Houston, Texas. The number of papers appearing on the program was large and well distributed over the field of science. To bring together papers of like interests, five sections were in session throughout the meeting.

The section devoted to geological sciences was very popular. The notable papers included: "The Big Springs of Texas," by R. E. Ryan, of Houston; "The Salt Domes and Gulf Coast Oil Fields," an illustrated lecture by Marcus Hanna, of Houston; "Leaves of Geologic History from the Topography around Houston," Donald C. Barton. Among the twelve other papers, one by W. T. Carter, of the U. S. Soil Survey, on the "Relationship of Texas Soils to the Geological Formations" was considered as an outstanding piece of work. The Section of Zoological Sciences contained twelve papers. Several of these were abstracts of longer papers, which are to be printed. Of outstanding worth was the paper "The Fleas of Texas and their Economic Importance," by M. A. Stewart, of the Rice Institute, and of unique purport was the paper by Karl Bleyl, of the Sam Houston State Teachers College, in which he describes a new remedy for snake bite, which is a serum taken from the snake itself. The Botany Section was largely given over to papers on the technical side of investigation into the relationships of cotton. Several papers on regional ecology in Texas were given.

The Physical and Chemical Sciences gave papers ranging from the chemical contents of grapefruit, a study in vitamins; a description of a gigantic permanent magnet, and up to cosmic rays. L. M. Mott-Smith, and L. G. Howe, of Rice Institute, told of measuring this mysterious ray at the altitude of twelve thousand feet in an airplane. The Educational Section was given over to archeology; papers on the present social and financial conditions of the world; on mental operations accompanying emotions and including papers on the comparison of the Texas Academy of Science with other state academies, by S. W. Bilsing, representative to the American Association for the Advancement of Science, and one by Clyde T. Reed, College of Arts and Industries, on "Science Clubs and the Junior Academy." The annual lecture, given at the banquet, was "Genetical Views of the Origin of Life," by Edgar Altenberg. Just before Dr. Altenberg's lecture, H. Y. Benedict, president of the University of Texas and also of the academy, made an announcement relative to the new McDonald Observatory which is to be built by the university somewhere in the state of Texas. The last session was the annual business meeting. Seventy-five new members were taken in and five new fellows created. It was announced by F. B. Plummer, of the publication committee, that Volume XV of the *Transactions* would be ready for distribution in a few weeks, and P. L. Turner, representative of the Southwest Press, stated that "The Bird Life of Texas" had reached the point where subscriptions were asked for. The new officers are: E. N. Jones, Baylor University, *president;* F. B. Plummer, *executive vice-president;* H. A. Wilson, Rice Institute, *vice-president of Section 1;* Colonel M. L. Crimmins, *vice-president of Section 3;*

H. B. Parks, San Antonio, *secretary and treasurer*. S. W. Bilsing was continued as the representative to the American Association Council and given the authority to represent the Texas organization at the next annual meeting.

Following the business meeting, three papers were given by members who were unable to attend on the first day. The best of these was a paper by O. M. Ball, supplementing his recent publication "The Eocene Plants of Texas." This paper was illustrated by lantern slides showing newly discovered and described specimens. One of them was a beautiful leaf recently found in a quarry in East Texas and has been named Warneri after S. R. Warner, of Sam Houston State Teachers College, who collected the specimen. S. R. Warner is a member of the academy and was in the audience and heard for the first time of the importance of his discovery and the fact that the plant was named for him.

H. B. PARKS,
*Secretary*

### THE OKLAHOMA ACADEMY OF SCIENCE

THE twenty-first annual meeting of the Oklahoma Academy of Science was held on November 25 and 26 at the University of Oklahoma, Norman. The meetings were divided into four sections and the number of papers presented in each section was as follows: Biology, 37; geology, 19; physical sciences, 22; social sciences, 29, making a total of 107.

The president's annual address was presented following the luncheon on Friday by Dr. Herbert Patterson, of the Oklahoma Agricultural and Mechanical College. The title of this address was "A Challenge to the Social Sciences." One hundred and fifty members and guests of the academy attended the annual banquet on Friday evening and Dr. Andrew Ellicott Douglass, professor of astronomy at the University of Arizona, gave an illustrated lecture entitled "Dating Prehistoric Ruins of the Southwest." Dr. W. B. Bizzell also gave a talk on "The Spirit of Adventure in Research." Dr. Douglass gave a second address at the general meeting of the academy on Saturday morning on the subject of "The Sun Spot's Cycle and the Cyclogram Method of Cycle Study."

One hundred and ninety members were registered and about 275 people attended the meetings.

The following officers were elected for 1933:

*President*, F. E. Knowles, Enid, Oklahoma.
*Vice-president*, Section A (Biology), Ralph D. Bird, University of Oklahoma, Norman, Oklahoma.
*Vice-president*, Section B (Geology), C. W. Tomlinson, Ardmore, Oklahoma.
*Vice-president*, Section C (Physical Sciences), Wm. V. N. Garretson, Stillwater, Oklahoma.
*Vice-president*, Section D (Social Science), O. D. Duncan, Stillwater, Oklahoma.
*Assistant Secretary-Treasurer*, Duane Roller, Norman, Oklahoma.

HORACE J. HARPER,
*Secretary-Treasurer*

STILLWATER, OKLAHOMA

## SCIENTIFIC APPARATUS AND LABORATORY METHODS

### AN APPARATUS FOR DETERMINING THE ABSORPTION OF CARBON DIOXIDE BY LEAVES UNDER NATURAL CONDITIONS

THE equipment described below was designed primarily for studies involving a large number of determinations of the photosynthetic activity of apple leaves under field conditions. The chief features are, first, a simple $CO_2$ absorption unit which can be made up of standard glassware and which is efficient, even though the air passes through the liquid at a rapid rate, and secondly, a light-weight, closely fitting leaf chamber made of cellophane, which is easily attached and held in place without cumbersome supports. The apparatus is essentially a simplification of that described by S. Kostytschew, K. Bazyrina and W. Tschesnokov,[1] and by Schandrel,[2] but involves less elaborate technique, so that a large number of determinations can be carried out at one time. An electric current is required to operate the pump.

The absorption unit is a modification of the Reiset tower used by Brown and Escombe[3] and consists of a glass tube, about 60 cm long and 3 cm in diameter, which is supported in an upright position. A glass Gooch crucible, with fused-in fritted glass disks, is attached to the lower end of the tower by means of thin-walled rubber tubing and serves to break the gas stream into minute bubbles. The size of the pores in the disks used was 100–120 microns, but finer grades of porosity down to 20–30 microns are available. The small end of the crucible is fitted with a rubber stopper, through which extends a short piece of glass tubing. A standard mercury filter with fused-in fritted glass plate may be used as a gas distributor instead of the Gooch crucible, but it is more expensive.

The upper end of the absorption tower is connected

[1] S. Kostytschew, K. Bazyrina and W. Tschesnokov, *Planta*, 5: 696–724, 1928.

[2] Hugo Schandrel, *Wiss. Archiv. für Landw. Abt. A Pflanzenbau*, 3: 529–560, 1930.

[3] H. T. Brown and F. Escombe, *Proc. Royal Soc.*, London, B 76: 29–111, 1905.

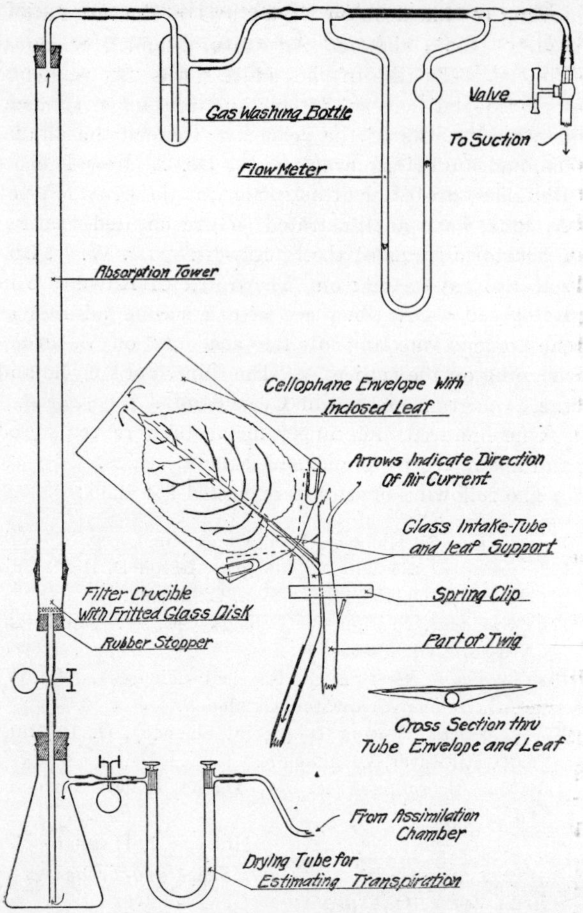


FIG. 1. Diagram of an absorption unit, and of an assimilation chamber.

by means of heavy rubber tubing to a flowmeter accurately calibrated with a Sargent wet test meter at different temperatures. The air passes through a dehydrating agent before it enters the flowmeter to avoid the accumulation of moisture in the capillary tube which has a bore of less than 1 mm and a length of 125 mm. An electric vacuum pump is used to pull the air through the system. By adjusting the sensitive gas valves, the mercury in the arms of the flowmeter can be kept at a definite level and the flow of air may thus be regulated to conform to a predetermined rate. The standard rate chosen for our preliminary tests was 100 liters per hour. The efficiency of the absorption unit is indicated by the fact that all carbon dioxide in the atmosphere is removed when passed through a column of 200 cc N/10 $Ba(OH)_2$ or KOH in a single tower at this relatively high rate, provided the solution remains sufficiently strong.

The reservoir containing the $CO_2$ absorbent consists of a 500 cc suction flask, fitted with a rubber stopper and a glass tube about 22 cm long. The glass tube touches the bottom of the flask, and its upper end, which extends above the stopper about 5 cm, is provided with a short piece of rubber tubing and a pinch-cock. A similar connection is found on the side arm of the suction flask.

A definite amount, usually 200 cc, of N/10 $Ba(OH)_2$ or N/10 KOH is allowed to flow from the protected stock bottle through a connected burette directly into the flask. To charge the flasks with the standard solution requires only a few minutes, after which all the pinch-cocks remain closed until the determinations begin. A large number of flasks may be filled in the laboratory to serve for many determinations in the field.

The leaf chamber, adopted as a standard after experimenting with many other types, consists of an envelope made from heavy-weight, moisture-proof cellophane. A special moisture proof paste must be used to seal the overlapping edges. The size may vary with the leaf to be studied. The envelope is slipped over a leaf which has previously been provided with a combination support and air intake. This consists of a glass tube which is bent as indicated in the diagram. It is held firmly in position against the stem by means of a spring clip so that the long arm passes on the under side of the leaf and supports it at an angle of about 30 degrees from the horizontal. A heavy-walled rubber tube attached to the glass support connects it with the side arm of the suction flask.

After the assimilation chamber is in place, the flaps on the open edge near the base of the leaf are bent back and held in place on the under side by means of paper clips. The corners of the envelope may also be folded back to reduce the size of the chamber to a minimum. The cross-section shows how the envelope fits about the leaf so as to avoid "dead air spaces" which might possibly interfere with the free supply of fresh air and carbon dioxide. The glass tube keeps the cellophane a few millimeters away from the under side of the leaf where the stomates are chiefly found on material we have used. The envelope with the enclosed leaf is easily held in place and may be adjusted to any plane, using the glass intake-support tube as an axis. It is thus possible to expose the leaf at a right angle to the sun's rays if desired. With some modification, the support and cellophane chamber can be used for two or more leaves or even for a whorl of leaves on a spur.

The supply of fresh air enters through the small opening which is left around the glass tube and the petiole. A thermometer may be inserted in this opening to record the temperature within the chamber. After passing over the leaf, the air is drawn to the absorption unit through the glass tube at the upper edge of the envelope. The single arm of the intake tube may be replaced by a Y-tube or a T-tube so that the air is withdrawn from the corners of the envelope, thus tending toward a somewhat better circulation of air over all parts of the leaf.

In spite of the rapid movement of air through the chamber (100 L. an hour), the temperature of the chamber when exposed to the direct sun will be from 6 to 10 degrees C. higher than the surrounding air. Condensation of the water vapor transpired by the enclosed leaf may occur on the relatively cool lower and shaded side of the envelope, but since little or no moisture is lost through the upper surface of the leaf, there is practically no accumulation of water on the corresponding exposure of the envelope. Excessively high and injurious temperatures, due to concentration of the heat rays in different parts of the leaf, are thus avoided. After several hours' use the cellophane becomes wavy and the moisture-proof coating may disintegrate, but this does not seem to interfere seriously with the transmission of light, nor does it have any noticeable detrimental influence on leaf activity. The wet cellophane becomes flaccid, but resumes its original stiffness when air dried.

The water transpired by the leaf in the chamber may be estimated by having the air pass through a dehydrating agent before it reaches the absorption tower. The weight of moisture adhering to the envelope must be added.

After all parts of the apparatus are in place, the stop-cocks on the suction flask are opened. The air is pulled through the system at the standard rate of 100 L. per hour, regardless of the size of the leaf. This should insure an ample supply of air containing "normal" amounts of $CO_2$, and it may actually provide the leaf with more $CO_2$ than it would have access to in relatively still air.

In our experiments, six to eight complete units, as described above, are attached to the same suction tank and are operated at one time. The air moving through each unit, of course, is governed by a flowmeter for each tower. All but two units are used to measure the carbon dioxide absorbed after the air has passed the leaf in the assimilating chamber. The remaining two units are used for control of the amount of carbon dioxide absorbed during the operations of filling the flask and titrating the solution, and also to determine the amount of carbon dioxide absorbed from an equal volume of "normal" air obtained within a few feet and at the same level as that which is passed over the enclosed leaves. The air used in these controls is made to pass through a cellophane envelope which is identical with that used on the leaves, so that the temperature of the gas entering the system is the same in all cases.

The running time has usually varied from one half to three hours, although the apparatus may be operated for longer periods by using a stronger solution for absorption. After each run, the liquid is allowed to flow back through the filter into the reservoir flask and the absorption tower is repeatedly rinsed with small amounts of distilled water until about 150 cc has been used in each case. Where the precipitate of barium carbonate is very heavy, suction may have to be applied to the flask, but this is unnecessary for periods not longer than one hour, or when potassium hydroxide is used as the absorbent. After the tower is thoroughly cleaned of adhering alkali solution, the flask is disconnected from the system and the pinchcocks are closed. Flasks contained fresh solution are put in place, after which the suction may be started for another determination.

The amount of carbon dioxide absorbed during the operating time is determined by titrating an aliquot of the solution in the flask, after adding barium chloride. The error introduced by the absorption of $CO_2$ during the operations of charging the flasks and titrating the unused alkali has been determined to be negligible in our experiments. The great dilution of the hydroxide solution caused by the use of liberal quantities of distilled water in rinsing minimizes the amount of carbon dioxide absorbed during titration. Where the flow is accurately regulated, the controls give identical results. The activity of the leaf with respect to the utilization or production of carbon dioxide is determined by the difference between the amounts absorbed by these control units and by the other units.

In agreement with Lundegardh, and others[4] the amount of carbon dioxide in 100 L. of "normal" air has been found by the use of the above apparatus to vary from as low as 38 mg to as high as 70 mg in a warm, unventilated greenhouse containing about 100 young vigorous apple trees growing in tubs. The former concentrations are more frequent on a clear mild day in a ventilated greenhouse during the morning hours, while the higher concentrations occurred at night. There may be appreciable variation from one hour period to the next, so that controls are essential for every determination.

The apparatus has been used to study the efficiency of apple leaves on plants grown under different conditions of nutrition. In some of our experiments, as high as 25 per cent. of the carbon dioxide contained in the "normal" atmosphere was removed by passing over a single leaf, but as a rule the amount removed was less than 10 per cent. The amount of carbon

[4] Henrik Lundegardh, "Environment and Plant Development." Trans. Eric Ashby. Edward Arnold and Company, London. 1931. p. 264.

dioxide absorbed during one-hour periods per 100 sq cm of healthy leaf surface exposed to the light varied from less than 1 mg to as high as 25 mg, with 2 to 10 mg the most frequent rate during the morning hours. In a few cases during daylight hours in the forenoon, the leaves actually increased rather than reduced the carbon dioxide content of the air. The respiratory rate is determined during the day by excluding light from leaves whose photosynthetic activity was established during the preceding hour, or by making determinations during the night.

In general, our preliminary results, obtained with the apparatus described, conform with those recorded by the Russian authors previously referred to, and they indicate that wide fluctuations in the activity of a given leaf from hour to hour and from day to day are to be expected, even though the temperature and other environmental factors are the same in successive periods. Nevertheless, a relatively active leaf seems to hold its rank compared to others under many varying conditions. The apparatus described should therefore be useful for many studies involving a knowledge of the leaf efficiency as influenced by a number of conditions or treatments.

A. J. HEINICKE
M. B. HOFFMAN
DEPARTMENT OF POMOLOGY,
CORNELL UNIVERSITY

# SPECIAL ARTICLES

## THE FUNCTION OF THE ADRENAL CORTICAL HORMONE AND THE CAUSE OF DEATH FROM ADRENAL INSUFFICIENCY[1]

THE functional significance of the adrenal cortex is unknown; practically all investigators of the problem agree upon this point. Various tentative hypotheses have been advanced to account for the function of these glands, but none of these hypotheses, or all of them taken together, have materially advanced the problem of cortical function.

We are of the opinion that data now in our possession, merely a brief outline of which will be presented here, explain in large measure the function of the adrenal cortex and the cause of death from adrenal insufficiency. The nature of the data is such that it is highly important to have in mind a clear picture of the type of experimental animal employed.

Bilaterally adrenalectomized dogs are used: they have well-healed wounds, are perfectly normal healthy animals at their peak weight. Any one viewing these dogs would be quite unable to distinguish them by appearance or behavior from control unoperated individuals. From the day of gland removal they are injected daily with adequate maintenance doses of the cortical hormone until ready for use. Some of the animals have been bilaterally adrenalectomized for nearly two years, others for lesser periods. In all cases, however, they were permitted to develop severe symptoms of insufficiency by withdrawal of extract, and then revived and returned to normal health by adequate injections of hormone. This is the routine procedure in the laboratory before any adrenalectomized dog is regarded as a fit subject for experimentation. Several of the older animals have passed through this routine eight to ten times. Our adrenalectomized dogs are, by all anatomical and physiological criteria employed, perfectly normal healthy animals, except that they lack adrenal glands. We reiterate and emphasize this point purposely. When an experiment starts, the cortical hormone is withheld and the animal allowed to become prostrate from insufficiency. Adequate doses of the hormone are then given and the animal returns to normal.

Study of such animals reveals some new and interesting data which, for the sake of brevity and clarity of presentation, will be given as bald statements. The more important points supporting these statements will be discussed more in detail later.

(1) The function of the adrenal cortical hormone is the regulation and maintenance of a normal circulating volume of fluid within the vascular system. In the absence of the hormone, fluid is continually lost from the circulation presumably by transudation through the capillary walls, with the result that the adrenalectomized animal is unable to maintain his normal blood volume, and eventually dies from circulatory collapse due to insufficiency of circulating fluid.

(2) Accompanying the progressive decrease in blood volume is a progressive fall of blood pressure to the death level. The decline in arterial pressure is apparently a direct result of the decreased volume of circulating fluid.

(3) The decrease in blood volume and blood pressure are not terminal phenomena, but first appear within twenty-four to seventy-two hours after discontinuing hormone injections and before active symptoms of insufficiency appear. Both volume and pressure steadily decline to the death point, which may not occur until eight to twelve days later.

[1] The expenses of this investigation, including the cost of enlarging this issue of SCIENCE to make early publication possible, have been defrayed by a grant from the Josiah Macy Foundation of New York.

(4) The manifestations and symptoms of adrenal insufficiency parallel in remarkable fashion the decline in blood pressure.

(5) Hemoconcentration, increased blood viscosity and the marked slowing of the circulation which invariably appears, are directly correlated with and chiefly dependent upon the decline in plasma volume and blood pressure.

(6) The heart rate varies inversely as the blood pressure, and the change in rate appears to be due to the progressively diminishing venous return to the right heart, and the effort of the heart to compensate for the greatly decreased quantity of fluid in circulation.

(7) The blood-urea and non-protein nitrogen also vary inversely as the blood pressure. The decreased renal function, so evident during adrenal insufficiency, we attribute to the changes in circulation previously mentioned, *i.e.,* diminished blood volume, decreased pressure, and presumably, therefore, to decreased filtration pressure and blood flow in the kidney.

(8) The increased viscosity of the blood is due to loss of fluid and increase of corpuscles per unit volume, and to the increase in plasma proteins due to hemoconcentration.

(9) Adrenalectomized animals, in the absence of the cortical hormone, are apparently unable to draw fluid back into the blood stream through the capillary walls. The accepted view that the osmotic power of the blood colloids is the chief factor involved in compensation needs further investigation. The blood colloids are proportionately increased in adrenal insufficiency, yet the animal does not dilute or compensate in face of a declining blood volume and arterial pressure.

(10) Following administration of adequate amounts of cortical hormone to prostrate adrenalectomized dogs, the blood volume, blood pressure and blood constituents all return to normal. The animal is able to dilute his blood and build up a normal blood volume, and all symptoms of adrenal insufficiency disappear.

(11) It is our opinion that all the manifestations, symptoms and physiological peculiarities, which have been described as occurring in adrenalectomized animals (see table on insufficiency), are merely results of a progressively failing circulation due to decreasing volume of circulating fluid, in an animal which is unable to compensate (as do normal animals) for its low blood volume and blood pressure by dilution.

(12) The striking similarity between the symptoms of adrenal insufficiency and those of traumatic or secondary shock, as reported in the literature for man, is too obvious to be ignored. The cardinal features of traumatic shock are likewise the cardinal features of adrenal insufficiency—*viz.,* depleted blood and plasma volume, lowered arterial pressure, hemoconcentration and inability to dilute the blood (uncompensated human cases). The really essential point in secondary shock is failure of the blood-diluting mechanism and loss of power to increase the blood volume. This is also the primary cause of the symptoms of adrenal insufficiency.

These statements require supporting evidence of an unequivocal nature. We believe that our data are sufficient to establish these contentions, and the main points will be briefly outlined here.

### BLOOD VOLUME

Fig. 1 shows the blood volume, hemoglobin, hematocrit and urea nitrogen changes in one of our

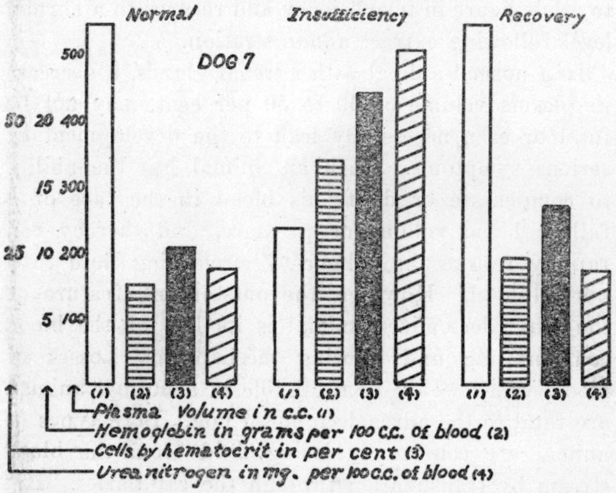


FIG. 1. The changes in plasma volume, hemoglobin, cells by hematocrit, and urea nitrogen in an adrenalectomized dog followed through a cycle of insufficiency. This animal had been adrenalectomized ten months previous and maintained in normal condition by adequate doses of cortical hormone.

experimental animals. The plasma volume of adrenalectomized dogs is invariably low. Losses of 40 to 50 per cent. of the plasma frequently occur. However, it is our opinion that the "vital-red" method of determining blood volume does not really gauge the extent of the plasma loss in an animal coming into insufficiency. The method is as good as any other now in use, but circulatory conditions are so peculiar in adrenal insufficiency that any of the present indirect methods for determining blood volume would be similarly inadequate.

We have strong evidence for the belief that our animals presenting volume readings indicating a plasma loss of 40 to 50 per cent. have really lost greater quantities. Data obtained by employing the "washout" method for blood volume determination reveal that the adrenalectomized dog loses 40–50 per cent. of his total blood volume within the first two or three days after withdrawal of hormone and before any evident symptoms of insufficiency appear. The animal eats normally, he is active and vigorous and to all appearances normal, yet his blood volume is greatly depleted. Accompanying this early diminution in volume is a small increase in blood urea, and a decline in arterial pressure of approximately 20–25 mm Hg.

The "washout" method of blood volume determination is apparently more reliable than the "vital red" method in so far as adrenal insufficiency is concerned. Unfortunately it necessitates sacrificing the animal. We do not yet know how low the blood volume actually sinks before death occurs. We are now investigating this point. But taking the "vital red" data as it stands, it is clear that the blood volume decreases to a low figure in insufficiency and returns to a normal level following extract administration.

In a normal animal with adrenal glands, a decrease in plasma volume of 40 to 50 per cent. may not be fatal or even necessarily lead to the development of serious symptoms. Such an animal has the ability to compensate or dilute his blood in the face of a falling blood volume or pressure, and thereby can rapidly restore the volume of circulating fluid to a normal level. However, the outstanding feature of the adrenalectomized animal is its loss of the blood compensating and diluting mechanism. Losses of blood, which would be negligible in a normal animal, are fatal to the adrenalectomized dog. Both types of animal are continually losing fluid from the blood stream by transudation through the capillaries. But whereas the normal dog continually dilutes and restores his blood volume, the adrenalectomized dog is unable to do so, and his blood fluids drain into the tissues and are lost from circulation. This point is discussed more in detail in the following section.

### Compensation or Dilution Following Hemorrhage, etc.

Further evidence supporting the contention that in adrenalectomized animals the blood volume progressively decreases to a level incompatible with life is furnished by bleeding experiments. Following hemorrhage, the normal animal with intact adrenal glands rapidly dilutes its blood by drawing fluid back into the blood stream to compensate for the decreased plasma volume. This power of compensation is remarkable, as any one will attest who has studied the problem. Normal dogs, weighing 10 to 12 kilograms, can withstand the loss of 40 per cent. of their total blood volume, or as much as 350 to 400 cc at one time, and within a period of a few hours or less, dilute to the extent of regaining their original volume. This compensation is due to withdrawal of water from the tissues. We have repeatedly removed 40 per cent. of the blood volume of normal unanesthetized dogs and cats, and observed that within three or four hours they were perfectly normal. Such observations are, of course, familiar to any student of hemorrhage.

The power of normal animals to compensate by dilution for lowering of blood volume is regarded as due to such reduction of blood pressure in the capillaries that the filtration pressure from within them no longer offsets the greater osmotic pressure of the plasma colloids as compared with the lymph, and consequently fluid passes into the blood stream. This mechanism of compensation, however, is probably not the sole factor involved, for we have evidence that the adrenal cortical hormone is vitally concerned in the phenomenon of blood dilution. In fact, our observations show that in the absence of the cortical hormone the animal lacks the ability to dilute its blood, even after slight or negligible blood loss. Following hormone administration, dilution again occurs.

Adrenalectomized dogs with well-healed wounds, and kept in perfectly normal condition by maintenance doses of extract, dilute their blood after hemorrhage, just as do normal unoperated animals. If extract is withheld for two or three days until the hormone content of the blood diminishes, the animals remain normal in all respects, except for decreased blood volume and pressure. They are vigorous and eat heartily. However, if small amounts of blood are removed, quantities which would be quite negligible to an animal with intact adrenals, an interesting phenomenon occurs. The blood pressure sinks to a very low level, where it remains unchanged for hours. No dilution occurs, and unless the cortical hormone is given, the pressure starts to decline further, and the animals die presenting all the classical symptoms of adrenal insufficiency. Following injection of the hormone, dilution promptly occurs, the blood pressure rises to normal and the animal returns to a normal condition, as evidenced by the changes in hemoglobin, hematocrit and plasma volume. We will cite one typical example.

An adrenalectomized dog (operated four months previously), weighing 10 kg and maintained in normal health by hormone, was taken off extract for several days. The dog remained normal in every respect; and the day he was bled he had eaten his full ration of 800 grams of kennel ration. His blood pressure had, however, declined from the normal of 106 mm Hg to 85 mm Hg. This decrease did not affect his vigor. A total of 40 cc of blood was withdrawn from the femoral artery over a period of one hour—an amount representing 5 per cent. of his normal blood volume. The animal's blood pressure fell from 85 mm Hg to 42 mm of Hg and the dog exhibited signs of prostration. He was able to walk back to his cage where he remained in a stuporous condition for 7 hours. At the end of this time his blood pressure remained unchanged at 42 mm of Hg. A few hours later it began to decline and an injection of extract was deemed necessary. Intravenous injection of an adequate amount of the hormone was given. Four hours later the blood pressure had risen to 60 mm and within 12 hours the pressure was 80 mm Hg. The dog was eating, and ran about the laboratory. Twenty-four hours after injection the pressure stood at 100 mm of Hg. Compensation or dilution had occurred, and the animal was again perfectly normal. Dilution never occurs in such animals, and death results, unless the hormone is injected.

In contrast to the type of experiment just mentioned, we can cite numerous experiments on bleeding normal dogs, both from our own experience and that of others, where large quantities of blood, 300 to 350 cc, are drawn at one time. The animals do not exhibit distress, but compensate by dilution extremely rapidly. The evidence seems clear that adrenalectomized animals are unable to dilute their blood, and can do so only when the cortical hormone is supplied.

The experiments upon hemorrhage also lend additional weight to our data on lowered blood volume in the adrenalectomized animal. Normal dogs of 10 to 12 kilograms weight can withstand relatively huge losses of blood without evident symptoms. A similar sized adrenalectomized dog, apparently enjoying equally good health, can not tolerate a loss as trivial as 50 to 75 cc, even when it is withdrawn over a period of an hour or two, without passing into a serious shock-like condition comparable to adrenal insufficiency prostration. The small quantity of blood removed from an adrenalectomized dog is of no significance to a normal animal possessing a diluting mechanism, but the loss of 50 to 75 cc by an animal which by all criteria such as vigor, activity and appetite is normal but which lacks power of compensation, and whose blood volume is already lowered, is fatal.

Another type of experiment showing the relation of the cortical hormone to the diluting mechanism is as follows: When the adrenalectomized dog, in severe insufficiency with a greatly lowered blood volume, a blood pressure of 40 mm Hg and a high blood urea, is injected intraperitoneally with 500 cc of normal saline, nothing happens and the animal dies. The individual is unable to tap the reservoirs of fluid because it can not dilute. However, if to such an injected dog hormone is administered, or fluid given by mouth, he revives in remarkable fashion. The blood pressure may rise 10 mm of Hg per hour for two or three hours until the pressure has risen to 70 to 80 mm Hg and the animal is restored to normal so far as vigor and appetite are concerned. The hormone enables the animal to utilize the injected reservoir of fluid in the body cavity, and dilution occurs very rapidly—more so than when such animals are not given fluids intraperitoneally.

### BLOOD PRESSURE

The importance of close observation of the blood pressure in adrenalectomized animals can not be overemphasized. The great hindrance has been the difficulty of making repeated determinations upon the same animal. The repeated daily arterial cannulation, necessary as a preliminary to the use of the mercury manometer on the unanesthetized adrenalectomized dog, is a technical impossibility. With the exception of Rogoff, who used the carotid loop, no other method has been employed. When consideration is given to the extreme sensitivity of adrenalectomized animals to anesthetics of any kind, to trauma or slight blood loss, it is easy to appreciate the difficulty of any prolonged study of blood pressure in such an individual over a period of several weeks or months.

We are using the direct intra-arterial method of Dameshek and Loman, which is extremely simple, highly accurate, and which makes it possible to determine the arterial pressure of an unanesthetized dog any number of times desired. The device has been repeatedly checked against the arterial cannulation method at high, low and normal pressures, using the two methods simultaneously in the same animal. The readings in mm of Hg are essentially the same in both instruments.

Two further points should be mentioned. Our animals are table trained especially for blood pressure work, and the pressures are determined directly in the femoral artery. The cortical hormone *per se* has no effect upon blood pressures. Slow or rapid intravenous injections of 30 to 40 cc of highly potent hormone does not raise the pressure in either the normal or adrenalectomized dog, except for a slight evanescent rise due to the traces of adrenalin present.

The resting arterial pressure of adrenalectomized dogs on maintenance doses of hormone is perfectly normal. It varies in different individuals from 100 to 115 mm Hg. After cessation of extract injections, the pressure progressively sinks day by day until the death level is reached. Fig. 2 shows the typical changes in arterial pressure in one of our cases. The symptoms of adrenal insufficiency parallel the decline in pressure. When the pressure is at a low level, in many cases as low as 45 to 30 mm of Hg, the animals exhibit severe symptoms and must be injected

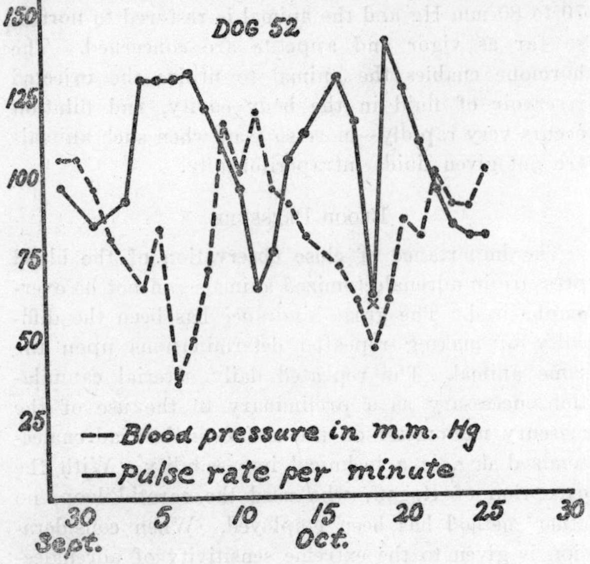


FIG. 2. The changes in blood pressure and pulse rate in an adrenalectomized dog followed through two cycles of insufficiency and recovery on extract. The significance of X is explained in the text.

with cortical hormone in order to prevent the pressure from sinking to the death level. Following injection, the pressure rises steadily and within 72 hours or less has attained the normal level and all symptoms disappear.

The decline in arterial pressure is one of the first departures from normal the animal off extract exhibits. Several days before the animal stops eating the pressure has fallen to 60 to 70 mm Hg. It is remarkable how active and normal such dogs appear with arterial pressures as low as they are. An arterial pressure of 60 to 70 mm of Hg is in general insufficient to produce noticeable symptoms in our dogs. It is only when the pressure sinks to below 60 mm that symptoms appear. We have observed several dogs, with arterial pressures as low as 36 to 39 mm of Hg, which were able to hop off the table and trot back to their cages. They were a bit wobbly on their feet, it is true, but nevertheless they were up and about.

The heart rate in general varies inversely as the blood pressure. When the pressure is normal, the heart is slow and steady. However, when the pressure starts to decline the heart rate speeds up and maintains a rapid rate so long as the pressure remains low. With a return to normal pressure, the heart rate decreases to normal. Fig. 2 illustrates these points. Some of our dogs show a precipitous fall in heart rate a few hours before death occurs. This is shown at X in Fig. 2. Following extract injection, the heart rate of such animals increases to a high figure and then declines to normal as the pressure returns to normal level.

Since the fall in blood pressure in the adrenalectomized dog is dependent upon the decline in plasma volume, the rise in pressure after extract administration depends upon the rapidity with which fluid is drawn back into the circulation and the blood volume increased. We have observed rises in arterial pressure of 10 mm of Hg per hour for the first two or three hours after injection, though generally the rise is around 5 mm of Hg per hour. When rapid dilution has occurred and the pressure stands at 65 to 70 mm of Hg, the rate of increase slows up. In all cases the pressure attains its normal level along with a normal blood volume by the end of 72 to 80 hours. The effect of the cortical hormone upon blood pressure is indirect, it raises the pressure by increasing the plasma volume, *i.e.*, the amount of fluid in circulation, and in no other way, so far as we have been able to determine.

### Blood Viscosity

The blood of adrenalectomized animals becomes increasingly viscous. Data obtained from two experimental dogs are shown in Fig. 3. The increased vis-

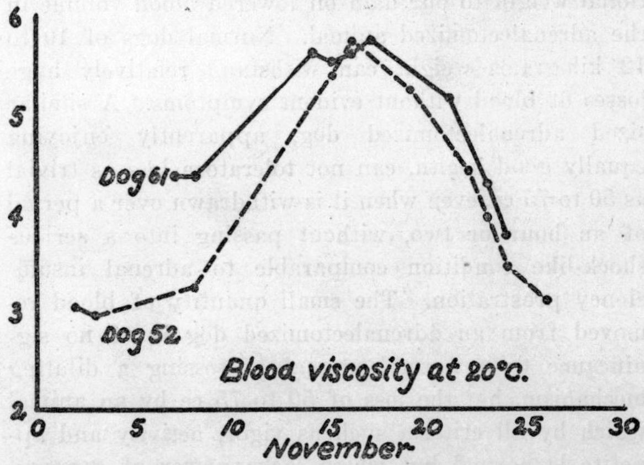


FIG. 3. Changes in blood viscosity of two dogs followed through a cycle of adrenal insufficiency and recovery after extract administration. The peak of the curve coincides with the point where extract was injected and when symptoms were most severe.

cosity is attributable in large part to (1) the increase of corpuscles per unit volume due to decreasing plasma volume, and (2) increase in plasma proteins due to hemoconcentration.

### Blood Urea and Non-Protein Nitrogen

One of the earliest changes from normality in the adrenalectomized dog deprived of extract is a rise in blood urea and non-protein nitrogen. This rise occurs simultaneously with the fall in arterial pressure, and an inverse ratio exists between the two, as a glance at Fig. 4 will show. When the blood pressure is normal,

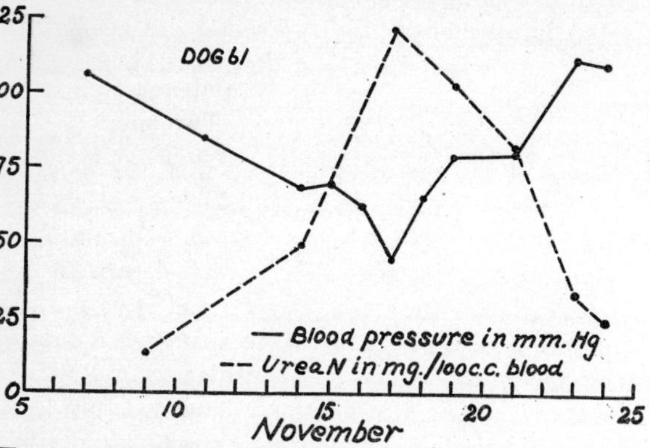


FIG. 4. Blood pressure and urea nitrogen changes in an adrenalectomized dog followed through a cycle of insufficiency and recovery on extract treatment.

the blood urea is low and at the normal level. When the pressure falls the urea rises and attains its peak when the arterial pressure is at a low level. Following extract injections the blood pressure slowly rises along with the blood volume, and the urea and non-protein nitrogen slowly falls.

Daily observation of blood urea and blood pressure reveals that, in general, the pressure starts to decline at approximately the same time as a detectable elevation of urea occurs, thus indicating that the rise in urea and non-protein nitrogen depends upon the falling pressure. However, we have observed several animals which showed a slight elevation of blood urea before the blood pressure had changed significantly. In such cases it seems likely that the blood flow through the kidneys is lessening as a result of a decreasing volume of circulating fluid.

When the animal exhibiting marked symptoms of adrenal insufficiency, with a very low arterial pressure, and a high blood urea, is given adequate injections of cortical hormone, the blood pressure invariably rises to the normal level before the blood urea sinks to its normal level. There is a lag of 24 to 48 hours after the normal pressure has been attained before the urea reaches the normal level. This lag is to be expected when we consider that the rise in blood pressure means that the animal is building up a normal volume of circulating fluid. The fall in urea occurs when the kidney function is resumed with consequent outpouring of urea.

The fact that the elevation of blood urea and non-protein nitrogen turns out to be dependent upon diminished blood flow through the kidney does not detract from the importance of the urea as a means of biological assay of the adrenal cortical hormone. The writers have long recognized that this method of assay is based upon a secondary phenomenon of adrenal insufficiency, namely, lowered renal activity. However, since the changes in blood urea are so easy to follow and so simple to quantitate, this method of assay retains its value.

## ADRENAL INSUFFICIENCY AND TRAUMATIC SHOCK

It is obvious that the conditions existing in adrenal insufficiency in animals are strikingly similar to those reported as occurring in traumatic or secondary shock in man. During the war detailed studies of traumatic shock were made on large numbers of individuals. In the following table we have listed the chief findings in adrenal insufficiency and traumatic shock and have arranged them for comparison. The signs and symptoms of the two conditions are very similar.

TABLE 1

CONDITIONS EXISTING IN ADRENAL INSUFFICIENCY (ANIMALS) AND TRAUMATIC SHOCK (MAN)

| | |
|---|---|
| 1. Blood volume | Decreased |
| 2. Blood pressure | Decreased |
| 3. Hemoglobin | Increased |
| 4. Hematocrit | Increased |
| 5. Red cell count | Increased |
| 6. Venous pressure | Decreased |
| 7. Rate blood flow | Decreased |
| 8. Blood viscosity | Increased |
| 9. Hemoconcentration | Increased |
| 10. Cardiac output | Decreased |
| 11. Venous return to R. heart | Decreased |
| 12. Heart rate | Increased |
| 13. Heart condition | Normal apparently |
| 14. Weak, fast pulse | Present |
| 15. Vaso constriction | Present |
| 16. Ability to dilute | Lacking |
| 17. Blood non-protein nitrogen and urea | Increased |
| 18. Alkali reserve | Decreased |
| 19. Basal metabolism | Decreased |
| 20. Blood sugar | Decreased in adrenal insufficiency<br>Normal or slightly above in traumatic shock |
| 21. Body temperature | Decreased |
| 22. Use vaso constrictor drugs | Ineffective |
| 23. Effect forcing fluids | Beneficial |
| 24. Vaso motor center | Normal apparently |
| 25. Sensitivity to painful stimuli | Decreased |
| 26. Sensitivity to cold | Increased |
| 27. Sensitivity to anesthetics | Increased |
| 28. Sensitivity to histamine | Increased in adrenal insufficiency, action unknown in shock |
| 29. Sensitivity to infections and toxins | Increased |
| 30. Urine volume | Decreased |
| 31. Sensitivity to hemorrhage | Increased |
| 32. Sensitivity to trauma and operation | Increased |

Blood sugar in insufficiency is generally lowered, whereas in traumatic shock it is either at the normal level or else slightly above. However, there is generally considerable laceration and tearing of tissue, together with blood loss in traumatic shock. These conditions may tend to raise blood sugar, for Aub has reported high blood sugars in shocked cats whose thigh muscles had been crushed. The cause of the low blood sugar in adrenal insufficiency will be discussed in a later paper.

It is the opinion of the writers that, since the essentials of adrenal insufficiency in experimental animals are very similar with those of traumatic shock in man, the two syndromes may possibly have a common origin—namely, some derangement of the adrenal cortex and deficiency of its hormone. In the adrenalectomized animal the glands have been extirpated, while in the shocked man they are still present, but the question arises—are the glands fully functional? If one may judge from the symptoms of traumatic shock the cortex would appear to be non-functional. In traumatic shock the individual is either unable to dilute his blood and increase his depleted blood volume (uncompensated cases) or else is able to partially do so, but only slowly (partially compensated cases) and must be aided by injecting fluids to increase the volume of fluid in circulation. The same condition exists in adrenal insufficiency in experimental animals. The animal lacks ability to dilute its blood in the face of a falling plasma volume and arterial pressure, and, in the absence of the cortical hormone, invariably dies. For some time the writers have been tempted on theoretical grounds alone to suggest that the secret of traumatic shock may possibly lie in the adrenal cortex, and that the cortical hormone may be found to be of benefit in controlling this syndrome in man.

Recently we have performed a set of experiments to test the relation between failure of the cortex and traumatic shock. The results are highly suggestive. Adrenalectomized dogs on maintenance doses of extract were used. The extract injections were discontinued for two days to permit the concentration of hormone in the animals to diminish. The dogs were still in perfectly normal condition and indistinguishable from normal dogs. They were lightly anesthetized with ether, the blood pressure determined and the testicles crushed in a vise by gradually increasing pressure. The recovery from ether was rapid and the animals were up and about within thirty minutes. The blood pressure was followed closely. One typical case will be cited. The arterial pressure dropped from 112 mm of Hg to 79 mm of Hg immediately after injury. One hour later the pressure stood at 54 mm of Hg. Two hours later it had risen to 67 mm of Hg. From this time on, however, the pressure slowly declined until at the end of eight hours it was 46 mm of Hg and the animal was prostrate and in profound shock. No dilution or compensation had occurred, except the evanescent rise during the first two hours. The dog was in such desperate straits that it was injected intravenously with adequate doses of extract. Two hours after injection the blood pressure rose from 46 mm Hg to 68 mm, and at the end of four hours from time of injection, the pressure was 74 mm of Hg. The dog was running about, was bright, energetic and ate his food in normal fashion. At the end of 48 hours the dog's pressure was 112 mm of Hg.

Control experiments where normal dogs with intact adrenal glands were similarly treated gave results as follows: Blood pressure before injury 135 mm Hg. (Animal under ether). Immediately after injury pressure 112 mm Hg, one hour later pressure 92 mm Hg. Animal ate meat eagerly. Two hours later pressure 92 mm, animal normal. Three hours after injury pressure 109 mm of Hg. The animal appeared perfectly normal at all times during the experiment.

A second set of somewhat similar experiments has been performed, in which profound surgical shock was induced in normal dogs by double adrenalectomy at one sitting. Immediately following completion of the operation, the blood pressure was normal. After twelve hours, the degree of shock was such that the animals appeared moribund. Blood pressure 35 to 39 mm of Hg, heart rate 200, femoral pulse so feeble it could barely be felt. The animals were conscious, but apathetic and quite insensitive to pain. The blood-diluting mechanism had completely broken down and compensation was lacking. Intravenous injections of adequate doses of the cortical hormone restored these profoundly shocked animals to normal life and vigor within 48 to 72 hours. These animals are alive and well at the present time, some three weeks after operation. Dogs similarly "shocked" and not injected with hormone invariably die within 48 hours.

These experiments lend considerable weight to our suggestion that the signs and symptoms of adrenal insufficiency, and of traumatic or secondary shock, are possibly due to one and the same thing, *i.e.*, failure of the blood volume and blood-diluting regulator mechanism, the adrenal cortex. The idea that the adrenal cortical hormone might prove of benefit in the treatment of human traumatic shock is advanced merely as a suggestion. Adequate proof can only come through clinical trial.

W. W. SWINGLE
J. J. PFIFFNER
H. M. VARS
P. A. BOTT
W. M. PARKINS

BIOLOGICAL LABORATORY
PRINCETON UNIVERSITY

# SCIENCE

VOL. 77 FRIDAY, JANUARY 20, 1933 No. 1986

*The American Association for the Advancement of Science:*
*The Constitution of the Stars:* PROFESSOR HENRY NORRIS RUSSELL ... 65

*Obituary:*
*Eliakim Hastings Moore:* PROFESSOR L. E. DICKSON. *Harlan Wilbur Fisk:* JOHN A. FLEMING. *Recent Deaths* ... 79

*Scientific Events:*
*Resolution on Technocracy of the American Engineering Council; The American Society for Testing Materials; The New York Botanical Garden; Officers of the Washington Academy of Sciences; Award of the Chandler Medal* ... 81

*Scientific Notes and News* ... 84

*Discussion:*
*Hamilton Red Beds in Eastern New York:* PROFESSOR GEORGE H. CHADWICK. *No Meteorite:* R. W. STONE. *More Fresh-water Medusae:* DR. WALTER C. KRAATZ. *"A Correlation Curiosity":* DR. LEONARD M. BLUMENTHAL. *How did Joule Pronounce his Name?:* PROFESSOR JOSEPH O. THOMPSON ... 86

*Scientific Books:*
*Hurst's Mechanism of Creative Evolution:* PROFESSOR T. D. A. COCKERELL ... 89

*Scientific Apparatus and Laboratory Methods:*
*Soy-bean Paste as an Emulsifying Agent:* DR. ADA M. FIELD, BEULAH H. ALEXANDER and ETHEL B. SYLVANUS. *Cellophane for Lantern Slides:* B. H. WALDEN. *The Radio-Mat:* DR. F. L. WELLS 91

*Special Articles:*
*Selection with the Magnet and Cultivation of "Reticulo-endothelial" Cells:* DR. PEYTON ROUS and DR. J. W. BEARD. *Relation between Oxygen Tension and Protein Synthesis in Certain Tissue Extracts:* PROFESSOR CARL VOEGTLIN, DR. MARY E. MAVER and DR. J. M. JOHNSON. *The Unique Nutritional Organs in the Embryos of the Top Minnows of the Mexican Plateau:* PROFESSOR C. L. TURNER ... 92

*Science News* ... 6

SCIENCE: A Weekly Journal devoted to the Advancement of Science, edited by J. MCKEEN CATTELL and published every Friday by

THE SCIENCE PRESS

New York City: Grand Central Terminal
Lancaster, Pa. Garrison, N. Y.
Annual Subscription, $6.00 Single Copies, 15 Cts.

SCIENCE is the official organ of the American Association for the Advancement of Science. Information regarding membership in the Association may be secured from the office of the permanent secretary, in the Smithsonian Institution Building, Washington, D. C.

# THE CONSTITUTION OF THE STARS[1]

By Professor HENRY NORRIS RUSSELL

PRINCETON UNIVERSITY

To number and name the stars is easy enough—or would be so if there were not so many of them; but to determine their real nature, and discover how and why they shine, is a task which, though well begun, is not more than half done.

## (1) THE PROPERTIES OF THE STARS

We have many ways of gaining information about the outside of a star. First and foremost, by collecting its light with a telescope and feeding it into a spectroscope, we learn that the stars, like the sun, are self-luminous incandescent bodies surrounded by atmospheres which contain the familiar chemical elements in a gaseous state. All the elements which are most abundant on earth have been found in the stars, and many of the rare ones—more and more as more powerful instruments can be applied—and few unidentified spectral lines remain, so that we can be sure that the stars are essentially similar in composition to our own world. No conclusion of science is more significant than this. The poet Stedman has expressed its meaning better in verse than any technical prose could render it.

> White orbs like angels pass
> Before the triple glass
> That men may scan the record of each flame,—
> Of spectral line and line
> The legendry divine
> Finding their mould the same, and aye the same,
> The atoms that we knew before
> Of which ourselves are made,—dust, and no more.

The materials of nature, and her laws, are the same everywhere. Upon this foundation we build.

[1] First Maiben Lecture before the American Association for the Advancement of Science, given at Atlantic City on December 30, 1932.

Applying these laws to our observations of the stars' light, we may calculate the temperatures of their surfaces—for the hotter an incandescent body is the more blue light it emits in proportion to red. Comparison with laboratory sources shows that the stars begin about where these leave off—very few having surface temperatures less than 3,000° and the great majority ranging from three up to fifteen or twenty thousand degrees (on the Centigrade scale). Some exceptional bodies may reach 50,000°. These conclusions are checked by other methods and entitled to confidence. At even the lowest of these temperatures, all but the most refractory chemical compounds are decomposed into their elements—which immensely simplifies the physical situation—and, higher up in the scale, the atoms themselves lose one or more of their outer electrons, becoming ionized and giving new and different spectra. The conspicuous differences between the spectra of the hotter and cooler stars originate from changes of this sort, combined with other and equally well-understood effects of temperature. When allowance is made for these, it is found that, despite the apparent diversity, the stars, or, at least their atmospheres, are remarkably similar in composition. The relative proportions of atoms of different kinds are very similar to those which are found in the earth's crust, with one important exception. Hydrogen, which forms but a small proportion of the earth's mass, is more abundant in the sun and stars than anything else. Helium is also abundant. It is reasonable, by the way, to suppose that these light gases escaped from our planet (which has not enough gravitative power to hold them) shortly after its birth as an independent body.

Finally, from the temperature and degree of ionization in stellar atmospheres, it follows that the pressure must be very low—something like a thousandth part of that of the air which surrounds us at sea-level. The pressures are different, of course, in different stars, but are always small.

Why we do not see down into regions of greater density and pressure was once puzzling; but it is now known that an ionized atmosphere, full of free electrons and charged atoms, will scatter light like a thin fog. This prevents us from seeing down deeper. The calculated temperature represents an average for the partly foggy layers toward the bottom, from which most of the observable light comes.

All this information could be obtained by spectroscopic means, if we knew nothing about the distances of the stars. Measurements of distance, which have now been made in various ways, for thousands of them, give us new data. The real brightness, or luminosity, shows a remarkably wide range. Our sun is not far from the middle of this range, and forms a convenient standard. Stars 100 times as bright are common. Many are known to be more than 1,000 times as bright, and a few give more than 10,000 times the sun's light. On the fainter side stars down to 1/100 and even 1/1,000 of the sun's brightness are common and a few are known which give but 1/10,000 of its light. Only the very nearest of these are visible to us, even with good-sized telescopes, so that there is not much chance of picking up the still fainter ones which probably exist. Very bright stars, on the contrary, can be seen at enormous distances, and our failure to find them indicates that very few such objects exist. There are, of course, various ways of measuring luminosity—with the eye, which is sensitive mainly to yellow and green light, with photographs, which work in the violet, and with heat-measuring apparatus, which is sensitive to all radiations alike. The corrections necessary to reduce measures on the other scales to the last (which is obviously the best for theoretical studies) can be calculated when the star's temperature is known.

If we know the luminosity and temperature of a star, we can at once calculate its size—its actual diameter in miles. Once more our results can be checked, by Michelson's beautiful interferometer method, and by various others, and it is found that the unavoidable assumption that the hazy indefinite lower atmosphere behaves like a hot solid surface, of standard properties, at a suitable average temperature, leads to reliable results. The stars differ less in diameter than in brightness. The general run of stars have diameters ranging from three or four million miles to about half a million (comparable with the sun's 866,000). Some are much larger, from ten million miles to 500 million in extreme cases, while a few are abnormally small, from 50,000 miles to 10,000 or even less.

Direct information about the interior of a star can be gained in only one way—by means of gravitation. Here, and here alone, the inner portions exert their full action, quite independent of their envelopement by great masses of matter. At ordinary interstellar distances, the mutual gravitation is quite negligible; but, fortunately, there are numerous binary pairs in orbital motion controlled by gravitation. For many such systems we can derive reliable values of the masses. These differ far less widely than the sizes or luminosities. The greatest mass so far measured is 113 times that of the sun, the least 0.18—a ratio of 700—as against 50,000 for the diameters, and more than 100,000,000 for the luminosities. Why this should be true is a problem for the theorist, which, as we shall see, has been successfully answered.

In density, the stars differ amazingly. Some stars have more than 100,000,000 times the sun's volume, and probably less than 100 times the sun's mass. The density of such a star is of the order of a thousandth part that of ordinary air. Those of smallest diameter are massive, and some of them have densities as high as 50,000 times that of water—almost a ton per cubic inch! How such tenuous bodies as the first can hold together and shine and how any material substances can be as dense as the second are other problems which have been satisfactorily solved.

These calculations tell us only the average density of the material inside a star. How much denser it is in some parts than others can be determined only in a few favorable instances—double stars whose components revolve in an eccentric orbit and, being separated by but a few diameters, are pulled out into ellipsoidal shapes by their mutual attraction. In this case the periastron (or point of closest approach) moves slowly forward at a rate which depends not only on the sizes and masses of the stars, but on the extent to which the density at the center exceeds the average. Only one system (Y Cygni) has so far been carefully studied. In this it appears that the concentration of density toward the center is large.

Barring this rare good fortune, all that we can find out observationally about a single star, in addition to its chemical (or atomic) composition, may be expressed by three numbers defining its mass, its radius and its luminosity. From these the density and the surface temperature may immediately be computed.

### (2) RELATIONS BETWEEN THESE PROPERTIES

These properties of the stars are not distributed at random, but are related among themselves in very striking ways. The simplest and perhaps the most important of these correlations is that between mass and luminosity, discovered by Eddington. Stars of large mass are always bright, and stars of small mass faint. A star of the sun's mass has nearly the sun's brightness; one of 4 times the sun's mass gives about 80 times as much radiation, and one of 16 times the mass 1,600 times as much, while one of ¼ the sun's mass radiates only about 1/200 as much heat.

Strangely enough, the size of a star seems to have very little influence on this relation. Red stars, fifty times the sun's diameter, and white stars only two or three times as big as the sun, if of the same mass, have nearly the same luminosity. Indeed, if a curve is plotted, representing the relation just indicated, with points corresponding to the data for individual stars, the deviation of the latter from the smooth curve averages hardly greater than the effects of the outstanding error of observation. There is but one exception. The stars of very small diameter, and very great density, are much fainter than others of equal mass—from 1/10 to 1/100 as luminous.

The luminosity and surface temperature (or the closely related spectral type) of a star are also correlated, but in a more complicated way, best illustrated by a diagram. Fig. 1, prepared from observations

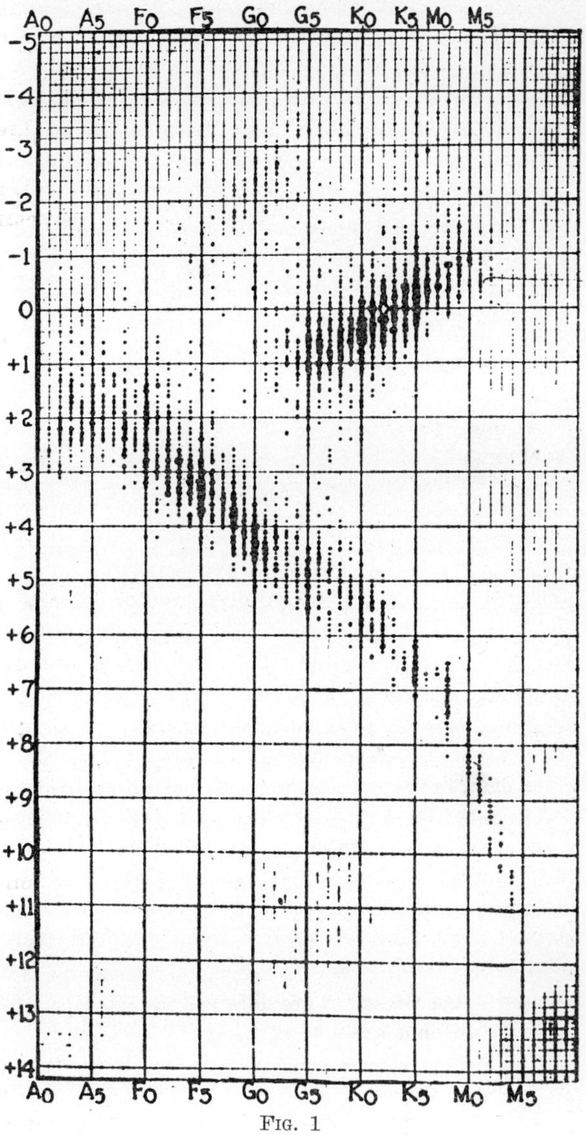


FIG. 1

of about 4,000 stars by Adams and his colleagues at Mount Wilson, shows the brightness (on the familiar scale of stellar magnitude) plotted against the spectral type—each dot representing one star. The points are very far from scattered at random. The majority of them congregate in a narrow band, crossing the diagram downward and to the right. Along this line, called the *main sequence,* we pass from bright, hot and massive stars, at the top, to faint, cool bodies of small mass at the bottom.

The hottest stars of all are not shown in the figure. They extend the sequence upward and to the left.

The sun belongs to this sequence, and is a fairly typical member. Though so different in brightness and in mass, these stars are fairly similar in size. A member near the top might be of 10 times the sun's mass, 4½ times its diameter, 1/10 its density, 800 times its luminosity and 2½ times its surface temperature. One near the bottom might have about ¼ the sun's mass, 3/10 its diameter, 9 times its density, 1/180 of its luminosity and half its surface temperature. There is an unbroken series of stars all the way between these types, and even beyond them, and the whole obviously forms a natural family. The great range in brightness within it arises mainly because the radiation from equal areas varies as the fourth power of the surface temperature.

A second sequence of stars is represented on the upper right-hand part of the figure. Hertzsprung's name of "giant stars" is very appropriate, for they are of gigantic size. Capella, which belongs at the lower left of this sequence, has in round numbers 4 times the sun's mass, 125 times its brightness, 14 times its diameter, 90 per cent. of its surface temperature and 1/700 of its density. A red giant at the upper end would have some 10 times the sun's mass, 1,500 times its luminosity, 150 times its diameter, ½ its surface temperature and less than 1/200,000 of its density. Here is evidently another natural family of stars. According to the data represented on our diagram, they are rather sharply separated from the main sequence, but Strömberg's calculations, based on other data, indicate that the gap is partially filled up.

A number of very bright stars are represented by scattered dots near the top of the diagram. These are the "super-giants" of which examples are found in almost every class of spectrum. A fourth important class of stars, the white dwarfs, would be represented by points in the lower left-hand corner. They are far fainter than those main-sequence stars of the same temperature, and so must be much smaller—indeed, their computed diameters range from 30,000 to 8,000 miles, no larger than the planets. Their masses, which can fortunately be determined in a few critical cases, are considerably larger than those of main sequence stars of the same luminosity, and their densities come out extraordinarily great, up to a ton per cubic inch, as was already mentioned. Few of these stars are known; but they are so faint that only those which lie very near the Sun (as stars go) can be adequately observed. There must be thousands of others, visible in great telescopes, but lost among the countless swarms of faint stars. This is typical of the effects of observational selection which meet the student of the stars wherever he turns, and demand eternal vigilance, lest they lead him astray.

### (3) The Problem to be Solved

The great task of theoretical astrophysics is to interpret these properties of the stars—individual and collective—by means of the general physical properties of the matter of which they are composed. Here we are greatly aided by the high temperatures of the stars. Chemical compounds are decomposed; hence we have to deal only with the properties of atoms, and of course of electrons and protons, and of light-quanta. Hence, the more we know about atoms, the more we can find out about the stars. The minutest things in nature give us the key to unlock the secrets of the greatest.

We must ask the physicist to answer three main questions:

(1) What is the *equation of state* inside the star—the relation connecting the pressure with the density and temperature?

(2) What is the *opacity of the material* which regulates the flow of heat from the intensely hot interior to the surface, and supplies the loss by radiation into space?

(3) By what processes, and according to what laws, is the *internal supply of heat* kept up, so that the star does not gradually cool down and go out?

We have now a satisfactory answer to the first question, and a fairly good one to the second; but only a beginning has been made with the third, though there is hope that we may know more soon. If we had this third answer we could predict, from general principles, what the stars ought to be like, and, if our knowledge were adequate and our reasoning sound, our predictions would agree with the facts. As things are, our partial knowledge enables us to interpret many of the most important properties of the stars, though not all.

### (4) First Success. The Mass-Luminosity Relation

Let us begin with the equation of state. Since the material is gaseous, we have by the familiar gas laws

$$p = R \varrho T/m \quad (1)$$

($p$ is the pressure, $\varrho$ the density, $T$ the absolute temperature, $m$ the average molecular weight, and $R$ a constant—$8.31 \times 10^7$ in c.g.s. units.) The density inside a star will be greater at some places, and less at others, than the mean. To get an idea what to expect, suppose we had an imaginary star of the sun's size and mass, and with uniform density throughout. The pressure at the center then comes out 9,800,000 tons per square inch, and the corresponding temperature, by the gas laws, is 11,500,000 $m$ degrees Centigrade. Under ordinary laboratory conditions, the molecular weight $m$ would vary enormously with the composition of the gas. But inside the star the atoms must be almost completely ionized, and the heavier an atom is the more parts it is split into. The *average* weight of one of these parts (which is what we need) is 0.5 for hydrogen, 1.3 for helium and about 2 for all the other elements, except the heaviest (which are too rare to be of importance). The general average thus depends almost entirely on the proportion of hydrogen inside the star. We shall see later that there is evidence that this is such as to make the value of *m* about 1.

For a homogeneous body of *M* times the sun's mass and *r* times its radius, the central temperature must be multiplied by $\frac{M}{r}$. If the body is not homogeneous, let *x* be the ratio of the density at any point to the mean density, and *y* the ratio of the pressure at this point to the pressure at the center of a homogeneous sphere of the same size and mass. A very simple calculation then shows that the temperature T is given by

$$T = 11{,}500{,}000 \frac{M}{r} \frac{y}{x} m. \qquad (2)$$

We can now calculate the temperature at any point inside the star, if we know what it is made of, that is, the value of *m*, and on what model it is built, that is, how the quantity *x* varies as we pass from the center to the surface. (If this is known *y* can be calculated.)

The density may increase greatly toward the center, making *x* very large there, but in this case *y* also increases. For example, there is a famous "model," discussed by Eddington, in which, at the center $x = 54$, that is, the central density is 54 times the mean density. But at the same point $y = 93$, so that the temperature is only 1.72 times as great as for a homogeneous sphere. Nearer the surface *x* and *y* both fall off, and the temperature decreases. It follows from this that, unless the central condensation is much greater than suggested above, the central temperature of the sun is about 15 or 20 million degrees. A generation ago no one would have dared to say much about the properties of matter under conditions so far removed from experience. But we know enough about atoms now to be sure of our ground.

At these high temperatures, the flying quanta of radiation, as well as the flying atoms and electrons, tend to drive the atoms which they hit outward and exert a powerful pressure. At 20 million degrees this radiation pressure amounts to 3,000,000 tons per square inch—enough to support a considerable fraction of the gravitational pressure inside a star. This was first realized by Eddington. If β is the fraction of the whole pressure which is carried by the gas, leaving $1 - \beta$ for the radiation, he derived the remarkable equation

$$\frac{1-\beta}{\beta^4} = 0.0033 \frac{y^3}{x^4} m^4 M^2 \qquad (3)$$

which enables us to compute the effect at any point in any star. The temperatures previously calculated must be multiplied by β. For the sun's center (with $m = 1$), $\beta = 0.97$ for the homogeneous model, and 0.997 for Eddington's model, so that the correction is small. For massive stars, it may be considerably greater.

The outcome of this discussion is that we have gained a good idea of the central temperatures of the stars. The value for the sun is probably 15 to 20 million degrees; for a faint star at the bottom of the main sequence, 12 to 15 million; for a bright star at its top, 25 to 35 million (allowing for radiation pressure). For the giant stars, the values are much lower, about 5 million for Capella and one million for a red star at the other end of the group.

For a star built on any given model, we can now find the outward temperature gradient at any point. This, with the opacity of the material, determines the rate of outward flow of heat—and the latter evidently supplies the radiation from the surface, which can therefore be calculated. The opacity arises mainly from the capture of radiation by atoms, which hold it for a moment before they re-emit it, and its law can be determined from the principles of quantum- and wave-mechanics. The researches of Kramers, Gaunt and others have now put the theory of opacity on an apparently reliable basis, though it is not yet exact. Passing over many details, it is found that the luminosity *L* of a star built on any model is given by the equation

$$L = C \frac{M^{5\frac{1}{2}}}{r^{\frac{1}{2}}} (m\,\beta)^{7\frac{1}{2}} \qquad (4)$$

where the coefficient *C* depends upon the model on which the star is built, but does not change rapidly with changes in this.

The equation shows that the luminosity of a star should depend but little on its size, and very greatly on its mass. For large masses, when β begins to diminish, the change is proportionately slower. This is an excellent qualitative description of the mass-luminosity relation, and numerical calculations show that the quantitative agreement is remarkably close. Eddington, who first worked the theory out, determined the constant *C* (which could not at that time be accurately calculated theoretically), from a single star, Capella, and found that the resulting formula represented the data for all reliably observed stars (except white dwarfs) in an almost uncanny fashion.

Theoretically, a star of given mass may have *any* luminosity, adjusting its size to suit. But to halve *L* multiplies *r* by 4, and reduces the surface temperature to 42 per cent. of its original value, so that any large change in luminosity, up or down, would place our hypothetical body outside the observed range of stellar surface temperatures. Within this range a rather small correction (carefully made by Eddington) serves to reduce the observed brightness of a star to the value it would have if shrunk or expanded so that its surface temperature was equal to the sun's. This correction hardly ever amounts to one stellar magnitude, while the observed range in brightness is fully 20 magnitudes.

Changes in the model on which we assume our star to be built do not greatly affect its luminosity. Eddington, Vogt and Biermann have discussed a large number of cases, and found that the effect very rarely exceeds one magnitude. Changes in the mean molecular weight, on the contrary, produce great differences. Recent discussions by Strömgren and Eddington agree in showing that stars of the same mass, size and density-model, differing only in the proportion of hydrogen which they contain, may differ in brightness by a factor of a thousand—more than seven magnitudes. With no hydrogen present, $m$ is about 2, and the central temperature high. This drives a rapid flow of heat to the surface. As the hydrogen percentage increases, $m$ falls, and so does the internal temperature, while the opacity gradually diminishes. At first the falling temperature prevails, and the luminosity diminishes. Finally, when the gas is almost all hydrogen, the opacity diminishes so rapidly that the escape of radiation becomes greater again. The minimum luminosity is reached with about 85 per cent. of hydrogen by weight. Agreement with the observed brightness is reached at a hydrogen content of 30 to 35 per cent., for the sun, Capella and Sirius, independently. There would also be agreement if about 99¾ per cent. of the gas were hydrogen; but this appears to be less probable. This interpretation of the mass-luminosity correlation is the first great triumph of the theory of stellar constitution. Strangely enough, it is almost *too* successful, for it shows that the observed facts result from very general properties of matter, almost independent of the internal constitution of the stars. Concerning the specific model on which they are built, it tells us practically nothing—but it does give us important information regarding the composition of the interior, which was wholly unexpected. Finally, we may note that this part of the theory does not even suggest why a star of given mass should have any particular size or surface temperature.

### (5) Second Success. The White Dwarfs

We have so far assumed that the familiar gas-laws can safely be applied to stellar material, even though it is much denser than any known gas. If the atoms were in their normal condition, this would not be true; they are bodies of known size, and would get jammed together at densities little greater than those of ordinary liquids, so that the material was no longer compressible. But, inside the stars, the atoms are highly ionized, and their remaining fragments, as well as the liberated electrons, are exceedingly small, so that there is no danger of their "jamming" even at thousands of times the density of ordinary matter. The realization of this led to the first intelligible interpretation of the white dwarf stars. It had been known for some time that all the data indicated that their densities must be enormous, but this conclusion was supposed to be physically impossible till Eddington pointed out that it was a natural consequence of the high ionization.

The later investigations of Fowler, Sommerfeld and other students of quantum theory show, however, that there is a limit to the degree to which a gas can be compressed. Nature abhors overcrowding, though she does not really abhor a vacuum.

Inside an atom the quantum laws provide only two places for electrons close to the nucleus, eight further out, and so on. Similar quantum restrictions apply to the free particles in a gas. Only a fixed number of *slow-moving* particles can be crowded into a given volume—say a cubic centimeter. To get more in we must add faster moving ones. This increases the average energy of a particle, and hence the pressure. Only the excess of the total energy of motion of the particles, above that tied up in this way, is available to count as heat. The lightest particles—the electrons—show this effect of "degeneracy" first. Being very numerous in the stars, they dominate the situation. When degeneracy has gone to the limit, the equation of state is

$$P = K_1 \rho^{5/3} \qquad (5)$$

Here $K_1$ is a constant (equal to $9.16 \times 10^{12}\,\mu^{-5/3}$, where $\mu$ is the average mass per free electron, which is 1 for pure hydrogen, and a little greater than 2 for heavy atoms). This equation is safe to use whenever it gives a considerably higher pressure than the perfect-gas law. For a density 1,000 times that of water, this happens when the temperature is less than two million degrees—while at ten million the gas-law is still a fair approximation. At intermediate temperatures the pressure gradually changes from one value to the other. The exact formula for the change has been worked out, but is complicated.

At extremely high densities, the velocities of the electrons become nearly as great as that of light, and the equation of state becomes

$$P = K_2 \rho^{4/3} \qquad (6)$$

where $K_2 = 1.23 \times 10^{15}\,\mu^{-4/3}$. The transition between this form and the last has also been accurately worked out. It is under way when the density is about two million times that of water.

We can now answer the question, What would become of a star which had lost heat by radiation until all possible sources of internal energy had been exhausted? There would be no more available heat in it, and the matter would therefore be in the degenerate state. The equation (5), together with the law of gravity, then enables us to work out in detail all the properties of the body, since (given the composition, and therefore $\mu$) there are no adjustable constants left. This has been done by Milne. A body of given mass settles down to a definite size and density. With 30 per cent. of hydrogen and a mass equal to the sun's, the radius comes out 1/62 of the sun's, making the diameter 14,000 miles, and the mean density 240,000 times the sun's. The central density is six times as great, or two million times that of water.

Smaller masses are of larger diameter—being less compressed by their own gravitation—so that the volume is inversely proportional to the mass. For large masses, the central density is so high that equation (6) becomes applicable. The compressibility increases, and the size of the body becomes still smaller. For masses greater than twice the sun's, practically the whole interior is in the second stage of degeneracy. The law of this state no longer assigns any limit to the possible contraction and any greater mass would presumably shrink until the protons and electrons themselves were "jammed." The resulting density can only be roughly guessed, but it is probably many billions of times the sun's, so that the shrunken mass would be only a few hundred miles in diameter!

Such bodies, whatever their masses, would be dead stars—cold on the surface, and quite invisible. But a star may be nearly but not quite dead, retaining a small amount of internal heat. In the deep interior this would contribute in but small proportion to the total energy and pressure, so that the inside of the star would be built very much as has been described. Towards the outside, there would be a gradual transition to more familiar conditions, and the degenerate core will be surrounded by an envelope of ordinary gas. The outer diameter should be larger, but not much larger, than has just been computed. The internal temperature will be much lower than that of a non-degenerate star, and hence the luminosity will be much smaller for a given mass than that of a normal star. Since the surface layers are composed of ordinary gas, the spectrum will differ little from that of a normal star.

Now these are exactly the properties which are actually exhibited by the white dwarfs, and there is no longer any doubt that these actually have degenerate centers. Milne points out that we should have not only white dwarfs with degenerate cores, but still fainter orange and red dwarfs, stages of approach to the dead "black dwarf." Such stars should be excessively faint, and only the very nearest of them would have any chance of being observed.

Of the few white dwarfs for which good data are available, four, by great good fortune, are components of visual binaries, and we can find their masses. These range from 0.85 to 0.37 times the sun's mass, and all lie within the interval for which even a completely degenerate mass finds a limit set for its contraction. It is possible that we do not find white dwarfs of large mass, because any such objects, if they existed, would be of such excessively small size that we could not see them at stellar distances, whatever their surface temperature.

A degenerate gas is known to be highly transparent to radiation. Hence, as Milne points out, the differences in temperature within it must be relatively small. The layer of non-degenerate gas near the surface is much more opaque, and acts as a blanket to keep the interior warm. Milne estimates that the temperature in the interior of the companion of Sirius does not exceed 15 million degrees.

The white dwarfs have, within the last few years, changed their rôle from most perplexing to the best understood class of stars. The present theory of their nature (which we owe to Milne) is the second notable triumph of the application of general physics to stellar constitution.

The properties of gas masses with degenerate cores have been the subject of lively discussion during the last couple of years, and a great deal of work has been done on the subject—notably by Milne and his colleagues at Oxford. To save a great deal of algebraic labor, he has worked on the assumptions that the rate of liberation of energy is uniform all through each mass (though differing from one mass to another), and that the opacity is constant in the gas phase, and also in the degenerate state, though much smaller. The transition between the two states is supposed to be sharp, but without discontinuity.

These assumptions do not lead to a close numerical representation of the properties of actual stars; for example, they give a change of luminosity with mass which is similar to, but only about 60 per cent. as great as, the actual change. However, they were not designed for this purpose, but to enable an exhaustive survey of the consequences of at least *one* set of assumptions to be made. The problem remains difficult, but Milne has solved it by methods of great mathematical elegance.

The results are interesting. For bodies of small

mass (less than about twice that of the sun), the size and brightness steadily diminish as the degenerate core grows larger. For large masses, the brightness increases slightly until the core is of about a quarter of the star's diameter, and then falls off. There is no great loss of light (exceeding a magnitude) until the core occupies most of the volume. All these configurations, except a few of very large mass, are smaller than those in which the center is just beginning to be degenerate. The latter diminish slowly, with increasing mass, from the size of Saturn to a little smaller than Uranus. The final completely degenerate forms are from one third to one fifth as big.

Milne has not yet extended his calculations to include the second stage of degeneracy, but it is clear that this would make the radii still smaller. His calculations, therefore, appear to represent transitions between ordinary stars and white dwarfs.

Professor Milne has expressed the opinion that the exact solution of certain equations might lead to much larger computed diameters, and hence to an explanation of main-sequence stars, and even giants, as bodies possessing dense, degenerate cores; but later calculations by Cowling are unfavorable to this view. If, however, Kramers' opacity law is substituted for the simpler assumption, keeping the same law of energy generation, Jeans has shown that bodies of large mass must inevitably be greatly concentrated toward the center. Further computations on this basis are to be desired; meanwhile the question whether actual stars (other than white dwarfs) may have degenerate cores must remain open.

### (6) Sources of Stellar Energy Synthesis or Annihilation of Atoms

So far we have considered only the escape of heat from a star, without inquiring how the supply is maintained. The rate of loss is almost incomprehensibly great. We can come nearest to realizing it by remembering that, according to the theory of relativity, heat, like other forms of energy, possesses mass. It is as proper to speak of a pound of heat as of a pound of ice; but a pound of heat is a very large amount—enough, in fact, to melt 30 million tons of rock and turn it into white hot lava. The sun radiates heat away into the depths of space at the rate of 4,200,000 tons per second—and the sun is a smallish star! Upon what vast stores of energy can it draw to keep going?

The first approximately adequate suggestion was made by Helmholtz, and developed by Kelvin. All parts of the sun attract one another strongly. If it was once larger than now and has contracted to its present size, the gravitational forces must have done an enormous amount of work during the contraction, which would necessarily reappear as some other form of energy. Part of this is doubtless still stored as heat in the interior. The rest, escaping to the surface, would maintain the radiation. The whole supply made available by contraction from a very large size may be calculated easily, though not exactly, since it depends on the way in which the density increases toward the center. On the most liberal assumptions regarding this it would suffice to keep the sun shining at its present rate for about 20 million years. Before the great extent of geological time was realized, this appeared to be an adequate explanation. But now we have conclusive evidence that the earth's surface has had very nearly its present temperature for 1,000 million years or more, which means that the sun has been shining about as strongly as at present through all these ages. Some greater supply must be sought, and the only present hope is in changes in the atoms themselves, involving a loss of mass.

Two principal suggestions deserve consideration. The first, and boldest is that, under certain rare conditions, a pair of the positive and negative charges out of which matter is built—proton and electron—may annihilate one another and disappear, leaving the whole amount of energy represented by their masses to escape, presumably as radiation of very high frequency, which inside a star would soon be absorbed, its energy reappearing as heat in the gas. Could such a thing happen, the annihilation of one per cent. of the sun's mass would keep it going for 150,000 million years. To consume the whole mass, if possible, would take much more than a hundred times as long, for as the mass decreased, the luminosity, and with it the rate of wasting, would diminish rapidly. The second hypothesis derives the energy from the transformation of hydrogen into other elements. The atomic weights of all the heavier elements (that is, of the separate isotopes of the complex ones) are very nearly integral multiples of the unit ordinarily used by chemists; but that of hydrogen is greater by one part in 130. If in any way hydrogen atoms could be broken up and their parts redistributed to form a heavier atom, the protons and some of the electrons condensing into the nucleus, and the remaining electrons forming the rest, there would be a loss of mass which would presumably escape as energy into the surrounding gas. Transformation of the sun's whole mass from hydrogen into other atoms would liberate heat enough to supply its present radiation for 100 billion years ($10^{11}$). This far more than meets all the demands of geology; but the maximum life, on this hypothesis, for the brightest known stars comes out less than one billion years, which is inconveniently short.

Radioactivity—which is a special case of the transformation of one heavy atom into others—also liberates energy at the expense of loss of mass. The known cases supply heat too slowly to keep the brighter stars going, and in too small a total amount to meet the requirements. Suggestions that heavier and more powerfully radioactive atoms than any known on earth may exist in the stars are purely speculative.

Very little can yet be said about the possibility of the annihilation of matter inside the stars; but that little indicates that it should not occur except at temperatures of many billions of degrees. More progress has been made in the discussion of the building up of heavier atoms out of hydrogen.

According to Heisenberg's new and very attractive theory, atomic nuclei are built up of protons and the recently discovered neutrons. The incorporation of a proton into a nucleus would in many cases change an atom of a known element into one of the following element ($Be^9$ to $B^{10}$, $B^{11}$ to $C^{12}$, etc.). The introduction of a neutron would change an atom into an isotope of the same element, but with atomic weight greater by 1. ($Li^6$ to $Li^7$, $B^{10}$ to $B^{11}$). By alternation of these processes the heavy elements might be built up, step by step. When a proton is built in, about 1/130 of its mass disappears and must be represented by heat liberated in the process. Building in a neutron probably liberates heat also.

At distances greater than 1/1,000 of the outer diameter of an atom, protons and nuclei repel one another. A fast-moving proton, rushing directly at a nucleus might, however, get so near it that attraction succeeded repulsion, and thus penetrate the nucleus and become a part of it. Neutrons would not be repelled, and would probably have a better chance of going in. We do not know enough about them yet to estimate the chances; but a tolerable idea of the probability of penetration of a proton can be obtained by means of wave-mechanics. The chance is greatest for the lightest nuclei, which have the smallest charges and repulsive forces. Calculations by Atkinson and Houtermans show that such penetrating collisions would begin to become important when the temperature of the gas rose above a few million degrees. Their predictions have been strikingly confirmed by the recent experiments of Cockcroft and Walton, who found, upon bombarding lithium with protons accelerated by a potential drop of 300,000 colts, that alpha rays—helium nuclei—were given off with a total energy corresponding to 16,000,000 volts. Evidently a proton penetrates a lithium nucleus (charge 3, mass 7) producing an atom of charge 4, and mass 8 (an isotope of beryllium) which breaks up into two alpha particles, charge 2, mass 4, while the energy represented by the loss of mass sets these in very rapid motion. The number of cases, per million atoms hit, in which this process occurs is of the order of magnitude predicted theoretically a year earlier.

There is then no room for doubt that the synthesis of heavier elements out of lighter ones and hydrogen may actually occur within the star and liberate great quantities of heat.

### (7) PROMISE OF THIRD SUCCESS. THE MAIN SEQUENCE

We have already seen that the interior of a star probably contains about 30 per cent. of hydrogen by weight. In the outer parts of the star a large fraction of the remainder are atoms of carbon, nitrogen and oxygen.

If the same is true in the interior (as appears probable), we may apply formulae recently given by Steenholt and calculate how hot the sun's interior should be to provide heat enough, by atom-building, to balance the outward leakage. Assuming that the central "furnace" contains one tenth of the sun's mass, and is 15 times as dense as the mean, we find that the necessary temperature is 15 million degrees if the active atoms are carbon, 21 million for nitrogen, and 28 million for oxygen. An increase of 30 per cent. in these temperatures would increase the rate of heat production a hundredfold; a decrease of 22 per cent. would diminish it in the same ratio.

The theory is still rough; but further refinements are not likely to alter the conclusion that, if the inside of the stars is at all like the outside in composition, a sufficient supply of heat for their needs will be developed if the central temperature is from 20 to 40 million degrees. The latter would suffice even for a very massive and luminous star.

Now we have already seen that the central temperature of the sun is probably 15 or 20 million degrees. We appear to have here, at last, an explanation why it is of its actual size. If it were twice as big it would be about half as hot inside, and far too little heat would be generated to keep it going; if it were half as big, far too much.

The same is true for the whole main sequence. The great white stars at the top radiate far more heat per gram than the red dwarfs at the bottom. They should therefore be hotter inside, especially as their lower mean densities diminish the chance of atomic collisions. Now there are eclipsing binary stars—whose diameters and masses can be found with considerable accuracy—which belong in all parts of the main sequence. If they are built on anything like the same model, the big white stars are actually hotter inside than the little red ones, to fully the extent demanded by theory.

If this theory is even approximately true, no star could reach an internal temperature as high as 100 million degrees, unless either all the hydrogen, or all the other elements from lithium to sodium, had been completely used up. It is noteworthy that there is no known star for which the data compel us to believe in so high a central temperature (as they do compel the belief that the sun's central temperature is several millions of degrees).

Another striking success of the theory of atomic synthesis is Atkinson's explanation of the relative abundance of the lighter elements in the sun. The strength of the spectral lines shows that lithium and beryllium are present in very small proportions in the sun's atmosphere. Boron is more abundant, and carbon, nitrogen and oxygen increasingly so. Now the lightest elements, if synthesis occurs, should be the shortest-lived, and we might expect that lithium and beryllium would be quite gone, having been all built up into heavier atoms. There is still helium there—plenty of it—but there is good theoretical reason to suppose that, though a proton might easily enter a helium nucleus, it would be very unlikely to stick there, so that the building of lithium would be slow. The lithium atoms thus made would not last long before they were in turn changed into beryllium, so the number present at any instant would be relatively small. The "lives" of heavier atoms would be longer, and they would therefore be increasingly abundant.

### (8) Unsolved Problems

Notable as the successes of this theory have been, it is still in a provisional stage. It can not yet treat quantitatively of the entrance of a neutron or an electron into a nucleus—though it has to assume that one process or the other must occur. Nor can it account for the presence in the sun and stars of the heavier metallic atoms, which would not be synthesized in appreciable amounts until after a very long time. Atkinson, who has discussed the matter very thoroughly, believes that some other process, not yet tractable theoretically, must have operated to produce them, and suggests that some of the heavy atoms thus built up may break down with liberation of helium, and thus supply material for further syntheses.

On the astrophysical side, the important sequence of giant stars remains unexplained. They radiate about as much heat, for equal masses, as the white stars of the main sequence; yet their internal temperature and density must both be much lower, unless the central condensation is exceedingly great. They are still a puzzle. It may be, as Atkinson suggests, that they are supplied by the conversion of hydrogen into lithium and other very light elements; or, as Milne believes, that they have small dense cores of high temperatures; or, as the speaker has suggested, that some unknown atomic or sub-atomic process is at work which is actually favored by low density. It is tempting to imagine that a proton or neutron may enter a nucleus and remain loosely bound there, but be liable to be drawn in deeper, with liberation of energy, after a time. Collision with another atom, during this waiting period, might knock the particle out, and prevent its permanent binding. But this is pure speculation, and need not be taken too seriously.

Despite these difficulties, good progress has certainly been made in interpreting the properties of the stars; and it is remarkable that so much success has been achieved while we are still ignorant of the density-model on which any star, except a few white dwarfs, is built. There is an intimate connection between this problem and the other incompletely solved problem of the source of stellar energy. Given either of them, we could deduce the other, provided that we knew the composition of the material at every point of the interior. "There's the rub"; for the composition involves the specification of the relative proportions of more than two hundred kinds of atoms, including the various isotopes. With regard to the internal temperature and opacity, all elements except hydrogen act very much alike, so that only the percentage of hydrogen is really important. But, when it comes to the liberation of energy, different elements, and even different isotopes of the same element, probably behave differently, and this would make prediction difficult, even though we knew the laws of atomic synthesis and disintegration exactly. To get anything that we can work with, we must cut the Gordian knot by assuming that the composition of all parts of a star's mass is the same. If this assumption was made solely to facilitate our analysis our position would be embarrassing; but, fortunately, there are good physical reasons to believe that inside a star there will be slow currents, mixing the gas and tending to make its composition uniform.

### (9) Model Stars. Vogt's Theorem

Material of exactly specified composition must have perfectly definite physical properties, so that, if the temperature and pressure are given, the density, the opacity, the rate of liberation of atomic energy, and so on, must be calculable by equations, which (whether we know them or not) are exact, and leave no room for ambiguity. If we knew these equations, we could calculate all the properties of stars of the given composition in the following way.

We may assume the star to be rotating so slowly

that it is practically spherical. (What happens otherwise is an additional problem, to be solved later, if we can.) The pressure will certainly be greatest at the center, since the overlying mass is greatest there, and the temperature, too, will be greatest, for otherwise heat would flow from the hotter parts to the center and could not be accounted for except by the grotesque assumption that the central material consumed heat instead of liberating it.

Start the calculations by guessing at any plausible values of the central pressure and temperature. Then the density, opacity and rate of heat-liberation are determined. Within a small sphere described about the center these quantities will change very little, so we may calculate the force of gravity at its surface, and the rate of flow of heat outward through it. From these we can find the outward gradients of pressure and temperature at the surface of our sphere, and so estimate their values at the surface of a sphere twice as big—which enables us to extend all our calculations to this second sphere. Proceeding thus, step by step, we may carry our calculations on as far as we please. This is known as the "method of quadratures." Though very laborious, it is powerful, and will solve a great variety of problems. Proceeding outward in this way, we find the temperature and pressure steadily decreasing—and incidentally calculate the mass inside each successive sphere, and the total outward flow of heat through it.

Finally, the pressure may fall to zero, denoting the outer limit of the mass. Knowing the radius and the heat flow, we can calculate what the surface temperature should be to permit the radiation of this amount into space. The temperature derived from our calculations should be 81 per cent. of this—to make allowance for the fact that the "surface temperature" is an average including hotter layers. This condition will usually not be satisfied—which means that we have made a false start with our guesses at the central temperature and pressure. By changing one of these—say the pressure—and repeating our calculations, we may succeed—usually after a great deal of labor—in getting a satisfactory solution—a model star, made of our given material, for which we know the mass, radius, luminosity, density-model, etc. Then we start with a new central temperature, repeat the whole process and get another model star,—and so on.

In this way, by a great but not impossible amount of calculation, we find out exactly what stars of the specified composition would be like.

One thing about them follows at once from the nature of the process of calculation. If we plot any two of their characteristics—say mass and luminosity —in a diagram, all the points representing our solutions will lie on a definite curve—that is, there will be an exact mass-luminosity relation. Similarly, if we plot luminosity against surface temperature, we will get a definite curve. These curves may be of complicated shapes, or even consist of two or more branches; but our points will be on lines, and never be scattered over an area in our diagram. In mathematical language, our model stars form a one-parameter family.

This is Vogt's theorem—the most important general proposition which has yet been established regarding stellar constitution. It has important practical applications. For example, the stars of the main sequence lie so close to one line on the diagram that they may all be of the same composition. The giants lie close to another line and may be similar in composition *inter se*. Indeed it is possible, though it looks unlikely, that the loci for the giants and main sequence may be two parts of the same curve. But the super-giants are represented by points which are apparently scattered here and there over a wide area in the upper part of the figure. Hence they can not all be of the same composition.

Vogt's theorem would fail for bodies cool enough to permit liquid drops to condense out of the gas—a contingency not to be feared in the stars—and also in the case of a star which derived its heat supply from gravitational contraction—for here the rate of heat production in a given part of the interior depends not merely on the temperature and pressure there, but also on the rate of shrinkage of the star as a whole. But its range of applicability is very wide.

A good many individual models of stars have been computed. In some of these, physically improbable assumptions were made to simplify the mathematical work—for example, that the rate of generation of heat per gram is the same in all parts of a star, though different in different stars. Such models, though of great value in the development of the theory, need not detain us here.

A curious class are the "point-source" models, in which it is assumed that all the heat is generated in one point at the very center—the rest of the star acting simply as a blanket to keep it from escaping. This is not so crazy as it sounds—it represents the limit of the quite plausible assumption that the heat is generated in a small central region of high temperature.

In some of these solutions, the density diminishes near the center—the matter being driven away by the enormous radiation pressure. Even with this extreme assumption, the luminosity for a given mass differs by less than one stellar magnitude from that of a model in which the heat-liberation is almost uniform—as Eddington first showed. Biermann, who has calculated several such models, concludes that they may be "finished off" into physically possible stars by replacing the point-source with a small, hot and very dense core—so dense that it is relativistically degenerate. This idea of a dense core was first suggested, long before, by Jeans, who showed that its existence was probable in stars of large mass.

The first calculations of stellar models with a law of heat-generation derived from theory (atomic synthesis) have recently been published by Steensholt. In the cases so far discussed, the density is less at the center than half way out to the surface. So much heat is produced in the inner regions, where the temperature is highest, that the point-source model is approached. Some of the theoretical models, therefore, have a partly empty center, others a very dense center. A great deal more calculation will be required before the subject is cleared up. The only observational data, on Y Cygni, indicate that in this star the central condensation is high.

### (10) Stability

The assumption that a star is in internal equilibrium, which has been the basis of the whole discussion, is justified by the observed constancy of the brightness, spectral peculiarities and other observable characteristics of the great majority of actual stars. But, before any theoretical model can be accepted as satisfactory, we must inquire what would happen to it if its equilibrium should be disturbed.

Possible disturbances may be of two kinds, mechanical, involving changes in the size or shape of the star, and thermal, involving changes in the rate of generation of heat inside, or loss from the surface.

The most important mechanical disturbance is a change in the size of the body. Suppose, for example, that a body, of low enough density to be gaseous throughout, were suddenly reduced to 9/10 of its previous diameter (remaining built on the same internal model). All parts of the mass, being nearer together, attract one another more strongly, and the internal pressure is increased. To maintain equilibrium, the temperature must rise, according to Lane's law, to 10/9 of its previous value in each part of the body—which means that a large amount of energy must be communicated to the gas. During the contraction, however, a great deal of work is done by the gravitational forces, and gravitational potential energy is lost. In the simplest case, when no changes occur in the atoms of the gas, and no compounds are present, an easy calculation shows that just half the change in gravitational energy would suffice to furnish the necessary heat. Hence the star can not actually contract unless some way is found to get rid of the other half. Radiation from the surface would ultimately bring this about, but the process is very slow. It would take the sun, for example, about 1½ million years to lose enough heat at its present rate to permit it to contract by 10 per cent.

If, by some hypothetical force, such a star should be rapidly compressed to (say) 90 per cent. of its present diameter, the freed gravitational energy would all appear as heat in the interior, the internal pressure would be too great to balance the weight of the overlying layers, and, the moment the constraint was removed, the body would begin to expand. When it reached its original size, all parts of it would be moving outward, and this expansion would overshoot the mark, carrying it to about 10 per cent. larger than normal. The internal temperature and pressure would then be too small, and contraction would ensue, to be followed by another expansion, and so on. The star would therefore show periodic changes in diameter, or pulsations, which would continue for a long time—though, after a great many oscillations, the "leakage" of heat from one part of the star to another might damp them out. The period of pulsation depends mainly on the density of the body. It would be a few hours for the sun, a few days for the yellow giants and many months for the enormous red giant stars.

If, however, the gas of which the star was composed became more heavily ionized at the higher temperature after the compression, part of the surplus energy would be used in bringing this about, and less would be left over to produce the pulsation—which would then be slower for the same density, but the body would still be stable, unless the ionization demanded more energy than the gravitational changes made available. In such a case, the pressure, after contraction, would be inadequate to sustain the load, and the mass would contract further and further, and never return to its original state. In a star made up wholly of one kind of atoms, there might be some chance of this—though not in all parts of the mass at once. But with a mixture such as is actually found in the stars there is no danger, especially as the abundant hydrogen is completely ionized except in a very thin skin at the surface.

The radiant energy and radiation pressure, by the way, adjust themselves so as to take up just their share of this gravitational energy—leaving the properties of the gas to determine the stability of the body.

A pulsating star should vary periodically in diameter, and also in surface temperature, brightness, color and spectrum. Now there are hundreds of stars—the Cepheid variables—which change in all these respects, repeating their variations regularly for thousands of periods. The pulsation theory gives a good account of almost all their properties—though it is not yet well understood why the rise in brightness should almost always be more rapid than the fall. They are brightest, and hottest outside, not when they are smallest (and hottest inside), but when they are rapidly expanding, as if the heating effect took time to work out to the surface. They are all super-giant stars, of exceptional luminosity, and their periods, ranging from a few hours to a couple of months, are in good agreement with their probable densities.

Forced changes in the natural spherical shape of a star would also lead to oscillations—of shape, this time, and not of size—but these would involve much smaller changes in internal energy, since some parts of the mass would be hotter while others were cooler, and are much less likely to lead to trouble.

One more type of disturbance must be noted. If a mass of the hot gas deep down should be suddenly raised nearer to the surface, it would expand to the degree permitted by the lowered pressure, and be cooled by a calculable amount. If the temperature gradient in this region is high enough, such a mass might find itself hotter than the surrounding gas, and therefore less dense, so that it would continue to rise of its own accord. In any such region, ascending and descending currents would be set up, and continued until the too-rapid change of temperature had been smoothed out. This effect would operate to change the model on which the star was built, and may cause a good deal of trouble to the theoretical calculator, but it is not likely to upset the stability of a star—though, if the convection currents are irregular, it might cause small irregular variability in brightness, as Rosseland suggests.

Thermal disturbances within a star have to do with the balance between the production of heat within it and the loss by radiation. They act slowly, because the store of heat already inside a star is so great. For example, the sun's interior contains, in the form of actual heat (disregarding potential energy of all kinds), enough to supply the present rate of radiation for some ten million years. If the supply of heat from subatomic sources were completely cut off, a slow contraction would ensue; if it were doubled, the excess would be consumed in forcing an expansion against gravity at the same rate. Even if 100,000 years' heat supply should be suddenly liberated (not at one point, of course, nor too near the surface), the effect would only be to increase the radius by about one per cent.—accompanied by pulsations about the new value. This expansion, by Lane's law, would lower the internal temperature. We have here an apparent paradox. A gaseous star, considered as a whole, has a negative specific heat; liberation of heat inside it cools it. The explanation is that the addition of this heat energy forces a much larger transfer of heat into gravitational potential energy—reminding one of the effect of a resisting medium in increasing the orbital velocity of a comet.

Suppose now that we have a star in radiative equilibrium—and that the hypothetical disturbing agency not only diminishes its diameter, but at the same time abstracts from it the excess heat freed by the contraction—so that there is no longer any tendency to pulsate about the new radius. Under the changed conditions both the income of heat from internal sources and the expenditure at the surface will be altered. If the two still balance, the new configuration will persist unchanged. If the income exceeds the outgo, the star will slowly expand, and return toward its initial state; it is secularly stable. In the opposite case, it is unstable, and will depart further and further from its original state. The condition for stability is therefore that the rate of heat production shall increase more rapidly, with increasing temperature and density, than the rate of outflow. It is easily verified that this also secures stability in event of a forced expansion.

These changes are unlike the mechanical pulsations in two respects. First, they are vastly slower, with a time-scale of millions of years (tens of thousands for the brightest giants), instead of days or months. Second, the return to "normalcy" is steady, without oscillations.

Heat-liberation by atomic synthesis increases very rapidly with the temperature, and satisfies the condition for stability; but heat production at a rate independent of pressure and density (such as arises from radioactivity) does not.

There is, however, another more subtle danger to which our star is exposed. Any disturbance is likely to set it pulsating. When smallest, it will be hottest inside, and the rate of heat production will be greater than the average. This tends to make the rebound a little greater than the contraction which preceded it, and so to build up the pulsation with steadily increasing amplitude. This effect has a long time-scale, like the last—as Jeans has shown—but it is ultimately serious. Eddington, who first pointed it out, suggests that it may be avoided by assuming that the heat-liberating process does not act instantly, but with a time-lag greater than the period of pulsation. This would "iron out" the irregularities and prevent trouble. Such a lag may easily occur in processes of atomic synthesis, provided that, as Atkinson suggests, the main liberation of heat occurs when the products at first synthesized break down.

An increasing pulsation need not necessarily grow till it breaks up the star altogether—it is entirely possible that, when the amplitude becomes considerable, secondary effects may slow up, and finally prevent, further increase of range. Stars for which the stability condition was not satisfied might then be started pulsating by the least disturbance, but the pulsation would increase only to a certain limit. The Cepheid variables behave in very much this way; they are never more than three or four times brighter at maximum than at minimum, and the change in diameter (derived from the observed radial velocities of the expanding or contracting surface) does not exceed 20 per cent. on each side of the mean. It is probable, though not proven, that these stars are actually unstable, in the sense here discussed, but that their pulsations are self-limited.

Jeans has shown that the tendency to pulsatory instability increases with the mass of a star. The Cepheids are among the most luminous, and hence presumably the most massive, of all stars. The period-luminosity relation among them—which has been so important in determining the distances of remote star-clusters and nebulae, may well represent the relation between the mass of a star and the density at which this instability begins to appear. A really satisfactory theory of the energy-supply of giant stars should explain this relation as a by-product.

### (11) History of a Star

The probable life-history of a star presents the most difficult problem of all. It is natural that the path of advancing knowledge regarding the physical constitution of the stars is strewn with the corpses of dead theories of their evolution. We are not far enough along yet to possess the basis for really constructive work on the subject.

The conclusions which can be drawn from our present limited knowledge depend greatly upon our assumption regarding the source of stellar energy. If the greatest available supply is the synthesis of other elements from hydrogen, a star's mass will change very little during its whole life. Beginning, we may imagine, with large radius and low density, it will at first have to draw on its gravitational energy and contract after the manner discussed by Kelvin, until it gets hot enough inside to start the process of synthesis. It will then approach a steady state, in which it will remain, with little change in size or other observable properties, until the active material —whatever it may be—is nearly exhausted. Then it will again begin to contract, and grow hotter inside, pausing again, perhaps, if some new energy-liberating process is "turned on" at a higher temperature. Finally, after all the available sources are exhausted, it will contract until degeneracy sets in at the center, and then pass through intermediate stages of the type discussed by Milne, into a state of great density. If its mass is small, it will be successively a white dwarf, a yellow dwarf and a black dwarf, finally extinguished. If its mass is large, it may contract to exceedingly small dimensions and be lost to all observation.

During this process its luminosity will increase slowly, till degeneracy sets in, and will fall rapidly as it becomes advanced. The maximum length of a star's life as a luminary—between the times when it gets hot enough on the surface to be visible, and when it reaches the degenerate stage—may be estimated by assuming that it was composed of almost pure hydrogen at the start, all of which becomes transformed. The result varies greatly with the star's mass, being $10^{11}$ years for the sun, and not more than 500 million for a super-giant of mass 50 times and light 10,000 times the sun's. This last figure is uncomfortably small; it makes the star's life shorter than geological time, and only four or five times longer than the interval during which light from the more distant nebulae has actually been on the way to our spectroscopes.

The relative lengths of time which a star will spend in different stages will depend upon the amount of transformable matter available to keep it going in each, and this, again, may depend on the breakdown of atoms formed in earlier stages or earlier in the existing stage (as Atkinson suggests). Knowledge of these is essential to any detailed prediction of the stages in which the stars will linger long, and in which therefore the majority of them will be found. Till this becomes available, we may well hesitate before pronouncing one star to be older or younger, in years, than another.

Suppose, for example, that there were many stars, of different masses, all composed of hydrogen and oxygen, or hydrogen and nitrogen, and all initially of very low density, and that the only process of atomic synthesis is that discussed above. They would perform "Kelvin contractions" till their central regions reached, approximately, the temperatures possessed by the various stars of the main sequence, and then would settle down with the corresponding radii, densities and surface temperatures. A massive star might become stabilized, with spectrum of class B, in a few hundred thousand years. A star of small mass might take scores of millions to reach a spectrum of type K or M; but, after they had done so, both would remain substantially unaltered for a long interval.

The white dwarfs show apparently definite signs of senility; but even here we must be on our guard against dogmatism in attributing this to greater age, for we do not know whether they started with the same composition as the others, or what has happened to them in the meantime. The fact that many of the known white dwarfs are components of binary systems, whose other members belong to the main sequence, suggests that, after all, they may not be much older than other stars—only more decrepit. If they have passed through such intermediate stages of contraction with very hot centers as have previously been described, it is hard to see how any hydrogen can be left inside them—though their atmospheres might still contain it, as their spectra indicate. But it is well to be cautious.

If annihilation of matter takes place within the stars on a large scale, their lives may be hundreds of times longer, and a star, during its history, may diminish greatly in mass and in luminosity. The possible life-histories may be much more complicated, depending on how much mass is lost by the consumption of various kinds of expendable material in different stages. The early stages of large mass and great luminosity will be relatively short, and the final faint stages of very long duration. Provided that any indestructible atoms remain, the final state is a black dwarf, as before.

The great problem of the longer or shorter time-scale may find its solution in another way. The theory of the expanding universe indicates that at a relatively recent time—something like $10^{10}$ years ago—the universe was probably either just beginning to expand perceptibly after a previous eternity of sluggishness, or very much smaller than at present, and expanding rapidly. The latter type of theory—adopted in different form by Lemaitre, Tolman and de Sitter—leaves hardly time enough for much change even in a massive star, and certainly none for a star of smaller mass. If such an epoch of intense cosmic activity occurred in the relatively near past, the stars may be indeed all of the same actual age, and may, with few exceptions, still be almost fresh from the mint—" in their first innings" as Eddington puts it. On Tolman's hypothesis, the universe previously to this "age of confusion" was contracting after a long history. It is perhaps permissible, and certainly attractive, to suggest that dense bodies like the white dwarfs may be survivors of this earlier world, which have come unscathed through the cataclysm.

Once again, we lack many data necessary for a definite solution. We do not know whence the stars arose, nor what their histories have been. But so much of the nature of the greatest material objects in nature has already been revealed from the study of the minutest that there is better reason than ever to hope, with Eddington, "that in a not too distant future we shall be competent to understand so simple a thing as a star."

# OBITUARY

## ELIAKIM HASTINGS MOORE

FOR forty years Moore has been a leading figure in the mathematical world. His fundamental researches have been recognized by many honors bestowed here and abroad. He played a leading rôle in the conversion of a local mathematical society into the present national one and in the initiation of the research journal of the nationalized society. He inspired and started on their research careers many of the younger generation. It is not possible to exaggerate Moore's profound influence on the development of mathematics in America.

He was born in Marietta, Ohio, on January 26, 1862. He graduated at Yale in 1883 and received his Ph.D. there in 1885. At the University of Berlin in 1885–86, he was most influenced by Kronecker, who like Moore had an abstract type of mind.

Young Moore taught at Yale for two years and at Northwestern University for four years. In 1902, President Harper selected Moore to initiate the department of mathematics at Chicago. With the effective support of two colleagues, Bolza and Maschke, who were seasoned research men, Moore began with great enthusiasm to develop a research center.

His plans matured so favorably at Chicago that Moore could extend his influence elsewhere. He took an important part in the conversion of the New York Mathematical Society into the American Mathematical Society and in making the latter truly national. Prior to 1899, the society published a single journal, its *Bulletin*. Moore was the first to foresee the rapid growth of research in mathematics in America and hence the need of an additional journal devoted exclusively to research. His influence was now so great that he was able to overcome the opposition to this expansion. Having been the father of the *Transactions* of the society, it was natural that he should serve as its editor-in-chief for the next eight years. Later he became president of the society. Ten years later (in 1921), he was elected president of the American Association for the Advancement of Science, the subject of his retiring address being "What is a Number System?"

Moore received numerous honorary degrees: Ph.D., Göttingen, 1899; LL.D., University of Wisconsin, 1904; Math.D., Clark University, 1909 (where he lectured on "The Rôle of Postulational Methods in Mathematics"); Sc.D., Yale, 1909; University of Toronto, 1921; Northwestern and Kansas Universities, 1927.

Since 1908, he has been associate editor of *Rendi-*

*conti del Circolo Matematico di Palermo.* In 1924, both the Mathematical Association of America and the National Academy of Sciences elected Moore a member of the American section of the International Mathematical Union.

Accounts of Moore's remarkable papers will appear in mathematical journals and in the "Biographical Memoirs of the National Academy of Sciences." The following classification of his papers shows that Moore devoted his first seven years of research largely to geometry, the next ten years to group theory and related topics, then six years to classical analysis, and his final twenty years to general analysis.

I. *Geometry.* Moore's first four papers (1885–88) were mainly on *n*-dimensional geometry. In 1900–04 and 1913 he wrote three more papers on geometry. More typical are his two papers (1902) on axioms of projective geometry.

II. *Groups.* When Moore came to Chicago in 1892, group theory was the fashion in the mathematical world. His twelve papers on groups (1893–1905) made fundamental advances. Moore's gift for abstract reasoning was especially effective in group theory. On the closely related topic of triple systems, he wrote four papers (1893–98). Also two papers on Kronecker modular systems (1897, 1907).

III. *Classical Analysis.* Although he was especially interested in improperly definite integrals, Moore published (in 1901) only two papers on them. His eight papers on real variables appeared in 1890, 1895–96, 1900, 1907.

IV. *General Analysis.* This subject is entirely Moore's own invention, and for the past twenty years he devoted his attention entirely to its development. In its final form, it is in MS. But with the aid of the Moore Fund (contributed by his many admirers), it is hoped that this MS. will soon be published in book form.

The oldest version appeared in 1909 in Vol. 2 of the Proceedings of the Mathematical Congress at Rome. Next came his New Haven Mathematical Colloquium in 1910. In all he published thirteen papers on general analysis (1909–22) and three closely related papers on linear integral equations (1912–13). To attempt to explain the nature of general analysis in a few words would be as futile as to do the same for Einstein. The inquisitive reader may well consult Bolza's introduction to Moore's general analysis in *Jahresbericht der Deutschen Mathematiker-Vereinigung,* 23 (248–303), 1914.

Moore's work easily places him among the world's great mathematicians. In America, his various accomplishments made him the leader. But he was a leader who was universally loved, and this was because he was at the same time a prince of a man.

L. E. DICKSON

## HARLAN WILBUR FISK

PROFESSOR HARLAN WILBUR FISK, of Kensington, Maryland, magnetician and chief of the section of land magnetic survey, Department of Terrestrial Magnetism, Carnegie Institution of Washington, died at the Washington Sanitarium, Takoma Park, Maryland, on December 26, 1932, after a brief illness. Professor Fisk was born at Geneva, Kansas, on September 25, 1869, and received his early scientific training at Carleton College, Northfield, Minnesota, where he came under the inspiring influence of Professor W. W. Payne. During the period 1899–1906 he held the professorship of mathematics at Fargo College (North Dakota) and was dean of the faculty during 1904–1906. He spent the summers of these three last years at Fargo as magnetic observer in the employ of the U. S. Coast and Geodetic Survey and in October, 1906, he joined the staff of the Department of Terrestrial Magnetism of the Carnegie Institution of Washington in the same capacity. He was successively advanced to the positions of magnetician and chief of the section of land magnetic survey. His field work, however, did not cease with his entrance into the department, for he carried out two detailed magnetic surveys of the Bermuda Islands in 1907 and 1922, respectively, and led a magnetic-survey expedition to British, Dutch and French Guiana in 1908. He also took part in various expeditions sent out by the department to investigate possible effects on the earth's magnetism due to solar eclipses, the most recent of these being on the occasion of the total solar eclipse of last August, when he was in charge of the three parties sent to New England by the department for this purpose. During the last few years he has been engaged in important researches of the secular variation of the earth's magnetism based largely on data obtained under his supervision by observers of the Department of Terrestrial Magnetism. These studies led him to suspect that secular changes in the earth's magnetism as observed on its surface might be the reflection of changes in the earth's interior. His work along these lines was internationally recognized.

Professor Fisk was a member of a number of scientific bodies, including the American Association for the Advancement of Science, Washington Academy of Sciences and the Philosophical Society of Washington. He was also an active member of the American Geophysical Union, being secretary of its section of terrestrial magnetism and electricity during the period 1929–1932. He is survived by his widow, Louie B. Hubbell Fisk, and four children, Clarence Wilbur, Marion Sarah, Willis Hubbell and Ernest Harlan.

Professor Fisk was a man of broad interests who took a leading part in the civic and religious activities of his community. He was held in the highest esteem by all his friends and colleagues because of his charming personality and sterling qualities of character.

JNO. A. FLEMING

## RECENT DEATHS

WILLIAM FRANKLIN EDWARDS, director of research for the U. S. Testing Company, New York City, formerly president of the University of the State of Washington, died on January 13, at the age of seventy-seven years.

DR. EDWARD N. BRUSH, professor emeritus of psychiatry of the University of Maryland and the College of Physicians and Surgeons in Baltimore, died on January 10 in his eighty-first year.

PROFESSOR JOHN GLAISTER, who held the chair of forensic medicine in the University of Glasgow from 1898 until 1931, when he was succeeded by his son, Professor John Glaister, has died at the age of seventy-six years.

CECIL FOWLER BEADLES, curator of the pathological department of the Royal College of Surgeons, London, died on January 3 at the age of sixty-six years.

DR. ELIE IVANOFF, of Moscow, specialist in artificial fecundation, who had many mammalian hybrids to his credit, died last year in Russian Turkestan, to which place he had gone, financed by the Soviet Government, for the purpose of producing hybrids between man and the chimpanzee, on which work he was engaged at the time of his death.

# SCIENTIFIC EVENTS

## RESOLUTION ON TECHNOCRACY OF THE AMERICAN ENGINEERING COUNCIL

THE following resolution was passed at the recent meeting of the American Engineering Council in Washington condemning the claims of technocracy:

The statements of a group of men organized under the name "technocracy" have received wide publicity through the press by reason of startling predictions which involve a complete overturn in our economic structure. These pronouncements, circulated as coming from engineers, have led to the belief that they represent practical engineering thought.

Many requests for information on technocracy have come to the American Engineering Council, which is the representative of national, regional and local engineering societies in the United States.

The council has endeavored to obtain from the promoters of the movement an authoritative statement of their findings and their program. It is significant that no information could be obtained beyond what has appeared in the press.

The accepted practice among engineers of presenting new developments to some engineering society for critical study and discussion has not been followed. The data and statistics brought forward in magazine and newspaper articles as a basis for speculative claims are open to question; some of the findings have been discredited or disproved by other investigations.

These statements and conclusions may have the serious effect of undermining public confidence in our present civilization, and they hold out an unwarranted promise of a quick solution of economic ills. The method of presentation has been marked by exaggerated, intolerant and extravagant claims. They have capitalized the fears, miseries and uncertainties due to the depression and have proposed a control which is, in effect, class dictatorship.

Contrary to these claims, there is nothing inherent in technical improvement which entails economic and social maladjustments. Indeed technology offers the only possible basis for continuing material progress. The volume of goods produced, distributed and consumed during the years 1928 and 1929 was not excessive. That volume may and should be surpassed upon the return of prosperity.

The alleged unmanageability of a machine economy has not been proved. Its dislocations are traceable to improper and unskilled use rather than to inherently harmful characteristics. Complete replacement of men by the machine is precluded by the law of diminishing returns. Instances are increasingly in evidence. Contrary to the pronouncements of technocracy, applied science holds the promise of better things to come in a society which fearlessly and intelligently meets its problems. It is the considered opinion of American Engineering Council that our present economic structure contains within itself the possibilities of progressive improvement and of the attainment of higher standards of living.

## THE AMERICAN SOCIETY FOR TESTING MATERIALS

THE thirty-sixth annual meeting of the American Society for Testing Materials will be held in Chicago during the week beginning on June 26. This week has been designated "Engineering Week" by the Century of Progress Fair authorities and Wednesday, June 28, has been designated "Engineers' Day."

The Hall of Science will house extensive exhibits of a technical nature both in pure and in applied science. They will be of special interest, since they will in general deal with processes and not merely products.

The fair opens officially on June 1 and will be in full swing during "Engineering Week." During this week and during the preceding week, designated "Science Week," special programs will be given in keeping with the aims and activities of the many societies holding meetings. On Engineers' Day, Wednesday, June 28, all the societies will join in an extensive program. Special trips and programs will be arranged at the fair. In the evening a dinner will be arranged at which will be present engineers and scientific men from this country and abroad. The society is taking an active part in plans for Engineers' Day and it is possible that some of the customary features of an annual meeting will be merged with the general plans.

The following organizations have signified their intention of participating:

American Association of Engineers
American Ceramic Society
American Foundrymen's Association
American Institute of Architects
American Institute of Electrical Engineers
American Institute of Mining and Metallurgical Engineers
American Society for Testing Materials
American Society of Agricultural Engineers
American Society of Civil Engineers
American Society of Heating and Ventilating Engineers
American Society of Mechanical Engineers
American Society of Municipal Engineers
American Society of Refrigerating Engineers
Institute of Radio Engineers
National Association of Practical Refrigerating Engineers
National Council of State Boards of Engineering Examiners
Society of Industrial Engineers
Society for the Promotion of Engineering Education
Western Society of Engineers

Among the technical features being arranged for the thirty-sixth annual meeting, there are the Symposium on Cast Iron, the discussion on Significance of Tests of Concrete and Concrete Aggregates, and an extensive report dealing with physical properties, corrosion-resistant data, etc., of light metals and alloys, in which field this committee functions.

## THE NEW YORK BOTANICAL GARDEN

NINE new corporate members of the New York Botanical Garden were elected at the annual meeting of the corporation held on Monday, January 9, at 2 P. M., in the office of Henry W. de Forest, president, at 165 Broadway, New York City.

They are: Joseph R. Swan, president of the Guaranty Trust Company; Arthur M. Anderson, a partner in J. P. Morgan and Company; Dr. William J. Bonisteel, professor of botany at Fordham University; Richardson Wright, author and editor of *House and Garden;* Raymond H. Torrey, nature study leader; Captain Henry B. Heylman, of Pelham Manor, known as a lover of trees; Robert H. Montgomery, owner of unusual collections of conifers and palms on his two estates, one near New York and one in Florida; George Arents, Jr., financier and owner of an estate in Rye, and Miss Mabel Choate, a daughter of the late Joseph H. Choate.

Arthur M. Anderson was elected as a manager to fill one of the vacancies caused by the deaths of Robert W. de Forest, Edward D. Adams and Frank K. Sturgis. Managers reelected to succeed themselves for three years are Henry W. de Forest, Clarence Lewis, Dr. Lewis R. Morris, N. L. Britton, founder and director-emeritus of the Garden, E. D. Merrill, director, and Henry de la Montagne, Jr., business manager.

In recognition of their gifts of important herbarium material, Frank W. Johnson and Kenneth K. Mackenzie were elected fellows for life. Mr. Johnson's contribution is of approximately 40,000 specimens of North American flora, while Mr. Mackenzie's gift of 60,000 specimens includes an especially complete collection of sedges, of which he has made a special study. Dr. Johnson is on the editorial staff of the P. F. Collier and Son Company, while Mr. Mackenzie is a practicing attorney.

In his annual report, Dr. E. D. Merrill, director, paid tribute to members of the staff and their assistants who have pursued their work diligently in the face of severe retrenchments both in salaries and money for equipment. He said:

> In spite of continued unfavorable economic conditions, in spite of reduced income, in spite of the fact that many suggested and desirable innovations could not be developed because of the financial situation, and in spite of the fact that in an attempt to balance the budget, salary reductions totaling $23,386 had to be made, definite progress has been made in various fields, and several important new projects have been developed. Much that has been accomplished has been due to the loyalty and interest of staff members who have maintained their morale in the face of discouraging circumstances.

An important innovation for the New York Botanical Garden the last year has been the establishment of the school for gardeners and special courses for professional gardeners, the first of its kind opened in this country. Dr. Merrill writes:

> Financial provision for the publication of the results of research by staff members should be made, if possible, to obviate the present discouraging outlook which is essentially to the effect that many researches, no matter how meritorious or how important, must remain unpublished. Staff members, while content with a limited income and an opportunity to prosecute scientific work, are no longer content when there is coupled the handicap of inability to publish the results of their researches.
>
> Lastly, the difficult period through which the institution has been passing during the past three years, and

the practical impossibility of making adjustments to meet the situation in reference to superannuated employes in the entire absence of any pension system, leads me to urge the establishment of an equitable contributory pension system just as soon as this becomes economically feasible.

## OFFICERS OF THE WASHINGTON ACADEMY OF SCIENCES

THE result of election of the officers for the Washington Academy of Sciences was announced at its annual meeting as follows:

*President*, Robert F. Griggs
*Non-resident Vice-presidents*, F. A. Vening Meinesz, Edward A. Birge
*Corresponding Secretary*, Paul E. Howe
*Recording Secretary*, Charles Thom
*Treasurer*, H. G. Avers
*Members of the Board of Managers* for the three-year term ending January, 1936: M. C. Hall, S. A. Rohwer
*Vice-presidents* representing the various affiliated societies of the academy:

Anthropological Society, N. M. Judd; Archeological Society, J. Townsend Russell; Bacteriological Society, N. R. Smith; Biological Society, H. H. T. Jackson; Botanical Society, C. L. Shear; Chemical Society, E. Wichers; Columbia Historical Society, Allen C. Clark; Electrical Engineers, E. C. Crittenden; Entomological Society, Harold Morrison; Geological Society, F. E. Matthes; Helminthological Society, G. Steiner; Mechanical Engineers, O. P. Hood; Medical Society, H. C. Macatee; Military Engineers, C. H. Birdseye; National Geographic, F. V. Coville; Philosophical Society, H. L. Curtis; Society of Foresters, F. C. Craighead; Washington Engineers, N. H. Heck.

At this meeting the affiliation of the Washington Section of the Institute of Radio Engineers with the academy was approved.

The new president, Professor Robert F. Griggs, is professor of botany at George Washington University. Dr. Griggs has been in charge of a number of expeditions to Puerto Rico, Guatemala, Texas and Alaska, the best known of which was the one to the Valley of Ten Thousand Smokes.

## AWARD OF THE CHANDLER MEDAL

DR. GEORGE OLIVER CURME, vice-president and director of research of the Carbide and Carbon Chemicals Corporation, has been awarded the Chandler Medal for 1933, according to an announcement made by Professor Arthur W. Hixson, of the department of chemical engineering in Columbia University, chairman of the award committee.

The Chandler Medal and Lectureship were instituted in 1910 by friends of the late Professor Charles Frederick Chandler, of Columbia University, pioneer in industrial chemistry and a founder of the American Chemical Society.

The aliphatic chemicals with which Dr. Curme has worked are open chain compounds, such as fatty acids, hydrocarbons, alcohols, esters and ethers. Of his work Professor Hixson writes:

Although the achievements of Dr. Curme are only now beginning to be recognized, it is of significant importance that his ideas and his thoughts as expressed to his intimate friends have changed but little in the fifteen years that have elapsed since he began this work. He saw clearly in 1915 and 1916, before anybody else appreciated the possibilities, just exactly what is happening to-day in the field of aliphatic chemistry and he predicted in those days the industrial use of these aliphatic compounds in quantities reaching into the millions of pounds per month, although at the time only test-tube quantities were available.

The achievements of Dr. Curme are many. His original work involved the production of acetylene, the thermo-decomposition of mineral oil inducted by sticking an electric arc beneath the surface of the oil. This was done in 1915–16.

Subsequently he has worked out practical methods for the production of ethylene glycol, ethylene dichloride, ethylene chlorhydrin, ethylene oxide, diethyl sulfate, dichlor ethyl ether and many other compounds. Most of this work has been patented.

Dr. Curme's greatest achievement has not been solely the working out of laboratory methods for making the compounds mentioned above, but in translating these laboratory applications to large-scale manufacturing processes. As is well known to-day, the production of ethylene glycol, ethylene dichloride, ethylene chlorhydrin and some of the other compounds mentioned runs into many millions of pounds annually.

More recently his early work in connection with the production of synthetic isopropyl alcohol and acetone has been commercialized and these products are now available on a large scale. He is considered one of the greatest living exponents of aliphatic chemistry.

The achievement that has attracted the most public interest has been the manufacture of synthetic ethyl alcohol, which was put into production in a large way during April, 1930, but the preliminary work for it had been done and the process well outlined over ten years ago.

Among the previous Chandler medalists are Dr. Leo H. Baekeland, president of the Bakelite Corporation, New York City; Dr. Irving Langmuir, associate director of research for the General Electric Company; Dr. Willis R. Whitney, director of research for the General Electric Company; Professor Moses Gomberg, of the University of Michigan; Professor F. Gowland Hopkins, University of Cambridge, and Professor James Bryant Conant, chairman of the Division of Chemistry of Harvard University.

The formal presentation of the medal will take place at Columbia University early in March, when Dr. Curme will deliver the annual Chandler lecture.

# SCIENTIFIC NOTES AND NEWS

F. TRUBEE DAVISON, assistant secretary of war in charge of aeronautics, was elected president of the American Museum of Natural History to succeed Professor Henry Fairfield Osborn at a meeting of the board of trustees held on January 9. Dr. Osborn, who has been president of the museum for twenty-five years, was elected honorary president. Mr. Davison has been a trustee since 1923, when he succeeded his father, the late Henry P. Davison.

DR. HERMANN WEYL, professor of mathematics at the University of Göttingen, who was the Thomas D. Jones research professor of mathematical physics at Princeton in 1926 and 1928, and Dr. James Waddell Alexander, professor of mathematics at Princeton University, have been appointed professors in the Institute of Advanced Study at Princeton. This brings the number of professorships in the faculty of mathematics to four, the appointments previously made being those of Dr. Albert Einstein, of Berlin, and of Dr. Oswald Veblen, of Princeton. Dr. Solomon Lefschetz, professor of mathematics at Princeton University, has been appointed to the Henry Burchard Fine chair of mathematics to succeed Professor Veblen. The school of mathematics of the institute jointly with the faculty of mathematics of Princeton University will issue the *Annals of Mathematics* under a board of editors selected from each of the two institutions.

DR. J. JACKSON, chief assistant at the Royal Observatory, Greenwich, has been appointed H. M. Astronomer at the Cape Observatory, South Africa, in succession to Dr. H. Spencer Jones, recently appointed Astronomer Royal at Greenwich.

DR. P. ZEEMAN, professor of experimental physics in the University of Amsterdam, and Dr. T. Levi-Civita, professor of mathematics in the University of Rome, have been elected foreign associates of the Royal Academy of Belgium.

WE learn from *The British Medical Journal* that on the occasion of the celebration of the tercentenary of the foundation of Dorpat University, fifty doctors, *honoris causa,* were created. These included Sir A. Smith-Woodward, of the Royal Society; Professor James Young Simpson, of the University of Edinburgh; Professor A. Birch-Hirschfeld, of Königsberg; Professor G. Liljestrand, of Stockholm, and Professor L. Martin, of Paris.

PROFESSORS F. A. F. C. WENT, of Utrecht, and F. F. Blackman, of Cambridge, have been elected corresponding members of the American Society of Plant Physiologists.

DR. GEORGE A. SOPER, consulting engineer, New York, has been made an honorary fellow of the Royal Sanitary Institute of Great Britain.

MANY tributes to Dr. William B. Coley, surgeon, were paid at a dinner recently held in the Waldorf-Astoria, New York City, in honor of his seventy-first birthday and his retirement from Memorial Hospital after twenty-one years' service. More than two hundred guests attended. Among the speakers were Dr. James Ewing, director of Memorial Hospital; Dr. Charles W. Mayo, of Rochester, Minnesota; Dr. John M. T. Finney, of the Johns Hopkins University; Dr. George Davis Stewart, of the American College of Surgeons, and Dean Frederick S. Jones.

PROFESSOR W. MANSFIELD CLARK, De Lamar professor of physiological chemistry of the Johns Hopkins University, was elected president of the Society of American Bacteriologists at the meeting held in Ann Arbor; Professor M. J. Rosenau, professor of preventive medicine and hygiene at the Harvard Medical School and professor of epidemiology in the Harvard School of Public Health, was named vice-president, and Professor James M. Sherman, professor of bacteriology and dairy industry and head of the department at Cornell University, was reelected secretary-treasurer.

DR. EDWARD SAPIR, Sterling professor of anthropology and general linguistics at Yale University, has been elected president of the Linguistic Society of America.

DR. JAMES RAMSAY HUNT, New York, was elected president of the Association for Research in Nervous and Mental Disease at the close of the recent annual meeting in New York. Drs. Charles Macfie Campbell, of the Harvard Medical School, and Earl D. Bond, Philadelphia, were elected vice-presidents.

THE Royal Astronomical Society of Canada has elected officers for 1933 as follows: *President,* Dr. R. K. Young, associate professor of astronomy, University of Toronto; *Honorary President,* Mgr. C. P. Choquette, Montreal; *First Vice-president,* Dr. Lachlan Gilchrist, University of Toronto; *Second Vice-president,* Dr. Ralph E. DeLury, Dominion Observatory, Ottawa; *General Secretary,* R. A. Gray, Toronto; *General Treasurer,* J. H. Horning, Toronto. Dr. R. K. Young gave the presidential address on "The Trend of Astronomy" at the University of Toronto on January 17.

DR. CARL H. LENHART has been appointed to fill the newly established chair of surgery at Western Reserve University, made possible by an anonymous gift of $300,000 in honor of Colonel Oliver H. Payne.

DR. ALBERT FISCHER, who has for several years been director of the laboratory for cellular physiology at the Kaiser Wilhelm Institute in Berlin, has returned to Copenhagen as director of the new institute for research in experimental biology established through the cooperation of the Rockefeller Foundation, the Carlsberg Foundation and the Danish government.

DR. W. L. SCHMITT left Washington on January 5 to join an expedition sponsored by G. Allan Hancock, of Los Angeles. An intensive zoological investigation of the fauna of the Galapagos Islands and the adjacent mainland is planned during the three months that the party will be in the field.

DR. ALFRED F. HESS, New York City, will give the Ingleby Lectures at the University of Birmingham in the summer term of 1933.

THE Terry Lectures at Yale University will be given by Professor Herbert S. Jennings, professor of zoology at the Johns Hopkins University, who in three addresses will speak on "What Outlook on the Universe does the Study of Biology Yield?"

THE annual Alpha Omega Alpha Lecture of the Jefferson Medical College, Philadelphia, was delivered by Professor Herbert M. Evans, of the University of California, on January 11, on "The Hormones of the Anterior Hypophysis."

PROFESSOR HUGH S. TAYLOR, chairman of the department of chemistry at Princeton University, will give a lecture on the evening of January 20 before the New York University Chapter of the Society of Sigma Xi on "The Concept of Speed in Chemical Reactions."

DR. CARLYLE JACOBSEN, of Yale University, spoke on January 16 before the psychological section of the New York Academy of Sciences on "The Effect of Lesions in the Frontal Lobe on Habit Formation." The address was illustrated by motion pictures of chimpanzees and monkeys.

THE Sigma Xi Club of the University of Florida held two meetings during the month of December. At the first, which was an open meeting, Dr. J. H. Brown, of the Johns Hopkins University, lectured concerning milk sanitation and public health. At the second, the department of biology entertained the club with a discussion of their research work and an exhibit of research apparatus, technique and collections of material.

DR. JAMES P. WARBASSE has inaugurated a discussion course on "Medical Sociology" at the Long Island College of Medicine. This is a required course for the students in their second year and is designed to stimulate them to realize the relationship of the physician not only to the profession but to society.

"THE Marquess and the Land Agent: A Tale of the Eighteenth Century" was the title of the presidential address of Professor G. N. Watson, professor of mathematics at the University of Birmingham, at a recent meeting of the Mathematical Association. The address consisted of a technical exposition of the researches of two eighteenth-century mathematicians, G. C. di Fagnano, Marchese di Toschi, and John Landen, on the rectification of curves. Their researches preceded the discovery of elliptic functions.

AT the annual conference of the Geographical Association which opened in London on January 4 at the London School of Economics, under the presidency of Dr. H. R. Mill, an exhibition of books, maps and appliances for the study of geography was given by Mr. G. A. German. A lantern lecture was given by Mr. J. M. Scott on "The British Arctic Air Route Expedition of 1930–31." Dr. Mill's presidential address was entitled "An Approach to Geography."

THE Rockefeller Foundation recently authorized a grant of $20,000 to the Biological Laboratory at Cold Spring Harbor, to be applied in support of its work in 1933.

MR. ELDRIDGE R. JOHNSON, of Philadelphia, has placed his yacht *Caroline* at the disposal of the Smithsonian Institution for an exploration of the West Atlantic Deeps, with sufficient funds to accomplish that end. This work has been placed in charge of Dr. Paul Bartsch, who has been busy for the past month gathering the necessary equipment and staff for such an undertaking. The exploration is to cover a period of four years. The first cruise set sail on January 17 from New York Harbor, and is intended to last until March 23.

DURING the months of January and February an exhibition of the "Atlas of the Historical Geography of the United States," a recent joint publication of the American Geographical Society and the Carnegie Institution of Washington, is being held at the house of the society in New York City. All the maps in the atlas are on display and a member of the society's staff is present to explain them to visitors. The exhibition is for the benefit of fellows and friends of the society and of teachers of history and geography in the schools of New York City and vicinity who may wish to familiarize themselves with the atlas.

THE annual report of the Gorgas Memorial Institute of Tropical and Preventive Medicine, covering the activities of the Gorgas Memorial Laboratory in Panama, for the period November 1, 1931, to October 30, 1932, has been made public. According to a summary given in the *Journal* of the American Medical Association, a study was made on the effect of mass treatment of malaria in a native population in

Panama, with quinine and plasmochin. In July, a station was established in the basin of the Tuira River, Province of Darien, where attention is being given to treatment of yaws with carbarsone and other drugs without the use of injection methods in an attempt to develop an oral treatment. Research was carried on in regard to the protozoologic, immunologic and pathologic features of malaria in Panama monkeys. Work was done to determine the susceptibility of local monkeys to trichinae, and whether they develop an immunity as do rats. Other investigations include those on the protozoa of the alimentary and genital tracts of the monkeys; anthropology and collection of skulls; genital tracts and uterine contents of monkeys and other animal life. Special studies on malaria in unprotected, insanitated areas were carried on in five river villages located on the Chagres River banks. Mass treatment for the entire population was given to prevent mosquito infection. The financial report disclosed that the total cash disbursements for the year were $47,484, an excess of $6,332 over the total cash receipts.

THE Field Museum of Natural History, Chicago, reports an attendance of 1,824,202 during 1932. In addition 700,000 persons, mostly children, were reached by the extension departments. The number of visitors exceeded the number in any past year and represented an increase of about 20 per cent. over 1931. It was the sixth consecutive year in which attendance exceeded one million, and during the last five years the museum has had approximately 1,000,000 more visitors than during the entire twenty-five years of its existence before occupying its present Grant Park site, to which it moved in 1921.

THE Board of Directors of *The Journal of Experimental Zoology,* at a recent meeting held in New York, voted to dissolve the corporation and turn over to the Wistar Institute the journal and all its assets. The modest endowment held by the corporation is to be held in trust by the Wistar Institute for the benefit of this journal. *The Journal of Experimental Zoology* has been published by the Wistar Institute since 1908. Its editors were the directors in a corporation which held title to the journal and the fund originally provided for its establishment. The editorial board will continue as it is and will be self-perpetuating. There will be no changes in editorial policy or publication management.

A "LANDING field" for birds traveling north and south has been provided by condemnation proceedings in the Federal Court as a result of which 8,240 acres in Dorchester County, Maryland, will be taken by the government at $14 an acre. The bird sanctuary is being established as a result of a treaty with Great Britain which provides for the care of migratory birds which travel from Canada.

# DISCUSSION

## HAMILTON RED BEDS IN EASTERN NEW YORK

AT the Toronto meeting of the Geological Society of America, the writer made the revolutionary announcement that the type Catskill red beds of the Catskill Mountain front had proved to be wholly of Portage age or older, thus much lower than the so-called "Catskill" reds farther west and actually *below* rather than above the Chemung. Extensive interfingering of heavy masses of continental red shales with upper and middle Hamilton faunal zones at the extreme east (Albany and Greene counties) was also reported. Subsequently[1] he has employed the name Kiskatom (kis′ ka tom′) red beds for this lower portion of the original Catskill group that belongs to the middle instead of the upper Devonian. This is the portion formerly falsely identified as "Oneonta"; the true Oneonta has been found to go much higher in the Catskill front and to correspond largely with the so-called "restricted Catskill" there.

Dr. Arthur G. Cooper's field work this summer, with which he has kept me informed, has shown that the top of the Hamilton (middle Devonian) goes even higher in the red beds than I had supposed. The publication of his results will be awaited with greatest interest, but meantime it seems wise to extend the term Kiskatom, following the original intention, up to the top of the middle Devonian reds, until such time as these may submit to subdivision in the field.

The entire classification of the upper Devonian from central Ohio to eastern New York has been rebuilt during the fifteen field seasons now closing. The correlations demanded by the field relations are extensively summarized in other publications now appearing. In general, the great thickening of all these sediments eastward carries the horizons higher and higher in that direction than was previously believed, diagonally across those overlapping facies that formerly were incorrectly used for correlation. From west to east the reds ("Catskill") are of successively older age, thus:

7. Cattaraugus (Bradfordian);
6. Blossburg (of Conrad; late Chautauquan but post-Chemung);
5. Montrose (of Vanuxem; upper Chemung or Wellsburg);
4. Catawissa (lower Chemung or Cayuta);
3. Catskill proper (of Enfield or upper Portage age);

[1] *Eastern States Oil and Gas Weekly,* September 2, 1932, Vol. I, No. 17, p. 7.

2. Oneonta (of Ithaca or lower Portage age);
1. Kiskatom reds (of Hamilton age).

Strictly speaking, the type Oneonta is only the upper Ithaca (Cincinnatus), but no name is yet available for the red equivalents of the lower Ithaca (Otselic), nor can we yet separate at east the Sherburne-Genesee horizons from these, though probably present. The original Catskill included 1 to 3, but in the later subdivision the Kiskatom was misidentified as Oneonta, while the term Catskill was restricted to 2 and 3, including thus the true Oneonta strata. To keep as close as may be to the intention of these writers, it is proposed to maintain the name Oneonta for all beds properly so correlated, meantime pushing the restricted term Catskill up to the still higher beds forming the peaks of all the true or eastern Catskills, whose age has been proved to be Enfield (upper Senecan). It is clear, however, that this name Catskill can no longer properly be used for those red beds farther west in Pennsylvania and New York that are of later and various ages, though they happen to possess the same continental facies.

Radical as these revisions may seem, that have put the "Portage" of Ohio far above the Chemung and the Catskill below the latter, it has nevertheless been our uniform experience that our mistakes were those of not going far enough. The field facts have forced us farther and farther from the long-accepted ideas. The future may force still greater departures. An indication of this is the unpublished field work of Mr. Charles E. Fralich, of Bradford, Pennsylvania (Torrey, Fralich and Simmons), on the Standish flags of the upper Genesee, showing a great eastward expansion of these and their equivalence to the "Sherburne" beds at Ithaca, formerly referred to the Portage.

GEORGE H. CHADWICK

CATSKILL, N. Y.

## NO METEORITE

IN the Pittsburgh *Gazette* of November 16, 1932, under the caption "Inspecting Sky Visitor," was a two column picture of a girl sitting on a table beside a large rock. Underneath it was the following statement: "A piece of a 200-pound meteorite, found two years ago by J. G. Shaw, Northside editor, in a field in Clarion County, is shown in the above photograph. Interest in the meteorite and the history of its fall to earth in a Clarion County oat field in 1896 was intensified by the promised display of Leonids, which were due shortly before daylight this morning."

I wrote at once to Mr. Shaw, the editor of *The North Side Ledger,* Pittsburgh, Pennsylvania, and under date of November 21 he replied that one night in August, 1896, a meteor was seen by people driving home. It appeared to land right beside them in a field about 150 feet from the road. The horses were so frightened that they ran away. A day or two later one of the party returned to the field and "found a boulder near where an oat shock had been set on fire and destroyed by either the sparks or heat from the yet warm meteorite. Nearly one half of it was found to be of iron composition and the remainder stone."

This is the stone now on exhibition in the office of *The North Side Ledger,* 715 West Diamond St., N. S., Pittsburgh. The iron portion was broken off years ago and is believed to be in the possession of a Mr. Swank, brick manufacturer, at Johnstown, Pennsylvania.

On receipt of Mr. Shaw's letter, I wrote to Professor Charles R. Fettke, head of the department of geology, Carnegie Institute of Technology, Pittsburgh, requesting that he examine the stone and give an opinion as to whether it is a meteorite. Professor Fettke's reply of December 7 is exceedingly interesting:

> I had an opportunity this afternoon to examine the so-called "meteorite" on exhibition at the office of J. G. Shaw, editor of *The North Side Ledger,* and found it to consist of a large boulder of medium-grained quartz sandstone. It is full of fossil plant fragments, largely compressed stems and branches, some of which are an inch or more in width. Carbonized plant tissues are associated with some of the fossils. The boulder has undoubtedly been derived from one of the sandstones of Pottsville or Allegheny age cropping out in the locality where it was found. A coating of limonite may possibly have occurred on the part which is said to have been removed and which is now owned by Mr. Swank, of Johnstown.

This proves that the stone in Mr Shaw's possession is not of meteoric origin. Possibly a small meteorite, maybe only an inch in diameter, struck and ignited the oat shock, and buried itself in the ground. It may be concluded that if a meteorite landed in Clarion County, Pennsylvania, one night in August, 1896, it has not been found.

R. W. STONE

PENNSYLVANIA GEOLOGICAL SURVEY

## MORE FRESH-WATER MEDUSAE

EVIDENTLY the rare and discontinuously distributed fresh-water jellyfish, *Craspedacusta ryderi* (Potts), is appearing from time to time in various parts of the country, and possibly oftener than reported in scientific literature. I am adding a record of the discovery of this medusa in Summit Lake, within the city of Akron, at about the same time as the discovery in Pennsylvania by Dr. Brooks.[1]

[1] SCIENCE, 76: 465, 1932.

Summit Lake is about two thirds of a mile long and a quarter of a mile wide in places. It is one of the chain of Portage Lakes. The other lakes, partly natural, partly artificial reservoirs, are south of the city. They are connected by channels and the Ohio Canal connects the waters of the others with Summit Lake. Some plankton and other aquatic work have indicated these lakes as satisfactory in their biota, though Summit Lake has been at times more or less polluted, and has a somewhat less varied fauna.

Craspedacusta has not appeared in any of the other lakes. All available specimens came from Summit from about September 6 to 17. The medusae were first seen and collected mostly by several persons living close to the lake shore. Collection was by buckets and dip nets from boats. The writer collected few himself, but obtained many others from the finders. In our own collection, we found scarcely any in sunny weather in midday, though this would supposedly be the best time for them to be near the surface, as recorded by several observers, as, for instance, Garman,[2] in Kentucky, who also noted calm water as most favorable. After I secured so few, local collecters said they took their large numbers at sundown. When finally we could get to collect at sundown, we found none, but the day was unusually cold and very windy, making the water very rough for a lake of this size. The water attains a depth of about 10 feet, where it was claimed most were collected.

Between 200 and 300 specimens were taken alive into the laboratory, but were probably overcrowded in collecting jars. They died off very rapidly, some disintegrating quickly. No exact date of their disappearance in the lake can be given, but certainly they were not seen over a period of more than half a month.

This is the second Ohio discovery. In 1926, also in September, Dr. R. C. Osburn, of Ohio State University, collected many medusae in an artificial pond near Coshocton, Ohio, about 58 miles southwest of Akron.

Dr. Brooks in his recent note on finding these medusae is mistaken in saying that seemingly his would make the fifth different locality for the medusae in the Western hemisphere. There will not be space for the citation of the records, most of which have been published in SCIENCE. My data on all these records, and papers of observers, indicate that there have been at least a dozen different localities in this country and one other in the western hemisphere.

WALTER C. KRAATZ

UNIVERSITY OF AKRON

[2] SCIENCE, 60: 477, 1924.

## "A CORRELATION CURIOSITY"

IN a recent issue of SCIENCE,[1] E. B. Wilson has obtained the probability that the three correlation coefficients correlating three variables should all be positive. Denoting the coefficients by r, s, t, it is stated that "the conditions on r, s, t are that they shall lie between +1 and −1 and that

$$1 - r^2 - s^2 - t^2 + 2rst \geqq 0."$$

It may be of interest to note that these conditions on r, s, t lead to a rather surprising formulation of the problem. Putting $r = \cos A$, $s = \cos B$, $t = \cos C$, we have (i) the angles A, B, C lie between zero and pi, and

$$\begin{vmatrix} 1 & \cos A & \cos B \\ \cos A & 1 & \cos C \\ \cos B & \cos C & 1 \end{vmatrix} \geqq 0$$

Now it may be shown that these two conditions imply $A + B + C \leqq 2\pi$, and the three angles satisfy the triangular inequality. The writer has shown that these relations are the necessary and sufficient conditions that three angles are the face angles of a trihedral angle. Hence, the problem is equivalent to finding the probability that three angles selected arbitrarily between zero and pi be the face angles of a trihedral angle.

Assuming that the distribution of points (A, B, C) in the cube with vertices (0, 0, 0), (π, 0, 0), (π, π, π) (0, π, 0) is of uniform density unity (an assumption that in terms of the variables r, s, t is different from the one made in the paper under discussion) it is found that the probability equals one-third.

LEONARD M. BLUMENTHAL

THE RICE INSTITUTE

## HOW DID JOULE PRONOUNCE HIS NAME?

IN the summer of 1897, while being conducted through the physics laboratory of the University of Edinburgh by Professor P. G. Tait, I chanced to tell him that at the University of Strassburg Professor Wilhelm Hallwachs, in speaking of Joule, had given the ou the sound of ou in you, and that after the lecture an English student had told him that the ou should have the sound of ou in out. And I asked Professor Tait whether he could tell me how the name should be pronounced. He smiled and said, "Well, I used to work with him and I can only say that he always called himself Joule," sounding the ou as in you.

The 1895 edition of the Standard Dictionary states that the ou is pronounced like u in rule, agreeing with Joule's own pronunciation, but the latest edition gives the ou the sound of ou in out. When I up-

[1] N. S., 76, No. 1979 (1932), p. 515.

braided Mr. A. G. Baker, publisher of Webster's New International, for the way his dictionary pronounced Joule, he defended himself by saying he had written to one of our leading American physicists, a man whom I deeply respect, and had been assured that the English physicists generally pronounced the name as though it were spelled Jowl. They doubtless do; they also says "figgers." But is not Joule himself the supreme authority as to the pronunciation of his own name?

JOSEPH O. THOMPSON
AMHERST COLLEGE

# SCIENTIFIC BOOKS

*The Mechanism of Creative Evolution.* By C. C. HURST. New York, The Macmillan Company; Cambridge, England, The University Press. Pp. 365. 1932.

BOOKS on genetics are so numerous that any addition might well seem superfluous. The repetition of the same facts, arguments and diagrams has become rather tiresome, and in pessimistic moments we sometimes wonder whether we are not witnessing the growth of a dogma. If we are thus somewhat inclined to be discouraged or bewildered, Dr. Hurst's book comes like a breath of fresh air. The problems of genetics and evolution are restated in an original and extraordinarily lucid way, with full attention to the latest work of the experimenters, and the last findings of the cytologists. The illustrations are nearly all taken from other works, but they are extremely good and well chosen. The print is large and distinct so that the book is easy to read. No attempt is made to shirk difficult problems, as the book is not written as a text for elementary classes. Hurst himself has been actively engaged in experimental work for over thirty years, covering the whole period of modern Mendelism.

The term creative evolution is adopted from Bergson, but interpreted in a biological rather than philosophical sense. It is pointed out that in biology A + B are not equivalent to the sum of A and B, but rather to X, an unknown or unpredictable quality. This may at first seem contrary to the Mendelian theory, which has enabled us in so many instances to predict the results of matings. But just as in chemistry sodium and chlorine unite to produce a substance differing from both in properties and appearance, so also the interactions of living units are continually giving results which could not have been foreseen in advance. A mind contemplating the nonliving universe could not be expected to predict life, the study of the lowest organisms would not lead one to expect the higher complex types, and least of all could the conscious and reflective mind of man have been surmised from a study of the beginnings of life.

We are charmed with the idea expressed by Tennyson in his "Flower in the Crannied Wall," and vaguely feel that somehow it contains the germ of all other life, but practically the conception is not valid. It is too much like saying that Tennyson's little poem is implied in the words it contains, which indeed would produce it sooner or later if arranged at random in all ways possible.

From such considerations Hurst develops a biological philosophy in contrast with the gloomy and deterministic prognostications of the physicist. Appealing to the past, with its story of increasing complexity and development, he imagines a future still more remarkable, but necessarily unpredictable by the human mind. Thus, like Wallace, he ends with metaphysical speculations which take us beyond the realms of experimental science, and will attract or repel according to the temperament and traditions of the reader.

All this, however, may be regarded as secondary to the main character and purpose of the book. Most of the chapters are devoted to a recital of the exact scientific facts in a manner wholly satisfactory to the mechanistically minded. There are said to be four great vital processes acting as random variables. These are mutation, transmutation, sex and natural selection. Especially valuable are the chapters dealing with transmutation and sex.

It has not been appreciated until recently how many "accidents" may happen to chromosomes, and how often those chance occurrences may give rise to new types. Closely related to those matters are the facts concerning polyploids, forms having various multiples of the basic number of chromosomes. The account of polyploidy is particularly clear and interesting, and from it we can see how new types, virtually new species, may arise independently at various times and places and yet be exactly alike. The same thing may happen after crossing, the hybrid progeny occasionally giving rise to new stable types which are fertile and remain constant. In other cases, as with cultivated fruit trees, perennial sunflowers, certain cacti, etc., a cross may give rise to new heterozygous strains which are then propagated vegetatively and so remain constant.

It is pointed out that the latest work of the experimenters is extremely hopeful for results of practical value. It has been shown that through the use of x-rays and otherwise the mutation rate can in certain organisms be enormously increased. While most of these mutations are detrimental, and very many lethal, among so many some will be advantageous under certain circumstances.

It is like a lottery, in which the chances for a prize are increased by the number of tickets taken, only in this case the cost of the tickets is very small, having no relation to the possible value of the prize. Add to this the discovery that virtually new species, and it is said even genera, may be produced through hybridization and we have a possibility of future results which we contemplate with amazement.

Even if we consider Hurst much too optimistic, the actual and unquestioned progress of recent years has reached a velocity which will surely take it somewhere. There is no indication whatever that we have reached the end of our rope.

Nevertheless, as Jacques Loeb used to say, the constancy of the characters of living things is amazing. Hurst puts it thus: "By far the greatest mystery in evolution is the continued existence of numerous species and even phyla whose genes have not mutated and whose chromosomes have not transmutated and whose characters remain the same to-day as they were thousands of millions of years ago." Actually, this is overstated. The ancient fossils, which look so much like living species, are not precisely the same. But the undeniable facts are sufficiently striking. The Foraminifera, the oysters, the oaks and the figs, have gone on under the same generic groupings for many millions of years, producing many specific types, but practically all these suggestive rather of a shuffling of the cards than the evolution of new genes. The experimentalist has accordingly proved too much. He has given us a picture of continual change, compared with which the actual stability of organisms in a state of nature contrasts very strongly. But here Hurst is able to introduce the ever-present principle of natural selection, which hews to the line and under most circumstances makes for stability rather than for change. Morgan's many Drosophila mutants rarely occur in the wild, because nature has no use for them.

But once in a very long while a new "star" is accepted by the manager of the play. I do not understand, in the light of all this, why Hurst, in his introduction, gives his blessing to the age and area theory of Willis. In part it is, of course, a truism, but as an actual picture of the distribution of life it is extremely fanciful. Other things being equal, of course the oldest type would be likely to have spread over the most country; but other things never are equal, and the actual distribution of any species is limited by many and complex factors.

There is this much to be said, the extent of distribution may often be taken as a measure of the stability of an organism. Thus the Painted Lady butterfly (*Pyrameis cardui*), which I saw in the midst of Africa, was quite the same insect which I could observe any day in summer at Boulder, Colorado. It must be an extremely constant type, but added to this is the fact that it is well known for its migratory habits. Very surprising are the results recently obtained by some botanists, who have discovered that certain representative species, in Asia and America, have similar chromosomes in spite of their long separation. These plants can be crossed and will produce fertile offspring.

From such facts and others Hurst undertakes to develop a precise criterion of species, to be determined by cytological and breeding evidence. Such "species" are apt to be more extensive than those commonly recognized, often including strikingly diverse plants which remain entirely separate in nature. It is not likely that botanists will follow this doctrine to its logical conclusion, which would, for example, compel us to unite the blue (*Aquilegia caerulea*) and yellow (*A. chrysantha*) columbines under one specific name. Probably we may use the term superspecies for these aggregates of cytologically similar types.

Another very interesting problem concerns the actual unit of life, which Hurst considers to be the gene. The genes multiply, keep their characters, unless they mutate, and are independent units. It is true that they cooperate to produce results in the cell or body, but this does not invalidate their essential integrity, which in very many cases has remained unchanged for ages.

The smallest units of life, concerning which we are just beginning to have some definite knowledge, may be essentially free genes. The diversity of the genes in higher forms of life could only exist where they were bound together in a cooperative system. Thus we may imagine the primitive genes, in the early days of the world, possibly mutating as often as genes do to-day, but the results were usually fatal. Then when they got into the same boat, as it were, and one could steer and another row, they could afford to be more diverse. Finally, in such a creature as man, they can take on all sorts of aspects, producing results which could never have been imagined in the beginning of things. It is more or less so with all of us. What might we not have become, could we have secured that job exactly suited to our potential talents!

After the book was in type, Hurst constructed a genetical formula for the inheritance of general intelligence in man, to which he attaches great importance. It is briefly explained in a long footnote (pp. 234–235). He recognizes ten grades of intelligence, following Woods, and, assuming that these represent different genetic formulae, gets statistical results closely agreeing with the theory. It seems improbable that ten such grades, independent of environmental influences, can be objectively recognized, and the least one can say is that the burden of proof is likely to be a very heavy one. Nevertheless, these matters can be scientifically investigated, and perhaps the expression of unconvincing opinions may lead to fresh light and ultimately to some basis of general agreement.

T. D. A. Cockerell

University of Colorado
December 4, 1932

# SCIENTIFIC APPARATUS AND LABORATORY METHODS

## SOY-BEAN PASTE AS AN EMULSIFYING AGENT[1]

In the United States the soy-bean (*Glycine hispida*) has been used chiefly for animal feeding and as a source of industrial products, but in the Orient it has long provided valuable staple foods for man. One property of importance in the preparation of foods and also for certain industrial processes is the stabilizing effect of soy-bean on oil-water emulsions. By substituting a cooked paste of soy-bean for eggs a salad dressing equal in quality to mayonnaise can be made.

Since lecithin occurs in soy-beans[2] we attempted to determine whether it contributed to their emulsifying action. Known additions of lecithin were made to other pastes of rather low original emulsifying power. The pastes were made by cooking corn starch, wheat starch or wheat flour with distilled water. Three samples of lecithin were used. Lecithins I and II were freshly prepared by extraction from egg yolk and soy-bean flour, respectively, while lecithin III was a commercial preparation of unknown age. The test consisted of preparing an emulsion under standardized conditions with each paste and noting the volume of oil which had been added when the emulsion began to "break." The experiment was then repeated with a duplicate sample of paste, into which lecithin had been dispersed before adding the oil. In a few cases the lecithin was dissolved in the oil itself. The amounts used, expressed as percentages of the weight of paste, were as follows: Lecithin I, 0.14 per cent. and 0.35 per cent.; lecithin II, 0.35 per cent.; lecithin III, 1.25 per cent., 2.5 per cent. and 5.0 per cent. In no case was there evidence that the lecithin greatly increased the emulsifying power of the paste; therefore the proteins of the soy-bean appear to be the chief stabilizing factor.

In preparing the mayonnaise-like salad dressing a paste was first made from sifted, finely ground flour, freshly milled from entire soy-beans of the Mammoth Yellow variety. The flour was mixed smoothly with five parts by weight of distilled water, boiled with stirring for two minutes over direct heat, cooked for fifteen minutes in a covered double boiler and cooled.

[1] From the Laboratory of Home Economics, University of California at Los Angeles.

[2] Hugh MacLean, "Lecithin and Allied Substances," "The Lipins," new ed., Longmans, Green and Co., 1927.

Weighed portions of this paste were beaten in the usual way with a hand or electric rotary beater, while a moderate stream of oil was added. Water was added as needed for thinning, and lastly the requisite amounts of acid, dry seasonings and coloring were incorporated. Two parts of paste to twelve or fourteen of oil and three of additional liquid will yield a product of satisfactory flavor and texture, but this does not represent the maximum capacity for oil.

Soy-bean paste as emulsifying agent in salad dressing has several merits. Among these are: (1) low cost, (2) ease of shipping and storing the beans, (3) heat sterilization of paste immediately before use, (4) the incorporation of rather a large volume of liquid for a given viscosity. Emulsions made with soy-bean appear to be less sensitive to low temperature storage than those stabilized by egg, but to be more sensitive to excessive amounts of seasonings, particularly salt. Further work is required on both of these points, however, as our observations were not conclusive.

Ada M. Field
Beulah H. Alexander
Ethel B. Sylvanus

## CELLOPHANE FOR LANTERN SLIDES

Referring to the article, "A New Use for Cellophane," in the December 16 number of Science, page 573, I would like to add one suggestion regarding the making of charts and tables on cellophane for lantern slides. The carbon paper should be cut twice the width of the lantern slide and folded so that the cellophane can be placed between the two carbon surfaces. With hard finish typewriter carbon paper the results are much more satisfactory with the carbon deposit on both sides of the cellophane.

B. H. Walden

Connecticut Agricultural
Experiment Station
New Haven, Conn.

## THE RADIO-MAT

All who are interested in the convenient device described by Dr. Warren in Science, December 16, 1932, p. 573, may be concerned to know that a device of this kind ready prepared for making slides is marketed under the name of RadiO-Mat, manufactured by the RadiO-Mat Slide Company of New York, and is obtainable from photographic dealers generally. In this laboratory we have made a large number of slides therewith. It is also possible to make legible projection material by simply typing the matter as one would a mimeograph stencil, on a blank piece of film. The ribbon can be left in, but it does not add greatly to the legibility and will smudge, as will a carbon under these conditions.

F. L. WELLS

BOSTON PSYCHOPATHIC HOSPITAL

# SPECIAL ARTICLES

## SELECTION WITH THE MAGNET AND CULTIVATION OF "RETICULO-ENDOTHELIAL" CELLS

THE supposition that certain highly phagocytic cells situated along the sinuses of the liver, spleen, bone-marrow, lymph-nodes and other organs have activities in common besides phagocytosis and constitute a physiological system, the "reticulo-endothelial system," has led to much discussion and experimentation. A host of functions, among them those of forming anti-bodies and bile pigment, are attributed to the cells in question. These attributions have been the easier because only oblique methods of test for them have been available.

Von Kupffer, the discoverer of the cells in the liver now classed as "reticulo-endothelial," observed that after the cells have taken up particulate material from the blood flowing by them, a greater or less proportion lose their hold on the capillaries and come away into the stream, new ones being provided by a proliferation and differentiation of the vascular endothelium. This happens irrespective of the character of the material phagocyted. We have taken advantage of the phenomenon to procure and cultivate the Kupffer cells.

A suspension of highly magnetic iron particles (the gamma ferric oxide of Baudisch and Welo[1]) in 7 per cent. gum acacia solution is injected into the circulation of a rabbit (or dog) on several successive days; and after two or three further days have elapsed—to give time for the particles ingested by blood leukocytes to be deposited—the animal is anesthetized and fluid is run directly through the liver, at first under low pressure to wash away the blood, then under high, with intermittent obstruction of the outlet tube and kneading of the liver to loosen and flush out the Kupffer cells. Warm Tyrode solution with 1/8 per cent. of gelatin for protective purposes[2] has proved as satisfactory a fluid as homologous serum. The Kupffer cells containing iron are separated from other elements by means of an electro-magnet, past which the suspension is slowly run, "washed" with gelatin-Tyrode solution while still held by the magnet, and plated in a culture medium consisting of this fluid, plasma and serum.

When first obtained in serum or Tyrode's solution and studied in the warm box the Kupffer cells have the general character of clasmatocytes, but they exhibit in addition special traits which distinguish them from those phagocytic elements of the spleen and of old inflammatory exudates which are supposed like them to be components of the "reticulo-endothelial system." It is plain that this "system" consists of elements differing from one another to no inconsiderable extent.

Kupffer cells proliferate *in vitro* despite an initial content of iron particles that is often large; and they retain their specialized character. Since this is the case experiments with cultures should throw light on the functions of the cells. Such experiments are under way.

It is obvious that the magnet can be utilized for the selective separation of the phagocytic cells of organs other than the liver.

PEYTON ROUS
J. W. BEARD

ROCKEFELLER INSTITUTE FOR MEDICAL RESEARCH
NEW YORK

1 Provided through the generosity of Dr. Oskar Baudisch.

2 Peyton Rous and J. R. Turner, *Jour. Exp. Med.*, 23: 219, 1916.

## RELATION BETWEEN OXYGEN TENSION AND PROTEIN SYNTHESIS IN CERTAIN TISSUE EXTRACTS

IN previous work[1] we showed that a marked decrease in oxygen tension below atmospheric tension under otherwise constant conditions of pH, temperature, concentration of substrate, etc., increases the degree and the rate of proteolysis in certain normal and malignant tissues. These results suggested experiments designed to show whether oxygenation of digests of tissues containing suitable protein split products would or would not result in enzymatic protein synthesis. Concentrated extracts of the following tissues in phosphate buffer (pH approximately 7.0) were used: Voluntary muscle of albino rats and rabbits, Jensen rat sarcoma and Walker rat carcinoma 256. The extracts were subjected to a preliminary period of digestion in an atmosphere of purified nitrogen, toluene being added to prevent bacterial growth. The digests were then treated with a current of purified oxygen from 2 to 4 hours. The mixtures were finally allowed to digest again in an atmosphere of nitrogen. The protein content was deter-

1 Carl Voegtlin and M. E. Maver, Public Health Reports, 47: 711, 1932; M. E. Maver, J. M. Johnson and Carl Voegtlin, Public Health Reports, in press.

mined by precipitation with trichloracetic acid,[2] and the total nitrogen was estimated in the precipitates by the micro-Kjeldahl method.[3] Simultaneous estimations were made of reduced and oxidized glutathione, the former being estimated by the iodometric method, using nitroprusside as end-point indicator, the latter being titrated after reduction with bismuth tartrate and $H_2S$. The total SH (SH glutathione, plus protein SH groups) was determined by iodine titration, and the pH by the glass electrode.

We found that oxygenation of digests of the muscle results in a relatively rapid protein synthesis, representing an increase of from 10 to 20 per cent. of protein nitrogen in terms of total nitrogen. Similar results were obtained with digests from the living portion of the Jensen sarcoma and Walker carcinoma, and likewise in a digest composed of papain plus fibrin and SH glutathione. Our results with these extracts indicate that the conditions favoring synthesis of proteins are (1) a relatively high oxygen tension; (2) a hydrogen-ion concentration not far removed from neutrality; (3) a relatively high initial concentration of SH groups attached to protein or glutathione which can give rise to a relatively high concentration of disulfides; (4) a sufficient concentration of suitable protein split products.

Small amounts of $CuSO_4$ added to the digests immediately before the oxygenation is begun may cause a temporary acceleration of protein synthesis, which, however, is followed by a resumption of protein cleavage.

These results obtained *in vitro* are of interest, as they suggest that variation in the oxygen supply of the tissues under physiological and particularly pathological conditions may exert a controlling influence on the equilibrium between cleavage and synthesis of tissue proteins. It may be that an inadequate $O_2$ supply to certain portions of malignant tumors favors necrosis and digestion of intracellular protein. On the other hand, in portions of tumors which are well supplied with oxygenated blood, conditions may be favorable for protein synthesis and therefore tissue growth. Further work is required before these deductions can be applied to other normal and malignant tissues. A detailed report of this investigation will be published in the *Journal of Pharmacology and Experimental Therapeutics*.

CARL VOEGTLIN
MARY E. MAVER
J. M. JOHNSON

NATIONAL INSTITUTE OF HEALTH
WASHINGTON, D. C.

[2] Seibert, *Jour. Biol. Chem.*, 70: 265, 1926.
[3] Koch and McMeekin, *Jour. Amer. Chem. Soc.*, xlvi: 2066, 1924.

## THE UNIQUE NUTRITIONAL ORGANS IN THE EMBRYOS OF THE TOP MINNOWS OF THE MEXICAN PLATEAU

DURING Cretaceous times the Mexican Plateau was isolated to some extent by the development of high volcanic ridges on the east, south and west and by desert on the north and the northwest. A fauna has developed here which is quite unique in some animal groups, and this is especially true in the case of the teleost fishes. While there has been some migration into and out of the plateau, for the most part the species upon the plateau do not exist elsewhere. In one instance, a family which is represented in North America elsewhere by a single species has bloomed in the isolation provided by plateau into many species.

It has been pointed out by Hubbs that most of the top minnows of the Lerma Valley should be separated into a single family, the Goodeidae. The classification is based principally upon the structure of the teeth and fin peculiarities. The family, as revised by Hubbs, contains the Genera Skiffia, Lermicthys, Charcodon, Balsadicthys, Goodea, Chapalicthys, Zoogoneticus and Girardinicthys. A study of the reproduction of seven of these genera reveals peculiarities that separate the group radically from all other top minnows and several features which are unique and undescribed. These features are the subject of this brief article, which is to be followed later by a more extensive illustrated description.

The course of reproduction in the lowland type of killifish (Gambusia, etc.) is characterized by the following features:

(1) Fertilization is accomplished by the transfer of spermatophores from male to female by means of a gonopod. Fertilization is internal. The sperm are stored by the female and serve for several succeeding broods of young.

(2) The ovarian follicle builds up a large yolk mass which is the sole means of nourishment for the embryo.

(3) The embryo remains within the ovarian follicle until hatched. It is then extruded into the intra-ovarian space and is born almost immediately. The yolk mass is almost entirely absorbed at birth.

(4) The gonads of the embryo are quite undeveloped at birth, no differentiation of ovary or spermary being discernible.

The contrast as shown in the reproduction of the highland type, Goodeidae, is indicated as follows:

(1) There are no spermatophores and there is no true gonapod in the male. In all genera, however, the anal fin has some short stiff rays at the anterior margin. Fertilization is internal, but apparently there is no storage of sperm.

(2) The ovarian follicle builds up a very small yolk

mass. There is an extensive degeneration of eggs after they have reached the maximum size.

(3) The embryo remains within the ovarian follicle until the small yolk mass is almost absorbed, in the meantime developing a group of nutritional filaments. A yolk sac also develops far past the limits of the yolk mass. The ovary develops a system of interfollicular canals and clefts.

(4) The embryo hatches and is left by a withdrawal of the ovary in the intra-ovarian space. The nutritional filaments develop into long finger shaped processes which are attached to the embryo at the proctodoeum. In at least four genera a wide space in the sub-mucosa of the embryonic gut extends out into the nutritional processes as far as the distal ends. The processes become liberally supplied with tissue spaces, sinuses and small blood vessels. While the embryos of all genera possess the nutritional processes there are structural differences that are constant in each genus.

(5) The embryo increases many times in volume while lying in the intra-ovarian space and after absorbing the small yolk mass.

(6) The embryo is born in an advanced stage with the gonads differentiated into recognizable ovaries and spermaries. The nutritional processes are still at their maximum point of development at birth. They are either broken off or absorbed within a few hours.

Reproduction in the lowland type of killifish is classified as simple ovo-viviparity, the egg, and later the embryo being retained in the ovarian follicle up to the time of birth. Reproduction in the highland type of top minnow is a two-phase process. The first phase, extending from fertilization to the point of the extrusion of the embryo from the follicle into the ovisac is an ovo-viviparity comparable to but shorter than the entire process in the lowland type. The second phase is a superimposed and genuine viviparity which is not comparable with any stage in the reproduction of the lowland type. The reproduction in the highland top minnows is therefore classified as ovo-viviparity with a superimposed viviparity.

The highland type of top minnows apparently arose from an ancestor much like the lowland type after viviparity had been established in the latter. The yolk sac developed in the latter type beyond the limits of the yolk mass is testimony that the ancestral type possessed a large yolk sac. The evolution of the reproductive peculiarities in the highland type from the condition which existed in its ancestral type would involve the following changes:

(1) Changes in the ovary to prohibit the full development of the yolk or to produce degeneration in the egg before it reached its full size.

(2) Earlier hatching of the egg.

(3) Retention of the embryo for a longer period in the intra-ovarian space.

(4) Development by the embryo of processes for absorbing food and oxygen from maternal ovary.

(5) Extensive changes in the somatic portion of the ovary, especially in vascularity, to furnish nourishment for the embryos.

(6) Interruption of the regular course of the germ cell cycle within the ovary due to the diversion of nutrition from the developing germ cells to the growing embryos.

The material for the above study was secured by an expedition financed by Northwestern University and the National Research Council. The writer was able to collect and to transport alive specimens of seven of the genera of the Family Goodeidae. All have proved to be suitable aquarium fishes and two (*Goodea bilineata* and *Zoogoneticus cuitzeoensis*) have produced an excellent breeding stock. Grateful acknowledgment is made to Dr. Isaac Ochoterena, of the National Institute of Biology of Mexico, and Mr. Quintin Rosas, of the Department of Forestry and Game, for courtesies in connection with the securing of collecting permits and to Mr. F. M. Riveroll, of the Department of Express, and Mr. F. C. Lona, of the National Railways of Mexico, through whose efforts shipments of live specimens were greatly facilitated.

C. L. Turner

Locy Zoological Laboratory
Northwestern University

## BOOKS RECEIVED

Beebe-Center, J. G. *The Psychology of Pleasantness and Unpleasantness.* Pp. viii + 427. 55 figures. Van Nostrand. $3.75.

Brolemann, H. W. *Faune de France.* Pp. xix + 405. 481 figures. LeChevalier, Paris.

*Bulletins of the National Research Council.* No. 87: Possibilities and Need for Development of Legal Medicine in the United States. By Oscar T. Schultz. Pp. ix + 135. $1.50. No. 88: Summary Information on the State Geological Surveys and the U. S. Geological Survey. Pp. 136. By M. M. Leighton. $1.00. No. 89: Report of the Committee on Sedimentation, 1930–1932. Illustrated. $1.00. National Research Council.

Franz, Shepherd Ivory and Kate Gordon. *Psychology.* Pp. xvii + 494. 143 figures. McGraw-Hill. $2.50.

Fournier, P. *Voyages et Découvertes Scientifiques des Missionnaires naturalistes français.* Illustrated. Le-Chevalier & Fils, Paris.

Logie, H. B., Editor. *A Standard Classified Nomenclature of Disease.* Pp. xvii + 700. Commonwealth Fund.

*Recent Social Trends in the United States:* Report of the President's Research Committee on Social Trends. Vol. I: Pp. xcv + 750. Vol. II: Pp. vi + 751–1568. McGraw-Hill. $10.00.

Reichenbach, Hans and Edward S. Allen. *Atom and Cosmos:* The World of Modern Physics. Pp. 300. 21 figures. Macmillan. $2.00.

*Report of the United States National Museum, 1932.* Pp. 177. Smithsonian Institution.

Saunders, Aretas A. *Butterflies of the Allegany State Park.* Pp. 270. Illustrated. University of the State of New York.

# SCIENCE

VOL. 77 FRIDAY, JANUARY 27, 1933 No. 1987

*The Depths of the Earth:* PROFESSOR REGINALD A. DALY ... 95

*A Program of Medical Care for the United States:* DR. C.-E. A. WINSLOW ... 102

*Obituary:*
*Ormond Stone:* PROFESSOR S. A. MITCHELL. *Arthur Gray Leonard:* PROFESSOR HOWARD E. SIMPSON. *John F. G. Hicks:* PROFESSOR RALPH W. HUFFERD. *Recent Deaths* ... 107

*Scientific Events:*
*Investigation of the Caribbean Region; National Fellowships at the Johns Hopkins University; Format of The Physical Review; The Journal of Chemical Education and The Chemical Leaflet; Dinner in Honor of Edward Bausch* ... 109

*Scientific Notes and News* ... 111

*Discussion:*
*Ether Structure:* PROFESSOR ALBERT P. CARMAN. *Energy of Urea Synthesis:* DR. H. BORSOOK and G. KEIGHLEY. *Heterosis: Specific not General in Nature:* F. A. COFFMAN. *The Production of Nutritional Anemia in White Rats:* ROE E. REMINGTON. *Mosquitoes Kill Live Stock:* DR. F. C. BISHOPP ... 114

*Scientific Apparatus and Laboratory Methods:*
*An Illuminator to Facilitate the Tracing of X-Rays:* C. A. BEVANS. *A Large Respirometer:* PROFESSOR WALTER B. BALCH. *New Fixing Fluids for General Purposes:* PROFESSOR ALEXANDER PETRUNKEVITCH ... 116

*Special Articles:*
*Variations in Visible Solar Light during Submarine Measurements:* PROFESSOR C. L. UTTERBACK. *Borreliotoses: Fowl-Pox, Molluscum Contagiosum, Variola-Vaccinia:* PROFESSOR ERNEST W. GOODPASTURE. *A Contribution to Vowel Theory:* PROFESSOR LEE EDWARD TRAVIS and ARCHIBALD R. BUCHANAN ... 118

*Science News* ... 8

SCIENCE: A Weekly Journal devoted to the Advancement of Science, edited by J. MCKEEN CATTELL and published every Friday by

THE SCIENCE PRESS

New York City: Grand Central Terminal
Lancaster, Pa. Garrison, N. Y.
Annual Subscription, $6.00 Single Copies, 15 Cts.

SCIENCE is the official organ of the American Association for the Advancement of Science. Information regarding membership in the Association may be secured from the office of the permanent secretary, in the Smithsonian Institution Building, Washington, D. C.

# THE DEPTHS OF THE EARTH[1]

By Professor REGINALD A. DALY
HARVARD UNIVERSITY

## INTRODUCTION

CHARLES LAPWORTH was one of the intellectual princes of our profession. He it was who discovered the "Secret of the Highlands." In another Scotland Yard he triumphantly illustrated the British genius for detective work. His penetrating eye saw in principle, and later Peach and Horne proved, the majesty of the Scottish thrusts. Thus a revolutionary idea became generally accepted. Yet a still more vital secret underlies the secret explained by the brilliant Lapworth. That further mystery, still unsolved to general satisfaction, is the cause of the clean-cut slicing and plastic shearing of the rocks when mountains are made. Clearly the data for solving the mystery must be sought under all the lands and seas—in the earth's vast interior.

There, too, is the condition for the isostatic rise of the crust when the regional ice-caps melted, or when continents lost weight by denudation and rose to renew their equilibrium. There ultimately is the key to the problem of former land bridges between continents and the key to paleogeographic problems in general. The petrologist also can not escape the necessity of thinking intensely about the third dimension, depth, as well as about the two dimensions of the maps. In short the geologist, however specialized, has to be a courageous soul and venture where angels can not tread. The equipped geologist shall know not only his six continents and the seven seas; he shall faithfully treasure every scrap of information that may come to him regarding the invisible and intangible, where lies the secret of secrets of all geological science.

[1] Presidential address read before the Geological Society of America, December 28, 1932. Somewhat abridged; illustrations and references omitted; to be printed in full in the *Bulletin* of the Geological Society.

To go down in imagination is an adventure, daring but thoroughly essential, for in depth is the seat of dominating energy and the origin of all rocks whatever.

Since the year 1900 discoveries and fertile hypotheses about conditions beneath the accessible part of our planet have been pouring into the literature and summarized in thick handbooks. The young science, geophysics, has become a giant with a giant's power to move, and then in a measure to fix, the foundations of geological thought. This evening I offer a speculative and of course tentative picture of the earth's interior in the light of the new geophysics, checked by facts of geology and by the possibilities of cosmogony.

### The Shells and Core of the Earth

In principle the picture is given in Tables I and II. The first shows the kinds, states and densities of the materials constituting a typical continental sector.

TABLE I

Earth-Shells in Continental Sector

(Crystalline Archean rocks at surface)

| Depth (km) | Material, with average density | |
|---|---|---|
| 0–30 | Granite and piezo-granite | SIAL (2.8) |
| | *Discontinuity* | |
| 30–40 | Granodiorite and piezo-phases | |
| | *Discontinuity* | |
| 40–60 | Piezo-gabbro.........CRYSTALLIZED SIMA (3.05) | |
| | *Discontinuity* | |
| 60–100± | Vitreous basalt (2.8–2.9) | |
| 100±–1200 | Vitreous ultrabasic silicate (2.9–4.5) | |
| | *Discontinuity* | |
| 1200–2900 | Vitreous silicate + oxide + sulphide (5.0–6.5) | |
| | *Discontinuity* | |
| 2900–6370 | Central core of iron (liquid?; 10.5–12.5) | |

TABLE II

Earth-Shells in Sector under Deep, Open Pacific

| Depth (km) | Material, with average density |
|---|---|
| 0–5.2 | Water (1.03) |
| | *Discontinuity* |
| 5.2–74.8± | Basalt and piezo-gabbro (CRYSTALLIZED SIMA; 2.95–3.05) |
| | *Discontinuity* |
| 74.8±–100± | Vitreous, femic basalt (2.85–2.9) |
| Below 100 | Shells as in Table I |

Table II similarly refers to the broad sector underlying the deeper part of the open Pacific Ocean. Somewhat different from either, at levels above the depth of 80 kilometers, would be any of the sectors capped by lofty chains of mountains or by oceans shallower than the deep Pacific.

This sketch of the earth's anatomy is based upon:

(1) The seismologists' determinations of wave velocities and changes of velocity in depth, with corresponding discontinuities of the material;

(2) The known composition of the upper part of the Sial;

(3) The dominantly basaltic quality of lava floods;

(4) The world-wide distribution of basaltic eruptives and the genetic association of basaltic magma with other observed igneous magmas and rocks (eruptive sequence);

(5) The necessity of assuming a distribution of densities to match the earth's moment of inertia and its mean density;

(6) The commonly accepted postulate that the earth's core is composed essentially of metallic iron, which, according to some high authorities, acts like a liquid against the weak, rapidly alternating stresses of earthquake waves;

(7) Experimental and seismological evidence as to the compressibilities of rock matter and iron, and the relation of the compressibilities to the speeds of earthquake waves;

(8) The observed and calculated thermal gradients in the planet;

(9) The probable distribution of radioactivity;

(10) The systematic differences of thermal conductivity among rocks, whether crystalline or vitreous;

(11) The probable origin of the earth;

(12) The composition of meteorites;

(13) The extreme weakness of the material below the depth of a few scores of kilometers (permitting isostatic adjustment);

(14) The facts bearing on orogenesis.

### An Earth Largely Vitreous

Here again are fourteen points. Not all of them make universal appeal and no treaty of Versailles is likely to bring peace soon in this other war of opinion. Full discussion of any of the points is out of the question, and whole fields of inquiry bearing on the nature of the earth's interior must be left untouched. Our time will be occupied chiefly with one fundamental assumption—that all but a small fraction of the 2,900-kilometer envelope of the planet's core is in the vitreous state. This implies the reality of a true crust, in the sense of a thin crystallized shell resting upon a series of non-crystallized shells; earth temperatures to correspond; strength nearly, if not quite, confined to the crust; and, because of the relations of density, potential instability for limited belts of the crust. The validity of this general idea is one of the most pressing and significant problems of earth science.

*Cosmogony and the Vitreous Shells:* First we observe that all the modern views about the earth's origin permit the hypothesis described. The erupto-tidal theory of Chamberlin and Moulton, the gas-filament tidal theory of Jeans and Jeffreys, the collision theory of Bickerton and Jeffreys, and the capture-collision theory of Hirayama and Van Anda all start with a gaseous earth. Chamberlin and Moulton argued for the rapid solidification of the young earth and for a tremendous increase of mass by the infall of planetesimals, the earth remaining crystalline except for subordinate, liquid pockets of quasi-eutectic composition. Yet it appears that these authors exaggerated the rôle of planetesimals in the earth's organization. Moreover, in any case the solar belch responsible for our globe may, by the erupto-tidal theory, have been big enough to retain the gaseous condition until the earth had attained practically its present mass. Jeffreys dates the segregation of the iron core at the gaseous stage—its most plausible explanation. He assumes that, after liquefying, the thick envelope about the core was "probably" made homogeneous in a chemical sense by thermal convection, and then by continued stirring was rapidly cooled and crystallized at great depth. However, it seems logical to think that the envelope itself was originally stratified, the intrinsic (chemically determined) density increasing with depth. If so, early thermal or other types of convection would cool only the outer part of the envelope about the core. Thus the initially high temperatures and non-crystalline character of all shells below the depth of a few hundreds of kilometers would be long preserved. Like the others, then, Jeffreys' cosmogonic scheme does not forbid belief that below a crust of moderate thickness the shells of the envelope are still too hot to pass out of the vitreous state.

*Seismology and the Earth-shells:* By general agreement the upper part of the Basement Complex (Archean terrane) is regarded as chiefly granitic. According to Sederholm's careful measurements in a regional sample (Finland), its average composition lies between those of average granite and average granodiorite. At depths greater than a few kilometers the Sial should be somewhat more basic because of an increased proportion of femic injections, and the lower half of the Sial may, in average, approximate granodiorite. There the density is doubtless increased still further by load metamorphism. Although these deeper rocks of the Sial are probably gneissic, their exact nature remains obscure. Hence there is some advantage in giving them the non-committal names of "piezo-granite" and "piezo-granodiorite."

Similarly, between the 40-kilometer and 60-kilometer levels the crystallized Sima, chiefly basaltic in chemical composition, is not likely to be gabbro or diabase, but denser rock. Its phases may be grouped under the name "piezo-gabbro."[2] The velocities of the earthquake waves are explicable if the Sial and crystallized Sima have the constitution described.

That the material just below the 60-kilometer discontinuity is vitreous basalt is an assumption at least permitted by studies of compressibility. Bridgman's pressure-volume curve for tachylite at 75° is relevant. It gives a rather close approximation to the compressibility of basaltic glass at pressures corresponding to depths of 60, 70 and 80 kilometers below the earth's surface. The density of the glass under these conditions is known within narrow limits. Taking the accepted value of Poisson's ratio at 0.27, the closely approximate velocity ($V_P$) of the longitudinal wave in tachylite at 75° and at the depths stated is found. Table III (col. 4) shows the result of such computation as well as the densities and elastic data. The expected high temperature of the glass at these levels is not allowed for in the calculation of wave velocity. Heating tends slightly to reduce compressibility and therefore wave velocity, but the correction required for this reason may be more than offset by proper correction for the difference between the high-pressure or static modulus of elasticity and the somewhat higher, seismically-effective or dynamic modulus for the same rock. Now the actual velocities of the longitudinal wave at the depths of 60, 70 and 80 kilometers within the earth have, according to the seismologists, the values shown in the last column of Table III. Comparison of this and the preceding column shows how well vitreous basalt meets the needs of the case. The agreement would be much poorer if crystalline peridotite were assumed at these depths, and is probably better than if vitreous peridotite be assumed.

TABLE III

DATA REGARDING A TACHYLITIC EARTH-SHELL

| Depth (km) | Volume compressibility | Density | Computed $V_p$ (km/sec) | "Observed" $V_p$ (km/sec) |
|---|---|---|---|---|
| 60 | $1.13 \times 10^{-6}$ | 2.80 | 7.4 | 7.8 |
| 70 | $1.07 \times 10^{-6}$ | 2.82 | 7.6 | 7.9 |
| 80 | $1.00 \times 10^{-6}$ | 2.85 | 7.8 | 8.0 |

[2] No important phase of this layer seems to be as dense and incompressible as eclogite.

Gutenberg's depth-velocity curve suggests only moderate chemical change between the 100-kilometer level and the discontinuity at 1,200 kilometers. Vitreous peridotite, perhaps merging into material like the average stony meteorite, would give the corresponding densities and wave velocities of Tables I and II, at these greater depths.

The meaning of each of the discontinuities, tentatively located by Gutenberg at 1,200, 1,700 and 2,450 kilometers of depth, is an unsolved problem. Goldschmidt supposes the changes of material to be in the direction from dominant silicate to dominant sulphide or oxide. The "observed" wave velocities seem to permit, though they do not compel, the idea of a vitreous condition for what Gutenberg calls the "intermediate layer," that between the 1,200-kilometer and 2,900-kilometer levels.

In conclusion, seismology has given results not unfavorable to our main thesis—non-crystallinity for all earth-shells below the thin crust. Experiments like those of Bridgman on liquids suggest that pressure alone can give the "glass" effective "solidity" in its reaction to the weak, short-lived stresses of earthquake waves. That the temperatures are high enough to prevent crystallization is a premise which would be strengthened if, as Oldham, Knott, Visser, Jeffreys and Gutenberg think, the earth's core acts as a true liquid against the stresses of earthquake waves; for presumably the temperature of the core would have to be exceedingly high to counteract the "solidifying" effect of the one to three millions of atmospheres of pressure upon the core material.

*Evidence from Thermal Gradients:* A review of the best data gives 1° C. per 36 meters or 28° per kilometer of depth as a good average gradient of temperature at the surface of the Archean complex. Extrapolation to depth is famously difficult. On any reasonable set of assumptions the gradient must, with increasing depth, become less steep: slowly near the surface and then faster to some moderate depth, where the rate of change becomes lower again. The troubles in calculating the gradients at depths greater than about 25 kilometers are numerous and of differing importance. There are two major troubles. One is connected with uncertainty regarding the distribution of radioactivity in the rocks; the other with uncertainty regarding the content of primitive, non-radioactive heat in those earth-shells which, through geological time, have actually felt the cold of outer space. Minor difficulties relate to the proper values to be assigned to the age of the earth and to the conductivity and specific heat of each of the outer earth-shells.

Because the crust has existed continuously since the Early Archean, all authorities assume strong concentration of radioactivity in the superficial shells. Jeffreys and others believe that the thermal output of the radioactive furnace is less than the heat lost by radiation from the surface, a large fraction of this squandered energy being an original endowment of the planet. Joly and Holmes, though also assuming much concentration of radioactivity in the crust, find the radioactive furnace efficient enough to endanger the continued existence of the crust, if unmoved.

According to Joly's well-known theory the crust persists, because periodically thinned by melting and then dragged over the earth's body; for both reasons the excess heat is supposed to have been rapidly conducted and radiated away. To this theory there are physical and geological objections, apparently fatal.

Holmes appeals to continental migration as the leading cause for the dissipation of the excess heat. The migration is thought to have been compelled by periodic convection and overturn of the whole 2,900-kilometer envelope about the earth's core. This bold suggestion implies that compression alone accounts for the downward increase of density in the envelope. Yet, as Williamson and Adams showed, mere compression of either basalt or peridotite could not give densities matching the earth's moment of inertia and mean density. There are other formidable objections to Holmes's theory, but here too time fails for their discussion.

Considering all the facts of the case, I think it most probable that no more than half of the heat radiated from the globe is of radioactive origin, the rest being original heat.

Holmes in 1915 and later Adams and then Jeffreys computed the temperatures to depths of 100 or more kilometers, on two assumptions: moderate heat of radioactivity, and little or no secular loss of heat from depths greater than a few hundreds of kilometers. Holmes deduced temperatures of 600°, 1204° and 1575° at the respective depths of 20, 60 and 100 kilometers. Both Adams and Jeffreys found considerably lower temperatures for the same depths.

All three sets of calculations are affected by the uncertainty as to the law of diminution of radioactivity with increasing depth, and all three ignore the possibility of thermal convection in the earth's body. The latter process would seriously affect the quantity of original heat to be dissipated in the course of time. While the single-step convection through the 2,900-kilometer envelope can not be assumed, Holmes has recently done good service in once more emphasizing (with Jeffreys) the possibility of convective transfer of primitive heat. If hot enough to be vitreous, the earth-shells at depth may reasonably be considered as infinitely weak (liquevitreous), whatever rigidity they exhibit against seismic and tidal stresses. In any of these shells convection is possible, provided: (1) the thermal gradient is steep enough; (2) the intrinsic (chemically determined) density is not far from uniform; (3) the shell is at least a few hundreds of kilometers thick; and (4) the viscosity is not many times higher than that of steel. Surface cooling establishes a thermal gradient in the topmost liquevitreous layer. Suppose this layer to be convectively overturned. The next shell beneath is chilled and thus has its own gradient steepened. Suppose it also to be convectively overturned. A third layer is then liable to the same change; and so on. These changes take much time, but it is conceivable that at long intervals original heat is brought from great depth to the base of the earth's crust. This speculative process, involving a slow, downward transfer of cold from shell to shell, may be briefly described as *delayed, tandem convection.* If such a mechanism has been at work, it is obviously wrong to postulate a fixed "initial" temperature for the outer earth, a temperature controlled wholly or essentially by the relation of melting temperature to pressure. For this reason the gradients calculated by Holmes, Adams and Jeffreys may be less steep than the true gradient.

Their assumptions of minor importance should also be examined. In each of the three calculations the thermal conductivity of crust rocks is taken at too high a value. Not enough allowance is made for the decrease of conductivity with increase of temperature; nor for the fact that the statically metamorphosed rocks of the crust, with the expected flat-lying schistosity, conduct heat in a vertical direction more slowly than the chemically equivalent but unlayered rocks (granite to gabbro) conduct heat. Moreover, Holmes (since 1929) and Jeffreys assume a vitreous state for earth-shells well within the layer affected by secular cooling, and should in their computations have allowed for the conductivity of vitreous rock, which, at ordinary temperature at least, is much lower than that of the equivalent crystalline rock. Again, all three calculations were based upon a too-low value of the specific heat, a quantity increasing with temperature and also with the change of state from crystalline to vitreous.

The net result of these minor errors also is to find the earth cooler in depth than it really is.

Until more is known about the cause of the distribution of radioactivity in the rocks and about the rôle of delayed convection, it is impossible for the mathematician to declare finally the existing thermal gradient in depth. My own tentative estimates of temperature give 760° and 1330° at the respective depths of 30 kilometers and 60 kilometers; below the 60-kilometer discontinuity, temperatures everywhere so high as to prevent crystallization. While these estimates appear compatible with the principles of earth physics, I dare to put them before you, primarily because they portray a vital part of a theory of the earth which seems best adapted to account for the facts of geology.

*Isostasy and the Vitreous Shells:* If the earth has a true crust resting on a succession of vitreous, because hot, shells, the weakness of the glassy material automatically explains the sensitiveness of the crust to glacial loads, and in general accounts for the condition of isostatic balance among the larger topographic features of the globe. Supposing radioactivity to be proportioned to the acidity of the crust, the thickness of the crust and the densities of the outer segments of the earth should vary systematically. The result is a scheme of densities different from those of the Pratt and Airy explanations of isostasy. The preferred scheme can not, of course, be described in exact figures; an indefinite range of choices within the limits set by my theory is admissible. Nevertheless, a reasonable set of choices seems to be indicated, and I have found that the corresponding arrangement of densities reduces the gravity anomalies about as well as the Airy hypothesis does and better than the Pratt hypothesis, so commonly used by geödesists. (Illustrative diagrams of the address here omitted). Hence the explanation of isostasy implied by the crust-substratum idea seems to have some support from the pendulum studies so far made.

*Evidence from Petrology:* Gravitative differentiation of magma is evident in certain intrusive sheets, laccoliths, lopoliths, dikes, thick extrusive flows, and probably in visible parts of a few batholiths. Year by year new examples are being discovered. It is surely not a wild idea to think that the earth, from the bottom of the crust to the top of the iron core, is also stratified according to intrinsic (chemically determined) density. As in differentiated sheets, the density of the envelope of the core should not be expected to increase uniformly with depth. The analogies mentioned suggest rapid changes of density at more or less widely spaced levels. Between any pair of those levels the intrinsic density may be nearly constant.

Because of their high density the deeper shells should not be eruptible into or through the crust. Normally the one layer that does erupt, as if emanating from a continuous earth-shell, is the basaltic. From the Pre-Cambrian to the present day it has delivered at the surface great masses of basaltic liquid in every continental and oceanic sector. This liquid issues alone or in direct association (inside the time limits of the petrogenetic cycle) with magmas of different composition. Thirty years ago the hypothesis that such basaltic magmas have come from local pockets of liquid in an essentially crystalline earth was held by some petrologists. But there is manifest difficulty in accounting for the pockets, whether as residuals of a planet once liquid, as locally developed eutectic solutions, or as local, radiothermal fusions. An increasing number of petrologists and geologists prefer the postulate that the erupted basalts originated in a world-circling, vitreous substratum.

Although not to be directly verified, this hypothesis has the advantage of explaining petrological and geodynamical facts more simply than any other yet published.

(1) In the first place, it enables us to understand why lava rises so high. The density relations expressed in Tables I and II are such that, if the crust is opened by a through-going fissure, the dead weight of the crust would tend to push up the substratum material at volcanic pipes to heights from three to six kilometers above sea-level.

(2) The hypothesis automatically accounts for the latent heat of the erupted, fluid basalts.

(3) Rising from a minimum depth of 60 kilometers, the basaltic liquid should be superheated. In fact the plateau-basalts, even after prolonged running and rapid radiation under the air, are still liquid to a degree apparently impossible if the flows started without superheat. If not superheated, could thin basaltic (diabasic, gabbroid) sills spread underground in their astonishing way?

(4) Without exception known to me, the earth's crust is basined where large volumes of basaltic magma were erupted at or near the surface, in the form of basaltic plateaus, or major cones, or lopoliths. The diameters of such structural basins measure hundreds of kilometers, a size suggesting that each erupted mass was transferred from a single, continuous earth-shell.

(5) The hypothesis seems to be the most adequate as a basis for deriving the origin of the 700 other species of post-Archean igneous rocks. Endowed with both latent heat and superheat, the erupted basaltic liquid is capable of melting and assimilating crust rocks, and these reactions, followed by differentiation of the syntectics, account for many of the non-basaltic species. On a particularly grand scale are the expected reactions and differentiations if large masses of the crust are thrust into, or founder in, the vitreous substratum.

The development of batholiths in orogenic belts was one of the earliest discoveries of earth science, and since Hutton's time has been accepted as proof of major, vertical displacement of melted rock. Why most batholiths are acid, granitic, is still a mooted question, but the best answer seems to be suggested by the twentieth-century proofs of extensive horizontal displacement of solid crust rocks towards each of the orogenic belts. This displacement is indicated by the arcuate ground-plans of the completed mountain-structures, by the nappe phenomena, and by the juxtaposition of geosynclinal facies originally distant from each other. Whether due to the earth's contraction or to the forceful, horizontal migration of independent blocks of continental size, each of the displacements involves an enormous addition of the solid material of the crust to the corresponding geosynclinal belt. The old view that this material or its equivalent volume of rock was locally piled up in excess on the earth's body, immediately giving each mountain-structure height to match, seems not to be in accord with the facts. For several young chains of mountains are still largely submarine, and others, somewhat older, attained their actual heights long after folding and thrusting had ceased. There appears to be only one alternative: the excess crust material sank into the earth's body at about equal pace with the orogenic paroxysm. In other words, the horizontal displacement of crust rock *towards* the geosynclinal belt was accompanied by vertical, downward displacement of crust rock *in* the belt. Such subsidence must be by downthrusting or downpulling, with the development of deep mountain roots; or by foundering of large pieces of the crust; or by both processes. If the material beneath the crust were crystalline and denser than the crust, neither downthrusting nor foundering on the required scale would be possible. Both are possible if the outer earth-shells are constituted as shown in Tables I and II.

Furthermore, it is worth noting that continental migration through the distances credited by Argand, du Toit, Heim, Holmes, Staub and Taylor, and even the horizontal displacements of the crust credited by Kober, who retains the contraction theory of mountain-building, are alike incredible unless the crust at each orogenic belt can sink deeply into a subcrustal layer. Hence, without assuming great weakness for this layer and also for it a density no greater than the mean density of the crust, both the contractionist and the migrationist are in trouble. Both are in still more trouble if they assume the horizontal displacement of crust rock to depend upon the horizontal scission, shearing, of strong crystalline rock from strong crystalline rock through the long distances and over the wide areas demanded. On the other hand, the resistance to such displacement is incomparably less if the crust moves over hot glass with the expected, little or no strength.

When there is strong horizontal displacement of the crystalline crust over the substratum, the crust yields at a geosynclinal prism. In part the roots of the mountain structure generated along that zone are due to downwarping of Sial and crystallized Sima. In part the local crust is broken into huge blocks, which founder in the substratum. This process may be called *major stoping*, to distinguish it from the ordinary *piecemeal stoping* at batholithic contacts. Major stoping means the local invasion of the crust by extraordinarily great volumes of substratum material, which at the higher levels loses much of its viscosity and becomes more typically magmatic basalt. Thus we have *abyssal injection* of the crust and that at maximum.

The foundered blocks and the deeply sunken roots of the new mountains are heated by the substratum, in which the temperature increases downwards from about 1,300° to a higher temperature, fixed by the thermal gradient (perhaps in average as much as 10° per kilometer of descent for some distance). There the immersed crystallines are selectively fused. The first of the secondary liquids melted out of the basic rocks are derived from the minerals that go into mutual solution at comparatively low temperatures. Sialic rocks will undergo this *pure-melting* at temperatures well below even the lowest temperature of the substratum. On account of viscosity true abyssal assimilation will be subordinate to pure-melting, but is also to be considered. All derived liquids are less dense than the basalt of the main abyssal injections and rise through it, to invade the mountain roots, which already inclose chilled, solidified apophyses from the basalt. These more salic bodies, due to the self-cleansing of the primary basalt, are bottomless in the sense of lacking floors of crystallized rock. For them the name *major abyssoliths* (Greek, *abyssos*, bottomless) is proposed.

Thus one important class of batholiths is speculatively explained, though in my opinion the word "batholith" should be defined without reference to its mode of emplacement.

The imagined mechanism implies that the magmas invading the mountain-structure during the prolonged petrogenetic cycle should be in the general *eruptive sequence* from basic to acid—the order actually observed. It involves also the important principle of *resurgency*, that is, the rise of both liquids and gases that had belonged to the now melted and assimilated parts of Sial and Sima.

In comparison with basalt, acid rock shows a greater volume change in melting and almost certainly has a smaller latent heat. Hence, if pure-melting of Sialic rock takes place at the substratum levels, and if the resulting liquid rises high into the mountain roots, it must be *superheated* considerably more than the primary basalt, risen to the same high levels. Have we here a partial explanation of the "caustic," replacing action of many batholiths on the intruded formations? I ask this even though we have so little field evidence of superheat in flows of rhyolitic lava.

Syntexis (pure-melting plus assimilation) is, then, supposed to be largely concentrated in the substratum itself, but should be expected also at all higher levels within the masses of primary liquid injected into the crust. Sediments as well as older igneous rocks will be so affected.

The suggested scheme implies a genetic classification of nearly all of the igneous rocks (here omitted).

*Some Objections:* Finally, a word about certain arguments against the crust-substratum hypothesis. That supposed to derive from the high velocities of earthquake waves below the 60-kilometer level has lost practically all its force since Bridgman measured the compressibility of tachylite. The objection that the hypothesis implies danger of general catastrophic foundering of the crust fails to recognize the strength of the crust as ample security against that danger. Jeffreys, Joly, Richardson and Kirsch are others who agree with this judgment. Foundering occurs only where the crust rocks are wholly immersed in the substratum, but immersion is difficult and needs the coarse brecciation of the crust at orogenic belts.

The repeated objection founded upon the high rigidity of the outer shells is likewise fallacious. The actual rigidity is relative to the smallness and periodic character of the stresses set up by the passage of earthquake waves, the wave of the body tide and by the elastic reaction of the globe to the Eulerian nutation. The stresses persist for the limited times because of the earth's viscosity, a quantity all the greater because the stresses are small, as Adams and Williamson found when experimenting on hot glass. In any case, the proof of rigidity gives no information about strength, so that there is no evident ground here for doubting the vitreous state of the basaltic substratum and of the shells lying between it and the iron core.

## CONCLUSION

We have briefly surveyed an old problem, weighted, as few others are, with fundamental meaning for geology. A problem it will long remain. Cosmogonic theory, seismological results, study of thermal gradients and of isostatic adjustment, like the multitude of facts of tectonics and petrology, all seem to support a thesis: Our planet is still too hot to crystallize at any depth greater than about 80 kilometers or 50 miles. But the support is not proof, nor is any theory of the earth to be absolutely demonstrated. As usual in the leading questions of science, we are pragmatists and search for the theory that works best. The thin-crust theory appears to work best. Yet the chief reason for putting it in the foreground is the fact that it can guide to fruitful research in the future. As never before, the geologist realizes the meaning of the ancient maxim, "deep calleth unto deep," the need of seeking in the shells and core of the earth explanation for the dramatic changes registered in its relief and visible rocks.

# A PROGRAM OF MEDICAL CARE FOR THE UNITED STATES

By Dr. C.-E. A. WINSLOW

PROFESSOR OF PUBLIC HEALTH, YALE SCHOOL OF MEDICINE; CHAIRMAN, EXECUTIVE COMMITTEE OF THE COMMITTEE ON THE COSTS OF MEDICAL CARE

In every field of human activity we are to-day facing one common problem—the problem of adjusting our social order to the altered conditions produced by a revolution in technology. "Neither do men put new wine into old bottles; else the bottles break, and the wine runneth out, and the bottles perish: but they put new wine into new bottles, and both are preserved."

The traditional relationship between a physician and his patient, for example, was admirably adapted to the conditions of a century ago. It was indeed one of the finest and most fruitful examples of human relationship which one could well imagine. The physician practiced an art over which he had complete control and mastery. In his head he could carry all the knowledge then in existence and in his black bag all the paraphernalia available for the healing of the sick. His profession was a priestly mission, not a business. He cared for all who were in need of his ministrations. Those who could pay nothing paid nothing and those who could contributed in proportion to their means for the support of an honored servant of society. The physician and his patients were neighbors and friends. They knew each other intimately and for a lifetime, and the adjustment between service and recompense in a given case was made almost automatically.

This is, of course, an extreme statement of the actual situation; but it represents an essential ideal which underlay the relation between the doctor and his patient at the dawn of the machine age. It is a relationship which still exists to-day. Most of us know physicians and patients who maintain contact on the same elevated plane. Yet it would be safe to say that such a relation is rare and is becoming more rare with the passing of the years. This is due first of all to changes in medicine itself. The old art is now also a new science. No longer can one man understand it or practise it by himself. There must be specialists and consultants of many and diverse kinds (some twenty-five such specialties are now recognized). There must be well-equipped and costly hospitals. There must be nurses. There must be laboratories and laboratory technicians. There must be physiotherapy, devices of numerous kinds and special experts to use them. There must be x-ray machines and radiologists.

Equally fundamental in their influence upon the older ideals of medical practise are the changes produced by technology in the general social order itself. The old neighborhood life has gone and with it the intimate and prolonged personal contacts which made the old relationship between physician and patient simple and easy of attainment. Still more deeply is this relationship affected by the subtle forces of a society dominated by the profit-motive in which as John Dewey has pointed out in "Individualism Old and New," old motives of social responsibility have disappeared and new ones have not yet been developed to take their place The physician finds himself half priest and half business man, a servant of society in a world which has ceased to recognize service except as measured by financial return, a business man in a field where the fundamental requirements of basic human need preclude the application of ordinary principles of economic individualism.

It is characteristic of the forces which dominate our civilization that the impulse which actually precipitated a broadly conceived study of this vital social problem was largely an economic one. It was primarily wide-spread complaint of the financial burden of illness on the one hand and legitimate dissatisfaction on the part of the professions and agencies furnishing medical service on the other which led to the formation on May 17, 1927, of the Committee on the Costs of Medical Care. From the first, however, the committee realized that it was impossible to consider costs without considering quality as well and it has set as its ultimate goal the "development of preventive and therapeutic services in such kinds and amounts as will meet the needs of substantially all the people" and the provision of such services "on financial terms which the people can and will meet, without undue hardship, either through individual or collective resources."

The committee, which made its final report on December 29 last, was composed of 48 members under the chairmanship of Dr. Ray Lyman Wilbur. Twenty-five of its members held the degree of doctor of medicine. Analyzed in another way, seventeen were private practitioners of medicine and dentistry, ten were representatives of institutions and special interests, six were public health workers, six social scientists and nine representatives of the general public. Funds for research were obtained through the generosity of eight foundations, and many other agencies have cooperated whole-heartedly in the conduct of special studies. An administrative staff was organized under the leadership of Harry H. Moore, whose vision has throughout been the inspiring force in the work of the committee. A brilliant research staff under I. S. Falk has been responsible for the actual conduct of the detailed investigations. The studies have been completed on schedule time (an almost miraculous result!) and have been published in 27 volumes.[1] The twenty-eighth and final volume, "Medical Care for the American People," is the report of the committee itself, signed by 35 of the 48 members of the committee. Minority reports were presented by two groups (one of eight physicians and an institutional representative, the other of two dentists) who find the report of the committee too radical; special minority statements were presented by a public health worker and a social scientist who find it too conservative.

In analyzing the findings of the committee it will be well to begin with one study which has received as yet but little attention but which should ultimately prove of far-reaching significance. This is Report No. 22 on "The Fundamentals of Good Medical Care," by Roger I. Lee and L. W. Jones. It gives us first an analysis of the number and kinds of illnesses to be cared for in the United States, second, an estimate of the amount and kind of medical care (home and office visits, laboratory tests, x-rays, days of hospital care, etc.) required by the average illness of each type. From these data the number of general practitioners, specialists, dentists, nurses, hospital beds, etc., needed for a given population are then computed. These analyses lead to the encouraging conclusion that a slight increase in medical personnel (with a considerable decrease in specialists), a very slight increase in nurses, and a considerable increase in dentists would be needed to meet the ideal needs of the American people for complete and adequate medical care. With proper organization they estimate that such complete care (preventive and curative, including effective health service and all nursing and hospital costs and charges for drugs) could be provided at an average cost of $36 per person per year.

The actual expenditure of the American people for medical care is to-day very close to this sum—$3,656,000,000, or $30 per capita; but the actual service rendered is very far from the adequate care which could be purchased for such an amount. The committee has obtained a remarkably clear picture of the existing situation. It has first of all (in Study 26) made a study of medical costs during a twelve-month period in nearly 9,000 families, representing various geographical areas and various economic levels; and it has supplemented this by intensive studies of community facilities in Shelby County, Indiana, the city of Philadelphia, the city of Detroit, San Joaquin County, California, the state of Vermont, and three representative southern counties (studies 6, 9, 10, 12, 13 and 23). These investigations reveal the following outstanding deficiencies in the present status of medical care.

A. *Maldistribution of facilities in various geographical areas.* These may be illustrated by the fact that in 1929 there was one physician to every 1,431 persons in South Carolina and one to every 571 in California; one dentist to every 5,274 persons in Mississippi, and one to every 990 persons in Oregon; one hospital bed to every 749 persons in South Carolina and one to every 154 in Wisconsin. Conditions in the Southern states are nothing less than appalling.

B. *Maladjustment of services in all areas.* In the rural areas, even where general practitioners are available, there is grave lack of hospital and laboratory facilities and of consultation service; and even in cities many physicians lack the hospital connections which would make the most effective work possible. On the other hand, the cities as a whole show a markedly excessive development of specialization. Forty-five per cent. of the physicians of the country have completely or partially limited their practise to a specialty, where we estimate that 18 per cent. would suffice for the real needs of the situation. Some patients suffer from lack of specialist service and some from too much.

C. *Waste in the provision of service.* There is wide-spread waste of time and of overhead costs in the rendering of service on an individual basis. About 40 per cent. of the average physician's income is consumed in overhead expense. The average physician also, particularly in the years immediately following graduation, wastes a large part of his time in waiting for patients, while the older man with unusual capacity in some particular field wastes much of his time in routine functions that a younger man could perform quite as well.

D. *Unwise expenditures for medical care.* Of the total of $3,656,000,000 a year now spent by the American people for medical care, 360 million dollars go for "patent medicines" and 125 million dollars for the services of cultists and irregular practitioners who

[1] The University of Chicago Press.

have never studied the human body and do not understand its working.

E. *Economic burden of emergency illness.* The average expenditure of $30 per capita per year does not seem exorbitant. It amounts to about 4 per cent. of the national income, less than we pay for household furnishings and supplies, less than half we pay for automobiles and only slightly more than we pay for recreation or for education or for tobacco, confections, ice cream and soft drinks. Such an average, however, gives no picture whatever of the actual situation. The other items mentioned can be predicted and budgeted; but sickness can not. Our studies bring out the astonishing fact that in the group of families with incomes under $2,000 a year (about half the population of the United States) one per cent. of the families spent over $500 in one year for medical care. It is this hundredth family (over one million of them in the United States in a given year) which contributes from one quarter to one half of its annual income to meet the emergency cost of illness which constitutes the critical economic problem in the field of medical care.

F. *Inadequate compensation for persons and agencies providing service.* One result of such economic maladjustment is that the compensation of the individuals furnishing service is on the whole inadequate and uncertain. The average net income of physicians in 1929 was $5,300, which may or may not be considered reasonable; but the median net income was only $3,500, and one third of all physicians had net incomes below $2,500. Private duty nurses were in a desperate situation even prior to the depression. Voluntary hospitals in many areas are now in serious danger of being forced to close their doors.

G. *Inadequate care of the sick.* The second result of economic maladjustment is that a shockingly large amount of illness is now actually uncared for (in spite of the potential adequacy of the resources at our disposal). The table below presents some of the most disturbing facts brought out in our study.

Clearly, the common catchword that "only the very rich and the very poor receive good medical care" is only half true. The very rich are reasonably well cared for (except for dentistry) and have slightly more special nursing than they need; but as one goes down in the economic scale the adequacy of care becomes less and less, except that the very low income levels receive more hospital care than those in the middle range. The lower half of the population (below $2,000 annual income) receive only a little over one third of the physicians' visits, less than two thirds of the hospital care, a little over one tenth of the dental care and a little over one tenth of the special nursing care required.

H. *Lack of preventive services.* Finally, there is everywhere a grave lack of the applications of modern medical science to the prevention of disease. We

| | Services received in families with specified incomes | | | | | | Services required by standards of good medical care |
|---|---|---|---|---|---|---|---|
| | Under $1,200 | $1,200–$2,000 | $3,000–$5,000 | $5,000–$10,000 | Over $10,000 | | |
| Physicians' home, office and clinic calls per person | 1.9 | 2.0 | 2.3 | 2.7 | 3.6 | 4.7 | 5.6 |
| Days of hospital care per person | 0.9 | 0.7 | 0.8 | 0.6 | 0.8 | 1.2 | 1.4 |
| Dental care, per person over 3 years of age | 0.1 | 0.2 | 0.2 | 0.3 | 0.4 | 0.6 | 1.0 |
| Cases receiving special nursing care per hospitalized case | 0.1 | 0.1 | 0.2 | 0.3 | 0.4 | 0.7 | 0.6 |

talk about preventive medicine and annual health examinations, but we do not practise them. As long as preventive services are immediately contingent on the payment of a fee for such services they can not be urged by the physician and they will not be sought by the patient.

So much for the defects in the operation of the general machinery for the provision of medical care to the American people. A second group of studies made by the committee deals with a very different picture found in certain special population groups where experiments have been made in providing medical care on a different basis through organized social planning. Reports have been presented on four different types of services of this kind—industrial medical services providing medical care for employees and their families, conducted by the Endicott-Johnson Company, the Homestake Mining Company and at Roanoke Rapids, North Carolina (Nos. 5, 18 and 20); university medical services at California, Cornell, Michigan, Oregon and Yale (No. 19); service provided for officers and men and their families at an army post at Fort Benning, Georgia (No. 21) and service provided by tax-supported physicians in the rural areas of Saskatchewan (No. 11).

It must not be inferred that the committee presents these instances as necessarily typical of industrial or military or other forms of organized medical care. The programs studied were chosen because they were believed to be good examples and they are significant, not necessarily as pictures of average organized practise to-day, but as illustrations of what organized practise can accomplish when properly safeguarded.

From this standpoint, the experiments reviewed are highly encouraging. They show us representative population groups which under an organized program are receiving a type of medical care which is free from practically all the limitations operating in the country as a whole. The beneficiaries of these services are receiving a far greater amount of medical care and medical care on the whole of better quality than corresponding economic groups in the general population. The expense of the service provided varies according to its completeness. The rural service in Saskatchewan which covers only home and office calls by physicians costs only about $2 per person per year. That at Homestake which does not cover dentistry or home nursing costs a little over $12. The highly developed and practically complete services of the Endicott-Johnson Company, the Fort Benning Post and the better equipped universities costs from $20 to $30 per person per year. In other words the actual cost corresponds very closely to the average expenditures of the general population at a corresponding economic level; but the service is something like twice as extensive. At Roanoke Rapids, for example, the mill population paid for their organized service $8.72 per capita per year as against $5.17 paid by the rest of the community (the latter being on a slightly higher economic level); the mill group, however, received three times as much hospital care, nearly twice as many physicians' office and home calls and ten times as many home nursing calls as did their fellow townsmen. At Homestake the organized group provided for $71,000 service which at current local rates would have cost $175,000.

The increased values obtained from organized service, in such instances as those cited, are not in any sense derived from exploitation of the professional personnel concerned but by elimination of waste time and needless overhead charges. The salaries of physicians in Saskatchewan and in the industrial and university service cited are well above the average for similar areas, and in general for the country as a whole.

The funds are obviously derived from various sources—from the tax levy in Saskatchewan and at Fort Benning, from the students in the universities, from employer or employee or both in the industries. In all instances, however, payment by the potential patient is on a fixed annual or monthly basis, so that the crippling burden of emergency illness is eliminated. Finally, as the Saskatchewan doctors and the industrial physicians testify with particular emphasis, the removal of the pecuniary inhibition in connection with a particular service makes it infinitely easier on both sides to offer and to receive medical care of a preventive and therefore really fruitful kind.

These investigations have, then, led the committee to its two major recommendations. The first of these is "that medical service, both preventive and therapeutic, should be furnished largely by organized groups of physicians, dentists, nurses, pharmacists and other associated personnel. Such groups should be organized, preferably around a hospital, for rendering complete home, office and hospital care." The chief difficulties which the committee believes can be overcome by group practise are listed as follows:

> The lack of coordination between general practitioners and specialists; the isolation of some practitioners from helpful contacts with their confrères and from hospitals and medical agencies; the lack of adequate supervision and control over the quality of some medical care; the enforced idleness of many physicians because of lack of patients; the difficulty experienced by patients in choosing qualified physicians; the unnecessarily large expenditure for overhead costs made by practitioners in individual private practice; and the increasing complexity of medical service which necessitates the use of ever-multiplying equipment, as well as a larger number and variety of subsidiary personnel.

Secondly, the committee recommends "that the costs of medical care be placed on a group payment basis, through the use of insurance, through the use of taxation; or through the use of both these methods." The argument here is, of course, obvious and inescapable. Only by distribution of costs over a period of time and over a group of families can the crippling economic burdens of emergency illness be avoided. Only by such distribution of costs on a fixed annual basis can the general use of preventive measures be brought within the range of practical possibility.

The ideal of the committee is the development in urban areas of community medical centers organized about existing hospitals. In some instances these would be city or county or town hospitals (particularly in rural areas). More often they would be voluntary hospitals, directed as our non-official hospitals are to-day by a lay board representing community interests. Practically all the physicians, dentists and private duty nurses in a community might be on the staff of one or another of the hospitals, and these staffs would be organized as those of our best hospitals are to-day, so that qualified chiefs of services would be responsible for the quality of service rendered. All professional policies would be directed by the professional groups concerned. Complete preventive and curative care of all types, in home, office and ward, would be provided for one fixed annual fee. The majority of physicians on the staff would be general practitioners and the individual would choose his own family physician with complete freedom among those available in the centers within his reach.

Such completely equipped centers might serve more than 50 per cent. of the American people who live in communities of over 15,000 or within reach of them. For smaller isolated towns (about 10 per cent. of the population) small branch hospitals could be used, affiliated with the larger centers for consultation service and for the handling of specially difficult cases. For the villages and rural areas (including slightly less than 40 per cent. of our population) still smaller "medical stations" should be established with one or two physicians, a dentist, a trained nurse-midwife and other public health nurses. They would rely upon medical centers or branches for facilities and service they could not themselves supply and would be visited at intervals by specialists from such centers.

The method of accumulating the collective reserves to pay for services would differ with local conditions. In remote rural areas the tax levy (as in Saskatchewan) would seem to be the only promising source. For the indigent in all areas the tax levy would necessarily provide, as it does (inadequately) at the present day. In industrial communities the employer might properly contribute his share, as he often does now. It seems highly desirable, however, for the development of a due sense of personal responsibility that as large a proportion as possible of the costs of medical care should be borne by those who are to receive that care—in other words, by payment from individual families through the medium of an insurance plan.

This is the method which has been universally adopted by the nations of western Europe (in contradistinction to the tax-supported state medical service of Russia and certain other countries of eastern Europe); and, in general, these nations have moved steadily forward from experiments with voluntary group purchase to programs of compulsory state insurance. The committee is nearly unanimous in recognizing that complete coverage of all those who require care can only be ultimately attained in the United States by a system of compulsory insurance. If and when such a program is adopted we trust that insurance for medical care may be sharply and completely separated from insurance covering wage losses due to illness, since we feel that the difficulties experienced in Europe have been largely due to confusion between these two different objectives.

The majority of the committee is not, however, prepared to recommend compulsory sickness insurance in any form at this time—chiefly for the following reason. We do not believe that adequate medical care can ever be provided by private physicians operating on a purely individualistic basis, and if the introduction of compulsory insurance crystallized and fortified the present system of medical practise, we believe that the dangers would outweigh the benefits. We should like, therefore, to see a period of experimentation with voluntary group purchase going hand in hand with the development of group practice so that when compulsion comes the public can contract with well-organized and well-established medical centers and their cooperating agencies. We can begin with industrial groups, church groups, neighborhood groups and other voluntary aggregations, while we are gaining experience in medical organization and in actuarial practise; and that this is not an idle dream is shown by experience in England, where something like six million people are now insured for hospital care in voluntary groups.

The report of the Committee on the Costs of Medical Care has already, in the brief time since its appearance, been subjected to very vigorous criticism. This is highly encouraging, since only platitudes receive easy and general acceptation. Many of these criticisms, however, are obviously made by those who have never read the report, since they condemn it for positions which it does not imply in any shape or form.

We have, for example, been charged in supposedly serious scientific quarters of advocating socialism and communism and of "inciting to revolution." Yet the entire program advocated by the communite is based primarily on group practise in voluntary hospitals and on group purchase by privately organized bodies of citizens. The tax levy is only brought in for rural areas where there is no other source of funds and for the support of the indigent which is already a universally accepted form of socialism. We believe that the policy we have proposed is the only way of forestalling a type of state action which has become almost universal in Europe and which will be inevitable here if such forms of voluntary group planning as we have suggested can not be successfully evolved.

A second ground of opposition to the report is that it advocates a type of group service called by the medical profession "contract practise" which may readily be made the agency of "unfair competition." Here, the whole question hinges on what is meant by "unfair competition." If a group of physicians render a substandard type of service there is certainly unfair competition with their professional confrères. If, on the other hand, a group of physicians is exploited through overwork or underpayment by an industry or some other agency organizing a group, there is unfair competition. Either of these conditions will injure both the public and the profession and should be strongly condemned. But if it be found (as it has often been found) that a group of physicians can receive ample compensation and yet furnish equivalent care to patients at lower cost than can their individual colleagues in the community, we have a different story. The advantages of group practise which accrue directly from the organized nature of that practise are clearly in the interest of both the profession and the public. No condemnation of "unfair competition" which is based only on such advantages can ultimately be maintained.

Opposition to the plans of the committee is also based on the fear of "lay control" of medical practise. The committee is quite at one with such critics in stating clearly that "lay groups organized for profits have no legitimate place in the provision of this vital public service." On the other hand, it is apparent that in a "vital public service" there are vital public interests at stake. Medicine can not to-day be practised without large capital sums invested in hospitals, laboratories and clinics; and the public must continue to have its voice in the management of such institutions. The combination of a lay board representing the public interests involved and a professional staff in full control of professional policies seems to offer the only rational solution of the problem.

Finally, there is the fear that group practice and group purchase would mechanize medicine and wipe out the essential personal relationship between physician and patient. There is no doubt that this has happened in some group practices, and there is no doubt that where it does happen it is destructive of the essential basis of good medical care. There is no reason, however, why it should happen. It does not appear to have happened in the university and industrial services we have studied or at Fort Benning. It does not happen in many of our best clinics where the appointment system is coming into use. In a properly organized medical center such as we have described the relation between family physician and patient (which has so largely disappeared from private practice in urban centers) could be restored to a new importance and dignity and freed from the constant inhibitions on both sides which are due to the intrusion of the element of pecuniary responsibility at every stage in what should be a free personal relationship.

The committee does not of course recommend the immediate completion of its program on any general scale or indeed in any given community. It does endorse the principles of group practice and group purchase as basic in any sound program of advance; but it recognizes that local differences—social, economic, geographical, psychological—will make widely differing applications of these principles desirable.

The committee recommends "that the study, evaluation and coordination of medical service be considered important functions for every state and local community, that agencies be formed to exercise these functions, and that the coordination of rural with urban services receive special attention." It urges experimentation in the direction of expanding existing institutions, hospitals, group clinics, pay clinics, industrial and university medical services and the like. To readers of SCIENCE it may be of particular interest to note the recommendation that

> The student health services, found feasible in certain universities, may be extended to other universities and academic institutions, and the services made available on a suitable periodic payment basis to faculty members and their dependents and to other university employees and their dependents. In "college towns" it may frequently be feasible to expand the university medical service into a community medical center which serves townspeople as well as students.

To quote again,

> The aim should be to adopt objectives which at present seem sound, and to develop definite and purposeful experimental methods of approaching those objectives, preserving, insofar as it is compatible with effective service, the maximum amount of local self-support, and self-control, and the greatest freedom, consistent with social welfare, for the professions and the agencies involved. Although too great decentralization of authority limits competence and threatens economic effectiveness, too great centralization of authority in any plan carries with it elements of ultimate weakness. Fortunately, we have retained in this country a wholesome local responsibility for medical service. This fact means that opportunities exist for trying out many plans under various and variable conditions. Where action can be limited to the city or county, we have several thousand experiment stations. If state action is necessary, there are forty-eight laboratories.

Experimental social planning along sound theoretical lines, but based on existing American institutions —this is the objective set before us for the solution of the economic problem of medical care.

# OBITUARY

## ORMOND STONE

### 1847–1933

AFTER living to the ripe age of eighty-six years, Professor Ormond Stone was instantly killed on January 17 near his home in Centreville, Virginia, when struck by an automobile while he was walking along the road. With his passing, the University of Virginia loses its oldest professor and astronomy a noted figure.

He was born in 1847 in Illinois and he received the M.A. degree from the University of Chicago. For five years he was at the U. S. Naval Observatory in Washington and left there in 1875 to go to the Cincinnati Observatory as director. When Leander McCormick, the son of the inventor of the famous reaping machine, gave to the University of Virginia the 26-inch refractor, the telescope was the largest and the finest in the world. In looking for a director, the distinguished astronomer Simon Newcomb recommended for the position the director of the Cincinnati Observatory. For thirty years, from 1882 to 1912, when he was retired on the Carnegie Foundation, Professor Stone directed the work of the McCormick Observatory. No photographic work was attempted, but valuable visual observations were made on double stars, variable stars, nebulae, the satellites of Saturn, etc. In addition, he observed three total solar eclipses, that of 1869 in Iowa, he was in charge of the Naval Observatory expedition to Colorado in 1878 and of the McCormick expedition to South Carolina in 1900.

Professor Stone was as much at home in the field of mathematics as he was in astronomy. He was the founder and the first editor of the *Annals of Mathematics,* later taken over by the American Mathematical Society.

The Vanderbilt fellowships at the University of Virginia attracted to the McCormick Observatory many capable young men. Among those now living who hold the degrees of doctor of philosophy from Virginia and who have attained prominent scientific positions are the following: Edgar Odell Lovett, president of Rice Institute; Heber D. Curtis, director of the University of Michigan Observatory; Charles P. Olivier, director of the Flower Observatory; Herbert R. Morgan, U. S. Naval Observatory; Ralph E. Wilson, Dudley Observatory; G. F. Paddock, Lick Observatory, and T. McN. Simpson, Randolph-Macon College.

The combination of a great telescope and skill as a mathematician brought distinction to the University of Virginia. Naturally the McCormick telescope did not long remain the largest in the world. Four years after its opening, the Lick telescope of 36-inch aperture was dedicated.

Professor Stone came of a prominent family. He was a brother of Melville Stone, for many years general manager of the Associated Press.

S. A. MITCHELL

## ARTHUR GRAY LEONARD

DR. ARTHUR GRAY LEONARD, professor of geology at the University of North Dakota and state geologist for thirty years, died at his home in Grand Forks on December 17, 1932. He was born at Clinton, New York, March 15, 1865. He graduated from Oberlin College in 1889, received the degree A.M. from his alma mater in 1895 and the Ph.D. degree from the Johns Hopkins University in 1898. He served as assistant state geologist of Iowa, assistant professor of geology at the University of Missouri and professor of geology at Western College before going to the University of North Dakota in 1903.

The wide range of Dr. Leonard's contribution to the knowledge of the geology of North Dakota is indicated by the titles of his numerous geological papers in scientific journals and the reports of the United States Geological Survey and the North Dakota Geological Survey on such subjects as lignite coal, clay, gravel and the possibilities of oil and gas. A complete list of his publications numbers over fifty.

Dr. Leonard's greatest contribution to the science aside from that as a teacher was his addition to the basic knowledge of the geology of lignite coal, its origin and the relation of the lignite-bearing beds to the geologic time scale.

HOWARD E. SIMPSON

## JOHN F. G. HICKS

THE many friends and former students of Dr. J. F. G. Hicks will regret to learn of his death on December 13, at his home in Portland, Oregon. At the time of his death he was teaching in the Institute of Technology Junior College in Portland. His health failed while he was doing research at the Bureau of Standards on paper deterioration (1929–1931).

Dr. Hicks was born in Philadelphia in 1884. He received his B.S. degree from the University of Pennsylvania in 1906, and his M.S. and Ph.D. degrees from the University of Illinois in 1916 and 1918, respectively.

Besides holding several industrial positions, Dr. Hicks held professorships in the departments of chemistry of Oregon State College, University of Nevada and North Pacific College. At the time of his death he was actively engaged in writing a textbook of chemistry.

RALPH W. HUFFERD

## RECENT DEATHS

CHARLES G. FAIRCHILD, formerly professor of physics at Oberlin College and later president of Rollins College, died on January 20, at the age of eighty-nine years.

DR. WINFIELD S. DUDGEON, professor of botany at Ewing Christian College, Allahabad, India, died at Ames, Iowa, on December 26, at the age of forty-six years. Professor Dudgeon had been spending a sabbatical year in the United States.

DR. JOHN H. STUMBERG, a member of the research staff of the Rockefeller Institute at Princeton, died suddenly on January 20, at the age of twenty-six years.

*Nature* announces the deaths of Professor Paolo

Enriques, professor of zoology in the University of Padua and president of the last International Congress of Zoology, and of Professor James Johnstone, professor of oceanography in the University of Liverpool, formerly director of the Marine Biological Station, Port Erin.

# SCIENTIFIC EVENTS

## INVESTIGATION OF THE CARIBBEAN REGION

ARRANGEMENTS have been made between Yale University and the Woods Hole Oceanographic Institution for a continuation of the cooperative program of marine investigations in the Central American seas, which was inaugurated by the Yale Oceanographic Expedition to the Gulf of Mexico on the schooner *Mabel Taylor* last year. The research ship *Atlantis*, belonging to the institution, is now being equipped for a three-months oceanographic cruise in the Caribbean, and is expected to leave Woods Hole at the beginning of February.

A series of observations will be made from Woods Hole to Bermuda and from Bermuda to Nassau, Bahamas, from which point the joint investigations take their start, with Professor A. E. Parr, curator of the Bingham Oceanographic Collection at Yale University, and a research associate of the Woods Hole Oceanographic Institution, in charge of the subsequent scientific work in the Caribbean waters.

The contemplated investigations will be chiefly concerned with the general oceanic circulation in the Central American seas, particularly as it affects the transportation of water from the inflow of the North Equatorial current through the passages between the Windward Islands at the southeastern end to the outflow of the Gulf Stream through the Straits of Florida in the North. Special attention will also be given to the problem of the origin of the cold bottom water in the isolated chains of deepsea basins extending through the Gulf and Caribbean region. It is hoped that the results of the coming cruise, combined with the observations from last year's expedition to the Gulf of Mexico, may prove sufficient to give a general outline of the oceanographic conditions throughout the Central American Seas on which further investigations can be based.

Along with the hydrographic observations, biological material will also be collected, and an attempt will be made to obtain an idea of the frequency of the larger deepsea animals by the use of a triangular otter trawl of much greater opening width than that of any gear previously employed for deepsea collecting.

## NATIONAL FELLOWSHIPS AT THE JOHNS HOPKINS UNIVERSITY

UNDER the National Fellowship Plan of the Johns Hopkins University, Baltimore, Maryland, three $1,000 fellowships for graduate study of chemistry at the university will be open to qualified students in colleges and universities this year. The three are the Francis P. Garvan Fellowship for New York, the H. A. B. Dunning Fellowship for Maryland and the Eli Lilly Company Fellowship for Indiana. The New York and Maryland fellowships have been endowed by their donors, while the Indiana fellowship has been renewed for a period of four years. The fellowships provide the student $1,000 annually for a period of four years.

The purpose of the National Fellowship Plan is described as "the selection and training of chemists who are especially fitted to contribute to fundamental chemical progress"; and, under the plan, thirty-two men, representing thirty-two states, are now pursuing research on the grounds at the Johns Hopkins University. Their work covers a wide variety of fields.

The fellowships, providing $1,000 annually for a period of four years, give the recipients an opportunity for fundamental training and original research in chemistry and related subjects. The four major branches of chemistry, inorganic, organic, physical and analytical, are studied, and an elective system of study is followed by the student. In addition to the fundamental curriculum, the students are given an opportunity for personal contact with leading European and American chemists, through a visiting lectureship which has been provided by Dr. A. R. L. Dohme, of Sharpe and Dohme, Baltimore.

The selection of the successful candidate is accomplished through state committees which evaluate the student's complete previous scholastic record, and his personal qualities as rated by his instructors. Students in the sophomore, junior and senior year of the colleges and universities of the designated state are eligible for the fellowships. The successful candidates will be notified on or before April 1, 1933, and will begin their work at the Johns Hopkins University in October, 1933.

## FORMAT OF THE PHYSICAL REVIEW

*The Physical Review*, together with the other journals published by the American Institute of Physics, has adopted a new style and format, with two three-inch columns on the page as in SCIENCE. It was chosen in a conference of all the editors. The advantages of the new format are said to be the following:

*Economy.* For a given amount of reading material,

less paper is used and fewer press operations are required. The saving is considerable.

*Readability.* The short line is recommended by authorities as being more easily and quickly read. This is based on reading tests. In proofreading this issue, the editorial staff accomplished the task with much less time and effort than heretofore.

*Adaptability.* The larger two-column page permits adapting cuts, tables and formulas either to the three-inch or the six-inch width. There is less waste white space at the sides of such material. The page is thus more uniform in appearance as well as more economical. Large cuts and tables may now be displayed properly instead of having to be turned lengthwise on the page.

*Convenience.* More material is presented on each page. Two open pages are the equivalent of three or more pages of the old format. Scientific reading requires frequent references to tables and figures. There will now be less necessity to turn pages in consequence.

*Bound Volumes.* Because of the more efficient use of paper, the bound volumes will be lighter. They will be slightly higher, but not too high for ordinary shelving. They will be thinner and so require less shelf space.

## THE JOURNAL OF CHEMICAL EDUCATION AND THE CHEMISTRY LEAFLET

*Industrial and Engineering Chemistry* reports that certain changes, in effect January 1, 1933, have been made in the editorial and business departments of the *Journal of Chemical Education* and *The Chemistry Leaflet*. A signed statement by Lyman C. Newell, chairman of the Division of Chemical Education, appears in the current issue of the *Journal of Chemical Education,* and is essentially as follows:

The withdrawal of financial support by the Chemical Foundation has necessitated certain changes in the editorial and business departments of the *Journal of Chemical Education* since its last issue. Neil E. Gordon has resigned as editor-in-chief and William W. Buffum as business manager. Otto Reinmuth is continuing as editor and Harvey F. Mack has been appointed business manager.

The impending reduction, and possible withdrawal, of the financial support which the Chemical Foundation so generously maintained for several years led to the appointment of a special committee at the Denver meeting of the division on August 22, 1932.

The special committee rendered its final report to the executive committee early in December, and the report was accepted.

When the special committee met on October 8 to consider the situation and formulate plans, it was learned that the Chemical Foundation could no longer grant financial aid for the *Journal of Chemical Education* and *The Chemistry Leaflet,* nor for the activities of the division. Prompt and drastic action was imperative. The result of meetings and conferences of the special committee is substantially as follows:

The ownership of *The Chemistry Leaflet* has been returned to Pauline Beery Mack, who convinced the special committee that she could continue its publication.

After extended efforts to find ways and means to continue the publication of the *Journal of Chemical Education* it was finally decided to accept the proposition of the Mack Printing Co., whereby the division shall continue to own and edit the *Journal of Chemical Education* and the Mack Printing Co. shall assume the business management and financial responsibility.

Neil E. Gordon's resignation as editor-in-chief has been accepted by the executive committee. The editorial office has been removed to Easton, Pennsylvania, where Otto Reinmuth continues to act as editor.

In accordance with a recommendation of the special committee, the supervision and general control of the affairs of the *Journal of Chemical Education* will be lodged in a board of publication. Many details are being worked out by this board in cooperation with the editorial and business departments. Further announcements of details will be made in future numbers of the *Journal of Chemical Education.*

*The Chemistry Leaflet* continues in the same style, but the *Journal of Chemical Education* has a new cover, page size, style and topography. The general editorial policy of each publication will not be altered.

## DINNER IN HONOR OF EDWARD BAUSCH

EDWARD BAUSCH, president of the Bausch and Lomb Optical Company, was the guest of honor on January 23 at the annual dinner of the Society of the Genesee, an organization of men and women who have lived in the Genesee Valley of New York State and who meet each year to honor an outstanding neighbor and renew old friendships. The annual dinners have been held in New York for many years and many notable men have been honored.

The speakers included Major General James G. Harbord, chairman of the board, Radio Corporation of America; Dr. Arthur L. Day, head of the Geophysical Laboratory, Carnegie Institution, Washington, D. C.; Dr. Rush Rhees, president of the University of Rochester, and Louis Wiley, business manager of *The New York Times.* President Elon H. Hooker was toastmaster.

A correspondent writes:

Edward Bausch is one of America's early microscope builders, starting when there were only eighteen microscopes in the entire country. He designed instruments and devised methods of producing them in sufficient quantities so that they could be sold at a low price.

Edward Bausch was born September 26, 1854, the oldest son of John Jacob Bausch, manufacturer of spectacle lenses and hard rubber frames. Edward built his first microscope while he was still in school. Before he completed his college course at Cornell University he was called home by his father to take over some of the responsibilities of the optical business.

The Bausch and Lomb Optical Company started manufacturing microscopes soon after Edward Bausch joined the company in 1874. Their microscopes won prizes at the Centennial Exposition in 1876 and were soon being produced in quantities for use in science courses in schools, and the laboratories of hospitals and research institutions. They added microscopic accessories and developed other scientific optical instruments until now they make thousands of different optical devices for use in science, industry, education and medicine.

Edward Bausch has been a leader in the invention of optical equipment and the development of mechanical means for producing it at a reasonable cost. He was born only a stone's throw from the Genesee River and has spent his long life building the enormous Bausch and Lomb Optical Company plant upon its banks. While his neighbors honor him for what he has done in the community as a man, the nation remembers him for his scientific achievements during this seventy-ninth year of a long and useful life.

# SCIENTIFIC NOTES AND NEWS

THE British Royal Astronomical Society has awarded its gold medal for 1933 to Dr. V. M. Slipher, director of the Lowell Observatory, Flagstaff, Arizona, for his spectroscopic researches on planets, stars and nebulae. Dr. Slipher has been invited to deliver the George Darwin Lecture this year.

THE University of Wales has conferred the degree of D.Sc. on Dr. Francis E. Lloyd, professor of botany in McGill University, and on Professor Robert Robinson, Waynflete professor of organic chemistry in the University of Oxford.

DR. C. JUDSON HERRICK, professor of neurology at the University of Chicago, was recently tendered a dinner given by a group of his colleagues in celebration of the twenty-fifth anniversary of his professorship.

DR. CHEVALIER JACKSON, professor of bronchoscopy and esophagoscopy at Temple University, has been awarded the medal of honor of the Italian Government by the King of Italy.

ACCORDING to *Nature* the Government of Ecuador has awarded the decoration of *Al Merito,* in the degree of Gran Oficial, to Dr. George Sheppard, state geologist to the Republic of Ecuador.

PROFESSOR WILHELM SCHÜFFNER, director of the Institute for Tropical Diseases, Amsterdam, has been awarded the Hans Aronson Foundation Prize.

THE Buchan Prize of the Royal Meteorological Society for 1933 has been awarded to David Brunt, for papers contributed to the *Quarterly Journal* and *Memoirs* of the society during the years 1927–31.

THE Bavarian Academy of Sciences has awarded the gold *Bene merenti* medal to Dr. Herman Strebel, in appreciation of the gift of his observatory at Ammersee to the State Observatory.

DR. WILLIAM H. PARK, director of laboratories for the New York City Department of Health, has been appointed to the Hermann M. Biggs professorship of preventive medicine at the New York University and Bellevue Hospital Medical College. The Biggs professorship was made possible by a memorial fund established shortly after his death in 1923 and recently increased to a total amount of $200,000 by a bequest of Mrs. Hermann M. Biggs and gifts from William R. Biggs and Mrs. Katherine Biggs McKinney, son and daughter of Dr. Biggs, and the Milbank Memorial Fund.

DR. A. B. LUCKHARDT, chairman of the department of physiology of the University of Chicago, has been elected honorary president of the International Anesthesia Research Society.

HOWARD COONLEY, president of the Walworth Company, New York, has been elected to the presidency of the American Standards Association for the year 1933. F. E. Moskovics, chairman of the board of directors of the Marmon-Herrington Company, Indianapolis, has been elected vice-president.

DR. CHARLES H. MAYO, of the Mayo Foundation, Rochester, Minnesota, has been elected president of the Minnesota Public Health Association.

DR. RALPH S. LILLIE, of the University of Chicago, was recently appointed an advisory trustee of the International Cancer Research Foundation.

L. V. COLEMAN, director of the American Association of Museums, has become a member of the American National Committee on International Intellectual Cooperation of the League of Nations.

MR. H. T. TIZARD, rector of the Imperial College of Science and Technology, London, has been appointed chairman of the Aeronautical Research Committee in succession to Sir Richard Glazebrook.

MR. C. F. A. PANTIN, of Trinity College, Cambridge, has been nominated to use the university's table at the Zoological Station at Naples.

DR. GREGORY SHWARTZMAN has received a grant from the Committee on Scientific Research of the American Medical Association for work on the "Rous

Agent" to be done in the Mount Sinai Hospital laboratories.

DR. EDWIN O. JORDAN, chairman of the department of hygiene and bacteriology of the University of Chicago, is spending the winter quarter in Jamaica, where he is conducting a special investigation under the auspices of the International Health Board of the Rockefeller Foundation.

PROFESSOR ROBERT REDFIELD, of the department of anthropology of the University of Chicago, in order to continue his field researches in Maya ethnology, is spending six months in southern Mexico.

EARL HANSON, of the department of terrestrial magnetism of the Carnegie Institution of Washington, has returned to the United States after spending eighteen months in the northern part of South America making surveys of terrestrial magnetism.

ABBÉ GEORGES LEMAITRE, professor of mathematics and of the history of the physical and mathematical sciences at the University of Louvain, has left Pasadena, where he has been conferring with Dr. R. A. Millikan, Dr. Albert Einstein and others, to return to Louvain. He will visit Washington and England on the way.

DR. F. BERNSTEIN, director of the institute of mathematical statistics of the University of Göttingen, is visiting the United States, more especially to study the work of Dr. William H. Park and Dr. Keresturi at the Willard Park Hospital on the B. C. G. method of combatting tuberculosis and of Miss Maude Slye, at the Sprague Memorial Institute of the University of Chicago, on the inheritance of cancer in mice.

LLEWELLYN N. EDWARDS, senior highway bridge engineer on the U. S. Bureau of Public Roads, sailed on January 20 for England where he plans to spend three months on research work. On February 15 he will read a paper on "The Evolution of American Bridges" before the Newcomen Society in London.

DR. L. B. TUCKERMAN, retiring president of the Philosophical Society of Washington, on January 14 delivered an address before the society entitled "From Material to Structure."

PROFESSOR WALTER S. RODMAN, of the department of engineering of the University of Virginia, spoke on January 12 on "Thomas Jefferson as a Scientist" before a combined meeting of the Virginia chapters of Sigma Xi and Phi Beta Kappa.

DEAN FRANK C. WHITMORE, of the School of Chemistry and Physics of the Pennsylvania State College, spoke before the Maryland Section of the American Chemical Society in Baltimore on January 20 on "Recent Work on Molecular Rearrangements."

DR. EUGENE C. BINGHAM, professor of chemistry at Lafayette College, will address the sections of the American Chemical Society in the Middle West on "Recent Progress in Rheology" at Indianapolis, Indiana, on February 1; at Dayton, Ohio, on February 2, and at Columbus, Ohio, on February 3.

M. W. STIRLING, chief of the Bureau of American Ethnology, gave a lecture on January 4 at Cornell University entitled "By Airplane to Pigmy Land."

DR. HARRISON S. MARTLAND, chief medical examiner for Essex County, New Jersey, will deliver the ninth Ludvig Hektoen Lecture of the Frank Billings Foundation on February 24. His subject will be "Recent Progress in the Medicolegal Field in the United States."

DR. MARIUS BARBEAU, ethnologist at the National Museum of Canada, delivered an address illustrated with motion pictures and lantern slides on "French Canada: Its Survival" before the Washington Academy of Sciences on January 12.

SIR T. CRISP ENGLISH will give the Hunterian Oration of the Hunterian Society, London, on February 27.

FRIENDS of Sir James G. Frazer have founded a lectureship in the University of Glasgow, a condition of the foundation being that Sir James Frazer, during his lifetime, should deliver in Glasgow one lecture each year. It has been arranged that Sir James Frazer will deliver his first lecture on March 3, 1933.

THE Royal Society Mond Laboratory at Cambridge will be opened by the chancellor of the university, the Right Honorable Stanley Baldwin, on February 3.

WESTERN RESERVE UNIVERSITY has received a gift of three hundred thousand dollars to found the Oliver H. Payne chair of surgery in the School of Medicine. Dr. Carl H. Lenhart has been appointed the first incumbent.

THE late Dr. William Sydney Thayer, of the Johns Hopkins University, left his collection of medical books to the Welch Library of the university and valuable prints to Harvard University.

BY the will of the late William J. Holland his collection of insects is left to the Carnegie Museum, on condition that a fund of $10,000 for making additions to it is set up. Should the Carnegie Museum not accept the bequest the collection goes to the U. S. National Museum.

DR. JAMES ALEXANDER URE, who died on November 20, bequeathed his estate to the University of Glasgow. The bequest, of the approximate value of £13,000, is to be used for scholarships and prizes in medicine, and especially for research on cancer and tuberculosis.

WE learn from the London *Times* that the British Association held on January 6 at Birkbeck College the usual meetings of organizing sectional committees to lay down the lines of the program of the Leicester meeting next September. As under a new statute the annual office of president of the association corresponds with the calendar year, occasion was taken to welcome Sir Frederick Gowland Hopkins, president of the Royal Society, to the chair. Sir Alfred Ewing, the retiring president, in introducing Sir Frederick Hopkins, said that there was no need for him to say how fortunate the association was in securing Sir Frederick Hopkins as president, a man already so preeminent as to be president of the Royal Society. Last year it had been, so to speak, the turn of that part of science which dealt with the constitution of non-living matter and with purely mechanical processes, which could certainly kill, but could not make alive. Now they turned, perhaps with relief and greater hope, to the still more difficult science of life, of whose fascinating problems no one could speak with more authority and clearer discernment than Sir Frederick Hopkins. One felt certain that in his hands the association would lose nothing of the public attention and interest its great annual conference continued to command. More than ever, he believed, the public wished to know about the advances of science, partly because these were now confessedly tentative and incomplete and partly because they might provide some guidance in the urgent perplexities of social affairs. Science had brought new powers and with them new dangers, grave dangers of which the community were scarcely yet aware. It was clearly the duty of science to point these out. After his installation Sir Frederick Hopkins said it was indeed no light task to continue the high tradition attaching to the presidency of the association and he would be well content if he could even approach the standard which Sir Alfred Ewing had so fully maintained.

AT a recent meeting of the directors of the American Chemical Society, the secretary was requested to express the very sincere appreciation of the society to the chemical industry for the aid it has given to *Chemical Abstracts,* and to send those whose agreements expire in 1932 the society's very sincere thanks. The secretary was further instructed to explain to the industry that while there is no hope of *Chemical Abstracts* being continued for any length of time with real efficiency without the continued help of the industry, the society feels that it must draw on its own reserves in 1933 rather than call for further help from the industry under present conditions. The proposal of the editor of *Industrial and Engineering Chemistry* to issue the "Analytical Edition" six times a year instead of four times, as at present, was approved by the directors. His proposal to issue the "News Edition" once a month, on the fifteenth, instead of twice a month, as at present, was not approved, and an additional amount was added to the budget to continue the "News Edition" as at present. It was also voted to defer the issuance of a new directory of the society.

PLANS for an arboretum comparable with the best in the United States are described in the report of the Arthur H. Scott Horticultural Foundation, prepared by John C. Wister, director, and issued as a supplement to the annual report of Swarthmore College. The purpose of the foundation is expressed as a desire "to help horticulture by visual demonstration which can be best realized by the planting in a public place of such trees, shrubs and flowers as can be used by people of average means living in the Philadelphia district." On the campus of Swarthmore the emphasis is placed on showy flowers that are suitable for planting in small gardens. There are at present about fifty kinds of lilacs, nearly fifty kinds of rhododendrons, fifty kinds of azaleas, over thirty kinds of cherries, about thirty kinds of apples, and over 100 kinds each of iris, peonies, daffodils and chrysanthemums—in all about 1,200 different plants. The largest project to be undertaken is the formation of the Scott Arboretum in the Crum Creek Valley, some one hundred and seventy-five acres of virgin timber and uncultivated river silt, which will be divided into four sections. One will contain only those plants, shrubs and trees native to Delaware County; a second area will have trees native to Pennsylvania but not native to Delaware County; a third will have plants and trees native to the North American Continent, and the final group trees which grow in this climate in other parts of the world.

THE next annual congress of the Royal Institute of Public Health will be held at Eastbourne from May 30 to June 4, under the presidency of Viscount Leverhulme. The scientific work of the congress will be conducted in the following sections: (1) State medicine and industrial hygiene; (2) women and children and the public health; (3) tuberculosis; (4) pathology, bacteriology, biochemistry and veterinary medicine; (5) climatology and hydrology. Delegates are being invited from the governments, the municipalities, the universities and other public bodies of Great Britain and Ireland and the British Dominions, as well as from Continental and foreign countries. Arrangements have been made with the railway companies for a reduction in the fares. The headquarters of the institute are now at 23, Queen Square, W.C.1.

*Nature* reports that the preparatory work of the organizing committee at Stockholm of the next World

Power Conference, which will take place in 1933 in Scandinavia, is proceeding steadily. The first plenary World Power Conference was held in London in 1924, the next in Berlin in 1930. There have also been sectional meetings with special programs, for example, at Basel in 1926 and London in 1928. The Scandinavian Conference will be such a special meeting, dealing with the energy problems of large industry and transport. Participation and collaboration of fifteen countries outside Scandinavia is assured and more than one hundred and seventy reports are announced. Some forty reports to be published at the meeting deal with problems of energy supply in large-scale industry, such as combined power and heat supply, the rôle of large-scale industry in national power schemes, etc. Many of the technical papers deal with the problems of long distance gas transmission, while other papers are devoted to more special power problems concerning the iron and steel industry, pulp and paper, and cement, sugar, textile and other steam heat consuming industries. Energy questions of transport provide the subjects for sixty-two reports; railway and marine transport, the peculiarities of city and suburban traffic are to be discussed with due emphasis on the new aspects which have been introduced by electric traction and Diesel engines.

# DISCUSSION

## ETHER STRUCTURE

IN SCIENCE for February 21, 1930, I proposed an explanation of the action of electric force and induction across a vacuum, that is, across the ether. The suggestion was to extend to the ether the conception used by Debye, that the dielectric properties of gases and electrolytes depend upon polarized ions or "dipoles" of the medium. The ether is thus to be conceived as having a structure, that is, with "ether dipoles" or polarized cells. From this we get directly the idea that an electric field produces linear arrangements of the ether dipoles, and this may have an effect on polarized light similar to crystal action. I have made an experiment to detect such possible effect. The electric field was between two aluminum strips 60 centimeters long and 1 centimeter wide and 0.5 centimeter apart. This condenser was in a high vacuum. The vacuum was so high that no discharge took place when the condenser plates were charged by a Holtz machine to approximately 30,000 volts. The electric field was horizontal. A beam of polarized light, with polarization plane at 45° to the horizontal was passed across the electric field. Not the slightest effect on the light could be detected when the field was put on and off. The analyzer was of the strained glass bar type ("Rayleigh Compensator") used by the late Lord Rayleigh in his experiment to detect a possible double refraction due to ether drift.[1] The sensitiveness was at least six seconds of rotation per centimeter beam length in the field. The field was about 60,000 volts per centimeter. Thus this experiment to detect an ether structure, like experiments for ether drift, gave a negative result. On a corpuscular light theory, the above experiment can also be interpreted as showing no electric moment of the light corpuscle or photon in the above conditions.

ALBERT P. CARMAN

UNIVERSITY OF ILLINOIS

[1] *Phil. Mag.*, p. 680, 1902.

## ENERGY OF UREA SYNTHESIS

IN the study of the energy change in the synthesis of urea from ammonia and carbon dioxide by liver slices we have found that synthesis of urea is accompanied by a definite and measurable increase in oxygen consumption. Our present facilities do not permit of precise measurements, but the results so far obtained suggest that one additional molecule of oxygen is used for every molecule of urea synthesized. Similar values were obtained with both glucose and d-1 lactate as fuel, and with and without ornithine. Comparison of the rates of synthesis of urea suggest that the fuel in this reaction is lactate or some product derived from it. It seems unlikely that more than a fraction of the specific dynamic action of protein can be accounted for by the superfluous energy released in the synthesis of urea from ammonia. Further experiments are in progress.

H. BORSOOK
G. KEIGHLEY

W. G. KERCKHOFF LABORATORIES OF THE BIOLOGICAL SCIENCES,
CALIFORNIA INSTITUTE OF TECHNOLOGY

## HETEROSIS: SPECIFIC NOT GENERAL IN NATURE

IN studies of hybrid vigor or heterosis in $F_1$ oat plants, variable results were obtained from different crosses. In the $F_1$ of some crosses nearly all the measurable parts are greater in the $F_1$ hybrid than in the larger parent. In other crosses possibly only one or two characters are noticeably increased. The difficulty of obtaining oat crosses in large numbers is a serious obstacle to studies of heterosis in oats, but it is believed that an increase of 10 per cent. over the larger parent may safely be considered a significant increase where small numbers are involved. Examples of these results are found in the cross Richland × Fulghum and Richland × Markton. In the first cross the $F_1$ plants averaged 13.2 per cent. taller, bore

17.5 per cent. more culms per plant, weighed 48.5 per cent. more, and yielded 35.2 per cent. more grain and 51.3 per cent. more straw on the average than the larger parent. In all other characters the hybrids were intermediate between the parents. In the second cross the $F_1$ plants yielded 18.9 per cent. more grain, and the grain-straw ratio was increased 33.8 per cent. over that of the larger parent. In all other characters the $F_1$ plants of this cross were intermediate in size between the parents. In other crosses other characters manifested the influence of heterosis.

Heterosis is commonly accepted as having a genetic basis and as such this increase in plant size is satisfactorily explained as being due to the bringing together in the $F_1$ of the growth factors present in both parents. The impression seems quite generally held that when heterosis occurs in an $F_1$ hybrid individual the increased size is of a more or less general nature, extending to all or most all the measurable parts of the hybrid organism. In the light of available knowledge it appears that this widely held conception may need some revision. Barring actual linkage, heterosis is a condition which more often has a rather high degree of specificity. In some crosses a number of the parts of the $F_1$ hybrid plant may show influence of heterosis, yet it does not necessarily follow that the parts are closely linked genetically. The fact that in some $F_1$ crosses only a single plant part shows the influence of heterosis, while in others there may be several showing increased size, definitely indicates lack of genetic linkage.

F. A. COFFMAN

BUREAU OF PLANT INDUSTRY
U. S. DEPARTMENT OF AGRICULTURE

## THE PRODUCTION OF NUTRITIONAL ANEMIA IN WHITE RATS

I HAVE read with interest the article entitled, "A Reliable Method for the Production of Nutritional Anemia in White Rats," by Robert S. Harris, which appears in SCIENCE for November 25. We have been feeding Klim to produce anemia in this laboratory for some time. At first[1] we reconstituted it by adding water, but for nearly two years now we have been feeding the dry powder, and have suggested it to a number of other laboratories.

Klim, being dried by a spray process, has less opportunity for metallic contamination than drum process milk powders. By purchasing in quantities of 500 pounds or more we have been able to standardize on the product of one plant, which runs quite uniform at 3 to 5 parts per million of iron and 1 to 2 parts per million of copper. This amount of copper corresponds very closely with that shown to be present in uncontaminated whole milk from different areas by Elvehjem and Steenbock and Hart.[2]

That Harris is able to produce a more pronounced anemia in a shorter time than we have reported[3] is probably due to a difference in method of handling prior to placing on the Klim diet. Elvehjem and Kemmerer[4] have shown that if young rats from the twelfth day, when their eyes open, do not have access to any supplemental food other than cow's milk, anemia develops very rapidly, whereas if allowed to partake of the usual solid breeding diet between the 12th and 21st (or 28th) day of age, development of anemia on a subsequent milk diet is much slower.

Harris' observation that there is an inverse relationship between rate of growth and hemoglobin is in agreement with the findings of other laboratories.

ROE E. REMINGTON

MEDICAL COLLEGE OF THE
STATE OF SOUTH CAROLINA

[1] Levine, Remington and Culp, *Jour. of Nutrition*, 4: 469, 1931.

[2] *J. Biol. Chem.*, 83: 27, 1929.

[3] Levine, Culp and Anderson, *Jour. of Nutrition*, 5: 295, 1932; and Coulson, Levine and Remington, *Amer. Jour. Public Health*, 22: 1141, 1932.

[4] *Jour. Biol. Chem.*, 93: 189, 1931.

## MOSQUITOES KILL LIVE STOCK

REPORTS of the death of live stock and even of man as a result of mosquito attack are current, but apparently few of these have been verified. It seems desirable, therefore, to record a recent outbreak of *Psorophora columbiae* Dyar and Knab, in Florida, which resulted in the death of at least 173 head of live stock and poultry.

This outbreak came suddenly and with great fury on the night of September 5 and continued for several days. The losses were most severe the first night, many animals being found dead or nearly so the following morning. Mr. T. E. McNeel, of the Bureau of Entomology, who investigated the outbreak several days after it occurred, made a careful check on reported losses in the vicinity of Miami and verified reports of the death loss of 80 cattle, 67 hogs, 3 horses, 1 mule, 20 chickens and 2 dogs. Reports of losses at other points in the vicinity of the Everglades have been recorded, but have not been checked. Mr. C. D. Mathews, chief of the Bureau of Dairy Inspection of Miami, stated that the milk supply from the Hialeah district was reduced by about 1,000 gallons a day from September 6 to 10 and had not returned to normal on September 20.

The death of the animals was attributed by many to blood loss. The manager of the Miami Soap Company, who received most of the dead stock, stated to Mr. McNeel that when the heads of the animals were cut off there was no flow of blood as normally occurs.

Dr. H. E. Miller performed post-mortem examinations on a number of the animals and stated that no mosquitoes were found in the air passages. While blood loss was no doubt an important factor, it is the writer's opinion that the death of the stock may have been due to the injection of a toxin by the mosquitoes as well as to the loss of blood.

In the case of the larger herds the cattle apparently protected themselves to some extent by bunching closely together, and those which had access to the canal stayed in the water up to their heads, and very little loss occurred in these herds. Smudges and applications of grease and oil were extensively used, and no doubt prevented greater death losses.

*Psorophora columbiae* is one of the smaller species of the genus. The eggs are laid on the soil and hatch quickly when submerged. Thus, great swarms of adults emerge almost simultaneously when egg-bearing areas are flooded. The species is usually of little importance as a pest of man. In this outbreak, however, it is reported that men who were making smudges and otherwise looking after stock had to wear heavy coats and blankets to protect themselves, and some of them stated that they were sick for several days from the bites of the mosquitoes.

F. C. BISHOPP

BUREAU OF ENTOMOLOGY
U. S. DEPARTMENT OF AGRICULTURE

# SCIENTIFIC APPARATUS AND LABORATORY METHODS

## AN ILLUMINATOR TO FACILITATE THE TRACING OF X-RAYS

IN studying x-rays of the organs of speech it is frequently necessary to make tracings of the films. Manufactured illuminators, intended for viewing films, are inadequate for tracing. They provide no surrounding board to which materials may be fastened; they are not convenient to work on; they heat up rapidly; and they are expensive.

The illuminator shown in the figure can be made cheaply and has none of these disadvantages. It consists primarily of an ordinary drawing board which can be tilted to any convenient angle by shifting the support (B). The strip (A) prevents objects from sliding off. A removable glass (D) of the appropriate size is set in the center of the board. Clear or opalescent glass may be substituted at will. (C) is a piece of clear glass between the bulb and the surface glass to deflect and absorb the heat. It, also, is removable to permit easy changing of the lamp. The tin reflector spreads at the sides to allow free ventilation. This illuminator has been used for several hours at a time without gettting hot.

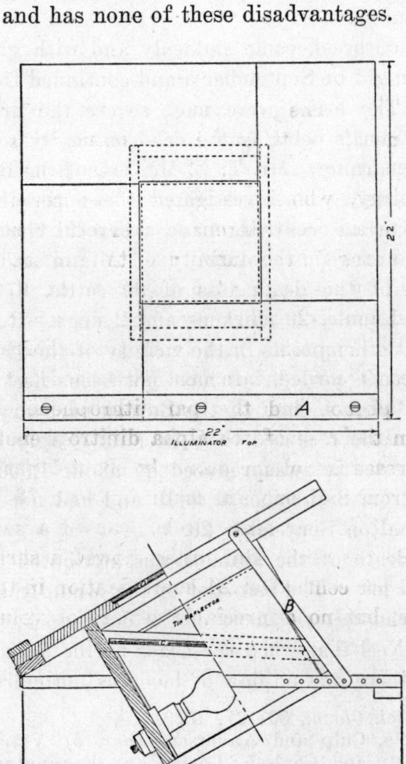


Masks of black paper, to cover all but the parts being traced, are provided and may be pinned to the board. By their use lines in the x-ray which seem to have been obliterated by overexposure can frequently be found and traced.

C. A. BEVANS

PHONETICS LABORATORY
THE UNIVERSITY OF CHICAGO

## A LARGE RESPIROMETER[1]

IN making some studies of the catalase, nitrogen and carbohydrate changes in asparagus roots after various treatments to break dormancy it was thought desirable to have some information on the respiration while these changes are going on.

Many difficulties were experienced in finding a respirometer which could be satisfactory. Nothing found in the literature described containers large enough to hold the plant roots which were being studied. The usual NaOH containers were too small to hold the amount of carbon dioxide given off in a 48 hour period, and more frequent weighing and measuring was not thought worth while.

After many different set-ups were made and several

[1] Contribution No. 113, Department of Horticulture, Kansas Agricultural Experiment Station.

different arrangements were tried, one which is herewith described (Fig. 1) was found satisfactory in

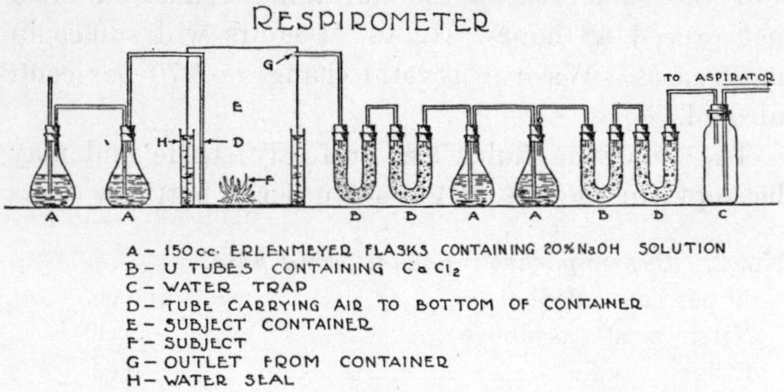


FIG. 1

every respect, including low cost for material and equipment.

The principal divergence from the customary respirometer is the subject container. This was made of galvanized iron. The air which has had the carbon dioxide removed in the pair of NaOH bottles (A) is drawn in at the top of the respiration chamber and carried to the bottom of the container in the metal tube (D). The air with the carbon dioxide of the asparagus respiration is then carried out of the container from the top through the opening (G). In this way there is a continuous change of the air in the container.

In using this container the greatest difficulty was experienced in making an air-tight seal which could be broken easily and frequently for examination of the asparagus root. Sealing wax, paraffin, grafting wax and similar materials had many objections. In no case could a tight seal be held for more than 12 hours, because the waxes withdrew from the galvanized iron container and the base, whether the base was metal or glass. To avoid this difficulty a base was made for the container, and in this base is a double-walled collar. The asparagus roots were set in this base. The side of the galvanized iron subject container fitted in between the walls. The double wall was then filled with water. No further trouble was experienced with air leaking through the container, and the respirometer has been in continuous operation for as long as 48 hours and no leaking has been detected.

An easy check for leaks is made by setting the respirometer up without putting a plant in the container. By introducing carbon-dioxide free air into the container and then passing the air through the entire apparatus the operator is able to take some carbon dioxide out at the aspirator, if there is any leaking in the system. None has been found after two interrupted 24-hour tests and one continuous 48-hour test.

This apparatus has the advantages of being easily and cheaply constructed, can be opened and closed easily and seemingly is satisfactory for measuring the amount of carbon dioxide given off by plants in the dark.

WALTER B. BALCH

## NEW FIXING FLUIDS FOR GENERAL PURPOSES

THE number of fixing fluids recommended up to date is admittedly very great. The excuse for the new formulae given here lies in the fact that all other fluids with which I am familiar, either harden the tissues too much or interfere with subsequent staining. Serial sectioning is often made very difficult, while macroscopic dissection becomes almost impossible. In addition, many fluids require prolonged washing. The duration of fixation is also often very limited, resulting in great inconvenience when one attempts to use the fluids on scientific expeditions. The new fluids recommended here represent the results of extensive experimentation extending over many years and are more or less free from the above-mentioned defects. Animals fixed in them remain soft and do not harden subsequently in 70 per cent. alcohol in which they may be left for many weeks. Washing is simple. All common stains may be used. Mallory's triple stain gives brilliant differentiation, though the picture is somewhat different from that obtained after fixation in Zenker's fluid. Complete penetration of all ingredients of the fluids is accomplished at the rate of one half millimeter per hour, but the nitric acid penetrates twice as rapidly. This was determined by an examination of pieces of liver at intervals of one hour. The surface of a smooth cut shows the fixed zone clearly. The penetration of paranitrophenol was determined by wetting the cut surface with ammonia and measuring the width of the zone in which the tissues turned yellow. Similarly, the penetration of cupric nitrate was determined with sodium sulfide.

The change in volume due to fixation was determined by measuring the displacement of water before fixation and after fixation. This was done by Dr. G. E. Pickford, who found an average swelling of about 10 per cent. in beef liver fixed for 24 hours in the phenol and the paranithrophenol mixtures, while in the case of the alpha dinitrophenol mixture the increase in volume was only about 5 per cent. A paranitrophenol mixture made up with 70 per cent. instead of 60 per cent. alcohol caused a swelling of about 20 per cent. Rat testes showed a shrinkage of about 5 per cent. after 24 hours fixation in the phenol mixture, but no appreciable change of volume after fixation in the paranithrophenol mixture. When transferred to 70 per cent. alcohol for 9 days, both showed an increase in volume; in the case of the testis fixed in the phenol mixture the increase amounted to about 13.5 per cent., in the case of that fixed in the paranitrophenol mixture to about 16 per cent. Transferred for 10 days into 80 per cent.

alcohol the first testis showed no further change in volume, while the second showed an increase to about 20 per cent. of its original size.

Phenol gives a peculiar elastic texture to the tissues, unlike anything produced by commonly used fixing fluids. Paranitrophenol comes nearest to phenol in this respect and, being stable in the mixture, is preferable where stability is desired. I have used both mixtures for arachnids, insects, myriapods, leeches, earthworms, flatworms, roundworms, older amphibian larvae and mammalian embryos. Professor J. S. Nicholas, of our department, is using my paranitrophenol mixture for rat embryos and fish in preference to sublimate or Bouin, while Professor W. R. Coe finds it very satisfactory for nemerteans. Macroscopic dissection of invertebrates and mammalian embryos fixed in either of these fluids is greatly facilitated.

No. 1. *Cupric-phenol fixing fluid.*

Stock Solution A.

| | |
|---|---|
| Distilled water | 100 cc |
| Nitric acid, c.p., sp.gr. 1.41–1.42 | 12 cc |
| Cupric nitrate, c.p., crystals $Cu(NO_3)_2 \cdot 3H_2O$ | 8 grams |

Stock Solution B.

| | |
|---|---|
| 80 per cent. alcohol | 100 cc |
| Phenol, crystals, c.p. | 4 grams |
| Ether | 6 cc |

The stock solutions are perfectly stable and may be kept in glass-stoppered bottles. For use take: Solution A—1 part, Solution B—3 parts. The mixture does not keep and must be used within a few hours. For the same reason the duration of fixation must not exceed 48 hours. 12 to 24 hours will suffice in most cases. Wash in several changes of 70 per cent. alcohol.

The following fluids are perfectly stable and may be kept for months in glass-stoppered bottles:

No. 2. *Cupric-paranitrophenol fixing fluid.*

| | |
|---|---|
| 60 per cent. alcohol | 100 cc |
| Nitric acid (as above) | 3 cc |
| Ether | 5 cc |
| Cupric nitrate (as above) | 2 grams |
| Paranitrophenol, c.p., crystals | 5 grams |

Duration of fixation not limited by time, except as to the minimum time required for penetration at the rate of one half millimeter per hour. Wash in several changes of 70 per cent. alcohol.

No. 3 to No. 6: These fixing fluids have the same composition as No. 2, except that in place of 5 grams of paranithrophenol they contain 0.5 gram of one of the following nitroderivatives of phenol: No. 3—orthonitrophenol, No. 4—alpha (2:4) dinitrophenol, No. 5—beta (2:6) dinitrophenol, No. 6—picric acid (2:4:6 trinitrophenol). Fixation and washing as in No. 2, but Nos. 5 and 6 require longer washing and leave the tissues yellow.

ALEXANDER PETRUNKEVITCH

YALE UNIVERSITY

# SPECIAL ARTICLES

## VARIATIONS IN VISIBLE SOLAR LIGHT DURING SUBMARINE MEASUREMENTS

WHILE making measurements on the intensity of some of the components of visible solar light beneath the surface of ocean waters, variations in the intensity of the incident light were found to be of such magnitude, on some days, that considerable uncertainties are introduced into the results if these variations are unaccounted for. These variations are not ones which depend upon zenith distance, but are occasioned by other circumstances. They are of particular importance when the depth of water is such that very small currents result in the submerged photoelectric cell. These variations occur on days when the sky is cloudless and the atmosphere very clear to the eye.

The time required to make a series of measurements of illumination intensity beneath the sea with a photoelectric cell to a depth of 50 meters, say, is an hour or more if one-meter intervals are chosen as unit layers of the absorbing medium. During this time the illumination intensity of the radiation incident upon the surface of the water changes slowly with the variation in the solar zenith distance. Also, the intensity of the visible light may vary within a few minutes by several per cent., even though there be a cloudless sky and a clear atmosphere. A study of these variations made during the summer of 1932 at the Friday Harbor (Washington) station of the Oceanographic Laboratories also show that a record of the total radiation intensity on a horizontal surface is not indicative of all changes which may occur in the illumination intensity.

Such variations are shown in Fig. 1. The total radiation was measured by means of an Eppley pyrheliometer connected to an Engelhard recorder. This instrument had recently been calibrated by Dr. Herbert H. Kimball in charge of solar radiation for the U. S. Department of Agriculture. The illumination intensity was measured by means of a calibrated photoelectric cell.

The curves in Fig. 1 are characteristic of the obser-

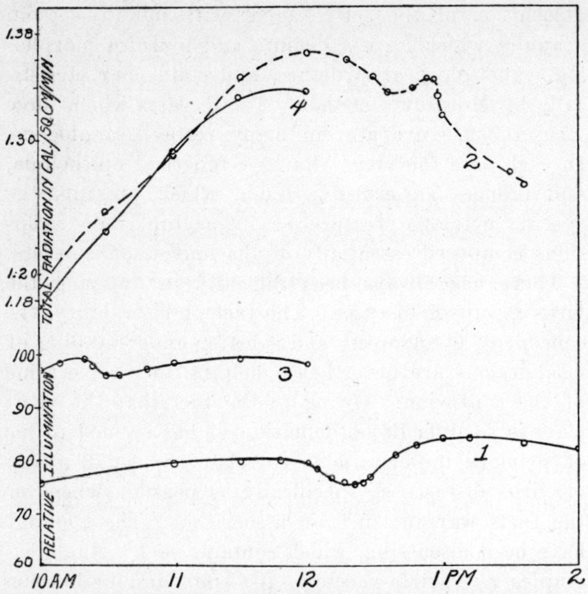


FIG. 1. Showing the variations in solar illumination intensity and total radiation.

vations. In making the observations the pyrheliometer and the cell were located near each other. Days were selected when there was no evidence of clouds or haze. The air in the region of the laboratories was entirely free from smoke. The days on which observations were made can well be called clear and cloudless.

Curves 1 and 2 were plotted from observations made on July 26, while curves 3 and 4 show the variations several days later. Curves 1 and 3 show the variations in the solar illumination intensity. Curves 2 and 4 show, respectively, the simultaneous variations in the total radiation. These data were selected from a series of observations to exhibit the magnitude and rapidity of the changes in illumination.

It is at once apparent from the illumination curves that on these days rather rapid changes are superimposed upon the changes due to zenith distance. Also, changes in illumination are not indicated by changes in the total radiation, although in curve 2 of July 26 a rather small but sudden change occurs in the total radiation at 11 A. M., and another more marked change between 12:40 and 1 P. M. Curve 4 shows only the gradual change in total energy, while simultaneous readings of illumination show a sudden change at about 10:20 A. M.

That a relation exists between radiation intensity and illumination has been shown by Kimball.[1] This relation is that radiation in calories per minute per $cm^2$ on a horizontal surface multiplied by 6,700 will give the illumination in foot-candles on a horizontal surface within $\pm 5$ per cent., the variation being characteristic of the position of the sun. This relation agrees, in general, with the present results, but does not account for the rapid changes found.

[1] H. H. Kimball, *Mo. Weather Rev.*, 52: 473, 1924.

In a study of the penetration of light into water, Shelford and Gail[2] did not take into account any variations in the incident light, although they apparently suspected variations to exist. In a later study, Shelford[3] *assumes* that, under a cloudless sky and a very clear atmosphere, the intensity of the visible solar light incident on the surface of water is constant between the hours of 10 A. M. and 2:30 P. M. Variations due to solar zenith distance and the smaller variations illustrated in curves 1 and 3 show that such constancy does not exist.

Poole and Atkins,[4] during a series of determinations of the penetration of the *total* visible light into the sea near Plymouth, found variations in the incident light with a bright sun, although they do not state that the sky was cloudless and the atmosphere clear.

It is evident that in making measurements of the absorption of visible light by ocean waters a knowledge of the variations in the incident light is quite necessary. The results of a study of the penetration of some of the components of visible solar light into the waters of Puget Sound and of Southern Alaska will be published soon.

C. L. UTTERBACK

OCEANOGRAPHIC LABORATORIES
UNIVERSITY OF WASHINGTON

## BORRELIOTOSES: FOWL-POX, MOLLUSCUM CONTAGIOSUM, VARIOLA-VACCINIA

THE judgment first expressed by Borrel,[1] that the specific granules of fowl-pox may well be the actual virus of this disease, a view later held by Lipschütz and by Paschen with respect to the specific granules of molluscum contagiosum and vaccinia, has received from recent studies strong support. Evidence has likewise accumulated which effectively upholds the view that the specific cellular inclusions (Bollinger bodies, molluscum bodies, Guarnieri bodies) of these three infections are composed essentially of colonies of the respective viruses which appear to be microorganisms and seem to require an intracellular environment in their hosts for their reproduction.[2,3,4,5]

[2] V. E. Shelford and F. W. Gail, *Pub. Puget Sound Biol. Sta.*, 3: 141, 1922.

[3] V. E. Shelford, *Pub. Puget Sound Biol. Sta.*, 7: 151, 1929.

[4] H. H. Poole and W. R. G. Atkins, *Jour. Marine Biol. Assoc.*, 14: 170, 1926; *ibid.*, 15: 455, 1928.

[1] A. Borrel, ''Sur les inclusions de l'epithelioma contagieux des oiseaux,'' *Compt. Rend. Soc. Biol.* 57: 642, 1904.

[2] C. E. Woodruff and E. W. Goodpasture, ''The Infectivity of Isolated Inclusion Bodies of Fowl-Pox,'' *Amer. Jour. Path.*, 5: 1, 1929.

[3] E. W. Goodpasture and C. E. Woodruff, ''A Com-

This evidence in substance may be summarized as follows: It has been demonstrated that the specific cellular inclusions of fowl-pox, molluscum contagiosum and vaccinia, namely, the Bollinger bodies, molluscum bodies and the Guarnieri bodies, are composed in large part of compact aggregations of enormous numbers of specific granules, respectively the Borrel, the Lipschütz and the Paschen corpuscles. There is good evidence that the great mass of these corpuscles if not all are regenerated within the infected cell. In the case of fowl-pox it has been proven that individual inclusions are totally and fractionally infective.[6] The corpuscles of fowl-pox, molluscum and vaccinia are demonstrably filterable. These granules, unlike the banal proteid granulations of cells, are not dissolved by dilute acids and they are resistant to tryptic digestion. They are likewise insoluble in lipoid solvents. In the case of the granules of fowl-pox and vaccinia there is agglutination in the presence of specific immune serum,[7] and in suspensions of virus centrifuged at high speed there is a marked parallelism between the concentration of specific granules and the concentration of virus. The vaccinia corpuscles have been found to increase in tissue cultures containing the virus. There is morphologic evidence of division of the granules by fission. Finally these granules react characteristically to certain staining methods, notably the silver method of Morosow, so that demonstration of them in preparations which contain them in considerable amount is thoroughly reliable in the hands of competent observers.[8] They are not readily or at all exhibited by the staining methods used to demonstrate bacteria. While the final demonstration of reproduction of these granules in the absence of tissue cells has not yet been attained, there is sufficient reason for judging that one is dealing here with a group of viruses which are micro-organisms and, in natural infections, obligatory cytotropes.

In the entire field of cytotropic viruses these are the only ones which present conclusive evidence of an association of the active agent with minute coccoid granules which have a definite and uniform morphologic and physical structure, and stain characteristically by Morosow's method. The diseases which these viruses cause are also in many respects analogous. In each case the virus attacks ectodermal epithelium, and induces an eruptive lesion which presents the specific cytologic feature of intracytoplasmic inclusions composed essentially of the uniform corpuscles.

There has always been difficulty in unifying the virus group of diseases. The fact of filterability, the concept of cytotropism and a better understanding of viral lesions are nevertheless helping to resolve some of the confusion. Owing to the fact that the virus class is so difficult of definition, it has seemed to me of primary importance to correlate any small group of virus diseases as specifically as possible whenever the facts warrant such an association. The group I have been discussing, which contains such notable examples as variola-vaccinia, fowl-pox and molluscum contagiosum, is at the present time separable from the general class of virus diseases into a more homogeneous one because of the presence of visible granules which have definite and similar characteristics and constitute an essential part of their analogous specific lesions. I therefore think it justifiable at this time to designate this group by generic and specific names on the basis of their specific granules, and I would suggest that fowl-pox be taken as the generic type. It was Borrel who in 1904 first discovered the specific coccoid granules of this disease, and later investigators have shown that they constitute the essential component of the cellular inclusions, that they are fractionally infective, and that the so-called Borrel bodies are filterable and specifically agglutinable by immune serum. It would therefore seem appropriate that Borrel's name should be associated with this group.

There is no adequate proof, however, that the granules of these diseases are viable, nor for that matter, that any cytotropic virus is a living thing; consequently a name which would at present classify these corpuscles among the living agents of disease might be misleading. One should rather choose a specific name which is non-committal as to the biological status of the agent.

I would therefore propose the name *Borreliota* as a generic title. The suffix *iota,* the Latinized name of the smallest Greek letter, has I am told by reliable authorities, an ancient and honorable usage signifying smallest particle. Translated in this sense the title Borreliota would mean the small particles or corpuscles of Borrel. The form Borreliota is either singular or plural.

The difficulty of applying specific terminology to

---

parison of the Inclusion Bodies of Fowl-Pox and Molluscum contagiosum,'' *Amer. Jour. Path.*, 7: 1, 1931.

[4] E. G. Nauck and E. Paschen, ''Der Morphologische Nachweis des Pockenerregers in der Gewebekultur,'' *Zentralbl. f. Bact.*, 124, (Orig): 91, 1932.

[5] E. W. Goodpasture, A. M. Woodruff and G. J. Buddingh, ''Vaccinal Infection of the Chorio-allantoic Membrane of the Chick Embryo,'' *Amer. Jour. Path.*, 8: 271, 1932.

[6] C. E. Woodruff and E. W. Goodpasture, ''The Relation of the Virus of Fowl-Pox to the Specific Cellular Inclusions of the Disease,'' *Amer. Jour. Path.*, 4: 713, 1930.

[7] J. C. G. Ledingham, ''The Aetiological Importance of the Elementary Bodies in Vaccinia and Fowl-Pox,'' *Lancet*, 525, Sept. 5, 1931.

[8] M. A. Morosow, ''Die Färbung der Paschenschen Körperchen durch Versilberung,'' *Centralbl. f. Bakt.*, I. Orig., 100: 385, 1926.

certain members of this group is apparent when one considers the fact that the virus of smallpox and that of cow-pox, while differing in certain important ways, are in reality to be considered modifications of the same virus, because they cross-immunize against each other. In other words there is not a specific difference between them, and this probably applies to other modified strains such as those of horse-pox, swine-pox, goat- and sheep-pox. It would therefore seem advisable to use not only a specific, but a sub-specific or variety name for the corpuscles of such related strains. I would therefore propose the following terminology:

*Borreliota variolae hominis:* specific corpuscles of small-pox (Paschen bodies, elementary corpuscles).

*Borreliota variolae bovis:* specific corpuscles of vaccinia (Paschen bodies, elementary corpuscles).

*Borreliota variolae equi:* specific corpuscles of horse-pox.

*Borreliota variolae porci:* specific corpuscles of swine-pox.

*Borreliota variolae ovium:* specific corpuscles of sheep and goat-pox.

*Borreliota mollusci:* specific corpuscles of molluscum contagiosum (Lipschütz corpuscles).

*Borreliota avium:* specific corpuscles of fowl-pox (Borrel corpuscles).

The acceptance of such a nomenclature based upon adequate experimental data would do much to attract attention to this related group as a whole, and would obviate the great confusion of terms now in use such as Borrel bodies, Lipschütz granules, Paschen corpuscles, elementary bodies and so on. At the same time the probability that the specific granules in question represent micro-organismal etiological agents would be duly recognized.

ERNEST W. GOODPASTURE
VANDERBILT UNIVERSITY MEDICAL SCHOOL

## A CONTRIBUTION TO VOWEL THEORY[1]

Two main theories of vowel production have been advanced, namely, the harmonic or steady state theory and the inharmonic or transient theory. The harmonic theory, advocated mainly by Wheatstone, Helmholtz and D. C. Miller, holds that the vocal cords generate a complex wave having a fundamental and a large number of harmonics. A wave at its source will contain all the frequencies that it will ever contain. The so-called resonating cavities (pharynx, mouth, nasal cavities, paranasal sinuses) will act to magnify those frequencies of the wave near the resonating frequencies of the cavities, the amount of amplification depending upon the damping constant of the cavity. The reinforced frequency bands determine the vowel quality.

The inharmonic or cavity tone theory, advocated mainly by Dodart, Willis and Scripture, holds that the wave or series of puffs from the vocal cords acts only as an agent for exciting the transient frequencies that are characteristic of the resonating cavities. Certain frequencies in the wave need not be present in the source but may be added by the resonating chambers. According to this theory, the vocal cords emit puffs of air, each puff setting the air in the above cavities into vibration, resulting in the so-called "cavity tones." The frequency of a cavity tone is determined by the natural frequency of the cavity, and is not dependent on any frequency aspect of the exciting or cord tone. This vibration of the cavity tone soon diminishes until it is started anew by a second puff. Here, as with the harmonic theory, the vowel quality is dependent upon the natural frequencies and damping constants of the vocal cavities.[2] The findings reported in the present paper tend to add weight to the inharmonic or cavity tone theory.

In order to delimit sharply the problem the head and neck of a cadaver was used to furnish the so-called resonating cavities and a pure sine wave as the force to act on these cavities. Our specimens (two male) presented normally extensive sinuses and normal nasal, oral and pharyngeal cavities (determined by sectioning the head after completion of the experiment). The soft palate was so fixed as to present an opening into both the nasal and the oral cavity which were patent. Both specimens had teeth. The source of the sine wave was a General Radio low frequency oscillator Type 377–B, activating a high-grade head phone. The waves were conveyed to the larynx or directly to the microphone from the head phone by a rubber tube 90 cm long and with a lumen 5 mm in diameter. For studying and recording the waves a Jenkins and Adair C6 condenser microphone with one additional stage of high quality amplification and a Westinghouse oscillograph were used. For all frequencies scouted, 120, 200, 300, 400, 500, 600, 700, 800, 900, 1000 and 1200 ~, the waves were studied first by holding the end of the tube carrying the sound directly in front of the microphone. With the exception of one frequency, 120 ~, all frequencies presented sine waves. Secondly, the waves were studied by placing the nose and mouth of the cadaver directly in front of the microphone after the rubber tube had been inserted through the trachea, into the ventricle of the larynx, just above the level of the vocal cords. The head was suspended from the ceil-

[1] This paper reports a part of a larger research program suggested by the late Dr. Henry J. Prentiss, head of the department of anatomy, University of Iowa. The program is now being kindly supported by Dr. E. M. MacEwen, present head of the department of anatomy.

[2] For a fuller discussion of vowel theories see H. Fletcher, "Speech and Hearing," 1929, Macmillan; and G. O. Russell, "The Vowel," 1928, Ohio State University Press.

ing by small wires in order to avoid the possible resonating effects which might come from supporting it on a table or platform.

For specimen No. 1 the sine waves of frequencies of 200 and 300 ~ and for specimen No. 2 the sine waves of frequencies 200, 500 and 900 ~ were altered in their passage through the specimen. Fig. 1 shows the

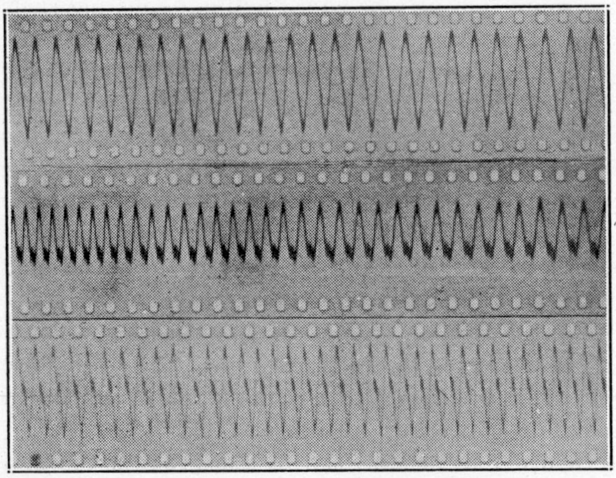

FIG. 1. Oscillogram of relatively pure sine waves (200 ~) led into the larynx of the cadaver. FIG. 2. Oscillogram of the waves emerging from the nose and mouth of the cadaver (specimen No. 2) when the waves depicted in Fig. 1 were being led into the cadaver's larynx. FIG. 3. Oscillogram of the waves emerging from the nose and mouth of the cadaver (specimen No. 1) when relatively pure sine waves of 300 ~ were being led into the cadaver's larynx.

relatively pure sine waves of a frequency of 200 ~ as they were taken directly from the end of the rubber tube. Fig. 2 shows the change produced in this frequency when the tube was inserted into the larynx of specimen No. 2. Fig. 3 shows the change produced in the sine waves of a frequency of 300 ~ by specimen No. 1.

There was a possibility that these changes might be due to the additional column of air imposed upon the vibrating diaphragm of the head phone by the cavities of the head and neck. This was tested by substituting a cardboard cylinder with a small input and output hole for the specimen. The waves emerging from this cylinder proved to be identical with those put into it. The possibility that these changes might be reflected waves was ruled out on the basis of the fact that all relationships between objects in the room were the same for the picking up of both the original input waves and those passing through the specimen. It appears that the alterations in the original waves emerging from the inserted tube occur during the passage of these waves through the cavities of the neck and head of the cadaver. Furthermore, the distortions are not a function of amplitude because the modified wave is smaller than the input wave.

With a more complicated original wave form, one might expect to obtain more striking structural changes in the waves as they emerge from the mouth and nose. We chose purposely the simple sine wave as the one to be modified, reasoning that any change produced in its form would be conclusive in regard to the point in question.

Because the recorded differences between the original waves and those emerging from the cadaver occur between the end of the inserted tube in the larynx and the nasal and oral openings, our results tend to support the cavity tone theory of vowel production. The resultant wave, being no longer pendular, must contain frequencies not present in the source and hence necessarily introduced by the cavities. Certain frequencies were not changed, probably because they did not excite the transient frequencies which were characteristic of the cavities. A close examination of the modified waves shows that a given wave may not be a perfect duplicate of its predecessor; *i.e.,* there is not absolute periodicity in the wave chain. This fits in well with Scripture's general conception of the inharmonic theory that each succeeding puff of air from the vocal cords changes the cavities' contents so that the cavities need not be exactly the same from puff to puff. If our input sine waves contained concealed harmonics, then our results are not so conclusive in favor of the inharmonic theory. However, it is thought that the waves emanating from the cadaver contained frequencies which were not present in the source.

It remains to attack the problem of vowel production with respect to both simple and more complicated input waves in relation to the condition, size and number of the so-called resonating chambers.

LEE EDWARD TRAVIS
PSYCHOPATHIC HOSPITAL
ARCHIBALD R. BUCHANAN
DEPARTMENT OF ANATOMY
UNIVERSITY OF IOWA

## BOOKS RECEIVED

BERLAND, LUCIEN. *Les Arachnides.* Vol. XVI, Encyclopédie Entomologique. Pp. 485. 636 figures. Lechevalier, Paris. 150 fr.

GLENN, OLIVER E. *The Sources of Error.* Pp. 127. Stratford. $1.50.

HILL, A. V. *Chemical Wave Transmission in Nerve.* Pp. ix + 74. 13 figures. Macmillan. $1.25.

MONROE, PAUL, EDITOR. *Report of the Educational Inquiry Commission, Government of Iraq.* Pp. 170. Government Press, Bagdad.

*Tôhoku Imperial University.* Science Reports. Vol. XXI, No. 4. Pp. 270. Illustrated. Maruzen, Tokyo.

VON ZITTEL, KARL A. *Text-book of Paleontology.* Vol. II: Vertebrates, Fishes to Birds. Revised by Arthur S. Woodward. Pp. 464. 533 figures. Macmillan. $7.50.

SPECIAL ISSUE CONTAINING REPORTS OF THE ATLANTIC CITY MEETING OF THE AMERICAN ASSOCIATION FOR THE ADVANCEMENT OF SCIENCE AND ASSOCIATED SOCIETIES

# SCIENCE

VOL. 77 | FRIDAY, FEBRUARY 3, 1933 | No. 1988

*The Atlantic City Meeting of the American Association for the Advancement of Science and Associated Societies:* DR. BURTON E. LIVINGSTON.
*The Meeting in General* 123
*Business Proceedings* 124
*General Officers of the Association* 126
*Membership and Financial Reports* 126
*Schedule of Proposed Meeting Places* 128
*The Secretaries' Conference* 128
*The Academy Conference* 128
*The Press Service* 129
*The Science Exhibition* 129
*The Ninth Award of the Association Prize* 130
*Henry Norris Russell, President Elect of the American Association* 132
*The Newly Elected Permanent Secretary* 133
*General Sessions of the Association* 134
*Scientific Sessions at Atlantic City:*
*Section A (Mathematics) and Related Organizations* 135
*Section B (Physics) and Related Organizations* 137
*Section C (Chemistry)* 139
*Section D (Astronomy)* 139
*Section E (Geology and Geography) and Related Organizations* 140
*Section F (Zoological Sciences) and Related Organizations* 140
*Section G (Botanical Sciences) and Related Organizations* 142
*Programs Related to both Section F and Section G* 145
*Section H (Anthropology)* 147
*Section I (Psychology)* 147
*Section K (Social and Economic Sciences)* 148
*Section L (Historical and Philological Sciences)* 149
*Section M (Engineering)* 150
*Section N (Medical Sciences)* 150
*Section O (Agriculture) and Related Organizations* 152
*Section Q (Education)* 153
*Organizations Related to the Association as a Whole* 154

SCIENCE: A Weekly Journal devoted to the Advancement of Science, edited by J. MCKEEN CATTELL and published every Friday by

THE SCIENCE PRESS

New York City: Grand Central Terminal
Lancaster, Pa. Garrison, N. Y.
Annual Subscription, $6.00 Single Copies, 15 Cts.

SCIENCE is the official organ of the American Association for the Advancement of Science. Information regarding membership in the Association may be secured from the office of the permanent secretary, in the Smithsonian Institution Building, Washington, D. C.

# THE ATLANTIC CITY MEETING OF THE AMERICAN ASSOCIATION FOR THE ADVANCEMENT OF SCIENCE AND ASSOCIATED SOCIETIES

Edited by Dr. BURTON E. LIVINGSTON

GENERAL SECRETARY

## THE MEETING IN GENERAL

THE Atlantic City meeting, which opened on Tuesday evening, December 27, and closed on Saturday, December 31, was the ninety-first meeting of the American Association. While not to be accounted among the largest meetings, this meeting was very successful in every way. Never before had the association met in Atlantic City.

Attendance was estimated as above 3,000. Since many of those who attend our meetings neglect to register, not having railway certificates for validation and not requiring either badge or General Program, it is increasingly difficult to secure anything approaching an actual count. Most of the societies that meet with the association are unable to furnish accurate information concerning attendance at their meetings. The actual registration was 2,066. Of these, 565 came from New York State, 238 were from Pennsylvania, and New Jersey, Massachusetts, the District of Columbia and Maryland sent 178, 177, 172 and 126, respectively. Other states that sent more than 30 were Connecticut (87), Ohio (63), Illinois (44), Virginia (40) and Michigan (34). There were 20 registrants from California, 23 from Maine, 4 from Florida and 2 from Washington. A peculiar aspect of this meeting is illustrated by the fact that only 8 persons registered as from Atlantic City.

This meeting was unusual in the manner of its preparation, for there was no local committee. Local arrangements were made through Mr. A. H. Skean, director of the Atlantic City Convention and Publicity Bureau, for whose very efficient and friendly help the association is deeply grateful. Many Atlantic City hotels furnished session rooms and other facilities, which proved highly satisfactory. The Haddon Hall Hotel was general headquarters, and it was unusually satisfactory. In the Municipal Auditorium unusually adequate space was provided for the science exhibition and the registration offices. Some of the general sessions were held there and also the sessions of several of the special scientific societies. The association is glad to express its appreciative thanks to Mr. Lincoln G. Dickey, director of the auditorium. The sessions of each society were in most cases held in the hotel that was designated as headquarters for that society, and many members were able to attend their society sessions without leaving the hotel in which they had lodgings. Meeting places were all situated on the Boardwalk and distances were not excessive; although taxicab rates were regarded as outrageously high, the taxi service was excellent. Jitney busses gave convenient and rapid transportation at a very reasonable rate.

It is a great pleasure to acknowledge with grateful appreciation the valuable aid given by the Bausch and Lomb Optical Company, the Spencer Lens Company, E. Leitz, Inc., the Eastman Kodak Company and the International Projector Corporation, who placed at the disposal of the association, for use at the many sessions, projection apparatus and microscopes valued at over $10,000.

This meeting encountered no cold weather, although there was considerable rain and mist or fog. Almost every one took exercise and found relaxation in walks along the Boardwalk, with the open sea on one hand and the hotels and shops on the other. It was indeed unusual to have all the meeting places almost within hearing of the perpetual roar and splash of the surf upon the beach.

The General Program, a book of over 200 pages, provided with summary and author index, was edited by Sam Woodley. Copies may be had on request addressed to the Washington office of the association.

Many of the lectures, addresses and scientific contributions given at this meeting, of which there were over 1,500, will appear in the pages of SCIENCE. Most of the technical contributions and some of the more general papers will be published in the journals devoted to the special sciences. In a number of instances those journals have already published abstracts. The American Association does not attempt responsibility for these publications, and any one interested in papers mentioned in this report or listed in the General Program may well write directly to the respective authors, to learn when and where their papers are to be published. But the forthcoming volume reporting Section K's symposium on "The Stabilization of Employment," which will be specially timely and authoritative, constitutes an exception to the general rule; it may be ordered from the Washington office of the association. (See Section M, in this issue of SCIENCE.)

Besides the American Association as a whole and its fifteen sections, about forty associated or invited organizations took part in the ninety-first meeting. These are named in the summarized reports farther on.

Dr. John J. Abel, of the Johns Hopkins University, was president for this meeting. His research work in some of the most difficult fields of pharmacology is known throughout the world and very many eminent scientific workers were guided and inspired by him in their earlier years. Dr. Abel led a symposium on Wednesday afternoon, under the auspices of Section N (Medical Sciences), on "Present Knowledge of the Hypophysis Cerebri."

The retiring president for the Atlantic City meeting was Dr. Franz Boas, of Columbia University, who is called the dean of American anthropologists. His retiring presidential address was given at the opening session Tuesday evening, on "The Aims of Anthropological Research." The address was published in SCIENCE for December 30.

The opening session of the meeting was held on Tuesday evening, at the Municipal Auditorium. Mr. A. H. Skean welcomed the association to Atlantic City, and Professor L. P. Eisenhart, of Princeton University, spoke some appropriate words of welcome for the State of New Jersey. President John J. Abel replied on behalf of the American Association and then introduced the speaker, Retiring President Franz Boas. The general reception was held in the Vernon room of the Haddon Hall Hotel, following the opening session.

Of less strenuous nature, but not less valuable than the scientific and business sessions, were the numerous dinners, luncheons, breakfasts and smokers, arranged by the various organizations, which were generally very well attended at Atlantic City. In addition to these, there were several field or inspection trips.

## BUSINESS PROCEEDINGS AT ATLANTIC CITY

By unanimous vote at the general session held on Thursday evening, December 29, Article 4 of the constitution was amended to provide for council representatives from the divisions. The amended article reads as follows: "The Council shall consist of the president, the vice-presidents, the permanent secretary, the general secretary, the secretaries of the sections, and the treasurer, of one fellow elected by each division, affiliated state academy and affiliated society, and one additional fellow from each affiliated society having more than 100 members who are fellows of the Association, and of eight fellows, two elected annually by the Council for a term of four years."

The executive committee met on Monday evening and Tuesday morning, also following the council sessions on Wednesday, Thursday and Friday mornings. The council met on Tuesday afternoon and Wednesday, Thursday and Friday mornings. Chairmen for these four sessions were, respectively: Dugald C. Jackson, Charles Zeleny, Burton E. Livingston and Dugald C. Jackson. Items of business were transacted as follows:

1. The privileges of the Atlantic City meeting were cordially extended to Dr. W. F. G. Swann, official representative of the British Association for the Advancement of Science.

2. The audited financial reports of the treasurer and of the permanent secretary for 1931–32 were accepted, also the permanent secretary's report on membership, as of September 30, 1932. (Some notes on these reports are presented in the next following section of this general report.)

3. Balanced budgets for 1932–33, proposed by the treasurer and by the permanent secretary, were approved.

4. The permanent secretary reported a bequest of $500 from Miss Luella Agnes Owen, of St. Joseph, Missouri, who died on May 31, 1932, after many years of membership in the association. The council expressed its great appreciation of this bequest and voted that it should be the nucleus of an endowment fund, the income from which is to be used for creating emeritus annual memberships in the association.

5. The council voted that the fees of all deceased emeritus life members be transferred from the general fund of life-membership fees to the Jane M. Smith fund, and that, in future, this transfer is to be made as emeritus life members become deceased. (The Jane M. Smith fund is a bequest of $5,000, the income from which is used annually for the establishment of emeritus life memberships. The principal is now increased to $7,500.)

6. William Matlack (M '78), William Fellowes Morgan ( M'78, F '32) and Nathaniel Lord Britton (M '78, F '82) were elected to emeritus life membership.

7. The sum of $300, of the treasurer's available funds (principally income from the Jane M. Smith fund for 1931–32) was appropriated for the three emeritus life memberships just mentioned.

8. The council appropriated research grants from treasury funds as follows: Henry B. Ward, a sum not to exceed $800; Charles F. Roos, $1,000; H. T. Stetson, $500; for allotment by the Committee on Grants, $700.

9. An appropriation of $1,000 from treasury funds was made as an honorarium for the executive secretary of the Committee on Foreign Guests at the approaching Chicago meeting.

10. An appropriation of $1,000 was made from the prize fund, for the Atlantic City prize.

11. For journal subscriptions of living life members for 1933, an appropriation of $1,539 was made from treasury funds, also an appropriation of $22 from treasury funds for rent and tax on the treasurer's safety-deposit box.

12. The council voted that $2,000 of the permanent secretary's funds now in the treasury be appropriated for use by the permanent secretary's office if and as needed.

13. Forty-nine fellows were elected by the council.

14. On recommendation of the Secretaries' Conference and of the executive committee, the council voted that members whose names appear in the fifth edition of "American Men of Science," which is about to be published, shall be elected to fellowship, if not already fellows; provided that if objection be raised against any name it shall be referred to the proper section committee for recommendation to the executive committee.

15. The council voted that non-members whose names occur in the fifth edition of "American Men of Science" shall be invited to join the association with the expectation of being elected to fellowship.

16. The council voted unanimously that, in view of information received from the American Medical Association, the membership of John R. Brinkley is discontinued.

17. The council voted that the Western Society of Engineers be invited to become officially associated with the American Association.

18. The committee on grants for research was asked to present a full report on the results of its study of the general question, How may the American Association best employ the funds annually becoming available for "research" or "for the advancement of science," so as to accomplish the most good?—It has been repeatedly suggested that these relatively small funds might perhaps better be employed in other ways than through individual grants in aid, and this entire question is open for discussion. It is desirable that thoughts and suggestions on this topic be sent to the permanent secretary for transmission to the committee on grants.

19. The council voted that the committee on the place of science in education be reorganized, with the following membership: Otis W. Caldwell (*chairman*), Karl T. Compton, E. R. Hedrick, Jerome Isenberger, Burton E. Livingston, Morris Meister.

20. The council voted with great regret to accept the resignation of Dr. Rodney H. True as secretary of the Committee of One Hundred on Scientific Research and expressed its keen appreciation of the valuable services rendered by Dr. True throughout his period as secretary of that committee.

21. The council accepted a report of the committee on source books in the history of science.

22. A report was accepted from Dr. Herbert Osborn, representative of the American Association on the Board of Trustees of *Biological Abstracts.*

23. The council named Philip Fox and Henry B. Ward as additional members of the committee on foreign guests for the Chicago meeting.

24. Dr. Philip Fox was elected executive secretary of the committee just mentioned.

25. The council accepted with thanks an offer of the sum of $500 from Dr. Duren J. H. Ward, of Denver, Colorado, for the purpose of organizing for the Chicago meeting a symposium on anthropological or sociological science as related to the advance of civilization.

26. Dr. Waldo G. Leland was named as a committee to organize the symposium just mentioned.

27. The council named Professor Roy E. Clausen (University of California) as chairman of the local committee on arrangements for the Berkeley meeting, to occur in the summer of 1934.

28. It was voted that the winter meeting of 1935–36 be at St. Louis, Missouri, provided satisfactory arrangements can be made.

29. The council elected officers at its session Friday morning. These elections have been published in SCIENCE for January 6.

30. The executive committee elected J. McKeen Cattell to succeed himself as its chairman, for the term ending with 1936.

31. The council accepted and adopted the following recommendation from the executive committee: In view of the approaching retirement of Dr. Henry B. Ward from the headship of the Department of Zoology of the University of Illinois, and in view of Dr. Ward's distinguished work for the advancement and organization of science, including his active participation in the work of the association and this executive committee, the committee regards it as fortunate that it is able to recommend him for election to the permanent secretaryship. It is understood that a portion of his time may be reserved for his research work.

32. In accordance with the recommendation just quoted, the council voted that the salary of the permanent secretary is to begin June 1, 1933.

33. Burton E. Livingston was nominated to succeed himself as a member of the Board of Trustees of Science Service, for the term ending in April, 1936.

34. Irving Fisher and W. F. Ogburn were appointed as a special committee to encourage and arrange for meetings of societies devoted to the social sciences in connection with the approaching Chicago meeting of the American Association.

35. The council adopted the following resolution of appreciation and thanks: At the close of the first Atlantic City meeting, which has brought together a large group of scientific workers and a wide variety of societies, effectively carrying out an extended program of over 1,500 scientific papers and discussions, the Council of the American Association for the Advancement of Science wishes to record its appreciation of the many excellent and efficient provisions made for the success of this meeting by the Atlantic City Convention and Publicity Bureau, and of the personal interest shown in caring for every detail by the director of the bureau, Mr. A. H. Skean, who, in addition to the usual duties of his position, has discharged in a large measure the functions of chairman of a local committee. Atlantic City contributed to the success of this meeting in many ways, especially through the unusually fine facilities of the magnificent Municipal Auditorium, made available through its director, Mr. Lincoln G. Dickey. The cordial thanks of the American Association and the scientific societies that met with it at Atlantic City are due to the several headquarters hotels, which provided so well for meeting places and society dinners. The Council further desires to acknowledge with hearty appreciation the services of the representatives of the press, who handled so effectively the large number of science news items that became available at the various Atlantic City sessions.

## GENERAL OFFICERS OF THE ASSOCIATION

The names of officers elected at Atlantic City have been published in SCIENCE for January 6, 1933. The names of the general officers for the ensuing year are shown below, for convenience of reference.

*President,* Henry Norris Russell, Princeton University.

*Retiring president,* John J. Abel, Johns Hopkins University.

*Permanent secretary,* Henry B. Ward, University of Illinois.

*General secretary,* Burton E. Livingston, Johns Hopkins University.

*Treasurer,* John L. Wirt, Carnegie Institution of Washington.

*Executive Committee:* J. McKeen Cattell (Garrison-on-Hudson, N. Y.), Karl T. Compton (Massachusetts Institute of Technology, Cambridge, Massachusetts), David R. Curtiss (Northwestern University, Evanston, Illinois), Philip Fox (Adler Planetarium and Astronomical Museum, Chicago), Joel T. Hildebrand (University of California, Berkeley, California), Burton E. Livingston (Johns Hopkins University, Baltimore, Maryland), Robert A. Millikan (California Institute of Technology, Pasadena, California), Henry Norris Russell (Princeton University, Princeton, N. J.), Henry B. Ward (University of Illinois, Urbana, Illinois), Edwin B. Wilson (Harvard School of Public Health, Boston, Massachusetts), A. F. Woods (U. S. Department of Agriculture, Washington, D. C.).

*Director of Press Service,* Austin H. Clark, U. S. National Museum, Washington, D. C.

*Executive Assistant,* in charge of Washington office, Sam Woodley, Smithsonian Institution Building, Washington, D. C.

## MEMBERSHIP AND FINANCIAL REPORTS

At the beginning of the year paid-up membership was 18,269 (the largest membership in the association's history) and it was 17,444 at the end; the net loss amounting to about 4.5 per cent. Paid-up memberships amounting to 1,397 were added during the year, but 315 of these were for only one half year. Twelve new life memberships were received during the year, and 20 additional ones have been received between September 30 and December 31.

Because names of members whose dues are not paid are retained on the roll until there is an arrearage for two years, it has been customary to employ "total enrolment" in appraising the growth of the organization, but those who are in arrears for a year or more ought not to be considered as *bona fide* members. There were 1,620 of these unpaid enrolments at the beginning of the year and 2,221 at the end; 789 of these were dropped on October 1, at the beginning of the present association year.

The audited report of the treasurer for the year 1931–32 is of special interest because of the Hector Edward Maiben bequest, from which the treasurer received $2,353.17 in cash, and securities appraised at $29,095.

The late Hector Edward Maiben was a sustaining member for about ten years before his death. A Nebraska farmer, with little formal education, but nevertheless very well educated through lifelong omnivorous reading, he was especially interested in the broader aspects of scientific research and in the advancement of knowledge. In memory of Mr. Maiben the Association Council has established the Maiben Lecture as an important feature of the annual meetings.

On September 30 the treasurer held endowment funds amounting to $200,774.83, according to cost or appraised values of the securities when acquired. He held also $35,010.81 of available but unappropriated fiunds accumulated in previous years, comprising $15,030 of permanent secretary's funds, $15,980.81 of treasury reserve and the prize fund of $4,000 (reserved for four annual prizes of $1,000 each, including the Atlantic City prize). The average rate of interest received in 1931–32 from the treasurer's funds was 4.8 per cent., a very satisfactory rate, for which the treasurer, the finance committee and the association are to be congratulated.

The permanent secretary's financial report for 1931–32 shows receipt of annual dues and entrance fees for the current year, amounting to $83,766.60. Delayed payments for earlier years and advance payments amount to $1,414.48. For life-members' journal subscriptions $1,548 was received from the treasurer. The amount paid to the publishers of SCIENCE for members' journal subscriptions was $52,601.09. Division allowances and allowances to affiliated academies amounted to $3,929. Circularization for new members cost $3,344.17. Travel expenses, *per diem* allowances and section expenses amounted to $4,799.16. Income from the New Orleans meeting was $8,658.51, and the cost of that meeting was $13,032.93. Corresponding items for the Syracuse meeting are $1,776.45 and $2,234.94. General expenses of the permanent secretary's Washington office amounted to $24,756.59.

At the beginning of the year the permanent secretary's generally available funds amounted to $22,-886.85, and these had been decreased to $14,849.50 at the end of the year. Additional permanent secretary's funds for special purposes (amounting on September 30 to $4,793.48) do not require special consideration here.

It is to be noted that the permanent secretary's reserve of generally available funds (which had been accumulated in past years, when income from dues, meetings, etc., surpassed outgo) was decreased by $8,037.35 in 1931–32. The reserve was planned to care for special projects or for depression periods and it has been a veritable life-saver, allowing the work of the association to be maintained as usual in spite of "hard times." Locally raised funds for recent meetings have fallen far short of covering the costs of those meetings, and research exhibits at the annual science exhibition have been increased in number and value, although that part of the exhibition produces expenses and gives no financial income. It is fortunate that this very important feature of the meetings might be continually enlarged and improved at New Orleans and at Atlantic City. The decrease in generally available reserves mentioned above is not to be regarded as a deficit in any real sense, for the association is not a commercial organization and any reserves that accumulate should eventually be used to insure excellent meetings and to further the work of the organization in other ways.

On September 30 the appropriable funds of the association were as follows:

| | |
|---|---|
| Permanent secretary's accumulated available funds | $15,030.00 |
| Treasurer's accumulated available funds | 15,980.81 |
| Treasurer's income for 1931–32 | 8,321.87 |
| Permanent Secretary's funds for specific purposes | 4,793.48 |
| Prize fund | 4,000.00 |
| Total | **$48,126.16** |

Appropriations made subsequent to September 30 are as follows:

| | |
|---|---|
| Research grants, from treasurer's funds: | |
| Henry B. Ward, not to exceed | 800.00 |
| Charles F. Roos | 1,000.00 |
| H. T. Stetson | 500.00 |
| For allotment, to be decided by the Committee on Grants | 700.00 |
| Honorarium for executive secretary of Committee on Foreign Guests at Chicago Meeting (Philip Fox) | 1,000.00 |
| Three emeritus life memberships (income mainly from Jane M. Smith fund) | 300.00 |
| Life membership journal subscriptions | 1,539.00 |
| Treasurer's safe-deposit box (including tax) | 22.00 |
| Atlantic City Prize | 1,000.00 |

Excepting the prize, which is derived from the prize fund, these appropriations are all from the treasurer's income for 1931–32, the balance of which may consequently be taken as $2,460.87, on December 31, 1932.

The executive assistant, Sam Woodley, of the Washington office, reported several important economies instituted during 1931–32, among which may be mentioned: a saving of over $1,000 in connection with the securing of nominations for fellowship, a saving of about $1,100 through the use of unsealed envelopes for billing and for circularization for new members (postage, 1½ cents instead of 2 cents), a saving of about $450 in connection with the editing of the General Program of the Atlantic City meeting, and savings of about $300 due to changes and modifications in office routine.

At the Atlantic City meeting a new endowment fund was started, consisting, at present, of $500, the recent bequest of Luella Agnes Owen. To this, it is hoped, additions may be made from time to time. The income from this fund is to be used for creating emeritus annual memberships.

By action of the council at Atlantic City, the fees of deceased emeritus life members are now added to the principal of the Jane M. Smith fund, increasing it from $5,000 to $7,500. On December 31, 1932, there were 53 living emeritus life members, including the three just elected to that honor.

## SCHEDULE OF PROPOSED MEETING PLACES

| | |
|---|---|
| Chicago, Ill. | Monday, June 19, to Friday, June 30, 1933. |
| Boston, Mass. | Wednesday, December 27, 1933, to Tuesday, January 2, 1934. |
| Berkeley, Calif. | Summer, 1934. |
| Pittsburgh, Pa. | Thursday, December 27, 1934, to Thursday, January 3, 1935. |
| Minneapolis, Minn. | Summer, 1935. |
| St. Louis, Mo. | Friday, December 27, 1935, to Thursday, January 2, 1936. |
| Rochester, N. Y. | Summer, 1936. |
| Washington, D. C. | Monday, December 28, 1936, to Saturday, January 2, 1937. |
| Denver, Colo. | Summer, 1937. |
| Indianapolis, Ind. | Monday, December 27, 1937, to Saturday, January 1, 1938. |

## THE SECRETARIES' CONFERENCE

The Atlantic City session of the Secretaries' Conference was held on Tuesday afternoon. It followed the Secretaries' Luncheon, which was provided by the American Association, and adjourned so that conference members might attend the first council session. Over thirty of the conference members were in attendance and the only regret concerning this session was that the time allowed for it was not as great as might perhaps have been profitably used in discussion. Dr. P. E. Brown is chairman and Dr. Mark H. Ingraham (University of Wisconsin) is secretary of this conference for 1933.

The Secretaries' Conference acts as a sort of standing committee of the association, to consider and to make recommendations to the executive committee and the council concerning relations between the association and the societies that meet with it. Its membership consists of (a) the secretaries of the association sections, (b) the secretaries of the associated societies and of other societies meeting with the association, and (c) the members of the executive committee. The Atlantic City session was mainly devoted to a discussion of the general problem concerning fellowship in the association, which followed a thoroughly studied report on this somewhat vexed question, presented by Dr. George T. Hargitt (Duke University), secretary of Section F. The conference recommended to the council that fellowship be retained as depending upon professional engagement in scientific work, not as an honor conferred for outstanding contributions or scientific eminence. It also recommended the discontinuance of the rather elaborate system by which fellowship nominations have been secured in recent years (at a cost to the association of about $1.50 per nomination, or over $1,000 per year, entailing much work on the part of members of the section committees and of the permanent secretary's staff). Constructively, it recommended that members not yet elected to fellowship whose names occur in the fifth edition of "American Men of Science"—which is about to be published—shall be eligible to fellowship unless objections are raised in individual cases. The council subsequently adopted this recommendation, adding that, in case of objections, these shall be referred to the proper section committee in each instance, for recommendation to the executive committee. Special arrangements may be required for fellowship nominations in some sections. Nominations may still be made by any three fellows, on blanks provided by the Washington office.

## THE ACADEMY CONFERENCE

The Academy Conference acts as a sort of standing committee of the American Association, to facilitate cooperation among the affiliated academies and between them and the association. This conference is composed of the academy representatives in the council of the association (one for each affiliated academy) together with three members representing the association as a whole. Academy affiliations with the A. A. A. S. are now 26 in number, as follows: Alabama, Colorado-Wyoming, Georgia, Illinois, Indiana, Iowa, Kansas, Kentucky, Maryland, Michigan, Nebraska, New Hampshire, New Orleans, North Carolina, North Dakota, Ohio, Oklahoma, Pennsylvania, St. Louis, South Carolina, Tennessee, Texas, Virginia, West Virginia, Wisconsin, Northwest Scientific Association.

The Academy Conference held its usual session on Tuesday afternoon, following the first session of the council. The members of this conference then dined together, at the annual Academy Dinner, provided by the American Association. The secretary of the conference, S. W. Bilsing (Texas Academy), was unable to be present on account of sickness in his family, and Miss Mary T. Harman (Kansas Academy) acted as secretary *pro tem.* For the ensuing year Howard E. Enders (Indiana Academy) is chairman of this conference and Emmett B. Carmichael (Alabama Academy) is vice-chairman. S. W. Bilsing was elected secretary for the ensuing 4-year term, to succeed himself. Dr. A. C. Walton (Illinois Academy) read a valuable paper on the practises of the affiliated academies in accepting papers for their programs and for their publications. A general discussion followed.

By special invitation, Dr. Otis W. Caldwell (Columbia University), chairman of the conference's committee on junior science organizations, read a report on the activities of high-school science clubs in New York City. Science clubs aid the advancement of science by starting at the beginning, as it were—aiming to discover and encourage young people who show capacity for later work in science, and to transmit to them at an early stage of their development some of the attitudes of mind and points of view of those who have led scientific advance in the recent past.

Following Dr. Caldwell's paper Dr. Enders spoke on pins adopted as insignia for the junior academies of Illinois and Indiana. The Academy Conference voted to recommend to the various state junior academies that pins of the type used in Illinois and Indiana be adopted, so that there might be uniformity in this respect among junior academies as well as distinguishing marks. Brief reports on junior academy work were presented from the following affiliated academies: Illinois, Indiana, Iowa, Kansas, North Carolina, Ohio, West Virginia, Kentucky, Alabama and Virginia.

A full report of the Atlantic City session of the Academy Conference will soon be sent to all conference members and to the secretaries of the academies that are affiliated with the American Association. Others may receive copies of the report for the asking, if they will send their requests promptly to the permanent secretary's office, Smithsonian Institution Building, Washington, D. C.

## THE PRESS SERVICE

(*By Austin H. Clark, director, A. A. A. S. Press Service*)

From the point of view of the Press Service, the Atlantic City meeting was the most successful in the history of the association. The Press Service desires most cordially to thank the members of the association and of the associated and affililated societies for the excellence and abundance of the material submitted in advance of the Atlantic City meeting, and also for the careful manner in which it was prepared. It desires also to express, to the many press representatives who took part in covering this meeting, the hearty and appreciative thanks of the association and its members. Especially gratifying was the fact that the great majority of the manuscripts and abstracts bore the date and hour of delivery, making it possible to provide them with release dates immediately upon receipt. This resulted in a very appreciable saving for the association, for the marking of release dates on papers submitted without the date and hour of reading means a considerable expenditure of time in searching through the manuscript of the program, and a corresponding outlay for clerical assistance. This year a minimum of clerical assistance was necessary at Washington in advance of the meeting, and none at all at Atlantic City. So large was the volume of excellent material sent in that all of it could not possibly be noticed in the press during the week of the meeting. But everything available for press notice will eventually be used.

## THE ANNUAL SCIENCE EXHIBITION

The science exhibition was arranged in the grand ballroom of the Municipal Auditorium. The committee on exhibition, and especially Dr. F. C. Brown, chairman of the committee and director of the exhibition, are to be congratulated on the extent, diversity and general excellence of this year's exhibits. It seems to this reporter that the Atlantic City exhibition was the most satisfactory one thus far held. There was an excellent research exhibition at the fourth New York meeting (December, 1916) but a continually improving series of efforts in this direction, with both commercial and research exhibits, had its start at the second Toronto meeting (December, 1921). The Atlantic City exhibition was the twelfth of the series.

A specially useful feature, introduced this year, was the Science Library, a collection of scientific books published in 1932; through the cooperation of 34 publishing houses over 300 volumes were thus available for examination. Another new feature of this exhibition was a series of short afternoon talks, at about 4:30 o'clock by men of science on their avocations or hobbies. David E. Smith (Columbia University) told about Oriental book collecting, Dayton C. Miller (Case School of Applied Science) talked on the development of the flute, illustrating his remarks by means of about 40 flutes selected from his collection of these instruments, which is the most complete in the world. C. N. Hickman (Bell Telephone Laboratories) spoke on the history of archery and showed, with demonstrations, how science may enhance the interest one has in that art. Austin H. Clark (U. S. National Museum, manager of the A. A. A. S. Press Service) spoke about butterflies and butterfly collecting. W. F. G. Swann (Bartol Research Foundation) illustrated cello playing as a pleasant hobby for a professional physicist.

The exhibition included exhibits as follows: U. S. Bureau of Entomology (Mexican bean beetles and surgical maggots); American Museum of Natural History (flattened skulls from Venezuela, new-type dinosaur from Montana, ultra-violet patterns of butterflies, muscular anatomy of the foot in bear, gorilla, chimpanzee and man, glass models of rotifers, etc.); Bartol Research Foundation of the Franklin Institute (recording instruments for study of cosmic rays, a cosmic-ray hodoscope); Bausch and Lomb Optical Co. (many types of microscopes and other apparatus for research and teaching); Charles Bittinger (color paintings of solar spectrum, eclipse corona, etc.); P. Blakiston's Son and Co. (several hundred scientific publications); Calibron Products, Inc. (physical apparatus); California Institute of Technology (x-ray fluoroscope and other research apparatus); Carnegie Institution of Washington (measurement of velocity of light, new photographs from Chichen Itza); University of Chicago Physical Laboratory (apparatus used in field study of cosmic rays); Hugh U. Clark and Leila G. Forbes (unrecorded manuscript map drawn by Henry Livingston, 1788, showing prehistoric Indian earthworks in Ohio); Clay Adams Company (biological models, charts and specimens for teaching); Columbia University, Botany Department (models of geometric cell forms); U. S. Coast and Geodetic Survey (automatic recording accelerometer); U. S. Bureau of Fisheries (research on vitamins in fish products, especially vitamin D in canned salmon and mineral content of oysters as related to prevention and cure of nutritional anemia); U. S. Bureau of Standards (unusual forms of familiar substances —water with excess of hydrogen isotope two, bubbles of mercury like soap bubbles, etc.); Fleischmann Laboratories (production of vitamin-D milk by feeding cows with irradiated dry yeast); Field Museum of Natural History (evolution of the horse, birds of western China and of Chile, the Mayan solar year, fossils from Labrador, reptiles and amphibians from Venezuela and from Solomon Islands, Asiatic mammals, etc.); Ford Motor Company (Johannsen gauges); R. Fuess, Inc. (apparatus for spectrum analysis, new meteorograph, etc.); General Electric Company (incandescent lamps for special uses); Gradwohl School of Laboratory Technique (parasites and parasitic diseases, etc.); Johns Hopkins University, Chemistry Department (models of molecules); Johns Hopkins University, Plant Physiology Department (radio-atmometers, especially newly developed black porous-porcelain spheres, and summer graphs of evaporation and sunshine); Kellogg Company (cereal preparations and Kaffee Hag); E. Leitz, Inc. (new colorimeter, new inverted microscope, Leitz ultropak, etc.); Lilly Research Laboratories and Johns Hopkins University (comparative studies on toad poisons); Linguaphone Institute (linguaphone courses in 18 different languages); McGraw-Hill Book Company (recent publications); Massachusetts Institute of Technology (portable Van de Graaff generator, evolved from old static machine, etc.); University of Missouri (purification of viruses); National Zoological Park (living Surinam toads); New Jersey Agricultural Experiment Station (solution culture and sand culture for growing standard plants); Rice Institute (Geiger-counter apparatus for cosmic rays, recording cosmic-ray electroscope, etc.); Smithsonian Institution (measurement of plant photosynthesis as related to light characteristics, $CO_2$ pressure, etc.); South Carolina Food Research Commission (vitamin contents of various foods); Spencer Lens Company (microscopes and other optical instruments); U. S. Public Health Service (nature and prevention of the disease pellagra); University Presses—Chicago, Oxford, Stanford, Yale (recent publications); D. Van Nostrand Company (scientific and technological books); University of Virginia (growth of nerves); Warren-Knight Company (lettering guides); Waukesha Motor Company (study of motor fuels); W. M. Welch Manufacturing Company (laboratory apparatus and equipment); Weston Electrical Instrument Corporation (electrical measuring instruments, etc.); Williams and Wilkins Company (scientific books and periodicals); Yale University, Institute of Human Relations (testing apparatus, alertness and personality tests, etc.).

The American Association is glad to express its appreciative thanks to all who took part in this record-making science exhibition at Atlantic City.

## THE NINTH AWARD OF THE ASSOCIATION PRIZE

Through the generosity of a member who prefers to remain anonymous the American Association has awarded the annual thousand-dollar prize eight times, and the Atlantic City award is the ninth. According to the rules, there is no open competition for the prize, but all papers appearing in the General Program of an annual meeting are automatically eligible, excepting invited papers presented at general sessions and presidential and vice-presidential addresses, which are not eligible. No attempt is made by the committee on prize award to select "the best" paper, since satisfactory comparisons are not possible between different fields of science. The prize is awarded simply to the author of some very notable contribution. The donor of the prize funds desires to aid and encourage younger authors rather than to honor older men.

The Atlantic City prize was awarded to Dr. Henry Eyring, of Princeton University, for a paper on "Quantum Mechanics and Chemistry, with Particular Reference to Reactions Involving Conjugate Double Bonds," which was presented before Section C (Chemistry) on Thursday afternoon.

### DR. HENRY EYRING AND HIS WORK

A chemist who thinks of chemical reactions in terms of contour maps, and of the speed of chemical processes in terms of the height of a mountain pass between one valley of reacting substances and the neighboring valley of reaction products, such is the recipient of the 1932 Prize offered by the American Association for the Advancement of Science. Had his subject been literature rather than science one might have attributed the development to vivid youthful impressions obtained when the young bachelor of mining engineering and master of science in metallurgy left the halls of the University of Arizona and crossed the Rocky Mountains to obtain the doctor's degree in chemistry in the University of California. We must, however, attribute the development to the impact of the newer ideas in mathematical physics upon a mind well trained not only in chemistry but also in physics and mathematics. His doctor's thesis in California was physical rather than chemical and dealt with ionization in various media produced by the alpha particles from polonium. Two years of post-doctorate effort as research associate to Professor Farrington Daniels in the University of Wisconsin brought Dr. Eyring into contact with the urgent problems of speed in chemical processes and in particular with the problem of molecular decomposition of nitrogen pentoxide, a process which apparently occurred at constant temperature at a velocity which was, to the first approximation, independent of its environmental medium.

As National Research fellow at the University of Berlin Dr. Eyring found in Professor M. Polanyi a kindred spirit with whom he could attack the problem of speed in chemical processes from a fundamental theoretical standpoint. There was a fortunate grouping of circumstances. Bonhoeffer and Harteck had just discovered para-hydrogen and were busily engaged investigating the velocities of interconversion of the ortho and para varieties. Such a problem was especially suitable to a quantum mechanical study for, at that time, the hydrogen molecule was the only one for which computation of the respective contributions of coulombic and interchange binding were available. Indeed, it was the existence of the non-classical interchange or resonance binding which was beginning to indicate the nature and magnitude of the valency binding. Briefly, Eyring and Polanyi explored the possible mechanisms by which para-hydrogen could be changed homogeneously into ortho-hydrogen and concluded that the easiest mechanism was that involving the interaction of an atom with a molecule. The problem resolved itself into a determination of the potential energy of a system of three hydrogen atoms at all distances $R_1$ and $R_2$ from each other. These energies, when plotted on a diagram with coordinates $R_1$ and $R_2$, gave a contour map of iso-energy lines representing a potential surface and consisting of two deep valleys separated by a saddle about 13 kilo cals. above the valley floors. It is this height of the mountain pass which is a measure of the activation energy of the process in question and determines the speed at which the reaction occurs. It was fortunate that simultaneous experiments in the Kaiser Wilhelm Institut gave Eyring confirmation of the approximate validity of his calculations and encouraged him to further enterprise.

The last two years have seen an extension of this method of approach to a wide variety of chemical problems. The rapidity of the development has made it necessary to make approximate and empirical assumptions which it will be necessary later to refine and make more precise. Dr. Eyring, however, impresses every one with the boldness of his approach to the undoubted difficulties which lie in his path. He justified his courage by the results presented at the Indianapolis meeting of the American Chemical Society in the spring of 1931, in which he showed that the element fluorine had a much lower rating as to reactivity than the previous chemical literature would indicate. Practically simultaneously von Wartenburg in Danzig showed that both molecular and atomic fluorine were relatively inert toward hydrogen at ordinary temperatures.

There were many problems at Princeton awaiting his arrival in September, 1931. During that year it had been shown in our laboratories that many molecules were adsorbed but slowly on surfaces important in technical catalytic reactions. With Mr. Albert Sherman, Dr. Eyring analyzed the problem of the speed of attachment of hydrogen to a charcoal surface and obtained results consistent with the concept of activated adsorption developed in Princeton and with the capacity of charcoal to induce the para-hydrogen conversion at its surface. The problem of mechanism in the photochemical hydrogen-chlorine combination which had occupied experimental investigators for a hundred or more years was also examined by the theoretical method and was shown to yield results identical in nature with those to which recent experimental investigations were tending, more especially in the direction of anticipating a lack of influence of water vapor on the velocity of the process. Recently, under the stimulation of the approaching Atlantic City meeting, Eyring dived down an entirely new avenue of investigation. It may be regarded as a by-path from his study of adsorption at charcoal surfaces, but it is a fundamentally new attack on problems of alternative organic reactions in a given system. At the moment, the reactions are most elementary in their nature, but in this new field it is necessary to walk first before one can run. There are many other fields still to be explored, and Dr. Eyring has the temperament to enlist active cooperation.

In the early days of quantum mechanics one imagined that it might be mainly concerned in its chemical aspects with atomic and molecular structure. It has been Eyring's privilege to show to those who were interested, not so much in structure, but in the speed and mechanism of chemical reactions that they also must concern themselves with these new developments of mathematics and physics.—*Hugh S. Taylor.*

## HENRY NORRIS RUSSELL, PRESIDENT ELECT OF THE AMERICAN ASSOCIATION

A truly encyclopedic knowledge of physical science is impossible at present, but Henry Norris Russell's scope approximates that. In the varied science of astronomy there are few fields to which he has not contributed. To physicists he is known for brilliant work in classification of spectra. He is a stimulating lecturer, to technical and lay audiences alike, and general readers are in his debt for regular accounts of astronomical progress. He took a leading part in preparing a general astronomical text. His acquaintanceship with scientific men is of the widest; on many committees he has strengthened liaison between diverse fields and assisted in formulating policies. Nor do these professional matters by any means exhaust his sympathy and energy.

He was born at Oyster Bay, New York, on October 25, 1877. His father, Alexander G. Russell, was born in Nova Scotia, of Scottish stock. His mother, Eliza Hoxie Norris, came of a line of New England sea-captains, and was born in Para, Brazil, where her father was temporarily resident as American consul. Both he and her mother showed strong interest in exact science.

At the age of 12, Henry Norris Russell came to the Princeton home of his mother's family. He took his A.B. at Princeton University in his twentieth year, late in the "golden nineties," which—it would now appear unjustly—have not been considered there a period of high intellectual attainment. Receiving his Ph.D. in astronomy from the same institution (under Young) in 1900, he spent 1902 through 1905 at Cambridge, England, first as research student at King's College, then as Carnegie research assistant at the observatory. He was recalled to Princeton as instructor in astronomy (1905) by E. O. Lovett, then head of the department; and in spite of other nations he remains at Princeton, as research professor, chairman of the department of astronomy, and director of the observatory. Among graduate students whom he and his colleague of many years, Professor Raymond Smith Dugan, have instructed are Joy, Shapley, Menzel, Dunham. Since 1921 he has been borrowed from Princeton for several months of every academic year by the Mt. Wilson Observatory as research associate.

Russell first attained general recognition by his work in the field of stellar constitution and evolution, about 1913. Starting from Hertzsprung's differentiation of red stars into giants and dwarfs, he organized the luminosity-type diagram—which shows relations between intrinsic brightnesses and the surface temperatures of stars. He gave physical interpretation to this now well-known picture by following lines suggested many years before by H. Lane and Sir Norman Lockyer. Subsequent developments in atomic physics, which could not have been foreseen, have invalidated Russell's theory, but the diagram itself has exercised controlling influence on the advance of stellar physics. He has continued contributing to this now very complex subject, and in the first Maiben lecture at the Atlantic City meeting of the A. A. A. S. he presented a critical summary of current knowledge. An earlier summary was given in a course of Lowell lectures in 1931. Early in 1923, as the direct result of arranging demonstrations of spectra for an undergraduate course, he became interested in the expanding subject of the relation of spectra to atomic constitution. In collaboration with F. A. Saunders he attributed the anomalous terms in the spectra of the alkaline earths to the joint action of two electrons, initiating the interpretation of complex spectra. He has taken an extensive part in the analysis of such spectra. Another series of papers deals with astrophysical applications of these principles and of ionization theory, culminating in a study of the composition of the sun's atmosphere (1929) and in studies of stellar spectra made in collaboration with W. S. Adams and Miss Moore.

In positional and dynamical astronomy, mention

may be made of his work on stellar parallax (published in 1911); on the photographic determination of the moon's place; and on dynamical parallaxes of double stars—the latest list by Russell and Miss Moore includes 1,777 objects. Photometric interests are represented by a discussion of the albedo of the planets and satellites (1916) and a series of papers on the determination of the elements of eclipsing variables (partly in collaboration with Shapley, then a graduate student). His war-work on airplane navigation also may be mentioned.

As first Terry lecturer at Yale, under the title "Fate and Freedom," Russell exhibited what future historians of the well-worn relationship of religion to science may describe as a last stand of the Calvinistic mechanist just before old dykes broke and the rising tide of indetermination blotted out his trenches—but he retires with honor since his thesis was that mechanism didn't matter. He has from time to time preached sermons in churches of various denominations.

Russell's honorary degrees are from Dartmouth—D.Sc., 1922—Louvain—Doctor, 1927—and Harvard—D.Sc., 1929. His medals include the gold medal of the R. A. S., the Lalande medal, the Draper, the Bruce and the Rumford. He served as vice-president of the mathematics-astronomy section of the A. A. A. S. in 1918, and as president of the American Philosophical Society in 1931–1932. He is a member of numerous other scientific societies and a foreign associate of the Royal Astronomical Society; he is chairman of the committee on stellar spectra of the International Astronomical Union, and a member of its committees on double stars, stellar parallaxes, stellar statistics, solar spectroscopy, stellar constitution and notations and units.

His work has been distinctly theoretical rather than observational. In 1908 he married Lucy May Cole, of New York; they have four children, of whom three are now in college. Travel is for him a ruling passion and he spent a sabbatical year with his family in Egypt and the Near East without visiting an observatory or reading an astronomical periodical.—*J. Q. S.*

## THE NEWLY ELECTED PERMANENT SECRETARY

Dr. Henry B. Ward, the newly elected permanent secretary of the association, is to retire next June from his position as professor of zoology and head of the department of zoology at the University of Illinois. The American Association is very fortunate in being able to secure the services of a man of Dr. Ward's attainments and experience.

He was born in Troy, New York, on March 4, 1865. Receiving the A.B. degree from Williams College in 1885, he taught science in the Troy high school for three years, after which he went to Harvard for graduate study, where he received the Ph.D. degree in 1892. He then studied in Germany, at Göttingen, Freiburg and Leipzig. At Leipzig, in the laboratory of the great zoologist and parasitologist, Rudolph Leuckart, Dr. Ward received the inspiration which determined the course of his whole future career. At that time Leuckart was at the height of his power and his laboratory was the world center for training men in the field of parasitology. Dr. Ward returned to the United States determined to devote his research activities to the field of parasitology and with the vision of an American laboratory where Leuckart's method would be used in training students.

After a year as instructor in the University of Michigan he was called to the University of Nebraska in 1893, where he served until 1909, continuing his researches on animal parasites and developing the first graduate center in the United States in the field of parasitology. He increased his interest in the medical relations of his subject, becoming dean of the medical school in 1902. In 1909 Dr. Ward was called to the professorship of zoology at the University of Illinois, where he has continued his researches, at the same time training many students in parasitology. In 1914 Dr. Ward started the *Journal of Parasitology,* which, through the 18 volumes which he edited, has been the only journal in the United States devoted to this subject. At Illinois, in addition to his work as head of the department of zoology, he has taken an active part in university administration and has served on important committees. During his summers he has carried out researches for the U. S. Fish Commission, especially on the conservation of salmon, and has repeatedly made field expeditions to the Pacific Northwest and to Alaska.

Dr. Ward has also taken an active part in scientific societies. From 1895 to 1922 he was secretary of the Society of the Sigma Xi. He has been president of the American Society of Zoologists, the American Fisheries Society, the American Society of Parasitologists and the Izaak Walton League. He has received honorary degrees from the University of Cincinnati and Williams College and is a member of many scientific organizations in this country and abroad. He has been deeply interested for many years in the organization and work of the American Association for the Advancement of Science, serving as secretary of Section F in 1900, as secretary of the council in 1901, as vice-president for Section F in 1905 and as a member of the executive committee since January, 1918. His knowledge of association affairs, his wide experience and his unusual executive ability admirably fit him for the important position of permanent secretary.—*W. W. C.*

## GENERAL SESSIONS OF THE ASSOCIATION

At the opening session, on Tuesday evening, Retiring President Franz Boas, of Columbia University, spoke on "The Aims of Anthropological Research," saying that anthropology attempts "to understand the steps by which man has come to be what he is, biologically, psychologically and culturally." Dr. Boas showed analytically and comprehensively how anthropologists are going about the accomplishment of that aim. His address has been published in full, in SCIENCE for December 30, 1932.

The general session on Wednesday evening was devoted to the eleventh annual Sigma Xi lecture, by Dr. Harlow Shapley, of Harvard University, on "Fact and Fancy in Cosmogony." The lecture was illustrated by means of lantern slides. It was pointed out that hitherto used theories of the origin of moon, planets, stars and the galaxy are becoming increasingly inadequate, through the rapid accumulation of highly dependable measurements and rigorous calculations of various sorts. For example, Harold Jeffries, who has been foremost in developing the Darwin hypothesis (that the moon is earth material drawn away by the tidal action of the sun) now thinks that the moon could not have been born from the earth. As to planet origins, the planetesimal hypothesis and related theories have failed to give general satisfaction. Dr. Shapley's suggestion was that we consider the possibility that moon, planets and sun may all be of the same age, having arisen in a secondary swirl or eddy of the parental spiral nebula that produced the local galaxy; thus the members of the solar system are merely survivors of that secondary swirl. As to the evolution of stars and galaxies, theories must remain very tentative indeed. Although we have much superficial knowledge of stars and reasonable explanations to suit, yet inside facts are still lacking. We have observations on more than 100,000 different galaxies, we estimate that ten times that number are within our present reach and we fancy that there are hundreds or thousands of millions; but whether our own galaxy is simple or complex we can not yet tell. There is no indication that our galaxy is of any special significance, either with regard to constitution or with regard to its position in the universe.

On Thursday evening Professor Dexter S. Kimball, of Cornell University, lectured on "The Social Effects of Mass Production." At the close of an enlightening discussion of various aspects of this subject, Dr. Kimball concluded, "If we shall achieve a semblance of economic freedom for all men, a high standard of life, security and delight in work, and leisure, it will be through much trouble and opposition, such as men have always encountered in winning political and religious freedom." The address appeared in SCIENCE for January 6.

Henceforth there is to be, at each annual meeting of the American Association, a Maiben Lecture, recently established by the council in memory of the late Hector E. Maiben, whose bequest to the association is noted on an earlier page (Membership and Financial Reports). The lecture is to deal authoritatively with some topic of great scientific interest and it is to be addressed to men and women of science in general rather than to special workers in the lecturer's own field. The first Maiben Lecture was given at Atlantic City, on Friday evening, by Dr. Henry Norris Russell, of Princeton University, who spoke on "The Constitution of the Stars." After discussing various lines of evidence, Dr. Russell concluded that atomic synthesis of heavier elements from hydrogen is probably the source of the heat and light radiated, the radiation representing the residual energy set free by the synthetic processes. The magnitude of this residue is enormous, by most human measures; the sun—which is a smallish star—radiates heat into surrounding space at the rate of 4,200,000 *tons* per second (and a *pound* of heat is sufficient to turn 30 million *tons* of rock into white-hot lava). This lecture was published in SCIENCE for January 20.

At a general session held on Tuesday afternoon at 4:30, Professor O. H. Caldwell, editor of *Electronics*, spoke on "Electrons at Work." His address dealt with the nature and operation of the electron tube and its many applications. Great industries are already built on the principle of the electron tube, those of radio apparatus and of talking pictures, for example. Electronics is now as important and adaptable in electric designing as is magnetic induction, and additional developments in this new field are rapidly emerging.

On Wednesday afternoon there were two lectures at 4:30, one by Dr. Carl C. Speidel, of the University of Virginia, and the other by Dr. Dayton C. Miller, of the Case School of Applied Science. Dr. Speidel's subject was "Nerve Growth and Repair," illustrated with 30 minutes of motion photomicrographs. Observations on growing tips of nerve fibers (in tadpole and salamander) under various sets of conditions were described, also the migration of early sheath cells (which showed interesting chemotaxes) and the whole process of formation of the myalin sheath. Nerve regeneration was discussed, with several case histories.

Dr. Miller discussed the evolution of the flute and of the musical scale, with sound illustrations produced from a number of instruments from his very extensive and comprehensive collection of flutes. This was a popular lecture, arranged in connection with the "hobbies talks" (see Exhibition, page 129).

The tenth annual Josiah Willard Gibbs Lecture, given under the joint auspices of the American Association and the American Mathematical Society, occurred on Thursday afternoon at 4:30. The speaker was Professor R. C. Tolman, of the California Institute of Technology. He discussed recent extensions of the principles of classical thermodynamics, which were most completely expressed by Gibbs. Possibilities for important differences between classical and relativistic thermodynamics were illustrated by means of applications of the newer principles, and it was emphasized that "we must no longer dogmatically assert that the principles of thermodynamics necessarily imply a universe which was created at a finite time in the past and is fated for 'heat-death' in the future."

Also on Thursday afternoon was given a popular, illustrated talk on "Personal Experiences in West Indian Hurricanes," by Dr. Melville T. Cook, of the Insular Experiment Station, Puerto Rico. Dr. Cook said that these hurricanes have been known since the first voyage of Columbus. Several of them generally occur each year, in the period from July to October, but most of them expend themselves at sea. Four have struck Puerto Rico since the American occupation. They progressed at from 8 to 12 miles an hour, but the rotary movement may exceed 150 miles an hour. The path may be as much as 150 miles broad.

On Friday afternoon there were two general lectures, one by Professor Russell W. Bunting, of the University of Michigan, and the other by Professor R. W. Wood, of the Johns Hopkins University. Dr. Bunting's subject was "Recent Developments in the Study of Dental Caries." He pointed out that this is the most common human disease of civilization, but that it is not generally common or very serious among uncivilized peoples. It is caused by a bacterium of the lacto-bacillus group, which is present only in small numbers, or is absent, in the mouths of persons with little or no dental decay. Some persons are immune and immunological study may sometime make prevention possible. Diet may be important, but conclusions are not yet possible in that respect. Oral cleanliness retards the progress of the lesions, but does not appear to prevent their inception. This disease requires much more study, with the correlation of findings in various fields of science.

Dr. Wood told, in his characteristically interesting way, how he had been able to solve the problem of a remarkable rose-purple film that covers the surface of some of the thin, concave gold sequins found in the tomb of King Tut-ankh-Amen, thus gaining a knowledge of what was apparently a secret of a very few Egyptian goldsmiths of Tut-ankh-Amen's time. Spectroscopic and magnetic examination showed that the film was mainly iron and that the gold beneath it contained iron as impurity. Numerous small globules stand out in high relief on these sequins, which shows that they were heated to a high temperature after having been hammered into shape, and that the original gold contained an impurity such as arsenic, which would give rise, on heating, to the small, superficial globules or bubbles just mentioned. The outcome of Dr. Wood's study is that these sequins were probably first hammered from nuggets of native gold that happened to contain both iron and arsenic, and then heated to a red heat to bring out the colored film, or perhaps the original gold contained only iron and the ancient goldsmith introduced arsenic by melting it in considerable bulk with orpiment.

## SCIENTIFIC SESSIONS

The following very brief account of the sessions of sections and societies that took part in the Atlantic City meeting have been prepared from reports furnished by the several secretaries and others, as indicated. In some instances the reports have been used with little or no alteration. In other instances these accounts are shorter than the reports. All accounts have been edited with as much care as was permitted by the very limited time that was available. To those who supplied the reports, which were indispensable, the general secretary wishes to express his hearty thanks and the appreciation of the American Association for that great service. It will be observed that the several scientific societies are arranged according to the respective association sections to which they are related. Several societies are shown as related to both Section F (Zoological Sciences) and Section G (Botanical Sciences), and the organizations of another group are shown as related to the association as a whole.

### SECTION A (MATHEMATICS)

(*Reports from C. N. Moore and W. D. Cairns*)

On Wednesday afternoon Section A joined with the American Mathematical Society and the Mathematical Association of America to listen to two highly interesting addresses presented by Dean L. P. Eisenhart, retiring president of the American Mathematical Society, and Professor E. R. Hedrick, retiring vice-president for Section A. Dean Eisenhart's address dealt with spaces admitting complete absolute parallelism. In the theory of infinitesimal parallelism, as proposed for Riemannian spaces by Levi-Civita and generalized by Weyl to affine linear connections, parallelism of vectors at distant points depends ordinarily upon a curve joining the points. However, in certain Riemannian spaces and linearly connected manifolds of order $n$ there are one or more fields of absolutely parallel vectors, that is, any two vectors of a field are independent of the curves joining the points of application of the vectors. But only in the case of Euclidean space of $n$ dimensions are there $n$ independent fields of absolutely parallel vectors.

Starting with $n$ independent fields of vectors, it is possible to define another linear connection with respect to which the fields are absolutely parallel, and thus we have linearly connected manifolds which are not Euclidean and which admit complete absolute parallelism. These ideas center around the researches of Weitzenböck, Cartan, Vitali, Hessenberg, König, Bortolotti and Eisenhart. Vitali suggested a Riemannian metric. In 1928 Einstein developed these ideas anew as the bases for a unified field-theory of gravitation and electricity. In 1925 Eisenhart pointed out the significance of this theory in connection with simply transitive continuous groups of motion of a Riemannian manifold. All these ideas have been fully developed by Cartan and Schouten in the geometry of the group manifold of any continuous group. Robertson studied the manifolds with complete absolute parallelism, admitting a motion of the space into itself.—Professor Hedrick prefaced his address by indicating its relationship to the addresses of Pierpont and of Dresden given at Nashville and published in the *Bulletin of the American Mathematical Society*, 1928. He then proceeded to discuss the three principal schools of the logical foundations of mathematics: the logistic, the postulational and the intuitional schools. A distinction was made between the intuitional method proper and certain logical ideas advocated by that school, in particular the objections to the use of the law of the excluded middle. Attention was called to recent work in which satisfactory logical systems have been created which do not satisfy that law, and the conclusion was drawn that much of mathematics may require reconstruction.—On Tuesday morning Section A and the American Mathematical Society joined with Section K and the Econometric Society to hear an address by Dr. W. A. Shewhart on probability as a basis for action. The ensuing discussion was opened by Professor E. V. Huntington and Professor Harold Hotelling.—On Wednesday evening a joint dinner for all the mathematical organizations was held at the Hotel Morton. The tenth Josiah Willard Gibbs Lecture, under the joint auspices of the American Mathematical Society and the American Association, was delivered by Professor R. C. Tolman on Thursday afternoon. Professor Tolman's address was entitled "Thermodynamics and Relativity." He pointed out some of the highly important modifications which take place in the conclusions of classical thermodynamics when we extend it on the basis of the relativity theory. He showed that in the new theory it is not necessary for a system in heat equilibrium to have uniform temperature, since at any point the temperature would depend on the gravitational field. Also in the new theory it is possible to have reversible processes at a finite rate and a succession of irreversible processes without a final state of maximum entropy.—A trip to Princeton University occurred on Friday, to inspect the new mathematics building, Henry Burchard Fine Memorial Hall, and a symposium on "Application of the Operational Calculus to Mechanics" was held in that building. The principal address of the symposium was delivered by Professor John von Neumann. He spoke first of the theorem due to B. O. Koopman, to the effect that the partial-differential equation of the probability-density in phase-space in classical mechanics leads to operational proper-value problems of the same type as those familiar in quantum mechanics. These operators can be handled by using the extension of the classical theory of Hilbert space, due to M. Stone, J. von Neumann and others.

On Tuesday evening and Thursday morning and afternoon the American Mathematical Society held sessions for the presentation of contributed papers. At the business meeting on Thursday afternoon the following officers were elected: *Trustees,* Dean L. P. Eisenhart, Professor W. B. Fite, Dr. Robert Henderson, Professor G. W. Mullins, Dean R. G. D. Richardson; *president,* Professor A. B. Coble; *vice-president,* Professor J. W. Alexander; *associate secretary,* Professor J. R. Kline; *librarian,* Professor R. C. Archibald; *member editorial committee of the Bulletin,* Professor D. R. Curtiss; *member editorial committee of the Transactions,* Professor F. R. Sharpe; *member editorial committee of the American Journal of Mathematics,* Professor E. W. Chittenden; *member editorial committee of the Colloquium Publications,* Professor Oswald Veblen; *members of council,* Professor G. D. Birkhoff, Professor G. A. Bliss, Professor L. M. Graves, Professor Einar Hille, Professor G. Y. Rainich.

The Mathematical Association of America showed a registration of nearly 300, 177 of these being members. Sessions were held on Tuesday afternoon and Wednesday morning. Mr. E. W. Marshall (Provident Mutual Life Insurance Company) discussed the educational aspects of the relation of mathematics and life insurance, outlining the mathematical requirements for the examinations for the Actuarial Society of America and the American Institute of Actuaries, and pointing out the deficiencies of college students as revealed by these; he discussed the qualifications of prospective actuaries aside from the mathematical background and made suggestions regarding the proper courses of study in college for actuarial work. Mr. Ralph Keffer (Aetna Life Insurance Company) considered the fundamental assumptions regarding mortality and the application of the theory of probability to the development of certain problems in life insurance; he discussed these from the standpoint of the individual purchaser of insurance, of the insurance company and of the state supervisory department, and he added a discussion of mortality investigations and of the limitations upon the interpretation of statistics. Professor J. A. Shohat (University of Pennsylvania) gave an account of the life and work of Dr. T. H. Gronwall, for the past five years until his death last May an associate in the department of physics of Columbia University. Professor Virgil Snyder (Cornell University) spoke of the successive congresses of mathematicians leading up to the international congress held at Zurich last September. Professor J. L. Walsh (Harvard University) gave a general theorem in interpolation series connected with his papers on the *Transactions of the American Mathematical Society,* 1932, and in the *Proceedings of the National Academy,* 1932.—The Chauvenet Prize, of $100, was awarded to Professor G. H. Hardy (University of Cambridge, England), for the best expository paper on a mathematical subject published in English by a member of the Mathematical Association in the triennium 1929–31. At the annual business meeting the following were elected: Professor Arnold Dresden, *president* for two years; Professors A. A. Bennett and E. B. Stouffer, *vice-presidents* for 1933; and Professors B. F. Finkel, W. L. Hart, E. V. Huntington and E. J. Moulton, *members of the Board of Trustees* for three years. The financial report showed a profit for the Mathematical Association of over $1,000, due largely to interest on endowment funds and the low cost of conducting the year's business. The Mathematical Association will meet at Chicago in the week of June 19, 1933, and at Cambridge, Massachusetts, in December, 1933, in affiliation with the A. A. A. S.

### SECTION B (PHYSICS)

(*Reports from A. L. Hughes, E. Monroe Harwood, Charles F. Brooks*)

At a session on Thursday morning the retiring vice-presidential address for Section B was given by Dr. Bergen Davis (Columbia University), which was followed by two invited papers, by Dr. A. W. Hull (General Electric Company) and by Dr. T. H. Johnson (Bartol Research Foundation). Dr. Davis, speaking on "The Conquest of the Physical World," discussed the efforts of man to control his environment from the earliest times and illustrated how his progress in this effort has been accelerated remarkably within the last few generations. In the realm of pure physics, the discovery of x-rays and radioactivity and the development of the quantum theory and the relativity theory are most important. The speaker dealt entertainingly with recent studies on the atomic nucleus, a phase of physics which may soon dominate the science. Dr. Hull spoke on "Characteristics and Functions of Thyratrons," in which many widely diversified applications of the thyratron were discussed. Dr. T. H. Johnson discussed "The Cosmic-ray Hodoscope," a remarkably ingenious device for recording visually the direction of cosmic rays passing through the apparatus.

At the sessions of the American Physical Society, held on Wednesday, Thursday and Friday, about sixty papers were presented. The activity in nuclear physics and in cosmic rays was reflected in a large number of papers on these and related topics. A symposium on "Cosmic Rays" attracted an audience of over six hundred. It was opened by Dr. G. L. Locher (Bartol Research Foundation), who discussed various types of cosmic-ray tracks and their interpretation. A paper by Dr. R. A. Millikan and Dr. H. V. Neher (California Institute of Technology) presented new types of cosmic ray electroscope recently developed by them. They found that cosmic-ray intensity at sea-level is independent of latitude and considered their results to be in accord with the view that cosmic rays enter the atmosphere as photons. Dr. A. H. Compton (University of Chicago) followed with a report of experiments in which he found that cosmic-ray intensity increases from the magnetic equator to the magnetic poles, this increase being barely perceptible at sea-level but more pronounced at an altitude of 20,000 feet. He considered these results to be consistent with the view that part, if not all, of the incoming cosmic rays are fast-moving charged particles.—Officers of the American Physical Society for the ensuing year are: *President,* P. D. Foote; *vice-president,* A. H. Compton; *secretary,* W. L. Severinghaus; *treasurer,* G. B. Pegram.

At the fourteenth annual meeting of the American Meteorological Society, on December 27 and 28, Dr. H. H. Kimball (Harvard University) delivered the presidential address, on "Recent Advances in the Theory of Meteorology and its Industrial Applications." S. P. Fergusson described the equipment and work of the Mt. Washington Observatory, and also showed that the barometers used at Cambridge, at Blue Hill, in Washington and at Toronto had varied from one another by only a few thousandths of an inch over a period of more than forty years. He recommended that a national standard barometer be set up. Dr. Wm. J. Humphreys (U. S. Weather Bureau) explained how specific humidity increases during a heat thunderstorm and decreases during a line thunderstorm. E. Monroe Harwood (Harvard University) reported a study of surface temperature of the western North Atlantic, from which it appears that the Gulf Stream varies but little in position and temperature.—Reports by a number of speakers, on the meteorology of the solar eclipse of August 31, 1932, aroused lively discussion. Dr. Charles F.

Brooks (Harvard University) pointed out that weather changes during the eclipse were similar to those accompanying the normal waning of the afternoon sun, but more rapid. S. P. Fergusson (Harvard University) described open-scale instruments, especially aneroid and mercurial barographs multiplying 6 and 7 times, also a portable anemograph and a large hygrothermograph. Jerome Namias (Harvard University) showed evidence of temperature change to a height of 700 m, and a marked sinking of a cloud during the eclipse. Charles H. Pierce and Harry Wexler (Harvard University) reported inflow of air aloft and outflow at the earth's surface, on the edges of the area of totality, in accordance with pressure changes induced by cooling. Dr. Bernhard Haurwitz (University of Leipzig, Harvard University and Massachusetts Institute) showed that changes in solar radiation, air temperature, pressure and wind were nearly what should be expected from computations. Professor Willis I. Milham (Williams College) offered results of observations on eclipse temperatures at Fryeburg, Maine. Dr. Oliver J. Lee reported that no pronounced effect of the eclipse on air temperature was noted above a height of 60 feet. —Professor P. R. Gast (Harvard University) showed that with the same intensity of light, tree seedlings grew little more than half as rapidly when the light came through a water screen that cut off infra-red radiation. Dr. G. A. Loveland presented evidence to the effect that windiness should be considered in forecasting minimum temperatures. K. O. Lange (Massachusetts Institute) told of instruction and research work in meteorology carried on at the Massachusetts Institute of Technology. J. C. Jensen showed some striking photographs that established the reality of ball lightning beyond doubt.—The society's membership decreased but little last year, and its financial condition remains satisfactory. Dr. Charles F. Brooks and William R. Gregg were reelected secretary and treasurer, respectively, and the following were elected councilors for 1933–35: Edward H. Bowie, J. E. Church, Chas. A. Donnel, Joseph B. Kincer and Chas. F. Marvin. The terms of President H. H. Kimball and Vice-President H. B. Hersey continue for another year. Among resolutions adopted at Atlantic City, one favored the inclusion of more research material in the *Monthly Weather Review*. Another favored courses in meteorology and climatology in institutions of higher education.

The fourth annual meeting of the Society of Rheology was its first as an affiliated society of the A. A. A. S. The program consisted of three symposia: (1) "Flow of Solids—Rocks, Metals and Cement"; (2) "Rheological Measurement"; (3) "Rubber and Association." Twenty-two papers covering a wide range of researches were presented. The scope of rheology was indicated, for example, by papers on "Flow of Igneous Rocks," by Robert Balk, "Plastic Deformations of Metals at Elevated Temperatures under Prolonged Loading," by A. Nadai, and "Rheological Properties of Cement," by Professor Eugene C. Bingham and Markus Reiner. This society and the Chemical Foundation have been sponsoring efforts, at the U. S. Bureau of Standards, aiming to establish the viscosity of water as the international primary standard for viscosity measurements. Dr. J. R. Coe, Jr., described the instrument that has been developed for that work. He has devised a method for improving the uniformity of bore of capillary tubes. The timing of flow in the ordinary sense is eliminated by an extremely accurate machine, which forces through the capillary a given quantity of water each second. Thus the only thing left to measure is pressure. Papers by Professor E. C. Bingham and Dr. W. P. Davey and their students, relating viscosities, association and temperature coefficients of homologous series of pure organic liquids and oils, were of fundamental importance. Professor S. S. Kistler presented a mechanistic theory of colloidal behavior which seems to explain thixotropic effects and other anomalies encountered in viscous and plastic flow.

The American Association of Physics Teachers devoted two sessions to eleven contributed papers, demonstrations of new apparatus and motion pictures, and reports of standing committees. In a session devoted to invitation papers, Professor H. B. Williams recommended that premedical students be given the fundamentals that constitute a well-rounded physics course. It is desirable to convince the student, by means of specific applications of physics to medicine, that he is already beginning his study of medicine while still engaged in physics. Professor D. L. Webster spoke on "Facing Reality in the Teaching of Magnetism," pointing out that, although physics deals mainly with realities, it is often necessary in its development to employ concepts that eventually prove to be unreal; in magnetism the pole is an example. It is a question whether such concepts should continue to be taught when it is possible to avoid them. Professor A. G. Worthing described the advantages of the objective tests of the reasoning type used at the University of Pittsburgh. The multiple-choice type of test is employed. Speaking on "Training in Physics," Dr. W. F. G. Swann emphasized the importance of teaching thoroughly the relatively few fundamental laws of physics, rather than attempting to cover the whole field less comprehensively.—Forty members attended the informal dinner held at the Ambassador Hotel on Friday evening.

At the business meeting it was voted to inaugurate

a quarterly journal, *The American Physics Teacher*, which is to be published by the American Institute of Physics under editorial supervision of the American Association of Physics Teachers.

### SECTION C (CHEMISTRY)

*(Report from J. H. Simons)*

Section C held four well-attended sessions jointly with the Mid-Atlantic Sections of the American Chemical Society. The retiring vice-presidential address for the section, by Dr. C. A. Browne (U. S. Department of Agriculture), was on "The Spontaneous Heating of Hay and Other Agricultural Products." Dr. Browne gave an extensive history of this subject and explained modern theories of spontaneous combustion. Twenty-eight contributed papers presented in many fields of theoretical, descriptive and applied chemistry and discussion was at times very lively. Among the papers presented was the one by Dr. Henry Eyring (Princeton University), on "Quantum Mechanics of Conjugate Double Bonds," which won the American Association Prize this year. An account of that paper is presented elsewhere in this issue of SCIENCE. Professor H. S. Taylor (Princeton University) discussed adsorption of hydrogen on oxide surfaces and differentiated between activated adsorption and adsorption of the van der Waal's type. C. E. Locoss and Professor A. W. C. Menzies (Princeton University) presented new data on the controversial topic of intensive drying as it influences certain physical properties. A paper on "Heat Capacities of Sixteen Normal Aliphatic Bromides" was given by V. Deitz, S. Goldheim and Dr. D. H. Andrews (Johns Hopkins University). Dr. M. L. Huggins (Johns Hopkins University) showed that his calculated values of interatomic and intermolecular distances were in remarkably close agreement with corresponding values obtained by experiment. Professor H. L. Johnston (Ohio State University) presented experimental results showing the amphoteric properties of silver hydroxide and the existence of $AgO^-$ in alkaline solutions. Dr. J. Bennett Hill (Atlantic Refining Company) discussed the consumption and production of petroleum products, the trends of gasoline manufacture and the desirable properties of lubricating oils. Following Dr. Hill's paper, Dr. M. R. Fenske (Pennsylvania State College) showed how by means of fractional distillations Pennsylvania oil could be distinguished from oils made up to have the same over-all physical properties. An improvement in the physical development of photographic films and plates was described by Dr. A. F. Odell (du Pont Viscoloid Company), who showed lantern slides developed in the new way. In this process development and fixation are performed at the same time and the resulting detail is remarkably good. "The Mechanism of Birth Shock in the Newborn" was the title of a paper by Dr. I. Newton Kugelmass (Fifth Avenue Hospital, New York City), who described a method whereby the loss of weight of human babies after birth could be reduced to a minimum. This loss of weight amounts to as much as 10 per cent. in human beings but it is much less pronounced in the animals studied.

### SECTION D (ASTRONOMY)

*(Report from Raymond S. Dugan)*

Section D held four sessions, from December 27 to 29, jointly with the American Astronomical Society. A group of papers headed by the address of the retiring vice-president of Section D, Dr. J. H. Moore, on "Solar Eclipse Problems," reviewed what had been learned during the few minutes of cloudless totality vouchsafed to itinerant astronomers. All agreed that the beginning of totality of the eclipse of August 31, 1932, was several seconds later than the prediction, and the discussion emphasized the necessity of agreement on what we mean by the beginning of totality.

The Lick Observatory expedition, at Fryeburg, Maine, encountered only moderate interference from clouds and secured excellent negatives of the flash spectrum on moving films. An outstanding picture of the corona was secured by the Georgetown University expedition, while the observers from Northwestern University obtained interesting data on temperature change at various heights above the ground. A film taken from a naval airplane showed the gradual darkening of the landscape as the shadow deepened.—Reports of the Leonid meteors of 1932 were given by Professor C. P. Olivier, director of the American Meteorological Society, and by P. M. Millman for the Harvard stations. On the morning of November 16, 430 meteors were observed visually at Oak Ridge, Cambridge, and ten of them were caught with cameras. The trails of two of these were interrupted by a synchronous shutter, with which the camera was equipped, and will give very accurate data concerning velocities. Five of the photographs are spectrograms, the first ones of Leonids ever secured. Dr. F. A. Melton and Dr. William Schriever showed some very convincing photographs taken from the air, of many elliptical scars in North Carolina and South Carolina, with parallel axes averaging nearly a half mile in length. These scars were attributed to the impact of a swarm of meteorites some four hundred miles in diameter.—In photometry, Dr. C. T. Elvey and J. S. Hall described their work with the photoelectric photometer, the former in measuring the intensity and outline of the *gegenschein,* the latter in observing stars in the infra-red.

A paper by Dr. Cecilia H. Payne showed the importance and difficulty of standardizing photographic photometry. In spectroscopy, Dr. V. M. Slipher presented further studies on the light from the sky itself; it is now possible to distinguish between scattered light from the stars, auroral light and what the author calls "cosmical radiation." Among the papers from Mt. Wilson was one by Adams and Dunham, describing their failure to find any evidence of oxygen on Mars, thereby setting a lower limit for the oxygen content of the atmosphere of that planet.—About eighty persons attended and for the most part stood faithfully by throughout the sessions. A lecture by Dr. Harlow Shapley on "Fact and Fancy in Cosmogony" was given at one of the association's general sessions, and Dr. Henry Norris Russell gave the Hector Maiben Lecture at another general session, on "The Constitution of the Stars."

### SECTION E (GEOLOGY AND GEOGRAPHY)

(*Report from Kirtley F. Mather*)

Section E held one session on Tuesday, in conjunction with the Geological Society of America. None of the other associated organizations related to this section were in session in Atlantic City, and the principal meeting of the Geological Society was held in Cambridge, Massachusetts, from December 28 to 30, but about thirty-five geologists and geographers attended the joint session in Atlantic City and ten papers were presented on the program. Professor W. H. Hobbs (University of Michigan), vice-president for Section E, presided. The address of the retiring vice-president, Professor Douglas Johnson (Columbia University) was entitled "The Rôle of Analysis in Scientific Investigation." Abstracts of all papers presented are to be published in the March issue of the *Bulletin of the Geological Society of America.*—Several geologists participated in a symposium on "Pleistocene and Recent Changes of Level along the North Atlantic Coast." Professor Thomas C. Brown (Fitchburg, Massachusetts) presented data indicating that the southward inclination of glacial lake terraces in central Massachusetts is less than two feet per mile and therefore does not correspond with the usual interpretation of the shore features along the coast of Massachusetts, New Hampshire and Maine. Mr. H. A. Marmer (U. S. Coast and Geodetic Survey) described the methods used by that organization in determining mean sea-level and emphasized the necessity for long-continued observations in order to exclude the large fluctuations due to atmospheric conditions. Professor William F. Cheney, Jr. (Connecticut Agricultural College) reported on statistical investigations of sea-level determinations which indicate that the Atlantic coast is rising in the vicinity of Portland, Maine, at a rate of approximately half a foot per century, is sinking at a rate of a few inches per century in the area between Boston and the southern tip of New Jersey, and is rising in the vicinity of Charleston, South Carolina, at a rate of slightly more than a foot per century.

### SECTION F (ZOOLOGICAL SCIENCES)

(*Reports from Geo. T. Hargitt, William H. Cole, H. B. Hungerford, A. I. Bourne, Horace W. Stunkard*)

Section F met jointly with the American Society of Zoologists on Wednesday, Thursday and Friday. On Thursday afternoon Section F adopted a resolution recognizing the great prospective value of a proposed compendium of methods for rearing and maintaining invertebrates, and endorsing a cooperative effort among zoologists toward the making of such a compendium. A committee, consisting of Professor J. G. Needham (Cornell University), Dr. F. E. Lutz (American Museum of Natural History, New York City) and Professor Paul S. Welch (University of Michigan), was named to consider ways and means and to further this project. The committee was authorized to add to its personnel.

On Thursday evening a dinner for all zoologists was attended by a hundred and fifty persons, following which was delivered the address of the vice-president for Section F, Dr. Charles Zeleny (University of Illinois), who spoke on "Genetics and Embryology." The address of Dr. Zeleny is to appear in SCIENCE.—This was the thirtieth annual meeting of the American Society of Zoologists, held from December 28 to 30, inclusive, with the largest attendance for several years. The program consisted of 213 papers, of which 76 were to be read, 17 were to be demonstrated and 120 were to be read by title. On Wednesday morning two simultaneous sessions were held, one in physiology and the other in embryology, with attendance of 70 and 100, respectively. Wednesday afternoon was devoted to the 17 demonstrations, including Dr. Robert Chambers' motion pictures of the developing sea-urchin egg. Due to the smallness of the room, this part of the program was not wholly satisfactory to all. At 4:30 on Wednesday, at a general session of the A. A. A. S., Dr. Carl C. Speidel gave an address on growing nerves, illustrated by motion pictures. The annual Biologists' Smoker was held on Wednesday evening, at the Ambassador Hotel, with about 500 in attendance.—Sessions for Physiology and Cytology were held on Thursday morning, with attendance of 130 and 100, respectively. At the afternoon business meeting a new constitution was adopted, 44 new members were elected and the following new officers: *President,* Charles Zeleny; *vice-*

*president,* J. H. Bodine. A special committee is to consider during the coming year the important questions of future policy of the society and changes in its organization. A resolution urging the appointment of a "person of proved scientific and practical acquaintance with the fisheries, regardless of the political party in power" was adopted. Following the business meeting sessions in physiology and miscellaneous subjects were held, with 150 and 30 in attendance.—On Friday morning the largest and most active session held by the society in recent years was devoted to a symposium on "Embryonic Determination," with invited papers by Dr. E. G. Conklin, Dr. R. G. Harrison, Dr. D. H. Tennent and P. Weiss. Over 200 persons attended and each paper was followed by a lively discussion. In the afternoon the Zoologists joined with the Naturalists, who had arranged a symposium on "Heredity and Evolution in Relation to Man."

The Entomological Society of America held its twenty-seventh annual meeting on Wednesday and Thursday. Thirty-four papers, dealing with research work in many phases of entomological study, were presented, some dealing with quite new fields of investigation. The annual address was given by Dr. J. M. Swaine, Dominion Entomologist (Ottawa, Canada), on "The Influence of Insect Life on Forest Development." An afternoon was devoted to a symposium on the influence of civilization on the insect fauna of North America. Forest regions, industrial regions, cultivated areas and purposeful introductions were considered by Dr. S. A. Graham (University of Michigan), Professor P. W. Claassen (Cornell University), Dr. R. C. Smith (Kansas State College) and H. S. Smith (University of California), respectively. Activities of civilized man were shown to have had a mighty influence on the insect population, increasing some species to destructive outbreaks in forests and fields and reducing others to a marked degree. In each case other living things, both plant and animal, were shown to have been very greatly influenced. Analysis of results following the introduction of parasites to reduce destructive insects emphasized the importance of anticipating probable consequences when any new insect factor is to be added to an environment.—Among papers of the general program that attracted special interest were a demonstration of radioactive lead arsenate in insect tissues, by Dr. David E. Fink (Takoma Park, Maryland), and an illustrated discussion of ultra-violet patterns in butterflies, by Dr. Frank E. Lutz and Richard Burlingame (American Museum of Natural History, New York City). It appears that the appearance of butterflies to one another is very different from their appearance to man.—This meeting of the Entomological Society was presided over by President J. J. Davis. Officers elected for 1933 are: *President,* R. E. Snodgrass; *first vice-president,* W. B. Herms; *second vice-president,* C. H. Richardson; *secretary-treasurer,* H. B. Hungerford.

The American Association of Economic Entomologists and its sections convened in the Viking and Tower rooms of the Haddon Hall Hotel, where the accommodations were excellent. The attendance was approximately 175. The Section on Plant Quarantine opened its program on Wednesday morning and continued throughout the day, the Section on Apiculture met on Thursday afternoon and the Extension Entomologists held their session on Friday morning. General sessions were held on Thursday and Friday. Many papers of timely interest were presented and a series of invitation papers were devoted to the present status of the codling moth problem. This association was shown to be in a healthy financial condition; 50 new members were added and approximately the same number were advanced from associateship to active membership. Officers elected were: *President,* Dr. W. E. Hinds (Baton Rouge, Louisiana); *secretary,* A. I. Bourne (Amherst, Massachusetts).

The American Society of Parasitologists held its eighth annual meeting on Wednesday, Thursday and Friday, under the presidency of Dr. Maurice C. Hall (U. S. Bureau of Animal Industry). The program contained 76 titles, contributed by 88 members, and 49 of the titles announced were presented either orally or by demonstration. Four sessions were devoted to the reading of contributions, arranged according to subject-matter. Seventeen papers dealt with susceptibility and resistance to parasitic infestations and others dealt with the morphology, cytology, physiology, development, life history, bionomics and control of various groups of protozoan, helminth and insect parasites. In the address of President Hall, entitled "Is Parasitology a Science?", an incisive analysis of the domain and methods of science was presented, showing the place of parasitology in the biological field; the speaker urged the increasing application of scientific methods to economic and social problems. The presidential address was followed by a demonstration session, at which refreshments were served. The demonstration program permits the presentation of many researches simultaneously, facilitates informal discussion between investigators and introduces a valuable personal and social feature. The annual dinner of this society was held on Wednesday evening, followed by a business session. In the year just closing the society had become incorporated and the *Journal of Parasitology* had been generously transferred to it by Professor Henry B. Ward, now permanent secretary of the American Association. This fine gift was appropriately acknowledged, and Dr. W. W. Cort, chairman of the editorial committee, reported for the committee and the editorial board. A vote of appreciation was given to the retiring secretary-treasurer, Dr. Norman R. Stoll. The following officers were elected for 1933: *President,* William H Taliaferro; *vice-president,* F. C. Bishopp; *secretary,* H. W. Stunkard; *treasurer,* Justin Andrews; *council members for four years,* N. R. Stoll and H. E. Meleney.

SECTION G (BOTANICAL SCIENCES)

(*Reports from S. F. Trelease, G. S. Avery, J. M. Arthur, N. M. Grier, W. A. Whitney, Harry M. Fitzpatrick*)

Section G met on Tuesday afternoon, in joint session with associated societies. Dr. E. D. Merrill delivered the retiring vice-presidential address for Section G, his subject being the interrelations between crops and civilizations. This address was followed by a memorial program celebrating the centenary of Julius von Sachs (1832–1897). Following introductory remarks by Dr. A. F. Blakeslee (presiding in the absence of Dr. H. L. Shantz), a paper by Dr. D. H. Campbell, on the Sachs text-book and its influence on botany in America, was read by Dr. G. J. Peirce. Dr. R. H. True spoke on "Sachs, the Man and the Teacher." Dr. C. E. Allen characterized Sachs as the last of the botanical epitomists. All these addresses are to be published in an early issue of the *Bulletin of the Torrey Botanical Club.*

The Botanical Society of America held a very successful meeting from Wednesday to Friday, with a membership attendance of over 200. The three sessions of the general section included a wide range of topics. Dr. G. H. Smith discussed the differentiation of mesophyll in deciduous trees. LaDema M. Langdon described fertilization, endosperm formation and stages of embryogeny for *Carya* and *Juglans,* as did Dr. E. Artschwager and Ruth C. Starrett for *Beta vulgaris,* emphasizing the time factor. Professor G. S. Avery, Jr., described marked increase in size of the upper leaves due to increase in size of all fundamental tissue cells caused by the "topping" of tobacco. Katherine Esau found that curly-top induces phloem degeneration in *Beta vulgaris.* Dr. E. B. Matzke emphasized the radial and bilateral symmetry of ten-, five- and three-stemmed flowers of *Stellaria media* and the importance of unfavorable nutrient conditions in causing androecial reduction. Professor D. S. Johnson reported on symmetry and curvatures of the sporocarp in *Marsilea* and *Pilularia.* Sister Mary O'Hanlon reported on a symbiotic fungus in the thalli of eight species of *Marchantia.* Dr. M. T. Cook discussed morphogenetic responses of certain dicotyledonous roots to invasion by nematodes. That certain Myxophyceae may tolerate temperatures as high as 852° C. was reported by J. J. Copeland, and thermal tolerance was suggested as a primitive character. Dr. B. M. Duggar and A. Hollaender found that the virus of tobacco mosaic was more resistant than certain bacteria and bacterial spores to monochromatic ultra-violet radiation. R. P. Wodehouse presented an "oil drop" theory of pollen-grain pattern formation. G. S. Torrey described his use of stereomicrophotography in botanical teaching. Wanda K. Farr demonstrated divisions of the epidermal layer of the cotton ovule after flowering, and suggested that daughter cells of such divisions may take part in the formation of fibers. The appearance, during stratification, of a fungus in the seed coats of *Symphoricarpos racemosus* and the time of differentiation of the floral axis in *Gladiolus* were described by Dr. Norma E. Pfeiffer. G. L. Church and Dr. E. C. Jeffrey noted the universal presence of polyploidy and sterility in several varieties of onions. They also reported chiasmatypy in a large number of somatic cells in plants, similar to that of the meiotic divisions. In meiosis in pollen-mother cells of *Digitalis ferruginea,* Sarah F. Wentzel showed the minute chromosomes retaining their individuality throughout the maturation divisions. Dr. I. J. Condit found that the diploid number of 26 chromosomes is constant in 31 additional species of *Ficus* of New or Old World origin. Development of the megagametophyte, endosperm formation and embryogeny in *Eragrostis major* were described by Dr. E. L. Stover. Dr. F. A. Varrelman described transitions between true stamens and carpels of stamen origin in *Malus spectabilis*—Twenty-eight papers were presented during three very interesting sessions of the Physiological Section of the Botanical Society and many of them provoked animated discussion. Dr. J. N. Spaeth, Alice M. Andersen and Florence Flemion presented five papers on seed germination. W. H. Tharp told of the production of more permeable seed-coats of barley by growing the plants in moist cages. Dr. W. E. Loomis discussed the daily growth of maize in relation to light and water supply. Professor O. L. Inman and Paul Rothemund described the decomposition products of chlorophyll isolated from the stomach contents of cows and sheep. Wanda K. Farr discussed the production of abnormal cotton fibers in relation to pressure variations within the boll. Dr. D. I. Macht told of the toxicity of diseased blood serum for the growth of lupine seedlings. L. P. Miller found that many compounds effective in forcing potato tubers increased respiration, without relation to increase in sugar content. O. W. Richards stated that considerable study of yeast cell division failed to reveal mitotic division.

Dr. A. W. Barton discussed the acidity of corn juices. Dr. J. S. Cooley and J. H. Crenshaw reported that wound dressings on apple trees, not usually toxic in the spring and summer, produced killing of tissue in the fall and winter. N. C. Thornton, describing effect of $CO_2$ on fruits and vegetables in storage, reported that high concentrations cause increased respiration in some tissues and decreased respiration in others; $CO_2$ was found to produce increased alkalinity of tissues. Evidence was presented by J. J. Copeland that certain strains of blue-green algae fix molecular nitrogen. Professor A. J. Heinicke discussed the influence of $CO_2$ supply, light, spraying and ringing upon photosynthesis in attached apple leaves. Dr. A. E. Hitchcock, Dr. William Crocker, Dr. P. W. Zimmerman, Professor C. G. Deuber and R. H. Wallace presented five papers on the toxic and anesthetic effects of various gases. The first three speakers showed slides and motion pictures illustrating the effects of carbon monoxide in stimulating the production of roots on stems and in anesthetizing plants. R. H. Wallace stated that neither ether nor chloroform would stop photosynthesis, except in lethal concentrations. Dr. F. E. Denny and Dr. J. M. Arthur presented the two concluding papers. Officers of the Physiological Section for 1933 were elected as follows: *Chairman,* L. Knudson; *vice-chairman,* J. M. Arthur; *secretary-treasurer,* E. F. Hopkins; *representative, National Research Council,* E. N. Transeau (alternate, F. E. Denny).—The session of the Systematic Section of the Botanical Society was devoted to a symposium on objectives and methods in field work. Dr. E. D. Merrill emphasized the importance of compiling for this purpose data in fields other than botany, such as information pertaining to economic uses and local names. K. A. Ryerson discussed the objectives of the plant exploration work of the U S. Department of Agriculture. Dr. E. T. Wherry elaborated the case of the box huckleberry as an illustration of the need of field work. Dr. F. W. Pennell showed the necessity of revising by field study all the herbarium concepts inherited from the past. A paper by Professor O. E. Jennings on cryptogams and field work concluded the symposium. On Thursday, following an illustrated lecture by Professor M. A. Chrysler, on the vegetation of the New Jersey pine barrens, a party of 22 spent most of the day on a field trip to those barrens and neighboring coastal marshes. Friday morning's session was mostly devoted to papers on the agrostology of Yucatan, and of Eastern Asia compared with Eastern North America, by J. R. Swallen and Y. L. Keng, respectively. Professor A. S. Hitchcock commented upon recent progress in American agrostology. Note was taken of a botanical map of Quebec by Fr. Marie-Victorin. Dr. C. R. Ball criticized certain trends in systematic botany. Alfred Rehder was elected *chairman* and C. A. Weatherby *secretary* of the Systematic Section.

The annual dinner for all botanists was held on Thursday evening, with an attendance of 230. President G. J. Peirce presided, and the retiring president, Dr. C. J. Chamberlain, delivered his address on the phylogeny and geographic distribution of the cycads. The address, illustrated with colored slides, included a witty and interesting account of field studies extending through many years. Announcement was made of the election of the following officers of the Botanical Society for 1933: *President,* E. J. Kraus; *vice-president,* G. E. Nichols; *secretary,* L. C. Petry; *treasurer,* H. A. Gleason; *member, editorial board, American Journal of Botany,* C. E. Allen.

The twenty-fourth annual meeting of the American Phytopathological Society was held from December 28 to 30. Nearly two hundred members were present and 112 papers were presented in eleven sessions. There were joint sessions with Section G, A. A. A. S. (the Julius von Sachs Memorial Program), and with the newly formed Mycological Society of America. The following officers were elected: J. C. Arthur, *president;* N. E. Stevens, *vice-president;* Carl Hartley, *councilor.* F. C. Meier, *secretary-treasurer,* and H. B. Humphrey, *editor-in-chief of Phytopathology,* continue. Forty-seven new members were elected, bringing the total membership now to 827.—The contributions presented at this meeting may be classified according to subject as follows: Diseases of miscellaneous crops (2 sessions), 15 papers; virus diseases of tobacco, 10 papers; soil treatment, seed treatments and sprays, 12 papers; diseases of forest trees, 9 papers; virus diseases, 11 papers; diseases of ornamentals, 11 papers; diseases of cereal crops (2 sessions), 20 papers; diseases of deciduous and small fruits, 13 papers; vegetable diseases, 11 papers. At the annual conference on extension work in plant pathology (held on December 28 under the chairmanship of R. J. Haskell) about 50 specialists took part in discussions of the following topics: use of lantern slides, film strips, motion pictures, photographic enlargements, colored plates and specimens with demonstrations and exhibits; use of radio (with demonstration), plant-disease schools and study classes, plant clinics, farm-and-home week programs, contests and clubs, agricultural trains and plant-disease surveys as a method of teaching.—A session on "The Outlook for Plant Pathology under Present Conditions," under the chairmanship of Professor H. H. Whetzel, considered changes in extension methods to meet changed economic conditions, the effect of present economic conditions on the prevalence of some plant diseases.—On December 28 was held the annual dinner, entertainment being furnished under the auspices of the pathologists of New Jersey, New York, Delaware, Pennsylvania and Harvard University.—Ten new or little known plant diseases were reported at this meeting: crown gall on *Carnegiea gigantea* (by Dr. Michael Levine); a sterile, but fungus-like, leaf spot on pineapple (by Dr. Melville T. Cook); a new sclerotial fungus from Texas (by D. C. Neal and R. W. Wester); a brooming of *Robinia pseudoacacia* (by Dr. Carl Hartley and L. W. R. Jackson); a *Nectria* canker of basswood (by D. S. Welch); *Nectria coccinea* on beech (by John Ehrlich); fig mosaic in California (by Dr. Ira J. Condit and Professor Wm. T. Horne); a new necrogenic virus disease of potatoes in California (by E. S. Schultz and W. P. Raleigh); a *Cytospora* canker of *Picea* (by C. J. Gilgut and Dr. O. C. Boyd). Other scientific contributions included descriptions of the perfect stages of *Sclerotium gladioli* (by Dr. F. L. Drayton) and of *S. oryzae* (by E. C. Tullis); the production of a fertile saltant of *Helminthosporium sativum* by ultra-violet irradiation (by Dr. F. J. Greaney and Dr. J. E. Machacek); acquired immunity to mosaic and spot necrosis in tobacco (by J. M. Birkeland); the toxicity of mercuric chloride-potassium iodide solutions (by W. P. Raleigh); the genetics of *Sphacelotheca sorghi* and *S. cruenta* (by Dr. H. A. Rodenhiser); the pathology of crosses between the loose and covered barley-smut fungi (by Dr. H. A. Rodenhiser and B. F. Barnes); the occurrence of apple scab on stored fruit (by C. O. Bratley); the virus diseases of dahlia (by Philip Brierley); *Sphaceloma* on sweet violets (by Professor L. M. Massey, Dr. R. P. White and Dr. A. E. Jenkins); a new fruit spot associated with apple measles (by Anthony Berg); bacterial cankers of *Prunus* in California (by E. E. Wilson); a tuber rot of potatoes caused by *Botrytis cinerea* (by Dr. Donald Folsom); and a bacterial blight of broad beans in Louisiana (by L. H. Person). Abstracts of the papers on the program of this meeting are printed in the January number of *Phytopathology*.

The ninth annual meetng of the American Society of Plant Physiologists, under the presidency of Professor D. R. Hoagland, was alternated with the sessions of the Physiological Section of the Botanical Society of America. Twenty-five papers were presented in the regular sessions of the society and 24 papers in joint sessions with Section G, the American Society for Horticultural Science and the Ecological Society of America. At the Plant Physiologists' dinner on Friday evening President Hoagland spoke on "Plant Physiology Problems," and Dr. W. W. Garner delivered the Stephen Hales address on "Response of Long-day and Short-day Plants to Relative Length of Day and Night." Professor Charles F. Hottes was elected Charles Reid Barnes life member of the society, and Dr. H. B. Vickery was awarded the Stephen Hales prize for outstanding contributions to the science of plant physiology, for his work on plant proteins. At the first session Professor J. N. Martin reported that most of the root reserves in sweet clover are stored in September after top growth is completed. K. H. Burnett and Dr. W. E. Loomis found that translocation from corn leaves was much more rapid in the afternoon than at night. J. D. Hartman emphasized the inverse relationship of turgor pressure and rate of cell wall hardening in determining the form of potato sprouts. Dr. F. M. Andrews reported on a technique for studying the viability of pollen. M. W. Parker found that the water soluble polysaccharides that form an important portion of sweet corn kernels resemble beta amylose. Dr. F. J. Veihmeyer and Dr. A. H. Hendrickson presented the results of extensive experiments showing that the wilting coefficient is a constant property of the soil and is not significantly affected by the species or condition of the plants used for its determination. At the Friday morning session Professor D. R. Hoagland and T. C. Broyer showed that accumulation of diffusible ions within a plant tissue is dependent upon the carbohydrate and oxygen supply of the tissue and has the temperature coefficient of a chemical reaction. Evidence that a quantum of blue light is as efficient in photosynthesis as a quantum of red light was presented by G. R. Burns. E. S. Johnston reported that normal tomato plants could be grown in light from which the infra-red waves had been removed. A close correlation between growth in corn and the total chlorophyll content of the plant was found by Professor H. B. Sprague and Normal Curtis. Dorothy A. Francis reported injury to plants by x-rays, but Professor C. A. Shull found that by the use of suitable filters and short exposures it was possible to obtain a stimulating effect. A passive rôle in water absorption was assigned to the roots of plants by Dr. P. J. Kramer. The thermal conductivity of oats increases with the moisture content, but is always very low, according to Dr. A. L. Bakke and Professor Harold Stiles.—At the joint session with the American Society for Horticultral Science, H. B. Tukey reported that when the abortive embryos of early varieties of cherries are transferred to a suitable nutrient medium they develop into normal seedlings without going through a rest period. High winter temperatures were found by Dr. Lee M. Hutchins to be the cause of prolonged dormancy in southern peach trees. Dr. W. E. Loomis pointed out that factors that change the course of plant development also alter the balance between growth and differentiation. Dr. Walter Thomas showed that the ratios between nutrients applied, nutrients recovered and effect on growth of apple might vary widely and pointed out the relation of his results to the philosophy of Holism. Dr. W. R. Robbins reported that sweet potatoes grown with deficient K showed less cambial activity and had a high length-diameter ratio. Results indicating that temperature factors are dominant over photoperiodism in the seeding of celery, cabbage and beets were reported by Professor H. C. Thompson. Dr. F. S. Brackett described the apparatus used at the Smithsonian Institution for studying photosynthesis and showed preliminary results on light and $CO_2$ studies which closely followed Blackman's law of limiting factors.

The newly organized Mycological Society of America held its first meeting, on December 28, 29 and 30, with Dr. Wm. H. Weston, Jr., presiding. A constitution was adopted and arrangements were made with the New York Botanical Garden for the publication of *Mycologia,* the official organ of the new society. The officers elected are: *President,* C. L. Shear; *vice-president,* C. W. Martin; *councilors,* H. S. Jackson and C. R. Orton; *secretary-treasurer,* H. M. Fitzpatrick; *editors,* G. R. Bisby, H. M. Fitzpatrick, E. B. Mains, F. J. Seaver, J. A. Stevenson and F. A. Wolf. The editor-in-chief for 1933 is F. J. Seaver. The naming of a historian was authorized. The vice-president is empowered to arrange for a summer meeting, which is expected to be primarily a fungus-foray.—On Wednesday afternoon the Mycological Society met in joint session with Section G, and on Thursday morning with the American Phytopathological Society. The Thursday afternoon session was devoted to the presentation of papers chiefly on the various aspects of sexuality in fungi. The papers on Friday morning were mainly on the Phycomycetes, while Friday afternoon's program was of a more miscellaneous character. Forty papers were given. A motion picture illustrating the life cycle of the Myxomycetes was shown by Dr. F. L. Howard, and Professor A. H. R. Buller and Dr. J. H. Craigie (University of Manitoba) showed photomicrographs of hand sections through living pycnia of Puccinia, showing fusion of pycniospores with trichogynous hyphae.

## PROGRAMS RELATED TO BOTH SECTION F AND SECTION G

(*Reports from J. W. Gowen and E. W. Lindstrom, Raymond Kienholz, W. P. Whiting, James E. Ackert, A. I. Ortenburger*)

The Biologists' Smoker, sponsored by the American Society of Naturalists in conjunction with the American Society of Zoologists, the Botanical Society and the Genetics Society, was held on Wednesday evening at the Hotel Ambassador, where a group of four hundred or more seemed to find the Pompeiian Grill Room a congenial place to renew acquaintances and talk over biological problems. The annual symposium of the American Society of Naturalists, on "Heredity and Environment in Man," was held on Friday afternoon with an attendance of approximately 250. Dr. H. H. Newman presented his critical evidence on the resemblances and differences of ten pairs of identical twins reared apart, in contrast with twins reared together. Body weight, general health and strength, condition of the teeth, mental and temperamental ratings were about twice as uniform in twins reared apart as in fraternal twins brought up together. From these facts it is concluded that, under such circumstances, the hereditary constitution received by each twin of the pair had about twice the effect of the differences in the environment in determining these characteristics. Dr. Barbara S. Burks presented a résumé of evidence for the relative effects of heredity and environment taken from studies on children in orphanages and elsewhere. As with the ancient Greeks, the modern evidence showed that human abilities cluster in family groups; that absence from school may depress tests for mental ability, but that ordinary environmental differences do not alter it; that differences between rural and urban intellects are to be attributed to the drainage of the mentally able from one locality to another, and finally that the home environment is closely related to the intellect of the family. Dr. A. Weinstein delivered a brilliant and searching analysis of facts and foibles in our present handling of human genetic problems. A fourth paper, by Dr. L. Hogben, on "Some Methodological Aspects of Human Genetics," was read only by title, but it will be published in the symposium series.—The following named officers of the American Society of Naturalists for 1933 were elected: B. E. Livingston, *president;* E. V. Cowdry, *vice-president;* M. Demerec, *treasurer;* E. W. Lindstrom, *secretary.* Dr. A. Banta was appointed chairman of a special committee to cooperate with the vice-president in arranging a special semi-centennial program for the next annual meeting. Thirty-seven new members were elected.—The annual Naturalists' Dinner was held on Friday evening, with President R. A. Gortner presiding. Dr. Gortner's presidential address "Others," which will be printed in SCIENCE shortly, was a forceful and penetrating analysis of relations between man and his natural resources; particularly with respect to his mineral resources, man is wastefully throwing away his heritage.

The Ecological Society of America, under the presidency of Dr. George E. Nichols, held sessions on Wednesday, Thursday and Friday. On Wednesday morning the ecological diagnosis of types of corn, the relation between yield of corn and environmental factors, the effect of vegetative cover on soil erosion and the vegetation of the Sonoran Desert were considered. The Wednesday afternoon session was devoted to papers on hydrobiology and aquiculture, with special reference to coastal waters. Among the topics presented was the interesting rôle of copper in the setting and distribution of the oyster; in brackish water a colloidal precipitate of copper oxychloride after ingestion initiates the attachment of the oyster larva after an average latent period of four minutes and twenty seconds. A brief account of the plans of the new hybrobiological laboratory of the State of Maryland, at Solomon's Island, in the lower Chesapeake Bay, was of general interest. Supplemental to this program was a field trip on Saturday to the oyster beds of Delaware Bay.—The ecologists' dinner was held on Wednesday evening, followed by the illustrated address of President G. E. Nichols, on "Photographic Records of Changes in Vegetation." Those attending the joint session with the American Society of Zoologists listened to a discussion of the distribution of amphibians and reptiles in the faunal areas of southern Arizona. It was shown that great variations in the vigor and fecundity of chinch bugs from year to year may be as responsible as are climatic fluctuations for their variation in numbers. A method of marking living snakes and unique data obtained thereby regarding their wanderings were presented. In the joint session with the Botanical Society of America papers on the following topics were given: effect of soil salinity on vegetation, invasion of grass range by shrubs when overgrazed, a new black porous-porcelain sphere for estimating drying influence of sunshine, spherical *versus* horizontal plane surfaces for measuring radio-atmometric effects, the edge of the forest in Alaska and reasons for its position as suggested by pollen analysis of near-by bogs, and epharmony in a New Zealand *Rubus*. The last mentioned paper has been sent by Dr. Leonard Cockayne, of New Zealand. The Ecological Society voted that a letter of greetings and appreciation be sent to Dr. Cockayne. A symposium on "Some Aspects of Forest Succession" included discussions by Dr. W. S. Cooper, Professor L. G. Romell, Dr. H. L. Shirley, Professor H. J. Lutz and P. B. Sears. A joint session with the American Society of Plant Physiologists and the Society of American Foresters was devoted to forest physiology and ecology. Among the subjects discussed were: the physiological activity of evergreens and green twigs in winter, the complementary effects of radiation and nitrogen intensities on growth of pine seedlings, relation of soil temperature to root development of pine seedlings, the reaction of chestnut bark to the blight disease, the distribution of Scotch broom in Virginia. An interesting field trip to the New Jersey pine barrens and plains was taken on Saturday.—The following are the officers for 1933: E. B. Powers, *president;* H. C. Hanson, *vice-president;* Raymond Kienholz, *secretary-treasurer*. C. F. Korstian was appointed associate editor of *Ecological Monographs*.

The Genetics Society of America, formed from the Joint Genetics Sections of the American Society of Zoologists and the Botanical Society of America (which have presented programs at recent annual meetings of the A. A. A. S.), held its first meeting at Atlantic City. Twenty-one papers were presented at the regular sessions, while an equal number were read by title and five were given by demonstration. A symposium on "The Progeny Test as a Means of Evaluating the Breeding Potentialities of the Individual" consisted of papers by Dr. H. D. Goodale and Dr. L. E. Kirk, which stimulated considerable discussion. One of the regular sessions was mainly devoted to chromosome analysis, including cytological studies by Dr. Edwin R. Helwig and H. Irene Corey, with genetic phases presented by Dr. Alexander Weinstein and Professor E. W. Lindstrom. A session devoted largely to the gene included papers on genic variability, multiple allelomorphs and the action of genes in development. A noteworthy contribution at this session was that of Dr. John W. Gowen and Elizabeth H. Gay, on "Gene Number, Kind and Size in Drosophila." By consideration of quanta of x-radiation absorbed in spermatozoa, mutations produced and size of chromosomes, it was concluded that the gene has a minimum of 14,380 loci and a size of fifteen protein molecules. Genic control of developmental processes was discussed by G. A. Lebedeff (*Drosophila virilis*), Dr. L. C. Dunn and D. R. Charles (mice), and Professor E. W. Sinnott (Cucurbita and Capsicum). Heredity in clones interrupted by sexual reproduction was discussed by Dr. T. M. Sonneborn, who has applied Mendelian methods to Protozoa, and by Dr. A. M. Banta and Thelma R. Wood, who found that recessive mutations accumulate in Cladocera after long-continued parthenogenesis. Dr. A. M. Banta's studies were presented also by demonstration. Cysticercus disease in rats and genetic factors in relation to malignant tumors were presented by demonstration and reading by Dr. M. R. Curtis, W. F. Dunning and Dr. F. D. Bullock. Sex-linkage and polymorphism in Mexican fishes were demonstrated by Dr. Myron Gordon.

The American Microscopical Society held its fifty-first annual meeting on Thursday. The following officers were elected for 1933: *President,* M. J. Elrod; *first vice-president,* R. J. Pool; *second vice-president,* J. J. Myers; *member of executive committee* (3 years), L. E. Noland. J. E. Ackert continues as secretary. The custodian, Dr. Henry B. Ward, reported that the Spencer-Tolles Fund is in excess of $16,500. Professors M. J. Elrod and J. E. Ackert were named to represent this society in the council of the American Association.

In the scientific program of the Phi Sigma Biological Research Society zoological papers predominated —several of them dealing with morphogenesis. A report on bat migration attracted considerable interest, as did the report of a European hydromedusa on the Maine coast. Three motion pictures were shown, one illustrating the possibilities of this medium for demonstrating plant zonation and successional relations. As usual, most of the contributions were from junior science students, who largely comprise the active membership of this society.

### SECTION H (ANTHROPOLOGY)

(*Reports from Carl E. Guthe and Dudley J. Morton*)

The American Anthropological Association, the American Folk-Lore Society and Section H presented a combined program on Wednesday, Thursday and Friday, and the American Association of Physical Anthropologists held meetings on Thursday and Friday. The opening general session of the A. A. A. S., Tuesday evening, was of particular interest to all workers in anthropology. At that session Professor Franz Boas, of Columbia University, retiring president of the American Association, spoke on "The Aims of Anthropological Research." The combined program mentioned above listed twenty-nine fifteen-minute communications, which dealt with various aspects of the comparative study of human cultures. Some of them reported upon results of research among specific cultures in Africa, the Near East, Australia and Oceania. Others were concerned with more general problems, such as motor habits, music patterns, prehistoric disease and culture parallels. However, as might be expected, the majority of the papers dealt with studies of North American Indian cultures. Seven papers discussed ethnological work among cultures found along the Atlantic Coast, on the Great Plains, in the Southwest, in California and on the Northwest Coast. On Wednesday morning seven papers presented reports upon recent archeological developments in Mexico, the Southwest, Texas, the Great Plains and the southern Mississippi Valley, and discussions centered around the relationships between Mexican and Southern United States cultures. Later in the week a series of papers described recent archeological work in Persia and Europe, including recent work in Jugoslavia, conducted by the American School of Prehistoric Research and associated organizations.—Following two papers on ballads and folk-lore, the major part of the Thursday morning session was devoted to a symposium attended by about sixty persons, on "Field Methods in Ethnology." The general approach to the problem was first discussed, and then the functional approach and the folk-lore approach were outlined.—The annual Anthropologists' dinner, held under the auspices of all four organizations, was served to sixty persons on Thursday evening. It was followed by Dr. William King Gregory's illustrated retiring vice-presidential address for Section H, on "The New Anthropogeny: Twenty-five Stages in Vertebrate Evolution from Silurian Chordate to Man." This address has been published in SCIENCE for January 13.—On Friday morning Section H held a joint session with the American Association of Physical Anthropologists, and on Saturday morning it joined with Section L, in a symposium on primitive linguistics.—The fourth annual meeting of the American Association of Physical Anthropologists was held under the presidency of Dr. A. H. Schultz. The program contained 23 papers and two evening addresses. A business session was devoted chiefly to reports on the encouraging progress of the census of human and anthropoid material in American collections. In the scientific sessions, papers were presented on many different phases of physical anthropology. Dr. W. K. Gregory, R. A. Miller, M. F. Ashley-Montagu and others discussed problems of human evolution; papers by Dr. A. Hrdlička, Dr. T. Michelson and Dr. B. Oetteking were interesting contributions to the study of human races; investigations of human growth were reported by Dr. C. B. Davenport, Dr. M. Hellman and C. E. Palmer; anthropometric methods were represented in the papers of Dr. T. D. Stewart and Dr. B. Oetteking. Among other subjects presented were anatomical variations in man and comparative studies on primates. The joint session with Section H and its allied societies was particularly stimulating. Its varied scope may be indicated by mentioning the splendid report presented by Dr. G. G. MacCurdy, on the recent discoveries of Neanderthaloid skeletons in Palestine, and the instructive motion picture of a chimpanzee by H. C. Raven. On Friday evening Dr. A. Hrdlička presented the most recent results of his intensive anthropological work in Alaska.

### SECTION I (PSYCHOLOGY)

(*Report from John E. Anderson*)

Section I held meetings from December 28 to 30. The vice-presidential address, on "The Historical Development of Response Psychology," was given by Professor Herbert S. Langfeld (Princeton University), at a joint dinner with Section Q on Wednesday evening. After outlining the history of response psychology Dr. Langfeld showed the increased significance of motor theories of consciousness. At this dinner, Professor Ernest Horn (University of Iowa), giving the vice-presidential address for Section Q on "The Problem of Meaning in Reading," emphasized the importance of semantic variations for studies of language development and of reading, and evaluated modern approaches to the problem of meaning. On Thursday afternoon, in the symposium on "Mental Development," Dr. Myrtle B. McGraw discussed the development of specific behavior during infancy and Dr. Edgar A. Doll discussed the psychological significance of cerebral birth lesions. In the remaining sessions twenty-seven contributed papers were presented, distributed as follows: Theoretical, 3; experimental, 5; physiological, 2; comparative, 1; child development, 3; effects of old age, 2; mental measurement, 7; abnormal psychology, 4.—Thorndike showed that a satisfying after-effect inserted in a series of mental connections strengthens the unrewarded connections in close proximity to it. Pratt demonstrated that new-born infants are sensitive to auditory stimulation. Miss Price showed motion pictures of infants reacting to a problem situation. Yoshioka demonstrated that young chimpanzees learn to make choice by position more easily than by brightness. Porter and Henninger reported a lack of positive relationships among measures of persistence. Luckiesh and Moss showed that nervous muscular tension incidental to reading decreases with an increase in illumination. Dwight criticized the use of the concept of organism. Maller showed the relationship between psychological measures and various socio-economic factors, while Anderson discussed the relation of socio-economic status to child care. Wechsler gave evidence that the decline in human capacities begins earlier than is currently maintained. Dr. Walter Miles showed the existence of a decrement in the performance of an industrial task as age increases.—In a joint session with Section Q, Kelley presented the results of a factor analysis of mental test scores, Hoke evaluated various techniques for eliminating cheating, Lamson reported on the high-school achievement of gifted children, and Courtis showed that means derived from cross-section studies give an inadequate picture of physical growth when compared with means derived from curves based on successive individual measures. Garvey obtained no evidence of sensitivity in the blind spot. Max and Joseph showed the absence of a relationship between handedness and heart action when the right or left arm did muscular work. Mitchell found that waking suggestion failed to affect relearning after short periods. Hunt discussed the meaning of pleasantness and unpleasantness. Johnson showed that sleep was not due to an absence of stimulation. Likert found a positive relationship between social attitudes and scholarship. Lotz discussed the relation between parent's emotional status and problem children's behavior. Tinklepaugh and Mitchell demonstrated the existence of monthly weight cycles related to menstruation. Macht and Davis showed that menotoxin, derived of menstruating women, which had been shown to be depressant for living plant tissues, sensitizes or depresses smooth muscle preparations according to dosage. Cowles presented a paper on a new pathology and treatment of the psychoneuroses, Burrow one on the fallacy of the senses and Feigenbaum one on equilibrium in normal and abnormal psychic apparatus.

### SECTION K (SOCIAL AND ECONOMIC SCIENCES)

(*Report from Harold Hotelling*)

A program of statistical contributions to the social sciences was held on Tuesday morning, with the chair occupied by Professor W. F. Ogburn (University of Chicago), vice-president for the section. Professor Herman C. Beyle (Syracuse University) presented his work on the construction of scales measuring political behavior, using the Thurstone psychophysical technique. Professor Ogburn analyzed the 1930 census data on family composition. Dr. Dorothy Swaine Thomas (Yale University, Institute of Human Relations) spoke on "Some Individual Biases in Observation." Quick and accurate estimation of the social status of a family is possible on the basis of living-room furniture, according to a paper presented by Professor F. Stuart Chapin (University of Minnesota). The type of mental abnormality known as schizophrenia was found, in an intensive study by Professor Robert Faris (Brown University), to result directly from loneliness. Case records showed that before commitment most of the patients had been cut off for long periods from intimate, sympathetic personal contacts; many city dwellers, lonely as solitary inhabitants of remote islands, develop this malady. Professor Wilson Gee (Institute for Research in the Social Sciences, University of Virginia) gave results of an intensive study of the changes in the population of a rural South Carolina township between 1900 and 1930.

The recently organized Econometric Society, affiliated with the A. A. A. S., held two joint sessions with Section K, one with Section A and the American Mathematical Society, and one with Sections A and K and the Mathematical Association of America. At the two first mentioned of these, President Irving

Fisher presided. Professor H. T. Davis (Colorado Springs) set forth an analogy of economic variables with an elastic mechanical system, using quadratic differential forms in his statistical analysis of economic series. Dr. Edward Thiess (Technical University, Hungary) developed the theory of a type of business cycle resulting from the interval between the beginning of a productive enterprise and its fruition. Mr. Carl E. Thomas (New York Federal Reserve Bank) read a paper on community expenditures and industrial fluctuations. Mr. John P. Norton (West Haven, Connecticut) proposed that contracts be made in terms of kilowatt hours instead of dollars, to gain stability. The rapid growth in the expectation of life in the United States was traced in a paper by Dr. Louis I. Dublin and Dr. Alfred J. Lotka (Metropolitan Life Insurance Company). They discussed recent changes in incidence of the principal causes of death, with tuberculosis taking a smaller toll than ten years ago and organic heart disease a greater one. Professor Truman L. Kelley (Harvard University) described the abysmal ignorance of elementary mathematics which he had found in students of statistics. His recital of shocking cases moved Dr. Arne Fisher to exclaim, "What right have those people in a university, a drag on the professors and the serious students?" Professor J. A. Shohat (University of Pennsylvania) urged that a statistical institute is needed for teaching and research, both in the mathematical theory of statistics and in economic problems which call for mathematical inquiry. Professor Charles A. Ellwood (Duke University) spoke on the uses and limitations of statistics in the social sciences. A paper by Professor John H. Cover (Chicago) dealt with liquidation and rehabilitation of the consumer and small business.—At one of the joint sessions with the mathematicians Professor Griffith C. Evans (Rice Institute) gave the retiring vice-presidential address for Section K, on "The Theory of Money." At the other joint session with the mathematicians Dr. Walter A. Shewhart (Bell Telephone Laboratories) spoke on "Probability as a Basis of Action," emphasizing the difference between a prediction based on assumptions considered with reference to probability theory and a prediction based on assumptions that are known to be satisfied. A spirited discussion by numerous members of the large audience followed the paper and the scheduled comments by Professor E. V. Huntington (Harvard University) and Professor Harold Hotelling (Columbia University). Dr. Max Sasuly (Brookings Institution) described a method of smoothing economic time series by moving averages.—The joint symposium on "Stabilization of Employment," in which Sections K and M took part, is summarized under Section M in this report.

SECTION L (HISTORICAL AND PHILOLOGICAL SCIENCES)

(*Reports from Joseph Mayer and F. E. Brasch*)

The historical and philological program at Atlantic City was probably the most significant in the history of Section L. Among those participating were Dr. William H. Welch, Dr. Harvey Cushing and Dr. Clark Wissler, and among the high lights of the sessions the following items were outstanding: China was pointed to as the mother of many scientific discoveries which are as a rule credited to Western learning, such as the principle of the circulation of the blood, the evolutionary hypothesis, and as possible source, by way of Syria and Persia, of the algebra of al-Khowarizmi. The reintroduction of Western learning into China to-day was apparently looked upon as the beginnings of an Oriental Renaissance.—Equally interesting was the presentation of data on the excellent examples of the dental workmanship of the old and new worlds in ancient time. The same materials, such as gold and silver, the same type of instruments and similarly successful surgical operations upon the teeth, as are used or as exist to-day were in evidence among the Etruscans in 1000 B.C. and among the Pre-Inca Indians of the new world. In fact, the successful transplanting and implanting of teeth discovered in those ancient times is now a lost art.—A most illuminating session was that on biography, in which it was clearly indicated that psychology, genetics and anthropology have much to contribute to a proper understanding of scientific biography. It was suggested, for example, that additional information required of every school child bearing upon physiology, heredity and environmental characteristics might be readily utilized for more properly developing the biographies of the great, and also for providing a cross section of what might be considered representative in a particular country or region at a given time.—The session on primitive linguistics provided additional interesting information, especially that bearing on the drum language of West Africa, the inference being drawn that by means of signals, beaten out upon specially constructed drums, messages quite similar in detail to written language are transmuted into sound and rhythm and communicated over a wide area. Especially interesting here was the suggestion that music and language are thus blended together, the signals representing thought communication at one time and musical scores at another.—The session on the history of medicine was especially outstanding. Among other things discussed was the famous Edwin Smith Surgical Papyrus, in which 48 surgical operations employed among the ancient Egyptians are minutely described. This papyrus, unknown until relatively recent times, provides an essential source book for ancient medical procedure.—The sessions were well attended, the one on History of Medical Science drawing an audience of more than 150, and the discussions were always significant and illuminating.

### SECTION M (ENGINEERING)

(*Reports from N. H. Heck, Howard Hotelling and Wm. F. Diehl*)

Section M took part on Wednesday in two joint sessions on the "Stabilization of Employment," with Section K and the Econometric Society. The Philadelphia section of the Institute of Radio Engineers arranged a joint session with Section M for Thursday afternoon. The retiring vice-presidential address for this section was given at the Thursday evening general session, by Professor Dexter S. Kimball, of Cornell University, whose topic was "The Social Effects of Mass Production." Dean Kimball's address has been published in SCIENCE for January 6. At the symposium on "Stabilization of Employment" invitation papers were given by Professor Irving Fisher, James W. Angell, Alvin Hansen, Dr. C. F. Kettering, Professor Dugald C. Jackson, Professor Walter Rautenstrauch, Elmer J. Working, Gerard Swope, Dr. H. L. Rietz, Leo Wolman, Dr. John Lyle Harrington, W. N. Loucks, Dr. Karl T. Compton and Royal Meeker. Fisher showed a close correlation between price changes and subsequent unemployment. Angell emphasized excessive post-war industrial expansion through bank credit as a principal cause of the present depression. Hansen ascribed the depression largely to great erratic international movements of capital while it was being attempted to maintain artificial high price levels. Kettering held that we suffer not from over-production but from inadequate distribution and that the necessity for continued constructive change must always be present with machines, so that we need not fear the latter. Jackson gave emphasis to the thought that the continuous, noncyclic contributions of research and invention to human welfare necessarily result in great social changes that require continued readjustment; undesirable features must be corrected, but the advantages of the machine age must not be lost. Rautenstrauch called attention to the fact that the capacity for energy conversion per man is now a hundred times as great as in pre-machine times; the resulting highly integrated social mechanism calls increasingly for scientifically designed control. Working showed how agricultural employment had maintained a remarkable degree of stability, as compared with industrial employment, but agriculture had to pay for this advantage by accepting earlier and more drastic price reduction. Swope held the view that workers must be assured of a minimum degree of employment, that adequate reserves should be established and maintained to this end, by cooperation of employers and employed, but without demands upon the state. Rietz's paper dealt with actuarial aspects of unemployment insurance. Wolman emphasized the inherent weaknesses of plans aiming to stabilize business through control of public works. Harrington and Loucks both discussed public works as an important factor in the stabilization of employment. Compton pointed out that legislation for the reduction and relief of unemployment is inevitable, being specially directed toward the improvement of facilities for cooperation among the various groups that are concerned. Meeker's witty talk, on "The Outlawry of Unemployment," concluded with the statement: "The abolition of both war and unemployment must be achieved if the good things of existing civilization are to be retained and another thousand years of Dark Ages is to be avoided."

The papers and the discussions that made up this important and timely symposium are being brought together and edited to form a book, which is to be published about February 25, 1933. The writing will be clear and readable. The subject is of interest to every one. The authors' names are assurance of reliability. The book may be ordered from the office of the permanent secretary, A. A. A. S., Smithsonian Institution Building, Washington, D. C. The price, $2.50 before publication, afterwards $3.50.

In the program of papers arranged by the Philadelphia Section of the Institute of Radio Engineers, an introductory talk by Professor Dugald C. Jackson, vice-president for Section M, was followed by three papers bearing on musical aspects of radio transmission and reception, with suggestions for improvement, which were presented by C. N. Weyl, A. V. Loughren and C. B. P. Aiken. Richard Kovacs gave a paper on electricity in the treatment of disease and in the alleviation of pain, presenting the history of this topic and emphasizing the evils of the attempted use of electric methods by medical quacks. F. Massa discussed recent developments in ribbon telephone receivers.

### SECTION N (MEDICAL SCIENCES)

(*Reports from W. W. Cort and Albert L. Midgley*)

The program arranged by Section N consisted of a series of symposia. All were well attended, with numbers varying from 50 to over 200, and interesting discussions developed at each session. The Wednesday morning symposium, on "Tuberculosis," was under the leadership of Dr. William H. Park, vice-president for Section N. In the first paper on this symposium Miss Lucy Mishulow discussed the value of culture methods of diagnosing tuberculosis by the use of the Bordet-Gengou and Lowenstein mediums. Miss Camille Kereszturi then outlined the results from a study of the value of the BCG vaccination in protecting young children in tuberculous homes against tuberculosis, concluding that this vaccine seems to have some protective value. Dr. M. C. Kahn gave a summary of his studies on the life cycle of the tubercle bacillus by the method of isolating single cells; his results on the modification of strains were particularly striking. The symposium ended with discussions by Dr. E. L. Opie and Dr. Park on the question of immunization in tuberculosis.—The Wednesday afternoon symposium, on the "Hypophysis Cerebri," was under the direction of Dr. John J. Abel, president of the American Association. At this meeting were present a large number of the most prominent workers in the United States in this field. The meeting had a very auspicious beginning in the presentation to Dr. Abel, by Dr. D. D. Jackson, of the Philip A. Conne Medal of the New York Chemists Club. Unfortunately, Dr. H. M. Evans, who was to give the first paper of this symposium, on the hormones of the anterior hypophysis, was unable to be present on account of illness; Dr. G. W. Corner gave a summary of Dr. Evans' results. Dr. P. E. Smith discussed the relationship between the pituitary and the gonads, showing a variability among different species of animals in the response to the anterior pituitary gonad-stimulating extracts and to the anterior pituitary-like hormone from pregnancy urine. Several different types of tests showed that the anterior pituitary-like hormone in human pregnancy blood reacted similarly to prolan and differently from true anterior pituitary extracts. Dr. E. M. K. Geiling gave a summary of the newer developments of the last few years in the study of the posterior lobe of the hypophysis cerebri, showing that a number of physiological properties of a heterogenous character have been ascribed to extracts prepared from this gland and emphasizing the importance of the possible rôle of the posterior lobe hormones as regulators of metabolites between the blood and the tissues. In the discussion Dr. Harvey Cushing drew on his wide clinical experience and pointed out the rôle of the various types of cells in the anterior lobe in relation to types of tumors and their resultant pathological pictures. Dr. Abel closed the discussion with an analysis of the difficulties associated with the preparation of active principles from this gland and their establishment as chemical entities. Other well-known workers in this field who took a part in the discussion were Drs. Kamm, Riddle and Collip.—The symposium on "Filterable Viruses and Filterable Virus Diseases" was held on Thursday. Dr. R. R. Hyde, the first speaker, defined filterable virus diseases as a group distinctly separated from those caused by protozoa and bacteria; their causative agents are very minute, cabable of passing filters with the most minute pores and producing well-defined and characteristic inclusion bodies. Dr. E. B. McKinley gave a classification of the various diseases which have been placed in the filterable virus group and discussed the characteristics of the causative agents, emphasizing their mode of reproduction. He pointed out that up to the present time, in spite of well-planned attempts, no one has been able to cultivate these viruses except in the presence of living tissue. Dr. E. V. Cowdry dealt with micro-incineration, a new technique for the study of viruses, especially application of this method to the study of the virus of yellow fever. Dr. Max Theiler gave a summary of recent investigations on the susceptibility of common laboratory animals to the virus of yellow fever, with an account of his own researches on the transfer of this virus to white mice and its localization in the brain; he pointed out the progress thus made possible in the development of a protective serum against yellow fever. Dr. T. M. Rivers emphasized particularly the pathology of the virus diseases, especially in relation to serum therapy. In the last paper on this symposium Dr. W. H. Park gave a general discussion of the epidemiology, prevention and treatment of poliomyelitis; statistical analysis of a thousand cases gave no evidence that the serum treatment had in any way influenced the development of paralysis or other results of this disease.—On Thursday evening there was a symposium on medical history, at a joint session with Section L, the American College of Dentists and the History of Science Society. Dr. William H. Welch presided. The first paper was the address of the retiring vice-president of Section N, Dr. H. T. Karsner, entitled "Mediaeval Guilds of Medical Interest." Dr. Karsner gave a very interesting account of the development and characteristics of the various guilds, such as those of the barbers, physicians and others that had relation to medicine. Dr. H. E. Sigerist gave an analysis of the Edwin Smith Surgical Papyrus, the oldest surgical writing known. According to his interpretation these writings were probably for the instruction of army surgeons, and showed no evidence of the pursuit of pure science. Dr. Harvey Cushing discussed the influence of the anatomical tables of Ercole Lelli, both on art and anatomy. The symposium closed with a discussion, by Dr. W. H. Welch, on the life and work of Antony van Leeuwenhoek, in honor of the tercentenary of Leeuwenhoek's birth.

The initial appearance of dentistry, through the American College of Dentists, in affiliation with the American Association for the Advancement of Science, marks a new era in dental history, in that a scientific program in this subject was offered in conjunction with those of other organizations in the field of science. This alliance has more than a passing significance, for, as was emphasized by this meeting, the dental profession has an important part to play in the promotion of research. By no means content to confine their activities to the mechanical and esthetic phases of the profession, workers in dental science are keenly alert to the importance and value of its biological aspects. The fellows of the American College of Dentists are greatly appreciative of this opportunity to present a program at Atlantic City.—The program, which had been arranged by a committee of which Dr. William J. Gies (Columbia University) was chairman, included both theoretical and practical discussions on a high scientific and intellectual level. There were sessions on Friday morning, afternoon and evening. It was opened by Dr. W. H. Park, vice-president for Section N. The need of dental research was discussed by E. H. Hatton (Northwestern University). The cause and prevention of mottled enamel, a preventable endemic lesion of the teeth, was discussed by F. S. McKay (New York) who showed how this disease points to a civic responsibility that closely allies dentistry with medicine and with the public health movement. A paper on the experimental production of typical dental caries in animals was given by Theodor Rosebury (Columbia University), who pointed out the importance of such experimental work in throwing light on the phenomena of tooth decay in man. Professor J. L. T. Appleton, Jr. (University of Pennsylvania) presented a new plan for the treatment and management of infected teeth, suggesting avenues of thought that should lead to progress in the eradication of dental foci of infection and consequently in the elimination of related disease conditions elsewhere in the body. An interesting discussion of dental and facial prosthesis, by V. H. Kazanjian (Harvard University), indicated a field of medicodental study that should give hope and encouragement to those afflicted with discomfort, disability and deformity through accident to or disease of the tissues of face and jaws. Orthodontic problems and the use of x-ray silhouettes in tracing facial growth, by B. Holly Broadbent (Western Reserve University), diet as related to the development of osseous tissues of jaws and face in the American Eskimo, by L. M. Waugh (Columbia University), aids offered by scientific research toward the improvement of dental restorations, by Wilmer Souder (U. S. Bureau of Standards), morphological change in mucous membrane of edentulous areas of the alveolar process, by W. H. Wright (University of Pittsburgh), were other topics discussed. On Friday evening there was a dinner session, at which three constructive papers were presented, as follows: "Status of Dental Research," by U. G. Rickert (University of Michigan), "Microscopic Research on Periodontal Diseases," by Rudolf Kronfeld (Loyola University, Chicago), and "Field Studies of Human Tooth Decay in Primitive Districts Providing Immunity," by Weston A. Price (Cleveland, Ohio). On Friday afternoon, at a general session of the American Association, Dr. R. W. Bunting (University of Michigan) gave an interesting lecture on recent developments in the study of dental caries.

### SECTION O (AGRICULTURE)

*(Reports from P. E. Brown, H. B. Tukey, H. C. Moore, Paul Moore)*

Section O and the American Society of Agronomy met in joint session on Wednesday, with Vice-president J. H. Gourley presiding. In the absence of the secretary, due to illness, Dr. R. P. Thomas (University of Maryland) served as secretary *pro tem.* The program consisted of a symposium of invitation papers on "Nitrogen in Relation to Crop Growth and the Use of Nitrogenous Fertilizers." The subjects discussed included nitrogen carriers in relation to plant growth, the use of ammonium and nitrates by plants, the effects of previous cropping on forms of nitrogen in soil, the rôle of microorganisms in the liberation and immobilization of nitrogen in soil, the occurrence of Azotobacter in peat soils, nitrogen fertilizers for cotton and truck soils, the assimilation of different forms of nitrogen by grasses and clovers, factors affecting the choice of nitrogen fertilizers, the use of nitrogen as a top dressing for wheat and reactions of ammonifying cultures of cottonseed meal. In the absence of Retiring Vice-president C. G. Williams, his address, on "Fifty Years of Experiment Station Work," was read by title only.

The twenty-ninth annual meeting of the American Society for Horticultural Science was held in four sessions, including a joint session with the American Society of Plant Physiologists. One hundred and sixty-two papers were presented, more than at any previous meeting in the history of the organization. Much interest was shown in the various phases of growth and nutrition of fruit trees, pruning and fungicides, stocks and vegetative propagation, small fruits, breeding and pollination, varietal behavior of fruits in cold storage, vegetable crops and ornamentals. The physiological view-point was dominant and many different questions of plant physiology received attention. The address of the retiring president, Dr. H. A. Jones (University of California), reviewed vegetable breeding at Davis, California. Dr. Laurenz Greene (Purdue University) was elected president for the year 1933.

The Atlantic City meeting of the Potato Association of America was opened on Thursday morning by President J. R. Livermore, who spoke on bud selection as a means for the improvement and development of better strains of seed potatoes. New developments in spraying were discussed by F. M. Blodgett (Cornell University), who reported maximum yields for a 4-year period from Rural potatoes in upstate New

York, secured by spraying 75–80 pounds of copper sulfate per acre, in the form of Bordeaux mixture, with pressure of about 400 lbs. As the amount of lime in the mixture was decreased, better yields were obtained. Dr. Harry L. Gui (Ohio Experiment Station, Wooster) described the life history of the potato scab-gnat and recommended corrosive sublimate or hot formalin as a seed-potato disinfectant; other control measures considered were crop rotation, addition of humus to the soil, and maintaining the pH value of the soil around 5.0 or less. Results of fertilizer tests at the Rhode Island Experiment Station were presented by Professor T. E. Odland, indicating the desirability of relatively high potash and low nitrogen content in fertilizer; variations in phosphorus content did not affect the yields as much as variations in nitrogen and potash content. A malnutrition trouble in potato plants in the region of Norfolk, Virginia, was described by R. L. Carolus; it caused stunted growth, yellowing of foliage and marked deficiencies in nitrogen and magnesium, accompanied by depressed yields, and it was associated with a low pH value and a low organic-matter content of the soil. Results of fertilizer placement tests, as conducted in Maine, Michigan, New Jersey and Virginia, were reported by Dr. W. H. Martin (New Jersey Experiment Station) and B. E. Brown (U. S. Department of Agriculture, Office of Soils Investigations).—Seed-potato certification problems were discussed at the Friday morning session. The committee on this subject presented standards for field and car inspections and urged their adoption in seed certification. The Potato Association voted its approval of these standards, which were also approved by the seed certification officials present. Legislative measures were discussed for protecting the certified seed industry. The Friday afternoon session was devoted to potato marketing problems. William Stuart presented a résumé of recent improvements in potato growing and marketing. Washing, grading and marketing potatoes in 15-pound sacks was the topic discussed in a paper by R. A. Porter (Elba, N. Y.). Daniel Dean outlined changes that have occurred in the potato industry of the United States in the past 60 years; rapid development of new potato-producing areas, such as those of Idaho, Aroostook County, Maine, and the South, has led to the use of better grading and marketing methods in the older potato districts. The work of the Interstate Potato Committee was described by A. E. Mercker (U. S. Bureau of Agricultural Economics), who stated that the committee has, in the last 4 years, enabled growers in the southeastern states to regulate their acreage so as to increase their profits.—The Potato Association adopted the following resolution:

*Whereas,* the Potato Association of America is indebted to the American Association for the Advancement of Science for certain services rendered and accommodations provided; it is therefore *resolved* that the association in convention assembled offers its sincerest appreciation to the American Association for the Advancement of Science for its cooperation in the planning of this annual meeting.

At a meeting of the Board of Governors of the Crop Protection Institute, held on December 28, Dr. W. C. O'Kane said that, notwithstanding the depression, the institute had been able to find much support, closing the year with as much productive work on hand as it had had at any time in its history. This year's work, on 16 research projects, was conducted mainly at the agricultural experiment stations of Washington, Iowa, Illinois, Ohio, Delaware, New Jersey, New Hampshire and Massachusetts. The secretary-treasurer, Paul Moore, reported receipts for the year of $44,198.54.

### SECTION Q (EDUCATION)

*(Report from Willis L. Uhl)*

Sessions of Section Q were held from December 27 to 29. Cooperative research, as conducted by the Middle States Association of College and Secondary Schools, was presented by Dr. E. D. Grizzell, and means for disseminating the results of research were discussed by Dr. Arthur B. Moehlman. Professor L. A. Pechstein summarized an investigation showing that personality topics are dominant in courses in psychology in high schools. The period of tenure of college teachers, reported upon by Professor Norman MacD. Grier, averages about seven years. Personality tests of teachers, reported upon by Dr. Gordon Hendrickson, showed no administrative values of such tests, and age, marital status and degrees held were apparently without significant bearing on test scores. That biological superstitions can be eliminated by specific teaching was reported by Professor Otis W. Caldwell. Regional differences in achievement among pupils in New York City were presented by Dr. J. B. Maller. The size of measurable error in college entrance requirements is greatest for foreign-language units, as reported by T. Ernest Newland and Charles McD. Morris. The attainments of students using a simplified typewriter keyboard were discussed by Dr. Willis L. Uhl and Dr. August Dvorak, who showed a saving of more than a year of the usual two year course. A symposium on general educational problems of mathematics and physics was led by Dr. E. R. Hedrick, Dr. W. B. Carver and Dr. F. K. Richtmyer. At a joint dinner with Section I, Professor Ernest Horn gave an address on the problem of meaning in reading, in which it was shown that the many different meanings of certain words and small groups of words introduce great difficulty in learning to read effectively.

ORGANIZATIONS RELATED TO THE ASSOCIATION AS A WHOLE

(*Reports from Jennie Hall, Edward Ellery, Howard Richards, H. R. Nelson, Agnes Z. Hill*)

The American Nature Study Society held its twenty-fifth annual meeting on Tuesday, Wednesday and Thursday. The sessions were of unusual interest, with attendance which varied from about 25 at the first session to 75 at the last. The Tuesday sessions were devoted to phases of service in knowing nature and to methods of stimulation and direction of interests in the phenomena of nature. The Wednesday morning session, under the chairmanship of Dr. Otis Caldwell (Teachers College, Columbia University), presented "A Socratic Discussion: The Responsibilities of Our Society." In the first half of the Thursday morning session the papers and discussions dealt with matters related to the development of nature training of teachers and children. Then an illustrated talk was given by Dr. H. C. Bryant (U. S. National Park Service), on the educational work carried on by the U. S. National Park Service, and Arthur N. Pack (Princeton, N. J.) showed unusually instructive and interesting motion pictures of "Grizzly Bears, Glaciers and Whales in Alaska." A business meeting was held on Wednesday afternoon. An exhibition of illustrative material was a feature of the meeting. The annual dinner of this society occurred on Wednesday evening, with an attendance of 60, followed by an entertaining illustrated lecture by Dr. G. Clyde Fisher (American Museum of Natural History, New York City), who spoke on his study of Crater Canyon, Arizona, and his airplane view of the recent solar eclipse.

The 33rd annual convention of the Society of the Sigma Xi was held on Wednesday. Two new chapters had been organized in the year just closed, one at Western Reserve University and one at Princeton University; also a new Sigma Xi club of 24 members, at Yenching University (Peiping, China). The society now has 60 chapters, with a total membership of approximately 12,000, and 31 clubs; the total membership of the society, including associates, is approximately 26,000. About 1,500 members and associates are added each year. An unexpended balance of about $3,000 over budget expenses was reported. Six of the chapters presented foreign scientists to their membership and public during the year; the chapter at the University of Minnesota has continued its plan of holding symposia, the last one being on "Evolution and Civilization"; its meetings were attended by a total of 12,700 people. The chapters at Pennsylvania, Colorado, Virginia, Wisconsin and Minnesota award research prizes; the Rochester Chapter holds an annual Sigma Xi Day, with a forenoon program for school children, an afternoon exhibition of current scientific research and an evening dinner with an address.—Professor A. O. Leuschner (University of California) was elected to the executive committee for five years, and Donald H. Sweet (Chicago) was elected to the alumni committee, for five years. The annual Sigma Xi dinner was well attended. The 11th annual Sigma Xi lecture, given under the joint auspices of the society and the A. A. A. S., was given by Professor Harlow Shapley (Harvard University) on "Fact and Fancy in Cosmogony."—New chapters were authorized at Duke University and at the University of California at Los Angeles. It was decided to hold a special meeting of the society in connection with the approaching Chicago meeting of the American Association. The semi-centennial meeting of Sigma Xi is to occur in 1936, at Ithaca, in connection with the Rochester meeting of the A. A. A. S., to be held in the summer of that year.

The Metric Association met on Thursday, under the presidency of Dr. A. E. Kennelly, with a program of several talks on the metric system and its progress in the United States, an inspection trip and a dinner. A resolution was adopted recommending to the United States Congress that the terms "metric yard," "metric quart" and "metric pound" be authorized for use by the United States Government as synonymous with meter, liter and half-kilogram.

The Gamma Alpha Graduate Scientific Fraternity held its annual council meeting and convention on Wednesday and Thursday, with more than 40 members present. A committee was appointed to consider ways and means by which Gamma Alpha might take more active part in the general program at winter meetings of the American Association. Officers for 1933 are: *President,* R. H. Wetmore; *secretary,* H. R. Nelson; *treasurer,* S. P. Miller; *editor,* C. F. Scofield; *recorder,* D. S. Welch.

Sigma Delta Epsilon, graduate women's scientific fraternity, held two sessions at Atlantic City. At the Wednesday morning breakfast, to which all women interested in science were invited, Dr. Abby Turner (Mount Holyoke College) discussed "Research in Women's Colleges, Its Trials and Joys." The following officers were elected for 1933: *President,* Edna Mosher (Adelphi College); *vice-presidents,* Janet Scott (*Chemical Abstracts,* Columbus, Ohio) and Mary Carlson (Northwestern University); *treasurer,* Katherine Jeffers (University of Missouri); *secretary,* Agnes Zeimet Hill (University of Wisconsin).

Pi Gamma Mu, an honor society in the field of the social sciences, held a luncheon on Thursday, at which the speakers were: Dr. Franz Boas (Columbia University, retiring president, A. A. A. S.), Emory R. Johnson (University of Pennsylvania) and Professor Harry T. Collings (University of Pennsylvania).

# SCIENCE

VOL. 77 FRIDAY, FEBRUARY 10, 1933 No. 1989

*The American Association for the Advancement of Science:*
*Some Thoughts on the Agricultural Experiment Station:* PROFESSOR C. G. WILLIAMS 155
*Quantum Mechanics and Chemistry with Particular Reference to Reactions Involving Conjugate Double Bonds:* DR. HENRY EYRING 158
*Obituary:*
*William Arnon Henry:* PROFESSOR FRANK B. MORRISON. *Recent Deaths* 160
*Scientific Events:*
*Conference on Spectroscopy at the Massachusetts Institute of Technology; The Fifth University of Michigan Greenland Expedition; The Fifth Pacific Science Congress; Engineering Week at Chicago; Award of the Nichols Medal* 162
*Scientific Notes and News* 165
*Discussion:*
*The Naming of the Subdivisions of the Wisconsin Glacial Age:* DR. M. M. LEIGHTON. *"Mescal Pits"—a Misnomer:* H. P. MERA. *Is Geology Easier for Boys than for Girls?:* KARL VER STEEG. *Brown Rootrot of Tobacco:* PROFESSOR T. R. SWANBACK and PROFESSOR H. G. M. JACOBSON 168
*Scientific Books:*
*Recent Zoological Text-books:* PROFESSOR A. S. PEARSE 169
*Scientific Apparatus and Laboratory Methods:*
*Improved Kymograph Recording:* DR. FREDRICK F. YONKMAN. *An Inexpensive Pyrometer for Temperatures up to 1000° C.:* DR. WILLIAM C. STADIE and DR. SYDNEY L. WRIGHT, JR. *Modification of the Backlin-Kirk Combustion Chamber for Microdetermination of Carbon and Lipoids:* WM. L. DOYLE 172
*Special Articles:*
*A Proof of the Law of Effect:* DR. EDWARD L. THORNDIKE. *Is Malignancy Due to a Process Analogous to Somatic Mutation?:* DR. M. R. CURTIS, DR. W. F. DUNNING and DR. F. D. BULLOCK 173
*Science News* 6

SCIENCE: A Weekly Journal devoted to the Advancement of Science, edited by J. MCKEEN CATTELL and published every Friday by

THE SCIENCE PRESS

New York City: Grand Central Terminal

Lancaster, Pa. Garrison, N. Y.

Annual Subscription, $6.00 Single Copies, 15 Cts.

SCIENCE is the official organ of the American Association for the Advancement of Science. Information regarding membership in the Association may be secured from the office of the permanent secretary, in the Smithsonian Institution Building, Washington, D. C.

# SOME THOUGHTS ON THE AGRICULTURAL EXPERIMENT STATION[1]

By Professor C. G. WILLIAMS

AGRICULTURAL EXPERIMENT STATION, WOOSTER, OHIO

IN so far as the United States is concerned, the first agricultural experiment station dates back only 57 years, Connecticut having the honor of establishing the first station in 1875.

It is of interest to note what called the experiment station into existence. In his first annual report, Director Atwater said: "There was bitter need of a better control of the trade in commercial fertilizers in the State. One of the chief arguments used in favor of the station has been that by its means a fertilizer control system could be introduced. The demand that its first efforts should be turned in this direction was imperative."

This report gives further proof of the reason for the existence of the station, in that 103 of its 108 pages are devoted to information regarding analyses, etc., of the commercial fertilizers on the market. Strange as it may now seem, there was a time when fertilizer manufacturers had a great deal of human nature about them of the unconverted sort. Some 200 samples were received and analyzed by the Connecticut station during this first year.

The questions put up by the Connecticut farmer of the seventies sound very much like those of the Mid-West farmer of 1932, as, for instance, "Are such and such brands of fertilizers of enough value to farmers in this county to warrant their purchase these hard times?"

For several years the staff of the Connecticut station consisted of the director and three or four chemists, whose principal work was to analyze fertilizers, soils, feeds and poisons. This does not mean that noth-

[1] Address of the president and chairman of Section O—Agriculture—American Association for the Advancement of Science, Atlantic City, December, 1932.

ing else was done, for it was during this early period that some of the most valuable agricultural research of the century was done by Director Atwater—in particular the discovery of the fixation of atmospheric nitrogen by legumes.

Just a word about the second agricultural experiment station, which was established two years later in North Carolina. Its staff consisted of a director, who was the chemist of the state board of agriculture, and three assistant chemists. Like the Connecticut station, its work for several years consisted principally of its analyses of soils, fertilizers and feeds and the examination of seeds.

In his first report Director Ledeaux says: "The Board of Agriculture has wisely refrained hitherto from ordering any field tests to be made at the station for the following reasons: (1) These experiments are very expensive. (2) They need to be conducted through a series of successive years to be worth anything. (3) Owing to the extreme diversity of soils in this state most results obtained would only benefit those farmers who lived near Chapel Hill, or had soil of similar character to ours."

The above statement is also repeated in the third annual report.

With a change in station directors the fourth year, we find the new director saying in his annual report: "Experience shows that chemical manures are used to best advantage only when their application is determined strictly by the results of experiments upon the land." However, no permanent field experiments were started by the North Carolina station until four years later, when a "strictly scientific station, not a model farm," to quote the language of Director Dabney, was established.

So much for the early setting of the agricultural experiment station.

The early distrust of field experiments, as voiced by Jordan, when at the New York station, Ledeaux and others was perhaps warranted. Attempts to draw conclusions from one or two years' work conducted on land that gave every evidence of a lack of uniformity, and without sufficient controls and replications, were very properly discredited.

At a later date—some 12 or 13 years ago—C. B. Lipman and Linhart, of California, gave perhaps the most severe criticism of field experiments made before or since. They concluded that "even when fertilizer experiments were properly planned and the results adequately studied by statistical methods, our present knowledge of the enormous variability of all soils and plants renders the data from any given fertilizer plot of value only on that plot, no matter how near the experimental one." And Lipman further concludes that such experiments are not worth "the large expenditure of money, time and energy involved."

In view of these and other criticisms of field plot work, the question arises, what is the attitude of present-day experiment station workers toward field plot experimentation? In order to secure definite information regarding this matter the following question was submitted to the agronomists of 15 representative experiment stations: "What has been the trend regarding field plot experimentation at your experiment station during the last 25 years? Has your station been increasing or decreasing this line of work in your state?"

These agronomists responded as follows:

From the Connecticut station: "There has been a marked increase in the amount of field plot work at this station during the last 25 years. In spite of the many weaknesses inherent in field plot work, still it can not be entirely dispensed with, and while our greenhouse and laboratory studies have also expanded we expect to continue field work."

From the North Carolina station: "During the past 25 years there has been a material increase in field plot experiments in this state."

From the California station: "In general our field plot work has increased quite materially during the past 25 years."

From the Kentucky station: "Twenty-five years ago this station had very little field plot work. At the present time we have in soil management, fertilizer and crops work approximately 2,900 plots. We do not have any sympathy with the idea prevailing in some quarters that field work has little or no value."

From the Michigan station: "The number of field plot experiments has greatly increased in recent years. We are very much interested in greenhouse experiments and laboratory studies. However to our mind the final test is the result given under actual field conditions."

From the Kansas station: "The general trend in this state at the present time is to increase the use of field plots in our soils experimental work. We believe that some types of work may be done successfully on very small areas and under greenhouse and laboratory conditions, but that field plots are also essential in many phases of our work."

From the Alabama station: "We have very definitely increased our experimental work using field plots as a means of securing more or less practical answers to more or less practical questions. It is our opinion that there is no other way to secure answers to many of our most important questions except through the use of field plots."

From the Minnesota station: "Minnesota has greatly increased the plot work with soils and crops out in the state, both on the sub-stations and on fields leased by the university. On the university farm plot work has been decreased as this soil represents only a very small part of the state."

From the Tennessee station: "We have quite materially increased our plot work in the last 25 years. I consider work of this kind very important; in fact I would not know how to get along without it."

From the Wisconsin station: "Our faith in the value of the field plot as a medium of experimentation is increasing rather than decreasing. The trend, however, is more and more in the direction of a combination of field, greenhouse and laboratory work."

From the New York station (Ithaca): "The soil at Ithaca lacks uniformity to a rather unusual degree. This difficulty has led us to substitute what we call 'frames' for ordinary field plots. We also use the greenhouse for certain experiments, but I think that the extent to which a greenhouse may be substituted for field experiments is rather limited. We have not curtailed in any way the work on our outlying experiment fields."

From the Illinois station: "The trend in plot experimentation was distinctly upward until the cost of operation began to be almost unbearable. We had our peak in the number of crops and soils fields in 1919—forty fields. I suspect the number will be smaller than it has been in the past. We are emphasizing our laboratory research more than used to be the case. We must find a good balance between the two."

From the Indiana station: "During the last 25 years the field plot experimental work of this station has increased many fold. All our experience tends to strengthen the view that the results of carefully conducted and long-continued experiments on a reasonably representative field of any distinct type of soil will apply to other areas of the same type wherever found under similar climatic conditions. We hope to add to our permanent experimental fields until we have one on every important soil type in the state."

From the Iowa station: "The area on which we are now carrying experiments is five or six times as large as formerly. Too much emphasis can not be put on the value of field plot experimental work in soils and crops."

From the Pennsylvania station: "There has been a continued increase in our field plot experiments year by year up to the present time."

Such is the testimony of representative agronomists of the United States.

The greater use which is apparently being made of field plots in the solution of soils and crops problems, as indicated above, is probably in large part due to improved methods in field experimentation. With more replications and controls, with a greater appreciation of the possibility of experimental error and a technique adapted to the measurement of such error, results are being secured to-day that were not to be had in some of the earlier work.

Not only have methods been improved in field plot experimentation, but there has been a general refinement in methods along all lines.

It is not so long ago that our workers with animals were content to use from one to five animals in feeding tests and to draw conclusions therefrom regarding rations and gains. Now, from 20 to 100 animals on each ration are regarded as quite essential, and the work must be repeated several times. Numbers, replications and controls are exceedingly important.

There is, I think, a rapidly growing tendency to break down departmental lines in research institutions in joint attacks upon research problems, both in planning and carrying them forward. Much more valuable results are to be had from such cooperation. And similar cooperative attacks may be and are being carried on between different experiment stations and between state stations and the Federal department of agriculture.

While many of our experiment stations got under way without any help from the Federal Government, the Hatch Act of 1887, the Adams Act of 1906 and the Purnell Act of 1925 have proved a great stimulus to research work. In the expenditure of Adams funds a higher type of research was insisted upon.

Some 7 per cent. of the projects of the agricultural experiment stations of the United States is listed by the Office of Experiment Stations as Adams projects, and 12 per cent. as Purnell projects. The latter act especially encouraged research in agricultural economics, home economics and rural sociology. Approximately one half of the projects supported by Purnell funds are in these three lines of work.

The field of the agricultural experiment station is an ever broadening one. Beginning largely in an effort to protect the agricultural public from fraudulent practices in the manufacture and sale of commercial fertilizers, feed stuffs, seeds, etc., the experiment station has taken over the vast fields of soils and crops, animal production, dairying, horticulture, forestry, agricultural and biological chemistry, plant and animal nutrition, plant and animal pathology, economic entomology, bacteriology, genetics, agricultural economics, agricultural engineering, home economics, food technology, rural sociology, textiles and clothing.

As one looks backward over these 50 years of experiment station work, he is impressed with the contribution the stations have made to our material progress—the hundreds of new varieties of farm and horticultural crops which have been developed;

The many new legumes which have been discovered and introduced, some of which will be found adapted to our widely varying conditions;

The discovery and development of economic methods for combatting insects and diseases which have made relatively certain the production of crops and animals which was previously a gamble;

The improved methods of breeding and feeding all kinds of live stock for increased production in milk, meat and eggs;

The economic use of commercial plant foods and soil amendments;

The invention of the Babcock test and its consequent influence on all dairy practices—not to mention other contributions.

Up to 10 or 12 years ago it was the fashion to descant upon the grave dangers confronting this country and the world at large from our rapidly growing population overtaking our production of food and fabric materials. We hear none of this to-day.

But back of and leading up to these practical results are more permanent contributions to our fundamental knowledge which will bear fruit in the decades to come, for our experiment stations have not been content with knowing "what," but have pressed on to the "how" and the "why."

What of the future?

The financial situation in which many of our experiment stations now find themselves is discouraging. A reduction of state appropriations is very general. What course Federal appropriations will take is uncertain at this writing, but in spite of our tremendous financial depression it is hardly conceivable that the Federal Government will scrap an organization which it has been slowly building up for the last 40 years.

A reasonable support of these institutions would seem to be assured.

# QUANTUM MECHANICS AND CHEMISTRY WITH PARTICULAR REFERENCE TO REACTIONS INVOLVING CONJUGATE DOUBLE BONDS[1]

By Dr. HENRY EYRING

FRICK CHEMICAL LABORATORY, PRINCETON UNIVERSITY

THE universally accepted conception of atoms as positive nuclei surrounded by electrons make it obvious that some sort of mechanics of such particles will properly describe their chemical behavior. The success of quantum mechanics in atomic physics where it gives quantitative agreement with experiment shows us clearly enough the general means to be employed. From this point of view it is convenient to regard the Schrodinger equation as our point of departure. Among the solutions of the Schrodinger equation which satisfy the supplementary quantum conditions only those which in addition obey the Pauli principle, *i.e.,* only those solutions which change sign when two identical particles are interchanged need be considered as having physical reality. Our scheme, though complete, is still much too difficult to proceed with. We must find other simplifying conditions. The first simplification is a familiar one. Because of the much greater mass of atoms than electrons the atoms travel relatively much more slowly so that in calculating the potential energy of any system from the Schrodinger equation we neglect the motion of the atoms without introducing serious error. The result is that we obtain a potential energy for the system under consideration as a function of the distance between the atoms, and this, as we shall soon see, provides just the necessary information for estimating rates of reactions. London was the first to point out that such a scheme probably provided a way for calculating activation energies. We next consider the nature of an activation energy. Consider the reaction $H_2 + I_2 = 2HI$. This is a well-known bimolecular reaction. For the rate of formation of HI, we can write

$$\frac{d(HI)}{dt} = f\,S\,e^{-E/RT}\,(H_2)\,(I_2).$$

The parenthesis around a formula indicates the concentration of that substance. Thus S $(H_2)$ $(I_2)$ is the number of collisions between molecules of hydrogen and iodine in concentration units and can be calculated from kinetic theory, while the expression $e^{-E/RT}$ is the chance that in a particular collision the two molecules collide with an energy E in a form to permit reaction. The energy E is called the activation energy and has for this reaction a value of 40,000 calories. The precision of activation energy measurements is seldom better than one large calorie; so that activation energies are ordinarily specified in large calories. The proper fraction f in our rate expression approaches one for most simple reactions.

[1] Based on a paper presented before the Section of Chemistry of the American Association for the Advancement of Science at its Atlantic City meeting for which the anunal prize of the association was awarded.

It is a steric factor which measures the probability of a collision being of a kind to permit reaction even though it is sufficiently energetic. The variations in f for different reactions is of a different order of magnitude than the variation in $e^{-E/RT}$ so that by far the most important quantity in determining rates of reactions is the activation energy. Similar considerations hold for other types of reactions, so that if we can calculate the activation energy for the different mechanisms we are able to answer the very interesting question as to which way the reaction will proceed. For example, the reaction just considered might proceed by the alternative mechanism,

$$I_2 = 2I$$
$$I + H_2 = HI + H$$
$$H + I_2 = HI + I.$$

But both theory and experiment agree in preferring the mechanism $H_2 + I_2 = 2HI$, while for the reaction of the other halogens with hydrogen, as well as in the conversion of ortho to para hydrogen, they again agree in indicating reaction by way of the atoms. In the border line case of the reaction of hydrogen with bromine, obtaining the correct results depends somewhat on the assumed ratio of coulombic to interchange binding. The other cases give results so clear cut as to be independent of assumed ratios of interchange to coulombic binding. The fact that the calculations indicate that fluorine should not react with hydrogen at room temperatures seems to have attracted considerable attention, probably because of the early erroneous experiments widely quoted in the literature. Experiments of von Wartenburg, as well as some unpublished experimental results of Kassel and the author, leave no question of the chemical inertness of the mixture in diffuse daylight at ordinary temperatures. As a matter of fact, the contrary result would be startling when one considers the strong homopolar bonds to be broken. There is certainly a correlation between increase in the strength of the bonds to be broken and increase in the activation energy of a reaction. This was noted experimentally and follows as a matter of course from our theoretical calculations.

Before proceeding further with a discussion of our results it is perhaps well to consider in a little more detail the method of calculation. The coulombic portion of the energy of a homopolar bond between a pair of atoms increases from 10 per cent. in the case of non-metals like hydrogen to 28 per cent. in the case of metals like sodium and is independent of the presence of other atoms. That is to say, the attractive potential just adds up for all atom pairs, no matter how many atoms are in the neighborhood of a given atom. The remaining part of the bonds, called the interchange binding, add up quite differently. The laws of addition up to and including eight electrons are now known as a result of investigations in this and other research centers and the indefinite extension to larger numbers of atoms only awaits a real need. The extension offers no more difficulty than that of being very tedious. The evaluation of the coulombic and interchange binding between atom pairs as a function of the distance between the atoms is accomplished by reference to curves constructed from spectroscopic constants. Empirical Morse curves are at present the most convenient for this purpose. Knowing the amounts of interchange and coulombic binding and the laws of addition it is then a simple matter to calculate the energy of any configuration, and so construct a surface which enables us to follow the mechanism of approach of two molecules until they reach a point where new bonds are as strong as old ones and we find a new pairing of the atoms taking place. Such potential surfaces in the simple cases involving three atoms consist of two long valleys corresponding to configurations of the initial and final substances separated by a saddle over which the system must pass. The height of this saddle measured from the initial valley floor is the activation energy for the forward reaction. For the reverse reaction the activation energy is measured from the floor of the other valley. The heat of reaction is of course the difference in the heights of the valley floors. In case of a reaction such as the unimolecular decomposition of $N_2O$ the initial region is a basin instead of a valley separated as before by a saddle from the final valley or valleys. The study of the kinetics of this reaction simply involves the study of a mass point on such a surface. Because of a change in multiplicity in the decomposition of $N_2O$ the reaction surface is a composite of two intersecting surfaces and some attention must be given to transition at the junction. With molecules containing more atoms, more dimensions are required for our surface, but the essential problem of finding the height of a saddle value measured from a valley or basin remains. In my first paper, with Professor Polanyi, these methods applied to the reaction between a hydrogen atom and a hydrogen molecule gave results in good agreement with the experimental activation energy found by A. Farkas.

Pelzer and Wigner, then, carrying the matter further, were able to show that the rates calculated, entirely theoretically, were in very good agreement with experiment; so that apparently in the reaction of a hydrogen atom with a hydrogen molecule we have for the first term a rather satisfactory detailed picture of a reaction.

In cooperation with Mr. A. Sherman these methods were then applied to the reaction in which the conversion of ortho to para hydrogen takes place on a surface. Again, so far as we can now judge, we find agreement with experiment. The process seems to be one in which a hydrogen molecule is split into atoms by two surface carbon atoms which are abnormally far apart, each hydrogen atom becoming attached to a surface atom. These hydrogen atoms are now apt to leave the surface with a different but similarly situated hydrogen atom by the reverse of the absorption process. The conversion is thus completed. The result that for the greatest ease of activated adsorption the carbon atoms should be from four to five times as far apart as the normal distance between the hydrogen atoms is a rather striking part of this picture. This would be achieved in lattices in which some positions are vacant and we should therefore expect the instability to heat treatment customarily found with very active surfaces. Since a particular distance of surface atoms favors adsorption of a particular type of molecule, preferential adsorption is to be expected. These calculations indicate that the conception sometimes held, that an equal distance between surface atoms and the atoms in the gaseous molecule favors activated adsorption, should be abandoned.

With Dr. Kimball an examination was made of the proposed mechanism for the hydrogen chlorine reaction

$$Cl + H_2 + Cl_2 = 2HCl + Cl.$$

The calculations indicated it to be far slower than the reaction

$$Cl + H_2 = HCl + H$$

and so the first reaction could be excluded. This seems to be in keeping with the most recent experimental opinion. Similar although rougher calculations indicated that water should not be helpful in this reaction which apparently contradicted experimental findings at the time but is apparently at present in agreement with experimental findings.

In a paper appearing this month in the *Proceedings* of the National Academy it is pointed out that the difference in zero point energy for compounds of two isotopes makes the lighter isotope more reactive, and so should assist in their separation. Whether or not this is the principal factor in enabling Dr. E. W. Washburn to preferentially electrolyze away the lighter isotope from water remains to be seen.

We thus bring to a new problem a considerable confidence in the essential correctness of our method. It was with this background that we considered the additions of hydrogen and bromine to butadiene. The details of the calculations together with certain extensions will be published elsewhere as a joint paper with Mr. Albert Sherman and Dr. George E. Kimball. The addition of bromine may be expected to occur in either of two ways:

$$Br_2 + H_2C = CH - CH = CH_2 \rightarrow BrH_2C - CH = CH - CH_2Br$$
$$\rightarrow BrH_2C - CHBr - CH = CH_2.$$

Taking explicitly into account in both cases the six electrons which change partners in the first reaction and using simply the methods already outlined we find for the first reaction an activation energy of 36.4 kilo calories, for the second an activation energy of 52 kilo calories. It thus seems sufficiently clear why 1–4 addition is to be expected. The sort of thing which might cause 1–2 addition to be preferred of course is to substitute for a hydrogen on 4 some group that introduces large steric effects. We hope to return to this aspect of the problem in the not too distant future. If the same calculations are made for the substitution of hydrogen to butadiene the activation energy for 1–4 addition is found to be 77 kilo calories and for 1–2, 113. Emphasis is of course not to be placed on the exact value of our figures, but their relative correctness seems reliable. The size of the calculated activation energies indicates, certainly in the case of hydrogen, that any addition can only occur catalytically. In the case of the addition of bromine the indication is less clear cut that the reaction must go by way of surfaces, but it certainly should be examined from that point of view. The factors which favor 1–4 addition in the gas phase will of course be less important for catalyzed reactions.

The significant point again seems to be at least qualitative agreement between theory and experiment. Very much remains to be done in the way of examining more closely the underlying approximations of this method with the idea of obtaining more precise results; but apparently even in its present unfinished form we have a surprisingly powerful tool with which to attack the almost endless variety of problems of chemical mechanism. Something is also gained by having a scheme into which the multitudinous experimental results may be fitted.

# OBITUARY

## DR. WILLIAM ARNON HENRY

DR. WILLIAM ARNON HENRY, one of the outstanding pioneers in the development of agricultural instruction, research and extension in this country, died at his home in San Diego, California, on November 24, 1932, from an attack of pneumonia.

The life story of Dean Henry, as he was usually called, is one to inspire youth and is typically American. Born on a farm near Norwalk, Ohio, on June 16, 1850, he was still in his early teens when his father was called into the Union army. Heavy responsibilities then fell upon the boy, which undoubtedly aided much in developing the great capacity for work which later characterized him. After a period of study in Ohio Wesleyan University, he had to interrupt his course to earn money by teaching school. He then entered the course in agriculture at Cornell University and through supplementing the funds he had saved, by doing whatever work he could find, he completed his course in 1880 and received the B.S. degree.

Immediately after graduation he was selected to take the position of professor of botany and agriculture at the University of Wisconsin. The "and agriculture" part of his title meant little, for there was no agricultural college, no experiment station and not even a department of agriculture in the university. He was to take charge of the university farm, which was badly run down, and to endeavor to develop the agricultural work so it would serve the farmers of the state.

Henry's career furnishes an outstanding example of a man whose far-sighted vision and keen judgment led him to make a radical change from his first specialty. Though trained as a botanist and horticulturist, when he became acquainted with Wisconsin conditions, he became convinced that live-stock farming and especially dairying offered the most general possibilities for success. He therefore threw his great energy into the development of dairying and other phases of the live-stock industry. Not only was his work one of the important factors in the development which made Wisconsin the leading dairy state, but also he gained an international reputation as an authority on live-stock feeding. He was granted honorary doctor's degrees by the University of Illinois, the University of Vermont and Michigan Agricultural College in recognition of his accomplishments and his services to agriculture.

At first Henry had practically no funds for research and indeed all facilities were most meager. With his magnetic personality, he soon interested some of the legislators in his work and secured a modest appropriation for investigations on the ensilage of fodders and the manufacture of cane-sugar from sorghum cane. This is of especial interest because it was the first definite state appropriation for research at the university. Henry later delighted in telling how one of the legislative leaders leaned across the aisle when the appropriation was under discussion, and remarked to his boon companion, "Let's kill this pup before it gets to be a dog." Only because of Henry's inspirational zeal and enthusiasm was he able to convince the legislators that it was wise public policy for the state to support agricultural investigations.

The investigations begun under this appropriation were instrumental in convincing farmers of the value of silage in live-stock feeding and resulted in there being more silos in Wisconsin than in any other state. Not only did he develop the agricultural work at the university, but also he literally "stumped the state," preaching scientific agriculture to the farmers on every possibility and winning them by his personality and clearly stated facts. Undoubtedly it was Henry who first "sold" the agricultural college and the university as well to the people of the state. He focused attention on the possibilities of the university as a service agency for the whole citizenry, using every means at his command—lectures, bulletins, press articles and interviews.

In these early days very few students were enrolled in the regular university courses in agriculture. Therefore, in an endeavor to interest farm boys in agricultural instruction, there was begun in 1885 under Henry's direction the first agricultural short course in America. The idea of giving at a university practical instruction to students who were not graduates of a secondary school met with ridicule and scorn on the part of many educators, but the short course was exceedingly successful and a somewhat similar plan has been adopted in practically every state.

He saw at an early date that an accurate and simple test for the butter fat in milk was urgently needed by the dairy industry, and stimulated the late Dr. S. M. Babcock to undertake the investigations which led to the invention of the well-known Babcock test in 1890. The same year he started the first dairy course in America in which practical instruction was given in the testing and manufacture of dairy products.

Burdened with numerous and exacting administrative and teaching duties, nevertheless he found time for research on many problems in animal production which were both of practical and scientific importance. He was among the earliest to study the effect upon the growth and development of farm animals of rations ample and deficient in protein and in minerals; the value of silage for live stock; the effect of various methods of preparing feeds for swine, and the value and use of dairy by-products in stock feeding. In his writings and addresses he continually emphasized the importance of efficiency in farming and he was a firm advocate of cooperative effort among farmers. As an author, Henry's lasting fame rests on "Feeds and Feeding," which for thirty-four years has been the most widely used text and reference work on live-stock feeding in the English language and is now in the 19th edition.

Energetic to the extreme, he never spared himself, but gave every ounce of his strength to the upbuilding of the agriculture of his state. Due primarily to this, his health at last broke under the strain, and in 1907 he retired from his university duties.

Few know that Henry was to a considerable degree responsible for the passage of the parcel post bill in 1912. Convinced of the value of parcel post to farmers, Henry worked for months in advocating the legislation. Appreciating the value of concerted action, he wrote to the agricultural editors of the country and asked them to announce a "Parcel Post Day" on March 1, 1912. On this day, all who were in favor of parcel post were asked to write their congressmen personal letters. As a result, the lawmakers at Washington were fairly deluged with a mountain of mail from all the rural districts.

After his retirement Henry spent considerable time in Connecticut, developing a large fruit farm with his only son, Arnon T. Henry. Later he took much pleasure in collecting rare plants for his residence on the west coast of Florida, and for the last several years resided in San Diego, where he indulged his early interest in horticulture and botany.

FRANK B. MORRISON

CORNELL UNIVERSITY

### RECENT DEATHS

EUGENE E. HASKELL, consulting hydraulic engineer, dean of the College of Civil Engineering at Cornell University from 1906 to 1921, when he retired with the title of professor emeritus, died on January 28, at the age of seventy-seven years.

PROFESSOR WILLIAM LISPENARD ROBB, head of the department of electrical engineering at Rensselaer Polytechnic Institute since 1902, died on January 26, at the age of seventy-one years.

DR. WILLIAM PHILLIPS GRAVES, professor of gynecology at Harvard Medical School since 1911, died on January 25, at the age of sixty-three years.

DR. VICTOR STERKI, assistant curator of zoology in the Carnegie Museum, Pittsburgh, died on January 25, at the age of eighty-six years. The Sterki collection of mollusca will be deposited in the museum.

SIR WILLIAM TAYLOR, president of the Royal Academy of Medicine in Ireland since 1927, died suddenly on January 29, at the age of seventy-two years. He was an honorary fellow of the American College of Surgeons and a past president of the Association of Surgeons of Great Britain and Ireland.

DR. MALCOLM EVAN MACGREGOR, in charge of the Wellcome Entomological Field Laboratories at Esher, Surrey, died on January 12, at the age of forty-three years.

PROFESSOR GUIDO TIZZONI, until four years ago professor of general pathology at the University of Bologna, has died.

THE death is announced of Dr. Albert Wigand, professor of meteorology at Freiburg, and of Dr. Karl Kreibich, professor of dermatology at the German University at Prague.

DR. HEINRICH MAHNKOPF died on December 20, 1932, aged forty years. He was a chief of division at the Prussian Geodetic Institute in Potsdam and Dozent at the Technische Hochschule in Berlin. Volume VI of the Publications of the International Latitude Service was recently completed and published under his direction. He succeeded Albrecht and Wanach in the work of the Latitude Service.

A CORRESPONDENT writes: "Miss Julia Irene Goodrich, known to many hundreds of biologists through the assistance she gave them in getting settled on their first arrival at Cold Spring Harbor, died January 21, at the age of fifty-seven years. Miss Goodrich was for twenty-seven years secretary to the director of what is now the department of genetics. She graduated from Smith College, showing especial proficiency in the classics and languages in general, like her uncle Chauncey Goodrich, who compiled a Chinese dictionary and translated the Bible into Chinese, and his son, L. C. Goodrich, lecturer in Chinese at Columbia University. Another uncle was professor of Latin at the University of Vermont. She was a member of the American Association for the Advancement of Science."

# SCIENTIFIC EVENTS

### CONFERENCE ON SPECTROSCOPY AT THE MASSACHUSETTS INSTITUTE OF TECHNOLOGY

THE Massachusetts Institute of Technology announces a Summer Conference in Spectroscopy in connection with its new Spectroscopy Laboratory. The arrangements are in charge of Professor George R. Harrison, and it is hoped that such a conference may become an annual summer event. On account of the air conditioning of the laboratory and the availability of summer cottages within commuting distance on the shore, this conference makes possible a combination of summer vacation with interesting scientific work under comfortable conditions.

The research facilities embrace five general subjects (1) quantitative measurement of spectrum intensities, (2) measurement of hyperfine structure, (3) analysis of spectrum series, especially with the aid of the newly developed mechanical analyzer, (4) vacuum spectroscopy of the ultra-violet, (5) quantitative chemical analysis by spectroscopic methods. In all these fields the laboratory possesses unexcelled, and in the second and fourth fields, unique, facilities. In addition to opportunities for conference and research, there will be graduate courses in spectroscopy, atomic and molecular structure and related subjects.

The plans provide for three groups: (1) scientists of recognized achievements in the field of spectroscopy, who will be guests of the laboratory, (2) graduate students who will be expected to pay moderate tuition fees, (3) industrial organizations which may send qualified representatives to work on spectroscopic problems of chemical analysis, or which may submit problems to be worked on by industrial research fellows under supervision of the laboratory staff, in accordance with contracts to be made with the Institute's Division of Industrial Cooperation.

Requests for information in regard to facilities or summer living arrangements and applications for admission to these activities should be addressed to Professor George R. Harrison, Department of Physics, Massachusetts Institute of Technology, Cambridge, Massachusetts.

## THE FIFTH UNIVERSITY OF MICHIGAN GREENLAND EXPEDITION

THE Fifth University of Michigan Greenland Expedition is included among the Second Polar Year Expeditions of 1932–33. This expedition is directed by Professor Ralph L. Belknap, who was second-in-command on earlier Michigan expeditions. With Evans S. Schmeling, aerologist, and Herbert Gardner, photographer and botanist, he sailed for Greenland on the *Morrissey,* Captain Robert A. Bartlett, master, which took the Peary Memorial Expedition to North Greenland last summer. His companions were landed with the supplies of the expedition on the neck of the Upper Nugssuak Peninsula in latitude 74°, while Dr. Belknap proceeded to Cape York to act as construction engineer in the erection of the Peary Shaft.

The expedition base is much the same as that of the Cornell Expedition more than thirty years ago and the station is located near the front of the Cornell Glacier outlet. Dr. Belknap, the director, rejoined his expedition on August 31 and the lumber used in erection of the Peary Shaft was then used to build the hut of the expedition, which has been named Peary Lodge. On September 18, Max Demorest, assistant aerologist, and Hansen, radio operator, with additional supplies, arrived from Upernivik on the little motor sloop *Saelen.* The *Saelen,* carrying letters on its return, was wrecked with the loss of all on board, so that relatively meager reports from Dr. Belknap have been received up to the present. However, a number of radio messages, relayed through various amateur stations, have indicated that the party is well, and that scientific work, particularly that in aerology, has been proceeding satisfactorily. The winter night, which arrived in early November, has since that time interfered with the upper-air studies.

When in February or March the light becomes better Dr. Belknap plans to make a somewhat extended penetration by dog sled of the inland ice and carry out various scientific studies including the upper air and sounding of the glacier. The expedition is expected to return in early October.

WILLIAM H. HOBBS

## THE FIFTH PACIFIC SCIENCE CONGRESS

ANNOUNCEMENT has been made recently by the National Research Council of Canada that plans have been resumed for holding in the coming summer the Fifth Pacific Science Congress, which it had been originally planned to hold last May. This congress will convene in Victoria and Vancouver, British Columbia, between the dates June 1 and 14, 1933. During the week following the sessions of the congress, excursions will be conducted through the western part of Canada.

The purpose of this series of congresses is to give opportunity for the discussion of scientific problems relating to the Pacific area, and to plan for the advancement of research upon these problems through the coordinated efforts of research institutions in the countries within the Pacific region. Previous congresses were held in Honolulu (1920), Sydney and Melbourne (1923), Tokyo (1926), and Batavia and Buitenzorg (1929). The congresses are organized under the immediate auspices of the National Research Council or corresponding scientific body in the country in which they are held, and are under the general sponsorship of the Pacific Science Association, which comprises scientific organizations from fourteen of the Pacific countries.

The program of the congress this year will include a series of general symposia upon the recent applications of science in forestry, agriculture and fisheries, also a general symposium upon the geological significance of the fiords in lands bordering on the Pacific Ocean, and a symposium for a discussion of the origin and antiquity of the American aborigines. Other sessions of the congress will be arranged in two general groups, one for the biological sciences and one for the physical sciences. In the former, provision will be made for the discussion of problems relating to agriculture, anthropology and ethnology, animal diseases, public health, botany and plant pathology, forestry, zoology, entomology and fisheries.

In the group for the physical sciences provision will be made for the discussion of problems of astronomy, geodesy and geography, geology and mineral resources, seismology and volcanology, oceanography, meteorology and terrestrial magnetism, and radio communications. The contributions to the program of the congress will consist mainly of specially invited papers.

The Government of the United States has been invited by His Majesty's Government in Canada to participate in this congress by the appointment of twenty-five official delegates to the congress from this country. These delegates will be named by the government. In addition the National Research Council of the United States has been authorized to extend an invitation to the learned organizations and institutions in this country to participate in the congress. Universities, societies and research institutions which may wish to appoint representatives to attend this congress are requested to communicate with the National Research Council.

W. H. HOWELL,
*Chairman, National Research Council*

## ENGINEERING WEEK AT CHICAGO

PLANS for the conference of engineers at Chicago, during Engineering Week, June 25 to 30, which is being sponsored by the Century of Progress Exposition, are making progress. Education will be an important theme of the conference, with the Society for the Promotion of Engineering Education taking an important part. In addition to its sessions some twenty of the national engineering societies will participate with sectional and national meetings.

On Sunday evening, June 25, when Engineering Week opens officially, the International Union of Pure and Applied Physics will have a joint session with Section M of the American Association for the Advancement of Science. A number of the engineering societies will participate with a program which is being arranged on the "Application of Physics to Engineering" by Dr. R. A. Millikan. On the evening of June 27, A. P. M. Fleming and H. Gough, of England, will address a similar joint session on "The Industrial Developments of the Century."

In addition to the individual activities of the various groups during the week, there will be a joint conference on Engineers Day. The program for this day includes a banquet at the Hotel Stevens. It is expected that there will be an attendance of more than 3,000. The program, which is not yet ready for announcement, will include addresses by distinguished American and foreign scientific men and engineers.

In addition to the educational exhibits at the Century of Progress Exposition, the sixth Midwest Engineering and Power Exposition will be held at the Coliseum during that week. At this exposition some 300 manufacturers will exhibit the latest developments in steam-generating equipment for power and process purposes. In addition there will be a wide range of equipment such as heating and air conditioning apparatus, water treatment and softeners for swimming pools and many other items of interest to engineers and superintendents of schools.

## AWARD OF THE NICHOLS MEDAL

AWARD of the William H. Nichols Medal of the New York Section of the American Chemical Society for 1933 to Dr. Wilder D. Bancroft, professor of physical chemistry at Cornell University, has been announced by Dr. Walter S. Landis, chairman of the Medal Committee. The medal will be presented at a meeting of the New York Section in the Electrical Institute Auditorium, Grand Central Palace, on March 10. "Protein Therapy" will be the subject of Professor Bancroft's medal address. Other speakers will be Professor W. Lash Miller, of the University of Toronto, who will narrate the achievements of Professor Bancroft, and Dr. Charles L. Parsons, of Washington, D. C., secretary of the American Chemical Society, who will discuss the personal aspects of Professor Bancroft's career. Dr. Victor K. LaMer, professor of chemistry in Columbia University and chairman of the New York Section, will preside.

In announcing the award Professor Bancroft's work is described as follows:

> Professor Bancroft's researches are derived from the work of Claude Bernard, French physiologist who sixty years ago advanced the view that anesthesia was due to a reversible coagulation of some of the proteins of the brain and of the sensory nerves. Although biologists, physiologists and medical men rejected Bernard's view, Professor Bancroft has demonstrated that it is of "enormous importance in physiology, pharmacology and medicine."
>
> Professor Bancroft's general conclusions are that in some forms of insanity a coagulation of brain and nerve protein occurs. In others, protein dispersion takes place. He points out that in manic depression and epilepsy a slight coagulation of protein has taken place in either all or a part of the brain. Therefore, he concludes that a chemical agent which has the opposite effect on proteins should work toward a cure.
>
> Through the use of these methods, Professor Bancroft's researches have indicated that the use of sodium rhodanate may cure narcotic addiction and that it may also be employed eventually as a treatment for hay fever.
>
> "If the brain is permanently abnormal," according to Professor Bancroft, "the thinking will be abnormal also and the patient will be called insane. The brain can be abnormal in two ways, by being too puckered or by being too mushy. There must therefore be two types

of insanity, a puckered type which will be helped by sodium rhodanate and a mushy type which will be helped by an anesthetic such as sodium amytal. These two types exist and can be helped in this way. Manic depressives and epileptics are of the puckered type; dementia praecox catatonics are of the mushy type.''

# SCIENTIFIC NOTES AND NEWS

DR. ALBERT EINSTEIN, who sails for Europe on March 15, will be the guest of honor at a dinner, given by friends of the Hebrew University in Jerusalem, at the Hotel Commodore, New York City. It is expected that a thousand men of science and letters will attend. It is planned to present to Dr. Einstein at the dinner a fund for the Hebrew University and for other organizations in which he is interested. The fund, it is hoped, will reach $100,000.

THE Edison Medal for 1932, awarded to Bancroft Gherardi, vice-president and chief engineer of the American Telephone and Telegraph Company, in recognition of his "contributions to the art of telephone engineering and the development of electrical communication," was presented to him by the president, H. P. Charlesworth, at the recent annual convention in New York City of the American Institute of Electrical Engineers. The principal speakers were Dr. Gano Dunn, of New York City, and Dr. Dugald C. Jackson, head of the electrical department of engineering of the Massachusetts Institute of Technology and chairman of the Edison Medal committee.

THE presentation of the Alfred Noble Prize to Frank M. Starr, of the General Electric Company, was made on January 23 at the opening meeting of the American Society of Civil Engineers. The prize, an award of $500, was presented by Arthur S. Tuttle, vice-president of the American Society of Civil Engineers, which is trustee for the memorial fund created in 1929 by friends of Mr. Noble. The award was made for a published paper, "Equivalent Circuits—II."

DR. WILLIAM BOWIE, of the U. S. Coast and Geodetic Survey, has been awarded, by the Royal Academy of Belgium, the Charles Lagrange Prize in recognition of his having effected the complete unification of the triangulation systems of Canada, the United States and Mexico. North America is the only continent having a single triangulation system.

MERLE RANDALL, professor of chemistry at the University of California, has been awarded a medal of merit by Charles University of Prague, in recognition of his contributions in research and the training of young men for careers in chemistry.

DR. GLADYS A. REICHARD, Barnard College, Columbia University, has been awarded the A. Cressy Morrison Prize by the New York Academy of Science for her monograph entitled "Melanesian Design: a Study of Style in Wood and Tortoise Shell Carving."

DR. EMIL ABDERHALDEN, professor of physiology at Halle, has been elected an honorary member of the Italian Society for Experimental Biology.

F. E. MATTHES, of the United States Geological Survey, has been elected president for 1933 of the Association of American Geographers, and S. S. Visher, of Indiana University, vice-president. The secretary, F. E. Williams, of the University of Pennsylvania, and the treasurer, R. S. Platt, of the University of Chicago, were reelected.

PROFESSOR GEORGE C. HUMPHREY, of the University of Wisconsin College of Agriculture, was recently elected president of the American Society of Animal Production.

AT the annual general meeting in London of the Royal Meteorological Society on January 18, Professor S. Chapman was reelected president. The Buchan Prize, awarded biennially for the most important original papers contributed to the society during the previous five years, was presented to D. Brunt.

DR. HARRY WOODBURN CHASE, president of the University of Illinois, previously professor of psychology and president of the University of North Carolina, has been elected chancellor of New York University to succeed Dr. Elmer Ellsworth Brown.

DR. WALTER H. EVANS, chief of the Division of Insular Stations of the Office of Experiment Stations, U. S. Department of Agriculture, reached the compulsory retirement age on February 1. During his forty-one years' service in the department, first as botanist and botanical editor of the *Experiment Station Record*, then as chief of the Division of Insular Stations of the Office of Experiment Stations, and for a time as acting chief of the office, Dr. Evans was responsible for establishing and developing agricultural experiment stations in Alaska, Hawaii, Puerto Rico, Guam and the Virgin Islands, and in promoting research, particularly in plant physiology and pathology, by the state experiment stations.

DR. CHARLES WEISS, formerly associate professor of applied bacteriology and immunology at Washington University School of Medicine, has been appointed director of the Clinical and Research Laboratories of the Mount Zion Hospital, San Francisco, California. He has also been appointed associate professor of research medicine in the Hooper Foundation of the University of California, and consulting immunologist to the University of California Hospital.

PROFESSOR W. S. NELMS, of the department of physics of Emory University, has been granted leave of absence for the coming spring quarter. He will spend the time at the University of Cambridge and the University of Berlin.

OTTO DEGENER, who is writing a comprehensive illustrated Flora of the Hawaiian Islands, has shipped a large collection of herbarium specimens to New York preparatory to its critical study at the New York Botanical Garden. This collection is the result of extensive botanizing on all the major islands of the Hawaiian Archipelago during the last ten years.

DR. J. DUFRENOY, director of the Station for Plant Pathology, near Bordeaux, is spending six months at Riverside, California, in the laboratory of plant physiology at the Citrus Experiment Station, investigating the cytological conditions associated with mottle leaf of citrus and other trees. He has been granted a fellowship by the Rockefeller Foundation for this investigation.

DR. OTTO HAHN, director of the Kaiser Wilhelm Institute of Chemistry at Dahlem and lecturer in chemistry (radioactivity) at the University of Berlin, will reach Ithaca in February, where he is this year non-resident Baker lecturer in chemistry. He will lecture for three months on his work on the chemistry of radium.

PROFESSOR J. J. R. MACLEOD, professor of physiology at the University of Aberdeen, and previously at the University of Toronto, is visiting professor at the Johns Hopkins University, where he is giving the Herter Lectures.

DR. ERNEST W. BROWN, professor of mathematics at Yale University, gave the second Arthur Lecture at the Smithsonian Institution on January 25. His subject was "Gravitation in the Solar System."

DR. HARVEY CUSHING, who last year retired as Moseley professor of surgery, Harvard University Medical School, delivered the fourth Harvey Lecture at the New York Academy of Medicine on January 19, on "Dyspituitarism: Twenty Years Later."

DR. IRVING LANGMUIR, of the General Electric Company, lectured on the adsorption theory at the Charlottenburg Institute of Technology on January 27. He was introduced by Professor Walther Nernst, with whom he was formerly a student.

CAPTAIN SIR HUBERT WILKINS, explorer of the Arctic and Antarctic, will lecture in the James Simpson Theater of the Field Museum, Chicago, at 3 P. M. on March 4. His subject will be "What I Have Discovered in the Arctic and Antarctic." He will relate his experiences on expeditions made by dog team, by airplane and by submarine. The lecture will be illustrated with motion pictures.

DR. F. G. DONNAN, professor of inorganic and physical chemistry at University College, London, gave the Ostwald Memorial Lecture of the British Chemical Society at the University of Liverpool on January 27.

PROFESSOR S. L. BOOTHROYD, of Cornell University, lectured at Lehigh University on January 11 under the auspices of Lehigh Chapter of Sigma Xi on "Meteors or Shooting Stars," describing some aspects of the work of the Harvard-Cornell Meteor Expedition to Flagstaff, Arizona.

THE Sigma Xi Club of the University of Florida held its annual banquet on January 18. Mr. H. H. Hume, director of the University Experiment Station, spoke on "The University of Florida in its Relation to the State as a Research Institution." He outlined many of the problems which are awaiting study and emphasized the university as constituting a disinterested agency for investigating these problems.

THE Sigma Xi Club of Montana State College held a public meeting on January 26, at which Dr. O. E. Sheppard, head of the department of chemistry, delivered a lecture concerning "Recent Developments in Chemistry," with a detailed discussion on the physics and chemistry of color production. This lecture was one of a series of three public lectures on "The Frontiers of Science" being given under the auspices of the club.

DR. D. B. JUDD, of the section of colorimetry of the Bureau of Standards, delivered three lectures on color vision at Bryn Mawr College on January 16, 17 and 18. A fourth meeting was devoted to a demonstration which included the blue arc phenomenon, the Purkinje after-image and examples of color transformation.

DR. JOHN H. PARKER, professor of plant breeding at the Kansas State College, Manhattan, gave the fourth series of annual lectures under the Frank Azor Spragg Memorial Fund, from January 24 to 27, at the Michigan State College. This memorial is in honor of Professor F. A. Spragg, who was in charge of plant breeding work at the Michigan Agricultural Experiment Station from 1906 to 1924.

DR. GEORGE SARTON, current Hitchcock professor at the University of California, was speaker on January 15 at the first meeting of the Singer History of Science Club, organized as a result of Dr. Charles Singer's recent visit of a year to the university and composed of faculty members and students interested in the history of science and its promotion as a field of scholarship. Dr. Sarton's address was on Simon

Stevin, sixteenth and seventeenth century Dutch mathematician, the first advocate of the decimal system for common use.

MEETINGS of the American Chemical Society are planned as follows: Washington, D. C., week of March 26, 1933; Chicago, Ill., week of September 11, 1933; St. Petersburg, Fla., March, 1934; Cleveland, Ohio, autumn of 1934; Eleventh Colloid Symposium, Madison, Wis., June 15 to 17, 1933; Fifth National Organic Chemistry Symposium, Cornell University, Ithaca, N. Y., December 28 to 30, 1933.

THE American Society of Mammalogists will hold its fifteenth annual meeting at the new Biological Institute, Harvard University, from May 10 to 13. Titles of papers must be filed before April 28 with the corresponding secretary, Dr. Robert T. Hatt, the American Museum of Natural History, New York.

A UNION OF GERMAN BIOLOGISTS has recently been formed, with Professor Lehmann, of Tübingen, as president.

MRS. FRANCES KINSLEY HUTCHINSON has given an estate of seventy-three acres at Lake Geneva, including a house on the property, with an endowment, to the University of Chicago for botanical work.

COLUMBIA UNIVERSITY and the Metropolitan Museum of Art will ultimately share in a trust fund of $150,000, bequeathed by the late William Fitz Randolph, of Glenbrook, Connecticut. The gross estate is valued at $601,073. After smaller bequests are paid, the two institutions are named as the residuary legatees.

THE new Royal Society Mond Laboratory of the University of Cambridge was opened on February 3 by Stanley Baldwin, as chancellor, who accepted the building for the university. The principal speakers were Sir Ernest Rutherford and Sir Robert Mond. The laboratory is an adjunct of the Cavendish Laboratory and will be directed by Professor Peter Kapitza, of Russia. It is reported that it will provide facilities for research into the magnetic properties of matter in the highest fields yet attained and for the study of properties of matter at lowest possible temperatures. Last year, when the need for greater accommodations became urgent, the council of the Royal Society offered the university a fund to build and equip the new laboratory. At the same time, through reorganization, accommodation of the scientific departments was made possible by a Rockefeller gift, which freed a site near the Cavendish Laboratory for the new building.

WITH appropriate exercises on the afternoon of January 14, the new museum building of the San Diego Society of Natural History, Balboa Park, San Diego, California, was opened to the public. The same occasion marked the fifty-eighth annual meeting of the society, which is the oldest scientific organization in southern California. The building is of concrete construction, with a frontage 220 feet long, and a wing 100 feet deep, and forms the first unit of what may eventually be a much larger museum plant. Provision has been made in the present structure for exhibition halls on three floors, a lecture hall, children's museum, administrative offices, workrooms and laboratories for all departments. The building represents an investment of about $175,000, which was raised by public contributions, largest of which was the gift of $125,000 by the late Miss Ellen B. Scripps, of La Jolla. William Templeton Johnson, of San Diego, was the architect. For the past sixteen years the museum collections have been housed in temporary exposition structures in Balboa Park.

PURDUE UNIVERSITY announces the completion, during the summer of 1932, of new laboratories for plant physiology and plant pathology in the School of Science. These laboratories are built around greenhouse units. The physiology laboratories are three in number, including elementary, advanced and private research laboratories. The pathology laboratory is in addition to those already in use in plant pathology and provides space for elementary study with rooms adjoining for research. Basements extend under most of the construction and will be equipped for controlled light, temperature and humidity research. New advanced courses will be offered both in plant pathology and plant physiology.

WALTER MERRITT SEWARD, who died on December 20, 1932, at the age of seventy-two years, formerly practiced medicine in New York, but for the past twenty years had been looking after a country practice in Brunswick County, Virginia, mostly on a charity basis. He had also been managing his timber lands in that county. A correspondent writes: "At the time Dr. Seward attended the Medical School of the University of Virginia, class of 1886, that school lacked proper clinical and hospital equipment. The lack of clinical and hospital equipment has since been supplied to the School of Medicine. But for some years, indeed since its inception in 1910, the School of Forestry at the University of Virginia has lacked an experimental and practise forest, which in a general way corresponds to clinical and hospital equipment in medical instruction. Dr. Seward's will leaves his forest of more than three thousand acres and more than two hundred thousand dollars in securities to the University of Virginia for the benefit of the School of Forestry. His bequest supplies the needed experimental and practise forest and greatly strengthens and enlarges the usefulness of the School of Forestry."

THE sixth session of the Allegany School of Natural History, in Allegany State Park, New York, will be held from July 5 to August 24, under the auspices of the Buffalo Museum of Science. Founded under favorable natural conditions in suitable location and surroundings, the Allegany School of Natural History offers courses for studies in botany, zoology and geology with emphasis on natural history. An instructor is provided for each class a full day each week and for a conference hour later in the week. In addition each student works out of class independently or with occasional direction for nearly two days. The courses offered are field zoology and field botany, the natural history of birds and nature study. The small classes and the plan of the schedule make it possible for the faculty to continue actively in research. There is an open-air museum, a nature trail, an Indian garden, a water garden and a fernery. Elsewhere in the park are hiking trails, swimming pools, bridle paths, baseball diamonds, tennis courts and a 120-acre lake with boating.

# DISCUSSION

## THE NAMING OF THE SUBDIVISIONS OF THE WISCONSIN GLACIAL AGE

AT the 1930 meeting of the Geological Society of America, held in Toronto, the writer presented a paper on "The Peorian Loess and the Classification of the Glacial Drift-Sheets of the Mississippi Valley," which was subsequently printed in the *Journal of Geology*.[1] In this paper he called attention to the fact that the evidence that the Peorian (Iowan) loess had been weathered before the Early Wisconsin drift had been deposited was not valid; that the only evidence of an interval was that of rapid deposition of loess. Therefore, two important conclusions were drawn; (1) the Peorian interval was not of interglacial magnitude but was intraglacial; and (2) the Iowan ice invasion was the first of the Wisconsin invasions.

Additional confirmatory evidence was found during the 1931 field season, and another paper was presented at the 1931 meeting of the Geological Society of America, held in Tulsa. This paper is to be published soon. In it the additional confirmatory evidence was presented, the importance of the "profile of weathering" as a criterion of interglacial intervals was emphasized, the post-Illinoian loesses were dated and their relationships, sources and conditions of deposition were discussed and a picture of the development and retreats and readvances of the major Wisconsin ice-fields was presented. New names for three of the subdivisions of the Wisconsin were proposed to replace those presented at the Toronto meeting and published in the *Journal of Geology*, which had been chosen with respect to the fields of ice accumulation rather than areas where the stratigraphic units may be studied, and which have since been found to be preempted. New names are, therefore, necessary.

The names which were withdrawn were Manitoban (Iowan), Quebecan (early and middle Wisconsin) and Hudsonian (late Wisconsin). The old name Iowan was retained, and the new names proposed were Tazewell, Cary and Mankato for the subdivisions shown in the following table. The name Tazewell is taken from Tazewell County, Illinois, where the Early Wisconsin deposits are well shown in their relations to the underlying Peorian loess. The name Cary is taken from a town in McHenry County, northeastern Illinois, where the Middle Wisconsin deposits are well displayed. The name Mankato is taken from Mankato, Minnesota, where the Late Wisconsin deposits are excellently displayed.

| *Age* | *Subdivisions* | |
|---|---|---|
| Wisconsin (Fourth) glacial) | Mankato | (Late Wisconsin) |
| | Cary | (Middle Wisconsin) |
| | Tazewell | (Early Wisconsin) |
| | Iowan | |
| Sangamon (Third interglacial) | | |
| Illinoian (Third glacial) | | |

M. M. LEIGHTON
ILLINOIS STATE GEOLOGICAL SURVEY

[1] Volume 39, No. 1, pp. 45–53, 1931.

## "MESCAL PITS"—A MISNOMER

SCIENTIFIC nomenclature has always been cumbered with a large number of inappropriate and inadequate terms, some due to a creeping in of temporary designations which were never intended to survive the laboratory stage and others due to a lack of understanding during early investigations in new fields. One of the newer scenes of effort in the field of Southwestern archeology has lately come to notice through the work of representatives of the U. S. National Museum, the Museum of the University of Pennsylvania and the Laboratory of Anthropology. The area in reference consists of the extreme southeastern part of New Mexico and the adjoining portion of southwestern Texas. Among the prominent features which distinguish one of the prehistoric cultures in this area, the principal habitat of which seems to be in the mountain ranges bordering the lower Pecos Valley on the west, are curious structures of open circular form, composed principally of small fragments of fire-cracked limestone. These circles occur abundantly in favorable locations from a point near Hope, New Mexico, in the foothills of the Sacramento Mountains, south throughout the Guadalupe and Davis Mountains for an as yet undetermined distance into Texas. The name "mescal pit" has been applied locally to this type of structure over a period of many years, and the use of this term has spread equally with the interest incited by the recent investigations. For the two field seasons of 1930 and 1931 the writer conducted expeditions for the Laboratory of Anthropology in the Guadalupe Mountains area, and during this time a number of "pits" were excavated or trenched. It was definitely determined that they were not pits, in any sense of the word; nor were they concerned especially with the preparation of mescal for food. Instead, they were found to be specialized refuse heaps. These circular mounds contained, in addition to the more obvious small cracked rocks, accumulations of ash, charcoal, food bones and other camp debris. As the term "mescal pit" is obviously a misnomer, and as it is likely to be perpetuated by usage, the writer feels that a designation more in keeping with the character of the structures should be chosen. Therefore the name "midden circle" is proposed. Further discussion of these circles, together with other archeological information gathered during the two seasons' work, will appear in a report now in preparation.

H. P. MERA

LABORATORY OF ANTHROPOLOGY
SANTA FÉ, NEW MEXICO

## IS GEOLOGY EASIER FOR BOYS THAN FOR GIRLS?

IN an article which appeared in the issue of SCIENCE, dated November 11, 1932, and written by Gragg Richards, of Detroit, Michigan, evidence based on statistics was introduced to prove that geology is an easier subject for men than for women. I have examined the grades of all the students who have taken my course in physical geology for the past seven years. They come from all the classes in college, ranging from 17 to 21 years of age, the larger proportion from the freshman and sophomore classes. Instruction consists of lectures, laboratory work and field trips. A standard college text-book is used, and students are required to supplement class work by outside reading; 10 to 25 readings constituting the usual number, the smaller figure being the minimum required. The average size of the laboratory section is about 25 and there is considerable personal contact between instructor and student, especially in the laboratory and in the field. The grades for the course are on the following basis: A—excellent, B—good, C—fair, D—unsatisfactory, F—failure. No conscious effort was made to follow a distribution curve. The group consists of 647 students, 254 men and 393 women. On the basis of A = 3, B = 2, C = 1, D = 0, the men show an average of 1.255 and the women 1.407.

| | Percentage | | | | |
|---|---|---|---|---|---|
| | A | B | C | D | F |
| Men (254) | 6.3 | 30.25 | 46.1 | 11.4 | 5.92 |
| Women (393) | 8.9 | 36.6 | 40.7 | 10.7 | 3.06 |
| Entire group (647) | 7.6 | 33.42 | 43.4 | 11.0 | 4.49 |

These statistics show clearly that the women are slightly better than the men, although the difference between them is so slight that one may consider them equal in ability. They also indicate that geology is as easy for women as for men. There is, in my opinion, based on eighteen years of experience teaching science, no marked difference in the ability of men and women.

KARL VER STEEG

COLLEGE OF WOOSTER

## BROWN ROOTROT OF TOBACCO

A FORM of brown rootrot of tobacco is due to the insufficient intake of calcium by the tobacco plant. The condition may be brought about by lack of available calcium, an excess of magnesium over calcium or the presence of appreciable amounts of ammoniacal nitrogen in relation to nitrate nitrogen. The foregoing findings were the results of researches carried on at the Connecticut Agricultural Experiment Station at New Haven and the Tobacco Substation at Windsor, Connecticut. Soil, sand, water cultures and field tests were made.

T. R. SWANBACK
H. G. M. JACOBSON

AGRICULTURAL EXPERIMENT STATION
NEW HAVEN, CONNECTICUT

# SCIENTIFIC BOOKS

## RECENT ZOOLOGICAL TEXT-BOOKS

IN reading the text-books which have been published during the latter part of 1932 a reviewer is impressed by certain facts which are perhaps worth mentioning: (1) Writers of text-books are unprogressive. They have at last given up Batrachia, Urodela and Anura; and use Amphibia, Caudata and Salientia, instead. But they cling to such archaic names as Platyhelminthes, Nemathelminthes, Trochminthes, Molluscoidea, Pelecypoda, Polyzoa and Infusoria. Even such a conservative institution as the *Zoological Record* has progressed to Platyhelminthia, Nemathelminthia, Ciliophora and Bryozoa. All biology does not have to be crammed into two great receptacles, morphology and physiology. Such a subject as psychology perhaps depends as much upon knowledge of the structure of neurones, tracts and areas as upon that of behavior, reflexes and reaction times; but two recent writers assert that psychology is (in the words of Octavius Roy Cohen) "nothing else but" physiology. The scientific name of an animal consists of the genus, species *and the name of the author;* but a student in elementary zoology has no chance to find this out. (2) A glossary should be a series of carefully considered, critical definitions of technical terms, instead of a list of careless, loose and inaccurate statements, such as a freshman might produce impromptu during an oral quiz. (3) Generic names are sacred and their spelling may not be changed to suit the whims of writers. Amoeba can not become ameba. (4) High-school teachers appear to be doing better teaching than university professors. Their texts are written for students to read and use; not for professional, backward-looking zoologists. Students in high schools are expected to solve problems, think and grow—not merely verify, draw, answer, pass and get credit.

*Animal Biology.* By LORANDE LOSS WOODRUFF. Macmillan, New York. $3.50. xii + 513. 1932.

This text-book presents zoology from "a general biological view-point." It is the work of a scholarly man who shows his general learning by frequent, apt quotations. Good judgment is shown in the use of technical terms; there are not too many, but enough are introduced to permit a student to gain some knowledge of zoological terminology. The book is well planned; the figures are well conceived and executed. The parts of the work that relate to general biological phenomena are well presented; though frequently stated in a teleological way. Those that deal with classification and newer knowledge in fields with which the writer is apparently not familiar are often uncritical and inaccurate. For example, Chapter III, on the physical basis of life, is admirable; Chapter VII, "Survey of Invertebrates" is not so well done; the part of the appendix which deals with classification is quite unprogressive; the glossary contains many questionable statements. On page 80 it is said that, "The Guinea worm, Filaria, is sometimes six feet long, and spends its adult life under the human skin and its youth in a Water-flea." Since the time of Reichard in 1759 the guinea worm has been placed in the Genus Dracunculus and it probably never reaches a length of six feet. Other examples of objectionable statements are, "the Earthworms, or Oligochaeta. . . . The largely sedentary and nocturnal life of earthworms renders special locomotor, respiratory, and sense organs unnecessary," (p. 81); "Absorption. The passage of nutritive and other fluids into living cells. . . . Alternation of Generations.—The alternate succession of a sexual and an asexual generation in the life history" (p. 473); "Chorion.—External embryonic membrane of Mammals. . . . Cloaca.—A cavity at the posterior end of the Vertebrate body. . . . Colony.—An aggregation or intimate association of several or many similar individuals to form a superior unit" (p. 476). Evidently the writer disapproves of the modern tendency to begin even generic names with small letters, for he begins even such words as Man, Bird and Butterfly with capitals. The topics discussed in the twenty-five chapters are: The scope of biology, cells, physical basis of life, metabolism, protozoa, metazoa, invertebrates, vertebrates, nutrition, respiration, circulation, excretion, reproduction, coordination, origin of life, continuity of life, fertilization, development, inheritance, adaptation, descent with change, biology and human welfare, and the development of biology.

*Manual of Animal Biology.* By GEORGE ALFRED BAITSELL. Macmillan, New York. $2.50. xiii + 382. 1932.

This is a laboratory manual intended to be used with Woodruff's "Animal Biology" and other standard zoological text-books, to which references are made throughout. It consists of two parts, "descriptive" and "laboratory directions" (which are also descriptive). The first part contains brief accounts of protoplasm, amoeba, euglena, volvox, paramecium, vorticella, grantia, hydra, obelia, starfish, earthworm, crayfish, insects, clam, frog and vertebrates in general, and vertebrate development. The second part, on detachable pages, contains laboratory directions concerning equipment, microscope, cells, green plants, fungi, protoplasmic movement, amoeba, euglena, volvox, paramecium, grantia, hydra, obelia, gonionemus, starfish, earthworm, crayfish, grasshopper, honey-bee, life history of moth, clam, chordates, vertebrates, tissues (epithelial, muscular, supporting), vertebrate skeleton, viscera, buccal and respiratory organs, enteron, vascular system, urinogenital system, nervous system, histology of nerves, tissue, vertebrate eye, spermatogenesis, oogenesis, fertilization, mitosis, and embryology of frog and chick. The method employed in each exercise is the observation of such structures as are described and the making of one or more drawings. Apparently no written notes are expected and no questions are asked. Twelve figures are presented.

*An Introduction to Zoology Through the Study of the Vertebrates with Special Reference to the Rat and Man.* By ZENO PAYNE METCALF. Thomas: Springfield, Illinois. $3.50. xx + 426. 1932.

This book has been written for agricultural students in general zoology and is presented in "three major divisions: (1) a general introduction; (2) the study of the detailed anatomy and physiology of a mammal, the rat, with comparisons from other groups of vertebrates; (3) the broader aspects of zoology. . . . Throughout this text-book the author has attempted to write on what he believes is the level that the average college freshman can attain. . . . It has not been written for zoologists but for beginning college students." The book appears to have been thoughtfully and carefully written. The figures are clear and appropriate. Classification receives little attention; morphology, physiology and the general aspects of biology and economic zoology are emphasized. The scope of the work is indicated by chapter headings in the three sections: (1) The field of zoology and the animal kingdom; (2) with special reference to the rat and mammals—general morphology and physiology; habits, external characters, general internal structure, integument, muscles, skeleton, locomotion, enteron, respiratory system, urinary system, circulatory system, metabolism, reproductive system, embryology, heredity, endocrine system, nervous system; and (3) distributional zoology, paleontology, evolution and history of zoology.

*Zoology.* By F. E. CHIDESTER. Van Nostrand, New York. $3.75. xii + 581. 1932.

In the preface of this book it is said that, "this text was written as a general survey for use by college students and to serve as a reference book by biologists. . . . Important features are the logical arrangement of facts about the animals within a group, a statement of the chief characteristics at the beginning of the discussion, and a summary of the economic importance at the end of each section. The newer physiology has been introduced and a bibliography checked by experts in each field is given at the end of each chapter." To the reviewer the book seems to be poorly organized and poorly written. It contains many questionable and inaccurate statements. For example, under the title "Characteristics" the following statements are made about Protozoa (p. 21): 1. Morphologically the simplest ones are equal to isolated epithelium. 2. Physiologically they are equal to the whole group of cells making up the human body. Protozoa are complete unicellular organisms and many have a brief multicellular phase. 3. Functionally they epitomize life processes. 4. Theoretically they are generalized cells. 5. Of practical economic importance, they cause many diseases. 6. As soil organisms protozoa are of doubtful importance.

Are the points enumerated characteristics and do they all mean something? In characterizing the vertebrates (p. 14) nothing is said concerning gill slits, but invertebrates (p. 16) are said to "lack gill slits or visceral clefts." "The term 'tropism' has long been used to indicate the reaction of an animal to some sort of stimulus," (p. 24) is an example of many loose statements. Two species of amoeba are said to occur in man (p. 26); whereas eight or more so occur. *Christispira,* a spirochaete, is affirmed to be "a large flagellate" (p. 29). The glossary contains many doubtful and curiously limited statements—*e.g.*: "*dentine,* the inner portion of a tooth; *lipoid,* a substance found in the nervous system which is dissolved by anesthetics or narcotics; *respiration,* oxidation of protoplasm releasing energy and producing carbon dioxide; *testis,* an organ in a male animal where sperms are produced." The twenty-two chapters are devoted to Introduction, Protozoa, Porifera, Coelenterata, Platyhelminthes, Nemathelminthes, Annelida, Trochelminthes, Molluscoidea, Echinodermata, Mollusca, Arthropods, Chordata, Cyclostomata, Pisces, Amphibia, Reptilia, Aves, Natural History of Mammals, Mammalia—Physiology, Social Life of Animals, and Evolution, Heredity, and Eugenics.

*The Essentials of Biology.* By JAMES JOHNSTONE. Longmans, Green and Co., New York. xv + 328. 1932.

"The intention of this book is to present a balanced account of the theoretical matter of animal biology. Botanical results are only noted in so far as they bear upon general biological science." The book is a thoughtful, philosophical consideration of modern science with special reference to biology. It is not a catalogue of facts to be learned, but a logical development of thoughts and relations. The statements made are carefully considered and mean something. At times they may be a little tiresome and abstruse, but the reader gains much and feels repaid. When scanning the book one wishes that college students in the United States could have more of the attitude of mind that would be essential for its use—more thoughtful consideration of the fundamental problems of science and less concern for memorized facts and propaganda. Johnstone's book may be read with profit by any student, young or old. It is in two parts and nine chapters, which indicate the contents: (I) THE INDIVIDUAL, (1) the Organism as a Natural Thing, (2) Organic Structure, (3) Organic Functioning, (4) Animal Behavior; (II) THE RACE, (5) Reproduction and Growth, (6) Development, (7) Heredity, (8) Transformism, and (9) the Evolutionary Career.

*Everyday Problems in Biology.* By C. J. PIEPER, W. L. BEAUCHAMP and O. D. FRANK. Scott, Foresman and Company, Chicago. $1.60. xxxiii + 686. 1932.

This is a biological text intended for use by high-school students in the ninth and tenth grades. It is a carefully considered, well-organized book written by experienced teachers. The student is stimulated to think about things biological, especially those related to man, and his capacity is continually increased. Topics are considered under twelve "units," presented as questions, in the following order: obtaining and using food, growth, reproduction, ecology, behavior, classification, economic biology, evolution and conservation.

A. S. PEARSE

DUKE UNIVERSITY

# SCIENTIFIC APPARATUS AND LABORATORY METHODS

## IMPROVED KYMOGRAPH RECORDING

SINCE the introduction of smoked, glazed paper for kymographic recording, numerous attempts have been made to obviate many of the disadvantages of this method. Of these attempts the most recent have been the successful efforts of Wichart, Thienes and Visscher,[1] and Patterson.[2] The former group of investigators employ cellophane coated with carbon sprayed from a pressure air gun, whereas Patterson delivers ink from quill pens against white, glazed paper. The former method allows for direct reproduction in the lantern by simple insertion between two glass plates but still retains the disadvantage of requiring carbonizing before and fixing after recording. Patterson's method simplifies preparation of a record which requires no shellacking but requires photographing for reproduction in the lantern.

More recently Warren[3] reported the use of cellophane as a transparent preparation, capable of receiving impressions from carbon paper in the typewriter or by pencil pressure. He cautions, however, against handling, which removes the carbon particles from the cellophane.

We have found cellophane an excellent recipient for India ink, which dries almost immediately and resists violent finger friction. Cellophane also takes red, blue and green ink (concentrated by evaporation to one half or one third volume), and thus allows for differential tracings to be made of any type of drawing, photograph or record.

We have further utilized the ink-taking properties of cellophane in keeping permanent records of physiological activity to be kymographically registered. Curved glass capillary tubes of very fine bore deliver ink to the cellophane, which is held in position on the kymograph drum by library paste or rubber bands. To afford less chance of breakage capillary tubes can also be bent to lead ink to the inner surface of ordinary steel writing pens, which are supported on light reed or aluminum recording levers. To render the record easily discernible, the drum is first covered with permanent white facing—either enamel or paper.

This type of cellophane record requires no smoking nor fixing. The ink will not rub off unless it is moistened with water or alcohol, in which case the cellophane will retake ink at site of removal. Any part of the permanent record, as suggested by others,[1, 3] can be placed between glass plates and used directly in the projection lantern. The economy of the method, obviating smoking, shellacking and photographing parts of records, is apparent.

FREDRICK F. YONKMAN

SCHOOL OF MEDICINE
BOSTON UNIVERSITY

[1] W. F. Wichardt, C. H. Thienes, M. B. Visscher, SCIENCE, 73: 99, Jan. 23, 1932.

[2] T. L. Patterson, Demonstration, The Federation of Amer. Societies for Exp. Biol. Philadelphia, April, 1932.

[3] K. L. Warren, SCIENCE, 76: 573, Dec. 16, 1932.

## AN INEXPENSIVE PYROMETER FOR TEMPERATURES UP TO 1000° C

THE use of an electrical muffle furnace in operations such as ashing of biological materials makes the control of temperatures up to 1000° C. highly desirable. Finding most manufactured pyrometers expensive we originally fashioned a simple thermocouple of chromel-alumel and calculated the temperature from e.m.f. as measured by a student potentiometer. Subsequently we used an inexpensive microvoltmeter procured through the Weston Electrical Instrument Corporation, Newark, N. J., who were kind enough to modify one of their standard instruments (Model 301) and equip it with a scale calibrated in centigrade degrees, the entire assembly making a direct reading pyrometer with a range up to 1000° C. accurate to ± 10° C. and obtainable at nominal cost.

No. 14 gauge pieces of chromel and alumel wires each about 3 ft. long were twisted together tightly for a distance of one inch. The twisted ends were protected from corrosion by means of a small silica test-tube packed with asbestos fiber. The free ends were insulated from each other by short lengths of silica tubing sufficient to bring the wires out of the back of the oven and were held in position far enough from the oven to avoid being heated by radiation. They were then connected to copper leads, which ran to the reading instrument. Changes of ambient temperature about this junction were not compensated for, and, for the accuracy desired, could be neglected. The modified microvoltmeter was made for us by the

Weston Electrical Instrument Corporation when we had furnished them with the following information: Nature of the thermocouple, range of temperature desired and total resistance in ohms of the thermocouple and its leads. Comparison of the readings of this instrument with the calculated temperature from e.m.f. measurements from room temperature to 1000° C. agreed to within ± 10° C. As the temperature of various points within the oven may vary by as much as ± 25° C., this accuracy is quite adequate.

WILLIAM C. STADIE
SYDNEY L. WRIGHT, JR.
THE JOHN HERR MUSSER DEPARTMENT
OF RESEARCH MEDICINE
UNIVERSITY OF PENNSYLVANIA

## MODIFICATION OF THE BACKLIN-KIRK COMBUSTION CHAMBER FOR MICRO-DETERMINATION OF CARBON AND LIPOIDS

IN the manometric determination of lipoids the combustion chamber is highly evacuated at the time it is to be removed from the Van Slyke manometer. In the original Backlin chamber[1] a stop-cock is present at the top of the combustion chamber which may be opened at this time to relieve this pressure which facilitates removal of the rubber connection to the manometer. At best this operation involves some risk of damaging the manometer. The chamber, as modified by Kirk,[2] has eliminated this stop-cock, thus necessitating removal of the rubber connection against the low internal pressure of the chamber. A simple method of reducing the hazards of such procedure is to add a three-way stop-cock (*cf*. diagram) in the

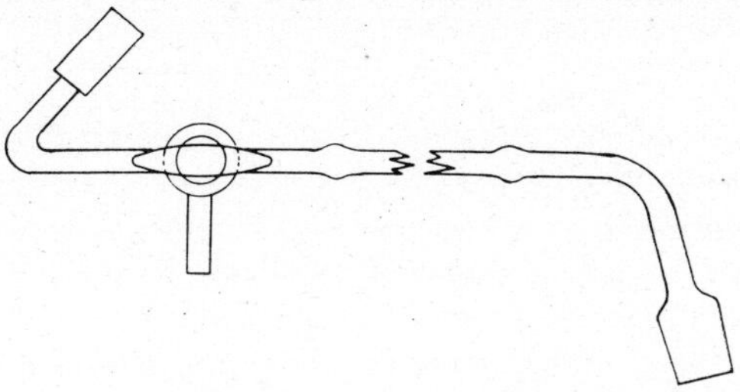

delivery tube of the chamber. After the upper cock of the Van Slyke absorption chamber has been closed this stop-cock may be turned to admit atmospheric pressure before detaching the delivery tube.

WM. L. DOYLE
ZOOLOGICAL LABORATORY
THE JOHNS HOPKINS UNIVERSITY

[1] E. Backlin, *Biochem. Zts.*, 217: 483, 1930.

[2] Peters and Van Slyke, "Quantitative Clinical Chemistry-Methods," Williams and Wilkins, 1932.

# SPECIAL ARTICLES

## A PROOF OF THE LAW OF EFFECT

PSYCHOLOGISTS and physiologists all agree that the behavior of man and of many other animals is modifiable by the experiences of life. He learns, so that the situation, S, which at first evokes, say, responses 1, 2, 3, 4 and 5 equally often, comes to evoke one response, say 4, always or ninety-nine times out of a hundred. The connection S → 4 has become enormously strengthened relatively to S → 1 or S → 2 or S → 3 or S → 5.

Concerning the forces producing learning there has been great disagreement. The writer (1898, 1914 and 1931) has maintained that the after-effects of a modifiable connection work back upon it, and that, in particular, a satisfying state of affairs accompanying or directly following a connection strengthens it. Troland maintained a similar doctrine.

The great majority of psychologists have maintained, on the contrary, that the strengthening of any connection is due to forces operating within the connection itself or prior to it. Repetition or frequency of occurrence, recency, intensity, finality or consummatoriness, tendency to attain equilibrium, and other features of the process have been alleged to be adequate to explain the strengthening of connections.

I have presented recently evidence from a variety of experiments to show that a satisying after-effect of a connection does in fact strengthen it under conditions equalized in respect of all other forces than the satisfying after-effect.[1] It is the purpose of this report to present an entirely independent experimental proof of the strengthening influence of a satisfying state of affairs upon the connection of which it is the after-effect and important new facts concerning the method of action of that influence.

We provide in an experiment a long series of situations to each of which several responses are possible, one of which is arbitrarily followed by a reward, any other being followed by a punishment. For example, a series of words is said by the experimenter, to each of which the subject may respond by any number from 1 to 10. If he says the number that has been chosen to be "right" he is rewarded; if he says any other, he is punished. So we have a long sequence of connections and after-effects, in the form Word 1 → number, reward or punishment, Word 2 → number, reward or punishment, Word 3 → number, reward or punishment, Word 4 → number, reward or punishment, etc.

[1] "The Fundamentals of Learning," E. L. Thorndike, 1932.

This series is repeated again and again. We quote the results for the first ten words in trials 1 to 4,[2] from a sample record.

| | Trial or round 1 | Trial or round 2 | Trial or round 3 | Trial or round 4 |
|---|---|---|---|---|
| catnip | 2 | 4 | 10 | 2 |
| cedar | 3 | 3 | 6 | 2 |
| chamber | 1 | 2 | 9 | 8 |
| chorus | 8 | 10 | 7 | 6 |
| dally | 4 | 8 | 5 | 4 |
| dazzle | C2 | 6 | 9 | 1 |
| debate | 9 | 7 | 2 | 5 |
| deduce | 5 | 2 | 2 | 2 |
| early | 4 | C5 | C5 | C5 |
| effort | 3 | 6 | C7 | C7 |

The time-intervals were as follows: One unit of the series from word to word or number to number took about 2.2 sec. The time from the announcement of "Right" or "Wrong" to the approximate mid-point of the word–number connection to which it belonged was about 0.5½ sec. The time to the mid-point of the next preceding connection was about 2.8 sec., to the next, 5.0 sec., to the next, 7.2 sec., and so on. The time to the mid-point of the word–number connection following the announcement of "Right" or "Wrong" was 1.7 sec. The time to the next following was 3.9 sec.; to the next, 6.1; and so on.

In such a series the rewarded connections are strengthened, but that fact is not our present concern. The fact to which I invite attention now is that the punished connections do not behave alike, but that the ones that are nearest to a reward are strengthened most. The strengthening influence of a reward spreads to influence positively not only the connection which it directly follows and to which it may be said to belong, but also any connections which are near enough to it. We may measure nearness in terms of time or in terms of number of connections or steps. Thus the punished connection *catnip* → *2* in Trial 1 preceded the reward for *dazzle* → *2* by about 11.6 seconds and by 5 connections or steps. The punished connection *cedar* → *3* in Trial 1 preceded the reward of *dazzle* → *2* by about 9.4 seconds and by 4 connections or steps. The punished connection *dally* → *4* in Trial 1 preceded the reward of *dazzle* → *2* by about 2.8 seconds and by one connection or step.

The amount of strengthening is measured by the percentage of repetitions in the following trial. For example, for the ten subjects of the experiment chosen as an illustration we find the following for punished connections alike in all respects save their proximity to a reward:

| | N | Percentage of repetitions in the following trial |
|---|---|---|
| One step removed | 4136 | 26.4 |
| Two steps removed | 2250 | 23.6 |
| Three or four steps removed | 1933 | 21.0 |
| Five or more steps removed | 1228 | 20.8 |
| Three or more steps removed | 3161 | 20.7 |

For 905 connections like these in all respects, save that a reward directly followed and belonged to them, the percentage of repetitions was about 50.

In such experiments the fact that a person responds to a word by a certain number makes him more likely to respond to that word at the next trial by that same number, even though the response was punished. The connection is strengthened more by being made than it is weakened by being punished. This has been indicated by Thorndike ('32, p. 112, and p. 280ff), and demonstrated by Lorge in articles to appear shortly in the *Journal of Experimental Psychology* and by the present series of experiments. The best measure of strengthening due to one occurrence of a punished connection at some specified proximity to a reward is then the excess strengthening over that due to one occurrence of a punished connection so remote from a reward as to receive zero influence from it. In the illustrative experiment those excesses are 5½ for one occurrence of a punished connection one step away from a reward, and 2½ for one two steps away.

We have made fifteen experiments, using various sorts of learning. The results show that a satisfying after-effect strengthens greatly the connection which it follows directly and to which it belongs, and also strengthens by a smaller amount the connections preceding and following that, and by a still smaller amount the preceding and succeeding connections two steps removed.

One occurrence of a rewarded connection produces an average excess strengthening of 22 (per hundred) with a probable error of 3. One occurrence of a punished connection next to and preceding a rewarded connection produces an average excess strengthening of 4 (per hundred) with a probable error of 0.4. A punished connection occurring after a rewarded connection receives an excess strengthening of about 5 (per hundred). A punished connection between two rewarded connections receives an

[2] In this experiment the series of words, each with its "right" number, was read to the subject first, so that correct choices even in the first round would be a matter of ability plus chance rather than of chance alone.

excess strengthening of 7½ per hundred. Punished connections two steps and 5 or more seconds away from a reward connection are influenced favorably by it.[3]

The proof that a satisfying after-effect strengthens directly the connection producing it, and also other connections in close proximity to it, is important, because it explains selective modifiability. It solves many problems for which the forces of frequency, recency and intensity are inadequate. It accounts for the true contentions of purposivism without recourse to mystical agencies.

The physiological explanation of the influence of a satisfying after-effect is as yet unknown, just as the physiological explanation of the influence of mere repetition of a connection is unknown. But we can now proceed to find out facts about the former which may lead us to a physiological explanation of it, and which are valuable in any case.

Thus, Dr. Rock has measured the effect of differences in the intensity of the reward. I have measured, though as yet very imperfectly, the effect of differences in the time-interval between the connection and its reward. I have measured the effect of differences in the relevance of the reward. Dr. Lorge is proceeding to measure the influence of an occurrence that is neither rewarded nor punished, so that we may compare the strengthening by it with the strengthening by various after-effects.

I can already frame a physiological explanation which demands little more from the nervous system than any doctrine of facilitation demands. And I venture to prophesy that the physiology of strengthening by the after-effects of a connection will be understood sooner than the physiology of strengthening by its sheer repetition.

EDWARD L. THORNDIKE

TEACHERS COLLEGE,
COLUMBIA UNIVERSITY

## IS MALIGNANCY DUE TO A PROCESS ANALOGOUS TO SOMATIC MUTATION?

MALIGNANT tumors develop in the walls of parasitic cysts of *Cysticercus fasciolaris,* the larval stage of *Taenia taeniaeformis* (*crassicollis*), the common tapeworm of the cat. Tumors have been produced experimentally by feeding rats *Taenia* eggs derived from cat feces. The shells of these eggs are digested off in the rat's intestine, and the oncospheres attach themselves to the wall of the intestine, work their way into the blood vessels of the gut wall and are carried to the liver by the portal circulation. They are strained out in the liver capillaries and grow rapidly forming clear vesicles, which about the seventh day become visible to the unaided eye.

At this stage some of the larvae have been transplanted to the subcutaneous tissues of other rats, but for the most part they have been allowed to continue their development in the liver. In either locality the growing larvae initiate considerable proliferative activity in the surrounding tissues which results in the formation of fibrous cyst walls. After from 8 to 27 months the cells of these cysts may show active and often atypical proliferation and may undergo malignant changes.

Most of the tumors produced have been polymorphous cell sarcomata, spindle cell sarcomata or a mixture of the two. The rarer tumors were of the following types: fibroma, chondroma, osteochondroma, chondrosarcoma, osteochondrosarcoma, fibrosarcoma, liposarcoma, adenoma and carcino-osteochondrosarcoma.

At the beginning of the present analysis (June, 1932) 52,223 rats from completed pedigreed matings had been autopsied. Of these 26,172 were infested with the parasite, 13,120 had survived the infestation for at least eight months (the minimum period of infestation observed in the case of a bearer of a *Cysticercus* sarcoma) and 3,285 had *Cysticercus* sarcoma. Besides these, 68 purchased animals and 316 of the unpedigreed descendants of purchased animals had the malignant complication of the *Cysticercus* disease.

*Taenia* eggs from cats obtained from various parts of the city and suburbs and others infested in the laboratory were equally effective in producing the disease and the associated malignant tumor, but rats showed marked strain and family differences in the proportion of individuals which developed both the disease and the complication.

Early in the experiments it was noted that the duration of the irritation (that is, the residence of the parasite in the liver) before the appearance of the malignant phase of the *Cysticercus* disease varied over a period of 19 months, which is half the maximum life span of our laboratory rats. Furthermore, the proportion of tumor bearers increased directly from the eighth to the twentieth month of infestation. It was also noted that usually only one cyst and in some of the early tumors only a small area of the cyst wall showed the malignant transformation, although the host might have had one to one hundred other cysts which were benign. Occasionally two or more apparently independent *Cysticercus* tumors occurred in the same host.

The clue to the explanation of the strain and family differences and to the variations in the duration of infestation appeared in the present analysis, when it was observed that in the 3,669 bearers of

[3] The detailed results for all the experiments will be published at an early date.

*Cysticercus* sarcoma there was a significant negative correlation ($-.527 \pm .008$) between the number of cysts in the liver and the duration of infestation with the parasite. It follows that if the bearers of *Cysticercus* sarcoma are distributed according to the number of parasitic cysts, a general decrease in the duration of infestation is observed with each successive increase in the number of cysts. Also the mean age at autopsy of these tumor bearers is parallel to the duration of infestation and in each case exceeds it by approximately two months, the average age at which the rats were infested. For each number of cysts the mean duration of infestation and mean age are slightly higher for females than for males, but in many cases the differences are not statistically significant. The essential factor is the duration of the irritation and not the actual age of the rat. This is shown when the tumor bearers are classified according to the age at which they were infested, for the mean age at autopsy rises proportionately with the age at which they were fed *Taenia* eggs; but the duration of infestation remains constant instead of decreasing directly with the age fed, as would be expected if age were the important factor. The mean duration of infestation not only became shorter but also became less variable with the increase in the number of *Cysticercus* cysts. This is shown by a gradual decrease in the standard deviations of the duration of infestation.

If the frequencies of rats infested with successive numbers of cysts are cut off at the mean period of infestation for tumor hosts with the corresponding numbers of cysts, and the percentage of tumor bearers among these is calculated, it is observed that the proportion of tumor bearers increases almost directly from 31.5 per cent. of the individuals with one cyst to 85.7 per cent. of those with 50 cysts. Above 50 cysts the number of rats in each group is small, since such large numbers of parasites are detrimental to the host. Nevertheless, in general the proportion of tumor bearers continues to increase with increase in numbers of cysts, and in several cases reaches 100 per cent. of the survivors of the *minimum* period of infestation. The males show a tendency to a slightly higher percentage of tumor bearers than the females, but in most cases the difference is not statistically significant.

If the different strains are considered separately, it appears that they all show the same general tendency to an increase in proportion of tumors with an increase in the numbers of parasites, but in some the increase is more rapid than in others. Furthermore, if in each strain the number of infested rats which reached the mean period of infestation for tumor bearers with the corresponding number of cysts is summed for the successive numbers of cysts, and the percentage of these which were tumor bearers is calculated, a marked difference is observed between certain strains. It can be demonstrated that this difference is determined by two factors, relative longevity and susceptibility to *Cysticercus* disease. That is, those strains which show a low proportion of tumor bearers show a low average length of life and a marked resistance to the *Cysticercus* disease, while the strains with a high proportion of tumor bearers show either a long average life span or a high degree of susceptibility to the disease.

Since an increase in the number of cysts, that is, an increase in the surface exposed to the irritant, decreases directly the time interval necessary for the onset of the malignant process and increases directly the probability of its occurrence until it becomes inevitable, it is apparent that *chance* is an important factor in the change of a normal to a *cancer* cell. Further, in the case of *Cysticercus* sarcoma hereditary factors influence the occurrence of malignancy only as they influence susceptibility of the individual to *Cysticercus* disease and longevity. Possibly when more is known about the etiology of other tumors for which there appears to be an inherited susceptibility and when the expression of genetic factors in the cells and tissues is better understood, it will be found that in the case of all neoplasms in all species the initial cell change occurs by a process analogous to somatic mutation and that hereditary factors determine this change only in so far as they influence longevity and the susceptibility of an individual to some specific irritant or condition which is favorable to mutation.

M. R. CURTIS
W. F. DUNNING
F. D. BULLOCK
INSTITUTE OF CANCER RESEARCH
COLUMBIA UNIVERSITY

## BOOKS RECEIVED

*Carnegie Institution of Washington.* Year Book No. 31, 1931–32. Pp. xix + 392. The Institution.

FREUDENBERG, K., Editor. *Stereochemie.* 6 Lieferung. Pp. 159. Franz Deuticke, Leipzig. M 18.

GOLDENWEISER, ALEXANDER. *History, Psychology and Culture.* Pp. xii + 475 + xii. Knopf. $5.00.

LOGSDON, MAYME I. *Elementary Mathematical Analysis.* Vol. II. Pp. ix + 188. 74 figures. McGraw-Hill. $1.75.

MERRIAM, JOHN C., and CHESTER STOCK. *The Felidae of Rancho La Brea.* Pp. xvi + 231. 42 plates. 152 figures. Carnegie Institution of Washington.

NOWLAN, FREDERICK S. *Analytic Geometry.* Pp. xi + 295. 159 figures. McGraw-Hill. $2.25.

RAYMOND, ALLEN. *What is Technocracy?* Pp. vii + 180. Whittlesey House, McGraw-Hill. $1.50.

*Tokyo Bunrika Daigaku.* Science Reports. Vol. I, No. 4: Pp. 41 + 59; Vol. I, Nos. 5–10: Pp. 61–131. Tokyo University of Literature and Science.

TURCK, FENTON B. *The Action of the Living Cell.* Pp. xi + 308. 17 figures. Macmillan. $3.50.

# SCIENCE

VOL. 77 — FRIDAY, FEBRUARY 17, 1933 — No. 1990

*Genetics and Embryology:* PROFESSOR CHARLES ZELENY ... 177

*Obituary:*
*Edwin Chapin Starks:* PROFESSOR F. M. MACFARLAND. *Herman Theodor Holm:* DR. A. F. WOODS. *Recent Deaths* ... 182

*Scientific Events:*
*International Vitamin Standards; The Morris Arboretum; The Proposed Everglades National Park; In Honor of Dr. Elihu Thomson* ... 184

*Scientific Notes and News* ... 186

*Discussion:*
*A New Mathematical Formula for Chemical Analysis in a Two Phase System:* PROFESSOR J. F. MCCLENDON. *Growth Retardation by the Partially Oxidized Sulfhydryl of Cysteine:* DR. FREDERICK S. HAMMETT. *Eocene Lagomorpha:* J. J. BURKE. *Blue Eyes for Brown:* DR. VILHJALMUR STEFANSSON ... 189

*Reports:*
*The Banting Research Foundation:* PROFESSOR V. E. HENDERSON and D. T. FRASER ... 192

*Societies and Meetings:*
*The Tennessee Academy of Science:* PROFESSOR JOHN T. MCGILL. *The Northwest Scientific Association:* J. W. HUNGATE ... 192

*Scientific Apparatus and Scientific Methods:*
*A Simplified Method of Staining Endospores:* ALICE B. SCHAEFFER and PROFESSOR MAC DONALD FULTON. *A Demonstration Jar for White Mice:* PROFESSOR C. REYNOLDS ... 194

*Special Articles:*
*Variability and Individuality:* DR. C. C. LITTLE. *The Mechanism of the Ionene Synthesis:* PROFESSOR MARSTON TAYLOR BOGERT. *The Vitamin D Potency of Egg Yolk from Irradiated Hens:* DR. GEORGE H. MAUGHAN and EDNA MAUGHAN ... 195

*Science News* ... 6

SCIENCE: A Weekly Journal devoted to the Advancement of Science, edited by J. MCKEEN CATTELL and published every Friday by

THE SCIENCE PRESS

New York City: Grand Central Terminal

Lancaster, Pa. — Garrison, N. Y.

Annual Subscription, $6.00 — Single Copies, 15 Cts.

SCIENCE is the official organ of the American Association for the Advancement of Science. Information regarding membership in the Association may be secured from the office of the permanent secretary, in the Smithsonian Institution Building, Washington, D. C.

# GENETICS AND EMBRYOLOGY[1]

By Professor CHARLES ZELENY

UNIVERSITY OF ILLINOIS

THE rapid rise of genetics has led to difficulties in relating its findings to those of embryology. The view has been expressed that progress in genetics is endangered by explorations in border fields. The problem has a general significance and seems to warrant discussion before a group of zoologists.

### INBREEDING AND OUTBREEDING

In treating these difficulties it may be allowable to take a theory of one of the necessary conditions of evolution and to apply it to the analogous realm of scientific progress. Among the numerous constructive contributions of genetics to the discussion of the factors of evolution is the support it gives to the view that periods of isolation alternating with periods of intermingling among groups are necessary for progress. Inbreeding and outbreeding are both essential. New hereditary constitutions are swamped by outbreeding, and their recessive genes are incapable of expression under the condition of free contact within a large population.

With progressive isolation, small, homozygous, closely knit populations are produced. Each establishes its own clear and definite racial qualities. Many of the groups die out because of inherent weakness. Others have innate vigor and continue to flourish under isolation for a considerable period of time.

For the latter, two roads are open. If they continue in isolation their homozygous constitution leads to stagnation and their incapacity for rapid response to changing environments dooms them to extinction. If, on the other hand, after they have established themselves under isolation and are no longer in

[1] Address of the vice-president and chairman of Section F—Zoological Sciences, American Association for the Advancement of Science, presented at the Zoologists' dinner, Atlantic City, December 29, 1932.

danger of being swamped by outbreeding, they break through the barrier separating them from their neighbors, they give and receive valuable contributions. A great variety of new gene combinations becomes available. A new period of isolation may establish some of these as promising steps in further evolution. So, with alternating cycles of inbreeding and outbreeding, rapid evolution is made possible.

This theory may be extended to the analogous conditions of scientific progress. The enthusiasm of a group in a special field may lead to isolation. Isolation favors the development of clearly defined concepts and of well-organized programs of investigation along the lines prescribed by these concepts. This favorable result, however, may be followed by the development of routines of procedure, leading, if the isolation be long continued, to eventual stagnation and sterility of the field in question.

From this sad fate the special science may be rescued by the stimulus of excursions into neighboring realms. The explorers may bring back many "wild and unusual" data that refuse to be confined within the corrals of the defenders of the home territory. Much confusion results. The situation is "viewed with alarm" by the home guard. But from these outside contacts new concepts arise which gain precision and clear definition in a new era of organized investigation. Thus alternating periods of isolation and of contact favor scientific progress.

### History of Genetics

Among the difficulties connected with the establishment of genetics were (1) the preoccupation of biologists with the interests and enthusiasms aroused by the publication of Darwin's "Origin of Species," (2) the introduction of a method of investigation unfamiliar to biologists, and (3) the inadequacy of knowledge of the processes of sexual reproduction.

Upon the rediscovery of Mendel's laws a small, compact body of active investigators extended his method to an ever-increasing number of species and to all details of somatic characteristics, including form, size, function and even behavior. The concept of stable units of heredity, or genes, was firmly established as a general law, and coordinately with it the law of segregation of the units of a pair in the formation of the gametes and the independent assortment of different pairs. Independent assortment was found to have exceptions. Linkage groups were recognized, and within a group there was discovered a certain percentage of breaking of the linkage, constant for any two pairs of genes. These percentages were shown to have a definite quantitative relation, such that the values in any linkage group could be arranged in linear order. And so, on and on, analyses of heredity data were made in terms of symbols, the genes, in a manner analogous to the atomic system of the chemists.

The investigators in genetics formed a compact body, the members of which had the same desire for demonstration of the universality of application of the gene concept. A very close inbreeding of ideas occurred, making the concept more and more well defined, unquestioned and all-sufficient. This isolation was of great importance from the standpoint of adequate development and demonstration of the gene concept. If the majority of geneticists had devoted their time from the very start to seeking points of contact with prevailing views in other biological fields, instead of devoting themselves to their knitting, the progress of the science of heredity might have been swallowed up in a morass of conflicting and imperfectly grounded speculations.

The next stage was not so profitable. Viewing with satisfaction the tremendous advance in "atomic explanation" of heredity and the ever-increasing number of individual cases to which it could be applied, geneticists tended to continue in isolation indefinitely on the ground of lack of sufficient data for an adequate approach to other biological fields. The fact that at its beginning the view of general significance of Mendel's results was a wild speculation, seemingly contrary to the bulk of previous observation, was forgotten. The need of stimulation by foreign ideas was lost sight of in the desire for retaining clearness of objective. In other words, the inbreeding was giving rise to a homozygous population of ideas, and genetics seemed destined to the stagnation and sterility of an exercise in gene sorting.

### The Cytological Frontier

From this stagnaton genetics was rescued temporarily by the older and continuing developments in cytology. The contacts here illustrate both extremes of functional relationship.

In the one extreme, two separate fields of biological inquiry develop independently to such an extent that the observations in one fit naturally into a common system with the other. No test is necessary. No independent demonstration is needed. For example, the law of segregation of genes fits naturally into the cytological observation of the separation of the chromosomes of a pair during maturation.

In an intermediate situation, observations in one field seem so obviously to be explained by those in another, yet without direct confirmation, that after the relation between the two is suggested, the confirmatory test may be applied at once. Test follows suggestion inevitably. For example, the law of independent assortment of different pairs of genes suggests independent assortment of different pairs of chromosomes. But such assortment of chromosomes could not be demonstrated until marked pairs were available for cytological observation. (Explanation of linkage of genes as due to location within a single chromosome also followed as a natural consequence of this hypothesis.)

At the other extreme, daring hypotheses of relationship are necessary. They must be *working* hypotheses, recognized as capable of test and therefore stimulating the invention of devices for test. A good example is the daring speculation on the cytological basis of linkage breaks, the view that the percentage of breaks in linkage is explained by the percentage of crossing over between the members of a pair of chromosomes. Its natural sequel is the view of a linear order of gene-containing chromatin granules within a chromosome and the accompanying exercises in chromosome map construction. When first formulated this hypothesis certainly was a daring speculation, but being accepted as a working hypothesis it was capable of test and has been substantiated in many different ways. The stimulus it gave to constructive work in genetics does not need review before this audience.

The success of the first excursions into the cytological realm led to similar ones concerned with deficiencies, translocations and many other phenomena of genetics. Continued success led to practical obliteration of the frontier, and now the terminology of the older genetics is fused with that of cytology, and the old symbols for units of heredity have become parts of chromosomes. Genetics, having incorporated cytology into its realm in this manner, entered upon a new program of sorting and rearranging genes and groups of genes. In place of the algebraic symbols of the old genetics, there were substituted the chromatin granules and chromosomal rods of the new, and these can be sorted and rearranged even more readily than the old symbols. The enthusiastic endeavors and striking advances in this field are commonplaces of recent genetics.

The cross between genetics and cytology was fertile, and the new period of inbreeding in the united realm has standardized concepts and procedures. The concepts are morphological ones and have now reached sufficient maturity so that they may be safely outcrossed with physiological and embryological ones.

## The Embryological Frontier

The wide gap between the genes as postulated units of heredity and their somatic expression in the adult can be bridged only by observations of embryological events. As at other frontiers, besides independent cultivation of the two fields in the hope that some obvious connection will appear, there should be coordination of experimental procedures, including materials from both sides.

Genetics supplies a technique for controlling hereditary constitutions. Experimental embryology supplies a technique for control of internal and external environments. From the embryological side a comparison can be made of two reaction systems, alike in all respects but one, and that one a single gene or a single component of the environment. A program of procedure based upon this possibility should throw valuable light upon the nature of genes and upon the physiological processes initiated by them. Study of time, place and nature of the changes in relative rates of physiological processes is of the greatest importance. In such a study the succession of events in the regeneration of an organ is a valuable aid and often yields clearer results than does a study of the more complex transformations of normal embryology.

Genetics made early contacts with embryology in the field of dominance, but for a long time evaded the issue by means of the presence-and-absence hypothesis. Multiple allelomorphs, the multiple effects of a single gene difference, the multiple factors concerned in a single somatic character, the effects of deficiencies and numberless other observations suggest intimate functional relations with embryology.

As examples, two embryological investigations will be outlined: the first is far from the frontier and concerns some observations on the development of serpulid worms; the second is near the frontier and concerns some observations on the bar-eye series of multiple allelomorphs in Drosophila.

## Serpulid Development

In all genera of serpulids the worm secretes a calcareous tube. There are two semicircles of gills, one on each side of the head. Each gill has a central shaft with thread-like pinnules on each side and with a terminal thread. The gills have a food-collecting as well as a respiratory function.

In the adults of one group of genera, of which Protula is an example, all the gills retain this typical gill structure.

In the adults of a second group, of which Apomatus is an example, the second gill from the dorsal side in each row has a terminal enlargement in place of the terminal thread. This acts as a plug, or operculum, for closing the mouth of the tube. Both of these modified gills retain the lateral pinnules and continue to have a respiratory and food-collecting function as well as the opercular one.

In the adults of a third group of genera, of which Serpula is an example, in place of one of the second gills there is an operculum without gill function. Its stalk is without the lateral pinnules, and the terminal enlargement is a simple cup with a notched edge. In place of the other second gill, there is a bud of embryonic cells, the rudimentary operculum.

In the adults of the fourth group of genera, of which Hydroides is an example, the relations of the structures are like those of the third group, but the functional operculum is a much larger and more complicated organ, having its terminal enlargement made up of two distinct cups, each with its own spines.

In their individual life cycles members of the fourth, or Hydroides, group pass through definite stages resembling closely the adult stages of the other groups. Emphasis is to be laid on the fact that these stages are passed through after the worms have completed the egg and free-living larval stages and after they have entered upon the sedentary mode of life in a calcareous tube. In each stage the function of the organs of the opercular series is the same as that of their adult homologues. The stages are not the transitory phases of a construction process. Furthermore, one stage is not, in any obvious sense, a necessary mechanical step in the building of the succeeding one. In fact, the transformation involves a radical destruction of parts of the preceding stage and the construction of strikingly different new parts. In some of the steps of the transformation the whole old organ is destroyed and is replaced by a new one.

The process warrants further description of the development of Hydroides. Soon after the free-swimming larvae settle down and secrete a limy tube, they form a right and a left row of gills, of the first, or Protula, type, without opercular modifications. After several days in this condition, the cells at the base of the terminal thread of the second left gill divide rapidly, forming an opercular enlargement, and the terminal thread is absorbed, but the stalk retains its lateral respiratory pinnules. The organ now has the general plan of the second gill of the second, or Apomatus, type. The opercular swelling continues its growth and forms a single cup with a serrated edge. The lateral pinnules are absorbed and the organ is a functional operculum of the adult third, or Serpula, type. In the meantime, the second right gill stops its growth, its terminal thread and lateral pinnules shrivel, and the stalk drops off at a definite cleavage plane near its base. The cells of the basal stub proliferate to form a small bud of embryonic character. At this point the whole opercular system, right and left, resembles that of adults of the genus Serpula. After a few weeks in this condition, a time during which new gills are added at the ventral edge of each branchial circlet, the functional operculum, in the position of the second left gill, drops off at a basal cleavage plane. The embryonic bud at the position of the second right gill now enlarges rapidly and develops into an operculum with a complicated double cup of the fourth, or adult Hydroides, type. At the same time, a bud of embryonic cells, the new rudimentary operculum, is developed in place of the lost functional operculum of the third, or Serpula, type.

According to the findings of genetics, the gene complement of the cells involved in the development of the second gill, right or left, remains unchanged throughout the life cycle of Hydroides. It is stimulated to respond in one way at one time and in another way at another time, or the physiological processes initiated earlier in the life cycle and involved in the opercular modification, affect the cells in these positions in different ways at different times. That the structural differentiation at any stage is not merely part of a sequence of necessary events in the erection of the adult structure is evidenced by the fact that regeneration of the removed functional organ (whether gill without opercular modification, gill with opercular modification, Serpula type of operculum or Hydroides type of operculum) gives a replica of the removed organ *without recapitulatory stages.* Thus an organ may be repeated in duplicate by appropriate stimulation either of the basal cells of the removed organ or of the prepared embryonic bud of the opposite side. Transplantation technique should yield further important results.

A stage in such a series is not the natural developmental consequence of the immediately preceding type of development of an organ. The change is a deep-seated one, involving other parts of the body and concerned with the time at which the gene complex is stimulated to activity.

The same genes stimulated by the different physiological agents of different periods of the life cycle give strikingly different somatic results at a particular point in the individual. In the same way, two exactly similar gene complexes of two groups of cells located in different parts of the same individual may at *one time* respond in different ways because the stimulating agents differ. The problem of differentiation of the individual, therefore, is one involving both time and place, though the gene complex is postulated to remain constant and independent of time and place.

From the standpoint of the recapitulation theory in its old form, the embryological facts find a ready explanation in terms of the supposed phylogeny of Hydroides. The problem may, however, be stated in other terms. How can one hereditary constitution give a juvenile organ different from its own adult organ but similar to the adult organ resulting from another hereditary constitution? The answer is not apparent, but two considerations may have a bearing upon the question: First, the differences in the opercula of the adults of the four groups of genera are similar to differences resulting from gene mutations in other animals. Second, changes in physiological processes resulting from environmental factors have been shown in many cases to resemble changes in physiological processes resulting from gene mutation without corresponding environmental change. May we not be justified in formulating the *working* hypothesis that gene mutation produces change in gene reaction similar to that produced in physiological processes by environmental change? And further, may we not be justified in hunting here for clues to the nature of gene action and even to the nature of gene structure?

Why does a gene complex express itself at the site of the second gill in different ways at different times in the life cycle? A gill without opercular modification, a gill with opercular enlargement, an operculum of the Serpula type and an operculum of the Hydroides type—these are not stages in the development of the adult Hydroides structure; but, as regeneration studies show, they are characteristically different and independent expressions of a single genotype at one and the same location in the developing individual. Certainly a more intimate study of the developmental processes in ontogeny will throw some light on the nature of the gene differences at the basis of differences in adult somatic expression. Such a study should pay special attention to regeneration and grafting technique in forms differing in a single gene or in a single environmental factor when all other hereditary and environmental factors are controlled.

### Multiple Allelomorphs

The second embryological investigation concerns the changes produced by a single gene mutation.

The different members of the bar-eye series of allelomorphs in Drosophila have characteristic differences in size of the eyes and in number of ommatidia as determined by facet counts. From the genetics side much is known of the normal rates of mutation, quantity and position effects within the gene or its immediate neighborhood, and acceleration of the rate of mutation under x-ray and radium treatment and at high temperatures.

The number of eye facets is strikingly affected by the temperature of the developing individual, and each mutant has its own temperature coefficient. In most of the members of the series the number of facets decreases with increase in temperature, but in infra-bar there is a reversal of the temperature effect. The characteristic adult somatic differences of several mutants thus may be simulated by one mutant when raised at different temperatures.

By appropriate transfers of larvae from one temperature to another at different times in different individuals, it is possible to locate in the life cycle the exact period during which temperature has a differential effect. This effective period comes in the third instar of the larva, has definite limits and is of short duration. The temperature of the developing individual at other times in its life cycle has no effect upon the number of facets in the adult eye. If we assume that the different physiological processes involved in the development of the eye have different temperature coefficients the differences in adult facet numbers of individuals raised at different temperatures are explained.

Changes in the bar-gene may be postulated to produce changes in the relative rates of the processes acting during the effective period and thus bring about changes in the temperature coefficients of the mutants and may even reverse the effect. A study of the nature of the difference in developmental processes produced by the different genes of such a series of mutations is likewise an avenue of approach to knowledge of the structure of the gene and the nature of gene action.

Since the circumstances connected with the production of the bar mutants make it possible to formulate a theory of difference between the genes of the series in terms of structural change, quantitative in some cases, and since the resulting somatic effects may be measured in terms of temperature effect upon an individual with unchanged genes, it seems worth while to postulate, for purposes of experimental test, theories of gene action in terms of relative rates of the physiological effects they produce.

### Conclusion

In conclusion, let us return to the original thesis, of the need of recurring cycles of inbreeding and outbreeding for sound scientific progress. Daring explorations on the embryological frontier of genetics, long considered by many geneticists as wild and dangerous speculations, are gaining ground as legitimate enterprises. Some of the results of these explorations are receiving attention. Both genetics and embryology are profiting by the functional contact. Fears that the "organizer" of the embryologist might destroy the gene or that the gene might inactivate the "organizer" are turning out to be groundless. Both concepts have passed their immature periods in isolation; they are now mature, and the union is a fertile one. It will serve no good purpose to brand the offspring as illegitimate.

# OBITUARY

## EDWIN CHAPIN STARKS

EDWIN CHAPIN STARKS, associate professor of zoology emeritus in Stanford University, died at his home in Palo Alto, California, on December 29, 1932. He was born in Baraboo, Wisconsin, on January 25, 1867, and spent his youth mainly in Chicago, where he received his early education, and afterward engaged in business. With an inborn interest in living things he was especially attracted by fishes, and early set about finding out all he could concerning them. He collected specimens of all that came within his range, mounted most of them in a remarkably skilful manner, and found out their names and relationships, searching all available libraries to do so. He entered into correspondence with Dr. Theodore Gill, of the U. S. National Museum, and with Dr. David Starr Jordan, then president of the University of Indiana. His eager inquiries received cordial welcome and prompt response from each of these great naturalists. To Dr. Gill may be traced his interest in the osteology of fishes, which later became his main field of study. Dr. Jordan encouraged him as he alone could, and the avocation of the boy and young man soon became the fixed ideal of his life. In 1893 he entered Stanford University as a special student in zoology, and quickly found a welcome in the enthusiastic group in that department under the guidance of President Jordan and Professor C. H. Gilbert. His definite purpose was to become a zoologist, an authority in the field of ichthyology, and nothing swerved him an instant from that goal. Things which did not bear directly upon this end he banished from his program without hesitation as useless distractions. The then existing major subject system at Stanford made possible a concentration of study and effort rarely found open to-day, especially for the so-called "special student," now almost standardized out of existence. He never took the trouble to fulfil the routine entrance requirements, and thus to become a regular student, nor to qualify for a degree. In such matters and in formal courses he was not interested. The privileges of laboratory, scientific collections and library, the sympathetic advice and guidance of able and inspiring teachers, the daily contact with a select number of ambitious associates gave him all the opportunities he desired. Equipped with an alert and naturally keen mind, and with powers of concentration far above the average, he soon justified the confidence placed in him.

In December, 1894, he accompanied Dr. Jordan and several other students on a zoological collecting trip to Mazatlán, Mexico, the first of many such field journeys in which his love of travel and adventure and of the study of living things in their natural surroundings was to have full range. The following summer he took part in an exploration of Puget Sound, headed by Professor Meany, of the University of Washington, in which the first systematic dredging in that body of water was undertaken. Back at Stanford in the fall, he again left in December, 1895, for southern waters, this time with Dr. C. H. Gilbert on the Stanford Expedition to Panama, where four months were filled with intensive field work upon the fishes of that region.

He was married in June, 1897, to a fellow Stanford student, Miss Chloe F. Lesley, who later also became a member of the faculty, and as associate professor of graphic art was retired in 1932. Their daughter, Dr. Dorothy J. Starks, is now an instructor in radiology in the Stanford University School of Medicine.

In 1897 he was appointed to an assistantship in the U. S. Biological Survey under Dr. C. Hart Merriam at Washington, where he spent two busy years. An opportunity to join the Harriman Expedition to Alaska in the summer of 1899 was eagerly seized, as it opened a new field of experiences and an excellent opportunity for acquaintance with the noted group of scientists taking part in it. On his return he became curator of the museum and assistant professor of zoology in the University of Washington. In 1901 he was called to Stanford as curator of zoology, was made assistant professor in 1907, and associate professor in 1927, in which capacity he served until his retirement in 1932.

In 1904 Professor Starks took part in a field trip for the U. S. Bureau of Fisheries in Oregon, under the leadership of Professor J. O. Snyder. In 1910 the Stanford Expedition to Brazil, headed by Professor J. C. Branner, gave him an opportunity to become acquainted with its northern and northeastern coasts and to make extensive collections of fishes there. A trip to Europe in 1907 to visit museums and to form personal contacts with zoologists, whom he had already known through correspondence and exchange of publications, was followed by a longer one with his family in 1913 and 1914, a part of which was spent in research in the Zoological Station at Naples and in museum work, the remainder in travel and in art studies.

The summers of 1909 and 1912 found him again on the waters of Puget Sound, in the former year as instructor in zoology at the Friday Harbor Marine Laboratory, in the latter as an investigator there. In the summer and fall of 1926 he made his last long collecting trip, a private one undertaken to the Philippines to secure certain forms for osteological study not otherwise procurable.

Throughout all these years and almost up to the very end of his life his scientific writings steadily appeared, the total number reaching more than eighty. Based upon each of the above expeditions were extensive reports dealing with faunistic and distributional results, either written by himself alone, or in collaboration with Dr. Jordan, Dr. Gilbert or others. The most notable of his many publications deal with the comparative osteology of fishes, in which he became a recognized authority. His careful analytical studies in this difficult field have thrown much light on the relationships of a large number of genera and families, and have furnished a solid basis for their classification. Not a little of the value of this series of studies is due to the unfailing cooperation of his wife, Mrs. Chloe Lesley Starks, whose superb artistic skill and accuracy provided his papers with illustrations not to be excelled anywhere.

Professor Starks was a life member of the California Academy of Sciences, to the *Proceedings* of which he contributed many important papers. He was also a corresponding member of the Zoological Society of London and a fellow of the American Association for the Advancement of Science.

As a teacher he was exceptionally gifted. His broad sympathy with students, his patience and clarity in exposition, his contagious enthusiasm, and his kindly humor won the affection and admiration of all his pupils. As a colleague he held a high place in the estimation of his faculty associates. His modest, retiring disposition led him to shun publicity, but his constant and generous hospitality within his own home drew around him a group small but unusually devoted.

Apart from his scientific work Professor Starks' interests were many and varied. Although a naturalist he found no pleasure in hunting or angling, but took the greatest delight in outdoor life, and in travel contacts with other places and peoples. He was an avid reader and his well-selected library gave evidence of his breadth of interest in the best in literature and art. His usual recreation was sought in his workshop, and from it issued from time to time artistic and beautiful products of his craftsmanship in wood and metal that were the wonder and envy of his friends. Photography and fine printing were also hobbies in which he excelled. His experiences and observations on each of his many expeditions were carefully recorded in separate journals, illustrated with sketches and photographs. Three of these, his own printing and binding, models of fine bookmaking, are highly prized by those of his friends who were fortunate enough to receive copies.

A broad appreciation of the beautiful in nature, in life, literature and art enriched his years. Upon his release from teaching responsibility he looked forward to continued activity in research and travel. But it was not to be. Never robust physically, an increasing cardiac weakness terminated his life after a short illness. His scientific writings will stand as a memorial to his exact and painstaking industry and high scholarship, his former pupils, his colleagues, and his friends will cherish still more the memory of a kind and joyous personality, sincere and faithful to the end.

F. M. MACFARLAND

STANFORD UNIVERSITY

## HERMAN THEODOR HOLM

DR. HERMAN THEODOR HOLM, who was on the staff of the Department of Agriculture for several years and who was connected with the department in various phases of scientific work for many years, passed away at Providence Hospital, after a brief illness, on December 26, 1932.

Dr. Holm was born in Copenhagen, Denmark, on February 3, 1854, and graduated under Warming from the University of Copenhagen in 1880. He was appointed to the Denmark North Polar Expedition in 1882 as botanist and zoologist under Admiral Garda and for some two years was icebound in Greenland. He added greatly to the botanical knowledge of West Greenland, and his extensive knowledge of altitude and circumpolar floras compelled attention of all interested in this subject.

On April 12, 1888, Dr. Holm landed in New York City, and as soon thereafter as possible applied for citizenship. He enjoyed telling that he was an American by choice and that we "could not help ourselves." Very soon after coming to this country he was appointed assistant botanist in the U. S. National Museum and occupied that position from 1888 to 1893, and was then appointed assistant pathologist in the U. S. Department of Agriculture. In 1897 he resigned this position, but, as above stated, he did much work for the department in connection with special botanical problems, drawing, and translating. For drawings that show the anatomy of plants he had no peer, and he read and translated all the Teutonic languages and many Latin languages. So wedded was he to his scientific work that some years ago he moved to an isolated farm in Maryland in order to have uninterrupted time for his work, but was finally persuaded to accept a position on the research staff of the Catholic University of America, where he was given ample room for his collections. Many of his papers were published in Germany. It seems regrettable that American botany should come to us through translation.

Although wedded to his profession Dr. Holm was

a gracious host. He gave many interesting small dinners and could cook on occasion. He took infinite pains to help good work, but for pretense and bad work his criticisms were devastating.

A. F. WOODS

U. S. DEPARTMENT OF AGRICULTURE

## RECENT DEATHS

JAMES M. WHITE, professor of architectural engineering and supervising architect of the University of Illinois, died on February 6, at the age of sixty-five years.

SAMUEL ANTHONY GOLDSCHMIDT, chemist, chairman of the Board of Directors of the Parsons Ammonia Company, died on January 29, at the age of eighty-four years.

DR. RONALD STEELE SADDINGTON, an assistant on the scientific staff of the Rockefeller Institute, died at the Rockefeller Institute Hospital on February 4, of an illness contracted three weeks ago while studying herpes. He was twenty-nine years old.

SAMUEL W. PHILLIPS, in charge of the erosion station of the Bureau of Chemistry and Soils of the U. S. Department of Agriculture at Zanesville, Ohio, was shot and killed by a burgler in his home on January 23. Mr. Phillips was in his thirty-ninth year.

SIR J. ARTHUR THOMSON, emeritus professor of natural history at the University of Aberdeen, died on February 12 at the age of seventy-two years.

SIR DANIEL MORRIS, scientific adviser in tropical agriculture to the British Colonial Office, previously from 1898 to 1905 imperial commissioner of the West Indies Department of Agriculture, died on February 9 at the age of eighty-eight years.

SIR FREDERIC G. HALLETT, secretary of the Imperial Cancer Research Fund and formerly secretary of the conjoint board of the British Royal College of Physicians and Surgeons, died on February 6. He was seventy-two years old.

THOMAS ALFRED COWARD, the British ornithologist, died on January 30, at the age of sixty-six years.

AUGUSTIN MESNAGER, civil engineer, vice-president of the Paris Academy of Sciences, died on February 6. He was seventy years old.

# SCIENTIFIC EVENTS

## INTERNATIONAL VITAMIN STANDARDS

THE international standards for vitamins A, B ($B_1$) and D, which have been allotted to this country, have been received by Dr. E. M. Nelson, Protein and Nutrition Division, Bureau of Chemistry and Soils, U. S. Department of Agriculture, Washington, D. C. These standards are made available to investigators in the United States through the generosity of the Health Organization of the League of Nations. Application blanks for obtaining the standards, which will be distributed for scientific purposes, can be obtained from Dr. Nelson. These standards were designed for the sole purpose of enabling investigators to express vitamin potency in units of universally accepted value. The quantities distributed are suitable only for assay with small laboratory animals, such as rats, pigeons and mice. In order to make the best use of these primary standards it is suggested that investigators give consideration to the possibility of making suitable secondary standards through the use of the material distributed.

Allotments of international standards have been deposited with Dr. E. Fullerton Cook, chairman of the U. S. Pharmacopoeia Revision Committee, 43rd Street and Woodland Avenue, Philadelphia, Pennsylvania, for distribution for research purposes and for the standardization of a U. S. Pharmacopoeia reference cod liver oil. The U. S. Pharmacopoeia reference cod liver oil, a secondary standard for vitamins A and D, is to be available to all applicants at small cost and is intended to serve particularly for establishing new and more desirable definitions for vitamin potency of U. S. Pharmacopoeia cod liver oil. The U. S. Pharmacopoeia reference cod liver oil will also serve as a suitable standard for all products for which claims for vitamins A and D potency are to be made. An announcement concerning this reference cod liver oil will be made by the U. S. Pharmacopoeia Revision Committee.

HENRY G. KNIGHT

## THE MORRIS ARBORETUM

APPOINTMENTS to the executive and scientific staffs of the Morris Arboretum of the University of Pennsylvania, at Chestnut Hill, have been announced.

Dr. Rodney H. True, professor of botany and director of the botanical gardens at the University of Pennsylvania since 1920, has been made director of the arboretum. Before going to Pennsylvania he was plant physiologist of the U. S. Department of Agriculture in charge of physiological investigations and also served at various times on the faculties of Radcliffe College, the University of Wisconsin and Harvard.

James Lambert, superintendent of the botanical gardens at the university for a number of years and a graduate of Kew Gardens in London, has been named superintendent of the arboretum, and the position of head gardener has been filled by the appointment of John Tonkin, who was head gardener under Miss Morris. James O'Neill, who also was in the employ of Miss Morris, will be custodian. A secretary, whose appointment will complete the executive staff, will be named later.

Four members of the faculty of botany have been appointed to the scientific staff. They are Professor Harlan H. York, pathologist; Associate Professor Edgar T. Wherry, ecologist; Associate Professor Conway Zirkle, geneticist, and Assistant Professor John M. Fogg, Jr., taxonomist.

Dr. York will carry on research investigations in connection with plant diseases, with particular reference to trees. Prior to becoming a member of the university faculty, Dr. York served as expert in charge of the research program in the forestry project of the New York State Department of Conservation.

As ecologist, Dr. Wherry will direct the study of plants in their relation to soil and atmospheric conditions and the relation of plants to each other in mixed plantings.

Dr. Zirkle, who is a former member of the research staff at Harvard University, will be associated chiefly with special studies of the reproductive processes in higher plants, particularly with reference to the processes concerned in inheritance.

Dr. Fogg will be in charge of the identification and grouping of the plants in the arboretum on the basis of their botanical relationship. It is the intention to assemble at Compton the most complete herbarium of woody plants that it is possible to collect from all parts of the world.

In addition to the executive and scientific staff, the organization of an advisory staff, which will include a landscape architect, a zoologist, a chemist and an engineer, has been recommended by the committee on administration of the arboretum, of which Dr. George Wm. McClelland, vice-president of the university in charge of the undergraduate schools, is chairman. The members of the advisory staff will be designated by the respective deans or department heads, subject to the approval of the committee on administration.

## THE PROPOSED EVERGLADES NATIONAL PARK

We are permitted to print the following memorandum addressed on January 7 by Dr. Wilbur, Secretary of the Interior, to Horace M. Albright, director of the National Park Service:

With the help of Dr. Fairchild and Judge Ritter, president of the association, and through the kindness of Mr. Henry L. Doherty, I was taken to Cape Largo, then by water through the Keys to Cape Sable, then to the mouth of the Shark River, up the Shark River through the Ten Thousand Islands to Everglades, and then along the Tamiami Trail, both west and east. The map of which I was sent a copy was most helpful. When additional copies are available, I should like to have them sent to Messrs. Doherty, Ritter and Fairchild.

This area has outstanding qualifications for national park status. It should be maintained as a water or marine park and a wide area should be taken in. Every effort should be made to keep this a primitive area. I think roads should not be built through it, but that the road which now goes down to the Middle Beach and the Cape Sable area, should be improved, and this region should be the southern entrance to the park. The northern entrance should be at Everglades. All visitors to the remote areas of the park should go by water. As few trails as possible should be built. These can be of simple construction, using elevated planks. This would avoid the mud with the change in tides, snakes, etc.

The protection of the park can be brought about by rangers with small boats, and by an autogiro. It is evident that the proper development of this park will not be costly and that the cost of its control and management can be kept down to figures that will be largely met by the usual reasonable entrance fees.

I need not describe the beauty of the mangrove forests, the unusual opportunities for education and inspiration as well as recreation, the marvelous bird flights, etc. These have been amply covered before.

The one thing that worries me most is the maintenance of a fresh-water supply into the upper reaches of the Shark and other rivers so that there will be no encroachment of salt-water. Such encroachment would destroy the most unique qualities of the park. This means that a wide area to the north must be kept in a virgin condition and that no cross canals interfere with the general drainage of water from Lake Okeechobee south.

It seems to me to need prompt action by Congress, so that large funds for the purchase of these lands can be obtained from private or state sources, and so that there will not be too many small areas to purchase. There is a tendency to bring into production land that should be allowed to remain in its primitive condition.

## IN HONOR OF DR. ELIHU THOMSON

Preliminary plans have been announced for a dinner on March 29, at which leaders in science, engineering and industry will honor Dr. Elihu Thomson, the distinguished engineer and inventor, upon the occasion of his eightieth birthday. The dinner is to be held at the Massachusetts Institute of Technology, of which Dr. Thomson was acting president from 1920 to 1922, and of which he is a life member of the corporation.

International in its significance, the dinner will bring together distinguished representatives of the electrical industry, to which Dr. Thomson has made so many important contributions, leaders from educational institutions, and officers of the various scientific academies, professional societies and technical organizations.

Preliminary plans for the tribute to Dr. Thomson provide for an afternoon conference on topics significant to the occasion. These include the historical development of the applications of electricity, the recent experimental trends and the latest theories of electricity and matter. In connection with this meeting, plans are being made for an impressive exhibit of many of Dr. Thomson's inventions and contributions in the electrical field.

The committee in charge of arrangements consists of the following:

Professor Dugald C. Jackson, head of the department of electrical engineering at the institute, *chairman;* Professor Gustav C. Dahl, of the same department, *secretary;* Dr. Charles G. Abbot, secretary of the Smithsonian Institution; Dr. James Rowland Angell, president, Yale University; Dr. William W. Campbell, director, Lick Observatory, and president, the National Academy of Sciences; Harry P. Charlesworth, vice-president of the Bell Telephone Laboratories, Inc., and president of the American Institute of Electrical Engineers; Dr. Karl T. Compton, president, the Massachusetts Institute of Technology; Dr. Harvey Cushing, Moseley professor of surgery, emeritus, Harvard University; Nelson J. Darling, manager, river works, General Electric Company; Alexander Dow, president, Detroit Edison Company; Dr. Paul D. Foote, director, Research Laboratory of the Gulf Production Pipe Line Companies; Honorable William C. Forbes; Professor Jeremiah D. M. Ford, Harvard University, president, American Academy of Arts and Sciences; Dr. Thomas S. Gates, president, University of Pennsylvania; Dr. George E. Hale, director, Mount Wilson Observatory; Nathan Hayward, president, the American Dredging Company; Dr. Frank B. Jewett, vice-president, the American Telephone and Telegraph Company; Dr. Arthur E. Kennelly, of Harvard University, president, the Union Radio Scientifique Internationale; John C. Lincoln, chairman, board of directors, the Lincoln Electric Company; Dr. Arthur D. Little, president, Arthur D. Little, Inc.; Dr. A. Lawrence Lowell, president, Harvard University; Dr. Roland S. Morris, president, American Philosophical Society; Dr. Calvin W. Rice, secretary, American Society of Mechanical Engineers; E. Wilbur Rice, Jr., honorary chairman of the board, General Electric Company; Andrew W. Robertson, chairman of the board, Westinghouse Electric and Manufacturing Company; Albert L. Rohrer, formerly of the General Electric Company; Clayton H. Sharp, vice-president and technical adviser, Electrical Testing Laboratories, and chairman, U. S. National Committee of the International Electrotechnical Commission; Ambrose Swasey, chairman of the board, Warner and Swasey Company; Gerard Swope, president, the General Electric Company, and Edwin S. Webster, president, Stone and Webster.

# SCIENTIFIC NOTES AND NEWS

PRESIDENT HERBERT HOOVER has been elected an honorary member of the British Institution of Civil Engineers.

BRITISH New Year's honors included the title of baron, conferred on Sir Thomas Jeeves Horder, senior physician to St. Bartholomew's Hospital.

A MEETING in memory of John J. Carty, vice-president of the American Telephone and Telegraph Company, who died on December 27, was held at Rollins College on February 9. The speakers were Dr. Frederick P. Keppel, president of the Carnegie Corporation of New York; Thomas A. Watson, who was associated with Alexander Graham Bell in the invention of the telephone, and Dr. David G. Fairchild, of the U. S. Department of Agriculture. Dr. Carty was a trustee of Rollins College.

THE Cameron Prize of the University of Edinburgh has been awarded to Dr. George F. Dick, professor of clinical medicine at Rush Medical College, Chicago, and Dr. Gladys H. Dick, fellow of the John McCormick Institute for Infectious Diseases, in recognition of their work on the etiology and treatment of scarlet fever. The award is made annually "to a person who, in the course of the five years immediately preceding, has made any highly important and valuable addition to practical therapeutics."

JAMES ORR ELTON, since 1921 manager of the International Smelting Company at Salt Lake City, has been awarded the James Douglas Medal for 1933 of the American Institute of Mining and Metallurgical Engineers. The award, the highest in the metallurgical field, was established in memory of Dr. James Douglas, who was largely responsible for the development of copper metallurgy in Arizona. The medal was conferred on Mr. Elton for his work in the treatment of smelter fume and in the production of electrolytic zinc; for the development of methods for preferential flotation of lead-zinc-silver ores and oxidized lead-silver ores; and for improvements in lead smelting. Presentation of the medal will be made at a meeting of the institute on February 22.

THE council of the British National Institute of Agricultural Botany has awarded the Snell Memorial Medal for 1932 to Dr. Kenneth M. Smith, entomologist of the Potato Virus Research Station of the University of Cambridge. The medal is given to

Dr. Smith in recognition of his valuable research work on the virus diseases of the potato.

THE Stephen Hales Prize of the American Society of Plant Physiologists has been awarded to Dr. Hubert Bradford Vickery, of the Connecticut Agricultural Experiment Station, for his work on vegetable proteins.

THE gold Paul-Ehrlich Medal has been awarded to Dr. Paul Uhlenhuth, professor of hygiene and bacteriology at the University of Freiburg, Baden.

THE Bernhard-Nocht Medal has been awarded to Dr. Hans Ziemann, professor of parasitology at the University of Berlin.

THE Swedish Medical Society has awarded the Gullstrand Gold Medal to Priestley Smith, emeritus professor of ophthalmology at the University of Birmingham, England, for his "ophthalmological researches, especially regarding glaucoma and the permanent growth of the lens."

DR. LOUIS MARTIN, subdirector of the Institut Pasteur and director of the Hôpital Pasteur, Paris, has been nominated Grand Officer of the Legion of Honor.

DR. FRIEDRICH VON MÜLLER, professor of internal medicine at Munich, celebrated on December 30 the fiftieth anniversary of his doctorate.

PROFESSOR EDWARD R. SCHWARZ, of the department of mechanical engineering at the Massachusetts Institute of Technology, has been elected to a fellowship in the British Textile Institute in recognition of his "notable contributions in the field of textile technology and research."

JOHN CLYDE HOSTETTER, director of research and development of the Corning Glass Works, New York, has been elected president of the American Ceramic Society, which opened its thirty-fifth annual convention in Pittsburgh on February 13. Mr. Hostetter succeeds Emerson P. Poste, consulting engineer of Chattanooga, Tennessee. Louis J. Trostel, of the General Refractories Company, Baltimore, has been made vice-president, replacing W. Keith McAfee, of the Universal Sanitary Manufacturing Company, New Castle, Pennsylvania.

CAPTAIN CHARLES M. OMAN has been appointed surgeon-general of the U. S. Navy, succeeding Rear Admiral Charles E. Riggs, whose term expired on January 19.

DR. RALPH HARTLEY WETMORE, assistant professor of botany at Harvard University, has been appointed director of the Botanical Laboratories.

DR. J. B. S. HALDANE has resigned from the Sir William Dunn readership in biochemistry at the University of Cambridge, to accept a chair in the University of London.

DR. NATHANIEL T. KIDDER was elected president of the Massachusetts General Hospital at the annual meeting of the corporation on February 1.

*Museum News* reports that an informal committee to advise on opportunities for service in building up Canadian museums has been formed by the Carnegie Corporation, following recommendation of Sir Henry Miers and S. F. Markham. The members of the committee are Eric Brown, director of the National Art Gallery, Ottawa; H. O. McCurdy, assistant director of the National Art Gallery; E. L. Judah, director of the Ethnological Museum, McGill University; J. C. Webster, of Shediac, New Brunswick, and Francis Kermode, curator of the Provincial Museum at Victoria.

DR. JAMES ANGUS DOULL, president of the Western Reserve University chapter of Sigma Xi, has announced the election of the following new members from the faculty of the School of Medicine: Dr. Carl H. Lenhart, professor of surgery; Dr. Claude S. Beck, assistant professor of surgery; Dr. Norman C. Wetzel, assistant professor of pediatrics; Dr. Rafael Dominguez, associate in pathology, and Dr. Carrol G. Barber, fellow in anatomy.

DR. HERMA PLANTENGA, specialist in plant pathology at the laboratory of Professor Dr. Johanna Westerdyk, at Baarn, Holland, is at present in the United States as a volunteer worker at the new division of plant pathology of the Rockefeller Institute at Princeton.

PROFESSOR N. I. VAVILOV, president of the Lenin Academy of Agricultural Sciences and director of the Institute of Plant Industry, Leningrad, is visiting the United States on his way from a trip to South America. Professor Vavilov is especially interested in the economic grasses and their relation to the development of civilization.

DR. ELLSWORTH HUNTINGTON, research associate in geography at Yale University, lectured before the Franklin Institute on February 9, on "A Theory of Civilization and Climate."

DR. CHARLES R. STOCKARD, professor of anatomy and director of the Experimental Morphology Farm at Cornell University, began on February 14 a series of lectures at the New School for Social Research, New York City, in which he will discuss "The Modern Analysis of Living Structures and Behaviors." Under this general heading, he will give fifteen weekly lectures.

THE twenty-fourth Kelvin lecture of the Institution of Electrical Engineers will be delivered by Sir Frank

Smith, secretary of the British Department of Scientific and Industrial Research, on April 27. The title of the lecture will be: "The Travel of Wireless Waves."

THE HENRY RUSSEL LECTURESHIP at the University of Michigan for 1933 has been awarded to Professor Walter B. Pillsbury, head of the department of psychology. The lectureship was established ten years ago by the late Henry Russel, who left $10,000 for the purpose. The income from the fund is divided into two sums, one being devoted to the lectureship and the other to the Henry Russel award. The latter will go to a faculty member, ranking not higher than assistant professor and showing promise of unusual talent.

AN inaugural banquet of the Smith-Reed-Russell Society of the School of Medicine, George Washington University, was held at the University Club on the evening of January 13, at which time guest speakers included Dr. Theobald Smith and Dr. Frederick F. Russell, two of the three investigators in honor of whom the society is named. Other speakers included the president of the university, Dr. Cloyd Heck Marvin, and Colonel Albert E. Truby, who received the key of the society for Walter Reed to transmit to Colonel Walter L. Reed, surviving son.

*Nature* reports that spring lectures at the Royal Institution are planned as follows: The session of public afternoon lectures at the Royal Institution was opened by Professor J. C. McLennan, who is giving an experimental course on the work on "Low Temperatures and Low Temperature Phenomena" with which he and the University of Toronto have been specially identified. A course on "Recent Advances in Genetics" is to be given by Professor J. B. S. Haldane, who recently returned to England from a visit to the United States. Later courses are by Sir William Bragg, who will review the progress in the past twenty years of the science of crystal analysis by x-rays, and Mr. A. R. Hinks, secretary of the Royal Geographical Society, on "Geography in the Public Service." Mr. Hinks will speak on the new one inch Ordnance Survey map, and the delimitation of national boundaries. Lord Rutherford will give a Saturday course on the "Detection and Production of Swift Particles." The course will be experimental, and as a part of his subject Lord Rutherford will describe the recent progress at the Cavendish Laboratory by Chadwick, Cockcroft and Walton and others. Sir James Jeans will give a course on "Modern Astronomy." The new Fullerian professor of physiology at the Royal Institution, Professor G. Elliot Smith, will give a course on the "Evolution of the Mind."

THE Federal Club, an organization of officials of the Federal Government and the government of the District of Columbia, having as its purpose the advancement of standards of administration and of personnel and the promotion of cooperation and efficiency in the business of government, appointed Dr. W. W. Stockberger, director of personnel and business administration of the U. S. Department of Agriculture, as member and chairman of its membership committee at a meeting held at the Cosmos Club in Washington on January 18. Other members appointed to this committee are E. C. Crittenden, chief of the electrical division of the Bureau of Standards, and E. C. Babcock, secretary of the United States Civil Service Commission. Albert K. Brown, Bureau of Fisheries, was elected a director, to succeed Commander H. A. Seran, Coast and Geodetic Survey, who has been detailed to duty at sea. Edgar B. Calvert, chief of the forecast division of the Weather Bureau, is now president of the club.

*Nature* states that the work, extending over the past two years, of various preliminary committees was brought to a conclusion on January 3 when the Institute of British Geographers held its first meeting and elected a council and officers. The initial membership is open to all present members of the staffs of university departments of geography in Britain; in the future, membership will be by election. With one possible exception, all universities, as well as a large number of colleges of university rank, in Great Britain have now departments of geography and there is thus an obvious need for coordinating the teaching and research work of their staffs and for permitting an exchange of views on matters of particular interest in the furtherance of the subject in the universities. The council and officers elected are: *President,* Professor C. B. Fawcett, University College, London; *Honorary Secretary and Treasurer,* Mr. A. A. Miller, Reading; *Honorary Assistant Secretary,* Dr. H. A. Matthews, Birkbeck College, London; *Council,* J. N. L. Baker, Oxford; Dr. R. O. Buchanan, University College, London; Professor H. J. Fleure, Manchester; Professor Ll. Rodwell Jones, London School of Economics; Professor P. M. Roxby, Liverpool, and Dr. S. W. Wooldridge, King's College, London.

THE London *Times* reports that a new scientific expedition to the Antarctic has been undertaken by Captain Riiser Larsen, who left London recently with several friends for the shores of Enderby Land. According to present arrangements, the exploring party will consist of Captain Larsen and two other men, who will join him and his friends in South Africa. From there they will board a tanker belonging to Consul Lars Christensen, and will make the 11-days trip to Enderby Land, which they expect to reach some time in February. There the three explorers will land with their supplies and 100 dogs, and for a year will make a close study of the coast of the Weddell Sea. Captain Larsen accompanied Amundsen's 1925 Arctic Expedition.

EARLY in January, according to *Museum News,* the Rochester, New York, Museum of Arts and Sciences was voted an additional $9,000 appropriation by the city council and will remain open. For a time the financial crisis in the city, which was receiving only a limited income from taxable property and had 50,000 welfare cases to care for, threatened to close the museum and Director Arthur C. Parker had tendered his resignation. With the added appropriation the museum is to continue its work; and at the request of the city museum board Mr. Parker has agreed to remain in charge.

THE committee of the American Psychological Association on Precautions in Animal Experimentation, consisting of Drs. C. P. Stone, E. G. Wever and C. J. Warden, *chairman,* desires to call attention to the following bills which have been introduced since January first to limit experimental work on animals: (1) New York Assembly, A. 63, proposing to prohibit any experimental work upon a living dog; (2) New York Assembly, A. 181, proposing to make it a misdemeanor to experiment or operate on a live dog for any purpose other than to heal or cure the animal; (3) Massachusetts Senate, S. 113, proposing to penalize certain experiments and operations on live dogs, and (4) Maine House, H. 217, proposing a fine for the practice of vivisection in schools supported wholly or in part by the state. Dr. Warden writes: "It is hoped that members of the American Psychological Association, residing in these states, will write letters of protest against the passage of these measures to the appropriate legislators. Bills of this kind are backed by powerful organizations whose efforts to obstruct scientific research must be met by active and determined resistance."

THE printed *Proceedings* of the Land Use Symposium, held at the summer meeting of the American Association for the Advancement of Science at Syracuse University, have just been issued. They contain all the papers presented at the meeting, which was well attended by economists, business men, research workers, foresters, agronomists, geographers and representatives of other earth sciences. Among the subjects treated in the *Proceedings* are the activities of the National Land Use Committee, Land Use and Agriculture, Land Use and Forestry, Land Use and Erosion, Land Use and Transportation, The Relation of Taxation to Land Utilization and Planned Land Use. The speakers included Dr. L. C. Gray, secretary of the National Land Use Planning Committee, Washington, D. C.; Dr. G. F. Warren, head of the Department of Agricultural Economics and Farm Management, Cornell University; Dr. F. P. Weaver, head of the Department of Agricultural Economics, Pennsylvania State College; Dr. Joseph S. Illick, head of the Department of Forest Management, New York State College of Forestry, Syracuse University; Mark Graves, director of the budget of the State of New York; Dr. Jacob G. Lipman, dean and director of the New Jersey Agricultural Experiment Station; Dr. Henry G. Knight, chief of Bureau of Chemistry and Soils, U. S. Department of Agriculture; Dr. Charles L. Raper, dean of the College of Business Administration, Syracuse University; L. R. Schoenmann, in charge of the Michigan Land Economic Survey. The *Proceedings* are arranged in a 60-page bulletin of standard book size, which can be procured from the Department of Forest Management, New York State College of Forestry, Syracuse, N. Y.

# DISCUSSION

## A NEW MATHEMATICAL FORMULA FOR CHEMICAL ANALYSIS IN A TWO PHASE SYSTEM[1]

OWING to the depression, the biochemist may be faced with a reduction in floor-space and budget, and, hence, one piece of apparatus may have to serve for a number of analytical procedures. I have shown[2] that the Bausch and Lomb micro-colorimeter may be used for the analysis of over 60 substances.

In many analytical procedures, the titration of a substance in water solution in the presence of large quantities of impurities leads to error which is greater the greater the ratio of the impurities to the "unknown."

In colorimetric analysis, colored impurities may often be ruled out by the use of monochromatic light that transforms the colorimeter into a spectrophotometer. Luminous, rarefied-vapor-tubes giving bright line spectra may be easily obtained, and color-filters used to filter out all bright lines except the one desired.

Impurities may not have worried chemists who were analyzing large samples of the unknown substance. But as the methods are adapted to smaller and smaller quantities of the "unknown" without a proportional reduction in the impurities, side-reactions which were insignificant in the older work become significant to the micro-chemist.

[1] From the University of Minnesota and Tohoku Imperial University.

[2] McClendon, "A System of Microchemical Analysis, Handbook of Experimental Chemistry." (1st ed., Japanese and English) Kyo-rytsu-sha, Tokyo, 1932.

A method that has long been used for getting rid of impurities is the extraction of the "unknown" from water-solution with $CCl_4$ or other non-miscible solvent. (Chloroform and $CS_2$ spontaneously decompose in storage and $CS_2$ is highly volatile and inflammable.) In case the partition-coefficient $CCl_4/H_2O$ is 200 or higher, some chemists have assumed that all the "unknown" is extracted with one extraction.

If the substance is colored, it may be determined directly in the colorimeter, and this is easier than getting it back into water to determine it by titration; and is just as accurate, if 10 readings of the colorimeter are made (finding the average being simply addition and moving of the decimal point). If the unknown solution is set at unit depth the colorimeter readings of the standard give the concentration of the unknown *directly,* without any calculation whatever (assuming the standard is in unit concentration).

In case the partition-coefficient, $CCl_4/H_2O$, is small enough to make repeated extractions necessary, the work becomes very laborious, owing to the fact that an infinite number of extractions are necessary to remove all the "unknown" from water-solution. If the partition-coefficient is known, the total "unknown" may be calculated from one extraction (knowing the ratio of volumes of the water-solution to the $CCl_4$). But the presence of impurities may alter the partition-coefficient to an unknown extent.

I have worked out a formula for calculating the total "unknown" from 2 extractions. It is not necessary to know the ratio of volumes of the water-solution to the $CCl_4$, but the ratio must be the same in the 2 extractions. The extraction is made in a separatory funnel and all the $CCl_4$-extract and none of the water-solution is removed. The funnel is stoppered and inverted and the water-solution in the hole in the stop-cock allowed to run back into it before admitting $CCl_4$ for the second extraction. If

$x$ = total,
$x_1$ = 1st extract and
$x_2$ = 2nd extract

the formula is:

$$x = x_1 + \frac{x_1 \, x_2}{x_1 - x_2} \quad \text{or} \quad x = x_1 + \frac{x_2}{1 - \frac{x_2}{x_1}}$$

J. F. McCLENDON

## GROWTH RETARDATION BY THE PARTIALLY OXIDIZED SULFHYDRYL OF CYSTEINE

IN the spring of 1930, I presented before the American Philosophical Society the experimental data leading to the postulate that growth by increase in cell number is regulated by a naturally occurring chemical equilibrium comprised of sulfhydryl as the accelerating portion and its partially oxidized derivatives as the retarding. The full report was published in *Protoplasma,* Vol. 11, pp. 383–411, in the same years.

At that time I recognized that complete validation of the postulate depended upon the demonstration of cell proliferation inhibiting properties by a partially oxidized derivative of the sulfhydryl group carried by a naturally occurring sulfur compound.

Since I had found that cysteine, cystin and glutathione (a cysteine-containing compound) all accelerated cell multiplication, and since these compounds occur naturally in living growing things, the obvious thing to do was to use a partially oxidized sulfur derivative of one of these compounds.

Such a derivative was not available nor had it ever been prepared, to my knowledge. I therefore gave this chemical problem over to Dr. Gerrit Toennies, chief of the chemical division of our institute. After three years of concentrated effort he has succeeded in producing and isolating a sub-oxidized sulfur derivative of cysteine, starting with cystin. This is a notable achievement. He himself will make the report of his method and the chemical properties of the product elsewhere. Suffice it to say here that his tests show the compound to be neither an SH combination nor cysteic acid, the completely oxidized sulfur derivative, but some intermediate stage.

For practical purposes, I had postulated in the paper referred to above that the compound must be water soluble, essentially neutral and fairly stable in aqueous solution for a reasonable period. Dr. Toennies has produced a compound which meets these requirements.

With the material which he has supplied me I have tested out its action on the growth of Hydra hydranths and the embryonic development of Crepidula eggs and larvae. Uniformly have I found that definite and marked retardation is produced by this partially oxidized sulfur derivative of cysteine, a naturally occurring sulfur-containing compound. The retardation is produced by a concentration of about one part per million sulfur in the sub-oxidized state. This concentration is of the same order of magnitude as that used for sulfoxide in previous experiments and which was found similarly retardative.

This finding, therefore, demonstrates for the first time the growth-inhibiting effects of partially oxidized sulfhydryl from naturally occurring compounds and thus puts on unequivocal foundation the postulate that growth by increase in cell number is regulated by the naturally occurring chemical equilibrium comprised of sulfhydryl and its partially oxidized derivatives.

Dr. Toennies' brilliant success puts in our hands a

compound of inestimable practical and theoretical value, the outcome from which no one can predict.

Frederick S. Hammett,
*Scientific Director*

Marine Experimental Station of the Research Institute of the Lankenau Hospital,
North Truro, Massachusetts

## EOCENE LAGOMORPHA

Among the discoveries made by the Carnegie Museum field party during the field season of 1932 which are of interest to the paleontologist was that of remains of Lagomorpha in the Upper Eocene of the Uinta Basin in northeastern Utah. This material will add considerably to our knowledge of the phylogeny of this group and will probably have considerable bearing upon Eocene and Oligocene stratigraphy as well.

Actually, the first discovery of Lagomorph fossils in the Uinta Eocene was made in 1923, when a Carnegie Museum field party, consisting of O. A. Peterson and J. LeRoy Kay, found a fragmentary lower jaw in Horizon C at Little Pleasant Valley, about six miles east and south of Myton, Uinta County, Utah. The poor condition of the specimen made it undesirable for a type, and its description was deferred, pending the discovery of better preserved diagnostic material. During the field season of 1931 members of our party obtained a single inferior cheek tooth of a Lagomorph from a horizon in the Duchesne Oligocene series very near the base of the latter beds, about two miles east of Randlett, Uinta County, Utah. In 1932 the Little Pleasant Valley locality near Myton was revisited and a number of excellent specimens, representing at least three species of Leporidae, were found in Horizon C of the Uinta Eocene series, approximately three hundred feet below the base of the Duchesne Oligocene.

This material is being studied by the writer at the present time and will be described shortly in the *Annals* of the Carnegie Museum.

J. J. Burke

Carnegie Museum

## BLUE EYES FOR BROWN

Few nowadays underrate the value of the press in the spread of knowledge. Cheering to certain minds will be in that connection extracts from a correspondence which began when *Collier's Magazine* for July 16, 1932, published in Freling Foster's column "Keeping Up With the World" the statement that:

> After a prolonged absence of sunlight, men on polar expeditions find that their eyes, irrespective of previous color, have turned blue.—*By C. G. Matson, Los Angeles, California.*

*Collier's* pays $5.00 for contributions such as Mr. Matson's. Under date of July 13 I accordingly tried to sell them the idea that:

> After a prolonged absence of sunlight, men on polar expeditions find that their eyes, irrespective of previous color, are still of the same color.

There came in reply a form letter, saying that my contribution was under consideration. Then, under date of September 7, Freling Foster wrote, declining (by inference) to purchase from me and defending Mr. Matson:

> This contribution was not only accompanied by confirmatory data but it checks with our reference books which describe how the human body is affected by the long polar night.
>
> One book that I can recall offhand is "Sunlight and Health," by Dr. C. P. Saleeby, which was published a short time ago by Putnam.

I checked up the reference and found that on pp. 59–60 of "Sunlight and Health" (N. Y., 1924) Dr. Saleeby says:

> Polar explorers record that, after prolonged absence of sunlight, all the eyes of their men are blue.

Dr. Saleeby did not mention the names of these explorers, and so I wrote him, quoting his own statement and asking further details. On November 24, he replied:

> I wish I could help you, but I know no other reference to the subject than the one which I refer to in my book—taken from the journal of Captain Scott, if I remember aright after all these years.

Here was a clue and I followed it up by writing to Frank Debenham, geologist of Scott's second expedition, now professor of geography in the University of Cambridge and director of the Scott Polar Research Institute. I gave a summary of the correspondence, adding:

> In the book itself I noticed no sign that Dr. Saleeby had relied . . . on the journals of Captain Scott. I am trying to make a rather thorough job of tracing down the belief or fact that eyes change color during the absence of the sun, and surely you at the Institute must have the best command of all the Scott material. I hope, then, that the Institute will be able to give me, first, proof or disproof that comes from the records of any member of the Scott expeditions and, second, any other evidence for or against that may be within your reach.

On December 18, Professor Debenham replied:

> Following up your query about the change of colour of eyes during the polar darkness, a phenomenon which I find it hard to believe, I wrote to our Dr. Levick. . . . I have certainly noticed no such effect.

Surgeon-Commander G. M. Levick, medical officer

and zoologist on Scott's 1910–1913 expedition, replied, December 15, to the institute:

With regard to my own eyes, I am rather a good example as during our last winter I spent six months with the rest of the northern party. . . . I noticed that my eyes had not changed in colour after this. I think that is the general experience.

VILHJALMUR STEFANSSON

NEW YORK, N. Y.

# REPORTS

## THE BANTING RESEARCH FOUNDATION

AT its recent annual meeting, the trustees of the Banting Research Foundation reviewed the work accomplished under its grants during the previous year.

The following changes have taken place in the trustees. Sir Robert Falconer has resigned, and in consequence Mr. C. S. Macdonald, president of the Confederation Life Association, was appointed chairman of the board; and Dr. H. J. Cody, president of the University of Toronto, was appointed vice-chairman. Sir William Mulock and Dr. Cody were joined as members of the board, representing the Board of Governors of the University of Toronto, by Dr. H. B. Anderson.

The following workers have received grants from the foundation during the past year: Miss A. M. Alley, McGill University, who has been working under Professor Babkin on gastric and salivary secretion; Dr. Maurice Brodie, McGill University, on poliomyelitis; Dr. H. H. Burnham, University of Toronto, on the vascular supply to the nasal mucosa; Dr. M. M. Cantor, University of Alberta, on the active principle of the adrenal cortex; Dr. H. A. Cates, University of Toronto, representing a committee studying the relation between parentage and the difficulties of childbirth; Dr. A. M. Davidson, University of Manitoba, on the diagnosis of skin diseases and their treatment; Miss Ruth Dow, McGill University, on the auditory area of the brain; Mr. G. T. Evans, McGill University, on the effect of lack of oxygen in exercise, high altitudes and anesthesia on the chemical changes in the heart muscle leading to failure; Dr. R. H. Fraser, University of Manitoba, on the diagnosis of tuberculosis; Dr. J. W. Gilchrist, University of Western Ontario, on the infections following childbirth; Dr. R. Gottlieb, McGill University, on the use of thorium dioxide in the diagnosis of abnormal conditions in the liver; Mr. H. C. Graham, Dalhousie University, on the excretion of uric acid; Miss E. R. Grant, McGill University, on the effect of starvation and exercise on the chemistry of muscle; Mr. J. M. Hershey, University of Toronto, working with Prof. C. H. Best, on the treatment of fatty degeneration of the liver; Mr. F. L. Horsfall, Jr., McGill University, on the fate of lactic acid in the body; Dr. E. E. Shouldice, University of Toronto, on the effect of operations on the intestinal canal; Mr. L. R. LeFave, Queen's University, on the diagnosis of typhoid fever; Professor D. Mainland, University of Manitoba and Dalhousie University, study of the human ovary; Mr. P. G. Mar, University of Manitoba, a study of a rare type of skin disease; Dr. D. R. Mitchell, University of Toronto, on the treatment of urinary infections; Dr. R. A. Moreash, Dalhousie University, on the damage to the liver which is supposed to be produced during the treatment of syphilis; Dr. J. M. McEachren, University of Manitoba, on cholesterol metabolism; Mr. S. Weinstein, University of Saskatchewan, on the oxidation of adrenalin; Dr. A. C. Abbott, University of Manitoba, on the thyroid gland; Professor H. D. Kay, University of Toronto, on experimental ricketts; Professor R. F. Shaner, University of Alberta, on the development of the tracts in the brain of the mammalian embryo; Mr. P. R. Macdonald, McGill University, on the innervation of the lacrymal gland. In addition, a detailed report was received from Dr. F. G. Banting on the work carried out in his department with the aid of funds received from the Banting Research Foundation, which resulted in the publication of eight communications dealing with the pathological changes due to the administration of excessive amount of vitamin D on the intestinal canal during acute intestinal intoxication, and with various methods in analyses required for the work that is being carried on in the department.

V. E. HENDERSON
D. T. FRASER
*Honorary Secretaries*

# SOCIETIES AND MEETINGS

## THE TENNESSEE ACADEMY OF SCIENCE

THE Tennessee Academy of Science held its fall annual meeting on November 25 and 26 at Vanderbilt University. In the absence of the president, Dr. A. Richard Bliss, Jr., of Memphis, Dr. Louis J. Bircher, vice-president, presided. Sixty-seven members registered and the average attendance of the public was unusually large.

Two morning and two afternoon sessions were well taken up in the reading and discussion of the thirty papers on the program, which by reason of the fact that the academy has not organized sections, were all given in the same room and were related to various branches of science—astronomy, physics, chemistry, botany, economics, physiology, genetics, pharmacology and pathology. Seventeen of the papers were by members of the academy teaching or pursuing scientific courses in universities or colleges. The institutions represented were the University of Tennessee, Vanderbilt University, George Peabody College, The Southwestern, Memphis, State Teachers College, Murfreesboro, Tennessee Polytechnic, Cookeville, Carson and Newman College, Jefferson City, Tennessee. Some of the other members contributing papers were R. M. Williamson, director of the U. S. Weather Service, Nashville, "A New Element in Meteorological Observation"; Dr. William Litterer, Tennessee state bacteriologist, "Six Cases of Rocky Mountain Spotted Fever in Tennessee"; Latimer Wilson, of Franklin, Kentucky, "Features of Galactic Structure"; Dr. Lucius P. Brown, formerly food commissioner of New York City, now a farmer of Spring Hill, Tennessee, "Problems of Taxation in Tennessee from the Standpoint of Economics"; John H. DeWitt, Jr., chief engineer of the Radio Station WSM, Nashville, "Vertical Radiators for Broadcasting Stations." Mr. DeWitt in discussing his subject described the steel tower recently erected near Franklin, Tennessee. This is the tallest radiator in the United States, and though 878 feet in height and having a diameter of 38 feet 370 feet above ground, rests on an insulated porcelain plate only about two feet in diameter.

At the Academy dinner, on Friday evening, Professor Bircher, presiding, read a report by President Bliss on "The Reelfoot Lake Biological Station," and Dr. W. G. Harrison, of Birmingham, Alabama, delivered an address on "The History of Medicine." Dr. Harrison discussed especially the contributions of physicians to science in early times and the contribution of scientists to medicine in modern times.

The following officers were elected for 1933: Francis G. Slack, associate professor of physics at Vanderbilt University, *president;* Charles W. Davis, professor of biology at Union University, Jackson, Tennessee, *vice-president;* John T. McGill, professor emeritus of organic chemistry, Vanderbilt University, *secretary-treasurer;* Jesse M. Shaver, professor of biology, George Peabody College, *editor;* Miss Eleanor Eggleston, assistant-librarian, Vanderbilt University, *librarian.*

The meeting of the academy in the spring of 1933 will be held at Walnut Log Lodge, Reelfoot Lake, Tennessee.

JOHN T. MCGILL
*Secretary-Treasurer*

## THE NORTHWEST SCIENTIFIC ASSOCIATION

THE ninth annual meeting of the Northwest Scientific Assocition was held at the Davenport Hotel, Spokane, Washington, on December 28 and 29, 1932. The attendance at the meeting was only slightly lower than that of the previous year, which marked the high point in attendance. In view of the prevailing financial conditions this year's large attendance was highly satisfactory. At the meeting this year, moreover, the out-of-town attendance was noticeably larger.

The presiding officer was Ivan C. Crawford, of the University of Idaho, the president of the organization. At the opening general session on December 28 an address was delivered by Dr. R. R. Parker, of the U. S. Public Health Service, Hamilton, Montana, on the subject "Tick Borne Diseases of the Rocky Mountain Region," and one by Dr. W. F. Thompson, of the University of Washington, Seattle, Washington, on the subject "A Deep Sea Fishery."

In addition to the general sessions, section meetings were held by the following sections: Botany-Zoology, Chemistry-Physics, Education-Psychology, Engineering, Forestry, Geology-Geography, Medicine-Surgery, and Social Science. The program of the Forestry section consisted of a symposium on "Forest Research Needs of the Inland Empire," papers on the progress and needs of research being given on each of the seven phases included, namely, silviculture, fire protection, tree diseases, insects, range management, utilization and economics.

At the business meeting on December 29 important amendments to the constitution were adopted relating to the enlargement of the number of trustees and outlining their duties. This makes possible a machinery for soliciting and caring for bequests, donations, etc., for the prosecution of research in the region. The association also accepted the invitation of the Pacific Division of the American Association for the Advancement of Science to affiliate with that organization.

The officers for 1933 are as follows:

*President:* Howard R. Flint, U. S. Forest Service, Missoula, Montana.

*Vice-president:* Thomas Large, Spokane, Washington.

*Secretary-Treasurer:* Otis W. Freeman, State Normal School, Cheney, Washington.

*Councilors:* Ivan C. Crawford, University of Idaho, Moscow, Idaho; E. E. Hubert, University of Idaho, Moscow, Idaho; Charles H. Clapp, State University, Missoula, Montana; J. W. Hungate, State Normal School, Cheney, Washington; E. F. Gaines, State College of Washington, Pullman, Washington.

*Executive Committee of Trustees:* F. G. Miller, Uni-

E. E. Hubert, editor of *Northwest Science,* the official publication of the association, was reappointed for the year 1933. Alfred L. Anderson, of the University of Idaho, will continue to serve as assistant editor.

The following were elected as chairmen of the various sections:

*Botany-Zoology,* A. L. Hafenrichter, State College, Pullman, Washington.

*Chemistry-Physics-Mathematics,* R. W. Gelbach, State College, Pullman, Washington.

*Education,* F. T. Hardwick, Whitworth College, Spokane, Washington.

*Engineering,* G. E. Thornton, State College, Pullman, Washington.

*Forestry,* F. G. Miller, University of Idaho, Moscow, Idaho.

*Geology-Geography,* E. T. Hodge, University of Oregon, Corvallis, Oregon.

*Medicine-Surgery,* R. E. T. Stier, Spokane, Washington.

*Social Science,* Claudius O. Johnson, State College, Pullman, Washington.

J. W. HUNGATE
*Retiring Secretary-Treasurer*

# SCIENTIFIC APPARATUS AND LABORATORY METHODS

## A SIMPLIFIED METHOD OF STAINING ENDOSPORES

IN our search for simple and efficient stains for routine bacteriological work, the Wirtz[1] method of spore staining proved far superior to others. Hansen's[2] and Möller's[3] techniques make use of steaming carbol fuchsin and an acid decolorizer. Dorner's[4] method, as recommended by the Committee on Bacteriological Technic of the Society of American Bacteriologists, involves the use of nigrosin. Muzzarelli's[5] and Abbott's[6] methods are each good, but even these resort to an acid decolorizer. Wirtz's method proved less complicated than these. Wirtz fixed air-dried smears in osmic acid, stained with malachite green, and used dilute carbol fuchsin as both decolorizer and counterstain. Spores were stained green, cells red. There was no blending of colors such as is often encountered with red and blue dyes.

We have eliminated fixing in osmic acid, shortened the time of staining and substituted aqueous safranin for the dilute carbol fuchsin. The malachite green is made up as a 5 per cent. aqueous solution, allowed to stand one half hour and filtered. This solution seems to be stable. The technique then is: Make films in the usual manner and fix by flaming three times. Flood with malachite green solution and heat to steaming three or four times within one half minute. Wash off the excess stain under the tap for about one half minute. Apply a 0.5 per cent. aqueous safranin solution one half minute. Wash, blot dry and examine. This procedure is evidently more simple than the original method. The whole staining time involved is less than two minutes, and a minimum of steaming is required. Within wide limits it is impossible to overstain or to wash too long.

Application of this method to thirty strains of sporeformers at different ages showed that agar slant cultures incubated at 37° C. for 24 to 36 hours always contain vegetative cells, sporangia and free spores. Thus a complete morphological description can be obtained at this time. Films from week-old cultures, recommended by the Committee on Bacteriological Technique,[7] tend to show excess of free spores and few vegetative cells or sporangia. The search for these structures in such films is time-consuming.

The part of a slant culture from which growth is taken affects the results of the spore stain. Films made from the butt end of a slant show more vegetative cells and fewer sporulated cells than films from the dried upper end of the slant.

The simplicity of the technique and the beautiful differentiation obtained with it should make this method useful for the identification of sporeforming bacteria.

ALICE B. SCHAEFFER
MAC DONALD FULTON

DEPARTMENT OF BIOLOGY
MIDDLEBURY COLLEGE

1 R. Wirtz, *Zentralblatt für Bakteriologie,* I Abt., Orig., 46: 727, 1908.

2 Hansen, cited by Buchanan, "Bacteriology," 3d ed., p. 153, 1930.

3 Möller, cited by Stitt, "Practical Bacteriology, Blood Work, and Animal Parasitology," 8th ed., p. 64, 1927.

4 W. C. Dorner, cited by Committee on Bacteriological Technic, "Manual of Methods," Leaflet IV, p. 11, 1932.

5 G. Muzzarelli, *Zentralblatt für Bakteriologie,* I Abt., Ref., 104: 484, 1932.

6 Abbott, cited by Stitt, "Practical Bacteriology, Blood Work, and Animal Parasitology," 8th ed., p. 64, 1927.

7 Committee on Bacteriological Technic, "Manual of Methods," Leaflet V, p. 5, 1930.

### A DEMONSTRATION JAR FOR WHITE MICE

A mouse in a closed vessel of known capacity is a favored way of showing roughly some of the effects of inhalation anesthetics. Motor excitement and depression may be noted, but not well, for in the limited space the mouse has nowhere to run. For this reason we have mounted a simple tread-mill in a 5 liter desiccator, so arranged that the number of revolutions is recorded on a slow kymograph. The apparatus is easily constructed without expense and permits a number of interesting experiments and demonstrations.

The wheel is a circle of screen wire just smaller than the inner diameter of the desiccator, thumbtacked to two light pieces of wood at right angles to each other. Its bearing is a piece of glass tubing about 2 cm long pushed through a tight hole where the sticks cross. The ends of the tubing are fused down until they fit freely, but without unnecessary play, a small finishing nail. With a washer below this makes a very freely turning wheel, and when mounted on a block at about 30° to the horizontal the mouse has no trouble and apparently a good deal of pleasure in running it.

The recording device is very simple. A piece of glass tubing about 18 cm long is put through a hole in a rubber stopper in the top of the desiccator. The ends of this tube are fused down to fit loosely a piece of iron wire. A short piece of rubber tubing is fitted over the lower end of the glass tube and tied securely around the wire. This makes a gas-tight joint, and also serves as a spring to resist rotation of the wire. Each end of the wire is bent at right angles. The lower bend is hit by a pin on the revolving wheel, the upper end is connected by a thread to a damped-down muscle lever. Thus every revolution of the mouse wheel, in either direction, is made to record on

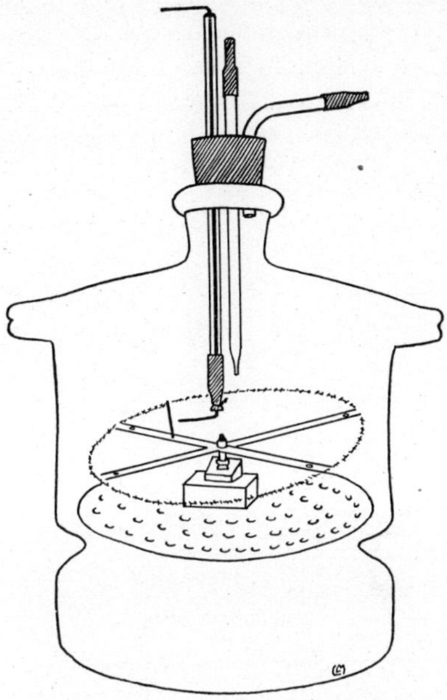

the kymograph, which of course also carries a suitable time tracing. Two other glass tubes through the rubber stopper allow gas or volatile liquids to be run in. An electrical contact is avoided in the recording mechanism because of the explosibility of several of the anesthetic mixtures.

C. Reynolds

Department of Pharmacology
Marquette University

# SPECIAL ARTICLES

### VARIABILITY AND INDIVIDUALITY

In 1920 the writer[1] published data which demonstrated that young animals of an inbred strain of mice showed a significantly higher percentage of growth of an inoculated tumor than did sexually mature individuals of the same strain. Strong[2] confirmed these results with different material and showed in addition that senile animals resembled very young animals in that they exhibited an increased tolerance of tumor implants as compared with that of young adults. These data were interpreted as indicating that the full expression of the genetic constitution of the individual was being assumed gradually during the period of infancy and adolescence, reached its most characteristic manifestation at the young adult stage and became less integrated and more decentralized during senility.

Warthin,[3] Child[4] and others have considered senility as a period of *involution,* and have looked upon individuality as a process directly measurable by the degree of manifestation of certain functions.

From evidence derived from a considerable mass of material it would appear that variability of a function or characteristic is a more fundamental indication of the nature of individuality than is the mean value of any physiological or morphological characteristic at any given time.

When, for example, variables of a genetic nature are reduced to a minimum for mammalian material by the use of closely inbred strains and when the

[1] *Jour. Exper. Zool.,* 31: 307–326, 1920.
[2] *Jour. Exper. Zool.,* 36: 67–134, 1922.
[3] "Old Age The Major Involution," Hoeber, N. Y., 1929.
[4] "Senescence and Rejuvenescence," Univ. of Chicago Press, 1915.

ontogenetic variables are to some extent controlled by the use of one sex and by the choice of some physiological function confined to a restricted period of the life cycle, the experimental conditions are simplified to a considerable degree.

Data derived from females of an inbred strain of mice (dbr) under investigation by Dr. W. S. Murray are available to show variation in litter size at various ages of the mother. When the coefficient of variation of litter size at successive 30-day periods of maternal age is calculated the following results are obtained.

| Age of mother in days | No. of litters | Mean litter size | Coefficient of variation |
|---|---|---|---|
| – 75 | 517 | 4.189 | 42.46 |
| 76–105 | 1298 | 4.985 | 38.81 |
| 106–135 | 1026 | 5.436 | 36.94 |
| 136–165 | 978 | 5.598 | 36.96 |
| 166–195 | 762 | 5.767 | 35.43 |
| 196–225 | 691 | 5.363 | 40.25 |
| 226–255 | 598 | 5.055 | 40.60 |
| 256–285 | 433 | 5.173 | 41.52 |
| 286–315 | 286 | 5.108 | 43.45 |
| 316–345 | 194 | 4.613 | 51.94 |
| 346–375 | 105 | 4.314 | 47.46 |
| 376–405 | 49 | 4.469 | 41.70 |
| 406– | 34 | 3.470 | 58.56 |

It will be noted that variation in litter size begins high, decreases, reaches a base level and then increases again as reproductive activity decreases and senility sets in.

A very similar result with, however, a shorter constant base level period was obtained for another inbred strain of mice (C 57). The slight difference between the two strains is probably a natural concomitant of the genetic characteristics which they each possess.

Looked at from the point of view of variation in physiological response to a constant stimulus, the work of the writer and of Strong on inoculated tumors already referred to, agrees in general with the data on litter size. In so far as somatic tissues are concerned there is good reason to believe that the age-variability relationship above described may be of general applicability.

The next question is whether a similar relative change in variability incidental to age applies also to the functioning of the germ cell. On *a priori* grounds there is no reason why the germ cell, as an organization, should not also show a durational phase in its various activities.

Data presented by Bridges[5] bear on this point. Using "crossing-over" between genes as an index and *Drosophila* as material he studied the relation of age to the absolute amount of crossing-over. He did not, however, analyze his data from the point of view of *variability* of the function of crossing-over in relation to the age of the mother. When his data for single cross-overs are studied with this point in mind certain suggestive and interesting results are obtained.

[5] Carnegie Inst. of Wash., Publ. No. 399, 1929.

The average variability in his two main tables shows the following distribution according to the age of the mother.

| Age period of mother from youngest to oldest | Percentage of variability in single "crossing-over" |
|---|---|
| 1 | 39.52 |
| 2 | 30.17 |
| 3 | 18.83 |
| 4 | 22.82 |
| 5 | 24.00 |
| 6 | 21.96 |
| 7 | 14.63 |
| 8 | 12.56 |
| 9 | 4.87 |
| 10 | 15.27 |
| 11 | 26.53 |
| 12 | 34.82 |

Again the very young and the very old females show the most variation. There is a secondary decrease in the third period but the primary stability seems to be in the ninth. While the evidence is not conclusive it supports the idea that very young and very old germ cells function more variably than do those of the middle-age periods.

This is an important conclusion and if substantiated by further data on different materials will lead us far towards a better understanding of various general evolutionary problems of prime importance.

(1) It might well develop that tendency to mutation, which in itself is an indication of variability, would be greater in very young and in very old germ cells.

(2) If this were true, domestication, in which very young and very old animals, protected from the competitive factor of natural selection, are used as parents, would provide a far greater chance for mutations to occur than would natural conditions.

(3) Similarly, somatic mutations would tend to be more frequent in very young or very old animals. Evidence that this is the case is to be found in the work of Strong,[6] Bittner[7, 8] and Cloudman,[9] who found genetic differences in spontaneous mammary

[6] *Jour. Cancer Research,* 13: 103–115, 1926.
[7] *Am. Jour. Cancer,* 15: 2202–2247, 1931.
[8] *Am. Jour. Cancer,* in press.
[9] *Am. Jour. Cancer,* 16: 568–630, 1932.

neoplasms produced by a single individual mouse. These various animals had very evidently reached a point where central physiological control of the variability of somatic cell variation had diminished to a stage where they no longer acted as individuals in the restricted sense.

(4) The origin of neoplasms as the result of the fundamental disintegration of a centrally controlled "individuality" would become more clearly established. Different types of neoplasms would naturally be expected to follow different age distributions—as they do—because the different tissues are organ systems of the body "age" physiologically at very different periods in ontogeny. As matters stand there seems to be sufficient evidence to conclude:

(1) "Individuality" in mammals and probably in all higher animals is a relative term with a well-pronounced durational phase.

(2) Within genetically comparable material, variability in form and function is greater in the very young and in the very old than it is in the height of reproductive efficiency.

(3) Measurements of simple increase or decrease in function are not sufficient to give a complete picture of the nature of individuality.

(4) Senility is not simply a "major involution" but rather a period at which the disintegration of individuality is the most interesting biological phenomenon. "Involution" as a concept suggests the opposite of "evolution." It would be much more accurate to consider old age as a period primarily of a type of physiological and morphological disintegration and incoordination.

(5) All studies of genetic characters in animals should consider the age factor as an important variable likely to influence fundamentally the justifiable conclusions as to the type and nature of the character under consideration.

(6) This applies not only to genetic characters and processes outside of the germ-plasm but to such characters and processes as mutation, crossing-over, and other chromosomal aberrations. It may be expected that variability in relation to age will be operative in all germ cells to a more nearly comparable degree than it will be in the somatic characters of various groups of organisms.

(7) There is, however, little likelihood of general mathematical values for such variation being immediately established since the genetic characters of strains and individuals would be expected to vary in so far as they affect the assumption and degeneration of "individuality."

(8) The existence of the durational phase in the development of individuality helps to bridge the gap which has existed between physiologic and theoretic genetics. It shows that geneticists must recognize and consider that factor before the gene-character relationship can become sufficiently definite to allow accurate evaluation of gene location, dominance and other genetic phenomena.

C. C. LITTLE

ROSCOE B. JACKSON MEMORIAL LABORATORY
BAR HARBOR, MAINE

## THE MECHANISM OF THE IONENE SYNTHESIS

IN a recent report[1] we described a synthesis of ionene that for the first time provides convincing evidence of the constitution of this interesting hydrocarbon, which has so lately risen to prominence in connection with studies of the structure of vitamin A.

Further work by Davidson and Apfelbaum, in these laboratories, has now thrown additional light upon the mechanism of this synthesis, in so far as the transition from a monocyclic tertiary alcohol (I) to a dicyclic hydrocarbon of ionene type (II) is concerned.

Manifestly, such a cyclization involves the elimination of a molecule of water, and this may be accomplished by the OH of the tertiary alcohol removing an H, either from the benzene nucleus, thus forming the second cycle, as shown in (A); or (B), from the adjacent $CH_2$ group, with production of the olefin (III), which then isomerizes to the dicyclic hydrocarbon (II), a type of rearrangement not at all uncommon in terpene chemistry:

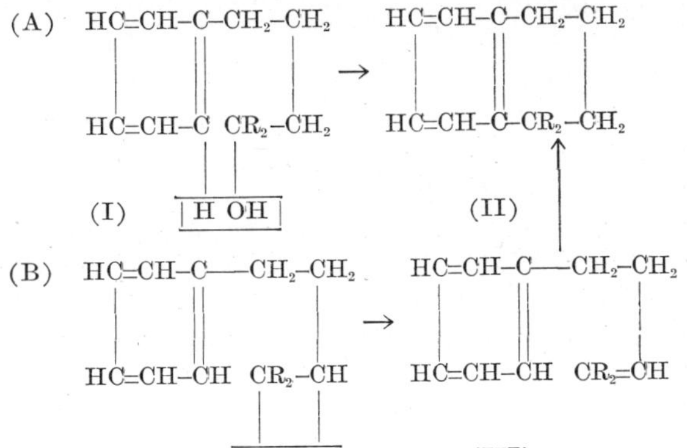


Since the next lower homolog (I) is much more easily prepared than the tertiary alcohol used for the synthesis of ionene itself, this was used in our experiments, as shown in the formulas above, and gave the corresponding lower homolog (II) of ionene.

That (B), rather than (A), represents what actually occurs in this cyclization is indicated by the following experimental facts:

[1] M. T. Bogert, SCIENCE, n.s., 76: 1977, 475, November 18, 1932.

(1) If heated with iodine as a catalyst, the tertiary alcohol (I) readily yielded the olefin (III).

(2) This olefin rearranged immediately to the dicyclic hydrocarbon (II) when digested with concentrated sulfuric acid.

(3) Treated with the proper concentration of sulfuric acid, or phosphoric acid, the alcohol (I) passed immediately to the olefin (III), which on longer treatment changed to the ionene homolog (II). Hence, either (III) or (II) was obtained, depending upon the duration of the treatment.

These reactions are now being extended and applied in manifold directions, for the synthesis of numerous polycyclic hydrocarbons and of derivatives not readily accessible by other methods.

MARSTON TAYLOR BOGERT
LABORATORIES OF ORGANIC CHEMISTRY
COLUMBIA UNIVERSITY

## THE VITAMIN D POTENCY OF EGG YOLK FROM IRRADIATED HENS

IN five experiments, tests were made to determine the relative antirachitic potency of egg yolk from irradiated hens. Four flocks of hens were used. (1) An irradiated flock of 350 hens had the usual laying ration containing one half per cent. cod-liver oil plus four hours daily access to the ultra-violet rays from one GE Model S-1 Sunlamp; (2) a non-irradiated flock of like size fed the same ration. (Both of these flocks averaged 62 per cent. production during the continuance of the experiment—five months). (3) A small farm flock (Exp. 1 and 2) was given a poorly balanced ration. These birds were producing from ten to twenty-five per cent. (4) Another farm flock of 150 birds, fed the laying ration (Exp. 4 and 5), completed the groups. Eggs were chosen from these hens after they had been in production about one month. They were laying about 50 per cent. daily.

The antirachitic potency of the eggs from these flocks was tested on different pens of rats, having a rachitogenic ration, Steinbock No. 2965. Different amounts of the egg yolk were fed, varying with the experiment. In three of the tests cod-liver oil was also fed the rats in order to make comparisons with the egg yolk.

The experiments confirmed the work of earlier investigators, showing that egg yolk contains appreciable amounts of vitamin D. The tests give clear evidence that irradiation of hens with ultra-violet rays will markedly increase this vitamin above the quantity normally found in eggs. A high vitamin D content may thus be maintained throughout the winter months.

[1] Aided by a grant from the Heckscher Research Foundation.

In the experiments where the quantity of egg yolk was 5 per cent. or more, that from irradiated hens prevented or cured rickets in rats almost as rapidly as exposure to a quartz mercury arc. Ten per cent. of such egg yolk in the rachitogenic diet was as effective as one half per cent. cod-liver oil, or radiations from the quartz mercury arc. These animals grew faster than the irradiated rats because in addition to the antirachitic factor the egg yolk supplied other necessary food ingredients.

Four per cent. egg yolk from the irradiated hens was more potent than one eighth per cent. of cod-liver oil in the rat diet.

While the non-irradiated hens had access to autumn sunshine (during November, 1931, the weather remained unusually fair in New York) the vitamin D content was sufficient to cure rickets. In this high-producing flock, as winter advanced and the hens had been in production longer and longer, the vitamin D content diminished to a low level, much below the amount necessary for satisfactory prevention or cure of rickets.

There seemed also to be a limited ability for hens to store vitamin D and to transfer it to the eggs when needed.

From the tests with farm flocks it was shown that eggs as ordinarily purchased contain varying amounts of vitamin D. Under the most favorable conditions the quantity may be quite adequate to prevent rickets in experimental animals. The season and the volume of production are at least two of the factors which determine the amounts.

GEORGE H. MAUGHAN
EDNA MAUGHAN
CORNELL UNIVERSITY

## BOOKS RECEIVED

FIELD, G. C. *Prejudice and Impartiality.* Pp. 116. McBride. $0.80.

FILIPETTI, GEORGE, WILLIAM DACHTLER and JUDSON BURNETT. *Operating Results of Manufacturing Plants in Minnesota, 1926–1930.* Bulletins of The Employment Stabilization Research Institute, University of Minnesota. Vol. I, No. 7. Pp. 101. 10 figures. University of Minnesota Press.

MACE, C. A. *The Psychology of Study.* Pp. viii + 96. McBride. $0.80.

REGAN, C. TATE and ETHELWYNN TREWAVAS. *Deep-Sea Angler-Fishes (Ceratioidea).* Report No. 2 of The Carlsberg Foundation's Oceanographical Expedition Round the World 1928–30. Pp. 113. 172 figures. 10 plates. Oxford University Press, London. 15 s.

REIGHARD, JACOB and H. S. JENNINGS. *Dissection of the Cat.* Revised by Rush Elliott. Pp. vi + 106. Holt. $1.95.

RIETZ, H. L. and A. R. CRATHORNE. *Introductory College Algebra.* Revised. Pp. xi + 328. Holt. $1.76.

SOUTHALL, JAMES P. C. *Mirrors, Prisms and Lenses:* A Text-Book of Geometrical Optics. Third Edition. Pp. xxiv + 806. 329 figures. Macmillan. $4.50.

# SCIENCE

VOL. 77 — FRIDAY, FEBRUARY 24, 1933 — No. 1991

*Recent Revivals of Darwinism:* DR. HENRY FAIRFIELD OSBORN 199

*The Value of the Determination of Free Energy Change for Organic Reactions:* PROFESSOR D. B. KEYES 202

*Obituary:*
*William Jacob Holland:* A. AVINOFF. *Recent Deaths* 204

*Scientific Events:*
*Danish Exhibit at the Chicago Museum of Science and Industry; The Herbarium of W. W. Ashe; Heckscher Grants at Cornell University; The American Journal of Science* 206

*Scientific Notes and News* 208

*Discussion:*
*Cortin and Traumatic Shock:* DR. NORMAN E. FREEMAN. *The Association of Termites with Fungi:* ESTHER C. HENDEE. *Anteprothrombin and Globulins:* IMOGENE P. EARLE and DR. PAUL E. HOWE. *The Relation of the Hypophysis to Experimental Diabetes:* DR. J. F. REGAN and B. O. BARNES. *Cancer Research:* DR. C. C. LITTLE 211

*Reports:*
*Appropriations for Grants in Aid by the National Research Council:* DR. W. H. HOWELL 214

*Scientific Apparatus and Laboratory Methods:*
*A Method of Outlining Cutaneous Nerve Areas:* PROFESSOR I. MACLAREN THOMPSON and DR. VERNE T. INMAN. *Cellophane Roll Films:* ROSS BONAR, FLOYD BONAR and PROFESSOR EARL C. H. DAVIES. *Silk Cellophane for Lantern Slides:* FREDRICK F. YONKMAN 216

*Special Articles:*
*The Relationship of Bacterium Granulosis to Trachoma:* DR. IDA A. BENGTSON. *The Action Current as Measure of Muscle Contraction:* PROFESSOR R. H. STETSON and H. D. BOUMAN. *Chemical versus Morphological Species Differences:* PROFESSOR S. C. BROOKS 218

*Science News* 5

SCIENCE: A Weekly Journal devoted to the Advancement of Science, edited by J. MCKEEN CATTELL and published every Friday by

THE SCIENCE PRESS

New York City: Grand Central Terminal

Lancaster, Pa. — Garrison, N. Y.

Annual Subscription, $6.00 — Single Copies, 15 Cts.

SCIENCE is the official organ of the American Association for the Advancement of Science. Information regarding membership in the Association may be secured from the office of the permanent secretary, in the Smithsonian Institution Building, Washington, D. C.

# RECENT REVIVALS OF DARWINISM[1]

By Dr. HENRY FAIRFIELD OSBORN

AMERICAN MUSEUM OF NATURAL HISTORY

BEFORE us are four recent volumes, the "Huxley Memorial Lectures," "The Causes of Evolution," by J. B. S. Haldane, "Problems of Relative Growth," by Julian S. Huxley, and "The Scientific Basis of Evolution," by Thomas Hunt Morgan, which bring us up to date in the latest British and American thought as to the nature and causes of evolution. They are popularly written and the chief impression they convey is their reversion to more or less pure Darwinism, especially surprising on the part of one of the authors, T. H. Morgan, who some years ago wrote a severe critique of Darwin's theory of adaptation.

We thus have presentations by a distinguished physiological chemist, by the leader of the experimental and genetic school, by an experienced zoologist, P. Chalmers Mitchell, and by one of the leading British authorities on animal life, Julian Huxley. The point of view shown in Julian Huxley's volume should be supplemented by his article in the recent edition of the "Encyclopaedia Britannica."

Preceding a critique of these volumes may we point out four historic explanations of the modes and causes of evolution.

### EMPEDOCLES–DARWIN HYPOTHESIS

This bit of absolutely inductive research has a 2,500 year speculative background because about 600 B. C., as described in my volume, "From the Greeks to Darwin," the Greeks began to speculate not only on the modes or kinds of evolution but on the hypothetical causes of evolution. Thus Empedocles of Agrigentum, a Sicilian town, anticipated what may be known as pure Darwinism, namely, that out of many kinds of accidents and variations more or less spontaneously occurring in animals, nature permits the survival only

[1] Address before the Osborn Research Club in the American Museum of Natural History, December 13, 1932.

of those which happen to fit in with the environmental times. This original very crude idea has come down through the ages of human thought, being modernized step by step until it finds its present refinement and up-to-date re-definition and re-statement in the four volumes before us. After many vicissitudes Darwinism is now once more flourishing.

### Erasmus Darwin–Lamarck Hypothesis

Similarly, the second great hypothesis as to the modes and causes of evolution, now known as Lamarckism, was adumbrated in Greek time because, as pointed out by Brooks in his "The Foundations of Zoology," the notion that bodily improvement, through the universally acknowledged individual adaptation which comes about through the skilful use of parts, as well as the counteraction of bodily degeneration through disuse of parts, has been discussed down through the centuries and reached its apogee in the mind of Erasmus Darwin, of Lamarck, its modernized ideas in the speculations of Herbert Spencer, and its mechanical climax in the writings of our own Cope. Relative to the ever-growing and verdant Darwinism, Lamarckism is decidedly moribund. It received its death thrust in 1880 when Weismann challenged every kind of evidence for the inheritance of acquired characters. It seems cowardly to attack a dying principle, but I may claim in self-defense that the Titanothere Monograph as well as the more recent Proboscidea Memoir give Lamarckism its final *coup de grace.*

### Buffon–St. Hilaire Hypothesis

The third great historic explanation of the nature and causes of evolution appears to have dawned upon the human mind at a relatively recent period, namely, that of the direct action of a favorable or unfavorable, or even of a new environment, on the body and indirectly on the germ as well, although it must be recalled that in all early speculations the sharp distinction which Weismann was the first to draw between the body cells and the germ cells was not clear. Nevertheless, the dictum of Buffon that the mammals of the New World were *dénaturés* as compared with their relatives in the Old World, followed by the violent physicochemical transformation involved in the speculations of Geoffroy St. Hilaire, fully foreshadows the modern speculations, experiments and observations not only on the final inheritance by the germ of the modifying influences of climate but also on the reaction of the germ and consequent origin of hereditary mutations under more or less violent physicochemical agencies.

### Aristotle–Driesch Hypothesis

The fourth great principle is purely speculative. It is not truly an induction from observed facts like the others. It is rather a deduction. Hydra-headed, it appears under new designations from the "entelechy" of Aristotle (384–322 B. C.) to the modern "holism" of Smuts or the "emergence" of C. Lloyd Morgan. Perhaps the most expressive designation is that of "vitalism," namely, that there is in life a mysterious self-perfecting principle, charmingly designated by Bergson the "élan vital." Needless to say, this is what the Latins called a *petitio principi;* it is begging the question and avoiding the difficulties by assuming the presence of this internal perfecting tendency. It is something like the assumption by older chemists of "phlogiston" as an explanation of the internal heat and of motion of the body.

Again, while stoutly maintaining that the entelechy of Aristotle and his successors is a theoretic assumption, we should by no means shut out the possibility of further observational or inductive demonstration that there is in life something in the nature of an internal perfecting principle. It is certainly rash at the present moment to deny the possibility of such future discovery. Certainly if there is an *élan vital* it should appear in the creative origin of new parts and organs, as, for example, in the beautiful eyes of the scallop *Pecten* which, as Bergson showed, present so many analogies to the human eye in the position of the lens and retina.

### Trends of Recent Thought

Unlike pure Darwinism, which is still greatly debated as an adequate explanation of evolution, and unlike Lamarckism, which is moribund except in the minds of a very few of its living advocates, the Buffon-St. Hilaire principle of direct environmental action both on body and germ is now universally admitted as one of the great causes of evolution. As shown in the experiments of Sumner, one of my former students, it is directly responsible for speciation in animals like *Peromyscus.* Sumner has positively demonstrated that modifications in color and form and proportion, traceable to the prolonged direct action of environment, are hereditary and therefore true germinal characters. Perhaps the best established zoological generalization of modern times is that subspeciation, and ultimately full speciation, is the inevitable result of prolonged change of environment especially visible in color, in proportion, and inevitable in habit which is the invariable precursor of change of form.

The three above principles—Darwinian, Lamarckian and Buffonian—rest upon both a purely speculative and a largely observational basis, and great zoologists, like Edward B. Poulton, who have devoted their entire lives to observations tending to establish pure Darwinism, firmly believe that the pure Darwin principle explains not only color evolution as seen in protective and aggressive mimicry, but that *all evolution of every kind is explainable by Darwinism.* This is very evident in the years of early correspondence which I enjoyed with Poulton, and our opposing views ripened into full presentation at the centenary of the British Association held in the British Museum a year ago.

My own position with respect to these three historic explanations has been frequently and clearly stated, but I may now briefly summarize it, namely, that pure Darwinism never sought to explain the origin of new characters. In fact, Darwin invariably used the word "chance" but open-mindedly declared that "chance" was a term which might simply express the ignorance of his time as to principles of origin which might subsequently be discovered. Since Darwinism is the only explanation of certain kinds of adaptations and since it is universally admitted that the survival of the fittest is a universal principle and that this applies to fitness in every organ of the body, we all gladly embrace pure Darwinism as one of the great factors of evolution.

As to Lamarckism, the case is quite different. The immediate inheritance by the next generation of the effects of individual adaptation is absolutely disproved, but in the age long or secular biomechanical adaptations of animals we do perceive a great principle which comes within the generic conception of Lamarckism, if not within the specific conception of Lamarckism which the great French naturalist advocated.

As regards the third great principle, namely, the direct action of environment, it seems to be no longer debatable. It is equally evident in every type of animal and plant which we may observe, but, like Darwinism, so far as we know at present it is confined to the modification of existing organs rather than to the origin of new organs, and even as regards the modification of existing organs, the direct action of environment is rather limited.

As a youthful observer I was first strongly impressed by Lamarckism and my early writings led to my classification with Cope as a neo-Lamarckian, but whereas Cope stuck to this explanation of the origin of all biomechanical adaptations to the very end of his life I soon abandoned it and took the speculative ground that there was an entirely unknown factor of evolution awaiting discovery. Fifty years of continuous and very close observation, often of the most laborious and tedious kind, aided by such a splendid assistant as William King Gregory, have only confirmed and strengthened my youthful conviction that the real underlying causes of evolution are entirely unknown, and my present feeling is that they are not only unknown but may prove to be unknowable. The universally and marvelously adaptive principle in the origin and development of biomechanical fitness may be something of the same nature as Newton's principle of gravitation. We may observe all its modes, workings and laws and be able to formulate them in detail even to the great test of prediction. But we may never know the underlying nature of the thing itself. As in gravitation so it may be in biology, some Einstein may succeed a Newton, and yet leave gravitation still in its simpler expression like,—the force that holds the moon in a constantly stable relation to the earth,—something unknown and unknowable, a fact which we can observe but never explain. That is my own present feeling about the whole evolution process.

Having dropped speculation very early in my biologic and paleontologic career, I settled down to the only absolutely safe course for a naturalist, namely, to continual and unremitting observation—day after day, night after night, month after month, year after year. I stick to observation as a shoemaker sticks to his last, through thick and thin, and all the generalizations which I have been able to make are in part confirming generalizations previously made by others, in part discovering entirely new principles hitherto unsuspected. I estimate that 90 per cent. of my time has been given to my own observation and less than 10 per cent. to reading the observations of others. In fact, I am somewhat ashamed of having done comparatively little reading. When I find some one has anticipated me I am only too glad to give him the fullest possible credit, but anticipations are rare because no one in the world has ever had the opportunity afforded me through the splendid financial resources of this museum and the dauntless corps of explorers, field collectors and coworkers who have built up the unrivaled collections in the department of vertebrate paleontology in the American Museum. Such actual documentary records of evolution as have never been accessible before to any naturalist or any observer, however keen, have opened the way to all which may be claimed as new discovery.

Recently Julian Huxley visited the Hall of the Age of Mammals and I showed him the small case two feet square which contains the entire fossil vertebrate collection of the Tertiary, of the year 1891. Then when I told him of the six great exhibition halls of the Life History of the Earth which will be overcrowded when all our existing collections are displayed in them, he was simply amazed. It is not the magnitude of these collections, but the exhaustive and refined way in which they have been assembled with extremely precise field records both as to locality and as to geologic level, which is of inestimable value. This minute observation of geologic sequence, first in America and then in the Tertiaries of India by Barnum Brown, has brought us to the point where we can demonstrate beyond refutation the absolute origins and continuous developments of new characters. Such observations were undreamt of by Buffon, by Lamarck or by Darwin.

# THE VALUE OF THE DETERMINATION OF FREE ENERGY CHANGE FOR ORGANIC REACTIONS[1]

By Professor D. B. KEYES

DEPARTMENT OF CHEMISTRY, UNIVERSITY OF ILLINOIS

IT is only within recent years that the importance of free energy determinations of organic compounds has been realized.[2]

The study of any chemical reaction resolves itself primarily into two fundamental questions: first, how nearly to completion does it go under various conditions, and second, how rapidly does it approach this limit in the presence of various catalysts. The answers to these two quesitons are to be found by means of free energy values.

The well-known formula $\triangle F.^\circ = -RT \ln K$ gives the relation between the equilibrium constant (K) and the change of free energy for the particular reaction under certain definite conditions. The value $\triangle F.^\circ$ is of more general significance than the value K and that is why this particular physical constant is usually sought. The factor R in the equation is the gas constant and T the absolute temperature

It is not necessary to determine the equilibrium constant directly under certain definite conditions in order to find $\triangle F.^\circ$ It is usually quite feasible to perform operations with various chemical equations in free energy terms, so that a numerical value of $\triangle F.^\circ$ is obtained.

It is sometimes quite expedient to use another well-known formula for the determination of $\triangle F.^\circ$ This is: $\triangle F^\circ = \triangle H - T \triangle S$.[3] In this case use is not made of the gas constant R and the equilibrium constant K, but the heat term $\triangle H$ and a change in entropy $\triangle S$. The term $\triangle H$ is a quantitative value of the heat given off or taken up during the reaction. This heat term is usually measured while the system is at constant pressure. The reaction, however, may be from one physical state to another and not necessarily chemical.

The change in entropy $\triangle S$ is made up of a series of $\triangle S$'s from the absolute zero up to the temperature existing at equilibrium for each constituent. For example, a solid in heating up from absolute zero to some higher temperature acquires an entropy value equal to the integral of the function $\frac{Cp}{T}$ over the temperature range, where Cp is the specific heat at constant pressure. When the solid changes from the solid state to liquid state the heat of fusion divided by the absolute temperature of melting will constitute the entropy change for that change in state. From then on the specific heat of the liquid is the determining factor until the boiling point of the liquid is reached and then the latent heat of evaporation must be taken into consideration. In this way it is possible to determine from specific heats and latent heat data the S for any particular chemical compound at any definite state and condition. The $\triangle S$ for a reaction is calculated from the S values of individual compounds in exactly the same manner as $\triangle F$. In other words, the $\triangle S$ value for the reaction is calculated by subtracting the sum of the S values of the reactants from the sum of the S values of the products.

It should be possible theoretically to measure the equilibrium constant of any chemical reaction and from this to obtain easily a $\triangle F.^\circ$ value. We would then have an answer to the question, what are the equilibrium conditions of the reaction, and thereby be able to determine whether or not the reaction was suitable for any particular purpose. Unfortunately, there are a great many practical difficulties that arise, especially with organic reactions.

Reactions studied by the equilibrium method have been those that, first, gave a measurable concentration of product and left a measurable concentration of reactant; second, involved relatively simple methods of analysis; third, had no complicating side reactions. With the exception of ionic reactions, as great a proportion of inorganic as organic reactions satisfy the first requirement—although that proportion is very small indeed. Analytical methods are much better developed for inorganic than for organic compounds. As for side reactions, the distinctive ability of carbon to combine with itself tends to cause much greater

[1] Read before the National Academy of Sciences, University of Michigan, on November 14, 1932.

[2] See American Chemical Society Monograph No. 60, entitled "Free Energies of Some Organic Compounds," by Parks and Huffman, recently published by the Chemical Catalog Company in New York.

[3] $\triangle F = \triangle H - T \triangle S$ under any conditions. $\triangle F = \triangle F^\circ$ when all reactants and products are under one atmosphere pressure.

difficulty with organic compounds. The reactions studied so far, then, have been largely inorganic.

It is well known that the equilibrium constant is determined by the ratio of the activities, and the activities in turn bear definite relations to concentrations of the substances present.

It can, therefore, easily be seen why it is difficult to obtain an accurate determination of the equilibrium constant directly whenever the equilibrium is such that some of these activities and the corresponding concentrations become extremely small. Such a condition quite often occurs when organic chemical reactions are considered.

Organic chemical reactions, on the other hand, are attracting considerably more interest in the industrial world to-day than do the inorganic chemical reactions, because our industries are developing much more along organic lines than along inorganic lines. This means, however, that the determination of equilibrium constants or better yet, free energy values, is becoming more and more important from the standpoint of the applied scientist.

It is interesting to note that in any of this work it is not only desirable but sometimes essential to investigate the catalytic situation involving the particular reaction and determine roughly the rate of reaction under certain definite conditions. This means that the determination of a free energy value for a specific organic reaction usually results in not only determining how far the reaction will go under certain definite conditions, but also how fast. In other words, studies of this kind usually give a fairly complete answer to the fundamental questions concerning the chemical reaction.

We may generally assume in most organic chemical reactions that it is impractical to measure the equilibrium constant directly and thereby determine the free energy for the reaction under certain definite and practical conditions. It is usually necessary to determine the $\Delta F.^\circ$ values for a combination of reactions which, added and subtracted from one another will result in the $\Delta F.^\circ$ value required as has been shown before.

Free energy change can sometimes be determined, especially in inorganic reactions, by setting up a reversible cell. The equation then becomes $\Delta F.^\circ = -nFE^\circ$. In this equation, n is the number of equivalents, the $F$ is a Faraday and the $E^\circ$ is the potential under standard conditions. In order to set up such a cell it is necessary that the electrons be mobile; that the atoms be capable of giving off and taking up electrons readily. This condition, especially of the carbon atom, is not common and therefore organic reactions do not readily lend themselves to this method of study.

The most practical methods of determining the $\Delta F.^\circ$ for organic reactions is the use of the entropy equation previously described. The reason for this is, the specific heats, latent heats, temperatures and heat change during the reaction can be measured usually with more accuracy than other physical constants.

Some preliminary results obtained by actual work of this character on certain interesting organic reactions in the industrial division of the chemistry department, University of Illinois, will be given below.

An attempt has been made to determine the $\Delta F.^\circ$ of the reaction between ethylene and water to produce ethyl alcohol. This reaction is particularly valuable because ethyl alcohol is the most important organic solvent at the present time. It is largely made by the fermentation of molasses, which involves rather large equipment cost. A study has been made of various synthetic methods during the last fourteen years, and it is believed that the action of water on ethylene has a most promising future.

The decomposition of ethyl alcohol to produce ethylene and water was first studied largely to determine what would be a satisfactory catalyst. The best catalyst found was aluminum oxide ($Al_2O_3$), impregnated with about 3 per cent. of phosphoric acid ($H_3PO_4$). Preliminary results indicated a decomposition of approximately 96 per cent. at 420–430° C. (700° K.), at a space velocity of 100. A small amount of aldehyde, ether and other by-products was found but not determined quantitatively. The $\Delta F^\circ_{700K}$, based on this 96 per cent decomposition, represented a value of +3,500 cal.

Parks and Huffman[4] indicate a value of +17,900 for $\Delta F.^\circ_{700K}$. Francis and Kleinschmidt[5] give a value for the same $\Delta F.^\circ$ of +7,650. Frost[6] indicates still another value for this physical constant of +6,008.

Our figure of 3,500 is undoubtedly low because the amount of undecomposed ethyl alcohol was probably less than the 4 per cent. indicated by the decomposition figures. There is no question, however, regarding the sign, and the probabilities are that the order of magnitude is also correct.

The difficulty with the direct determination proved to be the inaccuracy of methods of analysis pertaining to the products of the reaction.

Considerable time was spent in an attempt to improve these analyses, with unsatisfactory results. The method of attack on this problem at the present time is to divide the reaction into two steps: (1) The absorption of ethylene in concentrated sulfuric acid,

[4] A. C. S. Monograph, "Free Energies of Some Organic Compounds," 123, 1932.

[5] "Applications of Thermodynamics," *Oil and Gas Jour.*, 25: 118, 1929.

[6] "Hydration of Olefins to Alcohols," *Zhur. Pridkladnoikhim*, 3: 1069–76, 1930.

and (2) the production of ethyl alcohol formed from the ethyl acid sulfate by further dilution. The important physical data to obtain in this case are the partial pressures of the reacting constituents.

Another reaction that is of real interest both to the scientific man and the applied scientific man is the reaction between propylene and hydrogen sulfide to produce an alkyl acid sulfide. A direct determination of the equilibrium constant at 573° K. indicated a △ F.° of + 3,000 cal. There are no data in the literature that would indicate the accuracy of this determination.

Considerable polymerization of the propylene occurred in the presence of catalysts such as phosphoric acid on activated charcoal. A quantitative analysis of this polymer is extremely difficult.

The study at the present time is along two lines: (1) the development of a catalyst that will eliminate this and other side reactions, and (2) the determination of the △ F.° by means of heat capacity measurements. Both methods hold out some promise.

Still another reaction which is of interest to many is the reaction between ammonia and ethylene to produce ethylamine. A study was first made of the reaction itself in order to determine directly the equilibrium constant. A silent electric discharge was used in the place of a catalyst. At 298° K., △ F.° found from these data was approximately + 1,200 cal.

Again the difficulty was due to analytical methods, especially those involving the determination of the amount of ethylamine formed. There were indications of side reactions taking place. Unknown amines apparently were formed. Preliminary results do, however, agree with some rather qualitative work done on the reaction by Francesconi and Ciurlo.[7] It will, of course, be necessary to determine by what, if any, amount the equilibrium is displaced by the discharge.

Further work will be done in the hopes of improving the methods of analysis. If these fail, an attempt will be made to procure a catalyst that will eliminate the side reactions or the △ F.° will be determined by heat capacity measurements.

The author wishes to acknowledge the assistance of Messrs. M. Gallagher, H. R. Duffey and F. T. Barr, who have done the experimental work and who have contributed many worth-while ideas.

# OBITUARY

## WILLIAM JACOB HOLLAND

WITH the death of Dr. William J. Holland, which occurred on December 13, 1932, a distinguished figure in the world of science passed away. He was the dean of American entomologists, the author of innumerable publications in this field. But Dr. Holland was far more than an eminent entomologist of world-wide reputation—he was a naturalist of a universality of erudition which is but rarely found among scientific men of the present day. With a prodigious memory, a keen understanding of the diversity of scientific problems, he was at home in the manifold domains of learning. Above all, he was a man of outstanding intellectual and spiritual culture, and that is why his loss has created an irreparable void in the community with which he has been associated for nearly three scores of years and within the ranks of his fellow workers in the scientific field.

William Jacob Holland was born in Bethany, on the island of Jamaica, on August 16, 1848. His family was of Moravian extraction, residing for a long time in Salem, North Carolina. From there his father was sent as a missionary to the West Indies.

From early boyhood Holland was trained in studies of natural history. Upon graduation from the Moravian College and Theological Seminary at Bethlehem, Pennsylvania, in 1867, he received the degree of bachelor of arts from Amherst College in 1869. For a year after graduation he served as principal of a high school in Amherst, and the following year occupied the same position at Westboro, Massachusetts. Having been ordained into the Moravian ministry he entered Princeton Theological Seminary and concluded the course in 1874. Subsequently he joined the Presbytery of Monmouth and came to Pittsburgh as pastor of the Bellefield Presbyterian Church, which position he held until 1891. In the course of his pastorate Dr. Holland devoted much time to scientific studies. He went to Japan as a member of the United States Eclipse Expedition in 1887 and used this opportunity in a very profitable way for various biological investigations. In 1891 he was made chancellor of the Western University of Pennsylvania, now the University of Pittsburgh. In 1898 his friend, Andrew Carnegie, invited him to assume the responsibilities as director of the museum founded by this steel magnate. This office was held by Dr. Holland with signal success until 1922, when he became director emeritus of the Carnegie Museum. Under the administration of Dr. Holland the museum attained the rank of one of the most important scientific institutions of its kind on the continent. Dr. Holland performed the duties as vice-president of the Carnegie Hero Fund from 1904 to 1922, and upon his election as president of that body became a member of the Carnegie Corporation.

[7] Francesconi and Ciurlo, *Gazz. chim. ital.*, 53: 598, 1923.

Dr. Holland was an active member of the board of trustees of several institutions of higher learning, and carried on the duties of Belgian Consul for some years after the world war. He had the distinction of becoming the founder of the American Association of Museums in 1907, and remained president of the association until 1909. He was a member of scores of scientific societies, among them the Zoological and Entomological Societies of London, the Entomological Societies of America, Washington, New York, Cambridge, Germany, France, Russia and Brazil; the American Zoological Society, Royal Society of Edinburgh, American Philosophical Society and several foreign scientific academies. He was a councilor for the Association for International Conciliation, a member of the Academy of Natural Sciences, Philadelphia, the Pennsylvania Historical Society, Historical Society of Western Pennsylvania and Moravian Historical Society.

Dr. Holland was the author of numerous scientific treatises and books, notably of "The Butterfly Book" and "The Moth Book," which became sources of reference for specialists and were chiefly instrumental in stimulating a wide-spread interest in lepidopterology among amateurs in this country. He also wrote many scientific papers published by the United States Government and the Zoological Society of London. The Encyclopedia Britannica applied to him as to a leading specialist in the museum field for the preparation of a survey of the history of scientific museums. For the last thirty-four years he edited the *Annals* and *Memoirs* of the Carnegie Museum. Washington and Jefferson College, Amherst College, Dickinson College, New York University, Bethany College, St. Andrew's in Scotland and the University of Pittsburgh conferred degrees of honorary doctorate upon him.

One of the most significant scientific achievements of Dr. Holland was connected with the paleontological explorations of the Carnegie Museum which were directed by him in Utah, Wyoming, Montana and North Dakota. The finds of these expeditions resulted in many discoveries, including the celebrated *Diplodocus carnegiei,* the original skeleton of which is adorning the gallery of fossils in the Carnegie Museum, whereas nine replicas were presented to the leading scientific institutions in Europe and both Americas. In recognition of his contributions to science Dr. Holland received decorations from Belgium, Austria-Hungary, Italy, Russia and Spain.

In his busy life, Dr. Holland found time to attend to many public responsibilities of diversified nature. For instance, he took an active part in the development of the water system in the City of Pittsburgh.

Dr. Holland passed away amid his favorite labors, lending his concentrated attention, as throughout his life, to various problems of natural history advanced by recent investigations. Until the end he remained absorbed by the adventurous spirit of scientific research, responsive to the lure of exploring some new avenue of the ever-widening horizons of knowledge. He lived a life of exceptional usefulness. Endowed with a profusion of gifts, among which his linguistic abilities were by far not the least, he cultivated his native talents and molded them into a personality of unique qualities and values. A churchman, a leader in education, the father of the Carnegie Museum in Pittsburgh, a man of learning honored far and wide by academies, international congresses and universities, Dr. Holland will not only be mourned sincerely, but his achievements will also not fail to remain an inspiration challenging the best within us.

A. AVINOFF

CARNEGIE MUSEUM
PITTSBURGH, PENNSYLVANIA

## RECENT DEATHS

GEORGE P. ADAMSON, chemist and formerly director of research of the General Chemical Company, New York City, died on February 16. He was sixty-eight years old.

DR. CLARENCE HENRY ECKLES, chief of the division of dairy husbandry at the University of Minnesota, died on February 13, at the age of fifty-eight years.

DR. CARL L. CORRENS, honorary professor of botany at the University of Berlin and formerly director of the Kaiser Wilhelm Institute for Biology, has died at the age of sixty-eight years.

HORATIO WARD STEBBENS, associate professor of mechanical engineering at Stanford University, died at the Stanford Hospital in San Francisco on February 2, following an operation several days before. Professor Stebbens, who has been at Stanford since 1914, was graduated from the University of California and the Massachusetts Institute of Technology, and prior to teaching, had been connected with various engineering projects.

THEODORE SAUNDERS DUNN, associate professor of mining engineering at Stanford University, was killed instantly when struck by an automobile on the Stanford campus the evening of February 3. Professor Dunn was a graduate of the Missouri School of Mines, and besides having practical experience with a number of mining corporations, and serving as a captain in the engineers during the World War, had served on the faculties of the Missouri School of Mines, South Dakota School of Mines and Georgia School of Technology, going to Stanford in 1930.

# SCIENTIFIC EVENTS

## DANISH EXHIBIT AT THE CHICAGO MUSEUM OF SCIENCE AND INDUSTRY

Word has been received from Dr. Max Henius, of Chicago, that the Ways and Means Committee of the Danish government has approved the expenditure of fifty thousand kroner for exhibits for the Museum of Science and Industry in Chicago. These exhibits are to portray the contributions of Danish scientists to world progress. Dr. Henius, who has been director of the Wahl-Henius Institute in Chicago for many years, has already secured a large operating model of a brewery for the museum. He has also been very active in the establishment of the Dan-American Archives, which are a gift of the American people to the people of Denmark.

The exhibits from Denmark will consist of originals and replicas of the apparatus used by Denmark's great scientists and engineers from Tycho Brahe in the sixteenth century to Knudsen, Poulsen and Bohr—Denmark's leaders in modern science. Tycho Brahe was one of the first great observers of the motions of the sun, moon, stars and planets. The observatories which he built and the instruments which he devised form one of the most precious heritages of modern astronomy. A model of his great observatory at Uraniborg as well as models of his instruments will form part of this exhibit.

It is also fitting that Chicago, the home for so long of Dr. Albert A. Michelson, whose measurements of light won him the Nobel prize, should receive from Denmark examples of the work of Ole Römer. Römer invented the transit circle and by his measurements of the light from Jupiter he was able to pronounce for the first time that light traveled at a definite speed and not at an infinite speed as had been supposed. Römer in 1676 estimated the speed of light at 192,000 miles a second and Michelson in 1926 corrected this to approximately 186,000.

In the field of electricity Hans Christian Oersted ranks with Michael Faraday. His discovery of electromagnetism forms, together with Faraday's discovery of electromagnetic induction, the foundation of the age of electric power. During his great career Oersted founded both the Danish Society for the Propagation of Science and the Polytechnic Institute. Replicas of his original apparatus, of his electromagnet, and a copy of his essay on his great discovery will form part of the Danish gift to the Museum of Science and Industry. A bronze tablet commemorating the centenary of Oersted's discovery of electromagnetism has already been given to the museum by Dr. Neils C. Oatved, of Detroit, Michigan.

Among these exhibits will also be included an early model and a modern telegraphone, the invention of the Danish scientist Waldemar Poulsen. The telegraphone, which has recently come into use again in Europe for recording telephone messages when the party called is absent, is a device which records sound on an iron wire. Poulsen's principal contribution to scientific progress which will be shown among this group of exhibits was his production in 1903 of an oscillator which made continuous radio waves possible.

No exhibition of the work of Danish scientists would be complete without that of Niels Bohr. Although the atomic theory has changed since Bohr received the Nobel Prize for his work, the rise of atomic physics dates back to him and every new discovery in the field serves to emphasize the task that Bohr performed in directing the thinking of scientists all over the world along these lines. Hence the Museum of Science and Industry has asked that the Danish government include the work of Bohr in this gift of exhibits.

The exhibits from Denmark will be housed temporarily in the Hall of Science of A Century of Progress. Although the Museum of Science and Industry will be opened to the public in May, 1933, the decision has been made to loan the Danish exhibits to A Century of Progress for six months before placing them permanently in the museum.

Correspondent

## THE HERBARIUM OF W. W. ASHE

The University of North Carolina has secured the W. W. Ashe Herbarium, a collection very valuable for its large number of type specimens from the southeastern states. William Willard Ashe (1872–1932), a graduate of the University of North Carolina and Cornell University, was the first forester employed by the state of North Carolina. After eighteen years in forestry service for North Carolina he spent twenty-three years in the U. S. Forest Service. He was a keen observer and the qualities that carried him far in his vocation of forestry also made him an important systematic botanist. He is credited with 179 scientific papers, about one third of them in systematic botany. In these he published 510 new botanical names (including species, varieties and forms).

The acquisition of the Ashe Herbarium by the University of North Carolina was made possible through the generosity of Mr. George Watts Hill, of Durham, N. C. Most of it is unmounted; but Mr. Hill's gift made possible not only the purchase of the plants, but the cost of mounting them and the purchase of suitable herbarium cases. To assist in assembling and mounting the herbarium, the university has secured the services of Mr. T. G. Harbison, of Highlands, N. C. He was for years a collector for the Biltmore Herbarium, a collector for Sargent for over a quarter of a century, is the author of a number of papers on systematic botany, and as a friend and fellow collector of Mr. Ashe he is familiar with Mr. Ashe's signs and symbols. With Mr. Harbison's assistance the herbarium should be ready for the use of visiting botanists by summer.

Through the generosity of Mrs. W. W. Ashe the university is also the recipient of a large number of Mr. Ashe's reprints of botanical and forestry interest and a number of botanical journals and books.

H. R. TOTTEN

## HECKSCHER GRANTS AT CORNELL UNIVERSITY

THE Heckscher Research Council of Cornell University has announced that supplementary grants amounting to about $11,000 have been made for the continuance of eighteen scientific researches.

The allocation of grants followed a gift of $10,000 from the Carnegie Corporation made last autumn. A special gift of $1,000 made by Mrs. Harry Snyder, of Minneapolis, for the promotion of research in biochemistry and allied fields at Cornell was also allocated at this time to the continuance of researches assisted by an earlier gift from Mrs. Snyder.

The Heckscher Foundation for the promotion of research at Cornell was established by Mr. August Heckscher, a trustee of the university, in 1920 by a gift of $500,000. During the twelve years it has been in existence the fund has provided an income of $445,-000 for the support of 200 separate projects.

The following supplementary grants were made for the academic year, ending June 30, 1933:

Professor Wilder D. Bancroft: For researches in photochemistry.

Professor Samuel L. Boothroyd, '04–5, G: To continue work on meteors.

Professor T. Roland Briggs, '09, and Carleton C. Murdock, '12: For a study of the size and shape of colloidal particles with special reference to catalytic agents.

Professor L. M. Dennis: For investigation of rare elements.

Professor R. Clifton Gibbs, '07: For a study of line spectra in the extreme ultra-violet.

Professor Edwin F. Hopkins, '15: For a study of the physiological effect of iron and certain other elements in the ionized state.

Professor Earle H. Kennard, '13, Ph.D.: For research in theoretical physics.

Professor Robert Matheson, 06–7: For a study of culicid ecology.

George Maughan: To continue study of the effects of ultra-violet light on animal physiology.

Professor Leonard A. Maynard, '15, Ph.D., and C. M. McCay: To continue investigations on physiological effects of purified diets in herbivora, and to continue investigations on biochemical changes that accompany aging in the animal body.

Professor Ernest Merritt, '86: For study of the influence of the conditions of the upper atmosphere on the transmission of electric waves.

Professor Murdock: For work in x-rays.

Professors Edward L. Nichols and Ernest Merritt: For studies in luminescence.

Professor Jacob Papish, '21, Ph.D.: For a study of the occurrence, distribution and association of the rarer chemical elements.

Professor Otto Rahn: For studies of radiation from living matter.

Professor Hugh D. Reed, '99, Alan C. Fraser, '13, and George C. Embody, '10: For the purpose of undertaking genetical studies and related problems in fishes.

Professor Floyd K. Richtmyer, '04: For investigations in the laws of absorption of x-rays.

## THE AMERICAN JOURNAL OF SCIENCE

DR. RICHARD S. LULL, Sterling professor of paleontology and director of the Peabody Museum of Natural History at Yale University, has been appointed editor of *The American Journal of Science,* succeeding Dr. Ernest Howe, who died in December.

*The American Journal of Science and Arts* was established by Benjamin Silliman in 1818, and is an integral part of the educational activities of Yale University. This was the first serial scientific periodical in this country as Silliman was the first professor of science. At that time the scientist had only the irregular publications of a few scientific societies or academies in which to bring out with some promptness the results of his work.

As planned by Silliman *The American Journal* was to embrace all branches of science, "more especially mineralogy and geology"; including also "the ornamental as well as the useful arts." Papers on these last subjects appeared occasionally in early volumes, but more and more infrequently and finally, in 1880, "the Arts" was dropped from the title. The wide range of subjects was gradually somewhat restricted and after the 1890's articles outside of the geological field were more and more infrequent. The other subjects (as chemistry, physics, botany, etc.) still find a place in the abstracts of papers published elsewhere, or in the reviews of books in all lines of science.

The elder Silliman carried all the work of the *Journal* for some twenty years till his son, Benjamin Silliman, Jr., came in to assist him in 1838. A little later (1846), his son-in-law, James Dwight Dana, was also included in the editorial board. The last soon took upon himself the entire work and carried this on until within a few years of his death in 1895. For years previous to this he had had the assistance of his son, Edward S. Dana (whose name was included among the editors as early as 1875). From 1895 until 1925, the name of the younger Dana alone appeared as editor-in-chief. In 1925–26, Professor Alan M. Bateman rendered essential assistance until, through his efforts, Dr. Ernest Howe became editor in 1926.

The associate editors of *The American Journal* have been of importance in their support in many directions, especially by their contributions of abstracts of original papers published elsewhere. The list of associate editors from 1851 to the present time includes the names of many of the most distinguished scientists of the time, chiefly in this country.

At the time of the hundredth anniversary of the *Journal* in 1918 a number of lectures, certain of which were made the basis of a series of Silliman Lectures at Yale, were gathered together and published under the title, "A Century of Science in America, with special reference to *The American Journal of Science*, 1818–1918."

The ownership of the *Journal* passed to Yale University in 1926 through the gift from the editor and owner, Edward S. Dana. An endowment has been gradually accumulated, a large part of which has been given by the immediate descendants of the founder of the *Journal*.

# SCIENTIFIC NOTES AND NEWS

SIR CHARLES SHERRINGTON, Waynflete professor of physiology at the University of Oxford, has been elected an associate member of the French Academy of Medicine.

DR. H. SPENCER JONES, recently appointed Astronomer Royal at the Greenwich Observatory, formerly a fellow of Jesus College, Cambridge, has been elected to an honorary fellowship.

DR. GILBERT THOMAS MORGAN, director of the chemical research laboratory of the Department of Scientific and Industrial Research at Teddington, has been nominated to the presidency of the Chemical Society, London.

DR. NEVIL VINCENT SIDGWICK, university reader in chemistry at the University of Oxford, fellow of Lincoln College, Oxford, and member of the Advisory Council of Scientific and Industrial Research, has been elected a member of the Athenaeum Club, under the provision which empowers the annual election of a certain number of persons of distinguished eminence in science, literature, the arts or public service.

AT the annual dinner on February 22 of the American Institute of Mining and Metallurgical Engineers, the Saunders Medal, for distinguished achievement in mining engineering, was presented to Walter H. Aldridge, president of the Texas Gulf Sulphur Company, and the James Douglas Medal, for distinction in metallurgy, was presented to James O. Elton, manager of the International Smelting Company of Salt Lake City.

DR. FRANK C. MANN, of the Mayo Foundation, Rochester, Minnesota, has been awarded the William Wood Gerhard gold medal of the Pathological Society of Philadelphia for 1932. Dr. Mann also gave the annual conversational lecture on the evening of February 9. His subject was "Observation on Experimental Pathology and Pathologic Physiology of the Liver."

OIL paintings of Dr. Charles N. Gould and Dr. Charles E. Decker, commemorating their many years of active service in connection with the development of geological science in Oklahoma, were unveiled on February 8 at the University of Oklahoma. Thirty-three years ago Dr. Gould organized the department of geology at the university and eight years later organized the Oklahoma Geological Survey. For seventeen years Dr. Decker has taught paleontology at the university. He has also served as secretary-treasurer of the American Association of Petroleum Geologists, and as grand president of Sigma Gamma Epsilon. Dr. Irving Perrine, formerly a member of the faculty of geology, presided. Short addresses were made by a number of former students. President Bizzell, of the university, accepted the paintings, which were presented by Gamma Chapter of Sigma Gamma Epsilon.

DR. WALTER H. EVANS, chief of the Division of Insular Stations of the Office of Experiment Stations, retired on February 1, having reached the compulsory retirement age of seventy years. Dr. Evans was presented by his associates with a signed scroll and a watch, as an appreciation of his long and devoted service and as an expression of their high regard for him in their personal and official relationships.

A DINNER in honor of Dr. Francis M. Pottenger, Monrovia, California, retiring president of the American College of Physicians, was given by Southern California members of the college in Los Angeles, on January 12. Dr. David P. Barr, St. Louis, was the guest speaker.

DR. WILLIAM ALLEN PUSEY, emeritus professor of dermatology, University of Illinois College of Medicine, will deliver the Adolph Gehrmann Memorial Lectures at the Research and Educational Hospital of the college on March 1, 2 and 3, on "The History and Epidemiology of Syphilis." A dinner in honor of Dr. Pusey has been arranged by the university, to be given on March 2.

PROFESSOR GEO. J. MILLER, State Teachers College, Mankato, Minnesota, was chosen president of the National Council of Geography Teachers at its recent meeting in Washington. The next annual meeting will be held at Northwestern University on December 26 and 27.

AT the January meeting of the Pathological Society of Philadelphia, officers elected for the year 1933 were: Dr. V. H. Moon, *president;* Dr. Morton McCutcheon, *vice-president,* and Dr. Herbert L. Ratcliffe, *secretary-treasurer.*

PROFESSOR WARREN WEAVER, chairman of the department of mathematics of the University of Wisconsin, has resigned his post to accept permanent charge of the Natural Science Division of the Rockefeller Foundation, a post which he assumed temporarily during a year's leave of absence. His resignation has been accepted by the regents, and Professor M. H. Ingraham has been named chairman of the department.

DR. GEOFFREY DOUGLAS HALE CARPENTER has been elected Hope professor of zoology at the University of Oxford, vacant through the retirement of Professor E. B. Poulton, who had held the chair for forty years.

PROFESSOR K. BERINGER, of Heidelberg, has succeeded Professor Bostroem in the chair of psychiatry at Munich.

DR. FRITZ EICHHOLTZ, professor of pharmacology at Königsberg, has been called to Heidelberg.

MR. JOHN L. WIRT retired as bursar of the Carnegie Institution of Washington on February 1. Mr. E. A. Varella succeeds him and Mr. E. B. Biesecker has become assistant bursar.

WALTER G. CAMPBELL, director of regulatory work in the U. S. Department of Agriculture, resigned recently to become chief of the Food and Drug Administration, effective on February 1. The position of director of regulatory work has been abolished, thus completing the reorganization of the department's law-enforcement work started in 1923.

THE Committee on Scientific Research of the American Medical Association has awarded grants in aid to Dr. Philip B. Armstrong, of the Cornell University Medical College, to study the action of drugs in relation to the innervation of the heart; to Professor Wm. C. Rose, of the University of Illinois, for a continuation of his studies on the nutritive importance of the amino acids, with particular reference to the isolation of a hitherto unknown dietary essential present in certain proteins, and to Dr. C. C. Speidel, professor of anatomy in the University of Virginia Medical School, in support of his work on myelinated nerve fibers.

DR. DINSMORE ALTER, professor of astronomy at the University of Kansas, spent the first week of February in Tucson, Arizona, where he conferred with Dr. A. E. Douglass, director of the Seward Observatory, regarding a plan for a joint research into the problem of meteorological cycles.

DR. RALPH H. SMITH, entomologist in the University of California Citrus Experiment Station, visited the lower Rio Grande Valley of Texas during January. He conferred on citrus pest control problems and delivered two lectures on oil sprays. Dr. Smith also visited refineries and petroleum testing establishments in the southern and middle-western states.

DR. P. H. ROLFS, formerly dean of the College of Agriculture at the University of Florida, after twelve years' absence, is returning to take up his residence at Gainesville, Florida. In 1920 he was employed by Minas-Gerais to establish and conduct a state agricultural college. This work was completed in 1928. Since that time he has been serving the state as the technical adviser in agriculture.

DR. GEORG MASING, the German metallurgist, delivered the Institute of Metals Lecture at the annual meeting of the American Institute of Mining and Metallurgical Engineers. Professor George B. Waterhouse, of the Massachusetts Institute of Technology, delivered the annual Howe Lecture.

DR. THORNE M. CARPENTER, of the Nutrition Laboratory of the Carnegie Institution of Washington, gave two lectures in February at Columbus, Ohio, before the Ohio State Chapter of the Society of Sigma Xi. On February 9 he spoke on "The Development of Methods for Determining Basal Metabolism of Mankind" and on February 10 on "Problems and Factors in the Determination of the Basal Metabolism of Man."

PROFESSOR PIET VAN DE KAMP, of the University of Virginia, on February 9 spoke on "The Absorption of Light in the Galactic System," before a combined meeting of the Virginia chapters of Sigma Xi and Phi Beta Kappa.

DR. D. K. TRESSLER, chief chemist of the Birdseye Laboratories, Gloucester, Massachusetts, addressed a joint meeting of the Massachusetts State College Sigma Xi and Graduate Clubs on February 16 on "Recent Researches on the Preservation of Foods."

THE Federation of American Societies for Experimental Biology will meet at Cincinnati, Ohio, on April 10, 11 and 12.

THE American Association of Petroleum Geologists will hold its eighteenth annual meeting at Houston, Texas, on March 23, 24, 25.

THE American Public Health Association announces its sixty-second annual meeting, to be held in Indianapolis, Indiana, from October 9 to 12. It was in Indianapolis in 1900 at the twenty-ninth convention of the American Public Health Association that Dr. Walter Reed read a paper entitled "The Etiology of Yellow Fever—A Preliminary Note" indicating that the mosquito serves as the intermediate host for the parasite of yellow fever. At the coming meeting it is planned to honor the only living participant in the Yellow Fever Experiment, Dr. John R. Kissinger, at a special memorial session. The scientific program will discuss aspects of modern public health practice, from the viewpoint of the health officer, the laboratory worker, the epidemiologist, the child hygienist, the industrial hygienist, the nurse, the vital statistician, the health educator, the food and nutrition expert, the sanitary engineer.

THE Ohio Academy of Science will hold its forty-third annual meeting at Ohio University, Athens, on Friday and Saturday, April 14 and 15, under the presidency of Professor R. A. Budington, of Oberlin College. As in former years, the program will consist of one or two general sessions of the academy and sectional meetings, one or more for each of the seven sections. The general sessions will be devoted partly to business and partly to the discussion of scientific topics of general interest, probably by eminent invited speakers. Friday evening will be given over to the annual dinner at which will be given the presidential address. The section of chemistry will meet for the first time with Professor William Lloyd Evans, of the Ohio State University, Columbus, as the first vice-president. This section begins with an enrolment of sixty-eight members. The Central Ohio Physics Club will meet with the academy again this year, as in the past few years. The Ohio Academy of Science is sponsoring a series of weekly radio talks of fifteen minutes each beginning at 7:15 P. M. each Friday over the Ohio State University broadcasting station, WEAO, covering the four months from January to April.

AFTER annuities and legacies have been paid, the residue of the estate of the late Frederick G. Bonfils, editor of *The Denver Post,* is left to the foundation which he created in December, 1927, as "a corporation, not for profit, organized for charitable, benevolent, scientific, medical and public educational purposes." The value of the estate is said to be estimated at over $10,000,000.

DR. J. MIDDLEMASS HUNT, who held the post of honorary dean of the Liverpool School of Tropical Medicine for many years, has made a bequest of £20,000 to the University of Liverpool to provide for the endowment of the chair of tropical diseases of Africa.

THE Chemistry Club of the Georgia State College for Women, Milledgeville, Georgia, cooperating with the friends of Charles H. Herty, is awarding annually a medal for work done in the field of chemistry in the South. The purpose of the medal is twofold: (1) To give public recognition to worthy research workers in the colleges and laboratories of industry, whose real value is often unappreciated by their institutions. (2) To honor Dr. Herty, who has contributed a great deal to the development of the South, and who was born in a house which stood on what is now the campus of the Georgia State College for Women at Milledgeville. The award will be announced by May 1 of each year, and the medal will be presented at the May meeting of the Georgia Section of The American Chemical Society, which is invited to meet at Milledgeville. A modest allowance will be made to cover expenses of the winner to this meeting, where he will deliver an address.

*Museum News* reports that the Carnegie Corporation has made a grant of a fellowship to the New York Museum of Science and Industry to allow studies to be made, under the supervision of Professor Edward S. Robinson, of Yale University, of problems peculiar to museums of science and industry. One of the most important problems concerns the comparative mental reactions of young persons of various ages when dealing with exhibits operated by hand and when dealing with automatically operating exhibits which can be studied from a distance slightly beyond arm's reach or behind glass. Others are concerned with the question of what proportion of visitors, particularly young ones, pay attention to the descriptive labels placed on the exhibits and also to the social and economic interpretations on the walls above the machine or apparatus; also, the characteristic reactions of people in this museum as compared to people in art or natural history museums.

ACCORDING to *Museum News* the Museums Association of Great Britain has adopted regulations for gaining its museum curator's diploma. These regulations set forth two aspects of the education of the museum official of which the association takes cognizance. Competent knowledge (a) of at least one subject relating to museum collections and (b) of museum administration, methods and technique. Knowledge of a museum subject must be shown by an earned degree, diploma or certificate from one of a number of specified educational institutions. Knowledge of museum technique is determined by examination, and a panel of examiners is established by the association for this purpose. Attendance is required for one week each at an elementary, an advanced and a specialized course approved by the association. As a final test a candidate must submit a thesis on museum work and a concrete example of curatorial work. Candidates must have three years experience in a museum or art gallery before the diploma is awarded. Fee for registration is 10s 6d and for taking the diploma one guinea.

# DISCUSSION

## CORTIN AND TRAUMATIC SHOCK

A novel explanation of the "secret" of traumatic or secondary shock has recently been published in Science by a group of investigators from the Biological Laboratory of Princeton University.[1] The physiologic phenomena associated with death from adrenal cortex insufficiency have been compared with those found in traumatic shock. The analogy is a close one, as the authors have shown in a list of 32 particulars. Fundamentally, both conditions are characterized by a diminution in the volume of circulating blood, with a failure of the blood-diluting mechanism. The suggestion is made that "the signs and symptoms of adrenal insufficiency, and of traumatic or secondary shock, are possibly due to one and the same thing, namely, failure of the blood volume and blood-diluting regulator mechanism, the adrenal cortex." Because the "adrenalectomized animals, in the absence of the cortical hormone, are apparently unable to draw fluid back into the blood stream through the capillary walls" the writers suggest that "the accepted view that the osmotic power of the blood colloids is the chief factor involved in compensation needs further investigation."

There is only one dissimilarity among the 32 particulars which the writers have listed showing the analogy between adrenal insufficiency and traumatic shock. This discrepancy, as they point out, is the fact that in adrenal insufficiency the blood sugar is low, while in traumatic shock it is normal or elevated. They promise a discussion on this point at some future time. It seems possible, however, that this discrepancy may be of more moment than is realized at first glance. That the secretion of the adrenal cortex exerts a profound influence on the storage and utilization of carbohydrates has been realized for some time. The prepotent function of the cortex of the adrenal is considered by Britton and Silvette[2] to be the regulation of carbohydrate metabolism. They have found that the glycogen in the liver and muscles is lower after adrenalectomy than in extreme inanition, severe exhaustion, after strychnine convulsions or after exposure to cold. They state that "moreover, the muscle glycogen and blood glucose in cases of hepatectomy are not depleted more thoroughly than in animals showing more or less severe symptoms of adrenal insufficiency." It is therefore recognized that the glycogen stores and the blood glucose level are reduced in adrenalectomized animals. If the blood glucose level is reduced by insulin, as shown by Drabkin and Edwards in 1924,[3] certain physiologic reactions occur which are very similar to changes which the investigators have found to occur after adrenalectomy. In insulin hypoglycemia there is an actual loss of blood volume and a considerable concentration of the blood. These animals also show a decline in blood pressure and death from insulin "shock." Is it possible that the death from adrenal insufficiency may result primarily from the alterations in the carbohydrate metabolism which secondarily exert some influence on the blood hydration rather than through some hypothetical control over the mechanism of fluid exchange?

Some interesting experiments are reported by the authors to "test the relation between failure of the cortex and traumatic shock" and the results to them are "highly suggestive." Traumatic shock was produced in adrenalectomized dogs. Administration of cortin promptly resuscitated the dying animals. Control experiments were performed which demonstrated that a similar trauma did not produce shock in normal dogs. Such an experiment is very convincing proof that cortin is a specific therapeutic agent for the shock which is associated with the absence of cortico-adrenal hormone. But quite as specific is the glucose which is injected into animals in insulin shock. No one believes that traumatic shock and insulin shock are due to the same mechanism.

Again, other experiments were performed in which "profound surgical shock was induced in normal dogs by double adrenalectomy at one sitting. Immediately following completion of the operation, the blood pressure was normal." At this point the question may be raised as to their criteria of "profound surgical shock" resulting from operations at the close of which the blood pressure was *normal*. If such animals received cortin they recovered and were normal in 2 to 3 days. Dogs similarly "shocked" and not injected with hormone invariably died within 48 hours. The investigators have clearly demonstrated that the cortico-adrenal hormone is a specific therapeutic agent

[1] W. W. Swingle, J. J. Pfiffner, H. M. Vars, P. A. Bott, W. M. Parkins, Science, 77: 58, January 13, 1933.

[2] S. W. Britton and H. Silvette, *Am. Jour. Physiol.*, 100: 701, 1932.

[3] D. L. Drabkin and D. J. Edwards, *ibid.*, 70: 273, 1924.

for the shock which is associated with absence of the adrenals, but they have not reported experiments in which the effect of cortin has been assayed in traumatic shock. Always when they produced shock the adrenals were absent. Shock was never produced when the adrenals were present. They conclude, "the idea that the adrenal cortical hormone might prove of benefit in the treatment of human traumatic shock is advanced merely as a suggestion. Adequate proof can only come through clinical trial." Since it is known that deficiency of the cortico-adrenal hormone results in a lowering of the glycogen and blood glucose levels and since it is known that if the blood glucose level is reduced by insulin, there is a reduction in blood volume with blood concentration, the suggestion that the function of the adrenal cortex is the regulation of blood volume and blood dilution seems unnecessary. Although the analogy between deficiency of cortico-adrenal hormone and traumatic shock is a close one, no convincing evidence has been presented that the two conditions have a common etiology or that the cortical hormone is of benefit in the treatment of shock.

NORMAN E. FREEMAN
MASSACHUSETTS GENERAL HOSPITAL
BOSTON

## THE ASSOCIATION OF TERMITES WITH FUNGI

A SURVEY of the fungi associated with *Kalotermes minor,* a dry-wood termite, *Reticulitermes hesperus,* the common western subterranean termite, and *Zoötermopsis angusticollis,* the large damp-wood termite, has been made.

Fungi were found to be associated with each of the fifteen colonies of *K. minor,* twelve colonies of *R. hesperus* and twelve colonies of *Z. angusticollis* studied. They were isolated (1) from the exterior of the termites, (2) from the gut of the termites, (3) from the fecal pellets of *K. minor* and *Z. angusticollis,* (4) from the "frass" with which *R. hesperus* plugs up abandoned galleries, (5) from the wood of the inner surface of the termite burrows, and (6) from the wood 1 to 2 mm below the surface of the walls of burrows. Henceforth, in speaking of the isolation of a fungus from a termite colony, this designation is used to include not only the termites themselves, but also their fecal pellets, the frass and the wood enclosing their burrows.

Representatives of thirty-three genera of fungi and twenty undetermined fungi were isolated from the colonies of the three species of termites. A somewhat smaller number of fungi was associated with *K. minor* than with *R. hesperus* or *Z. angusticollis,* seventeen genera of fungi and four undetermined fungi being isolated from twelve colonies of *K. minor* as compared to twenty-five genera and eight undetermined forms from twelve colonies of *R. hesperus* and twenty-two genera and three undetermined forms from twelve colonies of *Z. angusticollis.*

The average number of fungi isolated from ten cultures made from each of twelve colonies of each of the species of termites was 4.91 for *K. minor,* 8.75 for *R. hesperus* and 7.25 for *Z. angusticollis.*

A smaller amount of fungous growth was present in the colonies of *K. minor* than in those of *R. hesperus* or *Z. angusticollis.* Furthermore, the wood containing the *K. minor* colonies usually showed little structural injury from fungous attack, while that enclosing the *R. hesperus* and the *Z. angusticollis* burrows usually showed decay. This is undoubtedly due to the fact that the wood containing the colonies of *K. minor* was drier and, therefore, less favorable to the growth of wood-destroying fungi.

*Penicillium* and *Trichoderma* were the genera of fungi most frequently isolated from the colonies of each of the three species of termites. There was no evidence of any specific relation between any fungus and a given species of termite.

Termites were placed upon pure cultures of a fungus, and were found capable of transporting large numbers of fungous spores and hyphae on their legs and bodies. Subsequent dissection revealed many entire and fragmented spores and a few fragments of hyphae of the fungus in the gut of the termites.

Fungi were more abundant on the inner surface of termite galleries than in the wood below the surface of gallery walls, only four cultures out of fifteen taken from wood 1 to 10 mm from the galleries of a colony of *K. minor* being positive as compared to sixteen positive cultures out of seventeen taken from the surface of gallery walls.

Twelve cultures made from the heartwood of a pole uninfested by termites were all negative. Seventeen out of twenty-seven made from the sapwood were also negative. In a termite-infested pole, of the same kind of wood and having a similar history of use, fourteen cultures taken at intervals throughout the diameter of the pole from wood adjacent to termite galleries were all positive. The same two fungi which were isolated from the wood near the exterior of the first pole were common throughout the diameter of the second pole in and near the termite galleries. Nine other fungi were also present in the termite-infested pole.

It seems evident, then, that termites may introduce fungi which were not previously present in the wood and that they may aid in the spread through the wood of these and of those already present.

The results of this investigation indicate that conditions in the burrows of *K. minor, R. hesperus* and *Z. angusticollis* are favorable to the growth of fungi and that fungi are present in the walls of the burrows and in the fecal pellets. Termites enlarge their burrows; they eat their fecal pellets. Fungi would seem, then, to be a common element in the diet of the termites. Further investigation, however, will be necessary to determine the significance of fungi as food for termites. Fungi may cause chemical changes in wood. Hence, the question whether their presence may render wood more available or more attractive to the termites also becomes a problem of interest.

A more detailed account of this investigation will appear later.

ESTHER C. HENDEE

ZOOLOGICAL LABORATORY
UNIVERSITY OF CALIFORNIA

## ANTIPROTHROMBIN AND GLOBULINS

IN a recent note[1] A. Fischer called attention to his work on the effect of the addition of heparin upon precipitation of proteins, especially of blood proteins, in an acetate-acetic acid solution at pH 5.0. With small additions of heparin there is an increased precipitation of casein, blood serum protein, or a precipitation of serum albumin. With increased amounts of heparin, precipitation may be inhibited or the precipitate dissolved. The addition of heparin to dialyzed serum albumin gives a flocculation at pH 5.0. These conclusions are similar to those previously published by Fischer in the *Biochemische Zeitschrift*.[2] Fischer concludes from his experiment that euglobulin is formed from serum albumin and suggests that euglobulin is formed in the liver through the combination of serum albumin with heparin.

We were interested in these findings of Fischer in connection with the blood of new-born animals. The serum or plasma of such animals does not contain euglobulin according to the ordinary methods of detecting it, and in some animals practically no pseudoglobulin I (if one wishes to recognize two pseudoglobulins). If euglobulin is formed by combination of heparin with albumin, it seemed possible that the failure to find euglobulin might in some way be connected with the concentration of heparin in the new-born blood. Furthermore, if euglobulin is formed by a combination of heparin with albumin, such a serum offers an excellent opportunity to test the fact. It is better than a purified serum albumin, because changes in the character of the protein through the removal of euglobulin and the purification of the albumin likely to occur in any purification process would be reduced to a minimum. The only change involved is the clotting of the fibrinogen.

Heparin preparations, both purified and crude, were presented to us by Hynson, Westcott and Dunning. The addition of heparin to new-born serum or to adult serum with an acetate buffer mixture according to the procedure of Fischer confirmed his results with regard to precipitation at pH 5.0, *i.e.*, a turbidity developed with the new-born serum where no precipitate had formed without heparin and a turbidity appeared with adult serum greater than that obtained without heparin. Furthermore, the pH for maximum precipitation was found to be different for the cow and horse. Additional amounts of heparin after the maximum turbidity was reached resulted in a decreased turbidity. However, the addition of a neutral salt or mixture of salts which precipitate euglobulin, such as 1.00 volume-molar sodium sulfate solution or of 1.425 volume-molar solution of potassium phosphate at approximately pH 7[3] to untreated new-born serum and to new-born serum to which heparin had been added failed to give a precipitation. The concentration of heparin used was that which gave the maximum turbidity at pH 5.0. Furthermore, the addition of 1.50 volume-molar sodium sulfate solution or of 2.025 volume-molar potassium phosphate at approximately pH 7, which precipitate both euglobulin and pseudoglobulin, gave equal precipitations with new-born serum in the presence or absence of heparin.

After these observations were completed a communication by Fischer and Schmitz[4] appeared in which they indicate that ammonium sulfate turbidity curves are not affected by heparin. These authors also state that the addition of herparin to serum and plasma from the same animal causes a difference in the distribution of albumin and globulin of plasma such that the albumin fraction of the plasma is decreased, while the globulin fraction is increased as compared to the corresponding fraction from serum. We have fractioned the new-born serum and plasma from the same animal, with and without the addition of heparin, at 0.75 molar and at 1.50 molar sodium sulfate. These concentrations are held to precipitate fibrinogen and total globulin, respectively, at dilutions of 1: 30. (No precipitate was obtained in the serum with 1.00 molar sodium sulfate, indicating an absence of euglobulin and fibrinogen.) Heparin was added in the concentration which gave the maximum turbidity at pH 5.0, in turbidity measurements such as Fischer has used, *i.e.*, 0.5 cc of a 1 per cent. solution of heparin was added to 0.5 cc of serum for each determination. No differences were obtained in the quantity of protein precipitated in serum or plasma in any concentration of salt.

[1] SCIENCE, 75: 443, 1932.
[2] A. Fischer, *Biochem. Z.*, 244: 464–485, 1932.
[3] Paul E. Howe, *Physiol. Rev.*, 5: 439–476, 1925.
[4] A. Fischer and A. Schmitz, *Naturwissenschaften*, 20: 471–2, 1932.

These results, while confirming Fischer's observations that heparin produces a combination in serum that is precipitated at approximately pH 5.0, does not substantiate his tentative conclusion that this combination is euglobulin or pseudoglobulin. Fischer's proofs of euglobulin have chiefly concerned procedures which depend upon precipitation at the isoelectric point; a sodium acetate buffer mixture, $CO_2$, dialysis. Precipitation near its isoelectric point is a characteristic of euglobulin; on the other hand, euglobulin, as it is ordinarily recognized, may be salted out with neutral salts. If the heparin-protein complex of new-born serum is euglobulin, it should have been precipitated at 1.00 molar sodium sulfate, or if only a partial combination the salting out might possibly have appeared at 1.50 volume-molar sodium sulfate. We realize that salting out is not an entire proof of a globulin. Salting out does, however, comprise one of the procedures used in differentiating and preparing euglobulin. Fischer's suggestion is exceedingly interesting, but its verification requires more evidence than isoelectric precipitation. It seems to us that this phenomenon observed by Fischer can be explained without assuming the actual formation of globulin.

IMOGENE P. EARLE
PAUL E. HOWE
BUREAU OF ANIMAL INDUSTRY
U. S. DEPARTMENT OF AGRICULTURE

## THE RELATION OF THE HYPOPHYSIS TO EXPERIMENTAL DIABETES

IT has been known since 1889 that removal of the pancreas leads to an increase in the blood sugar and appearance of sugar in the urine. Insulin, prepared from the pancreas, is effective in controlling the metabolism of sugar but does not cure the condition. Recently Houssay reported that extirpation of the hypophysis prior to removal of the pancreas was effective in preventing severe diabetes. It appears that we have confirmed this work. Two dogs did not survive long after the second operation, but in them the typical hyperglycemia did not develop. A third animal has survived over three weeks, during which time he has remained in good health. The tolerance for glucose is normal and the fasting blood sugar is within the normal range. No spontaneous glycosuria has occurred.

The animal shows certain symptoms which indicate complete removal of the hypophysis. Autopsy will show whether or not the hypophysectomy was complete and if there is accessory pancreatic tissue. This work is being continued at the University of Chicago.

J. F. REGAN
B. O. BARNES
PHYSIOLOGICAL LABORATORY
UNIVERSITY OF CHICAGO

## CANCER RESEARCH

IN the January, 1933, number of *The American Journal of Cancer* is an editorial on cancer research. In this the editor states that the prime needs of cancer research are first, *brains;* second, *time;* and third, *money.*

I should like to point out the obvious fallacy of any generalization of this type, even though it be made by one who for years has been connected with an institution utilizing each of the three components mentioned. In a field as complex as that of cancer research one institution may need primarily brains, another time for investigation and a third money. Furthermore, the primary need of any one institution engaged in cancer research may change from month to month or from year to year. It is also obviously true that no one component alone will result in progress. Brains without time or money result merely in theories. Time alone is obviously sterile. Money without brains or time is a material and impersonal factor. If each scientific man would avoid the field of generalization about the work of all others and would apply himself to his own problems in the way that he believes best, utilizing, in the proportions which he is able to find them and is able to develop them, the three elements of brains, time and money, more progress will result.

C. C. LITTLE
ROSCOE B. JACKSON MEMORIAL LABORATORY
BAR HARBOR, MAINE

# REPORTS

## APPROPRIATIONS FOR GRANTS IN AID BY THE NATIONAL RESEARCH COUNCIL

THE National Research Council wishes to announce that the research aid fund of which it has had charge for the past three years is to be continued during the present calendar year, 1933. The fund is administered by a special committee on grants in aid of research, which is composed of the chairman and treasurer of the council and of the chairmen of the council's seven divisions of science and technology. This committee will be ready to consider requests for grants of moderate amount from this fund for the support of the individual research work of qualified investigators in the fields of the natural sciences, who are citizens of the United States or of Canada.

Requests for grants from this fund will be acted

upon by the committee at two meetings during the year, in May and in December. It is requested that applications for grants to be considered at the meeting in May be filed with the council before March 15 and that applications to be considered at the December meeting of the committee be forwarded to reach the council before October 15, 1933.

The council has adopted the following policy for the administration of this research aid fund:

(1) Grants will be made in order to cover such expenses as the following: apparatus, materials and supplies, technical assistance, and field expenses.

(2) In general, grants will not be given for personal salaries or fellowship stipends, for expenses of publication, for the purchase of books, for travel to attend scientific meetings, or for research work of students under instruction.

(3) Preference will ordinarily be given to the support of investigations—(a) in which the problem and methods to be used are clearly stated, and in which definite results can be expected with the aid of the grant; (b) toward which the university or other institution to which the applicant is attached also contributes financially or through special support; (c) for which a grant of not more than $1,000 is requested.

(4) A report of progress should be made by the grantee to the Secretary of the Committee within a year after beginning the use of the grant.

(5) Periodical reports of expenditures from grants are expected, ordinarily, at the close of each quarter.

(6) The title to property purchased from grants will remain with the National Research Council until ultimate disposition of the property is made by the Council.

Correspondence in regard to applications for grants should be addressed to the Secretary, Committee on Grants in Aid, National Research Council, 2101 Constitution Avenue, Washington, D. C.

At its meeting in December, 1932, the committee on grants in aid made thirty-four grants for the support of individual research, as follows:

George E. Davis, Department of Physics, Iowa State College, development of improved methods of determining absorption spectra; Jacob Kunz, professor of theoretical physics, and J. T. Tykociner, research professor of electrical engineering, University of Illinois, determination of the magnetic moment of hydrogen; P. A. Ross, professor of physics, Stanford University, x-ray analysis and the Compton effect.

Charles B. Breed, professor of railway and highway transportation, Massachusetts Institute of Technology, cost of highway transportation; Wilber E. Harvey, assistant professor of metallurgical engineering, Lehigh University, combined effects of corrosion and fatigue upon welds; C. F. Hirshfeld, chief, research department, The Detroit Edison Company, in cooperation with H. Diederichs, professor of experimental engineering, Cornell University, determination of the temperature of the metal of a tube wall separating bodies of steam and water.

H. K. Benson, professor of chemical engineering, University of Washington, biochemical decomposition of sulfite waste; Cecil E. Boord, professor of organic chemistry, Ohio State University, synthesis of olefines; George A. Hulett, professor of physical chemistry, Princeton University, electrical conductivity of pure water; Wesley G. Leighton, assistant professor of chemistry, Pomona College, activation of surface phenomena in quartz by ultra-violet light; A. L. Robinson, assistant professor of chemistry, University of Pittsburgh, thermochemistry of dilute solutions; O. F. Stafford, professor of chemistry, University of Oregon, concentration of the $H^2$ isotope of hydrogen by the electrolysis of water.

Paul H. Dunn, fellow in geology, University of Chicago, correlation of Silurian strata in the Mississippi Basin; Ross L. Heaton, consulting geologist, Denver, Colorado, stratigraphy of the central and southern Rocky Mountain region.

Reginald D. Manwell, assistant professor of zoology, Syracuse University, effect of atebrine and rauwolfine on avian malaria; Eric Ponder, professor of general physiology, New York University, effects of intravascular lysins on red blood cells; Bret Ratner, clinical professor of pediatrics and lecturer on immunology, New York University and Bellevue Medical College, proteins and amino acids of milk; B. T. Simms, professor of veterinary medicine, Oregon State Agricultural College, salmon poisoning in dogs; Carl C. Speidel, professor of anatomy, University of Virginia, fundamental activities of nerves in the living animal; Maurice B. Visscher, professor of physiology, College of Medicine, University of Illinois, mechanical efficiency of heart muscle; Herbert U. Williams, professor of pathology, University of Buffalo School of Medicine, evidence of syphilis in mummified bodies from Peru.

William A. Cannon, lecturer in botany, Stanford University, derivation of oxygen by the roots of land plants; Henry J. Fry, professor of biology, New York University, mitosis in *Chaetopterus;* Ernst Gellhorn, professor of physiology, College of Medicine, University of Illinois, influence of metabolites and internal secretions on fatigue; Madeleine P. Grant, assistant professor of zoology, Smith College, thyroid secretion in amphibians and mammals; E. Raymond Hall, assistant professor of vertebrate zoology and curator of mammals, University of California, monographic study of the American weasels; Hans Jenny, assistant professor of soils, University of Missouri, ionic exchange of potassium on soil colloids; Harold Kirby, Jr., associate professor of zoology, University of California, flagellates in termites; C. R. Orton, professor of plant pathology, West Virginia University, natural dissociation of *Fusaria* in the soil.

C. W. Brown, professor of psychology, University of California, central nervous mechanism of emotional responses; Clarence H. Graham, assistant professor of psychology, Clark University, analysis of visual response by means of an electrical recording method; Harry F. Harlow, assistant professor of psychology, University of Wisconsin, effect of complete striate muscle paralysis upon learning and thinking; Truman Michelson, ethnologist, Bureau of American Ethnology, Smithsonian Institution, study of special data upon the ethnology of the Fox and Ojibwa Indians; William S. Webb, professor of anthropology and archeology, University of Kentucky, archeological survey of Kentucky.

W. H. HOWELL,
*Chairman, National Research Council*

# SCIENTIFIC APPARATUS AND LABORATORY METHODS

## A METHOD OF OUTLINING CUTANEOUS NERVE AREAS

IN 1928 we discovered that the cutaneous area supplied by a nerve may be rendered insensible to light touch by subjecting the nerve trunk to the influence of an alternating current; the area may be outlined by the procedure employed in cases of peripheral nerve lesions. Though we have not explored the literature to its depths, our efforts in this direction have failed to reveal a previous record of such a finding.

This indicated a new experimental approach to some of the problems of cutaneous innervation and sensation; such work has been pursued in this laboratory since 1928, and preliminary reports have appeared.[1] We did not intend to publish the technique apart from the results, but requests for an account of the method indicate that a brief note would place it at the service of others who might find it useful. We shall describe the apparatus used by us, suggesting some desirable modifications; others will occur to those who use the method.

The current from the 110 volt D. C. main was converted into an alternating current by a small Alexanderson alternator (Fig. 1); because of its noise this should be in another room than that wherein the observations are being made. The alternator may be driven by A. C. or by D. C.; Fig. 1 shows the latter arrangement. The frequency was controlled by a variable resistance in the circuit driving the alternator; it was estimated from the number of teeth and the r. p. m. of the alternator, this being ascertained by a Starrett speed indicator. The current strength was controlled by a system of variable resistances in the primary or input circuit (Fig. 1); our method of measuring it was unsatisfactory and need not be described; that this is unimportant is indicated below.

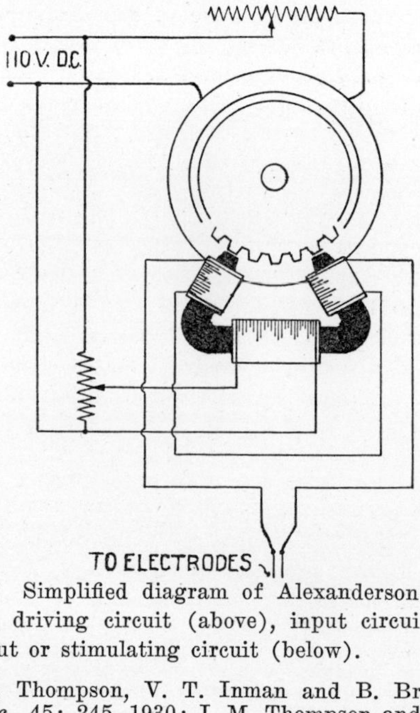


FIG. 1. Simplified diagram of Alexanderson alternator, with driving circuit (above), input circuit (left), and output or stimulating circuit (below).

We have applied the method systematically only to the nerves of the forearm and hand, to which the following account refers. Each nerve to be investigated was subjected to unipolar stimulation through the intact skin. We used metallic electrodes, padded with gauze soaked in a saturated solution of NaCl; subsequently we have found a 4 per cent. solution equally satisfactory. The large inactive electrode was applied to the opposite arm. The stimulating electrode (diameter about 1 cm) being placed on the skin over an appropriate part of the nerve trunk, somewhat as indicated by Hughson,[2] the current was *gradually* turned on by withdrawing resistance from the input circuit. With practice the nerve was soon "picked up"; this was evidenced by the sensation of flutter projected into its cutaneous area, as described by Hughson.[2] As the current was increased, testing with a von Frey hair revealed that at a certain level of current strength tactile sensibility disappeared in the area supplied by the nerve under stimulation, though remaining unaltered elsewhere; to this loss of sensation we apply the provisional term "masking" in preference to anesthesia. Manipulation of the electrode and of the current extended the masked area to a limit beyond which no further manipulation could extend it; it was then outlined on the skin as in the case of a peripheral nerve lesion, every precaution being taken to ensure that the subject received only tactile stimuli.

Fig. 1 shows no apparatus for measuring the frequency and strength of the current, that being unnecessary if one is merely outlining nerve areas: it is sufficient to manipulate the current (and the electrode) until the area is masked. If he so desire, the

[1] I. M. Thompson, V. T. Inman and B. Brownfield, *Anat. Rec.*, 45: 245, 1930; I. M. Thompson and A. Barron, *ibid.*, 48: 35 (Suppl.), 1931; I. M. Thompson, *Jour. Anat.*, 66: 148, 1931.

[2] W. Hughson, *Anat. Rec.*, 23: 371, 1922; *Johns Hopkins Hosp. Bull.*, 33: 338, 1922.

investigator may introduce suitable meters, etc., at appropriate places in the output or stimulating circuit. As a result of further work, we recommend a larger generator than that described above, yielding stronger currents at low frequencies. For the subsequent development of this field of investigation such a generator has been designed and installed in this laboratory, and will be described later; using it, satisfactory masking occurs with currents of about 100 to 300 cycles per second, 5 to 10 volts and 0.5 to 3 milliamperes. All our work on nerve areas, however, was done with the small alternator. Possibly currents generated otherwise may yield similar results.

The space available here precludes reference to the difficulties inherent in such a procedure; these will be discussed in a more detailed publication. The method is not easy, and demands practice and patience on the part of observer and subject alike. We have encountered one or two subjects who, for some obscure reason, possibly physiological or psychological, were unsatisfactory for such work, wherein the importance of reliable subjective responses is obvious. Outlining the same area on the same subject on different occasions has yielded reasonably consistent results.

The nature of the results is indicated in Fig. 2.

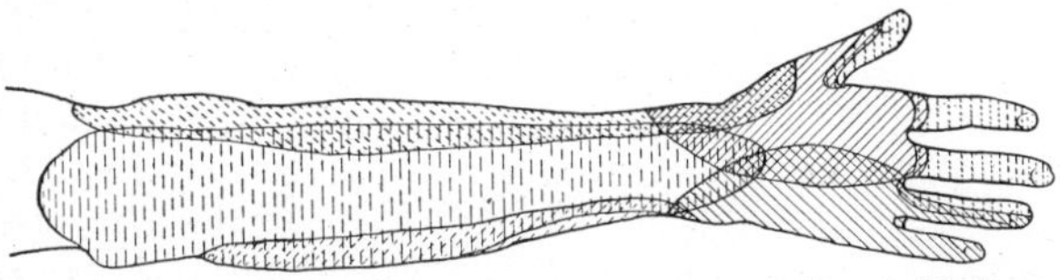

FIG. 2. A sketch of the dorsal aspect of the right forearm and hand of an adult male, showing the cutaneous areas supplied by various nerves; these are not labelled, for anatomists will recognize them. In this individual the median nerve supplied the entire dorsal aspect of the index and middle fingers. The extent of the overlaps is easily seen. In this person certain small areas on the back of the wrist were supplied by three cutaneous nerves: for example, that in the middle is seen to be supplied by the dorsal cutaneous nerve of the forearm, the radial and the ulnar.

So far as we know, ours are the first pictures of the *complete* innervation, *including overlap areas,* of any region of the body in single individuals. We have succeeded in estimating the size of these areas and in studying their variations; preliminary results have been presented by Thompson, Inman and Brownfield, and by Thompson[1]; a detailed analysis is being prepared.

I. MACLAREN THOMPSON
VERNE T. INMAN
UNIVERSITY OF CALIFORNIA
MEDICAL SCHOOL
DIVISION OF ANATOMY
BERKELEY, CALIFORNIA

## CELLOPHANE ROLL FILMS AND THE FIXING OF CARBON PAPER TYPING ON CELLOPHANE[1]

THE wide-spread interest in the use of cellophane for slide lanterns[2] seems to justify reference to the paper presented by the authors[3] before the Division of Chemical Education of the American Chemical Society, at Denver, Colorado, on August 24, 1932.

A cellophane roll film carrier was described for using the cellophane in rolls instead of slides. The device is fitted into any ordinary slide lantern with no modification of the lantern necessary. Any one interested in this device will find a scale drawing for one form of it given in the *Journal of Chemical Education.*[3] The cellophane roll film carrier will hold over 33 feet of 0.001 inch thick cellophane. This is equivalent to about 120 slides, yet forms a roll less than ¾ inch in diameter, and weighs less than one glass slide. The article also gives a description of methods of preparing the films, including colored pen work; also uses of such films, and methods of fixing carbon paper typing.

Typing on cellophane slides and films is done with carbon paper. Every one seems to have had trouble with smearing of such typing, but we have worked out a simple method which is so satisfactory that a roll film has been used over 400 times and still shows no evidence of smearing. A brief description of it may be of interest to readers of SCIENCE.

The procedure consists of passing the typed film through a suitable liquid and carefully blotting it between unglazed paper while it is still moist, care being taken that the blotting paper does not slide over the wet surface. The paper removes most of the liquid and the excess ink. The film is then placed between dry paper and pressed for several minutes to complete the fixing.

Of fifty chemicals tried, organic liquids for the most part, the most satisfactory for the purpose are: amyl acetate, ethyl acetate, methyl acetate, acetaldehyde, benzyl alcohol, iso-amyl alcohol, ethylene glycol monoethyl ether ("cellosolve") and a mixture of 75 per cent. di-ethyl ether and 25 per cent. ethyl alcohol.

Other liquids fairly satisfactory are: iso-butyl alcohol, iso-propyl alcohol, methyl-ethyl ketone, acetone, ethylene chloride, ethylene bromide, benzyl

1 Contribution No. 89 of the Division of Industrial Sciences of West Virginia University.

2 "Lantern Slides from Cellophane," John L. Wilson, *Jour. Chem. Educ.*, 8: 2212 (November, 1931); "A New Use for Cellophane," K. L. Warren, SCIENCE, 76: 573, (December 16, 1932); "Cellophane for Slide Lanterns," B. H. Walden, SCIENCE, 77: 91 (January 20, 1933); "The Radio-Mat," F. L. Wells, *ibid.*

3 "Cellophane Roll Films for Slide Lanterns" was sent to the *Journal of Chemical Education* on July 20, 1932, and appears in a somewhat abbreviated form in *Jour. Chem. Educ.*, 10: 92–94 (February, 1933). Since August numerous brief references to the paper have appeared in the daily press and periodicals.

chloride, nitrobenzene, di-ethyl aniline, pyridine, and carbon tetrachloride.

Results are much better when the chemicals of the first list are used.

Ross Bonar
Floyd Bonar
Earl C. H. Davies

Chemistry Department
West Virginia University
Morgantown, W. Va.

## SILK CELLOPHANE FOR LANTERN SLIDES

Recently Warren,[1] Walden,[2] and Wells[3] suggested the use of plain cellophane as a recipient of carbon in projection lantern slides. As a further suggestion, special du Pont Number 300 white silk cellophane takes ink directly from the typewriter ribbon without smudging and, after momentary drying, the record is permanent. If the original impressions are gone over for the second typing, legibility is enhanced. The cost of this special silk cellophane is less than one cent per slide.

Fredrick F. Yonkman

School of Medicine
Boston University

[1] K. L. Warren, Science, 76: 573, December 16, 1932.
[2] B. H. Walden, Science, 77: 91, January 20, 1933.
[3] F. L. Wells, Science, 77: 91, January 20, 1933.

# SPECIAL ARTICLES

## THE RELATIONSHIP OF BACTERIUM GRANULOSIS TO TRACHOMA

The question of the relationship of *Bacterium granulosis* to the etiology of trachoma has been discussed in a recent publication.[1] As stated in that article the organism of Noguchi "merits consideration as the etiological factor" in the disease. This view was expressed in spite of the accumulation of negative evidence of many workers, including the writer, and the doubts which have been expressed by some who have been the most sanguine in their expectation of the solution of the trachoma problem following the isolation of this organism with which a transmissible granular condition may be produced in monkeys. Such doubts are based on the failure of many investigators to isolate the organism from trachoma in different parts of the world and the considerable number of negative results which have been obtained in attempting to produce trachoma by inoculation of human subjects with the organism.

I reported that the granular condition originally induced with difficulty in *Macacus rhesus* monkeys by inoculation with cultures of *Bact. granulosis* was very readily transmissible and that transmission could be accomplished by merely rubbing a sterile swab over the affected conjunctiva and then rubbing it over the conjunctiva of a normal animal, thus demonstrating the fact that it is not necessary to excise tissue and to inject this subconjunctivally. In other words, as described by one worker, the granular condition may be described as one which is "highly infectious."

The question arose: "Is human trachoma as readily transmissible?" There are a number of clinicians who, after long experience with trachoma, still question the ready communicability of the disease. On the other hand, Taborisky[2] inoculated the conjunctiva of 5 blind subjects with the conjunctival secretion of trachoma cases and all acquired the disease.

In order to obtain a comparison between the granular condition induced in monkeys by inoculation with cultures of *Bact. granulosis* and that induced by direct transfer of secretions from trachoma cases, a series of monkeys was started in the early part of 1932 in which granular lesions were produced by repeated swabbing of secretions from trachoma cases in Rolla, Missouri. A number of attempts had previously been made to accomplish this without success. A granular condition which developed slowly was obtained in 2 monkeys and from one of these was transmitted to another monkey by repeated swabbing. As reported recently[3] two parallel series of monkeys (8 in each series) were then considered, one in which attempts were made to transmit the granular condition originally induced by inoculation with cultures of *Bact. granulosis* and the other in which attempts were made to transmit the granular condition originally induced by transfer from trachoma cases. Four monkeys in each series had been previously inoculated with a vaccine of *Bact. granulosis* with the idea that the test might show whether there were immunological differences in the two conditions. In the "culture" series 5 of the 8 animals developed the granular condition after one swabbing from an infected monkey, and one after two swabbings, and one died. In all these the granular condition occurred spontaneously in the uninoculated eye. In the "direct transfer" series all the monkeys were swabbed 3 times (on consecutive days) and one of the 8 developed a granular condition in both eyes, 6 remained unaffected and one died. Of the 6 unaffected, 5 have since been swabbed from infected monkeys, one a single time, one 2

[1] Ida A. Bengtson, *Pub. Health Rep.*, 47: 1914, September 19, 1932.
[2] J. Taborisky, *Graefe's Arch. f. Ophth.*, 123: 140, 1930.
[3] Ida A. Bengtson, *Pub. Health Rep.*, 47: 2281, December 9, 1932.

times and three 3 times (on consecutive days). In 4 of these lesions have developed gradually and in one of these the uninoculated eye has become affected. In neither series was protection afforded by the vaccine, since more were affected in the vaccinated than in the unvaccinated groups. Regarding the gross appearance of the lesions there was no great difference. The condition was rather less active in the "direct transfer" series than in the "culture" series. The results obtained indicate that the condition induced by direct transfer from trachoma in Missouri was less easily transmissible than that induced by inoculation of cultures of *Bact. granulosis.* Quoting from the report "Whether this difference is significant and whether it would constantly be true can not be said without further tests." It may be that as in other diseases certain strains of the organism concerned may be more virulent than others.

The results reported by Olitsky, Syverton and Tyler in SCIENCE, for January 6, 1933,[4] lend support to the view that *Bact. granulosis* is concerned in the etiology of trachoma. Of significance is the use of tarsectomized tissue in the experimental work carried out by these investigators. The chances for successful transmission of the condition to animals and for isolation of the organism concerned are without doubt greatly enhanced by the use of large amounts of material. The great amount of negative evidence in certain localities as reported in the literature and in unpublished work concerning which information has been received by the writer, may possibly be explained on this basis. It is apparent that most workers have not used tarsectomized tissue, which is difficult to obtain because many ophthalmologists consider the tarsectomy operation as of questionable value for the cure of trachoma.

Another phase of the problem is of interest. If the work of Olitsky and collaborators can be confirmed in certain other parts of the world where only negative results have been reported, using the sort of material and the methods employed by them and it is definitely established that *Bact. granulosis* is the etiological factor in trachoma, then the isolation of an organism which is non-filtrable and which grows on the ordinary culture media, from a disease which is characterized by the presence of inclusion bodies, takes on a certain significance. A revision of the rather generally accepted view of the nature of the infective agent in at least some of the group of diseases in which inclusion bodies occur (diseases usually classified as belonging in the "filtrable virus" group) would be necessary. As I reported in 1928[5] in a study of inclusion bodies in over 200 cases of trachoma these bodies were present in nearly 50 per cent. of the cases. More recently, Taborisky[6] has reported that observations during a period of 20 years justify the belief that there can be no trachoma without inclusion bodies at some period, if cases are followed from the beginning. As the result of the microscopical study I reported that the inclusion body in the early stages was composed of rod-shaped organisms. A photograph of a very unusual preparation is shown in this publication, in which the nucleus of an epithelial cell is surrounded by numerous rod-shaped organisms which morphologically at least could very well be said to correspond with *Bact. granulosis*, though identification on this basis is obviously impossible. The definite rod-shaped forms are seen very rarely. Usually the inclusion body appears as a more or less structureless mass, in which at a later stage very minute coccoid bodies staining reddish with Giemsa appear. Apparently the group of organisms forming the inclusion body is acted on by the living cytoplasm of the epithelial cell and transformed into these small bodies which are the "elementary bodies" of Halberstaedter and von Prowazek. These are visible when occurring in the cell, but it may be that they occur outside the cells also, in which case they are indistinguishable or very nearly so. The difficulty of cultivating such forms can be readily understood. As stated in an article now in press, these "elementary bodies" are probably for the most part non-cultivable and they may constitute the active infectious agent, the so-called "virus," while the rod forms which are cultivable occur only rarely. In a word the organism when developing in the tissues may occur in a different form than when growing on artificial culture media. The supposition offers an explanation of the difficulty of cultivating the organism unless large amounts of material are used, in which the chances of encountering the definite rod forms are increased.

IDA A. BENGTSON

NATIONAL INSTITUTE OF HEALTH
U. S. PUBLIC HEALTH SERVICE

[4] P. K. Olitsky, J. T. Syverton and J. R. Tyler, SCIENCE, 77: 24, January 6, 1933.

[5] Ida A. Bengtson, *Pub. Health Rep.*, 43: 2210, 1928; *Amer. Jour. Ophth.*, 12: 637, 1929.

[6] J. Taborisky, *Graefe's Arch. f. Ophth.*, 124: 453, 1930.

## THE ACTION-CURRENT AS MEASURE OF MUSCLE CONTRACTION

IT has been considered impossible to show a definite quantitative variation of the action-current with the contraction of human muscle. Upon contraction the oscillations of the oscillographic curve, which are always running even with resting muscle, coarsen and widen, but it is impossible to correlate changes of frequency or changes of amplitude with the degree of contraction, for the good reason that the oscillations during the contraction have no definite frequency and no definite amplitude; detailed study of the curve shows that the oscillations are extremely irregular. A significant measure of the action-current during contraction must be in terms of a summation of the current.

The planimeter measure of the area generated by the oscillographic curve during the contraction-disturbance is possible; but the method is tedious and inaccurate. But the summation of the action-current disturbances by a ballistic galvanometer is convenient and accurate; the action-currents have only to be amplified without distortion, rectified and photographically recorded.

An adequate method of measuring the action-currents from the muscle contraction is the less difficult part of the problem. There must also be some measure of the force of the contracting muscle. The group of muscle fibers must be isolated so that the contraction has a definite beginning and end in time; and the force that they exert must be measured in terms of some simple physical result. If the contraction is opposed by antagonistic muscles excess heat will be developed which it is impossible to measure.

The type of movement known as "ballistic," and familiar in many forms of skilled movement, like piano-playing and typing, can be made to fill these conditions. In the free (or "loose") movement of a skilled pianist, the flexor group actuates the forearm by a sudden pulse which has a uniform duration of about 45 sig.; it is quite unopposed by the extensors and sets the limb in motion with a very rapid acceleration, whereafter for three fourths of the stroke the limb swings free by momentum with a uniform velocity which is easily measurable; under proper conditions the length of the stroke varies with the velocity. It is easy to check such movements from the kymograph tracing; during the momentum phase the tracing is a right line which can easily be tested with a straight-edge; in a series of such strokes the ratio of the velocity to the length of stroke is fixed if they are ballistic. A skilled pianist can make such free and ballistic movements eight out of ten times.

Since the mass of the moving limb is constant and the path of the excursion can be made constant, the velocity of the ballistic movements becomes a measure of the varying force of the contractions. For the success of the study we found the choice of skilled pianists as subjects a vital point. The upper-arm was fixated so that the elbow joint was maintained in the same position to make the path of the excursion constant. The forearm was carefully supported so that a free, horizontal movement could be repeated without any influence of gravity, and the movements were recorded on a kymograph.

Electrodes of Ag or Zn shaped to fit the surface, wrapped in muslin wet with NaCl solution, were bound firmly with adhesive tape to the arm over the respective muscles. Under these conditions a series of movements were recorded and the corresponding contractions were registered from the ballistic galvanometer.

An actual series of strokes gave the ratios of excursion to velocity: .28, .26, .31, .31, *.23*, *.24*, .31, .28, *.35*, .26, .32. It is apparent that the fifth, sixth and tenth strokes are not free; and a check of the kymograph tracing with straight-edge confirms this. If the summated action-currents vary with the velocity, the ratio of velocity to action current should be fixed; the actual values in this case were: 1.0, 1.2, 1.1, 1.2, *1.7*, *2.0*, 1.4, 1.2, *0.9*, 1.1, 1.1. With the exception of the tense strokes, fifth, sixth, tenth, the values vary within 10 per cent., which is significant in physiological measurement.

When movements of this type occur against a fixed external tension, it was found possible to fit the results to an equation in which a constant (a) multiplied by the excursion plus a constant (b) is equal to the action-current (a Exc. + b = Ac. cur.). This indicates that a constant number of fibers is employed in overcoming the fixed resistance.

If a to-and-fro movement of this form is repeated in series in which both the beat-stroke and back-stroke are ballistic, the results are much more precise. A series of 25 movements with 3-inch excursion, a series of 25 with 5-inch excursion and a series of 25 with 7-inch excursion, all over the same path and at the same rate per sec., were recorded on the kymograph. In such series all the force exerted by the contraction of the flexor group of fibers and of the extensor group of fibers appears in the momentum of the to-and-fro movements; and the momentum varies directly with the length of excursion.

Parallel records were made by a ballistic galvanometer of the summated action-currents of the flexors and by a second ballistic galvanometer of the summated action-currents of the extensors. The sum of the summated flexor- and extensor-action-currents should be proportional to the length of excursion of the respective series of movements (which is an indicator of the force exerted). Thus in an actual case, the readings show a series of 2-in. excursion with a ratio to the sum of the action-currents of .86, and a series of 5-in. with a ratio of .86, and a series of 7-in. with a ratio of .83. When repeated in reverse order, the series give ratios: .83, .86, .85.

It is easy to make an ocular demonstration of this quantitative relation between action-current and muscle contraction by sending the amplified, rectified action-currents from rapid to-and-fro movements through a milliameter or a level indicator; the oscillating pointer will indicate a middle point for the series of contractions from a series of horizontal ballistic movements. The one important thing is to have a skilled pianist as subject capable of making the free ballistic movements. If the rate per sec. of the movements, as well as the path, is fixed, it is easy to see the shift of this middle point of oscillation of the indicator pointer with each change in length of excursion of the movement series, and approximate readings may be made to show the proportionality.

If the subject increases the rate per sec. of such a series of ballistic movements, the readings of the level indicator show some interesting relations. As the subject approaches his maximum rate, the amount of action-current indicated reaches a maximum; apparently the muscles are exerting their maximum force; from that stage on the increase in rate per sec. reduces the excursion proportionally. The maximum rate per sec. is achieved with the minimum excursion; in the final stage the excursion is very slight and the coordination is irregular and a "forced tremor" supervenes.

It is evident that there is a maximum number of available fibers for a given movement and when that number is in action the increase of rate of the repeated movement depends on reducing the excursion so that the flexor and extensor groups of fibers can each take up the momentum in reversing the movement of the limb; at last the coordination breaks down, the movements are irregular and a forced tremor is the result.

These results were obtained repeatedly with some four subjects. The maximum rate differs somewhat from subject to subject, but there are no essential differences in the quantitative relations of action-current and contraction. It is obvious that the findings fit the all-or-none hypothesis for the contraction of human muscle fibers.

R. H. STETSON
H. D. BOUMAN

PSYCHOLOGICAL LABORATORY
OBERLIN COLLEGE

## CHEMICAL VERSUS MORPHOLOGICAL SPECIES DIFFERENCES

THE writer has had the opportunity to make analyses of the sap of plants of the genus *Valonia* from many localities. Under current classification based upon morphology, these plants are referable to three or four different species. But, as has already been pointed out in the case of plants classed as *Halicystis ovalis* (Lyng.) Areschoug, chemical differences contravene morphological characteristics.[1] These chemical distinctions have since been utilized in segregating part of the genus *Halicystis* as a new species.[2]

Table I shows the relevant data in the case of genus *Valonia*. The new analyses in this table were made by the following methods: Halide was determined by titration with silver nitrate; it consists predominantly of chloride. K + Na was determined as total sulfate, K as chlorplatinate and Na by dif-

TABLE I

CHEMICAL CHARACTERISTICS AND ENVIRONMENTAL DATA FOR VARIOUS REPUTED SPECIES OF VALONIA

| Reputed species | Locality | Habitat | Depth | Water temperatures* | Composition of sap | | | | Condition of materials | Authority (See footnotes) |
|---|---|---|---|---|---|---|---|---|---|---|
| | | | | | K | Na | Cl | K/Na | | |
| | | | m | °C. | | | | | | |
| Valonia utricularis | Naples | On rocks | 0 | ? | 368 | 20.4 | 369 | (18.0) | = – | 4 |
| | " | " " | 0 | ? | 291 | 152 | 418 | 1.91 | = – | 5 |
| | " | " " | 0 | 18° | 372 | 266 | 639 | 1.43 | Fair (March) | – |
| V. macrophysa | Naples | On tunicates | 30 | 12° | 465 | 164 | 657 | 2.77 | Good (February) | – |
| | Dry Tortugas, Fla. | On masonry | 0 | 28° | 494 | 97 | 617 | 5.10 | Good (June) | 6 |
| | Bermuda | On coral rocks | 0 | 25° | 517 | 90 | 597 | 5.73 | – | 7 |
| V. ventricosa | Makahaa, Tonga | Under rocks | 0.3 | 25° | 497 | 125 | 619 | 3.97 | Excellent (Sept.) | – |
| | Main shore, Tonga | On sea weeds | 1.0 | 25° | 545 | 55 | 620 | 9.92 | " " | – |
| | Dry Tortugas, Fla. | Under rocks | 0.3 | 28° | 562 | 46 | 618 | 12.21 | " (June) | – |

* Water temperatures are only rough approximations.
+ Mean of four controls.

[1] S. C. Brooks, *Proc. Soc. Exp. Biol. Med.*, 27: 409–12, 1930.
[2] L. R. Blinks and A. H. Blinks, *Bull. Torrey Bot. Club*, 57: 389–95, 1930.
[3] A. Meyer, *Ber. Deutsche Bot. Ges.*, 9: 77–9, 1891.
[4] S. Camlong and L. Genevois, *Bull. Sta. Biol. Arcachon.*, 27: 309–21, 1930.
[5] E. Pantanelli, *Bull. Orto Bot. R. Univ. Napoli*, 6: 1–37, 1918.
[6] S. C. Brooks, *Protoplasma*, 8: 389–412, 1929.
[7] W. J. V. Osterhout, *Jour. Gen. Physiol.*, 5: 225–30, 1922.

ference. Data as to habitat, depth, and water temperature are germane, because of their possible physiological effects on different representatives of a single species. All plants were freshly gathered, and in good condition, except as noted.

The data relating to *Valonia utricularis* show that in this species there is relatively little selective accumulation of potassium: this species stands at the bottom of the list in so far as selective permeability is concerned. Meyer[3] regards his data as probably inaccurate, and this is almost surely the case with regard to the value for Na. All three analyses refer to plants from the same vicinity, and some seasonal differences are to be expected, as Camlong and Genevois have shown in the case of other marine algae.[4]

Plants usually referred to *V. macrophysa* Kütz have been collected for analysis from three stations: Naples, Bermuda and the Dry Tortugas Keys of Florida. The plants from the Golfo di Pozzuoli near Naples, where they grow at a depth of about 30 m, attached to tunicates, show less power of selective accumulation than do plants supposedly of the same species, which grow attached to rocks in shallow water in Bermuda and Florida. The former grew at a temperature which at the time of collection (January) was not far from 12°, while the latter were flourishing at a water temperature of about 28°. Some suggestion of a morphological difference is apparent, although Professor W. R. Taylor has been unable after careful study to find any certain difference. Yet in Florida the ratio of K to Na is about 5, while near Naples it is about 2.75. Other collections at Naples showed some variation from this figure, but the ratio of K to Na did not in any case exceed 3.17. The Bermuda plants resemble the Florida plants in all respects.

Are we here dealing with physiological variants, or with distinct valid species? If the habitats of the two types could be interchanged would their physicochemical characteristics change too!

The plants classed in the table as *V. ventricosa* present a still more puzzling situation. The two samples from Tonga tentatively assigned to this species may very well in one of the two cases be *V. forbesii* J. G. Aghard. Morphological characters said to distinguish the two species are most unsatisfactory, and field identification was impossible. Professor W. A. Setchell has kindly examined specimens of the Makahaa collection, and tentatively assigns them to *V. ventricosa*. The habitat of the plants collected at Makahaa was like that of *V. ventricosa* in the Dry Tortugas of Florida: under coral rocks on sand in about one foot of water or less at low tide. The plants along the main shore reef of Tonga grew on and among other algae in considerably deeper water. Yet the sap of these latter plants was like that of Florida specimens of *V. ventricosa,* while that of the former was much more like that of *V. macrophysa* Kütz from Florida and Bermuda.

These facts lead us to inquire whether physicochemical characteristics which are quantitatively well defined may not be valuable aids to the systematist. In some cases it is possible that environmental factors alone have produced the chemical differences noted. Yet it hardly seems likely that this is ordinarily the true explanation, any more than that it is the true explanation of morphological differences. Further study may well make chemical analysis an indispensable tool for the systematist.

My sincere thanks for their courteous generosity are due to the director and staff of the Stazione Zoologica at Naples, where part of this work was done, and to Columbia University and the Woods Hole Marine Biological Laboratory for granting me the use of the table supported by them. Different phases of the work were made possible by grants from the National Research Council, the Bache Fund of the National Academy of Sciences, which made it possible for Mrs. M. M. Brooks to collect samples for me at Tonga, and from the Board of Research of the University of California. For all these I wish to express my thanks.

S. C. BROOKS

DEPARTMENT OF ZOOLOGY
UNIVERSITY OF CALIFORNIA

## BOOKS RECEIVED

ALTER, DINSMORE. *Introduction to Practical Astronomy.* Pp. viii + 136. Crowell. $2.00.

EDDINGTON, SIR ARTHUR. *The Expanding Universe.* Pp. viii + 182. Macmillan. $2.00.

FALK, I. S. *Organized Medical Service at Fort Benning, Georgia.* Pp. x + 125. Publication of the Committee on the Costs of Medical Care: No. 21. University of Chicago Press. $.90.

FREUDENBERG, K. *Stereochemie, 7.* Lieferung. Pp. 157. Franz Deuticke, Wien. M. 18.

GUILD, C. ST. C. *Surveys of The Medical Facilities in Three Representative Southern Counties.* Pp. xvii + 179. 9 figures. Publication of The Committee on the Costs of Medical Care: No. 23. University of Chicago Press. $1.00.

HALE, HERBERT M., Editor. *Records of the South Australian Museum.* Vol. IV, No. 4. Pp. 161. Illustrated. Public Library, Museum and Art Gallery of South Australia, Adelaide.

HUXLEY, JULIAN and others. *Science in the Changing World.* Edited by Mary Adams. Pp. 286. Century. $2.00.

LEVEN, MAURICE. *The Incomes of Physicians.* Pp. ix + 141. Publication of The Committee on the Costs of Medical Care: No. 24. University of Chicago Press. $2.00.

MATTHEWS, BRYAN H. C. *Electricity in Our Bodies.* Pp. 108. 19 figures. George Allen and Unwin, London. 4s. 6d.

TÔHOKU IMPERIAL UNIVERSITY: *Science Reports.* Vol. XXI, No. 5. (Mathematics, Physics, Chemistry.) Pp. 208. Illustrated. Maruzen, Tokyo.

# SCIENCE

VOL. 77 FRIDAY, MARCH 3, 1933 No. 1992

*The Spontaneous Heating and Ignition of Hay and Other Agricultural Products:* DR. C. A. BROWNE 223

*Bread Quality of Wheat Produced in Aqueous Culture Media:* DR. W. F. GERICKE 229

*Obituary:*
*Recent Deaths* 232

*Scientific Events:*
*The School of Medicine of Rosario; Australian Fossils for the Harvard Museum; Administration of the Boulder Dam Project Area; New Pharmacopoeial Vitamin Advisory Board; The Washington Meeting of the American Chemical Society* 232

*Scientific Notes and News* 235

*Discussion:*
*Is it "Fair to Say that Hookworm Disease has almost Disappeared from the United States?":* DR. CH. WARDELL STILES. *Can a Publication be Camouflaged?:* DR. NEIL E. STEVENS. *The Age of Meteor Crater:* F. MARTIN BROWN. *Thorndike's Proof of the Law of Effect:* PROFESSOR R. M. OGDEN. *The Earliest Dated Dwelling in the United States:* DR. HAROLD S. COLTON 238

*Scientific Apparatus and Laboratory Methods:*
*A Home-made Electrically-driven Psychrometer:* J. F. TOWNSEND. *The Current Rotor:* DR. PAUL S. GALTSOFF and LOUELLA E. CABLE 242

*Science News* 8

SCIENCE: A Weekly Journal devoted to the Advancement of Science, edited by J. MCKEEN CATTELL and published every Friday by

THE SCIENCE PRESS

New York City: Grand Central Terminal
Lancaster, Pa. Garrison, N. Y.
Annual Subscription, $6.00 Single Copies, 15 Cts.

SCIENCE is the official organ of the American Association for the Advancement of Science. Information regarding membership in the Association may be secured from the office of the permanent secretary, in the Smithsonian Institution Building, Washington, D. C.

## THE SPONTANEOUS HEATING AND IGNITION OF HAY AND OTHER AGRICULTURAL PRODUCTS[1]

By Dr. C. A. BROWNE

U. S. BUREAU OF CHEMISTRY AND SOILS

THE production of heat, as a manifestation of vital activities, was associated at first almost entirely with the processes of animal life. This is not surprising when we consider the effect of the transpiration of large quantities of water from the immense leaf surfaces of growing plants which tends to keep their temperatures below that of the surrounding air.

The original observation of Lamarck[2] in 1777 that the fleshy spike or spadix of the flowers of *Arum maculatum* at a certain stage of growth was perceptibly warm to the touch first called the attention of scientific men to the heat-producing power of growing plants. Senebier[3] in 1800 confirmed this observation of Lamarck and at the same time noted the additional fact that this production of heat was especially pronounced in the presence of oxygen. The connection of this observation with the familiar oxygen respiration of animals was indicated later by the experiments of Saussure[4] in 1822, since which time the validity of a true respiration process by plants, in which oxygen is consumed and carbon dioxide evolved, has been universally recognized.

The intensity of this heat production by plants and its relation to oxygen consumption were examined by other investigators in succeeding years. In experiments by Kraus[5] in 1882 upon the spadix of flowers of *Arum italicum* a maximum temperature of 44.7° C.

[1] Address of the vice-president and retiring chairman of Section C—Chemistry, American Association for the Advancement of Science, Atlantic City, December, 1932.

[2] Lamarck, "Flora française." 1777.

[3] Senebier, "Physiol. végétale," III, 314. 1800.

[4] Saussure, *Ann. Sci. Nat.*, 21, 285, 1822; *Ann. Chim. et Phys.* (2), 21, 279, 1822.

[5] Kraus, *Abhandl. Naturf. Gesell. Halle*, 16, 1882.

was observed. During the production of this heat large quantities of carbon dioxide were evolved, and in a few hours a third or more of the dry substance of the spike (consisting of reserves of starch and sugar) was consumed.

If transpiration and the radiation of heat are retarded, as when the organs of plants are heaped together in large piles, the production of heat by vegetable cells becomes very apparent. The production of heat in piles of grain and in heaps of grass was probably observed by man in prehistoric times. It was also observed at a very early period that under certain conditions some plant materials, as hay or straw, might undergo so great an increase of temperature during spontaneous heating as to burst into flames. In later times, when men began to speculate as to the cause of things, the phenomenon of the spontaneous heating and ignition of plant materials was ascribed to the presence of an occluded fire or heat, and this explanation was retained by Bacon,[6] Boerhaave[7] and other philosophers until comparatively modern times.

The German botanist Goeppert[8] showed in 1830 that when a mass of barley grains was allowed to germinate in a wooden box, temperatures as high as 50° C. might be obtained. He did not differentiate, however, between the heat evolved by the respiration of the sprouting grain and that developed by the vital processes of adhering micro-organisms. This distinction was first clearly demonstrated by Cohn,[9] a plant physiologist of Breslau, who showed in 1890 that the first production of heat by the respiration of germinating seeds came to an end at about 40° C., which coincided with the thermal death point of the young plants. Cohn then observed after a short pause a second rise of temperature to about 65° C., which he attributed to the vital processes of thermogenic micro-organisms.

The maximum temperature observed in the most carefully controlled experiments upon the heating of plant materials by biological agencies does not usually exceed 70° C., which is about the thermal death point of most vegetating micro-organisms. This is some 160° C. lower than the temperature necessary for the ignition of hay, and the problem which has perplexed scientific men for so long is how to explain the great increase in temperature between the death point of the thermogenic micro-organisms and the point of spontaneous ignition.

6 Bacon, "Novum Organum." Translated by P. Shaw, 2 v. London. 1802.

7 Boerhaave, "A New Method of Chemistry." Translated from the printed edition by P. Shaw and E. Chambers. London. 1727.

8 Goeppert, "Ueber die Wärme-Entwickelung in den Pflanzen." 272 pp. Breslau. 1830.

9 Cohn, "Ueber Wärme-Erzeugung durch Schimmelpilze und Bakterien." Jahrg. Schles. Gesell., 68: 23–29. Breslau. 1890.

There have accumulated during the past fifty years many detailed accounts, by careful observers, of the visible phenomena of the spontaneous ignition of hay. These accounts all largely agree as to the main facts, so that the one specific instance which we have selected will be sufficient for general purposes of illustration. This typical case, related in *Liebig's Annalen* in 1873 by the German agricultural chemist Ranke,[10] is of classic interest, for its publication acted as a stimulus in drawing the attention of scientific men for the first time to a careful study of the complicated problem of the spontaneous ignition of hay.

A partial translation (by the author) of Ranke's original article is as follows:

On my estate Laufzorn, which is situated south of Munich about four hours by post near the Grünwald forest, a burning odor was observed on the morning of October 19, 1872, in the west corner of a large massively constructed barn.

In this section of the barn was stored a part of a crop of rowen that had been harvested upon the estate and unloaded in two adjacent piles, one of which contained about 22½ tons and the other about 15 tons.

This rowen had all been harvested in apparently well dried condition during excellent weather between the 5th and 10th of August. During the whole of September there was noticeable only the customary strongly aromatic odor of hay which increased in intensity until finally on the 17th and 18th of October a perceptible burnt odor began to be noticed. This empyreumatic burnt odor had become so strong on Saturday morning, October 19, that my manager was convinced the interior of the mow had caught fire. He determined at once to remove the hay as carefully as possible and in case fire should be discovered to extinguish it with a large quantity of water.

All available buckets, casks and other containers were accordingly filled with water upon the scaffold of the barn above the rowen and at 10: 30 A. M. the removal of the hay was very carefully commenced. . . .

As the removal now began to be pushed more vigorously from the top there were suddenly observed at a depth of about 5 feet several sparks. At the same time smoke and flashes of sparks were suddenly observed on one of the wagons, upon which the latest removed portions of rowen were being hauled from the barn. This was about 1: 30 P. M.

The entire mow and the loaded wagon were now drenched with water. The rowen that was now being hauled out was of a deep brown color and was spread out upon the grass near a pond situated behind the barn.

From now on the removal of rowen could be performed only with constant drenching with water, since almost every forkful as soon as it was taken out began to glow. It was also frequently necessary to pour water again upon the material which had been loaded since even the boards of the wagon repeatedly broke into flames. Even the rowen that had been spread out on the grass near

10 Ranke, "Experimenteller Beweis der Möglichkeit der Selbstentzündung des Heues." *Liebig's Ann. Chem. und Pharm.*, 167: 361–8. 1873.

the pond reignited repeatedly, so that it had to be extinguished three times. The material outside in the open broke out into actual flames, which was prevented inside the barn by the constant energetic drenching with water. It might be mentioned in this connection that on the following day the grass sod, upon which the removed rowen had been spread, was found to be completely burned. . . .

Finally after it had become dark the work of removing the burning material from the barn was completed. The burnt mass formed, as it were, the core of the pile and was estimated to have a diameter of about 11 feet at the top; it extended downwards to about 1½ feet from the floor where the diameter of the hot portion, however, had narrowed down to about 4 to 5 feet. The burned area extended backwards to within about 1½ feet from the rear wall of the barn.

The condition of the burnt mass was that of an actual carbon with a retention, however, of its original structure. The form of every spear of grass and of every flower could be plainly recognized. If this grass carbon was rubbed upon paper, the latter was colored black.

Ranke, acting upon a suggestion by Professor Buchner,[11] of the University of Munich, attributed the repeated spontaneous ignition of his hay to the strong absorptive power of the hay charcoal for atmospheric oxygen.

The pyrophoric carbon theory of Ranke was at once confronted with a serious objection, which was the difficulty of explaining the origin of the heat that is necessary to raise the temperature of the hay to the point of carbonization. When a pile of green grass begins to heat, the incipient elevation of temperature is commonly attributed to the oxidation of sugars by the action of enzymes in the plant cells and in the adhering micro-organisms that produce fermentation. The life of the plant cells and of the micro-organisms is, however, destroyed before the temperature reaches 80° C., and the activity of the oxidizing enzymes can hardly be supposed to exceed 100° C., which is some 50° C. below the temperature at which hay begins to carbonize and some 130° C. below the temperature at which hay ordinarily ignites. It is the bridging over of these large unexplained gaps in the increase of temperature in a heating haystack that constitutes the real problem of its spontaneous ignition.

It is not possible in the limits of space at our disposal to describe all the theories which have been proposed to explain this difficulty. Laupper,[12] the well-known Swiss authority upon the spontaneous ignition of hay, supposes pyrophoric iron, and not pyrophoric carbon, to be the causative factor. Others have supposed spontaneously inflammable gases, such as phosphine, to be responsible for the ignition. It has been also supposed by some that there are two kinds of heat production, one due to vital causes at low temperatures and one due to chemical causes at high temperatures. This conception, however, is baseless, for the entire production of heat, from the first rise in temperature to the point of ignition, is due to the effects of chemical reactions; therefore scientifically no differentiation can be made between vital heat and chemical heat.

In order to explain how a heating haystack can catch fire the German bacteriologist Miehe[13] assumed that pyrophoric carbon can be formed at the comparatively low temperature of 70° or 80° C. The following passage is translated from his original article upon the subject:

I believe that carbonization may indeed take place even at this temperature, for it must be considered that the action continues for a considerable time, even for months. The hay undergoes so to speak a dry distillation, in which the elements of the organic compounds are rearranged; new volatile compounds of simpler composition are set free and the material remaining behind approaches more and more the composition of pure carbon. That oxidations still take place above 75° and 80° has already been indicated by the experiments of Schlösing and of Boekhout and DeVries. The carbon is of an extremely fine porous character, each cell retaining its structure. It is plausible to suppose that such carbon may condense oxygen in a manner similar to finely divided platinum (platinum sponge). It would then, perhaps similar to platinum sponge, acquire a strong oxidizing power and perform oxidations that would be possible normally only at a much higher temperature. It could exercise this oxidizing effect either upon itself or upon the absorbed easily oxidizable gases, such as hydrogen, phosphine, volatile hydrocarbons (methane, ethylene, etc.), that are produced by the slow distillation or decomposition of the organic constituents of the hay. Such oxidations might perhaps take place even in undisturbed piles of hay after a certain interval of time when the ingress of oxygen was limited. The temperature would then slowly increase. Or, as seems more probable, the oxidations would develop only when an abundance of oxygen can enter, or in other words when the pile is torn open or when air passages are created intentionally or unintentionally. In fact, it is the general consensus of opinion (see Medem and other writers) that ignition is only produced when free entrance is given to the air by the insertion of poles, construction of air pits, opening up of the stack, etc.

The assumption of Miehe that pyrophoric carbon is produced at low temperatures has been adopted by other students of the problem. The supposition, however, is hardly tenable, for there are many cases

11 Buchner, *Liebig's Ann. Chem. und Pharm.*, 167: 361. 1873.

12 Laupper, ''Die Neuesten Ergebnisse der Heubrandforschung,'' *Landw. Jahrb. Schweiz Jahrg.*, 34: 1–54. 1924.

13 Miehe, ''Die Selbsterhitzung des Heues. Eine biologische Studie.'' 127 pp. Jena. 1907.

recorded where spontaneous ignition of hay has taken place without any evidence of carbonization and indeed within only a few days after it has been stored away, whereas Miehe supposes that the action continues "for a considerable time, even for months."

In 1929 the author[14] suggested as a possible solution of the problem of spontaneous ignition the formation, by micro-organisms under anaerobic conditions, of unsaturated unstable intermediary compounds which, in the sudden exposure of the interior of the fermenting mass of hay to the air, absorb atmospheric oxygen with so much avidity that the temperature is rapidly raised not only above the death point of the micro-organisms but even to the point of ignition of the hay. This spontaneous ignition may take place almost instantly, as James, Bidwell and McKinney,[15] of the Department of Agriculture, have observed in the case of heating horse manure, or it may take place more slowly, according to the rapidity with which the outside air gains access to the hot pocket in the interior of the hay. In other words, the micro-organisms that produce the incipient fermentation of the hay by enzyme action or otherwise are responsible for the preparation of the mine that may, or may not, later be sprung with the spontaneous ignition of the mow or stack.

The splitting-off of water from the organic constituents of plants is one of the most common reactions attending the deterioration of agricultural products, and one effect of this change, of great importance in the study of the problem of spontaneous ignition, is the accumulation of residues of greater and greater calorific energy. The significance of this reaction in plant life and in fermentation was pointed out as far back as 1870 by the German chemist, Adolph Baeyer,[16] who in a very suggestive article published in the *Berichte* of the German Chemical Society may be said to have blazed the way to an understanding of some of the reactions that take place in the decomposition of plant materials by micro-organisms.

Baeyer supposed that as a first step in this decomposition the elements of water are stripped off from the sugar molecule with the formation of unstable intermediary products, which, by the readdition of water and in other ways, finally give rise to lactic acid, alcohol, carbon dioxide and the other end-products of fermentation. The splitting-off of water from the carbohydrate molecules results in the removal of H and OH groups from the carbon chains and in the formation of unsaturated intermediary compounds with carbon atoms that are united by double bonds. These compounds are of a very labile reactive character and by the subsequent readdition and reelimination of water pass through various modifications before the final end-products of the fermentation are reached.

Since the time of Baeyer's classical paper there have been almost innumerable speculations as to the nature of the intermediary compounds which are produced in the fermentation of sugars. Among the most plausible of the theories which have been proposed is the one of Wohl[17] and Neuberg[18] that the first compound produced by the stripping-off of water from the sugar molecule is an unsaturated intermediary substance that breaks down immediately into two molecules of an enolic form of methyl glyoxal as shown by the following equation:

1.

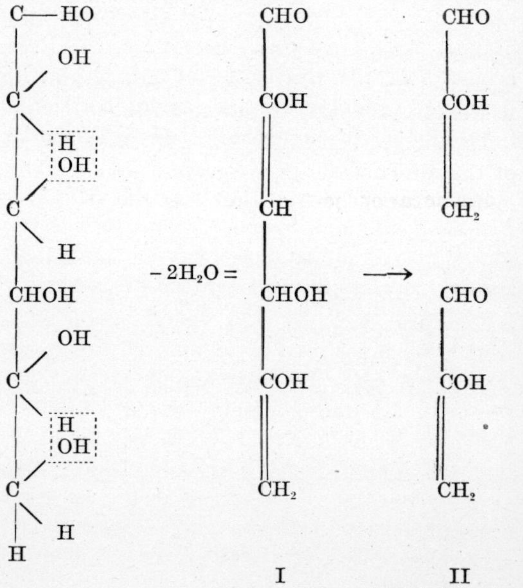


Sugar — I Intermediate — II 2 Mols. Methyl glyoxal enol

The unsaturated enolic form of methyl-glyoxal has not been isolated from fermentation mixtures, and it probably only exists momentarily. Methyl glyoxal itself ($CHO{-}CO{-}CH_3$) has, however, been detected in fermentation products, and this fact is a strong argument in favor of the Wohl-Neuberg theory of fermentation.

[14] Browne, "The Spontaneous Combustion of Hay." Tech. Bulletin No. 141, U. S. Dept. of Agriculture. September, 1929.

[15] James, Bidwell and McKinney, "An Observed Case of Spontaneous Ignition in Stable Manure." *Jour. Agr. Research*, 36: 481–5. 1928.

[16] Baeyer, "Ueber die Wasserentziehung und ihre Bedeutung für das Pflanzenleben und die Gährung." *Ber. Deutsch. Chemisch. Gesell.*, 3: 63–75. 1870.

[17] Wohl, "Die neue Anschauung über den chemischen Verlauf der alkoholischen Gärung." *Biochem. Zeits.*, 5, p. 45. 1907.

[18] Neuberg, "Zuckerumsatz der Pflanzenzelle." Handbuch der Biochemie, II Aufl. Bd. 2, Jena. 1925. For a full discussion of the Wohl-Neuberg and other theories regarding the fermentation of sugars see Oppenheimer's "Die Fermente," Bd. II, p. 1450, V Aufl. 1925.

A direct proof of the formation of unsaturated highly reactive enolic compounds in the decomposition of sugars has recently been furnished by Nelson and Browne,[19] of the Bureau of Chemistry and Soils, in the isolation of the so-called "glucic" acid

$$\begin{array}{c}\mathrm{COOH}\\ |\\ \mathrm{COH}\\ \|\\ \mathrm{CH_2}\end{array}$$

corresponding to the enolic form of methyl glyoxal. This acid is produced by the action of weak calcium hydroxide upon a dilute solution of glucose at 70° C. in the absence of air. The calcium salt of the acid deposits almost immediately; it absorbs oxygen from the air with the greatest avidity and with an intense evolution of heat. It is perhaps by the rapid oxidation of unsaturated highly reactive intermediary substances similar to this that the heat of a fermenting haystack is produced. In this connection it might be noted that Lange[20] has recently obtained evidence of the production by *B. coli* of an unsaturated very unstable highly oxidizable intermediary product, which is similar in some of its reactions to propiolic acid $CH \vdots C \cdot COOH$. It is possible that the acid detected by Lange is closely related to the glucic acid of Nelson and Browne.

The oxygen which is needed for the transformation of the intermediate unsaturated compound may come in part from the air; but it may also be supplied by the decomposition of water, in accordance with the simultaneous reduction-oxidation reactions which have been especially studied in Germany by Wieland.[21]

Tschirch[22] has proposed a modification of this reduction-oxidation theory to explain the spontaneous ignition of hay. He criticizes the hypothesis of the formation of pyrophoric carbon at 70° C., as suggested by Miehe, and as a substitute for this supposes that the ignition is due to the rapid evolution of oxygen from the organic constituents of the hay as a result of the action of reducing enzymes under anaerobic conditions. To quote from Tschirch's original article (author's translation):

If half-dried hay is packed tightly together in a thick layer, the most easily reacting oxydases are the first to become active. This first phase of the reaction is the first nondangerous stage that is associated with only a slight increase of temperature. It is an oxidation or combustion process that involves a consumption of oxygen. As soon as the oxygen is used up, however, the activity of the reductases sets in. They find points of attack in all the oxygen-containing constituents of the cell contents and cell membrane. . . . Cellulose, for example, contains 51 per cent. and aspartic acid 48 per cent. oxygen. The reduction process which advances rapidly with rising temperature is the second dangerous stage which sets in about 50°–70°. At these ranges of temperature the reductases apparently attain their optimum of activity. Very favorable conditions for their action exist especially in the interior of a haystack where all the oxygen is consumed by oxydases. The disintegration process reaches its maximum, therefore, in the interior of the haystack and can proceed here to complete carbonization, preceding which in a preliminary stage, there are first produced brown colored intermediary products, that still contain H and O, and which also constitute the basis for the color of "brown hay." The abundant supply of oxygen, that is suddenly made available in the reduction process within the firmly packed haystack, where no outlet is possible for the generated gas, leads finally as in so many other cases to an explosion, that is to say to a rapid combustion of the available carbon compounds, both those reduced as well as those still unreduced. The heat that is generated in the reduction process can not alone explain the ignition since this never mounts to the ignition temperature of cellulose. It is only the generation of oxygen and the occurrence of an explosion that explains satisfactorily the ignition.

The hypothesis of Tschirch has not met with general acceptance, principally for the reason pointed out by Hildebrandt[23] that the development of high temperatures in heating hay does not take place under the complete exclusion of the air, as would be expected if his explanation were correct, but only after atmospheric oxygen has gained access to the fermenting material.

There is not time, nor would it be altogether profitable in this connection, to discuss the possible rôle of the reductases, oxydases, peroxydases, catalases and other enzymes that are supposed to take part in the fermentation of plant materials. They play unquestionably a very important part in the chemical reactions which are involved in the spontaneous heating of plant materials, although not necessarily an indispensable part. The writer[24] described in 1929 a peculiar spontaneous decomposition of sugar cane molasses that was perfectly free from micro-organisms and enzymes, in which the sugars were gradually converted into dark-colored organic compounds of higher and higher carbon content. These changes, which are the result of obscure internal chemical reactions, can

19 Nelson and Browne, "The Properties and Chemical Constitution of Glucic Acid." *Jour. Am. Chem. Soc.*, 51, pp. 830–6. 1929.

20 Lange, "Production of an Unsaturated Compound by *B. coli* in a Synthetic Medium." *Proceedings* for the Soc. of Experimental Biology and Medicine, p. 1134. June, 1932.

21 Wieland, "Ueber den Mechanismus der Oxydations-Vorgänge." *Ber. Deut. Chem. Gesell.*, 45 (2606); 46 (3327); 47 (2085); etc. 1914, etc. For a full review of Wieland's theory see Oppenheimer's "Die Fermente," Bd. II, pp. 1283–95. 1925.

22 Tschirch, "Die Entzündung der Heustöcke." *Mitt. Naturf. Gesell. Bern*, pp. 133–137. 1917.

23 Hildebrandt, "Beiträge zur Frage der Selbsterwärmung des Heues," *Zentbl. Bakt.*, (II) 71: 440–90. 1927.

24 Browne, "The Spontaneous Decomposition of Sugar Cane Molasses," *Ind. Eng. Chem.*, 21: 600–6. 1929.

be explained only upon the basis of a progressive splitting-off of water from the sugar molecules, similar to those which have been previously described. As a result of this continual stripping-off of hydrogen and hydroxyl groups, residues are left which under certain conditions release their energy almost explosively in the "hot room" of sugar factories with the evolution of acid vapors, carbon dioxide and other gaseous decomposition products. A very high temperature is developed, with the result that the molasses froths and boils over, being finally converted into a porous carbonaceous residue.

We have so far considered only the heat evolution which results from the rapid oxidation of the unsaturated compounds that are produced by the splitting-off of water from sugar molecules. A certain part of the celluloses and hemi-celluloses of hay is hydrolyzed into sugar in the initial stages of the fermentation process, and the sugar thus formed must be considered as sources of heat producton in addition to the sugar originally in the hay.

There are in the hay, however, large quantities of insoluble cellular materials, such as cellulose, lignin and pentosans, which are not hydrolyzed in this way, but which nevertheless undergo decomposition in the anaerobic fermentation of hay by the same process of splitting-off of water. Analytical determinations show that these cellular components of the hay undergo in the process of sweating a continual loss of oxygen and hydrogen in the form of water, with the accumulation of unsaturated residues that become richer and richer in carbon. As this decomposition progresses, the hay changes in color first to yellow, then to light brown (the color of the so-called brown hay), then to dark brown and finally to black, the product in the last state approaching the composition of the so-called hay carbon. It is not pure carbon, however, and contains only from 50 to 70 per cent. of carbon, according to the degree of alteration which the cellular substance of the hay has undergone.

It can now be readily seen that with the formation and accumulation of unsaturated residues under anaerobic conditions in the porous cellular materials of hay the accidental entrance of air into the interior of the stack may bring about such a rapid absorption of oxygen at the points of unsaturation that the temperature may be quickly raised to the point of ignition. The reaction is perfectly similar to the familiar spontaneous ignition of cotton whose fibers have been coated with thin layers of an unsaturated vegetable oil, such as that of linseed. It is not necessary, therefore, to assume with Miehe, and other students of the subject, that ignition takes place only as a result of the formation of pyrophoric carbon or, according to Laupper, with the formation of pyrophoric iron. The unsaturated highly reactive decomposition products in a fermenting haystack are produced at comparatively low temperatures far below those necessary for the production of pyrophoric carbon or pyrophoric iron. Many spontaneous ignitions of hay have occurred when there was no blackening of the material, such as would be produced as a result of carbonization. The traces of iron compounds in hay no doubt act as catalysts in the process of spontaneous ignition, similar to the action of traces of iron and cobalt compounds in the spontaneous ignition of an oily piece of cotton, but such iron can not be regarded as the fundamental cause of the ignition.

The exact coincidence of all the conditions necessary for the spontaneous ignition of hay is fortunately of infrequent occurrence. If the hay is too wet it will not ignite; if the hay is too dry it will not ferment. If there is a constant unimpeded circulation of air through the interstices of the hay, the unsaturated intermediate substances are oxidized as fast as they are formed and there is no accumulation of those easily decomposable residues which by their final almost instantaneous oxidation raise the temperature in a few minutes from 80° or 90° to the point of ignition of the hay. The opening up of a hot haymow is, therefore, a hazardous operation and should only be done when every precaution has been taken to extinguish the conflagration that may immediately break out, such as happened in the case narrated by Ranke and such as has happened in so many of the other cases that have come under observation. The first quenching of the outbreak of fire with water does not remove the danger. The unstable rapidly oxidizable residues are still there and, with the evaporation of the water from the hot hay, may ignite spontaneously again and again, as indicated by Ranke, whose description of the phenomenon has been repeatedly confirmed by other observers.

Statistics show that spontaneous ignition of hay occurs almost exclusively in large mows and stacks. The large stack not only creates a better insulation against radiation of heat from the inside and a slower penetration of atmospheric oxygen from the outside during the precursory period of anaerobic fermentation, but it also offers a more favorable opportunity for creating somewhere in the mass of material the exact conditions of moisture, temperature and oxygen penetration that are necessary for spontaneous ignition. When fermentation begins there is an immediate migration of moisture from the warmer to the cooler zones of the stack; a cool section that was previously dry enough to withstand fermentation may acquire by condensation sufficient moisture from a contiguous hot fermenting zone to become a good medium for the rapid development of micro-organisms. In this way a single load of undercured hay in the center of a large mass of well-cured hay may start fermentations throughout the whole mass of material. With the migration of these fermenting zones from point to point there may finally be found somewhere a zone having the optimum conditions of moisture, temperature and air supply that lead finally to ignition. If this necessary coincidence of optimum conditions does not obtain, the stack, after several months of fluctuating changes of temperature, begins to cool down, with perhaps an occasional sporadic elevation of temperature at isolated points. The impeded penetration of air prevents the accelerated oxidation of the unstable organic residues; these are only very slowly oxidized and when the stack has finally approached the temperature of the outside air, these once highly oxidizable complexes are so sufficiently stabilized that the stack may be opened up without danger.

While this sketch of the chemical processes involved in the spontaneous heating and spontaneous ignition of hay is probably in general correct, there are many details of the problem that must be worked out under carefully controlled quantitative conditions. We need observations upon the production of heat, consumption of oxygen and evolution of carbon dioxide, water, etc., by large masses of fermenting hay in a respiration calorimeter, for it is only in this way that we can determine how much of the heat is produced as a result of anaerobic reduction-oxidation reactions and how much is produced by atmospheric oxidation. We need more observations upon the elementary analysis and heats of combustion of hay at various stages of spontaneous heating. We need further research on the nature of the solid, liquid and gaseous organic compounds that are produced in both the anaerobic and aerobic fermentations of hay, particularly of those elusive intermediate compounds which are the most difficult of all to detect. We need more knowledge of the phenomena of moisture migration and heat transference in large masses of hay. We need also more exact information as to the temperatures of ignition of hay at different stages of the fermentation process. When fundamental knowledge upon these and other points has been acquired we shall be able to visualize more clearly the details of the complicated reactions that take place in the spontaneous heating and spontaneous ignition of hay and other agricultural products and to arrive at the best practical means for reducing the enormous economic losses from this cause.

# BREAD QUALITY OF WHEAT PRODUCED IN AQUEOUS CULTURE MEDIA

By Dr. W. F. GERICKE

LABORATORY OF PLANT NUTRITION, UNIVERSITY OF CALIFORNIA

AMONG the causes of differences in the bread properties of wheats, those related to the quality of their proteins are of much interest to cereal chemists. Quality in flour as affected by the character of protein appears to be a very definite entity when expressed by baker's marks, and while the loaf of bread is and perchance always will remain the ultimate criteria of quality, nevertheless the concept "quality of protein" is still an intangible term, lacking a precise chemical definition. The interested trades feel a real need for simple and reliable tests of protein quality, which apparently may vary from season to season in accordance with the vagaries of climate; consequently experiments were designed to attack the problem from another angle, namely, by the water culture method, whereby specific treatment could be accorded the material selected for milling and baking operations.

Wheat protein is supposed to be identical in chemical composition among varieties. The fact of differences in the character of bread due to protein would, in lieu of differences in quantity thereof, be accounted for by differences in its physical character. It is known that the physical state of colloid particles varies with the nature of the medium surrounding them, and as plant sap is a more or less concentrated salt solution, it appeared as not improbable that variation in the quality of wheat protein might reflect certain features of plant sap. The fact of variation in the concentration and composition of plant sap with cultural treatment and also the differences in physical character of starches derived from the same source also were suggestive as to the type of experiment required to throw more light on the protein problem.

To obtain such data, the writer grew wheat in aqueous culture media on a scale large enough to provide samples for milling and baking operations. The plants were grown in a series of tanks filled with water, over which a seed bed was mounted, and which permitted production of a crop in culture media that could be altered at will.

Full description of the technique of crop production in a water medium by mass planting will appear in due season. As a preliminary note, however, it may be stated that the essential features of the method consisted primarily of (1) a seed bed mounted over and in contact with a water surface, so that the crop could be planted by mere broadcast scattering of the seed and grown to maturity without further replanting; and (2) the use of "fertilizing units," a single bottle per tank containing all elements required for growth of plants in water which being once applied requires no further attention and thus eliminates much of the tedium associated with classical water culture experimentation. The seed bed consisted of poultry netting stretched tightly over the top of the tanks. Burlap placed on the netting furnished support for the seed sown thereon. A thin layer of sawdust covered the seed to maintain the required moisture conditions for germination. With the sprouting of the seed, the roots penetrated the burlap and extended into the water and the plants grew to maturity in place as seeded. The "fertilizing units" contained ten elements, of which those required in relatively large amounts were supplied by the ordinary grade of fertilizer applied to land and those required in small amounts were supplied from equally inexpensive sources. Ordinary tap water was used. From 800 to 1,400 grams of dry grain was grown per reservoir, having 25 square feet of seedbed. The maximum yield obtainable per 25 square feet of water surface has not been determined, but apparently is decidedly larger than can possibly be obtained per equal area of soil surface.

Three sets each of an array of seven varieties were grown, two in water, one in soil. Of the former, one was located under glass, the other in the open field. The soil set consisted of plats in the open field. All samples grown in liquid media received similar treatment up to the heading stage. When that state of development was obtained, the solution of each reservoir was drained, the fertilizing units removed and fresh water supplied. Then the treatment was altered: One reservoir out of every set of two received a new fertilizing unit, thus reproducing therein for the final growth period the same culture medium in which all samples were started. The other reservoir received no salts, the crop being allowed to grow to maturity in a nutrient-free medium. Thus the length of the period during which nutrients were available for absorption was made to differ. In the one case, the salt content of the mature plant was expected to be low, as no nutrients were available for absorption during the latter part of the growth period. In the other case, it was expected to be high because all elements were available in relatively large quantities throughout the entire growth period. The soil-grown crop received a very heavy application of $NaNO_3$ at approximately the same growth stage as that at which the crop grown in liquid medium had the nutrients removed. The conditions in regard to the supply of nutrients in the soil-grown crop were in essence similar to those of the crop grown in liquid medium which contained nutrients throughout the entire growth period of the plants, save as to amounts of nutrients available which were assumed to be less in the soil than in the liquid medium.

From an agronomic standpoint, yield is an important consideration in growing a crop for investigations dealing with the bread quality of wheat. In field culture, variation in yield may or may not reflect itself in the baking properties of the flour. However, as these experiments were not designed to show the conditions under which such correlations are obtained—or failed to be obtained—no consideration will be given to the physiological properties of the culture media in respect to their effects upon yields, save in one aspect. With all varieties grown in liquid media, both under glass and out of doors, larger yields of grain were obtained from the reservoirs that did not contain any nutrients during the latter part of the growth period, than were obtained from those which contained an abundance of nutrients throughout the entire growth period of the plants. These results, at first consideration somewhat surprising, are, however, in full accord with the observed facts of nature, namely, that for a considerable portion of their growth, many plants rooted in soil thrive in a media low or nearly depleted of available nutrients, granted of course that the supply was adequate during their early growth stage. This condition exists because plants have a higher rate of absorption of nutrients than the soil has of making nutrients available.

Analyses of the crops revealed that the percentage of water soluble and also total ash in the plants grown in the liquid media varied with the treatments, and was higher in the cultures where nutrients were available throughout the entire growing period than where they were absent during the latter part of the growth period. Likewise, the ash of the grain varied similarly with the treatments, but it was of decidedly lower value than that of the straw. The grain harvested from the reservoirs in which the supply of nutrients was not restricted was not so well filled as was that obtained from the reservoirs in which nutrients were restricted. The filling of the individual kernels in a head of wheat appears to be largely a matter of adequate production of carbohydrates by the plant and its translocation into the kernels. It appears, therefore, that the failure of the grain to fill properly was, in part, due to the excessive absorption of some of the inorganic nutrients, and the consequent effect in the restriction of the production of carbohydrates. Within limitation, the amount of carbohydrates in wheat plants appears to be inversely related to that of the absorption of inorganic elements, but whether this relation applied to all elements expressed as total ash or only certain ones thereof, was not deducible from the data. The percentage of ash of the patent flour also varied with the treatments, but it was of decidedly lower value than that of the grain, the range being 0.4 per cent. to 0.7 per cent.

Milling and baking operations were performed according to the directions of Standard Mills for their experimental laboratories. Apparently the yield of the various mill products of wheat was not altered by the treatments. Only patent flour was used for the baking tests and the bread produced therefrom showed decided differences in quality, both as to varieties and the cultural treatments employed.

The data obtained are as yet too fragmentary to indicate how the nature of plant sap affects the colloidal state of the proteins and starches. Apparently the ash content of flour throws no light on the matter. The ash content of the straw varied from 3.5 to 17 per cent. among varieties and treatments, and while the quality of the bread did not vary correspondingly with that of the ash, it was evident that some type of relation did exist.

It soon became apparent that, in order to clarify this relation, it was necessary to differentiate two fractions of the total amount of each element absorbed, one on which yield was dependent, and one on which it was not. The fact that yield of grain was not restricted by the absence of nutrients in the culture medium during the latter growth period of the wheat plants indicated the arrival of a stage in their development when the absorption of nutrients no longer had nutritional functions. This growth phase was not identical with all elements. Neither was it fixed for any element, as conditions which affected the rate of supply of nutrients during the early growth of plants affected the time of arrival of that period. The crop-yielding power of various increments of any element absorbed by plants from the culture media varied with the time of their absorption; those which were absorbed early possessing greater power than those absorbed late. Corresponding to this difference in yielding power, other differences in the properties of the absorbed nutrients may be assumed. Among these are composition and concentration of plant sap. While the amounts of nutrients absorbed at maturity do not give a true picture of these properties of sap during growth, nevertheless they do indicate the direction of possible fluctuations in these characters. It appears safe to assume that the concentration of the sap of plants due to the nutrients on which yield is dependent is less than that due to nutrients which can not function causatively. The absorption, occurring too late, becomes excess because of the brevity of time remaining for utilization. The quantity absorbed too late to function causatively is superimposed upon that which functions causatively with corresponding effect on concentration of the plant sap.

By precluding the absorption of nutrients during the latter growth phase of wheat, the relation of the crop-producing value of varying quantities of an element to that of yields of grain can be determined. With some qualification, this relation can be expressed as a straight line function for all elements. At no period of the development of wheat will the absence of either nitrogen or phosphorus in the culture medium preclude reproduction, and the magnitudes of yield become a given multiple of the quantities of either of these elements absorbed during the early growth phases of the plants. This straight line relation is contingent on sufficient time subsequent to the absorption of the quantities in question to permit the plants to elaborate the materials into the maximum amount of product possible which is defined by the lowest percentage of the element in the composition of the mature product. Absorption of these elements occurring too late in the life of wheat to effect yield reflects itself in the composition of the plants, and is expressed for the specific elements in question by the degree it exceeds the minimum percentage obtainable in the mature product. But in the case of iron, calcium or potassium, the relation is not so simple because the absence of any one of these elements at certain growth phases will preclude reproduction, even though their presence in the medium at a former growth phase had resulted in considerable vegetative development. Only after certain minimum quantities have been supplied to bring the plants to such a state of development that the first increment supplied thereafter will effect grain production, are yields proportional to varying amounts of the element absorbed.

It is inferred from these relations between yields and quantities of various elements required that the physical properties of the plant sap arising from the truly nutritive quantities of each of the elements absorbed does not vary save by those factors which are part and parcel of growth. Changes are features of growth. A definite type of reactions or characteristics prevails, or follows one after another, in the constitution of plant sap with the circumstances of growth. But the plant is always exposed to secular forces which may intensify or lessen the rate of changes of the components of the truly nutritive character of plant sap. Nutrients which can not function productively thus become the cause of variation of the physical properties of plant sap because they are superimposed on those which define the type.

Wheat varieties vary more or less markedly as to the amount of an element required per unit weight of grain produced. Furthermore, the ash content of their straws varies with the elements absorbed. Subtracting the amount of nutrients required for any measure of yield of any variety from that of its ash, one obtains a measure of the quantity of material which caused secular variation in the plant sap. Better bread was obtained from wheats having a relatively large excess of salts in the straw beyond the minimum required for the yield obtained than from those having none or only a small excess.

# OBITUARY

## RECENT DEATHS

CHARLES WILFORD COOK, professor of economic geology at the University of Michigan, died on February 17 at the age of fifty years. He had been connected with the department of geology for twenty-five years and was well known for his work in economic, and especially in oil, geology.

DR. CHARLES SPENCER WILLIAMSON, head of the department of internal medicine of the University of Illinois Medical College, Chicago, died on February 15 at the age of sixty years.

*Nature* reports the death of Lieutenant Colonel John Stephenson, known especially for his work on the oligochaetes, from 1912 to 1920 professor of biology and principal of the government college at Lahore, India, and later until 1929 lecturer in zoology at the University of Edinburgh.

PROFESSOR ALFRED SCHAARSCHMIDT, head of the Institute of Chemical Technology at the Technische Hochschule, Charlottenburg, has died at the age of forty-nine years.

THE death is announced of Dr. Johannes Schmidt, the biologist and oceanographer of Copenhagen.

# SCIENTIFIC EVENTS

## THE SCHOOL OF MEDICINE OF ROSARIO

A CORRESPONDENT of the *Journal* of the American Medical Association reports that the board of directors of the School of Medicine of Rosario, Buenos Aires, recently resigned because the directors have had some difficulties with the students. The new board of directors has expressed a wish to nullify many of the regulations made by the previous boards for the management of the school. The School of Medicine of Rosario is dependent on the University of Litoral. The university controls seven medical schools and also other scientific centers. One of those centers, the Escuela de Agronomía y Veterinaria of the province of Corrientes, has more teachers than students. As a result of the economic conditions, the government recently reduced the yearly allowance of the University of Litoral, which in turn reduced the allowances given to the medical schools and scientific centers under its control. The medical school of Rosario could have met this deficit by reducing some of its expenses. There are, for instance, three courses on the same subject (psychiatry); many other subjects which are not strictly of a university nature could have been discontinued. However, in order to economize, the salaries of the professors were reduced. Drs. Ruíz and Hug, directors of the institutes of anatomy and of pharmacology of the medical school of Rosario, whose contracts expired, refused to sign a new contract at a reduced salary. Then the board of directors decided to eliminate the course of pharmacology. However, the students and some professors opposed dropping the course and finally they decided to continue it. The vacancies left by Drs. Ruíz and Hug were reported so that applications for the positions could be made. The monthly salary to be given professors in those positions is 500 pesos ($130) as directors of the institution and 300 pesos ($78) as professors, making a total of 800 pesos ($280) a month. However, this amount is more theoretical than real, because, owing to taxes, the salary is reduced to 700 pesos ($182). The full time professors of the medical school of Rosario had 1,300 and 1,500 pesos ($338 and $390), respectively, for their monthly salary. By giving them only 700 pesos the school saves 1,500 pesos a month, although the full-time system is sacrificed. Those full-time professors have devoted the past ten or fifteen years to laboratory research and now they are compelled to practice medicine or do other things for a living, while their places are taken by others who have not had so much experience. There were five full-time professors in the medical schools of Argentina. By the elimination of these two there are now only three (Drs. Houssay, Lewis and Elizalde).

## AUSTRALIAN FOSSILS FOR THE HARVARD MUSEUM

THE largest and most complete specimen of a plesiosaur ever discovered in Australia is included in the collections made by William E. Schevill, assistant curator at the Harvard Museum of Comparative Zoology. Mr. Schevill returned in December from an 18-months expedition to Australia, and a preliminary investigation of his findings is now in progress.

The most important discovery, it is believed, is the skeleton of the plesiosaur. It is about two thirds complete, making possible for the first time an accurate reconstruction. Previous finds in Australia have been only fragments. The Harvard specimen is now being prepared for mounting, although it will be some months before it is ready for display.

The remains of various species of Plesiosaurus have been found previously in Europe and America, and the present finding of a more complete example of the Australian plesiosaur will make possible important comparisons. The Australian specimen is known as "Kronosaurus queenslandicus."

Previous specimens have been found in England, Germany, the United States—New Jersey, Kansas and Wyoming. In some American examples, stones of various sizes, from a quarter of an inch to 4 inches in diameter, were found in the position of the stomach, and are supposed to have been swallowed as aids to digestion. The fossil remains at Harvard are being carefully studied for evidence of similar feeding habits among the Australian species.

Mr. Schevill's find was located on the ranch of R. W. H. Thomas, near Richmond in northwestern Queensland, which was a submerged area during the Cretaceous period. In addition to this skeleton, he has brought back a large number of specimens, including not only fossils but also a series of present-day animals. The entire shipment was made in 95 cases, weighing in all eight tons.

The Australian collection has been made as part of the museum's program of obtaining field specimens from every section of the world. Many of these will be arranged in "systematic collections," showing graphically the history of evolution. The exhibition collections are used as a supplement to text-books by Harvard University students in courses on zoology and paleontology.

## ADMINISTRATION OF THE BOULDER DAM PROJECT AREA

The Secretary of the Interior, Dr. Ray Lyman Wilbur, on February 15 approved the bills for administration of the Boulder Canyon Project area, introduced by Senator Hayden, of Arizona, and Congressman Arentz, of Nevada. The Secretary says:

> Hoover Dam is now under construction and storage of the waters of the Colorado River in the immense reservoir to be created thereby will begin, probably, early in 1935.
>
> This largest artificial reservoir in the world possesses great recreational and educational possibilities which should be conserved. The bill provides for the efficient and economical accomplishment of the purpose by entrusting this responsibility to the National Park Service, while the Bureau of Reclamation administers the area so far as it has to do with the primary purposes of the original legislation. In this way the building up of duplicating organizations is avoided.
>
> The bill also determines the limits essential to the project and definitely establishes the reservations. It vacates withdrawals heretofore made and restores about 1,400,000 acres to entry.

No claim of exclusive federal jurisdiction is made as to the new reservation and Secretary Wilbur announces that none will be. Accordingly, the laws of Nevada and Arizona, including those as to schools, taxation and elections, will not be disturbed in the new reservation set up by the bill.

As to the smaller federal reservation, heretofore established by order of Secretary Wilbur, at Boulder City, the bill proposes that Nevada shall have full rights of taxation therein after construction of the dam is completed; that Nevada shall immediately have the right, in the Boulder City area, to collect a property tax for school purposes and a mining tax, and to conduct schools.

The Secretary states the department does not propose to submit any estimates of appropriations during the fiscal years 1933 and 1934 for recreational development.

Secretary Wilbur considers the bill very important and urges its enactment at this session of Congress. He says of it:

> The bill replaces uncertainty with certainty, solves numerous existing administrative difficulties, makes possible orderly planning for the future and provides fully for the interests of the United States and of adjacent communities as to the development and use of this highly important area.

## NEW PHARMACOPOEIAL VITAMIN ADVISORY BOARD

The Board of Trustees of the United States Pharmacopoeia has announced the appointment of a Pharmacopoeial Vitamin Advisory Board consisting of

Dr. Lafayette B. Mendel, Yale University.

Dr. H. C. Sherman, Columbia University.

Dr. E. M. Nelson, Protein and Nutrition Division, Bureau of Chemistry and Soils, U. S. Department of Agriculture.

E. F. Kelly, Baltimore, Maryland, representing the United States Pharmacopoeia Board of Trustees.

E. Fullerton Cook, Philadelphia, Pennsylvania, representing the United States Pharmacopoeia Committee of Revision.

The appointment of this board has been the outcome of several pharmacopoeial conferences, held in New York during the past year, attended by vitamin experts in the United States, who have recommended a revised standard for the vitamin A and vitamin D potency of the official cod-liver oil. The same group has approved assay methods for both vitamins and these assay methods are proposed for official adoption.

Fifteen vitamin laboratories in the United States, one in London and one in Norway are now determining the vitamin A and vitamin D potency of a special "Reference Cod-Liver Oil," supplied by the U. S. Bureau of Fisheries. This oil will be available in a few months for distribution by the United States Pharmacopoeial Vitamin Advisory Board. A nominal charge will be made for this "Reference Oil" which will have known vitamin A and vitamin D activity, expressed in International Units. This oil will be distributed through the office of the Chairman of the U. S. P. Vitamin Board to be addressed at 43d Street and Woodland Avenue, Philadelphia, Pa.

## THE WASHINGTON MEETING OF THE AMERICAN CHEMICAL SOCIETY

LEADERS of science and industry will address the eighty-fifth meeting of the American Chemical Society in Washington during the week beginning March 26. Seventeen of the professional divisions of the society, embracing every principal field of chemistry, will hold sessions. The history of chemistry will be traced in exhibits at the Library of Congress.

Researches presented by workers in the Federal Service will bring to the attention of the nation contributions to science made by the government departments. Numerous committees in the District of Columbia are making arrangements for an extensive program of inspection of federal laboratories and scientific services, the aim being to convey knowledge of the development of Washington as one of the great science centers of the world.

Many of the leading industries as well as universities, colleges and other institutions will send representatives. Dr. Irving Langmuir, associate director of the General Electric Company, will give a public address on "Surface Chemistry" in Constitution Hall, 18th and D Streets, N.W., on Wednesday, March 29, at 8:30 P. M.

The formal sessions will open with a general program on Monday, March 27, following a meeting of the directors of the society, at which Professor Arthur B. Lamb, of Harvard University, president, will preside. Speakers at this general session and their topics will include:

Charles F. Kettering, chief engineer of the General Motors Corporation, Detroit, "The Relation of Chemistry to the Individual"; Harry L. Derby, president of the American Cyanamid Company, New York, "The Relation of Chemistry to the State"; C. M. A. Stine, vice-president of E. I. du Pont de Nemours and Company, Inc., Wilmington, Delaware, "The Relation of Chemical to Other Industry"; Professor Hugh S. Taylor, head of the department of chemistry, Princeton University, "Chemistry—its Interrelations with Other Sciences."

Agriculture and food, petroleum, biological chemistry, chemical education, medicinal chemistry, rubber, sugar, dyes, industrial and engineering chemistry, organic, and physical and inorganic chemistry are among the general fields to be covered at sessions of the professional divisions. The Division of Chemical Education, of which Professor Lyman C. Newell, of Boston University, is chairman, plans a symposium on "Recent Developments in Various Chemical Industries." The purpose of this symposium is to acquaint the chemistry teachers of the country with industrial developments.

The Division of Biological Chemistry, of which Professor J. B. Brown, of the Ohio State University, is chairman, will hold a symposium on "Anemia"; the Division of Agricultural and Food Chemistry, headed by Professor H. A. Schuette, of the University of Wisconsin, one on "Insecticides."

The Division of Industrial and Engineering Chemistry, of which Professor D. B. Keyes, of the University of Illinois, is chairman, will hold a symposium on "Glass" in conjunction with the Glass Division of the American Ceramic Society.

The Division of Physical and Inorganic Chemistry, of which Professor W. A. Noyes, Jr., of Brown University, is chairman, will hold six sessions, including a symposium on "Electrolytes," under the chairmanship of Professor Victor K. LaMer, of Columbia University, and a symposium on "Analytical Chemistry," under the chairmanship of Professor N. H. Furman, of Princeton University. The Division of Petroleum Chemistry, headed by F. W. Sullivan, of Whiting, Indiana, is arranging for two sessions, one being devoted to a symposium on "Properties of Hydrocarbon Mixtures." Other divisional meetings are scheduled.

A demonstration of dust explosions has been arranged by the Division of Chemical Engineering, Bureau of Chemistry and Soils, for Thursday, March 30, at Arlington Farm. The demonstration, which will be in charge of D. J. Price, will show in miniature what takes place when organic dusts explode under various conditions met in industry and how the hazards from these dusts can be largely minimized.

Special events include a visit to Edgewood Arsenal, called "the chemists' contribution to national defense." There will be a demonstration of chemical warfare weapons by the First Chemical Regiment and of airplane dispersion of smoke by officers of the Air Corps.

# SCIENTIFIC NOTES AND NEWS

THE School of Mining of Leoben will confer an honorary degree in mining engineering on President Hoover for his services to mining and technology and for his literary work. It was planned to confer the degree on March 2 in the presence of representatives of the government and all the Austrian universities. The diploma was to be received by Gilchrist Baker Stockton, the United States Minister.

DR. WALLACE W. ATWOOD, president of Clark University, who was an American delegate to the Pan American Institute of History and Geology meeting in Rio de Janeiro, reached New York on February 22. After the meeting, which ended early in January, Dr. Atwood went to Peru and Bolivia, where he studied the highland country for Incan and pre-Incan archeological information. Dr. Atwood was elected president of the institute for the meeting to be held in Washington in 1935.

DR. JONATHAN C. MEAKINS, director of the department of medicine at McGill University, has been elected president of the American College of Physicians and Surgeons for 1934.

DR. CHARLES EDWARD MUNROE, chief chemist for explosives at the United States Bureau of Mines, emeritus professor of chemistry at George Washington University, has been appointed honorary chairman of the committee making plans for the Washington convention of the American Chemical Society, which opens on March 26. Dr. Munroe, who is now eighty-three years old, is the sole surviving charter member of the society, formed in 1876.

PROFESSOR THOMAS C. ESTY, from 1922 to 1929 dean of Amherst College and for many years a member of the department of mathematics, has been appointed by the trustees to be the first vice-president at the recommendation of President Stanley King. Professor Esty will exercise the power and carry on the work of the president in the absence of Dr. King.

DR. WILLARD E. HOTCHKISS, formerly dean of the Stanford Graduate School of Business, has been appointed president of the Armour Institute of Technology in Chicago.

DR. VICTOR GOLDSCHMIDT, professor of mineralogy at the University of Heidelberg, celebrated his eightieth birthday on February 10.

THE council of the Physical Society, London, has awarded the tenth Duddell Medal to Professor Wolfgang Gaede, director of the Kaiser Wilhelm Institute of Physics at Karlsruhe, for his work on the design and production of high vacuum pumps.

THE Royal Dublin Society has awarded the Boyle Medal to Dr. Paul A. Murphy, professor of plant pathology at University College, Dublin.

DR. AUSTIN F. ROGERS, professor of mineralogy at Stanford University, has been elected to membership in the Mineralogical Society of France.

AT Columbia University Dr. Arnold Knapp has been retired with the title of professor emeritus of ophthalmology. Dr. Howard B. Adelmann has been appointed assistant professor of anatomy; Dr. Karl Meyer, assistant professor of biological chemistry, and Dr. Richard Thompson, assistant professor of bacteriology.

DR. LEWIS R. HILL has been appointed professor of bacteriology at Loyola University School of Medicine, Chicago, succeeding Dr. Emil Weiss, who resigned recently because of ill health.

DR. PAUL BLUM has been nominated professor of therapeutic hydrology and climatology at Strasbourg, and Dr. Cristol, professor of biological chemistry at Montpellier, in succession to Dr. Derrien.

IT was announced in SCIENCE last week that Captain Charles L. Oman had been appointed surgeon-general of the U. S. Navy. This appointment, like others made by the outgoing administration, has not been confirmed by the Senate.

CAPTAIN WILLIAM CHAMBERS has been transferred from the division of planning, Bureau of Medicine and Surgery, U. S. Navy, Washington, D. C., to duty as director of the American Scientific Mission, Port au Prince, Haiti, succeeding Captain Montgomery O. Stuart.

D. L. VAN DINE, until recently an entomologist with the Tropical Research Foundation in Cuba, has been appointed head of the Division of Fruit and Shade Tree Insects of the Bureau of Entomology, U. S. Department of Agriculture. This appointment relieves Dr. C. L. Marlatt, chief of the bureau, of the direction of federal investigations on the insect enemies of fruit.

DR. R. VON IHERING has been commissioned by the Federal Government of Brazil to study the prospects of fish culture in the reservoirs of the arid regions of Northwest Brazil (frontier of the states from Piauhy to Bahia). Biologists interested in limnology will be given transportation facilities for the study of subjects correlated with fish culture. Candidates recommended by their instructors can address Dr. R. von Ihering, cidade de João Pessoa, Estado de Parahyba, Brazil.

DR. JAMES ANGUS DOULL, professor of hygiene and public health in the School of Medicine of Western

Reserve University, has leave of absence to organize an epidemiological study for the Leonard Wood Memorial for the Eradication of Leprosy. Dr. Doull will sail on March 25 from Vancouver for the Philippine Islands, and will be absent from Cleveland for about six months. He will initiate studies on the frequency of leprosy in relation to diet, age, living conditions, contact with previous cases and other factors. These and similar studies will be continued over some years in the Philippines and possibly in other parts of the world.

DR. VICTOR NEHER, of the California Institute of Technology, is on his way to Peru, to make a further study of cosmic rays. He plans to fly over the highest peaks of the Andes, using one of the regular transport planes of Pan American Airways System specially chartered to carry his equipment.

DR. ROY W. MINER, curator of marine life at the American Museum of Natural History, sailed on February 24 to gather additional data, including motion pictures, of the Great Reef of Andros Island. He was accompanied by Chris E. Olsen, as artist. The object of the expedition is to add to the knowledge of such reefs and to enhance the display of great Bahamas coral reefs now in the museum.

PROFESSOR WILLIAM H. SELLEW, assistant director of the department of engineering research of the University of Michigan, has sailed for Germany, for a conference with Professor Planke, of Karlsruhe, an authority on air-conditioning methods.

DR. ALICE H. FARNSWORTH, associate professor of astronomy at Mount Holyoke College, is spending her sabbatical leave for the remainder of the year at the Perkins Observatory, Delaware, Ohio, pursuing special studies in spectroscopic problems.

KARL P. SCHMIDT, assistant curator of reptiles at Field Museum of Natural History, has returned to his post at the museum after six months of research on type specimens of reptiles in European museums, carried on under a fellowship awarded to him by the John Simon Guggenheim Memorial Foundation of New York.

AT its recent meeting the Committee on Scientific Research of the American Medical Association made grants to Dr. Ernest Carroll Faust, professor of parasitology, department of tropical medicine, Tulane University of Louisiana, for continuing his investigations on human strongyloidosis; to Dr. W. T. Dawson, professor of pharmacology at the University of Texas, for further work on the relations between chemical constitution and toxicity of cinchona alkaloids; to Dr. Jessie L. King and Miss Ethel Soule, of Goucher College, Baltimore, to aid in a study of the effect of cortical extract on adrenalectomized rats, and to Dr. John Guttman, of New York City, to continue his research in the laboratories of the New York Post-Graduate Medical School of Columbia University on the electric current produced by sound in the auditory apparatus.

DR. L. H. ADAMS, of the Geophysical Laboratory of the Carnegie Institution, retiring president of the Washington Academy of Sciences, delivered on February 16 an address on "The Basic Concept of the Physical Sciences."

THE third Joseph Henry Lecture before the Philosophical Society of Washington will be given by President Karl T. Compton, of the Massachusetts Institute of Technology, in the auditorium of the Cosmos Club on the evening of March 11. The subject of the address will be "High Voltage."

DR. ARTHUR H. COMPTON, professor of physics at the University of Chicago, gave a lecture on "Cosmic Rays" on February 22, at the Brooklyn Academy of Music, under the auspices of the department of physics and the Proctor Foundation of the Brooklyn Institute of Arts and Sciences.

PROFESSOR EDWARD KASNER, of Columbia University, gave three public lectures in January and February before the People's Institute. The titles of these lectures were "Numbers and Infinity," "Spaces and Dimensionality," "Geometry and Physics."

PROFESSOR H. S. JACKSON, of the department of botany of the University of Toronto, gave the annual Darwin anniversary address under the auspices of the Botanical Seminar of Michigan State College on February 14. He spoke on "Some Life Cycles of the Rusts in Comparison with those of the Red Seaweeds."

DEAN FRANK C. WHITMORE, of the Pennsylvania State College, spoke before the Central Pennsylvania Section of the American Chemical Society on February 15 on "Some Unorthodox Organic Chemistry," and on the same subject on March 1 before the Kansas City Section of the American Chemical Society.

DR. HARLAN T. STETSON, director of the Perkins Observatory of Ohio Wesleyan University, addressed the Chicago Astronomical Society on February 8 at the Adler Planetarium, on "The Correlation of Solar Activity with Radio Transmission." On February 14 he lectured before the Rittenhouse Astronomical Society at the Franklin Institute, Philadelphia, on "Some Coming Problems of Cosmic Astronomy."

ON February 17 Dr. Arthur D. Little broadcast a ten-minute talk on "Industrial Research," this being one of the series of scientific talks sponsored by General Electric Company in recognition of the electrical industry's debt to scientific research. In the afternoon of the same day, he spoke before the weekly colloquium of the Research Laboratory at Schenectady on "Some Professional Experiences."

PROFESSOR AUGUSTE PICCARD, of the University of Brussels, gave a Norman Wait Harris lecture at Northwestern University on February 15 on "Exploring in the Stratosphere."

SIR WILLIAM B. HARDY, director of food investigation, department of scientific and industrial research, gave the Trueman Wood Memorial Lecture before the Royal Society of Arts on February 22, on "Industrial Research with Biological Material."

AT the fifteenth annual meeting of Edison Pioneers on February 11, the formation of an International Edison Foundation was announced. The foundation, which has not yet been incorporated, plans to provide fellowships in physics and chemistry in universities of the United States and other countries. American graduate students will be sent abroad and foreign students will be brought to the United States to continue their education in physics and chemistry. Dr. Arthur E. Kennelly, professor emeritus of electrical engineering at Harvard University and the Massachusetts Institute of Technology, is chairman of a committee of three appointed to confer on the fellowships.

RECENT action of the Rockefeller Foundation has approved a grant for two years, ending July 1, 1934, for a sum not to exceed $20,000 to supplement the funds of the Ohio Wesleyan University for the maintenance of the scientific program of the Perkins Observatory.

A GIFT of £500 from the Rockefeller Foundation has been made to the Molteno Institute of Parasitology of the University of Cambridge, for the purchase of instruments and for assistance in connection with investigations carried on by Professor Keilin.

ACCORDING to the *Journal* of the American Medical Association the Thomas W. Salmon Memorial Committee of the New York Academy of Medicine announces that small grants are available to physicians and others who are engaged in research work in the field of psychiatry, mental hygiene and child guidance. Workers who are interested in receiving such grants may apply to the committee, 2 East One Hundred and Third Street, New York.

# DISCUSSION

## IS IT "FAIR TO SAY THAT HOOKWORM DISEASE HAS ALMOST DISAPPEARED FROM THE UNITED STATES?"

### I. INTRODUCTION

SINCE 1930 I have motored about 10,000 miles through the Gulf-Atlantic states, chiefly in the sandland districts. These trips have given an opportunity to compare present conditions with those of the earlier years of the century and to converse with people of all walks of life.

A striking point in these conversations has been the number of persons who believe that hookworm disease has been eradicated from this country and who cite as authority newspaper reports allegedly based on statements attributed to the Rockefeller Foundation.

The Thirteenth Annual Report (1927—for 1926) of the International Health Board of the Rockefeller Foundation contains in fact (pp. 5–6) the following paragraph:

> The diseases that the Board has chosen for special attention have been world-wide in their distribution and of great economic importance. Field research in the epidemiology of hookworm disease has *advanced knowledge* concerning the life history of the hookworm, both in its free-living larval form and in its adult relationship to the host, so that we now have a much better understanding of the disease. This knowledge has enabled *governmental agencies* to *delimit* the field of control work and to modify the methods of treatment and of prevention to such an extent that the former *administrative methods of control have been revolutionized. The results have been extraordinarily successful.* At the present time *it is fair to say that hookworm disease has almost disappeared from the United States* and is rapidly coming under control in many parts of the world. But the *great achievement* is not the social and economic rehabilitation of the more than six or seven million people who have been treated for the disease during the past ten or fifteen years; it is the development of administrative measures that will prevent millions yet unborn from ever suffering from its ravages. (Original not in italics).

Until recently I had no idea that so many people had taken the Foundation's report seriously, but during these recent trips I had to combat it so frequently that I wrote to Mr. Rockefeller, Jr., placed before him evidence as to the wide distribution of the disease in the Southern states, offered to motor with a representative of his selection in order to collect additional data for him, and urged him to take steps to modify the claim published by the Foundation. My letters were referred to the directors of the International Health Division, but up to date no retraction or modification has come to my attention.

### II. ANALYSIS OF THE FOUNDATION'S CLAIM

The three essential points in the claim are:

(1) *Important discoveries in the biology of hook-*

*worm:* On pp. 62–72 are cited observations (regarding: 1 temperature, 2 moisture, 3 soil, 4 fermentation, 5 water in bulk, 6 salt) in connection with which the thought arises whether these are the points of "advanced knowledge"; at least, these are presented in a way that the reader (if not familiar with the literature on the subject) might easily conclude that they are new discoveries.

All six are repetitions (in new localities) of observations made 25 to 40 or more years ago.

(2) *Revolutionized administrative procedures in control:* On pp. 62–72 of the report are cited four control measures (1 shoes, 2 sanitation, 3 education, 4 treatment), but by no stretch of the imagination can these be called new. According to p. 62 of the report the egg-count method "has revolutionized administrative methods of control of the disease."

Accepting this as the basis of the "great achievement" mentioned on p. 6, the point may be raised that only two Southern states (Alabama and Tennessee) have published surveys based on this technique while officials of the Boards of Health of five Southern states have informed me that they do not use the egg-count method.

The word "delimit" (p. 6) together with the discussion (pp. 62–72) seems to indicate that the so-called "Alabama Plan" is part of the revolutionized method of control. The "Alabama Plan" was indeed revolutionary but it was short lived. It was tried out in a few counties and was promptly abandoned.

A practical question arises, namely: What "governmental agencies" applied these "extraordinarily successful" administrative methods in counties which have no health unit? Only county, state, and national health agencies come into consideration. Of the sixty-seven counties in a certain Southern State, only four have full-time units; neither the State Board of Health nor the U. S. Public Health Service applied revolutionary methods in the sixty-three other counties. It is estimated that less than five per cent. of the rural population of this particular state has whole-time local health service; who served the other ninety-five per cent.? Surely neither part-time health officers nor county physicians could accomplish the "great achievement" claimed by the Foundation.

(3) *"It is fair to say that hookworm disease has almost disappeared from the United States."* Rather definite information is available which, unfortunately and to my profound regret, does not square with this enthusiastic claim. See III.

### III. Hookworm Disease in the Gulf-Atlantic States

In a recent publication (1932) I have summarized the hookworm situation as follows.

(1) The extreme case known as the "dirt eater" is much more rare now than from 1902 to 1910. (I have seen less than fifty in the past two years.)

(2) In general, the cases are much lighter than when the work first began in 1902.

(3) The disease has been reduced both in intensity and somewhat in extent, but

(4) The job has not been completed.

The fundamental problem in hookworm control is not a question of bookkeeping or microscopic examinations, but requires a change in the daily habits of hundreds of thousands of rural whites, Indians, and negroes.

In studying the prevalence and importance of hookworm disease three methods are used according to circumstances and the individual preference of the workers:

(1) *Diagnostic microscopic examinations:* Through courtesy of the State Boards of Health I was able to summarize the results of 121,388 recent (1929) examinations in Alabama, Arkansas, Florida, Georgia, Kentucky, Mississippi, Tennessee, Virginia, and West Virginia; 34,131 of the specimens (or 28.1 per cent.) were "positive."

(2) *Egg-counts:* Otto and Cort,[2] two leading apostles of the egg-count technique, have summarized evidence gathered (in Virginia, Tennessee, Kentucky, Florida, and Alabama) by themselves and "by several members of the International Health Division" and they conclude that hookworm disease has not almost disappeared from this country.

Havens,[3] of the Alabama State Board of Health (and an apostle of the egg-count method), says that "in the southern counties of Alabama—hookworm control—still is a major public health problem."

(3) *Symptomatic inspection:* During a motor trip of 5,524 miles[4] with one assistant I examined 18,649 white children in 98 graded schools, using the method of rapid symptomatic inspection (in which my personal theoretical error is about 17 per cent. as checked by the "smear method"); 6,063 of these children (or 32.5 per cent.) showed symptoms in harmony with hookworm disease; deducting 20 per cent. as theoretical error, the corrected estimate is 26 per cent.

In five rural schools in one county, I have more recently examined 429 white pupils, 266 (or 62 per cent.) of whom showed symptoms in harmony with hookworm disease; deducting 20 per cent. as theoretical error, the corrected estimate is 49.6 per cent.

### IV. Summary

In view of the foregoing (and other) data I am constrained to take issue with the hookworm experts

[1] Public Health Reports, Aug. 1, 1930.
[2] *Jour. Amer. Med. Assn.*, July 11, 1931.
[3] *J. Med. Assn. Alabama*, Jan., 1933.
[4] *Southern Med. Journ.*, 1932, 189–192.

of 61 Broadway, and to submit that their claim is not "fair," in fact, it has done harm in certain localities.

V. CONCLUSION

Not only a scientific but also a great moral and humanitarian issue is involved. It is to be regretted that the Rockefeller Foundation has not complied with a duty it owes to the rural children of the South, to the scientific world, to itself and to Mr. Rockefeller (Senior and Junior), frankly and publicly to modify its *ex cathedra* claim in harmony with facts.

Economics, education, welfare, health and even human life are involved.

CH. WARDELL STILES
WINTER PARK, FLORIDA

## CAN A PUBLICATION BE CAMOUFLAGED?

THE persistence of the faith that in some mysterious manner material may be distributed to the public without being published, by the mere device of mimeographing instead of printing, was again illustrated at the Atlantic City meeting. In at least two societies during discussions of the still vexed question of publishing abstracts, "mimeographed" as a substitute for "printed" abstracts were urged on the alleged grounds that "publication" would thus be avoided.

In his discussion "What is a Publication?"[1] Storer points out that the method used in reproduction has no bearing on the question of publication. He cites among other examples the experience of the Biological Survey with *Bird Banding Notes,* a mimeographed publication which when it was initiated bore a note on the first page of each issue—"Bird Banding Notes is not a publication and is not for general distribution." In spite of this, however, the scientific value of the contained matter soon became evident and the material was cited by other investigators. I am further informed by the Biological Survey that *Bird Banding Notes* is now being sent regularly to *Biological Abstracts* at the request of the editor of that review journal.

The *Plant Disease Reporter* is a case in point. This mimeographed serial was established in 1917, as a means of making readily available to working pathologists incidental information thought to be of transient rather than of permanent interest and which should be placed in their hands more quickly than was possible through any available printed medium. The result was a collection of mimeographed notes, the popularity of which was immediately attested by the material presented as well as by the demands for the *Bulletin,* as it was then called. In 1923, to still further emphasize the informal nature of the series, the name was changed to *Reporter.* In spite of this, the actual scientific value of the material included has been abundantly attested by its repeated citation in regularly printed scientific literature and by numerous reviews of its contents in the *Review of Applied Mycology* everywhere recognized as the standard review journal for mycological and plant pathological literature.

It is obviously possible for a group of workers in a limited field, for example, taxonomists, to bind themselves not to recognize species published by a particular method or for that matter in a special group of languages or in a particular color of ink. But general scientific matter disseminated in any form available for more or less permanent record is certainly scientifically published, whatever the method of duplicating employed.

NEIL E. STEVENS
BUREAU OF PLANT INDUSTRY
WASHINGTON, D. C.

[1] SCIENCE, n. s., 75: 486–487, 1932.

## THE AGE OF METEOR CRATER

IN SCIENCE,[1] Professor Blackwelder proposes that the Coon Butte crater in Arizona is of the Post-Tahoe epoch, some forty to seventy-five thousand years old. This decision is supported primarily by the evidence of the lake bed in the crater proper. However, in connection with the lake-bed a statement is made that I feel needs some correction. On page 559, Dr. Blackwelder states concerning a layer of rhyolitic ash in the lake bed: "The bed of volcanic ash is plainly the record of an explosive eruption somewhere in the south-western arid region. *No such eruption is known to have occurred since Pleistocene (late glacial) times.* If the age of this shower is ever determined it may afford important evidence regarding the age of Meteor Crater." (The italics are mine). It happens that the date of the shower mentioned is probably known accurately. At a meeting of anthropologists in Santa Fé during September, 1931, the Arizona University party reported the discovery of pit houses filled with ash, not too distant from the Meteor Crater. Wood was recovered from these and has been dated by Dr. Douglass, using his tree-ring calender. It had been buried by an eruption that took place in the neighborhood of 793 A. D. If the two showers are identical, then Barringer's dating of 2,000 to 3,000 years ago is probably the most acceptable of all.

Much supporting evidence for the inter-glacial dating is drawn from the formation and degradation of the talus slopes. I feel strongly that we can not draw analogies from the formation of talus where the only agents are those normal to a moist and colder climate. There is no doubt in my mind that the talus slopes were built up by the impact and explosion and not by the usual forces that disintegrate cliff faces.

[1] Vol. 76: No. 1981, pp. 557–560, December 16, 1932.

However, Dr. Blackwelder's evidence of the deeply corroded limestone blocks must be explained before a modern dating can be satisfactorily applied to the meteor fall. Whether or not sufficient heat could have been generated to partially calcine the blocks and thereby render them prone to rapid corrosion is debatable, but is still a possibility. If such calcining took place, the advanced state of corrosion might have resulted in a matter of months, even with little rainfall.

All in all, it seems that the date of the great meteor's fall is still much in doubt. Whether the fall was recent, as Barringer suggests, or ancient, as Blackwelder holds, depends upon which way you wish to interpret the known facts. I agree with Blackwelder that the layer of volcanic ash in the lake will play a great part in settling the point. Dr. Douglass' date on the ash fall that buried the timbers of the Arizona pit houses and subsequent similar information that will be massed in the near future will be keystones to the problem.

F. MARTIN BROWN
FOUNTAIN VALLEY SCHOOL OF COLORADO
COLORADO SPRINGS, COLORADO

## THORNDIKE'S PROOF OF THE LAW OF EFFECT

As one of "the great majority of psychologists" who have criticized Thorndike's "law of effect,"[1] for which he now presents a positive proof,[2] I venture to suggest that this law is insusceptible of proof except on premises which many psychologists, and also many biologists, will not accept.

The statement that a "satisfying after-effect strengthens directly the connection producing it" can be maintained only under the assumption that a course of behavior consists of a number of separate and discrete acts; whereas, if the fundamental premise of all behavior be Coghill's principle that "the behavior pattern expands from the beginning throughout the growing normal animal as a perfectly integrated unit,"[3] all end-effects are consummatory, and it is not permissible to rule them out of experiments such as Thorndike records. Furthermore, Thorndike's report that the effect of a reward is noticeable in the unrewarded results that occur in proximity to those that are rewarded supports the view that learning is a self-regulating process, the parts of which are not discrete acts, but members of the whole unit of action.

What Thorndike's experiments seem to demonstrate is the effectiveness of learning without recourse to "repetition or frequency of occurrence, recency, intensity." What they do not demonstrate is that conditions have been equalized in respect of "finality, or consummatoriness, tendency to attain equilibrium and other features of the process [that] have been alleged to be adequate to explain the strengthening of connections." They do not demonstrate inadequacy of these last-named features, because these features suggest a dynamic interpretation at variance with Thorndike's assumption that learning consists in strengthening connections between parts otherwise discrete and independent.

Thorndike, himself, suggests the necessary correction to his theory when he states that "a satisfying after-effect strengthens greatly the connection which it follows directly *and to which it belongs*" (italics mine). As has been pointed out by other critics,[4] it is not *pleasure* but *success* which stamps in the right action; and it may be said to do so because the whole process is from the beginning a "perfectly integrated unit." Although the process may be disrupted, so long as learning is taking place every achievement is a consummatory process, the end-effect of which is one of finality because equilibrium has been attained. The end-effect "belongs" to what has gone before because it is an integral part of the entire unit of action. It is therefore not an "after-effect" of this action.

R. M. OGDEN
CORNELL UNIVERSITY

[1] *Cf.*, *Psych. Rev.*, 20: 188 *ff.* 1913.
[2] SCIENCE, 77: 173. February 10, 1933.
[3] *Cf.*, G. E. Coghill, *Arch. of Neur. and Psychiat.*, 21: 989. 1929.
[4] *Cf.*, H. Cason, *Psych. Rev.*, 39: 440, 1932; M. H. Trowbridge and H. Cason, *Jour. of Gen. Psych.*, 7: 245, 1932; E. C. Tolman, C. S. Hall and E. P. Bretnall, *Jour. of Exp. Psych.*, 15: 601, 1932.

## THE EARLIEST DATED DWELLING IN THE UNITED STATES

ABOUT the year 660 A. D. some timbers were cut on the slopes of the San Francisco Mountains in Arizona and used in a dwelling. Twelve of these timbers, now a mass of charcoal, have been dated by tree-ring studies and have given us the earliest date for an American home. This dwelling is 124 years older than our previously dated oldest dwelling.

The site from which the charred timbers were secured was a rectangular pithouse (N. A. 1531), belonging to the period in Southwestern archeology known as Pueblo I.

Previous to this time the earliest dated dwelling in the Southwest was a pithouse occupied in 784 A. D. This belonged to the period called Pueblo II. We have now not only the earliest dated house but also the first reported date in Pueblo I.

These earliest dated pithouses were excavated by the Museum of Northern Arizona, Flagstaff, Arizona, under the direction of Lyndon L. Hargrave, Field Director and the timbers dated by John C. McGregor, curator of dendro-chronology.

HAROLD S. COLTON
MUSEUM OF NORTHERN ARIZONA

# SCIENTIFIC APPARATUS AND LABORATORY METHODS

## A HOME-MADE ELECTRICALLY-DRIVEN PSYCHROMETER

BECAUSE of the inaccuracies of the hair hygrometers used in our work, the need has developed for an accurate and convenient means of making humidity determinations in small enclosures where a sling psychrometer can not be used. For this purpose an electrically-driven psychrometer was constructed (see Fig. 1), using the thermometers from an old stationary psychrometer mounted on a frame to which is attached a small electric hair dryer. When the motor is running, air is sucked over both wet and dry bulbs, and readings may be taken after approximately two minutes.

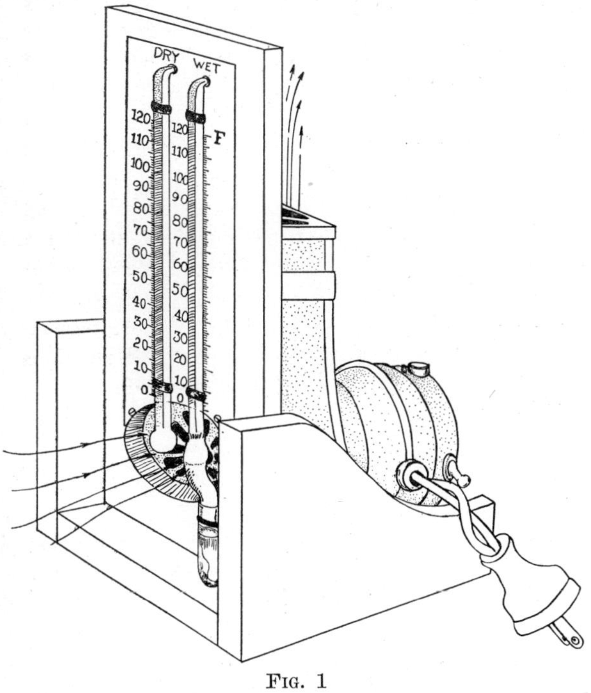


FIG. 1

Instruments operating on this principle are on the market, but those that have come to our attention are high in price and too large for our needs. This home-made instrument, the parts of which cost less than $10, was assembled for the purpose of testing its convenience for our work, but without attempting to perfect it as a precise laboratory instrument.

Many improvements are obviously desirable. The thermometers should be at least as accurate as those of a good grade sling psychrometer, and graduated on a scale to be read to one half degree F. The mercury columns should be easy to see under unfavorable conditions, as through the glass door of an incubator. For compactness the scale should cover only the usual temperature range of the work. A suitable suction device is of primary importance for furnishing an air current of as high velocity as possible, consistent with small size and freedom from excessive heating. As pointed out by Carrier and Lindsay[1], the wet bulb error may increase markedly at reduced air velocities. In assembling the instrument the thermometers should be so placed as to prevent evaporation from the wet bulb wick influencing the dry bulb, or either of the bulbs being influenced by motor heat. If the air is drawn over the bulbs from a direction other than that of the operator, the chance will be largely removed of influence from body heat or moisture when the instrument is used in the open laboratory.

The electric psychrometer was checked against a sling psychrometer under varying conditions and found in close agreement, particularly as to wet bulb temperatures. The discrepancies that occurred were such as might be ascribed to the character of the thermometers of the electric instrument, which were difficult to read with accuracy closer than one degree, and which showed errors in the dry bulb readings when checked in our chemistry department against an accurate laboratory thermometer. The influence of motor heat on the thermometers did not become apparent until some time after the maximum wet bulb depression, and then chiefly in enclosed spaces. An increase of one degree in both the dry and wet bulb readings was observed in a small incubator after five minutes' operation, but this would obviously make but little change in humidity determinations.

Our use of the instrument has been mainly in checking the hair hygrometers in our breeding cages and incubators. It has been found desirable to check each hygrometer individually under the usual conditions where it is kept. This avoids the possibility of disturbing the adjustment by handling, and makes it unnecessary to keep the hygrometer out of use for several hours for complete response to changed humidity conditions before an accurate test can be made. As some of the hygrometers have shown large errors in scale readings when calibrated over a wide range of humidities, and as it is not yet known whether these errors remain constant for any length of time, it has seemed best to make tests frequently and at the usual incubator humidity.

The electric instrument would appear to make practicable the use of a stationary psychrometer in

[1] "Temperatures of Evaporation of Water into Air," W. H. Carrier and D. C. Lindsay. *Trans. Am. Soc. Mechanical Engineers*, 1924, vol. 46, p. 739.

an incubator in which the air circulation is constant, by establishing the difference between the wet bulb reading at the regular incubator air velocity and the maximum wet bulb depression. This difference applied as a correction to the observed stationary wet bulb reading should give an approximate humidity determination. Frequent checking would be advisable to correct for any changes in air velocity or reduced evaporation from the wet bulb wick. If the incubator temperature and humidity vary only in narrow limits, a few readings at various points should form the basis of a simple chart for approximate corrections. If the air movement is not subject to variation by reason of material introduced into the incubator, the stationary psychrometer may be placed at any convenient point. Otherwise it should be located close enough to a fan to insure a constant current over the bulbs, regardless of changes of air circulation in the main body of the incubator. With low air velocities, it is particularly important that the thermometer bulbs be protected against any varying source of heat, as from the fan motor or the incubator heating elements. A stationary psychrometer has been in use in this way in an incubator for a short period with apparent success. The humidity determinations with this instrument may be more accurate, and certainly less erratic, than those obtained with our hair hygrometers, particularly in an incubator in which the frequent opening of the door tends to keep the hair instrument continually out of adjustment during the day.

For general use about the laboratory or insectary the electric instrument has advantages over the sling psychrometer in reducing the danger of breakage, and in ease of reading, as the thermometers may be read while the motor is running and the wet bulb held constant by the air current. Its special adaptability for use inside small enclosures makes it seem an instrument that is worth perfecting for entomological work.

J. F. Townsend
Agricultural Experiment Station
New Haven, Connecticut

## THE CURRENT ROTOR

Last summer, while engaged in a study of post-embryonic development of mackerel and other marine fishes at Woods Hole, Massachusetts, the authors used a simple device which enables one to change water without losing small organisms that live in the aquarium. The essential feature of the apparatus is a cylinder, A, of 60 mesh or finer monel metal screen suspended in a tank and rotated by means of an electric motor. Rotation of the cylinder when placed at one end of an oblong aquarium sets up a complex system of currents the direction of which is indicated

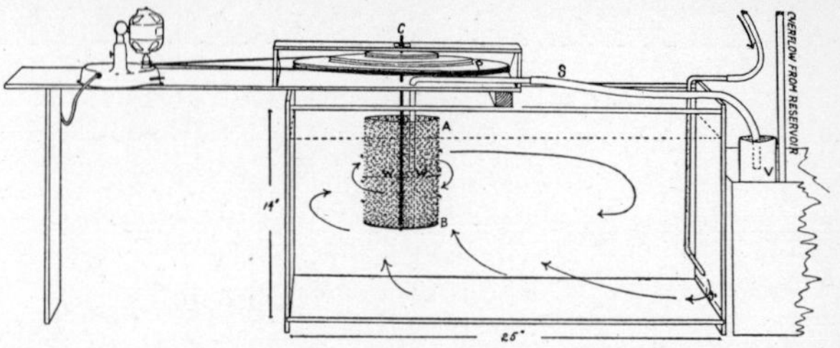


in the accompanying illustration. Strong circular currents are formed in the immediate vicinity of the cylinder, while at the far end the water moves very gently. There is also a noticeable upward motion from the bottom of the tank.

The speed of rotation and the corresponding strength of currents may be regulated by the speed of the motor controlled through a rheostat and by means of a set of pulleys of different diameters. The dimensions of the cylinder also affect the strength of the current produced and therefore should vary according to the size of the aquarium used. The cylinder shown here is 4 inches in diameter and 6 inches long. About one inch is left above water. The tank is $25 \times 15 \times 14$ inches. The bottom of the cylinder, B, is a celluloid or monel metal disk. Non-corrosive material should also be used for the suspension rod, C, and brace wires, W. The diameter of the pulley, P, is 12 inches.

The water can be withdrawn from the tank through a siphon, S, the upper end of which is placed inside the revolving cylinder. When the cylinder is in rotation small organisms never are actually drawn against its wall, because the centrifugal force throws them away from it. They are then caught up in the circular currents and soon find themselves in quieter waters at the far end of the aquarium. In this manner the water in the tank can be changed without losing its inhabitants.

When it is desirable to supply a constant flow of water this can be accomplished by placing the lower end of the overflow siphon, S, in a vessel, V, adjusted so that the top of it is level with the water in the aquarium. The water is introduced from a reservoir, in which it is kept at constant level. If necessary the water from a laboratory faucet can be filtered through glass wool to remove sediment and other foreign matter.

The revolving cylinder not only provides for changing water without losing small organisms that are kept in the aquarium, but also by setting the water in motion it prevents the accumulation of the organisms and their sticking to the bottom. In this respect it can be used instead of a plunger jar.

Paul S. Galtsoff
Louella E. Cable
U. S. Bureau of Fisheries

# SCIENCE

VOL. 77 FRIDAY, MARCH 10, 1933 No. 1993

*The Historical Development of Response Psychology:* PROFESSOR HERBERT S. LANGFELD 243

*Obituary:*
*John Belling. Recent Deaths* 250

*Scientific Events:*
*The Faculty of Medicine of Paris; Revision of the International Electrical Units; The Priestley Lectures at the Pennsylvania State College; The Sixteenth Session of the International Geological Congress* 251

*Scientific Notes and News* 254

*Discussion:*
*University Patents:* DR. ALAN GREGG. *The Coefficient of Correlation:* JOSEPH BERKSON. *Attempt to Confirm the Existence of a Filtrable Cycle of Bacteria by the Use of "K" Medium:* C. V. SEASTONE and MARY B. LAWRENCE. *Univalent Chromosomes of Tradescantia virginiana:* THE LATE DR. JOHN BELLING 257

*Special Correspondence:*
*University Expedition to Study the Natives of Central Australia:* PROFESSOR J. B. CLELAND 260

*Scientific Apparatus and Laboratory Methods:*
*A Universal Dilatometer:* R. HOLCOMB. *Permanent Slides for Use in Teaching the Howard Method:* J. D. WILDMAN 261

*Special Articles:*
*The Distribution of American Men of Science in 1932:* DR. J. MCKEEN CATTELL 264

*Science News* 8

SCIENCE: A Weekly Journal devoted to the Advancement of Science, edited by J. MCKEEN CATTELL and published every Friday by

THE SCIENCE PRESS

New York City: Grand Central Terminal
Lancaster, Pa. Garrison, N. Y.
Annual Subscription, $6.00 Single Copies, 15 Cts.

SCIENCE is the official organ of the American Association for the Advancement of Science. Information regarding membership in the Association may be secured from the office of the permanent secretary, in the Smithsonian Institution Building, Washington, D. C.

# THE HISTORICAL DEVELOPMENT OF RESPONSE PSYCHOLOGY[1]

By Professor HERBERT S. LANGFELD

PRINCETON UNIVERSITY

THERE are, I venture to say, few psychologists of the present day so thoroughly mentalistic that they do not incorporate some form of motor response in their psychological system. Where they differ is in the importance they attach to such responses and in the relation they believe exists between response and consciousness. The prevailing, and what might be considered the conservative view, is that response follows perception or ideas either as an effect or as an accompaniment and that such conscious states are only affected by response in so far as such response stimulates proprioceptors, which in turn set up an afferent impulse. According to this view, then, consciousness lies, as it were, between the afferent and efferent impulses and consequently occurs before the response. In a previous paper I have described a view which makes response an essential factor of consciousness.[2] It follows from this position that without response there would be no consciousness. No matter how many or how strong are the stimuli and the resulting afferent impulses, without the efferent impulses and specific response, either incipient or overt, an organism would have no awareness of a world; so far as that organism is concerned there would be no experience.

This view undoubtedly seems extreme to many scientists, but it does not in the least break with the past, nor is it new in any of its essential features. It is my purpose, then, in this paper to sketch briefly its historical development and to describe some of the more recent experimental findings which seem to support it. I should say, at the outset, that many of the authors of the past, especially those who wrote before the birth of experimental psychology, made but brief reference to such a view, and no one of them devel-

[1] Address of the vice-president and chairman of Section I—Psychology, American Association for the Advancement of Science, Atlantic City, December, 1932.

[2] H. S. Langfeld, "A Response Interpretation of Consciousness," *Psychol. Rev.*, 38: 87–108, 1931.

oped a consistent and thorough response theory. But it is fair to assume that even a chance remark from a respected philosopher or scientific man has often had a strong influence on the future of thought.

There are many of our present psychological concepts whose roots can be traced to the early Greek philosophers. In support of our present thesis we find Plato's identification of thought with inner speech. Inner speech, however, can as well be accepted by the mentalist as by the response psychologist, for the remark may simply mean that we hear ourselves think and need not necessarily refer to incipient response of the vocal organs. Therefore, unless we wish to force the interpretation of Plato's statement, one can only assume that at best it was merely a faint but nevertheless fruitful suggestion. Parmenides, before him, however, wrote in no uncertain terms. He does not even mention vocal response, but takes us at once to the gross movements of the organism. "For just as thought finds at any time the mixture of its erring organs, so does it come to men, for that which thinks is the same, namely, the substance of the limbs, in each and every man; for the highest degree of organization gives the highest degree of thought."[3] Not only did Parmenides plainly identify thought with motor response, but he even went further and, to recast the statement in modern terms, correlated degree of intelligence with degree of muscular coordination, which was the underlying idea in some recent investigations of the relation of intelligence scores to the speed of reaction.

Many centuries later, La Mettrie referred to the identification of thought, or as he called it "faculties of the soul," with the organization not only of the brain but of the entire body.[4] He further stated "that thought is so little incompatible with organized matter, that it seems to be one of its properties on a par with electricity, the faculty of motion, impenetrability, extension, etc."[5] This, the basis of his materialism, is a very general statement. A more specific reference to a response theory is his remark that "the brain has its muscles for thinking, as the legs have muscles for walking."[6] Such a phrase would be highly fantastic from any other point of view than a motor concept of thought, and even his sharpest critic would hardly accuse La Mettrie of phantasy or mysticism.

In much of the literature upon motor response, kinesthesis plays an important if not a leading rôle. There is, in such instances, it seems to me, a serious confusion, as I have explained elsewhere.[7] According to a thoroughgoing motor theory, perception is identical with the response system, not a consequence of it, and kinesthesis, being a perception, must therefore itself be identified with such response. The motor theory does not in any way depend for its verification on introspective reports of kinesthesis. Even if we never had a perception of the feel of our muscles, the motor theory would in no wise be invalidated. As a matter of fact, relative to the total perceptual experience of the individual, kinesthesis is a rarity and, further, it is obvious from what has just been said that for a psychologist to dwell upon the function of kinesthesis does not in itself class him as a response psychologist. If such were the case, there would be very few psychologists who do not fall under that category. In short, kinesthesis can as well fit into an afferent-perception-efferent-response theory as into a response or motor theory. And so when Erasmus Darwin stated in his "Zoonomia" that "the organ of touch is properly the sense of pressure, but the muscular fibres themselves constitute the organ of sense, that feels extension," he does not commit himself to any particular theory.[8] It is difficult for us to-day to interpret accurately this statement which, in the light of our finer distinction of terms, appears to us ambiguous, and this holds for several other authors I shall quote, whose descriptions are in sensory rather than motor terms. When, however, he further states that ". . . the whole muscular system may be considered as one organ of sense, and the various attitudes of the body, as ideas belonging to this organ," there can be little doubt that he attached much importance for consciousness to the motor side of the total organic response.

Professor L. Carmichael in his article on Sir Charles Bell[9] has shown how amazingly broad and prophetic were that scientific man's views on physiology and psychology. It is not surprising, therefore, to find that Bell was cognizant of the important rôle of muscular action in perception, especially in the experience of space. In his book on "The Hand"[10] he remarks that "without a sense of muscular action or consciousness of the degree of effort made, the proper sense of touch could hardly be an inlet to knowledge at all." Just as in one of the above statements of Darwin, so here it is not clear

[3] J. Burnett, "Early Greek Philosophy," 2nd edition, 1908, p. 202. The last clause is G. H. Lewis's translation in his "Biographical History of Philosophy," 1905, Parmenides, 51–52.

[4] La Mettrie, "Man a Machine," p. 128. Chicago, Open Court Pub. Co., 1912.

[5] *Ibid.*, pp. 143–144.

[6] *Ibid.*, p. 132.

[7] H. S. Langfeld, "A Response Interpretation of Consciousness."

[8] Erasmus Darwin, "Zoonomia, or the Laws of Organic Life," Vol. 1, Sect. xiv. London, 1794.

[9] L. Carmichael, "Sir Charles Bell: A Contribution to the History of Physiological Psychology," *Psychol. Rev.*, 33: 188–217, 1926.

[10] Sir Charles Bell, "The Hand," London, William Pickering, p. 195, 1833.

to what extent reference is made merely to kinesthetic sensations. Further, it is not safe to conclude that Bell believed the sensation of touch to be dependent upon motor experience. I am inclined to think, rather, that he had in mind touch localization. Certainly, when he stated that "it is to the muscular apparatus and to the conclusions we are enabled to draw from the consciousness of muscular effort, that we owe that geometrical sense by which we become acquainted with the form, and magnitude, and distance of objects," he is referring to the genetic theory of space based upon movement.[11] Although there may be some doubt from these earlier writings of Bell's adherence to the notion that movement is a *sine qua non* of touch perception, there is little possibility of mistaking his meaning in the article he wrote some twenty years later, entitled "On the Necessity of the Sense of Muscular Action to the Full Exercise of the Organs of the Senses."[12] The title itself is clearly indicative of his position, and Carmichael has pointed out that Bell believed that the stimulation of the sensory nerve was not sufficient for a perceptual experience. Something more is necessary, namely, muscular movement.[13] In other words, Bell held that the total afferent-efferent system is a true correlate of the perception.

Seven years before Bell wrote this last-mentioned paper appeared Baron von Holbach's English translation of the "System of Nature," the original of which was published in 1770. In it he expressed the view that consciousness depends upon organization and specific action. He speaks in the language of the time, but the thought is distinctly modern in that he emphasizes action patterns. "To convince ourselves," he wrote, "that the faculties called *intellectual* are only certain modes of existence, or determinate manners of acting which result from the peculiar organization of the body, we have only to analyze them: we shall then see, that all the operations which are attributed to the soul, are nothing more than certain modifications of the body, etc., etc."[14] This remark refers not only to the doctrine that the mental does not exist without the physical, but also that response is a necessary factor.

In the beginning of this same century, 1801, Destutt De Tracy, in his "Elemens d'Ideologie,"[15] expressed similar views of the direct relation of movement to the mental. He considered "it certain that we cannot conceive of any perception produced in us, even the most purely intellectual, without some kind of movement in some one of our organs." One might think from this statement that he was describing that relation of ideas to action, which later took the form of the ideo-motor theory: but from his further remarks that we can only regard action of thought and of sensing as a particular effect of the act of moving ourselves and that "this notion is worthy of serious consideration," it is clear that he was not thinking of the possibility of movement always following an idea, but rather of the dependence of the idea on the movement.

Of the work of the middle of the last century, Lotze's theory of local signs and his genetic interpretation of space perception have a significant bearing on the motor theory. His idea that spatial localization depends on muscular movement means that at least some quality of our mental experience is in direct relation to if not identical with response. It is true that Lotze spoke of "Muskelgefühl" and thus invited the criticism that sensations of movement can not by some magical alchemy become visual perceptions. We find here the old confusion, noted above, between kinesthesis or feeling of movement and the efferent impulse and the movement itself.

Alexander Bain described localization in terms very similar to those of Lotze, and unfortunately with the same confusion. He states: "An object seems to us to be up or down, according as we raise or lower the pupil of the eye in order to see it; the very notion of up and down is derived from our feelings of movement, and not at all from the optical image formed on the back of the eye." He comes very much closer to the present conception of the rôle of response when he writes: "And now, as to the *sensations,* or the proper mental elements of Sight. These are partly optical, resulting from the effect of light on the retina, and partly muscular, arising through the action of the various muscles. Nearly all sensations of sight combine both elements."[16] There is evidently here a direct reference to movement itself. Bain further specifically calls attention to the function of the organs of speech and believes that "a *suppressed articulation* is in fact the material of our recollection, the intellectual manifestation, the *idea* of speech."[17] He also combats the notion that the brain is the seat of sense impressions and believes emphatically that the total nervous arc is necessary for consciousness, a view which was later elaborated by Professor John

[11] Sir Charles Bell, "On the Motions of the Eye, in Illustration of the Uses of the Muscles and Nerves of the Orbit," *Phil. Trans. Roy. Soc. Lond.*, pt. 1, p. 167, 1823.

[12] Sir Charles Bell, "On the Necessity of the Sense of Muscular Action to the Full Exercise of the Organs of the Senses," *Proc. Roy. Soc. Edinburgh*, 361–363, 1842.

[13] L. Carmichael, "Sir Charles Bell: A Contribution to the History of Physiological Psychology," p. 209.

[14] Baron von Holbach, "System of Nature," English translation, Vol. 1, p. 53, 1835.

[15] Destutt De Tracy, "Elemens d'Ideologie," Paris, 3rd ed., Chap. xii, 1817.

[16] Alexander Bain, "The Senses and the Intellect," p. 246, 4th ed., New York, Appleton, 1894.

[17] *Ibid.*, p. 357.

Dewey.[18] In Bain's words, ". . . nervous action supposes currents passing through these completed circles, or to and fro between the central ganglia and the organs of sense and motion; and that, short of a completed course, no nervous action exists."[19] Continuing, he explains thought by the same nervous mechanism. After citing the example of persons who talk to themselves, he expresses the opinion so frequently quoted that "the tendency of the idea of an action to produce the fact shows that the idea is already the fact in a weaker form. Thinking is restrained speaking or acting."[20]

George Henry Lewes recognized the importance of the motor processes as shown in his statement that "every psychical fact is a product of sense-work, brain-work, and muscle-work,"[21] but one can not say that he ever held to a strictly motor theory of consciousness. His remark that ". . . in all cases an action of some kind results; directly or indirectly, every sensation is *completed* in an action; and thus Action is the pole-star of even the most wide-wandering Speculation"[22] is evidently a formulation of the ideo-motor theory.

It is difficult to evaluate Mach's contributions to the motor theory, for his statements are strangely contradictory. His "thought experiment," so far as we can judge from his description, remains entirely in the realm of ideas. In connection with space, both visual and tactual, he recognizes the importance of the muscles and shows in some detail how they contribute to breadth, depth, right, left, symmetry, etc. If he had throughout been consistent with his statement that "the will to perform movements of the eyes, or the innervation to the act, is itself the space-sensation,"[23] there would be no doubt that at least in spatial experience he was a thoroughgoing motorist, but he later states that it is hard to decide whether "the innervation itself is the space-sensation, or whether . . . the space-sensation is before or behind the innervation."[24] And further on he remarks, "In so far as we have spatial perceptions, these depend, according to our theory, on sensations. What is the nature of these sensations, and what organs are active in connexion with them, we must leave an open question."[25] When he comes to the problem of time, a phenomenon which he would have had little difficulty to explain in motor terms, he assumes a special time sense. In regard to music he clearly denies any function to the response mechanism, for he says, "Music can no more come into being merely through the motor sensations accompanying musical performances, than a deaf man can hear music by watching the movements of players."[26] It is evident from the above quotations that he started with a clear-cut motor concept and became less sure of it as he proceeded.

Georges Dubreuque in his article on "L'Intuition Motrice" in 1898 remarked that Condillac's great mistake was to omit from his statue the principal phenomenon which is necessary in the acquisition of sensation, namely, movement. He discusses in particular the perception of space and numbers which he believes require movement for their realization. His notion that the concept of numbers and such mathematical constructions as infinity have their origin in the response mechanism seems well founded on fact. Similar ideas regarding the origin of mathematical concepts have appeared in recent writings, such as that of Dr. P. Chaslin.[27] In reference to space Dubreuque remarks that it is quite possible to have the perception of an empty space, that is to say, a space without objects. For even though there would be no tactile or visual sensations, there would still be motor sensations.[28]

William James's dualistic view-point colored all his writings. It can not be said that he ever subscribed to a strict motor theory, even though he gave the motor processes a very important place in his psychology. Although not the originator of the principle of the ideo-motor theory, his name is usually associated with the theory, due to the prominence he gave it. But the ideo-motor theory, as its name implies, presupposes the existence of conscious processes before the response, and merely asserts that response is an invariable consequence of idea. It is only in so far as this theory emphasizes the necessity of response that it is a contribution to the development of the motor theory. The same qualification must be made in regard to the James-Lange theory of emotion. Here, too, a dualism underlies the concept. If we could stop with the bare statement that the bodily responses are the emotions, that is to say, identical with the consciousness of the emotions, we would be justified in claiming James as a motor theorist. But James went on to explain that it is our consciousness

18 John Dewey, "The Reflex Arc Concept in Psychology," *Psychol. Rev.*, 3: 357–370, 1896.

19 Alexander Bain, "The Senses and the Intellect," p. 355.

20 *Ibid.*, p. 358.

21 George Henry Lewes, "Problems of Life and Mind," Vol. 1, p. 147, 1874.

22 *Ibid.*, p. 145.

23 E. Mach, "The Analysis of Sensations," p. 129. Tr. by C. M. Williams, Chicago, Open Court Pub. Co., 1914.

24 *Ibid.*, p. 170.

25 *Ibid.*, p. 184.

26 *Ibid.*, p. 280.

27 P. Chaslin, "Essai sur la Mechanisme Psychologique des Opérations de la Mathématique Pure," Paris, 1926.

28 G. Dubreuque, "L'Intuition motrice," *Rev. Phil.*, 46, p. 291, 1898.

of these processes which constitute the emotions, in other words, that the afferent impulses back to the brain from the periphery are necessary for the consciousness of the emotion. Dr. Walter Cannon, it seems to me, was correct in rejecting this part of the theory, although on the basis of the motor theory I can not agree that the response as such is not an integral part of the physiological pattern of the emotions. It might be added that James comes very close to a motor theory when he stated that "no impression or idea of eye, ear, or skin comes to us without occasioning a movement, even though the movement be no more than the accommodation of the sense-organs; and all our trains of sensation and sensational imagery have their terms alternated and interpenetrated with motor processes of most of which we practically are unconscious."[29] This statement seems indeed to imply a step beyond the ideo-motor theory.

Hugo Münsterberg made a most signal contribution to response psychology with his action theory. For him the response is a necessary factor for consciousness in that the degree of openness of the motor channels is in direct relation to the degree of vividness of the mental process. Although Münsterberg did not identify response with consciousness, since he placed mental phenomena in another universe of discourse distinct from that of physiological processes, and although he was concerned particularly with the one attribute of vividness of consciousness, yet he and his pupils were primarily interested in the response phase of experience in their experimentation.

In 1899, Professor B. B. Breese, a pupil of Münsterberg, gave a very clear and concise exposition of the motor theory. In his own words, "Consciousness . . . depends for its existence and character upon the transference of sense stimuli into motor paths. This hypothesis considers the incoming, or sense stimulation, and the out-going, or motor innervation, as a single nerve process. There is no point of separation between them. The motor discharge is necessary in order that any central activity take place."[30] In experiments on retinal rivalry Breese found that the time of retention of the field before one eye was increased by the contraction of the muscles of the right or left side of the body respectively. From the results of his experiments on retinal rivalry he concludes that "in general, *inhibition of the motor elements tends to inhibit consciousness.*"[31] He is even more emphatic when he states that "the limitations of the motor adjustments become the limitations of thought,"[32] which means, if this is true, that we should expect to find a correlation between thought and muscular coordination. In regard to the inhibition of the spoken word during the learning of nonsense syllables by requiring the subject to count during the learning, Breese remarked that the increase of errors was not due to distraction but to the fact that the words could not find their natural expression in vocalization.[33] That is to say, the proper motor adjustment for the series was partially inhibited. Experiments recently conducted by Mr. Michael Blankfort in the Princeton Laboratory on the rôle of the motor processes in learning seem to confirm the assertion of Breese that the distraction was not the main cause of the increase of errors. In Blankfort's experiment the subject performed an act of skill with one hand, while the other hand merely carried out simple tapping movements during one series and remained idle during the other series. There was a greater transfer of training from one member to the other when the hand not performing the main task was idle. Check experiments indicated that distraction was not the cause of the difference. The explanation seems to lie rather in the fact that the other hand, when idle so far as a definite task was concerned, could carry out incipient responses similar to the movements of the hand performing the skilled movements, and was thus practising synchronously with the latter hand.

Josiah Royce believed in the close relationship of ideas and activity. Thought, for him, is "our consciousness of an act or of a series of acts adjusted to an object, in such a wise as fittingly to represent that object, etc."[34] He believed further that our mental images of an object can not be separated from our response. It is not clear, however, just where Royce places the motor process, but it is fair to assume that he did not unequivocally identify motor processes with consciousness.

Theodore Ribot throughout his writings insisted upon the importance of the rôle of movement in mental life. He has expressed himself most decidedly, perhaps, in his "Psychologie de l'Attention."[35] He asks if "the movements of the face, the body, the limbs, and the respiratory changes, which accompany attention, are as is usually asserted merely effects, signs." Are they not, on the contrary, he questions, "the necessary condition, the indispensable factors of attention"? He holds the second thesis, for, as he says, "if one suppresses all movement one entirely inhibits attention."[36] He argues for a motor theory of attention in terms similar to those used by James

[29] W. James, ''Principles of Psychology,'' p. 581, Vol. 2, London, Macmillan, 1901.

[30] B. B. Breese, ''On Inhibition,'' *Psychol. Rev. Monog.*, 3: 47–48, 1899.

[31] *Ibid.*, p. 58.

[32] *Ibid.*, p. 62.

[33] *Ibid.*, p. 58.

[34] Josiah Royce, ''Outlines of Psychology,'' p. 285, New York, Macmillan, 1906.

[35] Theodore Ribot, ''Psychologie de l'Attention,'' Paris, Alcan, 1906.

[36] *Ibid.*, p. 32.

for the emotions when he says that if a spectator at the opera could suppress all responses of the eyes, head, etc., what would remain of attention would be a very empty function, would in fact not be attention at all.[37] He further makes the emphatic statement that we must either assume elements of movement in all cases of voluntary attention or admit that an explanation of the mechanism is impossible.[38]

During the first decade of the present century a number of French psychologists incorporated the motor theory in their explanation of mental phenomena. B. Bourdon[39] attributes a secondary rôle to tactual and muscular sensations in the perception of form. As he uses the term sensation rather than response, it is probable that he had merely kinesthesis in mind. Dr. R. Nuel, on the other hand, is more explicit in his book on "La Vision." "The visual phenomena," he explains, "are entirely motor. There can be absolutely no question of visual consciousness in the infant before it has made bodily responses to visual stimuli."[40]

Dr. N. Kostyleff tries to break from an explanation of experience in purely mental terms by his theory of reflexes. For example, in discussing abstract ideas, he states that "it is only necessary to substitute for a psychological explanation the objective notion of reflexes in order that the general scheme of an objective explanation shall form a clear picture."[41] Throughout his writings Kostyleff makes constant use of the term reflex, and it is unfortunately not always clear what he means exactly by this expression. In fact, one gains the impression at times that it may be one of those magical phrases which are supposed to solve all psychological problems.

P. Souriau, writing about the same time as Kostyleff, implies an acceptance of the response theory so far as the emotions are concerned. For example, he remarks that the drop of the mouth which is a sign of sadness is without doubt the sadness itself.[42]

Professor Judd in a series of articles has explained the functional nature of the efferent response in a manner with which I find the theory I have expressed here and elsewhere to be in entire agreement. In criticizing the long-discarded innervation sensations, he makes it evident that the motor theory does not imply a direct representation in consciousness of the efferent impulse, but rather that consciousness is functionally dependent upon it. He rightly states that the advantage of the innervation theory was lost by calling the conscious processes innervation sensations. He regrets that no one had "asserted that the outgoing motor processes are indeed related to consciousness, but not in such a way as to arouse new sensations, etc."[43] In "What is Perception?"[44] he describes the function of motor tendencies in spatial perception and in the "Motor Processes and Consciousness" the unifying functions of such tendencies. "Unity of percepts," he writes, "and unity of ideas are . . . phrases which describe an aspect of consciousness dependent on motor tendencies."[45]

In the minds of the present-day psychologists, the motor theory is most closely associated with the names of Professor Washburn and of Professor Holt. Space does not permit a review of the many important contributions to the subject which Washburn has made, beginning with the book on "Movement and Mental Imagery."[46] Nor is such a review necessary in this place, since she has been extensively quoted in recent articles on response. Holt has not written so much directly on the motor theory, but the monistic view of consciousness and the identification of response with consciousness form the foundation of all his work. Perhaps the most concrete exposition of his view is to be found in the Supplement to "The Freudian Wish" on "Response and Cognition." To quote one phrase from this chapter, "The volitional element in behavioristic attention will be, . . . the process whereby the body assumes and exercises an adjustment or motor set such that its activities are some function of an object; are focused on an object."[47] He goes on to show that the behaviorists in describing objective action are describing consciousness.

Dr. Eugene Posch's psychology[48] is in close agreement with Holt's views. Posch explains the higher mental processes as well as the sensations in terms of verbal and postural response, muscle tonus and innervation. At about the same time as Posch, Dr. R. Müller-Freienfels published his views on the nature of thought and phantasy. He also stresses motor responses as essential to thought, but he does not

37 *Ibid.*, 37–38.

38 *Ibid.*, p. 73.

39 B. Bourdon, ''La perception visuelle de l'Espace,'' Paris, Schleicher Fréres, 1902.

40 R. Nuel, ''La Vision,'' p. 256, Paris, Doin, 1904.

41 N. Kostyleff, ''Les Substituts de l'Ame dans la Psychologie moderne,'' p. 194, Paris, Alcan, 1906.

42 P. Souriau, ''La perception des Faits psychiques,'' p. 56, *Année Psychol.*, 1907, 13.

43 C. H. Judd, ''The Doctrine of Attitudes,'' *Jour. Phil., Psychol. and Sci. Meth.*, 5, p. 682, 1908.

44 C. H. Judd, ''What is Perception?'' *Jour. Phil., Psychol. and Sci. Meth.*, 6, 36–44, 1909.

45 C. H. Judd, ''Motor Processes and Consciousness,'' *Jour. Phil., Psychol. and Sci. Meth.*, 6, p. 91, 1909.

46 M. Washburn, ''Movement and Mental Imagery,'' Boston, Houghton Mifflin, 1916.

47 E. B. Holt, ''The Freudian Wish,'' p. 178, New York, Henry Holt, 1915.

48 Posch published a book in Hungarian in 1915 which was finished in 1911. I obtained his views from an article entitled ''Umriss einer realistischen Psychologie,'' *Arch. f. d. ges. Psychol.*, 1923, 44, 191–243, in which he summarized the contents of his book.

consider them the exclusive condition of mental processes.[49] Posch states that he is in accord with Müller-Freienfels, except in so far as the latter retains a remnant of ideational elements in his theory. Posch affirms that "What one calls ideas, memory pictures, visual images, etc., can one and all be entirely resolved in attitudes, poses, etc., and must be, if one is to pursue a realistic psychology."[50] He holds to a strict monism and vigorously attacks the notion that mental qualities reside in the brain.

Professor J. F. Dashiell has given a clear account of the identification of the whole nervous arc with consciousness. He translates the thought experiment of Mach into motor terms. In his words, "if, now, we recognize that the process of thinking differs from any other trial and error activity mainly in degree of explicitness, are we not presented with another physiological conception of thinking, an alternative to the intra-cerebral conception. . . .?"[51] And on the subject of meaning he states that "it is my thesis that such abbreviated, anticipatory reactions aroused by a thing are that thing's meaning."[52]

The phenomenon of empathy, as described by Lipps, Vernon Lee and others, is a striking example of the function of the motor processes and can only, it seems to me, be explained by the motor theory. The work of neither of the above-named authors, however, did more than suggest to future writers the possibility of such an explanation. Dr. H. Friedländer, on the other hand, makes a contribution to both empathy and the motor theory in his description of the perception of weight when he states that, "The sensations in the arm, hand, and finger are almost entirely absent from consciousness and the object is filled with a 'sensory something' that appeared directly as the *weight* of the object. *This weight formed a unity with the visual appearance of the object.*"[53] It must be said, however, that Professor David Katz and his pupils, of whom Friedländer is one, can not be classed as motor theorists. It is true that we find many statements like the above which could well have been written by an adherent of the motor theory. Katz, for example, states that "we *produce* quasi through our muscular activities characteristics such as roughness and smoothness, hardness and softness; we are really the *creator of these qualities.*"[54] We also find them referring to movement as a form-giving factor and they give many results of their valuable researches which can well be interpreted according to the motor theory, but they always refer to kinesthesis in their own descriptions.

In England Professor S. Alexander is the chief exponent of a motor theory and many of his writings are based upon this concept. It would be difficult to find a clearer account than the following: "all knowledge from bare sensation up to the highest truth is revealed to our apprehensions and revealed through action."[55] And further, "The older writers used to say that afferent nerves conveyed sensations to the brain and mind, awakening there pictures which represent external things, upon which pictures we then behave appropriately. These pictures are mythology, and exist only in the fancy of theorists who are not content with facts. What the afferent nerves convey to the brain is nervous (or mental) excitement. It is the efferent or motor reaction (always in their continuity with the afferent process) in which these excitements discharge in virtue of which we apprehend the qualities of external things."[56]

Dr. M. J. Piaget emphasizes the importance of motor response in the development of intelligence. There are, according to him, three levels of mental activity of the child. The first is the "intelligence motrice," which occurs before or independent of language. There is a progressive accommodation of the organism to the objects of the environment due to the motor patterns and a reciprocal adaptation of the object to the organism, as when weight is felt as a force. The child is, however, ignorant of the real meaning of the motor activity. There is no active control, merely a passive acceptance. In the further development of the child there occurs the second level, egocentric thought and lastly rational thought.[57]

In Germany Dr. L. Grünhut has recently, in answer to the Gestalt theory, contended that we perceive form by running our eyes over the given visual stimuli. We do not merely open our eyes for possible sensations, but rather create our perception by allowing our eyes to wander over the object. We do not see isolated points, but through this active process we perceive a unity in a given manifold. In other words, he explains that the picture on the retina and the afferent impulses are not yet a perception. It is only through response that discrete points in space are formed into a coordinated whole.[58] In an article which has appeared this year, Professor F. M. Gregg

[49] R. Müller-Freienfels, "Das Denken und die Phantasie," p. 10, Leipzig, Barth, 1916.

[50] E. Posch, "Umriss einer realistischen Psychologie," p. 205.

[51] J. F. Dashiell, "Is the Cerebrum the Seat of Thinking?" *Psychol. Rev.*, 33, p. 18, 1926.

[52] *Ibid.*, p. 25.

[53] H. Friedländer, "Die Wahrnehmung der Schwere," *Zsch. f. Psychol.*, 1920, 83, p. 135. See also my article, "A Response Interpretation of Consciousness," p. 98.

[54] D. Katz, "Der Aufbau der Tastwelt," *Zsch. f. Psychol.*, Ergänzungs bd., 11, p. 260, 1925.

[55] S. Alexander, "Art and the Material," p. 19, New York, Longmans, 1925.

[56] *Ibid.*, pp. 20–21.

[57] M. J. Piaget, "Les trois Systemes de la Pensée de L'Enfant," *Bull. Soc. fr. de Phil.*, 28, p. 100, 1928.

[58] E. Jaensch and L. Grünhut, "Über Gestalt Psychologie und Gestalt Theorie," *Mann's Pädagogisches Magazin*, No. 1262, p. 134, 1929.

also applies the motor theory to explain certain of the phenomena which have interested the Gestalt psychologists.[59]

Professor M. Ponzo has expressed his general view in the statement that there is not only a concomitance of motor phenomena and mental states, but an invariable participation of motor response in all forms of mental activity.[60] He has described the rôle of response in his account of the experimental work of the Turin laboratory. Several of his examples are the following: Illusions of size of objects occur through changes in the motor response;[61] we understand better what is said by internal repetition or murmur of the words,[62] an observation which was also made some time previously by O. Jespersen;[63] each individual expresses himself in motor terms in a fashion as characteristic as are certain of his anatomical features.[64]

Finally, we have a successful attempt by Dr. E. Jacobson to detect directly the muscular response during mental activity by means of the action potentials. He found that the action patterns during silent thought correspond to those obtained when the words were actually spoken. He concludes that "during imagination, recollection and concrete or abstract thinking involving words or numbers, muscular contractions characteristically appear as specific components of the physiologic process of mental activity."[65]

We have seen from this brief historical sketch that the rôle of motor response in consciousness has been emphasized by many thinkers throughout the centuries, either directly or by suggestion through the reference to kinesthesis. Much of the discussion has been theoretical, or at best what Titchener after Brentano has termed empirical, but this is true of most of the fundamental theories of psychology until the nineteenth century. Since then a number of experiments have yielded results which seem to support the theory. It is fair to predict that in the future there will be less theorizing and more research of a nature similar to that of Jacobson. The theory itself must wait upon further experimental findings for its development and more precise refinement.

[59] F. M. Gregg, "Materializing the Ghost of Köhler's Gestalt Psychology," *Psychol. Rev.*, 39, 257–270, 1932.

[60] M. Ponzo, "Principes et Facteurs du Dynamism psychologie dans les Recherches de l'Ecole de Psychologie de Turin," *Jour. de Psychol.*, 27, p. 617, 1930.

[61] *Ibid.*, p. 630.

[62] *Ibid.*, p. 624.

[63] O. Jespersen, "Lehrbuch der Phonetik," p. 6, 2te aufl., Leipzig, Tuebner, 1913.

[64] M. Ponzo, *loc. cit.*, p. 641.

[65] E. Jacobson, "Electrical Measurements of Neuromuscular States during Mental Activities," vii, "Imagination, Recollection and Abstract Thinking Involving the Speech Musculature," *Amer. Jour. Physiol.*, 97, p. 209, 1931.

# OBITUARY

## JOHN BELLING

JOHN BELLING died on February 28, 1933, in San Francisco. He was born at Aldershot, England, on October 7, 1866, and taught in private and public schools in England, taking instruction meanwhile at London and Birmingham. In the university at the former place he received the degree of bachelor of science. In later life he was given the honorary degree of doctor of science by the University of Maine in 1922.

He lectured in the Horticultural College at Swanley, England, and later at Llandidloes, Wales, in 1900–01. Shortly after this he migrated to the British West Indies, where he became investigator in the Department of Agriculture. In 1907 he came to the Florida Experiment Station as assistant botanist and published important researches there on hybrid beans.

Shortly after the war he came to the Carnegie Institution of Washington as cytologist in the department of genetics, and was associated with Dr. A. F. Blakeslee in the investigation of the chromosomes of Datura. Here his genius in microscopy and his philosophic insight opened up a new field in the study of the behavior of chromosomes and in the interchange of segments between non-homologous chromosomes. Belling was subject to periods of depression during which he did some of his most brilliant work. Believing that it was important for him to have a change of scene he was transferred by the institution to Berkeley, California, where he worked in a corner of Professor E. B. Babcock's laboratory, continuing his fundamental researches on the structure of chromosomes in hyacinths and various lilies. In these investigations, under superlative technique, he believed he was able to see structures, which on account of their number and size, he identified with genes.

Belling was the author of a book on the use of the microscope, which has been eminently successful. A book on the study of the chromosomes has been written, but not published. After the sixth International Congress of Genetics, held in Ithaca last summer, a number of foreign delegates traveled to Berkeley to examine Belling's preparations showing the structure of the chromosomes, and to discuss with him his interpretations of them.

He married Miss Hannah Sewall, who died in 1926

without issue. He is survived by a brother, James Belling, of Cornwall, England.

CHARLES B. DAVENPORT

## RECENT DEATHS

EDWARD BRUCE WILLIAMSON, research associate in the Museum of Zoology, University of Michigan, died on February 28, at the age of fifty-five years.

DR. H. GREGG SMITH, associate in biochemistry at the State University of Iowa, died on February 26. He was thirty-four years old.

NATURE reports the deaths of Professor Johan van Baren, an authority on soil mineralogy, professor of geology and mineralogy in the Agricultural University of Wageningen, Holland, on February 7, aged fifty-seven years, and of Lieutenant-Colonel J. C. G. Kunhardt, formerly of the Indian Medical Service, who did valuable work on plague prevention in India and also in the advancement of the rubber industry, at the age of fifty-seven years.

# SCIENTIFIC EVENTS

## THE FACULTY OF MEDICINE OF PARIS

A CORRESPONDENT of the *Journal* of the American Medical Association writes that the Faculty of Medicine of Paris, having often complained of its cramped quarters, which in view of the constantly increasing number of students have became inadequate, received from the Rockefeller Foundation the offer of a gift of $6,000,000 for new buildings for the faculty of medicine, on condition that the French government furnish an equal sum. It was impossible to erect the new buildings on the present site along the Boulevard St. Germain, in the center of Paris, where real estate commands an enormous price. When a different site was sought, consideration was given to the site occupied by the Halle-aux-vins, on the bank of the Seine farther to the east. The Halle-aux-vins in that case would have been moved outside the city. The wine merchants refused to move. Attention was then given to a large unoccupied area south of the city, which was being used for a military aviation school. The suggestion of this site brought protests from the professors, students, medical libraries and the dealers in surgical instruments that had been grouped for centuries about the present buildings. This site was several miles away from the principal teaching hospitals. Attention was then given to a tract occupied by the Ste. Anne psychopathic hospital, located to the south in the vicinity of the University City. It was not long before protests were heard. Professors think the location is still too remote, and their opinion is shared by the merchants. Furthermore, it would be necessary to rebuild a much larger psychopathic hospital elsewhere; for it is now inadequate, owing to the increasing number of insane persons. The council of the faculty of medicine, according to the correspondent, is placed in an embarrassing position by the gift of the Rockefeller Foundation, especially in view of the state of the French treasury. The present buildings of the faculty of medicine are only fifty years old, and it would suffice to add further stories or erect annexes. In short, the council appears disposed to postpone until more propitious times the realization of the generous proposal of the great American philanthropist. Attention has been called also to the fact that the magnificent university buildings erected with the same aid but located too far from the center of the city are already revealing grave disadvantages by reason of their remoteness. The students are attending their lectures less regularly on account of the time required to go to and fro.

## REVISION OF THE INTERNATIONAL ELECTRICAL UNITS

THE Bureau of Standards reports that the third biennial meeting of the advisory committee on electricity and photometry established by the International Committee on Weights and Measures opened on January 31 at the International Bureau of Weights and Measures, at Sevres, near Paris.

The international committee has undertaken to revise the present international electrical units. It proposes to base the units directly upon absolute measurements in the electromagnetic centimeter-gram-second system, instead of defining them by means of the mercury-ohm tube and the silver voltameter. Redeterminations of the ohm and ampère by absolute measurements are in progress in several national standardizing laboratories, including the Bureau of Standards; at the meeting at which the bureau was represented by E. C. Crittenden, chief of the Electrical Division, plans were made for comparing the results found in different countries and for furnishing to all countries standards based upon the combined results.

The international committee likewise hopes to establish uniform units and standards throughout the world for the measurement of light. In this attempt it is collaborating with the International Commission on Illumination. A special committee on units and standards appointed by the latter commission, and consisting of representatives of France, Germany, Great Britain, Japan, the Netherlands and the United States, met in Paris on January 30 to prepare recommendations on photometry for the official advisory committee.

The bureau has proposed the establishment of a system of photometric units based primarily upon the intensity of the light given by a "black body" radiator at the freezing point of platinum. The adoption of such a basic unit must be supplemented by agreement upon a method for measuring lights differing from that of the basic standard in color. The flicker photometer, with proper allowance for the characteristics of individual observers, affords one of the most simple and practical methods for making such measurements. Its use has, however, not been viewed with favor abroad. Consequently, a basis for international agreement is being sought in spectrophotometric measurements of colored filters, from which standard values for transmission of visible light can be calculated by means of "visibility factors" which have already been accepted by the International Commission on Illumination.

In both of these projects the National Physical Laboratory of Great Britain and the Bureau of Standards have been cooperating. Mr. Crittenden therefore visited London on his way to Paris in order to compare experimental results found at the bureau with those of the British laboratory. These two laboratories have joined in proposing that the new units in electricity and in light be put into general use on January 1, 1935. An alternative proposal is that their introduction be deferred until 1937. The most important duties of the 1933 meeting are to choose between these dates and to agree upon a definite schedule for carrying out the series of comparisons and interchange of standards which will be necessary.

## THE PRIESTLEY LECTURES AT THE PENNSYLVANIA STATE COLLEGE

THE seventh annual Priestley Lectures at the Pennsylvania State College will be given at 7:30 P. M., on April 3, 4, 5, 6 and 7.

Two memorials to Joseph Priestley have been established by the faculty and alumni of the department of chemistry: 1. In 1919 the alumni of the department purchased the old Priestley residence at Northumberland, Pennsylvania, about seventy miles from the college. They have built near the house a museum to hold such Priestley relics as can be gathered together. The alumni have assumed responsibility for the maintenance of the whole property in recognition of Joseph Priestley's contributions to early American chemistry. 2. An annual series of lectures was inaugurated by members of the faculty in 1926, bearing the name of the Priestley Lectures. These lectures deal each year with the border-line between physical chemistry and some other branch of science.

In 1931, Phi Lambda Upsilon (honorary chemical fraternity) undertook the financial support of the Priestley Lectures. These lectures, therefore, now constitute a joint memorial to Joseph Priestley on the part of both the faculty of the Department of Chemistry and the Honorary Fraternity of Phi Lambda Upsilon.

This year's lectures deal with the border-line between physical chemistry and metallurgy. They will be given by Professor Eric R. Jette, of the School of Mines of Columbia University.

The former Priestley Lectures are as follows:

The first year's lectures dealt with the border-line between physical chemistry and biocolloids. They were given by V. Cofman, of the Experimental Station of E. I. Du Pont de Nemours and Company.

The second year's lectures dealt with the border-line between physical chemistry and metallography. They were given by Dr. S. L. Hoyt, of the Research Laboratory of the General Electric Company.

The third year's lectures dealt with the border-line between physical chemistry and medicine. They were given by Dr. H. B. Williams, head of the department of physiology of the College of Physicians and Surgeons, Columbia University.

The fourth year's lectures dealt with the border-line between physical chemistry and ceramics. They were given by Dr. Louis Navias, of the Research Laboratory of the General Electric Company.

The fifth year's lectures dealt with the borderline between physical chemistry and electrical engineering. They were given by Dr. John W. Williams, assistant professor of chemistry at the University of Wisconsin.

The sixth year's lectures dealt with the border-line between physical chemistry and biological chemistry. They were given by Dr. Victor K. LaMer, associate professor of chemistry of Columbia University.

## THE SIXTEENTH SESSION OF THE INTERNATIONAL GEOLOGICAL CONGRESS

THE International Geological Congress will hold its sixteenth session in Washington, D. C., from July 22 to 29.

The project of holding an International Geological Congress originated in connection with the Centennial Exposition of 1876 at Philadelphia. A Founders' Committee was formed in that year with James Hall, state geologist of New York and one of America's foremost geologists, as its president. The committee included T. Sterry Hunt, of Canada, as secretary, six other members from the United States and Canada, and one each from England, Sweden and Holland. Thomas Henry Huxley was the member from England. This committee asked the Geological Society of France to cooperate in preparing for a congress at the Paris Exposition in 1878 and the French society appointed an organization committee on July 27, 1877.

This meeting was the first of a series of fifteen congresses that have been held as a rule at intervals of from three to four years, in various countries of Europe and in Mexico (1906), Canada (1913), and the United States (1891). The preceding one was held in South Africa in 1929.

The International Geological Congress is regarded as a continuing organization for which the responsibility is passed on from the organization committee of one session to that of the next. Attempts have been made at various times to induce the congress to form an International Union or to affiliate with the International Research Council, but the preference of the members has been in favor of the more informal organization that has always existed.

However, the thirteenth session which met in Brussels in 1922 adopted a set of statutes consisting of twelve articles, which were essentially a formulation of the traditional practises of the congress and which were for the most part very general in character.

In general the meetings of the congress are financed by contributions from governments, organizations and individuals. The coming session was financed, in its early stages, by contributions from members of the organization committee. Subsequently, however, the Geological Society of America undertook to pay the expenses of organizing the congress, and has offered a liberal subsidy to reduce the cost of the excursions to participants.

One of the principal objects of the International Geological Congresses is to enable geologists to acquaint themselves, by personal observation, with some of the most significant and distinctive features of the geology of the country in which the congress is held. For this reason it is customary for the organizers of each congress to carefully plan and prepare a number of excursions to take place before and after the scientific sessions. On each excursion a special type of geology generally predominates. The nature of some of the excursions to be given in connection with the coming congress in Washington is indicated by the following summary descriptions of them:

Eastern New York and Western New England.
Mining districts of Southeastern and Central States.
Appalachian Valley in Virginia.
Paleozoic stratigraphy of New York.
Coastal plain of the Chesapeake Bay region.
Oil fields of Oklahoma and Texas.
Geomorphology of the central Appalachians.
Mineral deposits of New Jersey and eastern Pennsylvania.
Transcontinental excursion starting from San Francisco.

These excursions will take place before the sessions in Washington and last from 4 to 12 days. In addition, a committee of New York geologists has arranged a group of one and two day excursions in the vicinity of New York for those who do not care for the longer trips. There will also be short excursions from Washington during the session.

After the Washington sessions there will be two transcontinental excursions, each lasting thirty-one days. These will include a wide range of geologic features with some choice of side trips. There will also be two shorter excursions after the congress, one for glacial geology and one to study the iron and copper deposits and the pre-Cambrian geology of the Lake Superior region.

In the minds of the founders of the congress one of its principal functions seems to have been to bring geologists together so that they could standardize by international agreement certain methods and ideas. This is clearly formulated by the president of the Organization Committee of the first congress in his address of welcome where he says, "The dominant motif in organizing this congress has been the need, felt by all, of mutual agreement on geologic classification and nomenclature," though he goes on to say "We can not invoke here the law of numbers; no majority can impose convictions which the sense of truth alone can bring about." The inherent limitations to such activity in a rapidly growing science, except as regards the standardization of cartographic symbols, has become increasingly clear with successive congresses, so that the tendency has been more and more away from standardization and towards exchange of ideas.

Thus, out of the program of the first Congress which consisted of the following topics:

1. Standardization of geologic publications from the point of view of nomenclature and symbols.
2. Discussion of various questions relating to the limits and characters of some formations.
3. Representation and coordination of alignment features (faults and veins).
4. Relative value of faunas and floras from the point of view of the delimitation of formations.
5. Value of mineralogic composition and texture of rocks from the point of view of their origin and age.

two lines of activity have developed, one represented by the program of topics for discussion, the other by the commissions for organizing the knowledge in certain fields and increasing international agreement in them.

As a result of this development the organization committee of the sixteenth session has proposed the following topics for special discussion at the coming meeting:

Measurement of geologic time by any method.
Batholiths and related intrusives.
Zonal relations of metalliferous deposits.
Major divisions of the Paleozoic era.
Geomorphogenic processes in arid regions and their resulting forms and products.
Fossil man and contemporary faunas.
Orogenesis.
Geology of petroleum.
Copper resources of the world.

In proposing for discussion such a topic, for instance, as "Major Divisions of the Paleozoic Era" it is hoped that as a result of the formal papers presented and the discussion that accompanies them, a closer approach to agreement in this very controversial field will be reached; but there will be no attempt to formulate certain conclusions as representing the opinion of the congress as a whole.

The international commissions of the congress appointed at any session carry over to the next session, at which they are expected to present their reports. They may be and many of them have been continued from session to session. Those appointed at the fifteenth session are:

1. Spendiaroff prize.
2. Palaeontologia Universalis.
3. Lexicon of Stratigraphy.
4. Glaciers.
5. Fossil Man.
6. Crust of the earth.
7. Geophysics and Geothermics.
8. Map of Europe.
9. Map of the Earth.
10. Distribution of the Karroo (Gondwana) system.
11. International Map of Africa.
12. Sub-Commission of African Surveys.

The success of several of these which are charged with the preparation of definite publications depends largely on funds from outside sources. The Prussian Geological Survey, under the auspices of the committees of the International Geological Congress, has supervised the compilation of the geologic maps of Europe and of the World, which have been published and are sold through regular publishers.

Other commissions have fostered work in the fields with which they were concerned or provided for the publication of results in current journals. There are obvious difficulties in the way of effective action by a commission whose members are scattered over the entire earth, as is the case with most of these commissions. However, even when they can not produce definite results they promote international agreement in the fields with which they deal.

The organization committee of the eleventh session held in Sweden in 1910 decided that it was desirable for the congress to exert a more extensive and systematic influence on the development of applied geology. They, therefore, published a volume on "The Iron Ore Resources of the World." It has been the practise of the organization committee of most congresses since then to prepare a similar volume on the resources in some major mineral deposit. Volumes on coal, phosphate and pyrite, and gold have been published by previous congresses and the organization committee of the sixteenth session is preparing one on copper.

These volumes aim to describe the geology of deposits all over the world and as far as possible to estimate reserves. They have been found very valuable by those concerned with the mineral industries and have probably helped to secure financial support for the congress.

Not the least valuable function of these congresses, as of all gatherings of scientists, is to bring about personal acquaintance and friendship among those who attend and to afford opportunity for informal discussion. During the scientific sessions of the International Geological Congresses some formal entertainments as well as informal gatherings of groups and individuals provide for this, but the best opportunity is afforded by the excursions, on which the participants are constantly together for a number of days, and discuss many of their problems with the evidence before them.

Any one may become a member of the Congress For information address General Secretary, International Geological Congress, U. S. Geological Survey, Washington, D. C.

M. I. G.

# SCIENTIFIC NOTES AND NEWS

DR. ROBERT F. GRIGGS, professor of botany at George Washington University, Washington, D. C., has been elected president of the Washington Academy of Sciences.

GEORGE W. FULLER, of Fuller and McClintock, New York, has been elected chairman of the Engineering Foundation. He succeeds H. Hobart Porter, president of the American Water Works and Electric Company.

DR. SYDNEY CHAPMAN, chief professor of mathematics at the Imperial College, South Kensington, has been made president for 1933 of the Royal Meteorological Society.

CONRAD BECK, director of R. and J. Beck, scientific instrument manufacturers, London, has been elected president of the Royal Microscopical Society.

THE degree of doctor of science will be conferred by the University of Dublin on Professor William Lawrence Bragg, professor of physics, Victoria University of Manchester, and on Professor John Scott Haldane, fellow of New College, Oxford, honorary professor and director of the Mining Research Laboratory, Birmingham University.

DR. EMIL ABDERHALDEN, professor of physiology at Halle, has been elected an associate member of the Society of Biology at Paris.

A TESTIMONIAL dinner to Professor Charles W. Ballard, of the faculty of the Columbia College of Pharmacy, was tendered to him by the Pharmacy Alumni Association on March 9. Professor Ballard has been associated with the College of Pharmacy for twenty-five years. Among the speakers were Dean Henry V. Arny, Dean Emeritus H. H. Rusby, Professor Marston T. Bogert, Columbia University, and Edward Bocker, the New York City Department of Health.

JOHN J. KELEHER, a member of the staff of the New York Aquarium, has been awarded the gold medal of the New York Zoological Society in recognition of his thirty years' service. The presentation was made by Dr. Charles H. Townsend, director of the aquarium, who himself completed thirty years with the institution last November.

IN recognition of their outstanding contributions to medicine, thirteen leading physicians and research workers from ten nations have been elected to honorary fellowship in the New York Academy of Medicine. The number of honorary fellows is limited to fifty; at present there are thirty-five. The new fellows are: Charles Achard, professor of the Faculté de Médecine of Paris and permanent general secretary of the Académie de Médecine; Roberto Alessandri, formerly professor of surgical anatomy, now director of the surgical clinic at the University of Rome; Sir Charles Ballance, consulting physician at St. Thomas's Hospital and National Hospital for Paralysis and Epilepsy, London; Frederick Grant Banting, professor of medical research at the University of Toronto; Sir Henry Hallett Dale, secretary of the Royal Society and director of the National Institute for Medical Research, London; Otfried Foerster, professor of psychiatry and neurology, Breslau; Carl Gustaf Forssell, professor of radiology in the Medico-Chirurgical Institute and director of radiumhemmet, Stockholm; James Bryan Herrick, emeritus professor of medicine, Rush Medical College, Chicago; Cornelius Ubbo Ariens Kappers, professor of comparative anatomy of the nervous system at the University of Amsterdam; George Richards Minot, professor of medicine, Harvard University; William Gibson Spiller, professor of neurology at the University of Pennsylvania and consulting neurologist at the Philadelphia General Hospital; Alfred Vogt, professor of ophthalmology at the University of Zurich, and Karel Frederik Wenckebach, professor of medical pathology and therapy at the University of Vienna.

PROFESSOR B. NĚMEC, director of the Institute of Plant Physiology of the Charles University, Prague, Czechoslovakia, will celebrate his sixtieth birthday on March 12. A correspondent writes: "Professor Němec is a prominent plant physiologist, working on experimental cytology, caryology, anatomy, experimental morphology, physiology of fecundation, symbiosis, parasitism, plant pathology and regeneration. His 'statolit' theory is well known, as are his recent discoveries of artificially induced mixoploidy and polyploidy in plants by means of chloral hydrate. These discoveries were discussed by him at the fifth International Botanical Congress held at Ithaca in 1926. Professor Němec is a corresponding member of the American Botanical Society, and of many other learned societies, Czechoslovak and foreign. He is the president of the American Institute in Prague. Professor Němec took an active part in the work which resulted in the liberation of his country. He is now a representative of the National Democratic Party in the Parliament and is, at the same time, one of the most prominent members of Charles University."

ON the recommendation of Dr. Gregory and Dr. Sherwood, of the American Museum of Natural History, the executive committee of that institution has appointed Dr. William Beebe a member of the department of ichthyology, with the title of research associate in oceanography.

DR. SAMUEL E. POND has resigned from the University of Pennsylvania, where he has been assistant professor of physiology in the Schools of Medicine and Dentistry, to accept the position of technical manager at the Marine Biological Laboratory, Woods Hole, Massachusetts. Dr. Pond will be in residence in Woods Hole throughout the year, beginning on April 1. In addition to the direction of laboratory matters of a technical nature he will continue his researches on elementary calcification and the solid phases in ossified tissues.

DR. GEORGE KREEZER has resigned as Merriam research fellow at Cornell University to become research associate at the Training School at Vineland, New Jersey. This appointment was made possible by a gift recently made by friends of the Vineland Laboratory. It is anticipated that Dr. Kreezer will conduct a series of investigations of birth-injured children by the methods of physiological psychology.

F. S. BRACKETT has retired from the directorship of the Division of Radiation and Organisms of the Smithsonian Institution and becomes research and consulting physicist. Dr. C. G. Abbot, secretary of the institution, has assumed the directorship of the division and E. S. Johnston has become assistant director.

PROFESSOR JAMES H. BREASTED, of the Oriental Institute, University of Chicago, sailed from New York on February 4 for an inspection of field work in Persia.

DR. MORRIS S. VITELES, assistant professor of psychology at the University of Pennsylvania and director of personnel research in the Philadelphia Electric Company, has been elected a member of the board of directors of the Personnel Research Foundation.

DR. THOMAS STOCKHAM BAKER, president of the Carnegie Institute of Technology, Pittsburgh, who has been lecturing in Germany under the auspices of the Carl Schurz Society, arrived in New York on March 3.

DR. H. H. DONALDSON, of the Wistar Institute of Anatomy, addressed the Sigma Xi Society at the University of Pittsburgh on February 15 on "What We have Learned on the Growth of the Brain during the Past Forty Years."

DR. ANNIE J. CANNON, of the Harvard College Observatory, gave on February 15 an address on "Eclipsing Experiences" before the science seminar of the University of Maine.

DR. BAILEY K. ASHFORD, colonel, U. S. Army Medical Corps, retired, professor of mycology in the School of Tropical Medicine, San Juan, Puerto Rico, discussed acute uncinariasis at the Research Club of the department of medical zoology of the Johns Hopkins University School of Hygiene and Public Health on February 20. His discussion was based on case histories of individuals who came to his attention almost immediately after receiving exceedingly heavy infestations of *Ancylostoma duodenale* while wading in infected water in Puerto Rico.

RECENT visiting lecturers to the department of geology and geography, Northwestern University, and their subjects included: T. A. Hendricks, of the U. S. Geological Survey, "The Classification of Coal"; L. E. Workman, of the Illinois Geological Survey, "Subsurface Methods as Applied to Illinois"; C. W. Washburne, consulting geologist, "Structural Studies in the Oregon Coast Ranges"; Dr. G. R. Mansfield, of the U. S. Geological Survey, "Viewpoints in Geological Research"; Professor E. S. Bastin, of the University of Chicago, "Ores of Copper Lean in Iron and Sulphur."

THE fourth lecture to the faculty and students of the School of Medicine, The George Washington University, on the Smith-Reed-Russell Society series was given on February 23 by Professor Stanhope Bayne-Jones, of the Department of Bacteriology, Yale University Medical School, and chairman of the Medical Division, National Research Council, on "Bacterial Toxins." The next lecture in this series will be given by Dr. Maurice C. Hall, chief of the Zoological Division, Bureau of Animal Industry, U. S. Department of Agriculture, on March 16, on "Drama Anthelmintica." The regular faculty seminar for February was given by Professor George B. Jenkins, of the department of anatomy, who spoke on "Comparative Embryology of the Central Nervous System."

A GIFT of $100,000 for the general purposes of the Gray Herbarium of Harvard University has been received from Earl Willson Bemis, of Worcester, Massachusetts. The original collection was founded by the late Asa Gray and given by him to the university in 1864.

A GIFT has been made by E. R. Squibb and Son, New York, through the National Research Council Committee on Drug Addiction, of a fellowship of $700 for work in pharmacology to be carried on under the direction of Professor C. W. Edmunds, in the Medical School of the University of Michigan.

PLUTARCO ELIAS CALLES, of Mexico, has turned over his Santa Barbara hacienda to the Agricultural Department to be used as an experimental station.

THE Prussian Ministry of Public Instruction has granted permission to the various clinics, institutes and the like, to announce the maximum number of students that, in their opinion, can receive proper training and to reject the applications of students in excess of that number. In the dental institutes, such restrictions were introduced some time ago.

UNDER an amendment of the United States patent statute approved by the President May 23, 1930, which authorizes the issuance of patents to inventors or discoverers of distinct and new varieties of asexually propagated plants other than tuber-propagated plants, 39 plant patents had been issued by the United States Patent Office up to the end of October, 1932. The administration of the law is vested in the commissioner of patents, but, as provided for in the law, the Secretary of Agriculture is charged with the duty of determining for the commissioner of patents, upon his request, whether varieties for which patent applications are made are in fact distinct and new. The special researches necessary to such determinations for the information of the Commissioner of Patents are assigned to the chief of the Bureau of Plant Industry to carry out. "A plant patent," according to Dr. W. A. Taylor, chief of the Bureau of Plant Industry, "grants to the patentee the exclusive right to use, vend and asexually reproduce the new variety covered by the patent throughout the United States and Territories for seventeen years. Naturally, under the limitations prescribed in the statute, most of the alleged new varieties thus far considered are in the horticultural field, relatively few general field crops other than tubers being capable of asexual propagation on a commercial scale in temperate climates. The granting of a patent on a new variety in no way passes on its adaptability to climatic conditions or for special uses or on its economic value, nor does it determine the validity or otherwise of any varietal name which may be applied to the variety by the originator or disseminator.

THE London correspondent of the *Journal* of the American Medical Association writes: "It is striking that in the present period of industrial depression and unemployment, unprecedented both in intensity and in duration, the general health of the population has been remarkably good and has even improved. The registrar-general's statistical review for 1931, which has just been published, shows a death rate of 12.3 per thousand persons living, 0.9 above that for 1930. That rate, however, was the lowest ever recorded, largely because of the exceptionally mild weather in the early part of the year, when the greatest number of deaths occur. The higher rate for 1931 is a reflection of the more severe weather of the early part of the year. Infant mortality was similarly affected, the deaths of children under 1 year being 66 per thousand live births, against 60 in 1930. That year and 1928, however, are the only years that have shown a lower mortality than 1931. The death rate for cancer was 1,484 per million persons living, against 1,454 in 1930. But if allowance is made for the difference in the age constitution of the population (which is constantly becoming greater) the increase in the cancer rate becomes much smaller. Tuberculosis again furnished a new low record, 896 deaths per million living. Road accidents due to mechanical vehicles caused 5,892 deaths. The figures for the preceding four years were 4,452, 5,196, 5,752 and 6,342. The decrease in 1931 is the first that has occurred since 1921, the figures having steadily increased previously. The birth rate was 15.8 per thousand persons living, the lowest on record and 0.5 below that for 1929 and 1930."

# DISCUSSION

## UNIVERSITY PATENTS

NOTHING seems at first sight more reasonable and effective to provide funds for research work in colleges, universities and research institutions than the exploitation, under the protection of patent laws, of the results of research work. Apparently in increasing numbers the universities in this country are resorting to patenting—directly or through approved agencies—for the stated purpose of obtaining money to support research work done by members of their staffs.

Arguments in favor of such a policy seem to have been published rather more fully than other types of comment. Experience, however, is proving that this policy of patenting, so attractive when first contemplated, involves more numerous and more serious difficulties than were at first foreseen, even by those who opposed the policy on ethical grounds. It is not with the ethical or moral validity of universities exploiting patents for revenue that the present communication deals. I wish to call attention only to some of the problems entailed by the policy, at present spreading among universities in the United States and Canada, of taking or being party to the taking of patents for the purpose of obtaining revenue for research work to be done by their students or staff. If explicit definition can obviate misunderstanding it may be well to observe that it is patenting for revenue and not patenting to prevent exploitation by others which is under consideration. I bring forward the matter because, now that the advantages of this policy have been published, it seems reasonable to point out some of the disadvantages.

A professor in one of our large state universities visited not long ago a university whose declared policy it is to take out patents where possible for the research work of its personnel. The professor talked with a young staff member about his research work. It became apparent that what the professor had learned from his own research work would lead, if pieced together with what the young man had found out, to a distinct advance in knowledge, an advance very probably capable of being patented. Although the young man would have been delighted to have had an honorable part in an advance of knowledge and might have received a merited recognition for his share therein, and although science might have been advanced, the professor kept his mouth shut because he couldn't see why his work should be an integral part of a patent controlled for the exclusive benefit of another university. Perhaps it would be better if both universities went in for the patent business. Then the professor wouldn't have felt so resentful or so much at a disadvantage. He would have magnanimously given the young man his big chance by telling him what he needed to know. But of course there is just the possibility that another man would have kept silence, gone back to his own laboratory to confirm the young man's findings and purloined the patent not for his personal advantage of course but for his university. In such a case the young man, if he were as intelligent as he is educated, would learn to keep his mouth shut. I cite this little story from real life because it is such a nice illustration of what patenting for money has done in this instance to the advance of knowledge—for which, incidentally, the two states' funds are being in part devoted.

Some time ago in a well-known medical school a certain synthetic antiseptic was on trial clinically. The first reports were almost as brilliant as the color of the substance itself. The opportunity to patent the antiseptic would have meant an income for research of perhaps $100,000 a year. This entrancing possibility was not seized. Instead of that the clinicians of that school, devoid of proprietary interest, maintained a critical attitude and pursued their investigations, during which the earlier (and honest) enthusiasms paled because the stuff wasn't as good as they thought at first. As the dean remarked to me later, "Would we have cared to examine it as critically if it might mean the loss of a big income for our research work?" For politeness' sake one should quench such doubt by assurances that of course they would, or at least they wouldn't have taken out the patent until they knew that further investigation could not qualify their confidence.

In the dairy state of Ubique I know of an owner of a large milk products company. He is angry because the University of Ubique Research Associates, Incorporated, has taken out a patent for a process that could improve the nutritional value of certain milk products. He says: "I pay taxes to support the State University and its research workers, and as soon as they find something of use to me I have to pay them again for being successful. I'll be ——ed if they can have it coming and going. I'll bring counter suit if they try to sue me."

It is obvious that obtaining a patent is not complete protection. Some money has to be set aside to put teeth in it, *i.e.*, to punish infringements. Without the aid of newspaper files many medical scientists can recall a trial which is reported to have cost the defendants $80,000. Duly skeptical of such a figure, I should, however, assume that the patentees did not use all their takings that year for research. Shortly after the trial they were told by a spirited chief of one city health service that he was going to use their process anyhow and on a large scale, for which he proposed to pay them just one dollar and if they wanted to refuse this offer and bring suit, maybe they'd win, but the city was rich and had good lawyers.

When the patentees set aside large sums for the prosecution of infringements instead of the prosecution of research, there is no assurance of good feeling in the scientific or academic worlds. A well-known American patent for the treatment of an important infectious disease is protected in one country abroad by a clause which forbids its use in research directed to its improvement. An entirely honorable research organization in that country on consulting legal advice as to the probable consequences of using the material for research purposes was told that they would probably be supported by the courts but that the trial would cost upwards of $15,000. Having no funds to fight for the legal right to do research work they have left that field where the patentee desires it to be left. The only consolation that could be offered to them is that their research staff will be spared the waste of time upon the witness stand—a waste of time which has disgusted at least one scientist in this country to the point of deserting a field in which lawsuits may require his time.

The dean of one of our larger medical schools complains that one of his teachers is so busy controlling the product made under a patent held by the university that there is no time left for research or teaching. As a university interest it can't be disregarded, since there may be some money in it, so a competent investigator is now busy testing a commercial product. As long as there is a chance of the product being improved by some one else, he is likely to be tied down for some time to this one subject.

In justice to the universities now in the patent business, it should be admitted that no case has yet come to common knowledge of an appointment or promotion being accorded to a man because his mind runs to patentable and consequently profitable research. Surprise at such an event would, however, be a trifle naïve when the universities intentionally and officially encourage patents for revenue to support the research expenses they so badly need.

One neither moralizes nor speculates in restating the present tendency as being an assertion on the part of certain universities that they are disposed to encourage the means to extract legally and certainly from the public in this and other countries a contribution to their own research work, which is as they believe inadequately supported. They invoke the patent law to supplement what public appreciation fails to provide: they insist on a general and immediate contribution to maintain research which they can not guarantee will be of value equal to its cost. An excuse is provided for the first time for the public to leave research in the universities to "look out for itself."

I am not interested in discussing here the ethics or morality of the matter. The way it is working out is proving dangerous: it tends to shut off unselfish exchange of ideas and information, it tends to kill a critical and impartial attitude, it tends to introduce quarrels and bitterness and to consume time and funds in lawsuits. It may quite naturally influence the choice of university personnel and the choice of research problems. If, in addition, the policy of taking out patents for revenue be interpreted as a declaration of independence the public may quite cheerfully acquiesce and leave research work to earn its own way. Why should gifts intended for the general welfare play the rôle of capitalizing a business? And what becomes of the peculiar function of university research as contrasted with that of the shrewdly administered business enterprise?

ALAN GREGG

30 CAMBRIDGE ROAD,
SCARSDALE, N. Y.

## THE COEFFICIENT OF CORRELATION

IN a recent article describing a least-square curve fitting machine[1] the authors make use of the Pearson product-moment coefficient of correlation to test the agreement of the parameters obtained by use of this device with those obtained by an algebraic method. This use of the correlation coefficient to test the agreement of two methods of measuring the same quantity is frequently seen in the literature, but the soundness of the procedure is open to question.

The idea of correlation as conceived by Galton implies that there is such a measurable quantity as *degree of relationship,* and the coefficient developed by Pearson is taken to give this measure. In keeping with this idea it is argued that if two methods of measurement agree well, their results will be "closely related" and *vice versa;* hence the use of the coefficient. As a matter of fact, the correlation coefficient is more correctly understood, specifically as a particular parameter obtained in a least-square fit of a straight line to the data correlated, and its significance is not general, but varies with the character of the data to which the fit applies.

In the case at hand, it can easily be shown that the coefficient measures, in large part, something quite different from what is intended. The method of procedure when two instruments or methods of measurements are to be compared is as follows: A series of determinations over the entire range of instrument or method $x$ is made, and upon the same data determinations are made with instrument $y$. The corresponding measurements are then correlated. The coefficient may be given by

$$r=\sqrt{1-\frac{\sigma^2_{x.y}}{\sigma^2_x}}$$

Where $r$ is the coefficient, $\sigma_x$ is the standard deviation of the $x$ measurements, $\sigma_{x.y}$ is the partial standard deviation of $x$, for a fixed value of $y$. Now, in instances of this kind, the distribution of $x$ is not generally normal, but rectangular, *i.e.,* about the same number of measurements is made at each value of $x$. Under these circumstances $\sigma_x$ depends on the range of $x$, being given by $\sigma^2_x=\frac{R^2_x}{12}$ where $R_x$ is the range of $x$. Consequently, $r$ is greater the greater the range of the measurements made. That the method can easily lead to paradoxical results may be seen as follows. Suppose two instruments to be uniformly comparable over their entire ranges, one with the other. A series of measurements is made over the lower half of the range and correlated, yielding a particular value of $r$. The same procedure is repeated for the upper half and the same value of $r$ is obtained, appearing to give a good check of the measure of how well the two methods agree. But if now all the data are put together as a single series, the correlation will be greater. For instance, if $r$ was 0.5 in the first case, it would be 0.9 in the second.

This fallaciousness in the use and interpretation of the correlation coefficient creeps in in other instances than where methods of measurement are compared. For instance, it is present when a physical trait like height is correlated with age, and the age range is arbitrary. It also vitiates not a little of the use made of the coefficient by psychologists.

In passing, referring to the main topic of the article first mentioned, it may be noted that the idea of obtaining a least-square fit of a line on the principle of elastic bands stretched from the points to be fitted was mentioned at least as early as 1921 by L. J. Reed.[2]

JOSEPH BERKSON

ROCHESTER, MINNESOTA

## ATTEMPT TO CONFIRM THE EXISTENCE OF A FILTRABLE CYCLE OF BACTERIA BY THE USE OF "K" MEDIUM[1]

AN attempt has been made to confirm the results of Kendall reported in the *Northwestern University Bulletin* (xxxii, 5, 1931). Complete failure with 'K' medium made by us according to his directions, was

[1] Gains and Palfrey, "A Least-Square Curve Fitting Machine," SCIENCE, 76: 472, November 18, 1932.

[2] Lowell J. Reed, "Fitting of Straight Lines," *Metron*, Vol. 1, p. 3, 1921.

[1] A detailed account of the work appears in the *Journal of Infectious Diseases*, 52: 20. 1933.

followed by experiments with 'K' powder kindly sent to us by Dr. Kendall. A protocol suggested by him, using the Rawlins strain of *B. typhosus,* was followed exactly. At least five attempts in accordance with this protocol and many more based on the first reports of the medium were made.

In connection with the 'K' medium, many difficulties were encountered; for example, no uniformity of pH from tube to tube could be attained. It also occasionally develops a spontaneous turbidity without inoculation.

In summary we may state that persistent efforts to confirm Dr. Kendall's experiments have been uniformly negative.

C. V. SEASTONE
MARY B. LAWRENCE

HARVARD MEDICAL SCHOOL

### UNIVALENT CHROMOSOMES OF TRADESCANTIA VIRGINIANA

AN esteemed correspondent, in SCIENCE (Vol. 77, pp. 49–50), states that, in *Tradescantia virginiana,* "the apparently serially arranged, miscalled univalent chromosomes represent in reality a segmented pachytene in which the synaptic pairs are lined up, back to back." I have lately been studying the pachytene of this species, and also of *Rhoeo discolor:* and have succeeded in obtaining clear preparations. In Rhoeo, only the sub-terminal parts of the 12 chromosomes synapse; and are afterwards seen at diplotene to separate, leaving terminal junctions. Thus the 12 bodies seen in the rings appear to me to be these univalents attached at the ends. For if they were "pairs . . . back to back," there would be, I think, 6 of them. In *Tradescantia virginiana* (which is, in my opinion, rightly regarded as a tetraploid), 12 of the 24 chromosomes can be seen to have synapsed, at pachytene, with their 12 homologues; while their sub-terminal parts show synapsis between 4 chromosomes. These can be seen to separate at diplotene, except for their terminal junctions. The 24 bodies seen in rings, in chains, or singly, are, I think, the univalents. For if they were "pairs . . . back to back," there would be apparently 12 of them.

JOHN BELLING[1]

BERKELEY, CALIF.

# SPECIAL CORRESPONDENCE

### UNIVERSITY EXPEDITION TO STUDY THE NATIVES OF CENTRAL AUSTRALIA

IN August, 1932, an expedition to study the natives of Central Australia was organized by the Board for Anthropological Research of the University of Adelaide, in conjunction with the South Australian Museum. The expenses were chiefly met by a grant from the Rockefeller Foundation, administered through the Australian National Research Council. The situation chosen on this occasion was Mount Liebig, situated almost on the Tropic of Capricorn, 200 miles by track west of Alice Springs. The natives belonging to this portion of Central Australia have hitherto escaped contact with Europeans, save to a very superficial extent. By means of a preliminary survey by Mr. Kramer, of the Aborigines Friends Association, in whom these natives had complete confidence, over 130 aborigines, including men, women and children, were gathered together for observation. Their equilibrium had been a little disturbed by a raid from an adjacent tribe, in which 7 men had traveled 100 miles to secure two women, killing their common husbands and one of the women, and abducting the other.

The personnel of the expedition included amongst others Dr. T. D. Campbell, to whom much of the credit of its success is due, Professors T. Harvey Johnston, C. S. Hicks and J. B. Cleland, Dr. H. K. Fry, Mr. H. M. Hale, director of the South Australian Museum, and Messrs. N. B. Tindale and J. H. Gray. As on previous occasions, the natives submitted themselves to many kinds of tests, some of them very trying, without the slightest murmur or objection.

Their good humor and sense of fun were again shown to a striking degree. Not the slightest attempt was made by any native to abstract articles from the camp, even though they could very easily have done so and must have coveted many of the objects seen. Any article accidentally lost by the party was almost invariably found by the natives and returned; one member, whilst watching a corroboree at night, dropped, without knowing it, two postage stamps; these were picked up and returned to camp, evidently being recognized as something unusual.

As the expedition had only a short time at its disposal, the study of the natives had to be concentrated. In physical anthropology this is an advantage; the native readily tires and novelty soon wears off. It would be probably difficult to hold together a body of 100 natives for a period as long as a month; many would desire before then to go for a "walk about."

Professor Hicks with his assistants studied each day the basal metabolism of two fresh natives. This was accompanied by a close study of the pulse and respiration rates, and of the body and skin temperatures throughout the morning as the warmth increased.

[1] Died February 28, 1933.

The natives were weighed and measured according to the Du Bois linear formula method of determining surface area, as well as for standing and sitting heights. Blood pressures were also measured, and katathermometer readings and wet and dry temperature measurements were obtained to give a basis for computing cooling power. When these data and those obtained previously are worked out it is hoped that conclusions may be drawn as to whether there is a true racial variation in basal metabolism; and whether the specific dynamic effect of protein meals on these natives, living with so little margin above a bare sustenance, is the same as for civilized Europeans; and that other important information will be obtained.

Blood-grouping showed again that only Groups A and O occur amongst the Central Australian natives. Out of 84 examined, 32 belonged to Group O and 52 to Group A.

Dr. Fry found that the class system of the Pintubi, which composed the majority of the natives, was of the 4-class nomenclature, but with the additional recognition of the 8-class of the adjacent Loritja. The legends and songs in relation to five ceremonies were obtained, together with their translations. Conception stories and dreams were obtained from five mothers.

Three hundred photographs were taken, which included standard photographs of bust and full-length, and a number of others concerning ceremonial records, pathological data and special features. Complete plaster casts were secured of the busts, including the faces, of two old men, of two young men, of two adult women, of one young woman, and of one newly born male baby; and a face cast of one young woman.

Pathological observations were recorded. The presence in some subjects to a slight degree of boomerang legs, and in several instances a soft enlargement of the parotid glands on each side was noted. Almost without exception pediculi were present in the hair.

It is the custom amongst these people for the mother to kill at birth an infant who is born whilst she is suckling its predecessor. The new-born baby, whose plaster cast was obtained, had been killed by its mother and stuffed into a rabbit's burrow, almost at the moment of arrival of the expedition at Mt. Liebig. Next day members became aware of this event, and with the concurrence of the natives and their assistance the body of the baby was unearthed and a complete description of it obtained. The placenta was attached. Soil or ashes are placed in the baby's mouth to stop its cries before the mother kills it.

Dr. T. D. Campbell and Mr. H. Gray obtained further standard records of measurements of adults and children, together with samples of hair, outlines of hair tracts, notes on the teeth and on the color of the skin, hair and eyes, and special information as regards the curve of the spine, shape of the foot, etc. The peculiar rubbery texture of the soles of the feet was again seen in a number of natives, but not in all.

Extensive cinematograph records were obtained of ceremonies, of daily occupations, of collecting and preparing foods, of making weapons and utensils, and of the meeting of two friendly parties of natives. Various animal and vegetable foods used by these natives were collected.

A meteorological equipment was taken and a very useful set of climatic records was obtained. Other incidental studies, such as geology and physiography, helped in an appreciation of the natives' physical environment.

The expedition proved successful, and has emphasized the value of team-work and the amount of information that can be collected in a short period of time by an intensive study.

J. B. CLELAND

# SCIENTIFIC APPARATUS AND LABORATORY METHODS

## A UNIVERSAL DILATOMETER

SINCE the publication of Ostwald's work on "Volume Chemistry" in 1877, several papers have appeared, discussing from a theoretical and experimental point of view the change of volume which takes place during the process of neutralization of an acid by a base. Ostwald[1] first noticed the phenomenon and investigated its relation to the nature of the acid and of the base. His work was extended and confirmed by Ruppin.[2] The influence of the concentration was then studied by Tammann,[3] who worked with solutions of concentrations between 0.1 and 0.005 normal and who proposed an hypothesis to explain the change of volume. An extensive experimental investigation was later carried out by Miss Freund,[4] who concerned herself with the influence of temperature and of the concentration at higher concentrations than those with which Tammann had worked. During the course of a physico-chemical study of the process of neutralization, Cornec[5] determined the densities of mixtures of solutions of potassium hydroxide and

1 W. Ostwald, *Jour. prakt. Chem.*, 16: 385, 1877.

2 E. Ruppin, *Zeit. physik. Chem.*, 14: 467, 1894.

3 G. Tammann, *Zeit. physik. Chem.*, 16: 91, 139, 1895.

4 I. Freund, *Zeit. physik. Chem.*, 66: 555, 1909.

5 E. Cornec, *Ann. chim. phys.*, (8) 29: 490, 1913.

phosphoric acid and by plotting density against molecular composition, there were shown decided breaks in the density-composition curve corresponding to the salts $KH_2PO_4$ and $K_2HPO_4$. More recently Saslawsky and Standel[6] have determined the volume change upon mixing solutions of acids and bases not only at the neutralization point but also in a series of mixtures of the constituents in other proportions. While their work is not intended to be of an accuracy comparable to any of that previously performed, it is of value in that it covers the concentration range from about 2 to 12 normal.

All the above work was performed by determining experimentally the densities of the solutions of the acid and base, and of the salt formed upon neutralization, and from these values, calculating the volume change taking place upon the formation of the salt

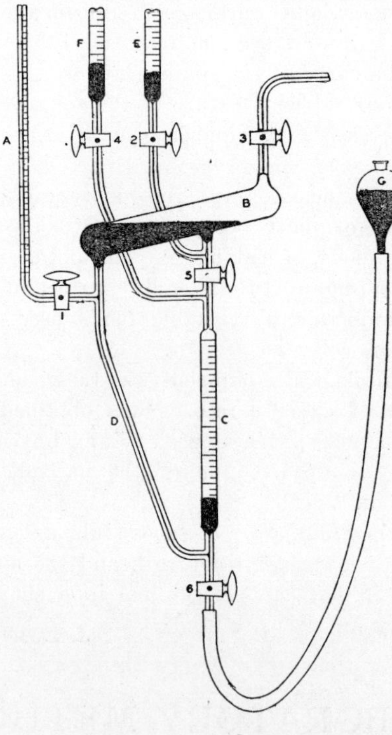


solution. As several of these investigators have pointed out, the value of the volume change so calculated depends upon the precision of the density determinations. Owing to the care necessary for the precise estimation of the density of a solution, even when allowing an error of $\pm 0.00005$, it was thought that a dilatometric method, whereby the volume change might be directly observed, would expedite the extension of this type of work. The changes of volume accompanying oxidation-reduction reactions and those reactions involving the formation of complexes, for example, have not as yet been studied although they have occasionally been utilized for other purposes.[7]

To this end an apparatus has been devised, as illustrated diagrammatically in the accompanying figure, with which it is possible to add known volumes of one liquid to a known volume of another, and, after equilibrium has been established, to read directly the volume change which has occurred. It is based upon a simple hydrostatic principle, which will be obvious after a description has been given of the method of use.

The apparatus, set in a thermostat at the required temperature, is filled with mercury from the reservoir G through stop-cock 6. Stop-cocks 1, 2, 3, 4 and 5 are opened and the mercury allowed to rise into the burettes E and F, into the capillary A, and into the outlet tube through stop-cock 3. All the stop-cocks are then closed. The burettes E and F are filled with the liquids under investigation, note being taken of the amount in E. In opening stop-cocks 4 and 6 and lowering the mercury reservoir, the liquid in F flows down to fill the burette C. The stop-cocks are then closed. On opening stop-cocks 2 and 6 the liquid in E flows through 2, bubbles up through the mercury in B and occupies the upper portion of the tube. Meanwhile the mercury flows through D to the reservoir. When the required amount of liquid from E has been transferred to B, the flow of mercury is reversed by raising the reservoir, sending mercury back up again into the burette E. The difference between the volume of the liquid remaining and of that originally present in E gives the volume transferred to B. Stop-cock 2 is now closed. By opening stop-cock 1 the position of the mercury in the capillary A may now be adjusted to a suitable portion of the scale, depending upon whether the alteration of volume to be measured is an expansion or a contraction. Stop-cock 6 is closed. The thread of mercury running from B to C through stop-cock 5 is removed by opening the latter till the liquid in C rises to the constriction just at the entrance to B. The apparatus is now in the condition depicted.

The level of the mercury in C is noted and also the volume of the closed-off system as measured at A. Portions of the liquid in C are allowed to pass up into B by opening and then closing stop-cock 5. To insure thorough mixing of the two liquids, the tube B is at a slight angle to the horizontal so that by rocking the apparatus sideways, the motion of the mercury layer sets up a turbulence in the liquid above it. Any volume change which occurs will be evident from the displacement of the meniscus of the mercury in the capillary A. Opening and closing stop-cock 5, observing the change of height of the mercury in C,

6 I. I. Saslawsky and E. G. Standel, *Zeit. anorg. allgem. Chem.*, 180: 241, 1929; 186: 171, 1930.

7 A. Benrath, *Jour. prakt. Chem.*, 80: 283, 1909.

and measuring the volume on A, gives a complete record of the changes of volume taking place upon mixing the two liquids. The outlet through 3 has been introduced for the purpose of discarding the solutions after use and for cleaning.

In the apparatus as built, the tube B has a volume of approximately 120 $cm^3$ with a length of about 20 cm and a diameter of about 3 cm. The burettes C, E and F are graduated for a volume of 50 $cm^3$ by 1/10 $cm^3$. The capillary A is graduated in millimeters over a length of 80 cm. To facilitate its mounting upon the frame of the apparatus, the capillary was wound into the form of a flat spiral with an average diameter of about 12 cm. Its volume after bending was calibrated with mercury in the usual way. One millimeter has a volume of 0.0021 $cm^3$.

Besides being of use in the study of neutralization and of other chemical reactions between solutions, the dilatometer should be of value for the investigation of volume changes under many other conditions. The expansions or contractions taking place upon dilution of concentrated solution have been incompletely studied. To date the phenomenon has been investigated with only a few of the many electrolytes,[8] with alcohol[9] and with a few other organic compounds. Solutions of substances in other solvents than water have been almost completely neglected. The relation between the miscibility of liquids and the accompanying volume change may perhaps be a fruitful source for information concerning the nature of the liquid state and of solutions.

Another form of dilatometer with which it is possible to measure directly the alterations of volume on mixing two liquids has just recently been described.[10] Its applicability to work of a general nature is limited in that the volume change is given on mixing the two liquids in only one proportion. It is obvious that with the dilatometer described above the value of the volume changes for a series of mixtures of the two liquids may be obtained in one experiment.

Further details concerning the design, construction and manipulation of the apparatus, as well as some of the results obtained by its use, will be published in more extended form elsewhere. This notice has been given for the description of a new type of dilatometer, constructed easily and at small cost, which may facilitate greatly the study of a fundamental property of liquids.

R. HOLCOMB

McGILL UNIVERSITY

[8] G. P. Baxter and C. C. Wallace, *Jour. Amer. Chem. Soc.*, 38: 70, 1916.

[9] F. L. Teed, ''Volume Alterations on and in Solution,'' London, 1926.

[10] J. H. Hildebrand and J. M. Carter, *Jour. Amer. Chem. Soc.*, 54: 3592, 1932.

## PERMANENT SLIDES FOR USE IN TEACHING THE HOWARD METHOD

MANY food analysts throughout the country are employing the Howard method[1] of testing various comminuted food products to determine the condition of the raw material as regards decomposition due to mold, and it frequently happens that analysts come to this laboratory for instruction in the technique of the method. In the course of his training it has been customary for an experienced analyst to check field by field with the student analyst in order to determine the ability of the student to recognize mold filaments of various types. However, a saving in time would result if, instead of using the standard Howard cell, permanent slides with clearly defined fields marked on them were employed.

The preparation of such slides has been accomplished in the following manner: Tomato pulp or catsup of rather thin consistency is used for the test material. One and one half per cent. (1.5 per cent.) of agar is added to the sample and dissolved by boiling. Before cooling, 4 to 5 per cent. of commercial formaldehyde is added.

The following method of delimiting the fields has been found most advantageous. Twenty-five perforations, each 1.31 mm in diameter, are made in colored cellophane, the holes being spaced about 1 mm apart and arranged in five rows of five holes each. This particular sized perforation was used since it is just slightly smaller than the field specified for use in the Howard method, namely 1.382 mm in diameter. A punch for making the holes can conveniently be made by cutting off a 0.052 inch drill at the upper limit of the twist and placing the shank in a suitable holder. By placing the cellophane over a hard fiber board it is readily possible with a hammer to make clean-cut perforations. A special die has been found useful in cutting the holes, although this is not necessary. The excess cellophane at the edge of the square is trimmed off, leaving a narrow margin of about 0.5 mm.

The cellophane mask is cemented to a clean microscope slide with the aid of balsam and covered with a cover glass. After the balsam is dry, a drop of the tomato agar preparation, previously softened in a boiling water bath, is placed on the cover glass and quickly spread out into a thin layer by means of a second cover slip. Excess pulp is removed after it hardens and the whole is sealed by ringing with balsam.

When ready for use, each field is examined for the presence or absence of mold filaments of the required length and a permanent record is made to accompany the slide.

J. D. WILDMAN

U. S. DEPARTMENT OF AGRICULTURE

[1] ''Methods of Analysis,'' Assn. of Official Agric. Chemists, pp. 400–401.

# SPECIAL ARTICLES

## THE DISTRIBUTION OF AMERICAN MEN OF SCIENCE IN 1932

For the fifth edition of the "Biographical Directory of American Men of Science" there have been selected by objective methods 250 of those not included in the earlier selections who are regarded by their colleagues as among the leading scientific workers of the United States. The methods used were the same as in the fourth edition; there and in the earlier editions they were fully described and their validity was discussed in detail.[1]

The primary object of the work, begun more than thirty years ago, was to secure a group for scientific study. Still earlier there had been selected by objective methods the thousand most eminent men of history, and measurements had been made of nearly a thousand students of Columbia University. Each of the three groups is suited to scientific study, owing to its sociological interest and to the availability of the material. At that time but little attention had been paid to the measurement of individual differences, the present writer having in 1885 invented the term and published the first quantitative work on the subject.

Arguments may be advanced for and against giving the names of the scientific men selected for study. Each of them is probably among our thousand leading research workers, but there are others who deserve to be included. The situation is the same as in election to an academy of sciences or appointment to a university position, except that the determination of scientific merit is more exact. We also have an analogous problem in the measurement of the ability of a child or a college student.

It is sometimes argued that all such determinations are undemocratic. Democracy, however, does not consist in reducing all to a common mediocracy, but in giving opportunity to each in accordance with his ability and fitness. We long have had school grades, college entrance examinations, requirements for the doctorate, qualifications for a university position, honorary degrees, and societies of limited membership. In so far as psychology is gradually developing quantitative methods to measure individual differences the results may at times seem harsh and inconsiderate of the individual; but in the long run truth is better than illusion.

While there are those who do not approve the selection of a group of leading scientific workers, others urge that the stars should be dropped when a position among the thousand is not maintained. The competition in the earlier selections was less severe, for in 1903 there were only about 4,000 Americans who had published research work, whereas now there are more than 20,000. It is also true that some men do not maintain the promise of their earlier work. A selection which is correct at the time within the limits of the probable error may not hold thirty years later. In order to make the situation definite and to supply information that may be of historical interest, there will be given in the new edition of the book an index number with the star, showing the edition in which the individual was added to the list.

As the number of entries in the book is now so large, it may be desirable to give the list of those to whom stars have been assigned in the fifth edition. The date of reference is approximately January 1, 1932, subsequent changes of address being given in brackets. The 250 names are as follows:

*Anatomists*

Edgar Allen, University of Missouri
George W. Bartelmez, University of Chicago
Edward A. Boyden, University of Minnesota
J. L. Bremer, Harvard University
Hal Downey, University of Minnesota
George B. Wislocki, Harvard University

*Anthropologists*

Ruth Benedict, Columbia University
Fay-Cooper Cole, University of Chicago
Ralph Linton, University of Wisconsin
Frank H. H. Roberts, Jr., Smithsonian Institution
Leslie Spier, Yale University

*Astronomers*

R. T. Crawford, University of California
Milton L. Humason, Mt. Wilson Obs., Carnegie Inst.
Hamilton M. Jeffers, Lick Obs., Univ. of California
Dean B. McLaughlin, Detroit Obs., Univ. of Michigan
Donald H. Menzel, Lick Obs., Univ. of Calif. [Harvard]
Herbert R. Morgan, U. S. Naval Observatory
H. H. Plaskett, Harvard College Obs., [Oxford Univ.]
R. F. Sanford, Mt. Wilson Obs., Carnegie Institution
E. C. Slipher, Lowell Observatory
Harlan True Stetson, Perkins Obs., Ohio Wesleyan Univ.
J. Q. Stewart, Princeton University
Otto Struve, Yerkes Observatory, University of Chicago
Ralph E. Wilson, Dudley Observatory

*Botanists*

H. A. Allard, U. S. Department of Agriculture
S. F. Blake, U. S. Department of Agriculture
John T. Buchholz, University of Illinois
Roy E. Clausen, University of California

[1] In order to prevent misunderstandings that occur, it may be stated here: (1) The present writer has devised the methods and compiled the returns, but, apart from casting one vote for the psychologists, has had no part whatever in the selections. (2) Residents of North America are included in the book, but only residents of the United States in the selections for the stars. (3) The applied sciences as such are not included. (4) When an individual is selected in more than one science, he is assigned to the science in which he stands highest. (5) The subject of research given in the book is usually, but not always, the subject in which the star has been assigned.

William S. Cooper, University of Minnesota
Otis F. Curtis, Cornell University
F. E. Denny, Boyce Thompson Institute
Carroll W. Dodge, Missouri Botanical Garden
J. Horace Faull, Arnold Arboretum, Harvard University
H. S. Fawcett, Citrus Exp. Sta., University of California
H. M. Fitzpatrick, Cornell University
T. H. Goodspeed, University of California
R. B. Harvey, University of Minnesota
Chas. F. Hottes, University of Illinois
D. F. Jones, Connecticut Experiment Station
Irving E. Melhus, Iowa State College
Raymond J. Pool, University of Nebraska
Alfred Rehder, Arnold Arboretum, Harvard University
William J. Robbins, University of Missouri
Karl Sax, Harvard University
Fred. J. Seaver, New York Botanical Garden
William Seifriz, University of Pennsylvania
Gilbert M. Smith, Stanford University
W. Randolph Taylor, University of Michigan
Sam F. Trelease, Columbia University

*Chemists*

Homer Adkins, University of Wisconsin
Rudolph J. Anderson, Yale University
Donald H. Andrews, Johns Hopkins University
F. Russell v. Bichowsky, Naval Research Laboratory
Arthur M. Buswell, University of Illinois
Wallace H. Carothers, E. I. du Pont de Nemours and Co.
George L. Clark, University of Illinois
E. J. Cohn, Harvard Medical School
Louis F. Fieser, Harvard University
N. Howell Furman, Princeton University
Reynold C. Fuson, University of Illinois
W. F. Giauque, University of California
G. E. Gibson, University of California
Henry Gilman, Iowa State College
Michael Heidelberger, Columbia University
Arthur J. Hill, Yale University
Charles D. Hurd, Northwestern University
W. A. Jacobs, Rockefeller Institute
John R. Johnson, Cornell University
Oliver Kamm, Parke, Davis and Company
M. S. Kharasch, University of Chicago
George B. Kistiakowsky, Harvard University
I. M. Kolthoff, University of Minnesota
Victor K. LaMer, Columbia University
Wendell M. Latimer, University of California
J. W. MacBain, Stanford University
Edward Mack, Jr., Ohio State University
Carl S. Marvel, University of Illinois
Leonor Michaelis, Rockefeller Institute
Thomas Midgley, Jr., Ethyl Gasoline Corporation
Julius Arthur Nieuwland, University of Notre Dame
John H. Northrop, Rockefeller Institute
W. Albert Noyes, Jr., Brown University
Linus Pauling, California Institute of Technology
Robert N. Pease, Princeton University
F. O. Rice, Johns Hopkins University
George Scatchard, Massachusetts Institute of Technology
H. I. Schlesinger, University of Chicago
Charles P. Smyth, Princeton University
C. M. A. Stine, E. I. du Pont de Nemours and Co.
E. C. Sullivan, Corning Glass Works
E. H. Volwiler, Abbott Laboratories
H. H. Willard, University of Michigan
John Arthur Wilson, Milwaukee, Wisconsin

*Geologists*

Ernst Antevs, Auburn, Maine
Donald C. Barton, Houston, Texas
Alan M. Bateman, Yale University
Kirk Bryan, Harvard University
Walter H. Bucher, University of Cincinnati
S. R. Capps, U. S. Geological Survey
Ralph W. Chaney, University of California
J. A. Cushman, Sharon, Massachusetts
C. N. Fenner, Geophysical Laboratory, Carnegie Inst.
Henry G. Ferguson, U. S. Geological Survey
Aug. F. Foerste, Dayton, Ohio [U. S. Nat. Museum]
Charles W. Gilmore, U. S. National Museum
Frank L. Hess, U. S. Bureau of Mines
G. F. Kay, University of Iowa
F. H. Lahee, Sun Oil Company
Morris M. Leighton, Illinois State Geological Survey
Chester R. Longwell, Yale University
H. E. Merwin, Geophysical Laboratory, Carnegie Inst.
Raymond C. Moore, University of Kansas
John B. Reeside, Jr., U. S. Geological Survey
Clarence Samuel Ross, U. S. Geological Survey
E. H. Sellards, University of Texas
W. T. Thom, Jr., Princeton University
Chester K. Wentworth, Washington Univ. (St. Louis)
Wendell P. Woodring, U. S. Geological Survey

*Mathematicians*

C. Raymond Adams, Brown University
A. Adrian Albert, Columbia University [Univ. Chicago]
Jesse Douglas, Massachusetts Institute of Technology
Lester R. Ford, Rice Institute
Tomlinson Fort, Lehigh University
Thornton C. Fry, Bell Telephone Laboratories
Lawrence M. Graves, University of Chicago
Mark H. Ingraham, University of Wisconsin
Rudolph E. Langer, University of Wisconsin
C. C. MacDuffee, Ohio State University
John v. Neumann, Princeton University
Oystein Ore, Yale University
Tibor Radó, Ohio State University
M. H. Stone, Yale University
Dirk J. Struik, Massachusetts Institute of Technology
T. Y. Thomas, Princeton University
J. V. Uspensky, Stanford University
Gordon T. Whyburn, Johns Hopkins University
D. V. Widder, Harvard University
R. L. Wilder, University of Michigan

*Pathologists*

T. Addis, Stanford University
S. Bayne-Jones, University of Rochester [Yale Univ.]
A. E. Cohn, Rockefeller Institute
Walter E. Dandy, Johns Hopkins University
Edward Francis, National Institute of Health
Evarts A. Graham, Washington University (St. Louis)
Alfred F. Hess, N. Y. Univ. and Bellevue Hosp. Med. Col.
Esmond R. Long, University of Chicago [Phipps Inst.]

K. F. Meyer, Hooper Foundation, Univ. of California
George R. Minot, Harvard University
Arnold R. Rich, Johns Hopkins University
T. M. Rivers, Rockefeller Institute
Carl TenBroeck, Rockefeller Institute
Augustus Wadsworth, N. Y. State Department of Health
Leslie T. Webster, Rockefeller Institute

*Physicists*

Samuel K. Allison, University of Chicago
J. W. Beams, University of Virginia
J. A. Bearden, Johns Hopkins University
Joseph A. Becker, Bell Telephone Laboratories
Robert B. Brode, University of California
Edw. U. Condon, Princeton University
David M. Dennison, University of Michigan
G. H. Dieke, Johns Hopkins University
Lee A. DuBridge, Washington University (St. Louis)
O. S. Duffendack, University of Michigan
Carl Eckart, University of Chicago
A. Ellett, University of Iowa
L. H. Germer, Bell Telephone Laboratories
R. Clifton Gibbs, Cornell University
Samuel A. Goudsmit, University of Michigan
Ross Gunn, Naval Research Laboratory
G. R. Harrison, Massachusetts Institute of Technology
William V. Houston, California Institute of Technology
J. C. Hubbard, Johns Hopkins University
Thomas H. Johnson, Bartol Research Foundation
Alfred Landé, Ohio State University
Otto Laporte, University of Michigan
Ernest O. Lawrence, University of California
Alfred L. Loomis, Tuxedo Park, N. Y.
F. W. Loomis, University of Illinois
Philip M. Morse, Massachusetts Institute of Technology
Otto Oldenberg, Harvard University
J. R. Oppenheimer, California Institute of Technology
A. G. Shenstone, Princeton University
Lewi Tonks, General Electric Company
L. B. Tuckerman, U. S. Bureau of Standards
Louis A. Turner, Princeton University
M. A. Tuve, Dept. Terrestrial Magnetism, Carnegie Inst.
G. E. Uhlenbeck, University of Michigan
H. C. Urey, Columbia University
William W. Watson, Yale University
Fritz Zwicky, California Institute of Technology

*Physiologists*

H. C. Bazett, University of Pennsylvania
G. H. Bishop, Washington University (St. Louis)
McKeen Cattell, Cornell University Medical College
Carl F. Cori, Washington University (St. Louis)
Edward A. Doisy, St. Louis University
J. G. Dusser de Barenne, Yale University
Wallace O. Fenn, University of Rochester
John F. Fulton, Yale University
Frank A. Hartman, University of Buffalo
Harry Steenbock, University of Wisconsin

*Psychologists*

John E. Anderson, University of Minnesota
Karl M. Dallenbach, Cornell University
J. F. Dashiell, University of North Carolina
Samuel W. Fernberger, University of Pennsylvania
Frank N. Freeman, University of Chicago
Clark L. Hull, Yale University
H. M. Johnson, Mellon Institute [American Univ.]
K. Koffka, Smith College
Mark Arthur May, Yale University
Donald G. Paterson, University of Minnesota
Edward Stevens Robinson, Yale University
Calvin P. Stone, Stanford University
Edward C. Tolman, University of California

*Zoologists*

Leslie B. Arey, Northwestern University
Robert A. Budington, Oberlin College
Asa C. Chandler, Rice Institute
Royal N. Chapman, University of Hawaii
C. H. Danforth, Stanford University
J. Frank Daniel, University of California
A. B. Dawson, Harvard University
L. V. Domm, University of Chicago
L. C. Dunn, Columbia University
Paul S. Galtsoff, U. S. Bureau of Fisheries
H. B. Goodrich, Wesleyan University
Frank Blair Hanson, Washington Univ. (St. Louis)
Selig Hecht, Columbia University
Leigh Hoadley, Harvard University
Davenport Hooker, University of Pittsburgh
Carl L. Hubbs, Museum of Zoology, Univ. of Michigan
Libbie H. Hyman, University of Chicago
W. A. Kepner, University of Virginia
George R. La Rue, University of Michigan
E. Carleton MacDowell, Sta. Exp. Evolution, Carnegie Inst.
James W. Mavor, Union College
A. L. Melander, College of the City of New York
Dwight E. Minnich, University of Minnesota
Ann Haven Morgan, Mt. Holyoke College
Charles Packard, Crocker Inst. Cancer Research, Columbia
Bradley M. Patten, Western Reserve University
Harold H. Plough, Amherst College
Alfred C. Redfield, Harvard University
W. A. Riley, University of Minnesota
Franz Schrader, Columbia University
C. C. Speidel, University of Virginia
H. W. Stunkard, New York University
C. V. Taylor, Stanford University
H. J. Van Cleave, University of Illinois
B. H. Willier, University of Chicago
Emil Witschi, University of Iowa
A. H. Wright, Cornell University

The 250 individuals whose names are given above have been selected from more than 20,000; consequently each of them stands first among more than eighty research workers, a somewhat severe selection. It is not feasible to give at this time the number and distribution of the some 22,000 entries in the edition of the directory now in press. 12,877 names in the fourth edition were distributed, according to the sections of the American Association for the Advancement of Science, as shown in the table.

TABLE I. DISTRIBUTION AMONG THE SCIENCES

| | |
|---|---|
| Mathematics | 756 |
| Physics | 991 |
| Chemistry | 2,561 |
| Astronomy | 239 |
| Geology and Geography | 903 |
| Zoology | 1,435 |
| Botanical Sciences | 1,187 |
| Anthropology | 111 |
| Psychology | 539 |
| Social and Economic Sciences | 23 |
| Historical and Philological Sciences | 37 |
| Engineering | 1,245 |
| Medical Sciences | 2,027 |
| Agriculture | 769 |
| Education | 54 |
| Total | 12,877 |

If the applied sciences are omitted (though all those included in the book were understood to have advanced science by research) and the classification adopted in these studies is used, the number is 9,785 and the distribution is as shown in the first column of Table II.

TABLE II. DISTRIBUTION AMONG THE FUNDAMENTAL SCIENCES

| | All | Women | Per cent. women |
|---|---|---|---|
| Mathematics | 756 | 61 | 8.0 |
| Physics | 991 | 28 | 2.1 |
| Chemistry | 2561 | 117 | 4.6 |
| Astronomy | 239 | 23 | 9.6 |
| Geology | 903 | 32 | 3.5 |
| Botany | 1187 | 119 | 10.0 |
| Zoology | 1436 | 130 | 9.0 |
| Physiology | 460 | 48 | 10.4 |
| Anatomy | 206 | 11 | 5.4 |
| Pathology | 396 | 28 | 7.1 |
| Anthropology | 111 | 11 | 9.9 |
| Psychology | 539 | 117 | 22.0 |
| Total | 9785 | 725 | 7.4 |

In the group of 250 there are three women. There are two in the National Academy of Sciences with about the same number of members. There are 725 women included in the book distributed (all of them being assigned to the twelve sciences) as shown in Table II. The percentage of women in each science is also given. It ranges from 2.1 per cent. in physics to 22 per cent. in psychology. The preponderance in the latter subject is due in the main to the large number of teaching and clinical positions open to women.

The average age of the 250 in the group is 42.9 years. Distinction is attained at an earlier age in mathematics and the exact sciences than in the natural sciences, the average age in the different sciences being as shown.

TABLE III. AVERAGE AGE IN THE DIFFERENT SCIENCES

| | |
|---|---|
| Mathematicians | 36.1 |
| Physicists | 36.0 |
| Chemists | 41.1 |
| Astronomers | 42.9 |
| Geologists | 49.4 |
| Botanists | 47.0 |
| Zoologists | 45.3 |
| Physiologists | 42.0 |
| Anatomists | 47.7 |
| Pathologists | 48.3 |
| Anthropologists | 41.8 |
| Psychologists | 44.0 |

In Table IV there is given under 1932 the distribution by states of the birthplace and residence of the 250 scientific men now added to the list. The numbers are multiplied by four in order to show comparisons with the earlier selections. There were 1,000 in 1903. The additions in 1910 were 269; in 1921 (the interval having been prolonged by the war) 351; in 1927, 250. The 601 names of 1921 and 1927 were considered together in the fourth edition of the directory. In the table all the figures are placed on the basis of a thousand entries, decimals being omitted.

While the numbers for most of the states are so small that they have only a limited validity, the general distribution of the scientific population in 1903 and its subsequent movements are clearly shown. Of the thousand scientific men of 1903, 134 were born in Massachusetts and 40 in Connecticut. This represents a birth rate of 108.8 per million population in Massachusetts, and of 86.9 in Connecticut, the population being based on the census of 1860. The birth rate is then reduced to about half in the surrounding states, being 47.2 in New York. There is a further reduction to one half in Pennsylvania, where it is 22.7, and this continues southward, the rate being 8.8 in Virginia, 5 in North Carolina, 2.8 in Georgia, 2.1 in Alabama, 1.3 in Mississippi and 1.4 in Louisiana. In the north central states the conditions are intermediate between New York and Pennsylvania and decrease southward.

The change in distribution of the birthplaces in the later selections is very significant for such a short period in the history of the nation. New England has lost its supremacy in the production of scientific men, the numbers from Massachusetts on the basis of a thousand, decreasing from 134 in 1906 to 100 in 1910, 80 in 1921–27, 72 in 1932. The corresponding figures for Connecticut are 40, 22, 27 and 16. The rural New England states fail even more in productivity. New York, New Jersey, Pennsylvania and Maryland also decrease. The gains are especially in the central

TABLE IV. Birthplace and Residence of Scientific Men Selected at Four Periods

| | Birthplace | | | | Residence | | | |
|---|---|---|---|---|---|---|---|---|
| | 1903 | 1910 | 1921–27 | 1932 | 1903 | 1910 | 1921–27 | 1932 |
| **North Atlantic** | | | | | | | | |
| Maine | 29 | 22 | 10 | 8 | 4 | 7 | 2 | 4 |
| New Hampshire | 15 | 11 | 12 | ... | 8 | 4 | 5 | ... |
| Vermont | 18 | 11 | 10 | 8 | 2 | ... | ... | ... |
| Massachusetts | 134 | 100 | 80 | 72 | 144 | 160 | 95 | 100 |
| Rhode Island | 5 | 15 | 2 | 4 | 8 | 11 | 7 | 8 |
| Connecticut | 40 | 22 | 27 | 16 | 43 | 60 | 33 | 56 |
| New York | 183 | 134 | 111 | 128 | 192 | 141 | 203 | 164 |
| New Jersey | 28 | 15 | 13 | 12 | 35 | 19 | 30 | 44 |
| Pennsylvania | 66 | 52 | 68 | 48 | 65 | 48 | 63 | 28 |
| **South Atlantic** | | | | | | | | |
| Delaware | 2 | ... | 3 | ... | 1 | ... | 2 | 8 |
| Maryland | 26 | 7 | 22 | 4 | 47 | 48 | 38 | 32 |
| District of Columbia | 3 | 4 | 5 | 8 | 119 | 97 | 128 | 76 |
| Virginia | 13 | 26 | 13 | 4 | 10 | ... | 5 | 12 |
| West Virginia | 1 | 7 | 7 | 4 | 3 | 4 | 3 | ... |
| North Carolina | 5 | ... | 8 | 4 | 6 | 11 | 3 | 4 |
| South Carolina | 5 | 11 | 7 | 4 | ... | ... | 2 | ... |
| Georgia | 3 | 4 | 5 | 8 | 1 | ... | ... | ... |
| Florida | ... | 4 | ... | ... | ... | ... | ... | ... |
| **South Central** | | | | | | | | |
| Kentucky | 8 | 7 | 8 | 4 | 3 | ... | 2 | ... |
| Tennessee | 6 | 7 | 7 | 4 | 3 | ... | 5 | ... |
| Alabama | 2 | 7 | 3 | 4 | 2 | ... | ... | ... |
| Mississippi | 1 | 4 | 3 | ... | ... | ... | ... | ... |
| Louisiana | 1 | ... | 2 | 8 | 1 | 4 | 2 | ... |
| Texas | 3 | 7 | 2 | 4 | 7 | 7 | 13 | 20 |
| Oklahoma | ... | ... | 2 | ... | ... | ... | 2 | ... |
| Arkansas | ... | ... | 3 | ... | ... | ... | ... | ... |
| **North Central** | | | | | | | | |
| Ohio | 75 | 86 | 81 | 72 | 34 | 37 | 33 | 40 |
| Indiana | 28 | 45 | 30 | 36 | 12 | 19 | 8 | 4 |
| Illinois | 42 | 52 | 75 | 88 | 63 | 104 | 86 | 96 |
| Michigan | 27 | 63 | 22 | 16 | 27 | 19 | 30 | 48 |
| Wisconsin | 35 | 41 | 40 | 20 | 23 | 48 | 18 | 28 |
| Minnesota | 4 | 19 | 23 | 32 | 13 | 11 | 30 | 36 |
| Iowa | 20 | 33 | 45 | 32 | 7 | 4 | 7 | 20 |
| Missouri | 14 | 19 | 35 | 40 | 21 | 22 | 13 | 40 |
| North Dakota | ... | ... | 2 | ... | 2 | ... | ... | ... |
| South Dakota | ... | ... | 5 | 8 | 2 | 4 | ... | ... |
| Nebraska | 2 | 4 | 10 | 20 | 9 | 15 | 3 | 4 |
| Kansas | 7 | ... | 18 | 32 | 5 | 7 | 8 | 4 |
| **Western** | | | | | | | | |
| Montana | ... | ... | 3 | ... | 2 | ... | ... | ... |
| Wyoming | ... | ... | 3 | 4 | 1 | ... | 3 | ... |
| Colorado | 3 | ... | 2 | 16 | 8 | 7 | 3 | ... |
| New Mexico | ... | ... | ... | 8 | 2 | ... | ... | ... |
| Arizona | ... | ... | ... | 4 | 2 | 4 | 7 | 4 |
| Utah | ... | ... | 5 | ... | ... | ... | ... | ... |
| Nevada | ... | ... | ... | ... | ... | ... | ... | ... |
| Idaho | ... | ... | ... | ... | ... | ... | ... | ... |
| Washington | 1 | ... | ... | 12 | ... | ... | 2 | ... |
| Oregon | ... | 4 | 2 | 4 | ... | 4 | ... | ... |
| California | 11 | 15 | 18 | 20 | 53 | 56 | 78 | 116 |
| **Territories and Dependencies** | | | | | | | | |
| Porto Rico | ... | ... | ... | ... | 1 | ... | 2 | ... |
| Alaska | ... | ... | ... | ... | 1 | ... | ... | ... |
| Hawaii | 1 | 4 | ... | ... | ... | 4 | ... | 4 |
| Philippines | ... | 4 | ... | ... | 3 | 7 | ... | ... |
| Panama | ... | ... | ... | ... | ... | 4 | ... | ... |
| **Foreign** | | | | | | | | |
| Canada | 34 | 33 | 30 | 36 | 2 | ... | 5 | ... |
| Brazil | ... | ... | ... | ... | 1 | ... | ... | ... |
| Cuba | ... | ... | ... | ... | 1 | ... | ... | ... |
| West Indies | 1 | ... | ... | ... | ... | ... | ... | ... |
| England | 25 | ... | 35 | 8 | 1 | ... | ... | ... |
| Scotland | 9 | 15 | 7 | 12 | ... | ... | ... | ... |
| Wales | 1 | ... | ... | ... | ... | ... | ... | ... |
| Ireland | 3 | 4 | 2 | ... | ... | ... | ... | ... |
| Germany | 19 | 22 | 12 | 36 | ... | ... | ... | ... |
| Austria-Hungary | 6 | ... | ... | ... | ... | ... | ... | ... |
| Austria | ... | ... | 7 | 4 | ... | ... | ... | ... |
| Hungary | ... | ... | ... | 8 | ... | ... | ... | ... |
| Norway | 1 | 4 | ... | 4 | ... | ... | ... | ... |
| Sweden | 3 | 7 | 5 | 8 | ... | ... | ... | ... |
| Denmark | 2 | ... | 2 | ... | ... | ... | ... | ... |
| Holland | ... | ... | 5 | 16 | ... | ... | ... | ... |
| Belgium | ... | ... | 2 | 4 | ... | ... | ... | ... |
| Poland | ... | ... | 3 | ... | ... | ... | ... | ... |
| Bulgaria | ... | ... | ... | 4 | ... | ... | ... | ... |
| Czecho-Slovakia | ... | ... | ... | 4 | ... | ... | ... | ... |
| Switzerland | 8 | ... | 8 | 8 | ... | 4 | ... | ... |
| Italy | 1 | ... | ... | ... | ... | ... | ... | ... |
| Spain | 1 | ... | ... | ... | ... | ... | ... | ... |
| Russia | 6 | 11 | 13 | 12 | ... | ... | ... | ... |
| Turkey | ... | ... | 3 | ... | ... | ... | ... | ... |
| Syria | ... | ... | 3 | ... | ... | ... | ... | ... |
| India | 4 | ... | ... | ... | ... | ... | ... | ... |
| Mongolia | ... | ... | ... | 4 | ... | ... | ... | ... |
| China | 2 | ... | ... | ... | ... | ... | ... | ... |
| Japan | ... | 7 | 3 | 4 | ... | ... | ... | ... |
| Siam | ... | ... | ... | ... | ... | ... | 2 | ... |
| Dutch E. Indies | ... | ... | ... | 4 | ... | ... | ... | ... |
| Australia | ... | ... | 2 | ... | ... | ... | ... | ... |
| South Africa | ... | ... | 2 | ... | ... | ... | 2 | ... |

west, the record for Illinois being 42, 52, 75 and 88. There are also large increases in other north central states: Minnesota, 4 to 32; Iowa, 20 to 32; Missouri, 14 to 40; Nebraska, 2 to 20; Kansas, 7 to 32. The more easterly states of Ohio and Indiana remain about stationary. Twelve states south of Virginia supplied only 35 men to the list of 1903; they show some improvement in the subsequent selections, 58, 57 and 44.

The residence[2] of leading scientific men in the different states follows in general their production, but certain regions produce more than they retain or obtain, while in others the reverse is the case. Massachusetts and Connecticut have had in residence even more scientific men than they have produced. This holds also for New York and of course in the greatest measure for the District of Columbia. Ohio and Indiana, on the other hand, have in residence less than half as many leading scientific men as they have produced. California gained greatly in the last arrangement, being surpassed only by New York and having a much larger percentage per million population.

On the list of 1903 there were 126 scientific men born in foreign countries, contributed in very unequal

[2] The scientific men were selected in 1903; the residence is of January 1, 1906, as given in the first edition of the directory.

measure by different nationalities, the number per million foreign-born population being: Switzerland, 68.9; England, 29.6; Germany, 7.1; Italy, 2.1; France, 0. The relative numbers of scientific men born abroad in the subsequent selections were 103, 144 and 172. There have been in the selections following the war a large percentage of scientific men who migrated to this country after having attained distinction at home.

Table V gives the institutions from which the 250 scientific men received their academic degrees. Harvard is still in the lead by a wide margin, having granted 19 bachelor's degrees, 39 doctorates of philosophy or science and 4 doctorates of medicine. Chicago comes next with a total of 42 degrees, followed by Columbia with 29. There then follows a group coming close together, Cornell, Princeton, the Johns Hopkins, Yale, Illinois, and California, with a drop to about half as many at Michigan and Wisconsin. These figures represent the situation for those who received their degrees on the average some twenty years ago. Since then the number of advanced degrees conferred by the state universities has increased with great rapidity. The 27 not recorded as having had a bachelor's degree had in practically all cases an equivalent education, in most cases abroad. Two men hold doctorates of both philosophy and medicine, leaving only 17 who do not hold one of these degrees.

TABLE V. THE INSTITUTIONS WHICH GRANTED THREE OR MORE OF THE DEGREES

| | A.B. or B.S. | Ph.D. or Sc.D | M.D. | Total |
|---|---|---|---|---|
| Harvard | 19 | 39 | 4 | 62 |
| Chicago | 13 | 28 | 1 | 42 |
| Columbia | 7 | 19 | 3 | 29 |
| Cornell | 9 | 11 | ...... | 20 |
| Princeton | 6 | 13 | ...... | 19 |
| Johns Hopkins | 2 | 10 | 6 | 18 |
| Yale | 5 | 12 | ...... | 17 |
| Illinois | 7 | 10 | ...... | 17 |
| California | 4 | 12 | ...... | 16 |
| Michigan | 8 | 1 | ...... | 9 |
| Wisconsin | 1 | 8 | ...... | 9 |
| Minnesota | 5 | 3 | ...... | 8 |
| Brown | 5 | 1 | ...... | 6 |
| Virginia | 2 | 4 | ...... | 6 |
| Amherst | 5 | ...... | ...... | 5 |
| Ohio State | 3 | 2 | ...... | 5 |
| Washington (St. L.) | 3 | 2 | ...... | 5 |
| Kansas | 4 | ...... | ...... | 4 |
| Pennsylvania | 2 | 2 | ...... | 4 |
| Stanford | 3 | 1 | ...... | 4 |
| Texas | 2 | 2 | ...... | 4 |
| Dennison | 3 | ...... | ...... | 3 |
| Iowa | 1 | 2 | ...... | 3 |
| Missouri | 3 | ...... | ...... | 3 |
| Nebraska | 2 | 1 | ...... | 3 |
| Swarthmore | 3 | ...... | ...... | 3 |
| Elsewhere | 82 | 4 | 2 | 88 |
| Total | 209 | 187 | 16 | 412 |
| Berlin | ...... | 3 | 1 | 4 |
| Toronto | 4 | ...... | ...... | 4 |
| Edinburgh | 2 | ...... | 1 | 3 |
| Leiden | ...... | 3 | ...... | 3 |
| Munich | ...... | 3 | ...... | 3 |
| Zurich | 1 | 2 | ...... | 3 |
| Elsewhere | 7 | 16 | 3 | 26 |
| Total | 14 | 27 | 5 | 46 |
| Grand Total | 223 | 214 | 21 | 458 |

In Table VI are given the institutions with which three or more of the scientific men are connected. Harvard has sixteen and California 15, followed by Chicago, Yale, Michigan, Columbia and Princeton. Seven of the men are connected with the Rockefeller Institute for Medical Research and six with the Carnegie Institution of Washington.

TABLE VI. INSTITUTIONS WITH WHICH THREE OR MORE ARE CONNECTED

| | |
|---|---|
| Harvard | 16 |
| California | 15 |
| Chicago | 13 |
| Yale | 13 |
| Michigan | 11 |
| Columbia | 10 |
| Princeton | 10 |
| Minnesota | 9 |
| Illinois | 8 |
| Johns Hopkins | 8 |
| Cornell | 7 |
| Rockefeller Institute | 7 |
| Stanford | 7 |
| Carnegie Institution | 6 |
| Washington (St. Louis) | 6 |
| Massachusetts Institute | 5 |
| U. S. Geol. Survey | 5 |
| Wisconsin | 5 |
| California Institute | 4 |
| Ohio State | 4 |
| Bell Tel. Labs. | 3 |
| Iowa | 3 |
| Pennsylvania | 3 |
| Virginia | 3 |
| Elsewhere | 69 |
| Total | 250 |

The movement from the universities to the research institutions, industrial laboratories and government service, which was notable shortly after the war, has apparently now ceased. In the list of 1927 fifteen of the 250 men were connected with the Carnegie Institution; nine with the Geological Survey; seven with the Bell Telephone Laboratories; six with the Department of Agriculture; five each with the Rockefeller

Institute, the Bureau of Standards and the American Museum of Natural History; four with the Eastman Kodak Company and three with the U. S. Health Service.

There have been selected by the average space allotted to sketches in biographical directories and encyclopedias the leading scientific men of the United States who died prior to the present century. There are not as many as a thousand reaching the standard of the 22,000 in the present edition of the directory; it is necessary to include large numbers of physicians and inventors. Preparations have also been made to select the thousand leading scientific men of the world now living and the thousand most eminent who are no longer living. A study of distribution among the sciences, in different nations and at different periods, supplies the beginning of a quantitative study of history. It is also proposed to print biographical sketches in a subsequent edition of the directory. Some further study has been given to family relationship among scientific workers. It is of interest to note the considerable number of sons of scientific men who have attained high standing in the course of the past twenty years.

The change in standing of a scientific man after a period of years gives in quantitative units (with a probable error attached) his gain or loss in the judgment of his colleagues. The efforts of a lifetime are condensed into a single informing and dramatic figure. Data have been published showing that men under forty years of age are likely to gain in reputation; between forty and forty-five to remain about stationary; after that age to lose and increasingly as they grow older. The average gains or losses yield information concerning the effects of different situations, for example, at one university or another, at large or small institutions, in research institutions, in industrial laboratories, in the government service, with much or little administrative work or teaching, etc. The data may ultimately give information concerning individual differences in relation to heredity and social influences. But this is one of many studies that the present writer has been unable to complete.

When the scientific men were arranged in 1903 in order of merit it was stated that the lists would not be published within twenty years. Nearly thirty years having now elapsed it may be useful to make public a list that has considerable historical interest. The order gives no information concerning the contemporary position, some of those near the bottom of the selection in 1903 having now risen to the top and some of those then at the top having dropped. In the fifth edition of the directory, to be published this month, the list will be given in full. There are here printed in the order of merit for each science the hundred men of science regarded in 1903 by their colleagues as the most distinguished, the number in each science being approximately proportional to the total number of workers. The names of those no longer living are given in italics with the years of birth and death.

MATHEMATICS: *Eliakim Hastings Moore*, 62–32; *George William Hill*, 38–14; W. F. Osgood; *Maxime Bôcher*, 67–18; Oskar Bolza; F. Morley; Ernest W. Brown; H. S. White.

PHYSICS: *Albert Abraham Michelson*, 52–31; Carl Barus; Edward L. Nichols; *Arthur Gordon Webster*, 63–23; *John Trowbridge*, 43–23; M. I. Pupin; *Ernest Fox Nichols*, 69–24; *Samuel Pierpont Langley*, 34–06; *DeWitt Bristol Brace*, 58–05; Elihu Thomson; *Robert Simpson Woodward*, 49–24; *Charles Proteus Steinmetz*, 65–23; *Henry Smith Carhart*, 44–20; Edwin H. Hall; J. S. Ames.

CHEMISTRY: *Ira Remsen*, 46–27; *Edward Williams Morley*, 38–23; *Oliver Wolcott Gibbs*, 22–08; *Theodore William Richards*, 68–28; *Edgar Fahs Smith*, 54–28; *John William Mallet*, 32–12; Russell H. Chittenden; Arthur Michael; *John Ulric Nef*, 62–15; *Harvey Washington Wiley*, 44–30; *James Mason Crafts*, 39–17; *F. A. Gooch*, 52–29; C. L. Jackson; *William Francis Hillebrand*, 53–25; *William Olin Atwater*, 44–07; Arthur A. Noyes; *Albert Benjamin Prescott*, 32–05.

ASTRONOMY: *Simon Newcomb*, 35–09; *Edward Charles Pickering*, 46–19; *Lewis Boss*, 46–12; W. W. Campbell; *Seth Carlo Chandler*, 46–13.

GEOLOGY: *Thomas Chrowder Chamberlin*, 43–28; *Grove Carl Gilbert*, 43–18; *Charles Doolittle Walcott*, 50–27; *Charles Richard Van Hise*, 57–18; *Samuel Franklin Emmons*, 41–11; W. M. Davis; *John Casper Branner*, 50–22; *Nathaniel Southgate Shaler*, 41–06; *Clarence Edward Dutton*, 41–12; *Raphael Pumpelly*, 37–23.

BOTANY: *William Gilson Farlow*, 44–19; N. L. Britton; *John Merle Coulter*, 51–28; W. Trelease; *Charles Edwin Bessey*, 45–15; *Lucien Marcus Underwood*, 53–07; L. H. Bailey; *Roland Thaxter*, 58–32; D. T. MacDougal; B. L. Robinson.

ZOOLOGY: *William Keith Brooks*, 48–08; *Charles Otis Whitman*, 42–10; *Alexander Agassiz*, 35–10; E. B. Wilson; H. F. Osborn; *Charles Sedgwick Minot*, 52–14; E. L. Mark; T. H. Morgan; W. M. Wheeler; *Samuel Hubbard Scudder*, 37–11; Chas. B. Davenport; *David Starr Jordan*, 51–31; Edwin G. Conklin; C. Hart Merriam; *William Healey Dall*, 45–27.

PHYSIOLOGY: *Henry Pickering Bowditch*, 40–11; W. H. Howell; W. T. Porter; *Samuel James Meltzer*, 51–20.

ANATOMY: *Franklin Paine Mall*, 62–17; *George Sumner Huntington*, 61–27; H. H. Donaldson.

PATHOLOGY: William H. Welch; W. T. Councilman; Simon Flexner; *William Osler*, 49–19; Theobald Smith; *Theophil Mitchell Prudden*, 49–24.

ANTHROPOLOGY: Franz Boas; *Otis Tufton Mason*, 38–08.

PSYCHOLOGY: *William James*, 42–10; J. McKeen Cattell; *Hugo Münsterberg*, 63–16; *Granville Stanley Hall*, 46–24; J. Mark Baldwin.

J. MCKEEN CATTELL

# SCIENCE

Vol. 77 — Friday, March 17, 1933 — No. 1994

*In Honor of Professor Einstein:*
*Greeting on Behalf of American Scientists:* President Karl T. Compton 271
*Address on "The Cosmic Parade":* Dr. Harlow Shapley 272
*Address by Professor Einstein* 274
*Obituary:*
*Olive S. Lammert:* Professor Mary Landon Sague. *Recent Deaths* 275
*Scientific Events:*
*Boulder Canyon Lake Wild Life Refuge; The Museums of Archeology and Geology at the University of Kentucky; Requirements for the License of Medical Students in New York State; The New Mexico Meeting of the Southwestern Division of the American Association for the Advancement of Science* 276
*Scientific Notes and News* 278
*Discussion:*
*Nature Sanctuaries—a Means of Saving Natural Biotic Communities:* Dr. Victor E. Shelford. *The Water Content of Medusae:* Professor Ross Aiken Gortner. *The Physiological Basis of the Twisting Habit in Plant Growth:* C. P. Haskins and C. N. Moore. *An Unusual Cretaceous Cirriped:* Dr. H. A. Pilsbry. *Stream Double Refraction Exhibited by Juice from Both Healthy and Mosaic Tobacco Plants:* Dr. William N. Takahashi and Dr. T. E. Rawlins 281
*Scientific Books:*
*Sinnott and Dunn's Principles of Genetics and Sansome and Philp's Recent Advances in Plant Genetics:* Dr. Albert F. Blakeslee 284
*Special Correspondence:*
*The Sixth Mendeleev Congress at Kharkov:* Dr. Victor Cofman 286
*Scientific Apparatus and Laboratory Methods:*
*Improving the Staining Action of Iron Haematoxylin:* Dr. Robert T. Hance. *A Device for Mounting Anatomical Preparations:* H. W. Schoenborn and Dr. C. P. Hickman 287
*Special Articles:*
*The Particle Size of the Virus of Equine Encephalomyelitis:* Professor A. P. Krueger, B. Howitt and Virginia Zeilor. *A New Process for the Synthesis of Phenanthrene and of Phenanthrene Derivatives:* Professor Marston Taylor Bogert. *The Formation of Semi-transparent Membranes from Cultures of Slime-producing Micro-organisms:* Dr. J. R. Sanborn 288
*Science News* 8

SCIENCE: A Weekly Journal devoted to the Advancement of Science, edited by J. McKeen Cattell and published every Friday by

THE SCIENCE PRESS

New York City: Grand Central Terminal
Lancaster, Pa. — Garrison, N. Y.
Annual Subscription, $6.00 — Single Copies, 15 Cts.

SCIENCE is the official organ of the American Association for the Advancement of Science. Information regarding membership in the Association may be secured from the office of the permanent secretary, in the Smithsonian Institution Building, Washington, D. C.

# IN HONOR OF PROFESSOR EINSTEIN[1]

## GREETING ON BEHALF OF AMERICAN SCIENTISTS BY DR. KARL T. COMPTON, PRESIDENT OF THE MASSACHUSETTS INSTITUTE OF TECHNOLOGY

It is a pleasure for me to have the privilege of greeting Professor Einstein on behalf of American scientists. There is first the pleasure of renewing a personal contact made with Professor Einstein on the occasion of his first visit to America shortly after the war, when he delivered a series of lectures on relativity at Princeton University. Going farther back, there is a second personal connection which Professor Einstein knows nothing about, but which I venture to say has been duplicated by many of my fellow American scientists in some such way as the following.

Some years ago, when my fiancée was debating with herself as to whether she was doing wisely in joining me in the great adventure, we were being entertained in the home of her most admired and respected friend, the pastor of her Methodist church. After dinner this man, who was by nature a poet rather than a scientist, asked me to explain to him in simple language Einstein's theory of relativity, and listened with apparently absorbed interest to my efforts to present this in non-technical language. The next morning he said to my fiancée, "I approve of your young man in all but one respect: he has no sense of humor. I asked him to explain to me Einstein's theory of relativity and he really tried to do it. You are taking a long chance in marrying a man who has no sense of humor." So I suspect every American physicist or mathematician has at one time or another been in a quandary as to whether he should engage upon the hopeless task of an attempted explanation, or whether he should find wisdom in cowardice by stating that he

[1] Address at a dinner under the auspices of the American Friends of the Hebrew University in Palestine, given at the Hotel Commodore, New York City, on March 15. Besides Professor Einstein, Dr. Compton and Dr. Shapley, the speakers included Dr. O. C. Kiep, German consul general; Dr. Solomon Lowenstein, executive director of the Federation for the Support of Jewish Philanthropic Societies in New York City; James Marshall, a vice-president of the American Friends of the Hebrew University in Palestine, and Dr. Nathan Ratnoff, director of Beth Israel Hospital, in New York City. Sol M. Stroock, chairman of the board of the Jewish Theological Seminary, presided. Professor Einstein spoke in German, his address being translated at its close.

did not understand the theory himself, which was very likely to be true.

The third reason for personal gratification lies in the fact that my first real research work in physics, which was my doctor's thesis at Princeton, constituted, I believe, the first reasonably conclusive experimental proof of the famous Einstein photoelectric equation and through it the correlation of the frequency of light, the contact potential characteristic of any metal illuminated by the light, and the kinetic energy of electrons ejected from the metal under the influence of the light. It was this work which was refined in certain particulars by Millikan four years later to give the most accurate experimental determination of that famous constant of modern physics known as "Planck's constant."

Professor Einstein's interpretation of the rôle of Planck's constant in phenomena which involve the interaction of radiation and matter has been the real foundation of all the marvelous development in spectroscopy and atomic structure, which is the outstanding achievement of physical science in the past twenty years—perhaps because big things are more spectacular than little things, or perhaps because people like to talk and to hear about things which they sense vaguely but do not understand, or perhaps for some other reason which I can not analyze, the public fancy has been taken much more with Professor Einstein's contributions to the theory of relativity than with his contributions to atomic physics and radiation. While the former contributions have been far more extensive, I believe that public opinion should not lose sight of the fact that Professor Einstein's basic contributions to the development of the quantum theory have probably been of even greater influence in effecting the development of the physical sciences than his great general theory of relativity.

Perhaps any attempt to estimate the relative importance of these two great contributions which Professor Einstein has made to twentieth century science is futile because the estimate may be different if gaged on the minute scale of the instantaneous condition of an atom or by the enormous scale of the universe as it is extending through all the ages. This contrast, however, will at least serve to emphasize the great range of interest and of application of the work of Professor Einstein.

It is needless for me to say that all American scientists are delighted with the new arrangement under which Professor Einstein will be regularly one of us. We are delighted not only because of the prestige which his presence will give to our institutions, but also because of the interest and stimulation which his presence will arouse in our young American scientists, who will see in him an ideal which unconsciously beckons them to "go thou and do likewise." Finally, we are delighted with the new arrangement because those of us who have had the privilege of coming to know Professor Einstein personally appreciate him as a person and are glad on personal grounds to have him as an associate. In this welcome we include also the most effective of all his colleagues, Frau Einstein.

## ADDRESS ON "THE COSMIC PARADE" BY DR. HARLOW SHAPLEY, DIRECTOR OF THE HARVARD COLLEGE OBSERVATORY

I AM requested to describe the universe of which our guest of honor is a part and concerning which he busies himself at times. I am asked to tell the story of a world that contains electrons, galaxies, space, comets, politics, slush and after-dinner speakers. I am to describe a universe that spreads throughout more than a million, trillion, trillion, cubic light years, that has existed for some thousands or millions of millions of years—and I have for this descriptive job ten minutes, minus the time taken by the introducer. You should pardon me if here and there I am rather brief with minor details. Indeed, I shall consider chiefly the grosser cosmos and not bother much with the intricacies of the atom or the private life of electrons.

As interpreters of the world we do not know how good we are, nor how bad. We must leave to future generations to say just where we went wrong. I suspect that if any attention whatever is paid to the science and scientists of the first third of the twentieth century it will be to the fundamental deductions and to the pioneer observations (crude as they are). I suspect that we are too near the front in this battle of nature's secrets against test-tubes, spectroscopes and mathematical analysis to realize how much we pursue current fads, how enthusiastically we over-interpret fragmentary observations of fragments. But even at this close range we can see the oncoming mortality of practically all current theories, both of the microcosmos and of the macrocosmos. There is an over-population of hypotheses; they crowd and cancel one another. New observations add to the slaughter. Within the past year, almost accidentally, we stumble upon fundamentals like the neutron and the positron, entities that had not been explicitly included in the atomic models and pictures of the preceding years. But brave hypotheses are necessary to guide, transiently; the observations stand for a while; the good measures, in fact, are essentially permanent; and the enthusiasm back of it all, the will to know and the willingness to fumble as we learn to know—they are eternal.

Leaving the fascinating though uncertain world of the atom and the molecule, let us accept matter as proved though not defined and gaze into the ominous astronomical world.

To picture for you most easily this universe of stars which stretches quite beyond reason, space and time and imagination, let me parade the cosmos before you, bit by bit. You are for the occasion transformed into super-cosmic beings, brought in for this show, let us say, from a place that lies beyond the bounds of our space-time and from an epoch preceding the beginning of time—impersonal spectators, you are looking us over. While you cosmics sit before me, smoking or fiddling with the spoons or thinking or perhaps just sitting, I start the sidereal parade with a waving of nebulous banners and a blare of celestial trumpets; for the first body ushered in is nothing less than Number Three. That is, Planet Number Three—dear old earth herself. On the return trip there will be less trumpeting, I surmise, when Number Three appears. Number Three, ladies and gentlemen, is one of the funniest things I can show you; the only place in the universe, so far as I am aware, where demagogues rule, where man destroys man, where imbecility of various sorts is bought and sold in the open market. It is, however, also the abode of ideals, altruism, reasoning thought.

Numbers One and Two are Mercury and Venus in this numbering of the planets outward from the local star. The star itself, one of thousands of millions, is a hot, radiant turmoil of mixed gases. If our star, the sun, were reduced in scale so that its million-mile diameter is but six inches (about that of this microphone) the planets on the same scale would be the dimensions of coarse sand grains and bits of gravel and of much the same importance. Number Three, a small sand grain, is fifty feet away and plodding its yearly trip about the sun in a circular orbit with astonishing monotony. How we all cling to that rocky fragment, holding on desperately, not physically of course, because gravity takes care of that; but holding on temporally, in time, for just as many turns as possible. Sixty, seventy, eighty whirls, and we let go —that is our portion on this merry-go-round that has already whirled dreamily about the sun a few thousand million times with scarcely any evidence of running down.

The furthermost of the planetary sand grains now known is Pluto, about five city blocks from this microphone sun; to the nearest star neighbor it is some three thousand miles.

But enough of this part of the parade; enough of Number Three with its superficial whiff of atmosphere, splash of ocean and smear of biology. We turn attention to phenomena more fundamental than planets.

A long interval now passes before you cosmic spectators—a parade of nothingness. Interstellar space is passing, the phenomenon, or lack of phenomena, that incites sober men to cosmogony, that leads thoughtful men to strange comments concerning space and time, infinity and eternity.

But look closely and you will see that the emptiness is not completely empty. In every cubic yard of interstellar space are a hundred atoms that have been ejected violently and driven from the hot atmospheres of stars. But these hundred atoms per cubic yard do not alleviate the stark emptiness. There are a trillion trillion times as many atoms in a cubic yard of the atmosphere in this room. Interstellar space is effectively a vacuum.

In addition to the few hurrying atoms and molecules, space is everywhere permeated with the weak radiation of all stars. The light of a thousand million stellar sources pours at the rate of fifteen thousand trillion pulses per second through every cubic inch of interstellar space. And, in spite of this, almost complete darkness prevails. Is it any wonder that scientists dream dreams when they seek to interpret the universe as a whole—its meaning in space and in time?

Coursing also through this pseudo-emptiness are occasional lost planets and comets, and frequently high-speed cosmic meteors, which record themselves as shooting stars when they strike and expire in our earth's protecting atmosphere. We have recently proved at the Harvard College Observatory the prevalence outside our solar system of these minute stony fragments from past explosive catastrophies. The speeds of meteors frequently exceed a hundred miles a second. Their significance in cosmogony is deep, their source is obscure and intimately tied up with the origin of the phase of the world that now exists. But numerous as they are, they do not relieve the essential vacuity of space.

The procession moves on and we pass before you stars of all sorts—giant spheres, a million times the volume of our own star; dwarf, shrunken suns that appear to be perishing from exhaustion of their radiant energy; stars of various temperatures and stages of evolution; double stars, triples, stars in groups, clusters and clouds. You will note that the chemistries are much alike from type to type, that the chemical elements of stars are the same as the elements of the flying meteors and of the crust of the earth. You will note also that regardless of the region of space or interval of time from which I select the sample stars for this procession, the same gravitational principles operate, the same laws of radiation prevail as those familiar now in the solar system—a common universal chemistry and common laws.

As the procession of stars goes by we do not see

any little planets or moons. They may be there, though invisible, but after all that's not an important matter.

The parade goes on, and now appear the nebulae, some bright and some dark, the most spectacular part of the pageant. For the bright nebulae are of weird form, of vast dimensions, agglomerations of radiant gases and of meteoric grains of sand and iron. And the dark nebulae are impressive because of the secrets they conceal by hiding great portions of the universe; impressive also because they originate, possibly, from exploded planets and stars or from earlier disrupted universes. Are they the materials from which eventually new stars and galaxies will arise?

In the procession that I have to this point passed before you were, first, the minor bodies, such as the planets and comets of the solar system. Next came a sample of interstellar space and its thin content of radiation and of stellar débris. Then the stars, singly and multiply, and the diffuse nebulosity, bright and dark, which may be star plasma or the wreckage of stars or, in a long-time universe, may be both.

We now rise to a higher order in the pageantry that passes. Here are not stars but great systems of stars which we call galaxies or, if they are remote and therefore hazy and indistinct and unresolved, we misname them nebulae or nebulous stars. Also in great variety the galaxies go by, some gigantic, some so dwarfish that they may contain but a few thousand million ordinary stars; some are spherical, most of them flattened, and more than half show that their population of stars is arranged in spirals.

These common spiral galaxies occur singly, doubly, in close confused triples and multiples, and in clusters and in great clouds and streams, which we term supergalaxies, sometimes millions of light years in extent.

A few of these galaxies have been observed with the spectroscope. There is a startling red shift of their spectral lines. Interpreting that red shift in the normal way as a recession of the galaxies, we are led to the concept of the expanding universe, a scattering of the galaxies, a lowering of the density of matter in space. We are led to the speculation that the origin of the present phase of the universe occurred not much more than three thousand million years ago, disturbingly recent to the orthodox astronomer. We are led to remarkable preliminary speculations connecting the theory of relativity with the recession of galaxies, from which we deduce evidence for a spherical finite world.

Finally, at the end of the procession, we try to exhibit the metagalaxy, the all-inclusive universe of galaxies; but the display is poor because, with a reach of only a hundred million light years, our sample possibly is misleading. We note, however, three conspicuous features:

(1) Exceeding non-uniformity in the distribution of matter.

(2) No evidence that our own galaxy is significantly placed with respect to the millions surrounding.

(3) No suggestion that in our deepest exploration we anywhere approach a boundary to the universe.

The cosmic parade is finished. I now retransmute you from super-cosmic beings to primates on Planet Number Three; and I leave with you the thought that, although in the last twenty years our knowledge of the sidereal world has more than doubled, the list of things we want to know has trebled or quadrupled, leaving us relatively more ignorant than heretofore, but making us also keener than ever to attain that spiritual satisfaction that only the struggle to comprehend can give.

## ADDRESS BY PROFESSOR EINSTEIN

LET me first give expression to my delight and gratitude for the wonderful reception which has been given to me in this festive hall by so prominent and distinguished an assemblage. But this honor, at so serious a time, would depress rather than exalt them, if it were not for the redeeming consciousness that, by this visit, I could be of service to two institutions which are very close to my heart—the University in Jerusalem and the Jewish Telegraphic Agency.

Let us fix our eye first upon Palestine. It should fill us with pride and joy that our work of upbuilding is made possible, to a great extent, by liberal gifts, and that those whose hearts and hands have achieved this upbuilding have imposed upon themselves a hard lot in order to serve a high ideal. We may therefore say that this work rests upon the shoulders of the best of our people. It is because of this that it has until now wonderfully withstood all the difficulties of trial and affliction and stands to-day more sound and promising than many settlements in lands more favored by nature. If the speed of growth does not satisfy some of our hot-headed and impatient brethren, let us remember that in social structures as well as in organisms the most worth-while are not those which grow and mature most rapidly.

As old as the plan of the upbuilding work itself is the plan for the establishment of the Jewish University in Jerusalem. This is not to be wondered at in a people who have for nearly two millennia treasured as the highest good the pursuit of the spiritual for its own sake. So it was that soon after the war, on one of the most beautiful spots of the country, the university was founded. Originally, it was not intended primarily as an institution of instruction but as a center of research.

The sympathetic interest which this work, together with the library in Jerusalem, had aroused among intellectual Jewish elements was universal and strong, and there arose great-hearted givers who made possible the realization of the university, in which efficient and devoted scientists were already busy and are still busy. In spite of many diseases of infancy through which such a new institution, exposed to so many varying influences, must pass, the university has to-day already demonstrated its vitality and the Palestine work can not longer be thought of without it.

With gratitude may be mentioned here Mr. Felix Warburg, and not less the American Jewish Physicians' Committee. The Jewish people will never forget their help on behalf of the university.

I am convinced that it is especially fortunate for the university that Mr. Weizmann has decided to put his abilities at its disposal and to found and direct a department for agriculture. His great experiences in the field of chemistry and administration and, last but not least, his rare knowledge of men will be of great usefulness for the university; his fascinating personality will also lend it new attractiveness. I believe in a sound and beautiful development of the institution in the next few years.

The significance of the University in Jerusalem for the Jewish people will be heightened by the fact that the Jews in eastern Europe are being barred from the sciences and the practise of scientific professions. In the course of the years, I have heard and read much that is sad regarding this spiritual misery, and, it is, unfortunately, not easy to say where the western boundary of this eastern Europe is to be sought. In any case, this boundary is indefinite and the psychical misery of the Jews is not lighter than the physical.

Many talented Jews are lost to culture because the way to learning is barred to them. It will be one of the foremost aims of the University in Jerusalem to alleviate this misery. May it contribute to the attainment by the Jewish people of a spiritual and moral height which will be worthy of its past.

The task of the Jerusalem University just referred to leads us to our second chief object, the Jewish Telegraphic Agency. The Jewish people belongs among the most oppressed national minorities; it is a national minority in all places whither its wandering staff has led it. It belongs among those peoples who must suffer to an especially high degree from the prevailing disease of an exaggerated nationalism. This nationalism is a grave danger for the entire western civilization, which at one time had its origin in Greece; behind it are powers inimical to life. To combat it is the inescapable duty of every well-intentioned and perceiving person of our time.

We Jews have to suffer from this scourge not only as one of the oldest branches of our western culture, but also as a people which is scattered over the entire world and is, therefore, regarded as nationally alien everywhere. In order not to be crushed, at this time, by inimical powers in its environment, this people requires living cohesiveness, solidarity.

Such a living cohesiveness is possible only if we are kept objectively informed about the lot of the Jews in all countries. This, the Jewish Telegraphic Agency has been doing for a decade and a half in a graphic and objective manner, and, in so doing, it has performed an important service to the Jewish people. To support this private enterprise in times of economic crisis is a self-evident duty of self-preservation. It is also part of the struggle for justice, whose significance transcends merely Jewish interests themselves. As director of the Jewish Telegraphic Agency, Mr. Jacob Landau has earned commendation which we joyfully acknowledge this day.

As I, myself, am no nationalist, the meaning of a people, in my opinion, lies in this—that it achieves something for humanity. I shall not bring up the question regarding the Jewish people here and now, but will only emphasize that this point of view must always be our guide in everything Jews undertake. The only worthy attitude of an individual as of a nation is this—to serve a greater whole and to strive for improvement and ennoblement.

# OBITUARY

## OLIVE M. LAMMERT

MARCH 5, 1894–OCTOBER 9, 1932

OLIVE M. LAMMERT, professor of chemistry at Vassar College, graduated from Vassar in 1915. From the time of her graduation until her death, except for two years of graduate work, she was a member of the Vassar department of chemistry. In 1919, as Sutro fellow from Vassar, she began graduate work at Columbia University; she received the doctorate in 1924.

The topics of her series of researches (presented in ten journal articles with J. L. R. Morgan) were a logical consequence of the initial one, the study of the effect of light upon the electrical conductance of solutions of the alkali halides in acetophenone. Professor Lammert's appreciation of the increasing importance in many fields of the determination of hydrogen-ion concentrations led her to organize at Vassar a course on this subject which is probably unique and has become an important unit in the work offered by the department. For the past six years she has been collaborating with J. L. R. Morgan in preparing a reference text-book on physical chemistry.

The independence of thought and the initiative shown in her great creative ability, her broad philosophical outlook, her persistence in carrying out detailed work, her highly developed experimental skill and her great resourcefulness made her work that of real genius. In all she did her boundless enthusiasm, her deft precision and her clarity of thinking were such that, as a former student writes, "she will always be more than a teacher—she will be the inspiration that carries us on." To her rigorous teaching she brought the gay touch of a keen sense of humor and the charm of a rare personality, the combination making "her classes memorable."

Her keen insight and balanced judgment made her a trusted, valuable member of important committees. These same qualities, together with her constructive sympathy and understanding, brought students to her constantly for aid in personal problems as well as in chemistry, and she, whose generosity was unlimited, was never too busy to help them, giving to many "one of the best parts of college life."

For all who knew her the words of Professor Reed, whose beautiful tribute appeared in the *Vassar Quarterly,* are true: Professor Lammert's death "has overwhelmed us at the college with a sense of tragic loss. She was brilliant, and gay and magnanimous; her presence radiated a sort of energy that made us all glad to be alive; she had a warm heart overflowing into actions of unforgettable kindness; and she was only thirty-eight."

A clear thinker, an indefatigable searcher for extreme precision, an exceedingly well-informed scientist and a marvelous manipulator, Professor Lammert is indeed a loss to physical chemistry.

MARY LANDON SAGUE

VASSAR COLLEGE

## RECENT DEATHS

DR. ARTHUR HOLLICK, paleobotanist of the New York Botanical Garden, died on March 11, at the age of seventy-six years.

JOHN L. STONE, professor emeritus of farm practise in the New York State College of Agriculture, Cornell University, died on March 8, at the age of eighty-one years.

RALEIGH DUDLEY MORRILL, associate professor of experimental engineering at New York University since 1926, died on March 11. He was forty-eight years old.

DR. HENRY GEORGE MEHRTENS, acting dean of the Stanford University School of Medicine, died on February 28, after a short illness from heart attacks. He had been connected with the Stanford faculty since 1915, and acting dean of the Medical School since the beginning of the present college year following the retirement of Dr. William Ophüls. Dr. Mehrtens received his medical training at Stanford and had been house physician in the Lane Hospital in San Francisco since 1915. He was professor of medicine, specializing in neuropsychiatry. Dr. Robert E. Swain, acting president of the university, said: "The death of Dr. Mehrtens is a very serious loss to Stanford University, to medical education and to medical science. An accomplished scientist and scholar at an early age, he was an effective teacher, and during the present year as acting dean of the university's medical school has devoted unselfish and effective service to its work."

HURON H. SMITH, curator of botany in the public museum of Milwaukee, Wisconsin, was instantly killed when the automobile in which he, his wife, and the father and mother of Mrs. Smith were riding was hit by a Milwaukee road passenger train at a crossing one half mile south of Glenview, Ill., early in the evening of February 25. Mr. Smith had been curator of botany at the public museum in Milwaukee since 1917. He was recognized as an authority on Indian life, on flowers and trees. He was made a member of the Menominee tribe of Indians several years ago. E-we-ona-ginka, medicine man of the Winnebagos, confided all his closely guarded secrets to Mr. Smith because he could find no young man of the tribe worthy to be his successor. Mr. Smith was a member of the Wisconsin Archeological Society, the Milwaukee Horticultural Society and honorary member of the State Forest Association. He was a fellow of the American Association for the Advancement of Science. He obtained his arts degree from DePauw University in 1905 and was an instructor in dendrology at Cornell University from 1905 to 1907 and obtained his master's degree from that institution. He was a tree specialist and dendrologist with the Field Museum, Chicago, from 1907 to 1911, and assistant curator of botany from 1911 to 1917.

# SCIENTIFIC EVENTS

## BOULDER CANYON LAKE WILD LIFE REFUGE

THE great artificial lake to be created by the Hoover Dam on the Colorado River will become a refuge and breeding ground for wild birds and animals under an executive order signed by President Hoover on March 3. The new reservation will be known as the Boulder Canyon Wild Life Refuge. Superimposed on part of the land and water area withdrawn for the Boulder Canyon project for river regulation, flood control, irrigation, domestic water uses and power development, the new wild-life refuge will cover a total of about 620,000 acres, approximately 132,000 acres of which will be a vast artificial lake on that part of the Colorado River, in Arizona and Nevada.

Administration of the refuge will be by the Department of Agriculture, through the Bureau of Biological Survey, subject to use by the Department of the Interior for its primary purposes. Paul G. Redington, chief of the Bureau of Biological Survey, in a statement issued on March 7 said that the flooded area will be wholly in the Lower Sonoran Life Zone, with the hot summer and mild winter climate of the mosquito and creosote bush country providing a breeding ground for many interesting birds and mammals of the southwestern desert region, and a winter resort for many northern migratory birds. Mr. Redington writes:

> It was a paradise throughout the year for Arizona quail, roadrunners, thrashers and other birds. In winter, swans, snow geese, many ducks, some shorebirds, waders and a host of other smaller migrant birds found a congenial resort in the Virgin and Colorado River Valleys, the natural outlet of the Great Basin. When this area becomes a great lake, with curving bays and deep inlets cutting back into side valleys and gulches, it will again be a great attraction for northern waterfowl and provide cover and food for the resident birds that are pushed back from the middle of the valley.
>
> The refuge will be an oasis in an otherwise arid country on one of the southward bird-migration routes, a way station from Klamath Lake Refuge, Oregon, to the Gulf of California. The Federal Bear River Refuge, on Great Salt Lake, lies 400 miles northeast, the Salton Sea Refuge is 225 miles to the south, and the Fallon Migratory Bird Refuge in Nevada is about 350 miles northwest. The new refuge, therefore, should prove a valuable resting spot and winter resort for many waterfowl that now seek congenial waters beyond our southern border.
>
> Beavers, muskrats and otters will be the main local aquatic mammalian fauna, but the protected area will also provide homes for antelope-squirrels and chipmunks, as well as for little desert foxes, gray foxes, raccoons, and other interesting animals of the region.
>
> The value of this new refuge in the Southwest is greatly enhanced by its geographic position, and a more favorable place for preserving and enjoying the close presence of aquatic and other wild life could not be found in the whole region. Within the new refuge it is unlawful to hunt, trap, capture, wilfully disturb or kill any wild animal or bird of any kind whatever, or to take or destroy the nest or eggs of any wild bird.

## THE MUSEUMS OF ARCHEOLOGY AND GEOLOGY AT THE UNIVERSITY OF KENTUCKY

THE University of Kentucky reports the opening on March 7 of two museums on the campus, the Museum of Archeology and the Geological Museum. The archeological museum, which is housed in a building of its own, will be opened to the public each Tuesday and Thursday afternoon from two to four o'clock, and the geological museum will be open daily.

The archeological museum was prepared with the purpose of depicting prehistoric human life in Kentucky, and has reproduced ancient graves, ossuary pits and other evidences of prehistoric races in the exact manner in which they were unearthed. Horace Miner, senior student, has been appointed curator under the supervision of Professor W. S. Webb, head of the department of anthropology and archeology.

The archeological museum occupies a small building which faces the side of the administration building and which was formerly occupied by the library. The basement floor is devoted to offices and a large lecture room for class work, and the museum proper is entered through a wrought iron grill, designated and executed in the College of Engineering under the direction of Stephen Saunier, instructor in the forge shop. It has as its motif Indian artifacts, such as shells, arrow heads, pipes and other accoutrements, which have been reproduced in the grill work in an intricate pattern.

The whole outlay of the museum tells a story of prehistoric life in Kentucky. Some of the features are the burials which have been reproduced with skeletons, artifacts and even the earth deposits around the burial ground. Professor W. S. Webb, head of the department, has placed there his private collection.

The geological museum is on the second floor of the administration building and was arranged by the department of geology in conjunction with the Bureau of Mineral and Topographical Survey. In it an attempt has been made to emphasize the rocks and minerals of economic and commercial importance in the state, together with other features of commercial and scientific interest.

Professor A. C. McFarlan is director of the Bureau of Mineral and Topographical Survey and David Young is curator of the geological museum. In this exhibit much attention has been paid to the Kentucky caves and a representation of cave material and typical cave phenomena has been prepared. Fossils of the animals and plants which lived in this region in past geologic ages and whose remains are now found preserved in the rocks of the state are well represented.

## REQUIREMENTS FOR THE LICENSE OF MEDICAL STUDENTS IN NEW YORK STATE

REQUIREMENTS of the New York State Education Department for the admission of American or European medical students studying abroad to New York medical licensing examinations have been announced by Dr. Ernest E. Cole, acting commissioner of education. These requirements are in harmony with regulations recently promulgated by the Federation of State Medical Boards of the United States. The federation has announced that students proposing to study medicine in Europe will be subject to the following regulations for admission to the various state medical licensing examinations:

1. No American student matriculating in a European medical school subsequent to the academic year 1932–1933 will be admitted to any state medical licensing examination or to the examination of the National Board of Medical Examiners, who does not, before beginning such medical study, secure from a state Board of Medical Examiners or other competent state authority, a certificate endorsed by the Association of American Medical Colleges or the Council on Medical Education and Hospitals of the American Medical Association showing that he has met the premedical educational requirements prescribed by the aforementioned associations.

2. No student, either American or European, matriculating in a European medical school subsequent to the academic year 1932–1933 will be admitted to any state medical licensing examination, or to the examination of the National Board of Medical Examiners, who does not (a) present satisfactory evidence of premedical education equivalent to the requirements of the Association of American Medical Colleges, and the Council on Medical Education and Hospitals of the American Medical Association, and graduation from a European medical school after a medical course of at least four academic years, and (b) obtain a license to practise medicine in the country in which the medical school from which he is graduated is located.

### NEW MEXICO MEETING OF THE SOUTHWESTERN DIVISION OF THE AMERICAN ASSOCIATION FOR THE ADVANCEMENT OF SCIENCE

THE thirteenth annual meeting of the Southwestern Division will be held from Monday to Thursday, May 1, 2, 3 and 4, at Las Cruces, New Mexico. The host institution will be the New Mexico College of Agriculture and Mechanic Arts, the post office address of which is State College, New Mexico.

Officers of the division are: Charles T. Vorhies, University of Arizona, *president;* F. E. E. Germann, University of Colorado, *vice-president;* Edwin F. Carpenter, Steward Observatory, University of Arizona, *secretary-treasurer.* Officers of the New Mexico Association for the Advancement of Science are: S. B. Talmage, *president,* New Mexico School of Mines, Socorro; H. C. Graham, *vice-president,* State Teachers College, Silver City; H. G. Fisher, *treasurer,* New Mexico Museum, Santa Fe; E. R. Harrington, *secretary,* High School, Albuquerque.

The general meetings will include the opening session on Monday morning; a symposium on problems relating to erosion, on Tuesday evening; and the annual banquet at which the retiring president of the division will deliver his address, on Wednesday evening. In addition there will be a luncheon symposium devoted to the historical interest of the region, in Old Mesilla, near Las Cruces, site of the signing of the Gadsden Purchase of 1853. The John Wesley Powell Lecture, now partially endowed by recent vote of the executive committee, will be delivered, probably on Monday evening, May 1, by Aldo Leopold, consulting forester, of Madison, Wisconsin.

Las Cruces lies at an elevation of 3,800 feet on the El Paso-Albuquerque branch of the Santa Fe Railroad, 40 miles north of El Paso.

Excursions and entertainment are being planned by the local committee under the chairmanship of Professor D. S. Robbins. Thursday, the last day of the meeting, has been set aside for the excursions. The points for which visits have been definitely planned are (1) White Sands, a large area of drifting dunes of gypsum sand, about 40 miles from Las Cruces; (2) the Jornada Experimental Range, about 23 miles from Las Cruces, and (3) El Paso, 40 miles southward, for its mining and metallurgical industries, its cement and electrolytic copper plants, several oil refineries, and, across the border, Juarez.

## SCIENTIFIC NOTES AND NEWS

THE bicentenary of the birth of Joseph Priestley occurred on March 13. He was born in Yorkshire and came to the United States on June 4, 1794, living in Northumberland, Pennsylvania, until his death on February 6, 1814.

DR. HUGO DE VRIES, the distinguished Dutch botanist, celebrated his eighty-fifth birthday on February 16.

DR. FRANK BURR MALLORY, until his retirement in 1932 professor of pathology in the Harvard Medical School, having reached the age of seventy years, has also retired as chief of the department of pathology at Boston City Hospital. Dr. Mallory has been connected with the hospital since 1891.

SIR ROBERT HADFIELD, metallurgical engineer, managing director of Hadfield's Limited, Sheffield, has been elected an honorary member of the Academy of Sciences at Leningrad, in recognition of his work for metallurgy. The Soviet Ambassador in London, I. Maisky, gave a luncheon in honor of the occasion on February 28.

DR. ARTHUR E. KENNELLY, emeritus professor of electrical engineering, Harvard University, was elected to membership in the International Committee of Weights and Measures at its meeting in Sèvres, France, at the end of January.

PROFESSOR MARSTON T. BOGERT, of the department of chemistry at Columbia University, has been elected president of the Columbia Chapter of Sigma Xi to succeed Professor Donald E. Lancefield. Professor Harold W. Webb, of the department of physics, has become vice-president, succeeding Professor J. J. Morgan, and Professor Arthur W. Thomas, of the department of chemistry, has been named secretary-treasurer to succeed Dr. G. Marshall Kay. Membership in Sigma Xi was granted to 115 candidates, including 17 faculty members.

DR. H. LUDENDORFF, director of the Astrophysical Observatory at Potsdam, has been elected president of the German Astronomical Society, to succeed the late Dr. Max Wolf, of Heidelberg.

*Nature* states that at the annual meeting of the British Royal Astronomical Society held on February 10, the following officers were elected: *President,* Professor F. J. M. Stratton; *Vice-presidents,* Sir Arthur S. Eddington, Mr. John Evershed, Dr. H. Knox-Shaw and Dr. W. J. S. Lockyer; *Treasurer,* Mr. J. H. Reynolds; *Secretaries,* Mr. W. M. H. Greaves and Dr. W. M. Smart; *Foreign Secretary,* Professor Alfred Fowler.

DR. DAVID RIESMAN has been elected professor of the history of medicine in the University of Pennsylvania, filling a newly established chair.

DR. J. HENDERSON SMITH, plant pathologist of the department of mycology at the Rothamsted Experimental Station, has been appointed head of the recently organized department of plant pathology, to succeed Dr. W. B. Brierley, now professor of agricultural botany at Reading University, formerly at the head of the department of mycology at Rothamsted.

*Museum News* reports that N. D. Riley has been appointed keeper of the department of entomology of the Natural History Museum (British Museum) in succession to E. E. Austen. H. G. Blair has been appointed deputy-keeper of the department. W. P. Pycraft has retired from the post of assistant keeper in the department of zoology of the Natural History Museum (British Museum).

ACCORDING to *Industrial and Engineering Chemistry,* George P. Gray, for the past two years director of the California Soil Improvement Committee, has become associated with the Colloidal Products Corporation, San Francisco, to assist in the continuation of the company's research program on the investigation of spreaders and fixators in their relation to spray material.

JOHN R. HEWETT, editor of the *General Electric Review* for nearly twenty years, has retired because of ill health.

DR. GUSTAV ZECHEL, of the department of anatomy of the College of Medicine, University of Illinois, has received a grant from the American Medical Association for the purchase of a microcinematographic apparatus which will facilitate his studies on the growth of malignant cells. Dr. Arthur Knudson, professor of biochemistry, and Dr. Lloyd H. Ziegler, professor of neuropsychiatry of the Albany Medical College have been allotted a grant for the study of the remote effect of rickets.

H. A. BENDIXEN, of Washington State College and Experiment Station, has received a grant from the Oberlaender Trust of the Carl Schurz Memorial Foundation, under which he will study problems of dairy manufactures and travel in Scandinavian countries, Germany and Russia for one year. During the year's leave of absence Dr. N. S. Golding, associate professor of dairying in the University of British Columbia, will serve in his place as associate professor of dairy husbandry.

PROFESSOR KNUT LUNDMARK, director of the University Observatory, Lund, Sweden, has been spending several weeks studying the collection of nebular photographs at the Steward Observatory of the University of Arizona, and Dr. Sture Holm, of the Lund Observatory, has been spending two months on photometric investigations with the three-foot reflecting telescope of the observatory.

AN Associated Press dispatch states that Professor Auguste Piccard is planning a balloon ascent to study cosmic rays in the stratosphere this summer, starting from the grounds of the World's Fair at Chicago, provided that arrangements for financing his ascent can be made with American balloon and metal manufacturers.

SIR HENRY H. DALE, director of the National Institute for Medical Research, London, will deliver the Dohme Lectures at the Johns Hopkins Medical School on April 20, 21 and 22.

DR. CURT STERN, of the Kaiser Wilhelm Institute for Biology in Berlin, delivered a lecture at the University of Kansas recently on "The Structure of the Chromosomes." He is now engaged in a tour as a speaker for Sigma Xi, honorary science fraternity. Following his address at the University of Kansas, he went to the University of Missouri.

DR. J. E. ACKERT, dean of the division of graduate study and professor of zoology and parasitologist at Kansas State College, Manhattan, addressed the Snow Zoological Club at the University of Kansas on February 21, on "Host-Parasite Relationships between Chickens and their Intestinal Nematodes."

DR. EDWARD MELLANBY, professor of pharmacology at the University of Sheffield, will deliver on June 8, 13 and 15 the Croonian Lectures on "Nutrition and Disease—the Interaction of Clinical and Experimental Investigations."

THE Romanes Lecture at the University of Edinburgh will be given this year by Dr. Heinrich Wieland, professor of chemistry at Munich.

THE Stuart McGuire Lectureship series at the Medical College of Virginia, Richmond, will be held on April 25, 26 and 27. Dr. Ronald T. Grant, of the department of clinical research, University College Hospital Medical School, London, will give three lectures on "The Pathology of Endocarditis" and a fourth lecture on "The Arteriovenous Anastomoses in Human Skin"; Professor Louis Hamman, of the Johns Hopkins University, will lecture on cardiac burgh will be given this year by Dr. Heinrich Wieversity, will hold a clinic.

THE second annual Sigma Xi Day of the Rochester Chapter was held at the University of Rochester on February 22. The principal event was the evening lecture, on "Lung Injuries of Industrial Importance resulting from Dust Inhalation," delivered by Dr. Cecil K. Drinker, head of the department of physiology at the School of Public Health, Harvard University. In addition, the program included a morning lecture intended especially for children, a series of seven lecture-demonstrations of current scientific research by members of the chapter and a formal dinner. "Light—Where it Comes from, Where it Goes" was the title of the children's lecture, given by Dr. Brian O'Brien, professor of physiological optics at the University of Rochester.

MEMBERS of the science faculty of Ohio University have organized a Sigma Xi Club. Officers elected for the current year are: *President,* Professor F. H. Krecker, head of the department of biology; *Vice-president,* Dr. F. B. Gullum, associate professor of chemistry, and *Secretary-treasurer,* Dr. D. B. Green, assistant professor of physics. Members are: Professors Paulsen, Anderson and Patrick, of the department of psychology; Professors Stehr, Rowles, Frey and Krecker, of the department of biology; Professors Morton, Reed and Starcher, of the department of mathematics; Professors Gullum and Clippinger, of the department of chemistry; Professors Heil and Green, of the department of physics, and Professor Clark, of the department of civil engineering. Meetings will be held bi-monthly throughout the year. The subjects of papers to be presented during the current year are: "Radio Thermy," "Principles of Biologic Control," "The Goal Gradient Process of Learning," "Concepts of Infinity," "A Study of Stresses in Arches by Means of Small Models," and "Relation of Clumping to Resistance to Toxic Substances in Invertebrates."

THE department of geology and geography of Northwestern University announces the continuation of its exchange arrangement with the University of Cincinnati, initiated last year. Early in March Dr. Nevin M. Fenneman, professor and head of the department of geology and geography, University of Cincinnati, gave four lectures at Northwestern University, and Dr. J. T. Stark, associate professor of geology, Northwestern University, will give a similar series of lectures at the University of Cincinnati. Professor Stark's lectures will deal principally with the geology of the Precambrian rocks of the United States and with the methods used in interpreting their structure and genesis; they will be delivered at Cincinnati during the week of March 20. The lectures given by Professor Fenneman dealt chiefly with problems of regional physiography. The subjects of these lectures were as follows: "The Middle Rocky Mountains," "The Appalachian Peneplains," "The Southern Rocky Mountains" and "The Grand Canyon District." In addition, Professor Fenneman spoke on the night of Thursday, March 9, before the Geological Society of Chicago on "Cyclic and Non-Cyclic Erosion."

ACCORDING to *Nature,* progress has been made in the discussion of the proposal to institute an international congress of the ethnological and anthropological sciences. Arrangements are now being made for a preliminary conference for further discussion to be held in Basel on April 20, 21 and 22. Invitations to the conference are being issued by the Royal Anthropological Institute of Great Britain, while the local arrangements are in the hands of Dr. Felix Speiser, director of the Museum of Ethnology, Basel. The conference will be welcomed on behalf of the City and the Education Committee, and its sessions will be held in the Burgeratsaal. The subjects for discussion are the scope of the proposed congress and its relation to existing congresses of like character, such as the International Congress of Americanists and the International Congress of Prehistoric and Protohistoric Sciences; constitution and procedure, and the date and place of the first meeting. On this last point, it has been suggested that meetings should take place in years alternate to those of the Prehistoric and Protohistoric Sciences Congress and coinciding once in every four years with the European meetings of the Americanists' Congress.

THE thirteenth annual summer term of the American School of Prehistoric Research will open in Prague on June 28, and close in Berlin on August 21. Dr. V. J. Fewkes, who last year conducted the expedition to Yugoslavia sponsored jointly by the school, the Fogg Art Museum of Harvard University and Peabody Museum of Harvard, will again be in charge as associate director for the summer term. The program will consist of a study of museum collections, field excursions, conferences, excavations (including field technique) and examinations. Requests for further information should be addressed to Dr. George Grant MacCurdy, director, Old Lyme, Connecticut.

THE department of biology of the College of the Pacific at Stockton, California, will open a Marine Biological Station on the Pacific Coast. Courses in elementary and advanced biology will be offered during the regular summer session. Students may spend three additional weeks at the station to carry out research in invertebrate zoology. Facilities will be offered for intensive laboratory work in biology and zoology. Student living quarters will be established close to the station at a low rate, and the cost of board will probably not exceed the amount charged at the college. It is hoped eventually to establish a permanent Pacific Biological Marine Station with courses continuous throughout the year.

*Museum News* states that the Adler Planetarium and Astronomical Museum, on Northerly Island, Chicago, will complete the lower floor and install additional ventilating machines in the next two months in order to take care of crowds expected at the time of the World's Fair this summer. In order to make the additions the planetarium is closed for the two months. During the fair lectures will be given every hour instead of twice a day.

*Nature* reports that Sir Dugald Clerk, who died on November 12, bequeathed £3,000 to the Institution of Civil Engineers; £2,000 to the Royal Society; £1,000 to the Royal Institution; £1,000 to the Royal Society of Arts; £1,000 to the Institution of Mechanical Engineers; £1,000 to the University of Glasgow; £1,000 to the University of Leeds; £1,000 to the University of St. Andrews; £1,000 to the University of Manchester; £1,000 to the University of Liverpool. The residue of the property is to be divided into thirty-one parts; three of these parts are to go to the Institution of Civil Engineers; two to the Royal Society; one to the Royal Institution; one to the Royal Society of Arts; one to the Institution of Mechanical Engineers; one each to the Universities of Glasgow, Leeds, St. Andrews, Manchester and London.

# DISCUSSION

## NATURE SANCTUARIES—A MEANS OF SAVING NATURAL BIOTIC COMMUNITIES

ONE of the characteristic things about organisms is their fluctuations in abundance from time to time. A community is an assemblage of plants and animals—a living thing which after a period of stress will never be exactly the same again. A nature sanctuary is a community or community fragment covering a certain area within which the fluctuations in abundance and other natural changes are allowed to go on unmodified and uncontrolled. Such areas afford opportunity for the study of the dynamics of natural biotic communities.

Outside of modern ecology there has been little or no tendency towards the development of specialists in the entire life of natural communities. The trend of research and education is toward specialization on particular objects or particular organisms. Perhaps one reason why nature study has been unsuccessful is because it is not the study of nature but of single natural objects or groups of objects which constitute a small part of any natural assemblage of organisms. Often this has resulted in the emotional protection of animals singled out by popular prejudice. In general, from a philosophical and practical view-point, the unmodified assemblage of organisms is commonly more valuable than the isolated rare species. However, because the significance of the unmodified assemblage is popularly ignored, the whole is commonly sacrificed in the supposed interest of the rare species. Usually neither need be sacrificed in any large natural area.

The nature sanctuaries are surrounded by areas in a less natural state, called buffer areas of partial protection. In a buffer area the vegetation is only slightly modified by man. It is a region of partial protection of nature and is zoned to afford suitable range for roaming animals under full protection. Since nature sanctuaries are areas in which natural forces are allowed free play, they may be classified with regard to the organisms now missing from the primeval community which once occupied the same area.

(1) First-class nature sanctuaries include areas of original vegetation containing all the animals which are historically known to have occurred there. (2) Second-class nature sanctuaries include (a) second growth areas approaching maturity with animals as in the first-class type and (b) areas of original vegetation from which not more than two important species of animals are missing. (3) Third-class nature

sanctuaries include areas modified to a greater degree than second-class ones.

(1) *Research reserves* of the National Park Service are essentially nature sanctuaries. They recognize two additional divisions of a park: (a) a greater part of the park open to the public and traversed by trails and roads, and (b) an area of development, hotels, etc. (2) *Natural areas* in the U. S. Forest Service sense are partial nature sanctuaries but primarily floral. (3) *Primitive areas* and *wilderness areas* in the U. S. Forest Service sense are primitive only in human transportation and conditions of living. Vegetation may be cut over and various animals wanting. (4) *Research area* and experimental area usually imply modification (except in the National Parks).

Except in desert and tundra, first-class nature sanctuaries are not available outside the national forest and national parks, and in rare instances in state and provincial parks. Buffer areas may serve as recreation areas, game reserves, etc. They are areas of partial protection not always available on all sides of natural areas. Reserve areas in the national parks and national forests are probably too small to serve as true nature sanctuaries. They have not been selected with reference to animals, and no buffer area of protection within which animals will not be disturbed is ordinarily set aside.

Nature sanctuaries are essential if any of the original nature in North America is to be saved for future generations for scientific observation of, among other things, the important phenomena of fluctuation in abundance of plants and animals, their social life, etc. Due to lack of knowledge of these fluctuations custodians view each change in abundance with alarm and desire to apply remedies immediately; hence, constant pressure must be exerted on government agencies to prevent the current popular idea of "control" and "improvement" from entering into the management of national parks, provincial and state parks and other reserves containing natural areas suitable as nature sanctuaries with buffer territories. The experiment of leaving areas essentially alone, which was so successful in a few of our parks, is worthy of repetition. In general much control activity is useless because it is applied to animals at their maximum abundance and barely hasten the natural decline.

The Ecological Society of America urges a subdivision of all but the small reserves into sanctuaries, buffer areas of partial protection and areas of development for human use where this is one of the aims of the reserves. A further aim of the society is to promote adequate scientific observation bearing on the fluctuations in abundance, to stimulate cooperation between the controlling agencies in charge of game and vegetation reservations in order that more logical units be developed and better methods of administration adopted.[1]

VICTOR E. SHELFORD
*Chairman of the Committee for the Study of Plant and Animal Communities, Ecological Society of America.*

## THE WATER CONTENT OF MEDUSAE

MY accuracy has been questioned by Bateman,[1] who writes that "Gortner's statement that medusae contain 99.8 per cent. water is contradicted."

The statements which he criticizes are as follows:

> As I write these lines there lie before me two sheets of paper. One is the photograph of a large Medusa (jellyfish) from the Atlantic Gulf Stream which was photographed immediately after being removed from the water and being placed upon the open pages of a magazine. The Medusa, as removed from the water, weighed in excess of 500 grams. In the photograph one can read the distorted print through the more or less transparent outer portion of the umbrella, but the central portion of the Medusa which measured approximately 10 × 12 cm was sufficiently dense and opaque to prevent the print underneath from showing in the photograph.
>
> The other sheet of paper is the opened pages of the magazine upon which the Medusa had been allowed to dry after being photographed. These pages simply appear as though they had been wetted and then dried. No noticeable film is discernible on the surface of the pages. The print is clear-cut, and even exposing these pages to ultra-violet light results in extremely slight fluorescence. The weight of these pages exceeds by less than 0.45 gram the weight of the pages before the Medusa was dried upon them. Less than 0.10 per cent. of dried residue from the large Medusa including the salts, etc., in the adherent sea water and all of the inorganic constituents of the living organism![2]

In the discussion to this paper (p. 702) I pointed out that I was dependent upon the statement of the collector as to the weight of the living medusa, but that I had myself confirmed the dry weight, also that on other occasions I had personally made somewhat similar observations. In another connection I have stated that "in some instances, as in the case of the jellyfish, only an insignificant fraction of the organism is composed of organic material, as little as 1 per cent. of the jellyfish being organic matter."[3]

Bateman's flat contradiction of my statement rests, in so far as I can ascertain, on his acceptance of the data of Krukenberg[4] (who reports 4.60 per cent.

[1] Full details of nature sanctuary plans will appear in the society's official organ, *Ecology*, early in 1933.

[1] J. B. Bateman, "The Osmotic Properties of Medusae," *Jour. Exper. Biol.*, 9: 124–127. 1932.

[2] R. A. Gortner, *Trans. Faraday Society*, 26: 678–704. 1930.

[3] R. A. Gortner, "Outlines of Biochemistry," N. Y. (1929). *Cf.* pp. 227–8.

[4] C. F. W. Krukenberg, *Zool. Anzeiger*, 3: 306. 1880.

solids in *Rhizostoma cuvieri,* 4.20 to 5.80 per cent. in *Aurelia aurita* and 3.70 to 4.25 per cent. in *Chrysaora hyoscella*) and the observations of Moebius[5] (who reports 2.06 to 2.10 per cent. in *Aurelia aurita*), and the non-acceptance of my data. It is somewhat surprising that Bateman does not report independent data of his own, since he used a large *Cyanea* in his own studies.

Unfortunately, I can not designate the species for which I have personal data, since no zoologist was available at the time the organism was secured. A photograph of the organism as secured, and as later dried down on a sheet of paper 23 × 30 cm has, however, been published.[6] This medusa was not *Gonionemus* sp., as Bateman erroneously assumes. In no place have I made any statement as to the water content of *Gonionemus.* Perhaps I am in error in wording my statements so that they might be interpreted as applying to all medusae, but I have said "a medusa,"[2] "one species of jellyfish (*medusa*),"[6] "the organism may contain," etc., and have recognized that the physiological condition of the organism, *e.g.,* presence of egg masses, etc., may make for a higher solid content. However, I still believe, from my own observations, that some salt-water medusae have a water content exceeding 99 per cent. and hope that investigators having access to such material will reinvestigate this question, for it is those organisms with the low solid content which present the interesting physiological problems.

ROSS AIKEN GORTNER
THE UNIVERSITY OF MINNESOTA

## THE PHYSIOLOGICAL BASIS OF THE TWISTING HABIT IN PLANT GROWTH

IN connection with the interesting paper of Dr. William Seifriz in a recent number of SCIENCE[1] on the spiral habit of growth, correlated with the twisting of the stem or trunk of many plants, considered as a result of physiological rather than environmental conditions, it was thought that it might be of interest to add a bit of evidence which has been obtained in this laboratory.

In the course of an experimental program on the genetic effect of x-rays, an investigation has been undertaken of the physiological abnormalities of seedlings of the citrus fruits grown from irradiated seed. It is hoped at a later time to publish the results in full, but two seedlings are of interest at the moment. From the time of sprouting, these young plants showed a decided tendency to spiral in a counterclockwise direction. Both plants twisted so markedly that the trunk was bent from the vertical and the leaves, during early life, were crushed against the stem. After six months the habit was abandoned, and the later growth was normal. Both plants showed some evidence of tissue inversion and other characteristic x-ray injuries during early life.

The seeds used in the work were obtained from a citrus experiment station, and represented a normally quite stable seed bed stock. Before treatment, they were soaked in distilled water for fifteen minutes and left in a moisture-saturated atmosphere for twelve hours. They were then dried on filter paper and were given doses of 2,400 roentgens of radiation from a thick-walled tungsten-target Coolidge tube operated at 200 k.v.p. and 30 ma. current. The seeds were then planted in flats in a mixture of sand and peat moss and maintained in a greenhouse, protected from wind and from sharp temperature change. Since the source of light was the sun, since undue mechanical shock was avoided for the seedlings, and since but two of the entire group showed any tendency to twist, it seems logical to assume tentatively that in this case a typical spiral growth, resulting in extreme twisting of the stem in a developing tree, was the result of a physiological rather than an environmental condition —possibly x-ray induced abnormal mitoses.

C. P. HASKINS
C. N. MOORE
RESEARCH LABORATORY
GENERAL ELECTRIC COMPANY
SCHENECTADY, N. Y.

## AN UNUSUAL CRETACEOUS CIRRIPED

THE decision of the International Commission on Nomenclature (Opinion 118) that *Scalpellum gabbi* Wade[1] is a *nomen nudum,* on account of the extremely cautious wording of Wade's account of it, seems to make some further action necessary to place this rather unusual barnacle on a satisfactory basis. Wade figured the carina and an upper lateral plate. These are not known to belong to one individual, and it is even possible that they do not belong to the same species; but it happens that the carina was selected by Charles Darwin as the essential plate in diagnoses of fossil species of Scalpellum, most of which are known by detached plates. Wade's figures of the carina are ample for the recognition of the species, which is quite peculiar among Cretaceous forms for the subcentral position of the umbo. Only four other Cretaceous species, all European, have this advanced form of carina. It may be doubted whether Scalpellum developed this type of carina so early, and it may turn out that these Cretaceous species belong to

5 K. Moebius, *Ibid.*, 5: 586. 1882.
6 R. A. Gortner, *Gamma Alpha Record,* 22: 42. 1932.
1 SCIENCE, January 13, 1933.

1 U. S. Geol. Surv. Professional Paper 137, p. 191, plate 62, figs. 3, 4, 6, 7.

the less evolved Smilium group, a question which can be settled when specimens are found with plates in place. I propose to restrict *Scalpellum gabbi* Wade to the carina represented in his plate 62, figs. 3 and 4. The figures are inverted.

H. A. PILSBRY
ACADEMY OF NATURAL SCIENCES,
PHILADELPHIA

### STREAM DOUBLE REFRACTION EXHIBITED BY JUICE FROM BOTH HEALTHY AND MOSAIC TOBACCO PLANTS

IN previous papers[1,2] we reported that juice from tobacco plants infected with tobacco mosaic virus exhibits a stream double refraction characteristic of sols containing rod-shaped particles. Juice from healthy tobacco plants did not show double refraction. The juice was always obtained by freezing the tissues, followed by thawing, pressing and centrifuging.

Since the publication of these results we have found that centrifuged juice from unfrozen, macerated, healthy leaves regularly exhibits stream double refraction, and juice pressed from healthy tissues which have been frozen, thawed and pressed may sometimes show stream double refraction if uncentrifuged.

After juice from unfrozen, macerated, healthy tobacco leaves was subjected to Vinson's[3] safranin—Lloyd's reagent treatment for purifying tobacco mosaic virus—the purified preparation failed to show stream double refraction; however, purified virus from unfrozen mosaic leaves exhibited strong stream double refraction and, like the unpurified virus, could usually be diluted with 200 parts of water before double refraction disappeared. These results apparently indicate that all the detectable doubly refractive material was removed from the healthy juice, but that none was removed from the infective juice by the purification treatment, and suggest the possibility that much or all of the doubly refractive material in the juice from diseased plants may be different from that in juice from healthy plants. However, the present evidence is insufficient to warrant conclusions as to whether the virus particles are or are not responsible for all or part of the double refraction exhibited by juice from diseased plants.

WILLIAM N. TAKAHASHI
T. E. RAWLINS
DIVISION OF PLANT PATHOLOGY
UNIVERSITY OF CALIFORNIA

1 *Proc. Soc. Exper. Biol. Med.*, 30: 155–157, 1932.
2 SCIENCE, 77: 26–27, 1933.
3 *Phytopath.*, 22: 29, 1932.

## SCIENTIFIC BOOKS

*Principles of Genetics; A Text-book, with Problems.* By E. W. SINNOTT and L. C. DUNN. McGraw-Hill Book Company, New York. Second edition, xvi + 441. 1932. $3.50.

*Recent Advances in Plant Genetics.* By F. W. SANSOME and J. PHILP, with foreword by SIR DANIEL HALL. P. Blakiston's Son and Company, Philadelphia. x + 414. 1932. $4.00.

THE two publications cited above are of interest from the light they throw upon the rapid evolution of genetics within recent years, entirely apart from the information which they may lay before the student. It was not so long ago that genetics was concerned chiefly with 3 : 1 ratios or modifications of such ratios. The original concept of the gene was independent of its location in the chromosome and the intimate behavior of chromosomes was of relatively little interest to geneticists. Cytologists seemingly had tired of working out the alteration of generations in lower forms and the relatively few who remained in the field of cytology appeared interested in the structure of chromosomes and their behavior in nuclear division without much concern as to what differences in structure and behavior mean to the organism and its offspring. A change has taken place in the attitude of geneticists toward cytology which has been especially marked within the last half dozen years. Chromosomal behavior has become the foundation upon which modern genetics is now being built as is shown by the two texts under review.

The American text by Sinnott and Dunn is a revised edition of their 1925 publication. Two new chapters have been added, one on the contribution of genetics to evolutionary theory, and one on the relation between genetics and development. The chapters on the application of genetics in plant and animal breeding, on inheritance in man and on the problems of eugenics have been eliminated. The treatment of biometric methods has been rewritten by D. R. Charles and placed in an appendix. Among the topics which have received new or extended treatment may be mentioned the induction of mutations by radiation; recent analysis of chromosomal changes; segmental interchange between chromosomes; the cytological demonstration of crossing-over; mapping of genes in chromosomes by cytological methods; chromosomal and genic balance; and the physiological interpretation of the facts of heredity. At the end of each chapter are given a dozen or more reference problems aimed to stimulate the student in extending his grasp of the subject under discussion by study of original sources in the literature. In addition there is in the appendix a list of over 400 problems based on the text, a large proportion of which demand calculations from data presented. The problem method seems to have met with success at the hands of the authors since the number of problems given is increased over the earlier edition. They should help the student to a more thorough grasp of the subject as is the case with "original" problems in text-books of geometry. They should thus make teaching easier for most teachers. It would not be surprising, however, if a demand should have arisen for a set of answers to be sold only to teachers as has been the case with the problems in texts on mathematics. The authors are recognized investigators and experienced teachers in the adjoining fields of botany and zoology. Their association in the Connecticut Agricultural College as well as more recently in Columbia University has given them an experience and sympathy in applied as well as in fundamental problems of their subject. As one would expect, their text has profited by their experience and appears to be a well-organized and balanced treatment of the principles of genetics which is presented in a form admirably adapted to the classroom.

The English publication by Sansome and Philp is a marked contrast to the American text. Its scope and manner of presentation is not adapted to the generalized undergraduate course in genetics. It is intended, however, primarily for the teacher and the research geneticist and by them will be found a valuable and stimulating book. Its title would suggest that the organisms discussed are plants only. This is in the main true, but a treatise on plants could not be good genetics if it gave no reference to Drosophila, which the authors apparently classify as a banana plant product. The subject-matter is further restricted to the more recent advances in plant genetics; those mainly of the last ten years. A balanced treatment even of this limited period is not attempted and certain topics such as sex, chimeras and the mathematics of inheritance and populations receive little or no consideration. The main purpose appears to be to acquaint the reader with the last words about chromosomes in relation to genetics. In some cases the last word literally had not yet been spoken since there are frequent references to papers in press. The authors might well have had added the subtitle "Chiasmotypy and its effect upon genetic phenomena," since much space is given to this still rather controversial theory. There can be no doubt, however, of the importance to geneticists of an understanding of the early stages in the reduction divisions. This has been hitherto largely a *terra incognita*. Fortunately, it is beginning to be explored through direct cytological observation and we are no longer confined to genetic evidence as to what has happened at this stage. Polyploidy and segmental interchange are discussed in considerable detail, especially in relation to the species problem.

The difference in view-point between the American and the English books may be seen by a couple of examples. Sansome and Philp devote eight pages to the various hypotheses advanced by different investigators to account for speltoid wheats and fatuoid oats because they obviously are a chromosomal problem tied up in some way with the polyploid nature of these species. These abnormal types are apparently not mentioned by Sinnott and Dunn, probably because they felt it wiser in presenting the principles of genetics in a text-book to concentrate upon the phenomena about which there was general agreement. In the English book there is an extensive bibliography of 47 pages placed in convenient position for reference at the end of the text. In the American book the citations are fewer in number and grouped at the end of the chapters to which they refer. This arrangement is doubtless an advantage for the student working over the pages for the first time but is inconvenient for general reference.

The English book is an outgrowth of the association of the two authors in the John Innes Horticultural Institution. It is only a dozen years ago at the Toronto meeting of the $A_3S$, that the leader of this institution denied that we had any knowledge of how species have arisen in nature, though he expressed the belief that any day the mystery of species might be solved. Bateson was the godfather of modern genetics and outstanding as a leader in genetic thought but, although at Toronto he confessed his conversion to belief in chromosomes, like so many of his day he never really came to think of genetic problems primarily in terms of chromosomal behavior. It is of interest, therefore, to see the John Innes Institution taking such a leading part in making chromosomes and their activities the basis of modern theories in genetics. In the book discussed, which in no small measure is an embodiment of recent investigations at this institution, the formation of new species in a number of plants has been shown to be a relatively simple chromosomal phenomenon.

The book is not a text for elementary students since it treats in large measure of unsettled problems and is not easy reading. It is a useful publication, however, and can be recommended strongly to advanced students and research workers since it brings together the most recent investigations in the modern field of cytogenetics.

ALBERT F. BLAKESLEE

CARNEGIE INSTITUTION
COLD SPRING HARBOR, N. Y.

# SPECIAL CORRESPONDENCE

## THE SIXTH MENDELEEV CONGRESS AT KHARKOV

ONE of the largest gatherings of chemists that have ever taken place was witnessed recently at Kharkov, capital of the Ukraine Soviet Republic, where some 3,000 chemists, from different parts of the U. S. S. R., and several foreign guests met at the sixth Mendeleev Congress. Since the death of the great chemist, the congress bearing his name has been held on an average of every three years. The last one met in Kazan in 1928, and the next in 1934 will coincide with the centenary of the work of the famous founder of the periodic table of elements. It will take place in Leningrad at the same time as the proposed international congress of pure and applied chemistry and will give an opportunity to many European chemists to become acquainted with their Russian colleagues.

The Kharkov Congress differs from similar gatherings in the division of its organizations into "columns" and "brigades," each studying some special problem in connection with the second Five Year Plan. Side by side with classical divisions into biochemistry, electrochemistry, colloid chemistry, there were special sections dealing with catalysis, raw materials (organic and mineral), chemical equipment, plant control, etc.

The first three days were devoted to general surveys in the more important subjects and to a review of the relations between chemistry and socialist reconstruction by Zatonski, formerly professor of physical chemistry and now an important figure in the Ukrainian government. Later the congress divided into columns and brigades. The outcome of their discussion was embodied in a number of resolutions, which were organized and coordinated by another smaller conference to be convened in Moscow on December 1 and will serve as a basis for development of the chemical program of the second Five Year Plan.

There were upward of five hundred reports presented at the congress, which makes it impossible to deal even superficially with their subject-matter. The titles of the papers read at the general meetings will indicate the range of the subjects covered: "The Application of Wave Mechanics to Chemical Problems, Including Recent Theories of the 'Spinning' Electrons," by George Roumer; "Electrostatic Theories of Valence," by G. K. Carkin; "The Structure of Complex Compounds," by T. A. Kazarnovski; "The Theories of Catalysis," by B. Roginski; "The Theories of Adsorption," by A. Frumkin; "Chemistry and Metallurgy," by E. I. Orlov; "Utilization of Raw Materials," by A. C. Fersman; "Chemistry and the Harvest Problem," by K. N. Sokolovski, and "Chemical Equipments," by S. L. Schipkin.

As examples of specific discoveries in the field of applied chemistry, one may mention the interesting researches of Madame Yermolyeva, of the Bach Institute of Biochemistry (Moscow), who found that traces of certain ferments obtained from decomposing bacteria will act as preservatives for caviar. These ferments have certain or all the properties of the bacteriophage, since they are able to destroy bacteria and to liberate more ferments in so doing.

A new process in aluminium technology, depending upon the special condition existing in the U. S. S. R., where petroleum refining and aluminium metallurgy can be developed side by side upon a large scale, has been worked out by E. A. Kazanovski (Moscow). It depends upon the production of aluminium chloride by the action of chlorine on impure bauxite or upon kaolin; the resulting chloride is used as a catalyst in the cracking of petroleum. From the residue on the cracking process one may recover hydrochloric acid and eventually regenerate chlorine, while the remaining bauxite is electrolized to give metallic aluminium.

An achievement to which Russian chemists point with pride is the manufacture of synthetic rubber from alcohol, the latter being obtainable from sawdust. An exhibition of chemical products, which was held at Kharkov at the time of the congress, included many objects from synthetic rubber (tires, goloshes, tubing, etc.) side by side with others made from the usual natural rubber and from rubber obtained from the roots of the Caucasian plant Tau-Saghiz (*Scrozonea Saghiz*). There were other exhibits showing various raw materials and also dyestuffs and pharmaceuticals, indicating a distinct advance in Russian fine-chemicals manufacture.

The congress was mainly remarkable because of the great interest shown in its proceedings not only by the participating chemists but also by the general public. This was due largely to the publicity given to technical matters in the Soviet press.

A number of foreign guests attended the conference. These included Dr. R. E. Liesegang, of Frankfurt, Professors Kurt Hess, Pitch and Klages, of Berlin, Dr. Giacomo Fauser, of Italy, Professor N. C. Greenwood, of Melbourne, Australia, Dr. V. Cofman and J. G. Crowther, London. The guests were presented with a beautiful set of photographs of eminent chemists, excursions were organized to the newly built dam on the Dnieper and the extensive electrochemical plants for the manufacture of aluminum, steel, etc., which are nearing completion, and most of the foreign chemists remained to witness the brilliant November celebration in Moscow.

VICTOR COFMAN

LONDON

# SCIENTIFIC APPARATUS AND LABORATORY METHODS

## IMPROVING THE STAINING ACTION OF IRON HAEMATOXYLIN

Iron haematoxylin, the most useful stain available to the cytologist, has during the past few years caused a great deal of trouble for a number of microscopists through its erratic behavior. Sometimes the desirable crisp black and white contrasting stain would be obtained, but more often it was not. The cytoplasm would retain the stain with the resulting muddy appearance seen all too often of late years. Stock solutions became turbid and lost their staining action in a few weeks.

Three years ago it occurred to the writer that if neutral solutions were essential to blood stains, neutrality might be a factor in the successful use of iron haematoxylin. Our distilled water was known to be slightly acid (about pH 6.6). A trace of sodium bicarbonate was added to a fresh 0.5 per cent. solution of haematoxylin. The straw-colored solution changed at once to the rich dark red wine color recognized as typical for an aged sample of this stain. Sections stained in this solution differentiated perfectly.

This 0.5 per cent. solution remains clear for about six months or occasionally longer and stains well as long as it is clear. These results have been obtained equally with haematoxylin crystals of pre-war Gruebler make or with the recent C. P. product of McAndrew and Forbes of America. After a solution of 0.5 per cent. haematoxylin becomes turbid the staining action is uncertain and the solution should be discarded. Even though six months should mark the functional life of the solution this does not seem serious in view of the successful behavior of the stain during this period.

Inasmuch as there appears to be a rather wide latitude in the quantity of bicarbonate that may or should be added to the solution of stain, it has not seemed worth while to determine the exact quantity added nor the pH obtained. In practise, to a liter of solution a very small quantity of sodium bicarbonate is lifted on the point of a scalpel and dropped into the solution. This rule of thumb procedure has never failed to work, although the quantities of alkali added must have varied considerably.

The making of a 0.5 per cent. solution is greatly facilitated by preparing (according to the directions given in Kingsbury and Johannsen's "Histological Technique") a 10 per cent. stock solution of haematoxylin dissolved in 95 per cent. alcohol. This solution keeps indefinitely and 5 cc of it in 100 cc of water gives a staining solution of the proper strength. To this solution the sodium bicarbonate is added.

This procedure has been in use for three years in this and neighboring laboratories and has given uniform results.

Robert T. Hance

University of Pittsburgh

## A DEVICE FOR MOUNTING ANATOMICAL PREPARATIONS

A simple and convenient method for mounting anatomical preparations is as follows: A plate is made by melting hard paraffin and pouring it into a form (as a box top, etc.) where it hardens to form a plate from one fourth to one half inches in thickness. During the process of melting, enough lampblack is added to give the mixture a deep black color, which is, of course, an advantage where a dark background is desired. To prevent curling of plates after immersion in preservative, two glass rods are embedded parallel to each other, one on each side of the plate, just before the process of hardening is begun. These rods may be of various diameters, but we have found that those from 5 to 8 mm in diameter are quite satisfactory. The length of the rods will depend upon the length of the plate as they are placed lengthwise within the plate (Fig. 1 a a). Before the rods

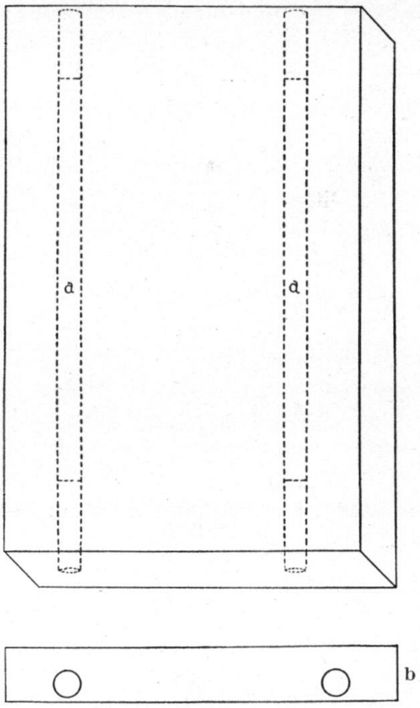


Fig. 1

are dropped in the melted paraffin a loop or two of heavy twine is wrapped around each end of each rod so that the rods will be suspended near the middle of the plate after it hardens (Fig. 1 b). Care must be taken to smear the inside of the box form with glycerine so that the hardened plate can be removed easily from the form.

The addition of some beeswax and resin to the paraffin-lampblack mixture will increase to a considerable extent the rigidity of the plate, although these constituents are not absolutely necessary.

Before the plate has hardened, and is still plastic, the anatomical specimen is pressed down slightly into the soft plate to hold it in position and is fastened there with thread looped around the parts of the specimen, passed through holes, and tied at the back of the plate. Necessary labels are now attached.

When completed, the preparation is immersed in a preservative in a museum jar. Such preparations will last for an indefinite time.

H. W. Schoenborn
C. P. Hickman
DePauw University

# SPECIAL ARTICLES

## THE PARTICLE SIZE OF THE VIRUS OF EQUINE ENCEPHALOMYELITIS

A most interesting epidemic of acute encephalomyelitis occurred among horses and mules in various local districts of California during the summer and fall of 1930, 1931 and 1932. Bacteriological and pathological studies of the disease were conducted by Meyer, Haring and Howitt and these workers have reported elsewhere[1,2,3] the salient characteristics of the virus and its effects on animals. In this work they recorded the filterability of the virus through Berkefeld V and N candles. However, filtration experiments utilizing the usual forms of candles, furnish no adequate basis for estimating the particle size of the virus because many factors other than mechanical sieve action have been shown to condition the filterability of a microorganism through such filters.

In order to obtain some idea of the virus particle size filtration experiments were performed with the acetic collodion gel ultrafilter series described by Krueger and Ritter[4] which possess the advantage of uniformity and low adsorbing surface area. The pore sizes of these membranes depends upon the percentage of nitro-cellulose dissolved in the glacial acetic acid and have been estimated by testing the permeability both to colloidal sols of known particle size and to water under certain standard conditions. The two methods of estimation give figures of the same order of magnitude with a relatively small constant difference between them. Manegold and Veit[5] have shown that this difference may be materially reduced by basing the pore size calculations from water permeability data upon the assumption of a random pore distribution as contrasted to parallel capillary bundles such as we had assumed to exist in the membranes. The result is a practical coincidence of the two pore size curves.

During the past year and one-half we have used different materials in making the membranes and have made minor alternations in the technique of preparation. The pore sizes of the series necessarily

Ultrafiltration of Suspensions of Encephalomyelitis Brains

| No. | Dilution of original supernatant from 20 per cent. brain suspension | Per cent. collodion (Ultrafilter) | Bacterial cultures from filtrate | Animal inoculation filtrate |
|---|---|---|---|---|
| 1 | Undiluted | 3.0 | 0 | Typical disease |
| 2 | Undiluted | 3.0 | 0 | Typical disease |
| 3 | 1: 2 with saline | 3.0 | B. subtilis | Typical disease |
| 4 | 1: 2 with saline | 3.0 | B. subtilis | Negative |
| 5 | Control undiluted | Unfiltered | 0 | Typical disease |
| 6 | Control 1:2 with saline | Unfiltered | 0 | Typical disease |
| 7 | 1:2 with broth | 3.0 | 0 | Typical disease |
| 8 | 1:2 with broth | 3.0 | 0 | Typical disease |
| 9 | Control undiluted | Unfiltered | 0 | Typical disease |
| 10 | Control 1:2 with broth | Unfiltered | 0 | Typical disease |
| 11 | Undiluted | 4.0 | 0 | Negative |
| 12 | Undiluted | 4.0 | 0 | Negative |
| 13 | Control, undiluted | Unfiltered | 0 | Typical disease |
| 14 | Control, undiluted | Unfiltered | 0 | Typical disease |
| 15 | Undiluted | 3.5 | 0 | Negative |
| 16 | Undiluted | 3.5 | 0 | Negative |
| 17 | Control, undiluted | Unfiltered | 0 | Typical disease |
| 18 | Control, undiluted | Unfiltered | 0 | Typical disease |
| 19 | 1:2 with broth | 3.5 | 0 | Negative |
| 20 | 1:2 with broth | 3.5 | 0 | Negative |
| 21 | Control, undiluted | Unfiltered | 0 | Typical disease |
| 22 | Control 1:2 with broth | Unfiltered | 0 | Typical disease |

[1] K. F. Meyer, C. M. Haring and B. Howitt, "The Etiology of Epizootic Encephalomyelitis of Horses in the San Joaquin Valley, 1930," Science, 74: 227–228, 1931.

[2] C. M. Haring, J. A. Howarth and K. F. Meyer, "An Infectious Brain Disease of Horses and Mules." (Encephalomyelitis)," University of California Agricultural Experiment Station Circular 322, August, 1931.

[3] B. Howitt, "Cross Immunization Experiments with Poliomyelitis Virus and that of Encephalomyelitis in Horses," *Proc.* Soc. Exp. Biol. and Med., 29: 118–120, 1931.

[4] A. P. Krueger and Ritter, "The Preparation of a Graded Series of Ultrafilters and Measurement of their Pore Size," *Jour. Gen. Physiol.*, 13: 409, 1930.

[5] E. Manegold and K. Veit, "Über Kapillarsysteme, XI," Kol. Zeitschr., Bd. 56, H. 1, 1931.

have had to be re-determined and do not correspond to the previously reported series. A description of the present membranes will be reported elsewhere.

In the present experiments the test material used was a 20 per cent brain suspension in normal saline freshly prepared from guinea-pigs which had been killed at the height of the disease. The suspension was centrifuged at low speed to remove coarse tissue particles and was then filtered under low negative pressures through sterile membranes of various pore sizes. The filtrates were tested for the presence of the virus by inoculating 0.3 cc. intracerebrally into guinea-pigs.

The table appended shows that the virus traverses a 3 per cent. membrane but is retained by a 3.5 per cent. membrane. The usual bacteriological tests for the detection of microorganisms were applied to the filtrates with negative results. Our data would indicate an approximate particle size of 500 $\mu\mu$ for the virus as it exists in brain suspensions. Under like conditions of preparation and filtration it is of the same order of magnitude as the causal agent of poliomyelitis[6] an analagous disease of man and is apparently ten times the size of the hoof and mouth disease virus particle.[7] Dilution does not appear to render the virus more finely dispersed, as by elution from carrier particles for example, nor to affect the filter pore surfaces so that the particles pass more readily.

A. P. KRUEGER
B. HOWITT
VIRGINIA ZEILOR

## A NEW PROCESS FOR THE SYNTHESIS OF PHENANTHRENE AND OF PHENANTHRENE DERIVATIVES

FOLLOWING up the researches on ionene lately communicated,[1] Davidson and Perlman have now succeeded, in these laboratories, in applying the knowledge gained in the ionene field to the development of a new process for the synthesis of phenanthrene and of its derivatives.

By the well-known Grignard reaction, 1-phenethylcyclohexanol-1 (I) was prepared from phenethyl magnesium bromide and cyclohexanone. When this tertiary alcohol (I) was treated with concentrated sulfuric acid, it split out a molecule of water and condensed to the same octahydrophenanthrene (III) as Bardhan and Sengupta[2] obtained from 1-phenethylcyclohexanol-2 (IV), and like it gave a good yield of phenanthrene (V) when dehydrogenated by heating with selenium.

Bardhan and Sengupta appear to assume a direct cyclodehydration between the OH of the alcohol and an H of the benzene nucleus. But, as we have shown in the ionene group (see the above reference), such condensations may proceed rather through the formation of the olefin first, which then rearranges by cyclization. That this is the case here also, Davidson and Perlman have now proven by heating the alcohol (I) for one minute with 50 per cent. sulfuric acid, when the olefin (II) was obtained. The same olefin was prepared by distilling the alcohol with a crystal of iodine. Treatment of this olefin with concentrated sulfuric acid rearranged it to the octahydrophenanthrene (III). These reactions indicate that the structure of the olefin is that shown in the formula (II), and that such an olefin could be formed by dehydration of either our alcohol (I) or that of Bardhan and Sengupta (IV). If this is really the mechanism of the condensation, as we believe it to be, it is clear why the same octahydrophenanthrene results whether the OH on the cyclohexane nucleus is in Position 1 (I) or 2 (IV).

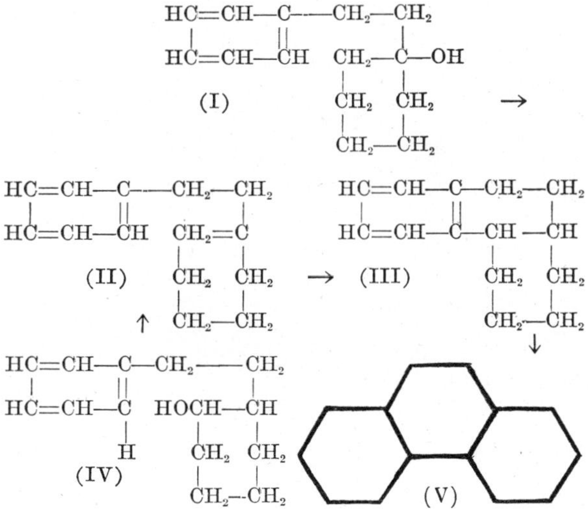


We believe that this synthesis has certain advantages over that of Bardhan and Sengupta, in that it starts with a simpler initial material, cyclohexanone instead of the potassium derivative of its ethyl carboxylate, and involves fewer steps. The investigation therefore is being extended in various directions, by using other carbonyl compounds in place of cyclohexanone and and other Grignard reagents instead of phenethyl magnesium halides.

MARSTON TAYLOR BOGERT
LABORATORIES OF ORGANIC CHEMISTRY
COLUMBIA UNIVERSITY

[6] A. P. Krueger and E. W. Schultz, "Ultrafiltration Studies on the Virus of Poliomyelitis," *Proc.* Soc. Exp. Biol. and Med., 26: 600, 1929.

[7] P. K. Olitsky and L. Boez, *Jour. Exp. Med.*, 45: 673, 1927.

[1] Bogert, SCIENCE, n. s., 76: 1977, 475, November 18, 1932.

[2] *Jour. Chem. Soc.*, 1932, 2520.

## THE FORMATION OF SEMI-TRANSPARENT MEMBRANES FROM CULTURES OF SLIME-PRODUCING MICRO-ORGANISMS

THIS article presents a brief description of a procedure developed at this laboratory for the successful production of semi-transparent sheets resembling parchment from cultures of slime-forming micro-organisms.

The investigations of Beijerinck[1] and Harrison[2] have made important contributions to fundamental knowledge of the viscous fermentations. These authors considered an appreciable number of causal species and described the formation of specific slimy materials. As a result of this work, attention has been directed to numerous groups of slime-forming bacteria, including the levulan-forming types, the producers of dextran, the cellulan-yielding group and those forming the nitrogenous slimes or mucins.

Concerning the class of nitrogenous slimes, stringiness in cultures of marine bacteria (Sanborn[3]) was developed to a degree of cohesiveness which permitted the drawing out of the slimy substance into fine, continuous filaments. Preliminary experiments showed that, with the aid of a coagulating bath, it was possible to convert these filaments into flexible threads. While such films proved to have little economic value, the results obtained were sufficiently arresting to justify the investigation of other slime-forming groups along similar lines.

In a recent article on the microorganisms involved in the formation of pulp and paper mill slimes, the author[4] has emphasized the filamentous and yeast-like fungi in addition to the bacterial groups. The slimes formed by this diversified flora were heterogeneous, and variously designated to indicate the major types. Of all the viscous materials produced in the carbohydrate media provided, the gelatinous, cellulose-like masses formed by certain species of Oidium and Monilia, possessed the most promising qualities. These organisms built up abundant, doughy surface growths which became tough and leathery after several weeks. Development was rapid in glycerol and potato decoction, resulting in the formation of thick, rubbery mats in the shallow layers of this medium. Dextrin or glucose may be substituted for glycerol.

The growths were collected and subjected to treatments, the purpose of which was to convert the slimes either into strands or into comminuted masses. The material could then be brought into uniform suspension and deposited upon the sheet-forming substratum. The formation of the sheet, due, in all probability, to the coalescence of the slime particles, was readily achieved. In one case the material was digested in zinc chloride and regenerated in the form of strands, in water. According to the other method the growth was comminuted directly by agitation, without digestion. This more direct procedure, now employed exclusively, yielded sheets of lighter color and greater transparency than could be produced by the former method.

Immediately following their formation, the sheets were treated with a lubrication emulsion to give them flexibility, resilience, and sizing qualities. The process was completed by drying in a steam hot plate sheet dryer. A more complete account of these slime sheets will occur in a later article.

J. R. SANBORN

INTERNATIONAL PAPER COMPANY
GLENS FALLS, N. Y.

[1] van M. W. Beijerinck, *Folia Microbiologica*, 1: 377. 1912.

[2] F. C. Harrison, *Trans. Roy. Soc. Can.*, 2 Ser. 4 Sec. 11: 71, 1905; F. C. Harrison, *et al.*, *Can. Jour. Res.*, 3: 449, 1930.

[3] J. R. Sanborn, *Jour. Bacteriol.*, 23: 350, 1932.

[4] J. R. Sanborn, *Jour. Bacteriol.* In press. 1933.

## BOOKS RECEIVED

ADAMS, ROGER and JOHN R. JOHNSON. *Elementary Laboratory Experiments in Organic Chemistry.* Revised. Pp. xiii + 363. 20 figures. Macmillan. $1.90.

CARNEGIE FOUNDATION FOR THE ADVANCEMENT OF TEACHING. *Twenty-seventh Annual Report.* Pp. vi + 174. The Foundation.

COOLIDGE, HAROLD J., JR. and THEODORE ROOSEVELT. *Three Kingdoms of Indo-China.* Pp. 231. Illustrated. Crowell. $3.00.

DORDILLON, RENE I. *Dictionnaire de la Langue des Iles Marquises.* Pp. 598. Institut D'Ethnologie. Paris. 87 fr.

GALLOWAY, J. J. *A Manual of Foraminifera.* James Furman Kemp Memorial Series, Publication No. 1. Pp. xii + 483. 41 plates. Principia Press.

HAWELKA, ROBERT. *Vierstellige Tafeln der Kreis-und Hyperbelfunktionen, sowie ihrer Umkehrfunktionen im Komplexen.* Pp. 109. 9 figures. Vieweg & Sohn, Braunschweig.

HEALD, FREDERICK D. *Manual of Plant Diseases.* Second edition. Pp. xii + 953. 259 figures. McGraw-Hill. $7.50.

HOSKINS, R. G. *The Tides of Life.* Pp. xi + 352. Illustrated. Norton. $3.50.

JONES, DONALD F., Editor. *Proceedings of the Sixth International Congress of Genetics, Ithaca, New York, 1932.* Vol. II. Pp. xvi + 405. Brooklyn Botanic Garden.

LEE, ROGER and LEWIS W. JONES. *The Fundamentals of Good Medical Care.* Pp. xv + 302. University of Chicago Press. $2.50.

LEVY, H. *The Universe of Science.* Pp. xiii + 224. Century. $2.00.

MONOD, THÉODORE. *L'Adrar Ahnet.* Contribution à l'étude archéologique d'un district saharien. Pp. 202. Institut D'Ethnologie, Paris. 37 fr.

RANEY, M. LLEWELLYN. *The University Libraries.* Vol. VII of The University of Chicago Survey. Pp. xv + 250. The University of Chicago Press. 12 vols., $30.00 a set.

SØRENSEN, WILLIAM. *Descriptiones Laniatorum.* Pp. 221. 29 figures. Levin and Munksgarrd, København. Kr. 12,50.

WALLIS, GRACE A. and WILSON D. WALLIS. *Our Social World.* Pp. xv + 378. 58 figures. McGraw-Hill. $1.60.

WIESNER, BERTHOLD and NORAH M. SHEARD. *Maternal Behavior in the Rat.* F. A. E. Crew and D. Ward Cutler, Editors. Pp. xi + 245. Illustrated. Oliver and Boyd, London. 12s, 6d.

# SCIENCE

VOL. 77 | FRIDAY, MARCH 24, 1933 | No. 1995

*Thermodynamics and Relativity:* PROFESSOR RICHARD C. TOLMAN ... 291

*Studies in Nuclear Physics:* DR. JNO. A. FLEMING ... 298

*Obituary:*
*Timothy E. Wilcox:* WILLARD W. EGGLESTON. *Recent Deaths* ... 300

*Scientific Events:*
*Report of the Council for Chemistry; The Yale North India Expedition; Anniversary of the Philadelphia College of Pharmacy and Science; Award of the Lamme Medal to Edward Weston; Elections to the Royal Society* ... 300

*Scientific Notes and News* ... 303

*Discussion:*
*The Law of Maximum Normal Nutritive Value:* DR. E. B. FORBES. *The Law of Effect:* PROFESSOR EDWIN G. BORING. *Is the Spelling Amoeba Sacrosanct?:* PROFESSOR M. F. GUYER. *More Ohio Medusae:* DR. WALTER C. KRAATZ. *Faraday's Diary:* PROFESSOR W. F. MAGIE ... 306

*Scientific Apparatus and Laboratory Methods:*
*Recent Developments in Gravity Apparatus:* DR. WILLIAM BOWIE ... 308

*Special Articles:*
*New Hardy Seedless Grapes:* DR. A. B. STOUT. *The Occurrence of Rotenone and Related Compounds in the Roots of Cracca virginiana:* DR. E. P. CLARK. *Effect of Temperature on Eversporting Eye Color in Drosophila melanogaster:* DR. JOHN W. GOWEN and E. H. GAY ... 310

*Science News* ... 6

SCIENCE: A Weekly Journal devoted to the Advancement of Science, edited by J. MCKEEN CATTELL and published every Friday by

THE SCIENCE PRESS

New York City: Grand Central Terminal
Lancaster, Pa. Garrison, N. Y.

Annual Subscription, $6.00 Single Copies, 15 Cts.

SCIENCE is the official organ of the American Association for the Advancement of Science. Information regarding membership in the Association may be secured from the office of the permanent secretary, in the Smithsonian Institution Building, Washington, D. C.

# THERMODYNAMICS AND RELATIVITY[1]

By Professor RICHARD C. TOLMAN

CALIFORNIA INSTITUTE OF TECHNOLOGY

## (1) INTRODUCTION

WE have met to do honor to the memory of Josiah Willard Gibbs. By the labors of this master, the classical principles of thermodynamics were given their most complete and comprehensive expression. As the subject for the tenth memorial lecture, it seems appropriate to discuss the extensions to these classical principles which have since been made necessary by Einstein's discovery of the special and general theories of relativity.

The need for an extension of thermodynamics to relativity arises in two ways.

In the first place the classical thermodynamics was —perhaps unintentionally but nevertheless actually— only developed for systems which were tacitly assumed to be at rest with respect to the observer, and further investigation is necessary for the treatment of thermodynamic systems which are moving relative to the spatial coordinates in use. This further investigation must be carried out with the help of those principles for the intercomparison of measurements—made by observers in uniform relative motion to each other— which form the subject-matter of the special theory of relativity.

In the second place, the older thermodynamics tacitly assumed that the behavior of thermodynamic systems could be described with the help of ideas as to the nature of space and time which we now know to be approximately valid only for a limited range of space-time and in the absence of strong gravitational fields. The considerations of the classical thermody-

[1] The tenth Josiah Willard Gibbs Lecture, delivered at Atlantic City, December 29, 1932, under the auspices of the American Mathematical Society, at a joint meeting of the society with the American Physical Society, and Section A of the American Association for the Advancement of Science.

namics were thus actually limited to the treatment of small enough systems and weak enough gravitational fields so that the deviations from this kind of space time could be neglected, and the Newtonian theory of gravitation could be applied as a close enough approximation. In order, however, to investigate the thermodynamic behavior of large portions of the universe as we may wish to do in connection with cosmological problems, and in order to obtain, even in the case of small systems, more precise expressions for the thermodynamic effects of gravity, it becomes necessary to extend thermodynamics to general relativity, and make use of the more valid ideas as to the nature of space and time and the more precise theory of gravitation which Einstein has now provided.

### (2) THE CHARACTER AND VALIDITY OF THERMODYNAMICS AND RELATIVITY

In carrying out these proposed extensions of thermodynamics to relativity, it proves possible to combine the known principles of thermodynamics with those of special and general relativity in a very natural manner with only small and apparently rational additions in the way of new hypothesis. Hence the character and validity of the system of relativistic thermodynamics that we obtain is largely dependent on the character and validity of the two component sciences.

In character, the classical thermodynamics may be regarded as a macroscopic, phenomenological science, which has no actual need for that interesting kind of support that can be furnished by the microscopic atomic considerations of statistical mechanics, but which attempts to treat the gross behavior of matter with the help of those generalized descriptions of the results of numerous gross experiments on the mechanical equivalent of heat and on the efficiency of heat engines, which we call the first and second laws of thermodynamics.

As to the validity of thermodynamics, we have feelings of great confidence, on account of the extensive experimental verification which exists, not only directly for the two laws themselves, but for an extraordinary number of consequences which have been drawn from them—often by elaborate but logical trains of deductive reasoning. Further additions to the principles of thermodynamics may be found, such as the newer so-called third law of Nernst and Planck, but we can not escape the conviction that, so long as the human mind retains its present ideas of rationality, these additions are likely to prove—as in the case mentioned—supplementary rather than destructive.

Relativity, a science which changes as it does our very ideas as to the nature of space and time, has much more fundamental and far-reaching implications than thermodynamics and can not be so easily characterized. There are, however, certain similarities between the two sciences which may be emphasized.

In the first place, at least in its present stage of development, relativity must also be regarded as a macroscopic theory dealing with ideas as to the nature of space and time which have been directly derived from macroscopic experiences. Indeed, in view of Heisenberg's uncertainty principle and the great difficulties which have been encountered in all attempts to construct a satisfactory relativistic quantum mechanics, we may even doubt whether these ideas as to space and time are even suitable for microscopic considerations. This, however, offers no difficulties if we are to combine with another macroscopic science such as thermodynamics.

In the second place, although we are often inclined to be specially impressed by the wonderful conceptual content of the theory of relativity, we may here emphasize its not negligible character as a phenomenological or descriptive science.

Thus the first of the two postulates of the special theory of relativity may be regarded as a generalized description of many failures to detect the absolute velocity of the earth's motion. And the second postulate may be regarded as a mere empirical statement of that constancy in the velocity of light, which is specially clearly demonstrated in the case of distant double stars by the lack of any effect from the changing motions of the members of the doublet on the time needed for their light to reach the earth.

Turning, moreover, to the two postulates necessary for the general theory of relativity, the principle of equivalence may be regarded not unfairly as a reasonably generalized description of Galileo's discovery that all bodies fall at the same rate. The principle of covariance, however, is on a somewhat different footing, since, as first pointed out by Kretschmann—given sufficient mathematical ingenuity—any physical law whatever could undoubtedly be expressed in covariant language the same for all coordinate systems, so that the principle of covariance can imply no necessary physical consequences. Nevertheless, as emphasized by Einstein, the actual phenomena of physics must themselves be independent of the choice of coordinate system which is a conceptual introduction on the part of the scientist which may be made in any way that may suit his convenience or please his fancy. Hence the actual employment of invariant forms of expression in searching for the appropriate axioms of physics is desirable in order to avoid the introduction of unsuspected assumptions which might otherwise be insinuated by the use of special coordinates. We can then also, somewhat facetiously, emphasize the phenomenological character of the principle of covariance, by regarding it as a generalized description of the familiar phenomenon, that the purely conceptual activities of man—in inventing imaginary coordinate systems—are likely in first approximation to have no immediate effect on the laws of physics.

As to the validity of the theory of relativity, we have to rely on three different kinds of evidence.

In the first place, we may put its agreement with a great range of diverse facts from different branches of science, which as isolated phenomena can often be attractively explained in terms of pre-relativistic notions, but which as a whole have only been successfully correlated with the help of the theory of relativity.

In the second place, we must put those special observations which distinguish as uniquely as may be between the predictions of relativity and those which would result from other points of view. Here we have in the case of the first postulate of special relativity the demonstration of the Lorentz contraction by the Michelson-Morley experiment and all its now numerous repetitions, if we may include the extensive work of Professor Miller as demonstrating this contraction at least as the primary effect. And we also have the remarkable demonstration of Einstein's time dilation by the beautiful experiments of Kennedy and Thorndike. In the case of the second postulate of the special theory, we have as most important the precise analysis of double star orbits by de Sitter. And turning to the general theory of relativity, we have the entirely satisfactory results of the three crucial tests provided by the rotation of the perihelion of Mercury, the bending of light in passing the sun, and the shift in the wave-length of light originating on the surface of the sun and on that of the companion to Sirius.

Finally, as a third kind of evidence, for judging the validity of relativity we must not neglect the bearings of that wonderful internal coherence of the theory, with its simple foundation and elaborate but logical superstructure, which so well attests the genius of Einstein. Although such qualities can of themselves provide no guarantee as to correspondence with external phenomena, we can, nevertheless, regard them as indicating that such correspondence—when found for our present limited range of observation—is likely to persist over a much wider range of possible experience.

Like all parts of science, the theory of relativity will presumably be subject to future modifications and additions, such for example as might be provided by a successful unified field theory. Nevertheless, just as the Einstein theory has retained the Newtonian theory of gravitation as an exceedingly satisfactory first approximation, we may expect at least for a long time that such changes will here—as well as in the case of thermodynamics—be supplementary rather than destructive.

The character of the two sciences of thermodynamics and relativity, which we are going to combine, is thus sufficiently similar that we may have no hesitations, on that score, and may expect the resulting relativistic thermodynamics to be itself a macroscopic theory suitable for use in the description of the gross phenomena of the external world. And the validity of the two component sciences is sufficiently established so that for the present we may concentrate attention, as we shall in what follows, on the rationality of that small amount of additional hypothesis which we must introduce to effect the combination.

### (3) THE EXTENSION OF THERMODYNAMICS TO SPECIAL RELATIVITY

We are now ready to consider the actual procedure adopted in the extension of thermodynamics, first to special relativity and then to general relativity. The extension to special relativity, so as to obtain a suitable thermodynamic theory for moving systems, was made by Planck[2] and by Einstein,[3] as early as the year 1907, in that brilliant period of development which was initiated by Einstein's publication of the elements of special relativity only two years previous.

(*a*) *Special Relativity and the First Law of Thermodynamics.* In order to appreciate the nature of this extension, let us begin by seeing what happens to the first law of thermodynamics when the extension is made.

In the classical thermodynamics for systems at rest with respect to the observer, we have found it important to distinguish two ways in which there can be an interchange of energy between a system and its surroundings, namely, through the flow of heat into the system from its surroundings and through the performance of work by the system on its surroundings. Making use of this distinction, and making use of the principle of the conservation of energy, which requires that any alteration in energy content can only result from interchange with the surroundings, we then write the first law of thermodynamics in the form given by the equation (1)

$$\Delta E = Q - W \qquad (1)$$

where $\Delta E$ is the increase in the energy of the system which accompanies the influx in heat Q and the performance of work W against external forces.

In *form* this equation can be taken over without modification into the thermodynamics of moving sys-

[2] Planck, Berl. Ber. (1907) p. 542; *Ann. der Phys.*, 26: 1, 1908.

[3] Einstein, *Jahrb. f. Rad. u. El.*, 4: 411, 1907.

tems, in the first place since the special theory of relativity has done nothing to upset the principle of the conservation of energy, and in the second place since we shall still wish to distinguish between the energy transfer W corresponding to work done against macroscopic external forces and the other modes of transfer which we call the flow of heat Q.

In the application of this equation to moving instead of stationary systems, however, an important difference—which would not have been suspected in prerelativistic days—now arises on account of the relations between mass, energy and momentum made clear by Einstein's work. To illustrate this difference, let us consider—as we usually do in thermodynamics—only very simple systems consisting of a given amount of thermodynamic fluid or working substance which exerts a pressure on its surroundings.

If such a system is *at rest,* the only way it can do work on its surroundings is by a change in volume under this pressure, and the application of the first law equation (1) then gives us simply

$$dE_o = dQ_o - p_o dv_o \qquad (2)$$

where the subscript $(_0)$ has been added to indicate that the quantities involved are all referred to coordinates in which the system is at rest.

If such a system is *in motion,* however, its momentum will in general change with its energy content even though we hold the velocity constant, owing to the special relativity relation which associates mass with energy. Hence in applying the first law equation to moving systems, even in the simple case of constant velocity, we shall have to include, in addition to the work done against external pressure, the work done against the external force involved in the change in momentum. We must then write in general

$$dE = dQ - p\, dv + \vec{u} \cdot d\vec{G} \qquad (3)$$

where the last term is the scalar product of the velocity of the system $\bar{u}$ and its change in momentum $d\bar{G}$. Moreover, in making use of this equation we must employ the special relativity relation connecting the momentum of the system with its energy flow

$$\bar{G} = \frac{E + p\,v}{c^2}\bar{u} \qquad (4)$$

where c is the velocity of light, and the term $\frac{E\bar{u}}{c^2}$ gives the momentum due to the transport of the energy of the system as a whole, and the term $pv\bar{u}/c^2$ corresponds to the additional flow of energy resulting from the work done on the moving volume by the action of the external pressure.

With the help of these two expressions for the first law (3), and for the momentum of a moving system (4), we can then obtain transformation equations which will give us expressions for all the quantities, involved in the application of the first law to moving systems, in terms of the analogous quantities as they would be measured by a local observer moving with the system. In accordance with the known equations for force, and the Lorentz contraction for moving volumes, we are already provided by the special theory of relativity with the simple transformations for pressure and volume

$$p = p_o$$
$$v = v_o\sqrt{1 - u^2/c^2} \qquad (5)$$

Furthermore, considering first an adiabatic acceleration in which the velocity of our system is changed without flow of heat or change in internal condition as measured by a local observer, and then considering more general processes in which flow of heat is permitted, we readily obtain as the transformation equations for energy and heat the two expressions

$$E = \frac{E_o + p_o v_o}{\sqrt{1 - u^2/c^2}}$$
$$dQ = dQ_o\sqrt{1 - u^2/c^2} \qquad (6)$$

This gives all the apparatus necessary for the application of the first law of thermodynamics to moving systems. It is to be specially noted that so far no new assumptions, beyond those already present in the mechanics of special relativity, have been introduced into our systems of thermodynamics, except, if you wish, our procedure in still giving the name heat to that part of the energy transfer which does not take place through the work done against macroscopic external forces.

(*b*) *Special Relativity and the Second Law of Thermodynamics.* Let us now turn to the more characteristically thermodynamic considerations involved in the application of the second law of thermodynamics, and examine the fate of this principle when the extension to special relativity is made.

In the classical thermodynamics the full content of the second law could be conveniently condensed into the very simple expression

$$\Delta S \geqq \int \frac{dQ}{T} \qquad (7)$$

where the left-hand side gives the increase in the entropy content S when a system changes from one state to another, and the right-hand side is to be obtained by dividing each element of heat dQ absorbed by its temperature T, and summing up for the whole process by which the system changes from its initial to its final state.

The sign of equality (=) in this expression applies to reversible processes which take place with that highest possible efficiency, which would just be sufficient to permit a return *both* of the system and its surroundings to their original state. And the sign of inequality (>) applies to those less efficient, actual processes which we ordinarily encounter in nature. With the help of the relation of equality we can then calculate the entropy of any system by considering an ideal reversible process by which it could be brought from its standard state to the state under consideration. And with the help of the two relations of equality and inequality, we codify all that extraordinary range of information as to the equilibrium and efficiency of physical-chemical processes which is subservient to the second law.

In making the extension to special relativity, it was found possible to take over this expression for the second law of thermodynamics as a postulate without any change at all in form. And this was evidently a rational thing to try to do, since it preserves the constancy of entropy for purely mechanical processes, makes the increase of entropy for reversible thermal processes dependent on the transfer of energy in forms other than work, and retains with the help of the sign of inequality those opportunities for irreversibility and spontaneous increase in entropy which lie at the heart of thermodynamic considerations.

In applying this expression to moving systems we must of course substitute values for entropy, heat and temperature which are appropriate for a moving system, and hence shall desire transformation equations which will permit us to calculate these quantities in terms of the analogous quantities which would be directly measured by a local observer traveling with the system in question.

In the case of heat, we are already provided by the application of the first law with the transformation equation

$$dQ = dQ_0 \sqrt{1 - u^2/c^2} \tag{8}$$

In the case of entropy, we are then directly led by the postulate itself to the conclusion that the entropy of a system must be an invariant for the Lorentz transformation

$$S = S_0 \tag{9}$$

owing to the possibility of changing the velocity of a system by a quasi-static reversible adiabatic acceleration, which leaves the internal state and proper entropy $S_0$ unaltered on account of the quasi-static character of the acceleration, and leaves the entropy S unaltered on account of the reversible and adiabatic character of the acceleration. This invariance of entropy is, moreover, in evident agreement with the statistical mechanical interpretation which relates the entropy of a system to the probability of its state, a quantity which could hardly be a function of the velocity with which the observer happens to be moving past the system.

Finally in the case of temperature, by combining the requirements of the postulate itself with the two transformation equations already obtained, it is evident that we are now necessarily led to the relation

$$T = T_0 \sqrt{1 - u^2/c^2} \tag{10}$$

in order that the postulated law (7) may apply to the description of a given change in state both from the point of view of a local observer moving with the system and from the point of view of other observers with respect to which the system is in motion.

(*c*) *Discussion of the Extension to Special Relativity.* This completes all that is necessary for the extension of thermodynamics to special relativity.

It will be seen that the additions in the way of new hypotheses, beyond what is already contained in the special theory of relativity and in the classical thermodynamics, have really been very small and apparently rational. Indeed, it seems fair to say that these additions consist solely in the assumption that the second law of thermodynamics, as expressed in the usual well-known form given by (7) will not break down when we turn to the consideration of moving systems, and that the quantity dQ occurring in this expression must still be interpreted as that part of the energy transfer which can not be considered as work done against macroscopic external forces.

It should also be noted that the results which are given by this extended theory are entirely coherent with the accepted body of theoretical physics. For example, the application of this theory to determine the dynamical properties of a moving enclosure filled with black-body radiation leads to the same results as were originally obtained by Mosengeil[4] from strictly electromagnetic considerations. And the transformation equation given for heat (6), which we have regarded as derived from an application of the mechanics of special relativity to the behavior of a portion of fluid, agrees with that which can be derived from electromagnetic considerations for the Joule heating effect in a moving electrical conductor. Most important of all, however, it should be noted that the extension has been so devised that any predictions, which we make with its help as to the behavior of a given system moving with a *constant* velocity u, will completely agree with those which would be made with the help of the classical thermodynamics by a local observer who moves along with the system in question.

It is important to emphasize these qualities of rationality and coherence, since our judgment as to the validity of this extension of thermodynamics must be largely based thereon. Any direct test of the extension would for the present be out of the question,

[4] Mosengeil, *Ann. d. Phys.*, 22: 867, 1907. The results of Mosengeil were employed by Planck in his method of obtaining the extension of thermodynamics to special relativity.

since all the various thermodynamic quantities for moving systems were found to differ from the analogous ones for stationary systems only by terms of the order of $u^2/c^2$ or higher, and we could only expect differences of this practically undetectable order for any thermodynamic theory of moving systems that might be proposed.

The usefulness of the extension consists partly in the ease with which we can now treat problems by simple thermodynamic methods which would otherwise involve complicated kinetic theory or electromagnetic considerations, as in the case of the moving enclosure filled with radiation. The usefulness of the extension depends mainly, however, on the increased insight which we now have into the nature of thermodynamics and thermodynamic quantities. Thus the invariance to the Lorentz transformation for entropy and for the ratio of heat to temperature provided by the special theory of relativity prove essential for the further extension of thermodynamics to general relativity to which we must now turn.

## (4) THE EXTENSION OF THERMODYNAMICS TO GENERAL RELATIVITY

In the general theory of relativity, the space-time continuum in which physical events take place is regarded as characterized by the formula for interval

$$ds^2 = g_{11}\,dx_1^2 + 2\,g_{12}\,dx_1\,dx_2 + \ldots + g_{44}\,dx_4^2 = g_{\mu\nu}\,dx^\mu\,dx^\nu \qquad (g_{\mu\nu} = g_{\nu\mu}) \tag{11}$$

where $x_1$, $x_2$ and $x_3$ are the three spatial coordinates that are being used, $x_4$ is the temporal coordinate, and the $g_{\mu\nu}$ are the ten gravitational potentials. The dependence of these gravitational potentials on the distribution of matter and energy is given by Einstein's ten field equations

$$-8\pi T^{\mu\nu} = R^{\mu\nu} - \tfrac{1}{2} R g^{\mu\nu} + \Lambda g^{\mu\nu} \tag{12}$$

where $T^{\mu\nu}$ is the energy-momentum tensor, $R^{\mu\nu}$ and R are obtained from the Riemann-Christoffel tensor by contraction, and $\Lambda$, the so-called cosmological constant, is a quantity which is observationally known in any case to be exceedingly small when expressed in reciprocal square centimeters, and may well be zero. Finally, the motion of free particles and light rays in this space-time continuum is determined by the equation

$$\delta \int ds = 0 \tag{13}$$

with ds greater than zero for material particles and equal to zero for light rays.

The results predicted by these fundamental equations of general relativity are in satisfactory agreement with all the facts that are now at our disposal, and in particular agree with the astronomical observations which have furnished the three crucial tests of relativity.

In order to include thermodynamics within this framework, we must now inquire into the analogues in general relativity of the ordinary first and second laws of thermodynamics.

(*a*) *The Analogue of the First Law in General Relativity.* In the case of the first law the procedure to be adopted is clear. In the classical thermodynamics the first law was an expression of the principle of the conservation of energy as applied to small stationary systems in the absence of a gravitational field, and in relativistic thermodynamics we must evidently use as the analogue of the first law the more general energy-momentum principle provided by relativistic mechanics.[5]

This principle can be expressed by the very simple *tensor* equation

$$(T^{\mu\nu})_\nu = 0 \tag{14}$$

and may be regarded as an immediate result of Einstein's field equations (12), since the tensor divergence of the expression there given for the energy-momentum tensor $T^{\mu\nu}$ can be shown to be necessarily identically equal to zero. For purposes of computation it is often more convenient to rewrite this equation in the *tensor density* form

$$\frac{\partial \mathfrak{T}^\nu_\mu}{\partial x^\nu} - \tfrac{1}{2}\,\mathfrak{T}^{\alpha\beta}\frac{\partial g_{\alpha\beta}}{\partial x^\mu} = 0 \tag{15}$$

and to obtain an insight into the nature of the principle, it is sometimes useful to rewrite it in the form of an ordinary divergence as expressed by the non-tensor yet nevertheless *covariant* equation

$$\frac{\partial}{\partial x^\nu}(\mathfrak{T}^\nu_\mu + \mathfrak{t}^\nu_\mu) = 0 \tag{16}$$

where the pseudo-tensor density of potential energy and momentum $\mathfrak{t}^\nu_\mu$ is defined for *all systems* of coordinates in such a way that we can substitute $\partial\mathfrak{t}^\nu_\mu/\partial x^\nu$ for the second term of (15).

To remind us of the physical significance of these familiar equations of relativistic mechanics, it will be recalled that the equations reduce in the absence of a gravitational field to the ordinary principles of special relativity for the conservation of the energy and momentum directly associated with matter and radiation. In general, however, in the presence of gravitational fields, it will be evident from the third form (16) in which the equations have been written that they will lead to conservation laws only when we include—along with the energy and momentum directly associated with matter and radiation—the potential energy and momentum of the gravitational field, which corresponds to the presence of the pseudo-tensor density $\mathfrak{t}^\nu_\mu$ in the equation in this form (16).

This general result proves to be of great importance

[5] Tolman, *Proc. Nat. Acad.*, 14: 268, 1926; *Phys. Rev.*, 35: 875, 1930.

for relativistic thermodynamics by permitting—even in the case of isolated systems—an increase in the energy directly associated with matter and radiation at the expense of the potential energy that we assign to the gravitational field. For example, if we consider a system composed of a perfect fluid having the proper macroscopic density of energy $\rho_{00}$ and proper pressure $p_0$ as measured by a local observer at the point of interest, and having no flow of heat, it is known that we can write

$$T^{\mu\nu} = (\rho_{00} + p_0)\frac{dx^\mu}{ds}\frac{dx^\nu}{ds} - g^{\mu\nu} p_0 \tag{17}$$

as an expression for the energy-momentum tensor. And if we substitute this expression into the above equations of relativistic mechanics, we can obtain for any infinitesimal element of the fluid of proper volume $\delta V_0$, the relation

$$\frac{d}{dt_0}(\rho_{00}\,\delta V_0) + p_0\frac{d}{dt_0}(\delta V_0) = 0 \tag{18}$$

From one point of view there is nothing surprising about this result since it merely states that a local observer who examines the behavior of an element of the fluid small enough so that the gravitational "curvature" of space-time can be neglected will find the rate of change in energy content related in the expected way to the work done against the external pressure. From another point of view, however, as this same equation can be applied to each one of all the elements into which the total fluid of the system can be divided, the result may seem somewhat surprising, since it leads to the possibility of systems in which the proper energy of every element of the fluid may be simultaneously decreasing or increasing, according as the system is expanding or contracting. Moreover, since it is this proper energy immediately associated with matter and radiation which determines the possibilities for entropy increase, we shall later find in relativistic thermodynamics an escape from certain restrictions imposed in the classical thermodynamics by the usual form of the principle of the conservation of energy.

Just as in the previous case of special relativity, we note that the extension of thermodynamics to general relativity involves, so far as the first law is concerned, no new hypothetical material beyond that already contained in relativistic mechanics. And we may now turn to the relativistic analogue of the second law of thermodynamics.

(*b*) *The Analogue of the Second Law in General Relativity.* To guide us in obtaining a suitable postulate to serve as the relativistic second law of thermodynamics, we must make use of the two fundamental ideas of general relativity which are expressed by the principles of covariance and equivalence. In accordance with the principle of covariance, our postulate must be expressed in covariant form the same for all coordinate systems, to avoid the danger of being influenced in its selection by a spurious simplicity when referred to some particular system of coordinates. And in accordance with the principle of equivalence, our postulate must reduce to the thermodynamic requirements of special relativity, when applied to an infinitesimal element of fluid using natural coordinates for the point of interest.

These two principles have been sufficient to lead with considerable confidence to the expression[6]

$$\frac{\partial}{\partial x^\mu}\left(\phi_0\frac{dx^\mu}{ds}\sqrt{-g}\right)\delta x_1\,\delta x_2\,\delta x_3\,\delta x_4 \geqq \frac{\delta Q_0}{T_0} \tag{19}$$

as the appropriate postulate to take as the relativistic analogue of the ordinary second law of thermodynamics. The quantity $\phi_0$ in this expression is the proper entropy density of the thermodynamic fluid under consideration as measured at the point of interest by a local observer; the quantities $dx^\mu/ds$ are the components of the macroscopic "velocity" of the fluid at that point; and the other quantities on the left-hand side of the expression have their usual significance. The significance of the right-hand side of the expression is more difficult to grasp, and will be specially treated in a forthcoming article by Professor Robertson and myself.[7] The quantity $\delta Q_0$ may be taken as the heat—measured by a local observer at rest in the fluid at the point of interest—which flows into an element of the fluid having the instantaneous proper volume $\delta V_0$ during the proper time $\delta t_0$ where these quantities are so chosen as to make

$$\delta V_0\,\delta t_0 = \sqrt{-g}\,\delta x_1\,\delta x_2\,\delta x_3\,\delta x_4 \tag{20}$$

and the quantity $T_0$ is taken as the temperature ascribed to this heat by the local observer.

The two signs of equality (=) and inequality ($>$) in the expression refer respectively to the two cases of reversible and irreversible processes, and in applying the principle to irreversible processes we are to regard an increment in coordinate time $\delta x_4$ as positive when taken in the direction to correspond to a positive increment in proper time $\delta t_0$ as measured in the ordinary manner by a local observer.

To show the agreement of this postulated expression for the relativistic second law with the principle of covariance, we have merely to note that it is a tensor equation of rank zero—both sides being scalar invariants—and hence is true in all coordinate systems if true in one. To show its agreement with the principle of equivalence we must see what it reduces to in natural coordinates for the point of interest. Intro-

[6] Tolman, *Proc. Nat. Acad.*, 14: 268, 701, 1928; *Phys. Rev.*, 35: 896, 1930.

[7] Tolman and Robertson, submitted to the *Physical Review* for publication.

ducing such coordinates x, y, z, t, *and making use of the transformation equations for entropy, heat and temperature provided by the special theory of relativity,* we find, however, that our principle then reduces to

$$\left[\operatorname{div}(\phi\bar{u}) + \frac{\partial\phi}{\partial t}\right]\delta x\,\delta y\,\delta z\,\delta t \geqq \frac{\delta Q}{T} \qquad (21)$$

where $\phi$, $\bar{u}$, $\delta Q$ and T are now the quantities referred to our present coordinate system which we ordinarily designate as entropy density, velocity, heat absorbed and temperature. And we see that this result does relate the change in the entropy of the element of fluid, instantaneously contained in the coordinate range $\delta x\,\delta y\,\delta z$, to the absorbed heat and temperature in the way

$$\frac{d}{dt}(\phi\,\delta x\,\delta y\,\delta z)\,\delta t \geqq \frac{\delta Q}{T} \qquad (22)$$

which is required by the second law of thermodynamics in special relativity.

At the present stage of observational knowledge, our belief in the validity of the proposed postulate is primarily based on this agreement with the two principles of covariance and equivalence. In addition, however, it may be emphasized that the principle has been chosen so as to be simply the immediate covariant re-expression of the special relativity form of the second law (21); and past experience has shown, notably, for example, in the cases of the fundamental formulae for space-time interval and geodesic trajectory, that these simplest possible covariant generalizations when feasible are likely to be correct. Furthermore, it may be remarked that the conclusions which have so far been drawn from this extension of thermodynamics to general relativity appear—at least after due reflection—to be reasonable and illuminating.

It must be emphasized, nevertheless, that these qualities are not sufficient to prove the validity of the postulate, since other covariant expressions might be found which would also reduce to the special relativity law in natural coordinates. Hence the postulate must be regarded as a real generalization with a range of validity to be finally determined only by the correspondence between observation and prediction.

*(To be concluded)*

# STUDIES IN NUCLEAR PHYSICS

By Dr. JNO. A. FLEMING

ACTING DIRECTOR, DEPARTMENT OF TERRESTRIAL MAGNETISM, CARNEGIE INSTITUTION OF WASHINGTON

## STUDIES IN NUCLEAR PHYSICS

THE Carnegie Institution of Washington announced on February 2 in a lecture by Dr. M. A. Tuve before the Franklin Institute on "The Atomic Nucleus and High Voltages," the results of the past year's work at the high-voltage laboratory of its Department of Terrestrial Magnetism in Washington. This program of investigations constitutes the present expression of a long-continued policy of the department of undertaking laboratory studies of the basic physical phenomena which underlie all large-scale manifestations of magnetism and electricity, as complementary to its field and observatory operations and theoretical investigations. These laboratory studies are now directed toward studies of the simplest cases of the interaction at close distances of the known primary material particles—the electron and proton, which have both electric charge and magnetic moment—and their simplest combinations.

During the past year Dr. Tuve and his colleagues, L. R. Hafstad and O. Dahl, have obtained results covering a variety of experiments in nuclear physics, including a verification of the existence of the recently discovered neutron, observations on the resonance-disintegration of aluminum by polonium alpha-particles, and studies of the disintegration of lithium and boron, using high-speed protons from a high-voltage tube. The Van de Graaff type of electrostatic generator, a simple metal sphere charged to a high voltage by a silk belt, was tested, developed and used for the atomic disintegration-studies. A special building is now under construction at the department to house a large (2-meter) generator of this type which was built at the department and tested during May, 1932. This equipment promises to give an intense source of artificial neutrons, this being one of the most interesting of its numerous potentialities. It will provide 10 microamperes or more of protons or helium-ions having energies above 1,500,000 electron-volts.

The existence of the non-classical phenomena at present explained on the neutron-hypothesis was verified in the department's laboratory last September by a repetition of the main features of Chadwick's experiments. Using a 3-mc polonium source bombarding beryllium, recoil-nuclei of nitrogen were found to produce a maximum of nearly 50,000 ions in the 15-mm ionization-chamber of a valve-counter of the type used by Chadwick. Recoil-nuclei were observed with this instrument and with the FP-54 pliotron connected to a small chamber and used in the same way as Pose has used the duant electrometer. The range of the recoil-protons was found to be about 44 cm in agreement with Chadwick's result. Several thousand stereoscopic photographs were made with the neutron-source mounted in a Wilson cloud-chamber, as in Feather's experiments, and the recoil-nuclei were identified and measured. Disintegration-phenomena in the chamber were not definitely assigned to neutrons because of the weakness of the source, but will be studied shortly using a much larger quantity of polonium. The absorption of the beryllium neutrons by one inch of lead, measured by counts of recoil-protons, was found to be about 55 per cent., in disagreement with Chadwick's 13 per cent. (measured by nitrogen-recoils), but agreeing with the value published in October by Thibaud and La Tour.

As a necessary safeguard to the validity of results with the high-voltage technique, as well as by reason of their intrinsic value, it was decided two years ago to carry out certain experiments using radioactive sources. One feature of this program was the development and test of instruments and methods for nuclear observations. The limits of sensitivity of the FP-54 pliotron have been investigated, and it has been utilized for measurements on high-speed protons produced by disintegrations and by neutron-recoil. A single-tube circuit using an FP-54 in an evacuated case achieves a charge-sensitivity limited only by the statistical fluctuation ($\pm 640$ e) of the grid-current ($10^{-15}$ ampere) of the tube, and the latter imposes a usable limit with this device not inherent in a true electrometer, although the much higher voltage-sensitivity is an advantage in many applications. Because of this fluctuation the minimum steady current theoretically observable is approximately $3 \times 10^{-19}$ ampere (2 electrons per second), and by actual test a current of $5 \times 10^{-18}$ ampere (30 electrons per second) is directly measurable in a time of several minutes. On the basis of experience with a cloud-chamber similar to that described by Blackett, an improved form was constructed, which has several important advantages over the usual form utilizing a piston and a liquid seal. A large-diameter flexible metal "sylphon" bellows is used, giving a chamber entirely free from leakage, with resulting constancy of expansion ratio and gas composition, which can be oriented vertically or in any other direction at will. A modified form of mercury spark-lamp provides sufficient illumination to enable the use of cinema positive film, with a very considerable gain in resolving power and contrast over the usual negative emulsion. A valve-counter of the type described by Wynn-Williams and Ward was developed, which is simple in construction and singularly insensitive to external disturbances, operating satisfactorily in the presence of the noise and electrical disturbances produced by the Van de Graaff generator. The useful amplification of such a device being limited solely by the noise-level of the early stages, this factor was investigated. The resulting amplifier has a noise-level comparable to the theoretical noise-level due to the Johnson effect (thermal agitation of electrons in a resistance) of the plate-impedance of the input-valve.

One problem of importance in radioactive research which was selected for attack is that of resonance-disintegration of the nucleus. Using the FP-54 in the same way as Pose has used the duant electrometer, Mr. Hafstad has studied the resonance-disintegration of aluminium. This work is only partially completed, but has progressed to a point where there can be no doubt of the existence of the phenomenon. Steudel's failure to observe it is not surprising in view of the geometry of his apparatus, and in contradiction to his results Mr. Hafstad finds that the "disintegration-yield" in his experiments, on the basis of an absolute calculation, checks Pose's high value. Details of the sharpness of resonance and other features are still under investigation.

Having experimented in this laboratory since 1926 with high voltages from spark-excited Tesla coils applied to vacuum-tubes, chiefly by reason of the lack of funds for a more suitable voltage-source, we were glad to adopt the inexpensive electrostatic type of generator for high voltages in air devised by Dr. R. J. Van de Graaff a year and a half ago. A generator of this type was built by the department a year ago, using a 2-meter aluminum sphere, charged by a 6-inch silk belt, and potentials as high as 2,000,000 volts were obtained in tests out-of-doors. Sufficient laboratory space not being available for immediate use of this generator, a 1-meter generator was assembled, and this has been used with a 23-section cascade-type vacuum-tube formerly used in the Tesla coil work. One interesting feature is the focusing action of such a tube, which approaches 100 per cent. for currents of 0.5 microampere of hydrogen- or helium-ions at 600 kv, although there is only a 2-cm diameter hole down the 5-foot tube. A hollow-anode, low-voltage arc (suggested by Dr. E. S. Lamar) is used for the ion-source, mounted inside the sphere and with the necessary power supplied by generators driven by the silk belt which charges the sphere. With this apparatus the disintegration of lithium and boron by high-speed protons has been investigated. With a very thin mica window on the tube near the target, the alpha-particles produced by the disintegrating nuclei have been identified and recorded by the linear amplifier (valve-counter) mentioned above. Lithium is found to give two ranges of alpha-particles in approximately equal numbers, the shorter range being just under two centimeters. The disintegration-yield from boron is roughly twenty times that of lithium at 600 kilovolts, and the majority of these alpha-particles have a range of nearly 3 cm, with a much smaller number having a longer range. Preliminary measurements indicate that for boron about 4,000,000 protons are required to produce one disintegration at 600 kilovolts. These results are in approximate agreement, both as to ranges and disintegration-yields, with those recently reported in *Nature* by Cockroft and Walton.

Dr. Tuve's lecture will be published in the *Journal of the Franklin Institute.*

# OBITUARY

## TIMOTHY E. WILCOX

BRIGADIER-GENERAL TIMOTHY E. WILCOX, retired Army surgeon, living in Washington, D. C., died on December 10, at the age of ninety-two years. He was born at North Litchfield, New York, on April 26, 1840. He graduated from Union College in 1861 with an A.B. and received the A.M. degree in course.

A brief tour with McClellan's army ended with typhoid fever. His medical studies were resumed and he received M.D. from the Albany Medical College in 1864. He was immediately appointed assistant surgeon of the 6th New York Heavy Artillery. He attended Jefferson Davis during his detention at Fortress Monroe after the Civil War. He was appointed assistant surgeon in the regular army in May, 1867, retiring as brigadier-general in April, 1904. In November, 1898, he went to Cuba as lieutenant-colonel chief surgeon and was honorably discharged in May, 1899.

General Wilcox was a born naturalist. Everything was fish to his net—plants, animals, minerals, insects, worms, reptiles, fossils, etc. The National Museum and other museums received many rare specimens from him. The fossil horns of a tiny deer and those of a primeval ox are in the National Museum. The snake *Tontilla Wilcoxii* Stejneger was from Arizona. *Townsendia Wilcoxiana* Wood was discovered at Camp Supply, Indian Territory, in the seventies. *Primula Wilcoxii* Wood (?) was from Fort Boise, Idaho. *Panicum Wilcoxiànum* Vasey was collected in Nebraska, *Quercus Wilcoxii* Rydberg and a cactus from Fort Huachuca, Arizona. His article in *Nature* in 1879–80 calling attention to the absence of angle worms around Boise, Idaho, caused much comment. He was author of occasional notes and papers in medical and other journals. From 1917 he was nearly blind, but his mind was clear to the end.

General Wilcox belonged to Phi Beta Kappa, Alpha Delta Phi, the Cosmos Club, Biological Society of Washington and the National Geographic Society. He joined the Torrey Botanical Club in 1880, being proposed by Dr. Alphonso Wood. In 1930, after 50 years membership, he was made a life member of the club.

WILLARD W. EGGLESTON
BUREAU OF PLANT INDUSTRY
WASHINGTON, D. C.

## RECENT DEATHS

W. ALBERT MANDA, of Orange, New Jersey, a well-known horticulturist, died on March 15, at the age of seventy years.

GILBERT CHARLES BOURNE, emeritus professor of zoology and comparative anatomy at the University of Oxford, died on March 9, at the age of seventy-one years.

DR. ROBERT INNES, formerly astronomer for the Union of South Africa, died suddenly on March 14, at the age of seventy-one years.

WILLIAM CAWTHORNE UNWIN, the British engineer, died on March 17, at the age of ninety-four years.

*Nature* records the deaths of Dr. C. A. Barber, lately lecturer in tropical agriculture at the University of Cambridge, aged seventy-two years; of Sir Benjamin Gott, chairman of the Commission on Educational and Cultural Films, and formerly head master of the Cheltenham School of Science, aged sixty-seven years, and of Mr. J. J. F.-X. King, the Scottish entomologist, aged seventy-seven years. Mr. King had presented his main collection of British insects to the University of Glasgow. The university is now to receive under his will the portrait of Mr. King painted by Forrester Wilson and the remainder of his collections, together with his library of books on natural history.

# SCIENTIFIC EVENTS

## REPORT OF THE COUNCIL FOR CHEMISTRY

IN its report for 1932, according to a summary given in *Nature,* the Federal Council for Chemistry refers with regret to the necessary postponement of the ninth International Congress of Pure and Applied Chemistry and the eleventh conference of the International Union of Chemistry, which were to have been held in Madrid in 1932. The next meeting of the union will take place in the spring of 1934 in Madrid, and not in Switzerland, as previously arranged. During the year, the Verein Oesterreichischer Chemiker and the Svenska National Kommitten för Kemie were elected members of the International Union. The report refers to a conference on chemical documentation, held in Paris in October, 1932, and indicates that the Federal Council and the Division of Chemistry and Chemical Technology of the U. S. National Research Council are in complete agreement with regard to certain criticisms of the activities of the International Committee dealing with the reform of biochemical nomenclature. The efforts of the British Standards Institution to extend the use of the words "British Standard" to include "chemical substances used in manufactures, photography or philosophic research and anti-corrosives" were supported by the Federal Council. The Board of Trade agreed to the institution proceeding with an application to register provided that it was in a position to submit support from the appropriate trade association or similar body. The report says: "In October, a committee consisting of Dr. E. F. Armstrong, E. R. Bolton, Dr. L. H. Lampitt, Professor G. T. Morgan, Emile Mond, Professor J. C. Philip, Sir William Pope, J. Davidson Pratt and D. Rintoul was appointed 'To consider how the resources of the various bodies concerned with the professional and scientific welfare of chemists can be most economically and efficiently utilized.' This committee has met on several occasions, and will present, early in 1933, a report on its findings for consideration by the Federal Council."

## THE YALE NORTH INDIA EXPEDITION

THE last chapter of one of the greatest geological events in the earth's history, resulting in the elevation of the Himalayan mountains, was witnessed by prehistoric man, according to evidence uncovered by the Yale North India Expedition, led by Dr. Hellmut de Terra, research associate in geology at Yale University. The expedition, which also included Mrs. de Terra, Professor G. E. Hutchinson, of the department of biology, and Mr. G. E. Lewis, paleontologist, has just returned to New Haven after spending the past fifteen months in the Himalayas.

Traces of prehistoric man in the form of knives, scrapers and other implements and the remains of a mammoth, whose former existence in the Himalayas has been hitherto unsuspected, comprised two of the more important finds made by the expedition. The geographical, geological and zoological information obtained is expected, it is said, to change present ideas about the early history and origin of the world's highest mountains.

Dr. de Terra has issued a statement in regard to the exposition in which he says:

> The paleolithic implements and the mammoth were found in formations that had been thrown into earth folds during the upheaval and indicate that prior to that time the southern Himalayas were considerably lower in altitude. The rise of the Himalayan range must have continued into historical times. The present high relief of the mountains is a recent achievement and ancient man looked upon a Himalayan range of quite a different appearance from that which modern man sees. We have found proof that prehistoric man in Northern India must have witnessed the last great mountain-making event, which resulted in the present great height of the Himalayas and neighboring high ranges.

The collections made by the expedition have just arrived at New Haven, where most of them will be placed in the Peabody Museum of Yale University. The members of the expedition will complete their investigations here by further study of the finds and their relation to their environment.

## ANNIVERSARY OF THE PHILADELPHIA COLLEGE OF PHARMACY AND SCIENCE

THE one hundred and twelfth anniversary of the founding of the Philadelphia College of Pharmacy and Science was celebrated on February 23 with a special convocation at which the honorary degree of master of pharmacy was conferred upon Dr. George Denton Beal, one of the directors of the Mellon Institute of Industrial Research at Pittsburgh. Dr. Beal then delivered at the exercises an address on "Advances in Pharmacy through Scientific Research," in which he reviewed the relation of pharmacy to other sciences and pointed out many instances of the ways in which the practise of pharmacy has stimulated research and scientific advancement not only in pharmacy but also in chemistry, bacteriology, biology and physiology.

The evening of Founders' Day at the College was featured by a testimonial banquet to Professor Frank Xavier Moerk, who is completing his fiftieth year as a member of the teaching staff at the Philadelphia College, where he is at the head of the department of analytical chemistry and is one of the executive officers of the faculty. Dr. Lewis C. Scheffey, 1915, Philadelphia physician who is president of the Philadelphia College Alumni Association, acted as toastmaster.

A feature at the testimonial banquet was the graphic portrayal by undergraduates in the dramatic society of outstanding events in Professor Moerk's career. This dramatic presentation was arranged by Registrar John E. Kramer, 1925. Felicitations of the board of trustees were extended by Professor Joseph W. England, 1883, its chairman, who is head of the scientific department of the Smith, Kline and French laboratories. Dr. Henry V. Arny, 1889, dean of

Columbia University College of Pharmacy, greeted Professor Moerk as one of his most distinguished students. For the faculty of the Philadelphia College, Dean Julius W. Sturmer spoke of his many years' association with Professor Moerk. An address was also made by Dr. B. Franklin Stahl, trustee of the college.

Presentations were made by Henry Brown, of Scranton; Frank P. Kelly, Jr.; Arthur Osol and James Q. Mackey.

The climax of the evening was the unveiling of an oil portrait of Professor Moerk which was presented to the Philadelphia College by his colleagues and other friends. Dean Charles H. LaWall, 1893, made the presentation. The portrait was painted by Mrs. Mary Sturmer Jones, the daughter of Dean Sturmer. The portrait was accepted for the college by President Wilmer Krusen.

Professor Moerk responded with a recital of some of the events of his career and an appreciation of the testimonial tendered him.

In addition to the personal good wishes extended by the more than three hundred friends who were present at the banquet, Professor Moerk received hundreds of telegrams and letters from all parts of the world. Mrs. Moerk sat enbanked in a veritable bower of floral tributes.

## AWARD OF THE LAMME MEDAL TO EDWARD WESTON

The 1932 Lamme Medal of the American Institute of Electrical Engineers has been awarded to Dr. Edward Weston, Montclair, New Jersey, "for his achievements in the development of electrical apparatus, especially in connection with precision measuring instruments," and will be presented at the summer convention of the institute, which is to be held in Chicago from June 26 to 30, 1933.

Previous awards of the Lamme Medal of the American Institute of Electrical Engineers have been made to Allen B. Field (1928), Rudolf E. Hellmund (1929), William J. Foster (1930) and Giuseppe Faccioli (1931).

A correspondent writes:

Mr. Weston, through his thorough fundamental knowledge of and his ability to observe and analyze chemical and physical phenomena, made important improvements in the quality and speed of electroplating, which contributed materially to the present practice in electrotyping, and nickel-, gold- and silver-plating. He also developed practical and economical methods for electrolytic copper refining.

Although the dynamo had been invented some years earlier, it had not come into practical use, and batteries were used in plating processes, placing serious limitations upon future developments. He, therefore, began the study and construction of dynamo-electric machines, and in 1875 became a partner in the firm of Stevens, Roberts, and Havell, of Newark, N. J., which engaged in the manufacture of such machines for electroplating, electrotyping, electric lighting, etc. This business was incorporated in 1877 as the Weston Company, and was consolidated in 1881 with the U. S. Electric Light Company, of which Mr. Weston served as electrician until 1888.

Mr. Weston had filed his first application for a U. S. patent on dynamo construction in 1876, and later received many patents in this field, his improvements causing phenomenal increases in the efficiency of these machines. He also invented new devices for starting, controlling and protecting them, and thus put their operation upon a practical basis.

From 1875 to 1886, he engaged in intensive development of both incandescent and arc lighting, doing notable work in the search for methods of making suitable incandescent filaments and arc light carbons.

As he had earlier been handicapped by the lack of generators suitable for use in electroplating, he now encountered, in all his researches, great difficulty in making the necessary electrical measurements with the clumsy, slow-acting instruments then available. Consequently, he soon developed and built for his own experiments a set of more practical instruments. His friends promptly wanted some of the same types, and he was soon spending much of his time on further developments of measuring equipment.

In 1883, he decided to relinquish his other interests and devote all his time to the research and development necessary to produce accurate and convenient electrical instruments. He established the Weston Electrical Instrument Company, of which he was vice-president and general manager from 1888 to 1905, and president from 1905 to 1924, when he became chairman of the board, a position which he still holds.

## ELECTIONS TO THE ROYAL SOCIETY

The council of the Royal Society, London, agreed to recommend for election as fellows the following seventeen candidates:

Blackett, Patrick Maynard Stuart, lecturer in physics, Cambridge University.

Collip, James Bertram, professor of biochemistry, McGill University, Montreal.

Crompton, Rookes Evelyn Bell, electrical engineer.

Dawson, Harry Medforth, professor of physical chemistry, Leeds University.

Doodson, Arthur Thomas, associate director of Liverpool Observatory and Tidal Institute.

Gough, Herbert John, engineer, National Physical Laboratory, Teddington.

Hammond, John, senior assistant, Animal Nutrition Institute, Cambridge.

Holmes, Gordon Morgan, physician to the National Hospital for Nervous Diseases, Queen Square, London.

King, Harold, chemist, National Institute for Medical Research, Hampstead.

Lennard-Jones, John Edward, Plummer professor of inorganic chemistry, Cambridge University.

McLeod, James Walter, professor of bacteriology, Leeds University.

Parkes, Alan Sterling, physiologist, Foulerton Student of the Royal Society.

Salisbury, Edward James, Quain professor of botany, London University.

Smith, Bernard, district geologist of H. M. Geological Survey.

Thompson, William Robin, superintendent of Farnham House Laboratory of the Imperial Institute of Entomology, London and Farnham Royal.

Tyndall, Arthur Mannering, Henry Overton Wills professor of physics, Bristol University.

Wedderburn, Joseph Henry, Maclagan professor of mathematics, Princeton University.

# SCIENTIFIC NOTES AND NEWS

A testimonial dinner to observe the eightieth birthday of Professor Elihu Thomson, of the Thomson-Houston and General Electric Companies at Lynn, Massachusetts, will be held in the Walker Memorial of the Massachusetts Institute of Technology on Wednesday evening, March 29. In the afternoon there will be a conference relating to the theoretical and experimental aspects of modern electricity, as well as to certain of its historical aspects, with particular reference to Professor Thomson's achievements.

The honorary doctorate of the University of Paris will be conferred on Dr. Harvey Cushing, who retired last year from the professorship of surgery at Harvard University and as surgeon-in-chief of the Peter Bent Brigham Hospital.

Dr. Alfred Newton Richards, since 1910 professor of pharmacology in the University of Pennsylvania, will be awarded the Kober Medal by the Association of American Physicians during its annual meeting in Washington, D. C., on May 9, in recognition of his work on diseases of the kidney. Dr. Rolla E. Dyer, of the U. S. Public Health Service, Washington, is the Kober lecturer for 1933. He will deliver the lecture on March 25, at Georgetown University.

At the annual meeting of the American Society of Parasitologists, honorary foreign membership was voted to: Professor H. A. Baylis, Natural History Museum, London; Professor Dr. E. Martini, Institut für Schiffs- und Tropen-Hygiene, Hamburg; Professor Edmund Sergent, director of the Institut Pasteur d'Algérie; Professor Etienne Sergent, chef du service antipaludique à l'Institut Pasteur d'Algérie, and Professor K. I. Skrjabin, Institut d'helminthologie de l'Ecole Veterinaire, University of Moscow.

Dr. Witmer Stone, of the Academy of Natural Sciences of Philadelphia, has been elected an honorary member of the British Ornithologists Union.

Dr. Emil Witschi, professor of zoology at the State University of Iowa, has been elected to membership in the Academy of Sciences at Halle.

Dr. Edward H. Cary, Dallas, Texas, president of the American Medical Association, was the guest of honor at the annual dinner of the *Rhode Island Medical Journal* in Providence on February 20, which was attended by nearly two hundred physicians. Dr. Frederick N. Brown, editor of the journal, was toastmaster. A briefcase and a Texas flag were presented to Dr. Cary, who was introduced by Dr. Norman Darrell Harvey, president of the Rhode Island Medical Society.

Arthur W. Dean, Winchester, chief engineer of the Massachusetts Department of Public Works, was elected president of the Boston Society of Civil Engineers at its eighty-fifth annual meeting on March 11.

William O. Moseley, Jr., Traveling Fellowships of the Harvard Medical School, to enable students who have attended the school to continue the study of medicine in Europe, have been awarded to Dr. Stanley J. G. Nowak, instructor in surgery; to Dr. Charles V. Seastone, Jr., research fellow in bacteriology and immunology, and to Dr. Neil L. Crone, interne at the Massachusetts General Hospital.

The Committee on Scientific Research of the American Medical Association has made a grant to Professor F. H. Pike, Columbia University, for the continuation of his work on the effects of combined experimental lesions of the central nervous system.

Dr. Hiram W. Kostmayer, professor and head of the department of gynecology, Tulane University Graduate School of Medicine, New Orleans, has been appointed acting dean of the school, succeeding the late Dr. Henry Daspit.

Clarence E. Libby, for several years associate professor of forestry chemistry at the New York State College of Forestry in Syracuse, has been appointed professor and head of the department of pulp and paper manufacture.

C. K. Morse, superintendent at the Nebraska School of Agriculture in Curtis, will take up university agricultural extension work in Lincoln in September.

Dr. Lorin A. Thompson, head of the department of psychology at the Ohio Wesleyan University, has been appointed director of the summer session, which after a lapse of twenty-five years is to be opened again. Professor Allen C. Conger, of the department of zoology, will continue as director of the summer school at Lakeside, a summer resort, under the auspices of the Methodist Episcopal Church.

Dr. J. Needham, of Gonville and Caius College, Cambridge, university demonstrator in biochemistry since 1928, has been appointed Sir William Dunn reader in biochemistry in place of Professor J. B. S. Haldane, who has accepted the chair of genetics at the University of London. Dr. Needham was visiting professor of biochemistry at Stanford University in 1929.

W. W. Kay, assistant lecturer at the University of Manchester, has been appointed lecturer in chemical pathology, and C. A. McGaughey, assistant lecturer in bacteriology, lecturer in veterinary bacteriology and hygiene.

Dr. Ernest G. Pringsheim, professor of botany at the German University at Prague, has been called to the University of Frankfurt.

Kenneth Headlam-Morley has been appointed secretary of the British Iron and Steel Institute in succession to Mr. G. C. Lloyd.

Dr. J. F. McClendon, professor of physiological chemistry at the University of Minnesota, who has for the past twelve months been studying the relation of iodine to goiter in Japan, China, Italy and Switzerland, will arrive on the *Aquitania,* which leaves Southampton on March 29.

Dr. Thomas H. Johnson, of the Bartol Research Foundation of the Franklin Institute, sailed on March 15 for Mexico, Panama and Peru, where he will make measurements of the directional distribution of the cosmic radiation. The work is jointly supported by the Carnegie Corporation through the Department of Terrestrial Magnetism of the Carnegie Institution of Washington and by the foundation.

Harlan H. Zodtner and Frederick A. Greeley, of the Astrophysical Observatory of the Smithsonian Institution, sailed on March 4 for Suez, taking with them about six tons of equipment for installing a solar radiation station on Mount Saint Katherine, Sinai, Egypt. The authorities of the Saint Katherine Monastery on Mount Sinai have agreed to construct the observatory and trails. The expedition, financed by John A. Roebling, is expected to continue three years, cooperating with the solar radiation observatories at Montezuma, Chile, and Table Mountain, California. Mount Saint Katherine was selected after about twenty months of exploration by Mr. and Mrs. A. F. Moore. It is about 8,500 feet in altitude.

Dr. Henry C. Sherman, Mitchill professor of chemistry at Columbia University, will be the principal out-of-state speaker at the annual meeting of the West Virginia Academy of Science, to be held at Fairmont State Teachers College, Fairmont, West Virginia, on May 5.

At its meeting on March 9, the Geological Society of Chicago was addressed by Professor Nevin M. Fenneman, of the University of Cincinnati, on the subject "Cyclic and Non-cyclic Erosion."

Dr. Allen O. Whipple, professor and head of the department of surgery of the College of Physicians and Surgeons of Columbia University, recently gave a series of lectures at the School of Tropical Medicine at the University of Puerto Rico.

The twenty-fourth course of Lane Medical Lectures will be delivered by Dr. J. C. Drummond, professor of biochemistry, University College, London, on the evenings of April 3, 4, 5, 6 and 7, at Stanford University School of Medicine, San Francisco. The general title of Professor Drummond's lectures is "Recent Advances in the Biochemical Study of Nutritional Disorders." Professor Drummond will also give a lecture at Stanford University on April 11, entitled "General Survey Lines of Future Progress."

The third International Congress for Experimental Cytology will take place in Cambridge (England) from August 21 to 26, 1933. There will be general discussions concerning the following problems: Cell respiration and cell metabolism; Cell form and function as demonstrated by recent advances in tissue culture; The electro-physiology of the cell; Entwicklungsmechanik and Explantation, and The cultivation of animal and plant viruses.

The third expedition from the University of Michigan in a biological survey of the Maya region in Central America in cooperation with the Carnegie Institution of Washington sailed from New Orleans on March first. The party consisted of Dr. L. C. Stuart, of the Museum of Zoology, herpetologist, and Mr. C. L. Lundell, of the University Herbarium, botanist. The objective is the great savannah area lying beyond Lake Peten in the Province of the Peten, Guatemala, where detailed studies and collections of the fauna and flora will be made. It is anticipated that headquarters will be established at La Libertad in the heart of the savannah and the work carried on from that base for about four months. The first expedition in what is planned as a twenty-year project to ascertain not only the present biological conditions but the environment under which the great Maya civilization rose and declined took place in 1931 to the region of Uaxactun far to the north in the Peten district where the Carnegie Institution has been excavating for some years. The second in 1932 was an elaborate series of explorations and studies of the cenotes and aguadas of the Yucatan peninsula, with Chichen Itza as the headquarters. The work is supported by the Carnegie Institution of Washington and the University of Michigan.

THE Laboratory of Anthropology at Santa Fe offers for the summer of 1933 twelve fellowships in field training. Four appointments will be made in archeology, working under the direction of Dr. F. H. H. Roberts, of the Bureau of American Ethnology, on Pueblo sites in Arizona. Four scholarships in ethnology are available for work under the direction of Professor Ralph Linton, of the University of Wisconsin, on the Wichita of Oklahoma. Four scholarships in linguistics are offered under the direction of Dr. Harry Hoijer, of the University of Chicago, conducting research on the Apache language in Arizona. The Fellowship Committee consists of Alfred M. Tozzer, *chairman,* Edward Sapir and Neil M. Judd.

ACCORDING to *Industrial and Engineering Chemistry, The Chemical News,* founded in 1859 by the late Sir William Crookes and for many years a publication of some importance, has apparently ceased publication. The issue for September 23 was the last weekly number and it bore a notice of change of frequency to a monthly issue, but only the October number appeared and that was late. In that number, however, the editor indicated some hope for a reorganization which would enable weekly publication to be resumed in November. However, according to *Chemistry and Industry,* the company formed under the name "The Chemical News, Limited" has now gone into liquidation and consequently the world's oldest English weekly chemical journal has come to an end. For years British and American investigators, especially in inorganic and analytical chemistry, published their results in this journal which, being a weekly, afforded means for prompt publication. Many of the discoveries of new elements were announced in its pages and for seventy-three years *The Chemical News* recorded in some form continuous progress in chemistry and allied sciences.

THE London correspondent of the *Journal* of the American Medical Association writes that at the invitation of the University of London, the Universities of Oxford and Cambridge and the Royal Colleges of Physicians and Surgeons have appointed representatives to consider, with those of the University of London, the present defects of the medical curriculum and to make suggestions for reform. The University of London was led to take action by a recommendation of the board of the faculty of medicine, which has been giving consideration to various criticisms of the medical curriculum. Representatives of the conference include Sir Farquhar Buzzard, regius professor of medicine, University of Oxford; Dr. W. Langdon Brown, regius professor of medicine, University of Cambridge; Dr. A. M. H. Gray, dean of the Faculty of Medicine, University of London; Lord Dawson of Penn, president of the Royal College of Physicians; Sir Holburt Waring, president of the Royal College of Surgeons. At the first meeting, Lord Dawson was elected chairman. The conference intends to call evidence and to review the whole course of medical education.

THE Grand Canyon National Monument, established by proclamation on January 6, is about fifty miles down the river from the point on the south rim from which tourists usually view the canyon, providing a number of new views. The proclamation covers 392 square miles and includes land already withdrawn by the Federal Government for study as to the best use to be made of it. The area is about 500 miles by motor from Los Angeles, and about 50 miles as the bird flies from Grand Canyon Village on the South Rim. Toroweap Point has an elevation of 4,750 feet, although the outer rim just above the point has an elevation of 6,500 feet. Looking downward from Toroweap Point it is 3,000 feet to the Colorado River, which appears to be a slender and seemingly insignificant ribbon of silver from this height. A huge cinder cone of volcanic origin with the mythological title of "Vulcans Throne" is also included in the monument.

THE National Park Service at Yellowstone National Park is again making preparations to distribute bison, grizzly bears and black bears to preserves, zoos, zoological gardens and parks. While the buffalo shipments will not be made until November and December, when weather conditions are more favorable, requests for bears will be handled as soon as received and the animals can be captured. It is announced that these animals will not be disposed of as pets. They are distributed primarily for purposes of exhibition and to maintain a balance in the Yellowstone Park animal world. Whereas the Park Service makes no direct charge for any of these animals, advance payment of from $55 to $70 for a buffalo, and $75 for a bear is necessary to cover the cost of crates, transportation from the point of capture to Gardiner, Montana, cost of feed, and expenses incidental to the shipment. Buffalo will be sent only as yearlings or older. In the case of a yearling the cost f.o.b. Gardiner, Montana, is approximately $55, the animal weighing 1,000 pounds crated; while for a full grown buffalo, which weighs about 2,000 pounds crated, the cost is approximately $70. All animals are shipped express collect. Should the charges in connection with shipment amount to less than the sum remitted, a refund of the balance will be made. Requests should include information as to the number, sex and approximate age of the animals desired.

THE *Journal* of the American Medical Association reports that at a meeting of a class at the Prussian Academy of Sciences in Berlin, a preliminary report was presented by Dr. Richard Walzer, of Berlin, on a recently discovered manuscript by Galen. The manuscript, which is entitled "On Medical Empiricism," furnishes a complete Arabian translation by Hubais of the work that is known in the Occident only through a few scanty fragments. "On Medical Empiricism" is by no means a polemic against empirical medicine but rather a manual in which the eminent Greco-Roman physician for didactic reasons permits the advocates of unsupported theories to present their views, the mode of presentation being that first the dogmatizing physician attacks the empiricist and then the empiricist is given ample opportunity to defend his position. This manuscript, along with the "Subfiguratio Empirica," will be an important source of information with regard to the empirical medicine of antiquity, which, in the main, has been known only through the polemical attacks of its opponents. The manuscript contains, furthermore, some new material on the history of philosophy, especially on skepticism, and a new fragment of the writings of Democritus and of the Cynic philosopher Diogenes. Likewise the antecedents of Hellenistic empirical medicine will be clarified by Walzer's discovery.

# DISCUSSION

## THE LAW OF MAXIMUM NORMAL NUTRITIVE VALUE

EVIDENCE has been accumulating for many years, but especially during the past quarter century, which is in harmony with the conclusions of the writer and his associates (1) that, in a critical sense, foodstuffs can not be evaluated individually; (2) that net energy values of individual foodstuffs are fundamentally variable, and hence are not practicable standard measures of reference, and (3) that the most nearly logical, single, conventional measure of whole nutritive value is the net energy of the nutritively complete ration.

The time, therefore, seems propitious for the formulation of a principle underlying these ideas—which may be called "The Law of Maximum Normal Nutritive Value" and which may be stated as follows:

> An individual foodstuff expresses its normal and most characteristic nutritive value, for a given kind of animal, under specified conditions governing nutritive requirement, only as it is a part of a ration which is qualitatively complete and quantitatively sufficient, for the conditions existing—except as it may express the same value by virtue of the capacity of the animal temporarily to protect itself from food nutrient deficiency by drafts upon the nutritive reserves of its own body, or as it may express even higher apparent value, under certain pathological conditions, or during undernutrition, by virtue of the protective or body-sparing capacities of nutrients.

It is true that a foodstuff may seem to have a greater value when added to a markedly deficient ration than when added to a more nearly perfect one, if the entire supplementing effect of the combination is, illogically, credited to the supplementary food; but this is only because the supplement is thus credited with more than its own value, since, logically, each component of the more nearly perfect ration should be credited with greater value than it has in the less nearly perfect ration. Manifestly, there is no scientific method of apportioning the nutritive value of a diet among its components.

From the critical point of view of the principle stated foodstuffs can not be compared with each other, as to nutritive value, except with reference to a constituent, or a quality, or a capacity which they have in common—which, obviously, constitutes an incomplete and therefore imperfect basis of comparison.

This position may seem extreme, but is finally inescapable. The experimenter has only to choose between a voluntary adoption of this logically correct point of view, and a forced acceptance of the same attitude, after having been driven from one fundamentally untenable position to another until no choice remains.

A reason for the frequent failure of investigators adequately to observe this principle, in nutritional studies, is apparently the fact that, under many conditions, especially in short-time periods of experimental observation, nutritive deficiencies are, for the time being, completely masked by drafts upon the reserves of the animal body. Experimenters, therefore, often overlook the fact that under some other conditions the same deficiencies would unquestionably affect apparent nutritive values.

Fundamental nutritive requirements may be considered, in a sense, to be satisfied, from one source or other, so long as life continues—if not from the food, then necessarily from the body.

It is sometimes only through the accumulation of discordant experimental results during the course of years that the effects of failure adequately to recognize the principle to which we call attention become apparent.

In spite of the simplicity and obviousness of the foregoing expressions, the experimenter in the field of nutrition will realize that the point of view is exacting and that its full observance would require very much more knowledge of the details of nutrition than is now possessed by any one.

The experimenter can only strive toward finality of results by planning his rations in consideration of the most that is known as to nutritive values of foodstuffs and nutritive requirements of animals—which, in a few words, and in most relations, signifies that in nutritional investigation rations should be complete, perfect and sufficient, in all characteristics except the single one upon which evidence is sought.

Information which would be most helpful, in relation to the whole subject of measures of nutritive effects and requirements, is detailed knowledge of specific nutritive deficiencies in relation to the utilization of food, and as to the extent of the protection, and the time element in the protection, of the animal, from food nutrient deficiencies, which may be afforded by drafts upon its own nutritive reserves.

E. B. FORBES

PENNSYLVANIA STATE COLLEGE

## THE LAW OF EFFECT

THORNDIKE[1] has just come out with an unusually striking demonstration of the law of effect, the principle that in learning a "satisfying after-effect strengthens directly the connection producing it," and Ogden[2] has hurried forward to say that after all a dynamical account of such relationships is preferable and that the retroaction of satisfaction simply means that a total temporal integration is most firmly established when it has completed itself. The time may come when the scientific world can do without the concept of cause-and-effect, or may remake it so that a cause can be subsequent to its effect. However, I do not believe that we are yet forced to any such novel view in theoretical psychology. There are at least four possibilities from which to choose:

(1) Success stamps in the preceding action retroactively—which is what the law of effect seems casually to mean, though it may be interpreted as (3) below.

(2) Success is the consummation of a process that is stamped in as a whole, so that the first part of the process actually is affected by a later part—which is, I think, nearly what Ogden means.

(3) Organization of a content, being potentially learning for ultimate reproduction, leaves a trace which persists to be affected by subsequent events. I believe that this view is really Thorndike's.

(4) "Retroactive facilitation" is actually the absence of subsequent inhibition: all mental organization would lead to memory but for the subsequent destruction of the traces, and success provides conditions for minimal destruction. This view is derived from the experiment of Jenkins and Dallenbach.[3]

The difficulty with the first two views is that, simply conceived, they imply the reversibility of time, the dependence of the present upon the future. The temporal Gestalt has, it seems to me, clear value as a scientific concept, but not in the form of (2). With such sensible and plausible alternatives as (3) and (4), why should we refuse, as Ogden does, to discuss the interrelation and mutual effects of the parts of the total integration?

EDWIN G. BORING

HARVARD UNIVERSITY

[1] E. L. Thorndike, SCIENCE, 77: 173–175 (February 10, 1933).

[2] R. M. Ogden, SCIENCE, 77: 240 (March 3, 1933).

[3] J. G. Jenkins and K. M. Dallenbach, *Amer. Jour. Psychol.*, 25: 605–612 (1925). *Cf.* W. S. Hunter, "Foundations of Experimental Psychology," 599–605 (1929).

## IS THE SPELLING AMOEBA SACROSANCT?

I HAVE received two or three blue-pencilled copies of a statement made in SCIENCE of February 10 of the current year (page 170) to the effect that: "Generic names are sacred and their spelling may not be changed to suit the whims of writers. Amoeba can not become ameba." Inasmuch as I am one of the illiterate who have dared to use the spelling "Ameba" in a recent book, presumably to the corruption of the youth of the land, my curiosity has naturally been aroused, and I have followed up the matter a bit bibliographically. I find that the original spelling was *Amiba,* a name given by Bary de St. Vincent in 1822. Ehrenberg admits this in a paper in 1830, although he impiously changed the spelling to Amoeba and uses this form of spelling in his well-known monograph of 1838. Surely Ehrenberg had no more right in 1830 to lay profane hands on what is "sacred" than we have to-day, so the *oe* form should have no better standing than the *e* form among zoological ecclesiastics! But then why use the term at all? Taxonomists have agreed, I believe, in accordance with the "International Code of Zoological Nomenclature" to accept the generic nomenclature set forth in the tenth edition of Linnaeus' "Systema

Naturae," and in that edition (1758) Linnaeus termed the creature in question *Volvox chaos,* later changing it to *Chaos protheus* in his twelfth edition. Thus the past nomenclature of Ameba seems to have been almost as protean as the creature itself. I suspect, however, that most of us will go on using the term Ameba or Amoeba, as our respective judgments may dictate. As to Paramecium, since the original spelling was with an *e* and not an *oe* or an *ae,* the correct form is obviously Paramecium.

M. F. Guyer
University of Wisconsin

## MORE OHIO MEDUSAE

In my recent communication on an occurrence of fresh-water medusae at Akron, Ohio,[1] I made reference to the approximate number of such discoveries in the United States. Since I stated mine was the second such occurrence in Ohio, I must make this correction. I inadvertently overlooked others of recent dates.

In September, 1930, some medusae were found in Vermillion River, some in a quarry near Ashland, and in October, 1931, some in a quarry near Toledo, all localities in northern Ohio. These were reported in an abstract by Mr. Robert L. Baird, of Oberlin, Ohio.[2]

Walter C. Kraatz
University of Akron

## FARADAY'S DIARY

In a recent review of Faraday's Diary (Science, Jan. 13) I pointed out that one of the most important experiments in electromagnetic induction, described in the First Series of Experimental Researches, noted as read on November 24, 1831, is entered in the Diary under date of December 26. I ventured to suggest that the date in the Diary must be wrong. After correspondence with Mr. Thomas Martin, the editor of the Diary, I am convinced that it was right. Mr. Martin permits me to say on his authority that considerable additions were made to the First and Second Series of the Experimental Researches in Electricity after the papers were read and before they were published.

No question of priority is involved, and I make this correction only for the sake of historical accuracy.

W. F. Magie

# SCIENTIFIC APPARATUS AND LABORATORY METHODS

## RECENT DEVELOPMENTS IN GRAVITY APPARATUS

The greatly increased interest taken in the use of geophysical methods in searching for buried geological structure, has resulted in an increased use of gravity apparatus for determining the value of g. For several decades the Von Sterneck invariable pendulum apparatus, or some modification of it, was used by geodesists for determining gravity. The observations were planned to meet the needs of physicists and chemists working in laboratories, and to enable geodesists to determine the figure of the earth or isostasists to study the distribution of densities throughout the earth's crust.

As gravity stations have become more closely spaced, it has been found that there is a definite relation between the gravity anomalies and the density of the rock close to the stations. This relationship is indicated in one way by large differences in anomalies for stations close together, of which there are several notable examples.

The Coast and Geodetic Survey, having had many calls for gravity surveys, assigned E. J. Brown, one of its field engineers, to the task of modernizing its pendulum apparatus, which had been in use since the early nineties. Brown finished his work about a year ago and the apparatus, named after him, has since been given a very severe test in the field, during which about seventy stations were established. The results have been in every way satisfactory. With the Brown apparatus one station a day can be observed, provided the distance between stations is not excessive, while with the old apparatus of the Coast Survey it was impossible to observe satisfactorily more than five stations per month.

The essential features of the Brown apparatus are:

(1) The receiver supports are about in the same horizontal plane as the knife edge on which the pendulum swings. This arrangement greatly reduces the flexure of the apparatus.

(2) The oscillations of the pendulum are made to actuate a photoelectric cell and the impulses are amplified until they operate the chronograph pen. With this arrangement the time signals sent from the Naval Observatory by radio can be compared directly on the chronograph sheet with the oscillations of the pendulum and a chronometer is not needed as an intermediary timepiece.

(3) Another very important feature of the Brown apparatus is that most of the auxiliary parts of the gravity equipment are installed permanently in an automobile truck. These parts include the chronograph, radio apparatus used for receiving the signals, switchboard, batteries, etc. The only important part

[1] Science, 77: 87, 1933.

[2] *Ohio Jour. Science*, 32: 323, 1932.

of the apparatus that needs to be taken out of the truck on arrival at a new station is the pendulum receiver.

(4) The pendulum receiver is designed in such a way that the pendulum can be clamped in a safe position without removing it, after observations have been made at a station. The receiver containing the clamped pendulum is then placed in an automobile truck and carried to the next station. At the new station the apparatus can be set up and the pendulum released and started in operation within a few minutes. A few electrical connections between the case and the apparatus installed in the truck and the erection of a short antenna completes the necessary arrangements. Ordinarily, the receiver remains evacuated during a whole season, and this helps to maintain a more uniform temperature of the pendulum.

There are several other novel features in the Brown apparatus, but they are of less importance than those mentioned. A brief account of the apparatus will be found in Transactions of the American Geophysical Union, dated June, 1932.

The Brown apparatus at the time of this writing is being used for a gravity survey in Cuba. It is expected that observations will be made at approximately seventy stations in that island, which were selected by the geologists of the Atlantic Refining Company of Cuba. The work is being done by the cooperation of that company, the Coast and Geodetic Survey, the Naval Observatory and Professor Richard M. Field, of Princeton University, chairman of the Committee on Geophysical and Geological Study of Oceanic Basins and their Margins of the American Geophysical Union.

Another new gravity apparatus, called the Lejay-Holweck Gravimeter, is receiving to-day a great deal of attention. This apparatus consists of a base on which is mounted a vertical frame that supports rigidly a short thin strip of elinvar extending vertically upward. Attached to the upper end of the elinvar strip is a bob of quartz whose coefficient of expansion is close to zero. The whole apparatus can be carried in a small box or case and is easily transported by hand.

The bob supported by the elinvar strip oscillates under the combined action of gravity and the elasticity of the strip. The mass of the bob is such that it is almost exactly balanced by the elastic force of the strip. By means of this arrangement the pendulum is given a very long period and in consequence is very sensitive to variations in the pull of gravity. This makes it unnecessary to have a very exact time control for measuring the periods of oscillation. It is stated that the apparatus is one hundred times more sensitive than the ordinary gravity pendulum and, therefore, an error in time may be tolerated that is one hundred times as great as that permissible with the usual pendulum apparatus.

In the *Comptes Rendus* of the Academy of Sciences of January 3, 1933, is a short article by Dr. Lejay telling of a gravity survey that had been made by him in the northwestern part of France. Forty determinations were made with the Lejay-Holweck apparatus in the two months of October and November, 1932. During two weeks of that period no observations were made. As an indication of the rapidity with which the observations were carried on, it is stated that on October 7, 1932, and again on October 11, observations were made at three stations. On each of several other days two stations were established. The average distance between the stations in this survey was about 40 kilometers. During the period, observations were made in Paris on three different dates and the range in the values of gravity at that station was only one part in a million. It is stated by Lejay that wherever he found it impracticable to find a stable support for his apparatus he preferred to secure what he considered a fairly accurate determination with an uncertainty of about two parts in a million of gravity rather than to delay the progress of his work. An accuracy of two parts in a million is really quite satisfactory for most purposes to which gravity data are applied. During the 7,000 kilometers traveled in an automobile during this gravity survey the pendulum did not change.

Lejay states that as a result of his campaign in northwest France one may be assured that it is possible for a single observer without any assistance and without great fatigue to complete one station per day, provided a means of rapid transportation is at the disposal of the observer.

It is understood that the computations for the topographic and isostatic reductions of the gravity stations in France will be made shortly. It will be of interest to learn the results, for until now there have been but few gravity stations in France for which the isostatic anomalies are available.

The Brown and the Lejay-Holweck types of apparatus are the only new ones known to the writer with which extensive and successful field work has been done. Other types of gravity apparatus are in the process of development. One is the apparatus of Fred E. Wright, of the Geophysical Laboratory of the Carnegie Institution of Washington, which is based on the use of horizontal helical springs to balance the pull of gravity on a weight at the end of a lever arm supported in a horizontal position by the torsion of the springs. Wright has developed his apparatus to the point where he was able to make some tests with it outside of the laboratory. No definite information is available as to the character of the results obtained during these tests.

An apparatus has been in the process of development at the office of the Geodetic Institute at Potsdam, Germany. This one has as its essential feature the balancing of a column of mercury against a fixed volume of gas. No definite reports of progress are available, but the writer has been led to believe from conversations and correspondence that the apparatus gives promise of being quite effective.

A new type of gravity apparatus has recently been developed in Norway. A description of the apparatus and of the methods employed in its use is contained in articles by K. Wold and G. Jelstrup, which appeared on pages 269 to 279 of *Gerlands Beiträge zur Geophysik*, No. 36, 1932.

It is well known that one or more of the petroleum companies of this country have been working on gravity apparatus and methods, but no information regarding them is in print. It is known, however, that a method has been employed whereby the oscillations of a pendulum kept swinging at a central field base station are transmitted by radio to surrounding stations at which they are compared directly with the oscillations of the field pendulums.[1] With such a method the required accuracy can be obtained by a short series of observations and any number of gravity parties can operate simultaneously in the field within a reasonable distance of the base. This method should be very effective in making an intensive gravity survey of a comparatively large area, but for the usual gravity work the expense of operating the base station with the transmitting apparatus would scarcely be justified.

It may be said without question that notable progress has been made recently in the improvement of gravity methods and apparatus, and it is very probable that even further advance will be made in the very near future. Gravity surveys will undoubtedly play an ever-increasing part in geophysical and geological studies designed to disclose buried structure, a matter of great importance in the search for petroleum, water and minerals. Anticlines, domes, synclines and masses of heavy rock or ore may be indicated by the values of gravity at stations located immediately above or very close to them.

William Bowie
U. S. Coast and Geodetic Survey

[1] This method was suggested by C. A. Heiland in 1927 in a paper given before the Section of Geodesy of the American Geophysical Union. See Bulletin No. 61 of the National Research Council, pp. 66–71.

# SPECIAL ARTICLES

## NEW HARDY SEEDLESS GRAPES

A project[1] in breeding grapes which has for its aim the development of hardy seedless clons of merit has now given 28 seedlings that bear seedless or near-seedless fruits and that are hardy in the climate of central New York. One of these plants has already been reported,[2] but most of them fruited for the first time in 1932.

Seedless grapes of various types occasionally arise directly from seeded grapes, presumably either by mutation, by segregation or by some particular combination of complementary factors. Such plants usually bear viable pollen and hence they may be employed as pollen parents in crosses with seeded plants in the effort to take advantage of any hereditary values which seedlessness may possess in obtaining more seedless individuals among the offspring.

The new seedless grapes thus far obtained in this project are all the progeny of hardy seeded grapes crossed with the tender seedless varieties Sultanina, Rose Sultanina and Black Monukka. According to the investigations of Goodspeed,[3] Susa[4] and Pearson,[5] in these seedless grapes fruits are for the most part produced only after pollination and fertilization, and hence the parthenocarpy is stimulative rather than spontaneous.

Vines of the tender seedless grapes are grown in the courts between greenhouses at the New York Botanical Garden, where they frequently flower at the time when the pollen can be used on hardy grapes in bloom at Geneva. Rather large numbers of seeds (several thousand) were obtained in the crosses, but a large percentage of the $F_1$ died in the nursery or vineyard, evidently because of tenderness inherited from the vinifera parent. Of the seedlings that survived some have seeded fruits and some have seedless or near-seedless fruits.

The occurrence of seedless grapes in considerable numbers in the $F_1$ generation of these crosses is a matter of importance to the practical results of the breeding effort. The occurrence of both seeded and seedless individuals in this generation is a result of significance in considering the heredity of seedlessness. It appears that seedlessness of the type here concerned is not a simple character in inheritance and that in these crosses one or both parents are hetero-

[1] By permission of the authorities of The New York Botanical Garden the writer has cooperated with the Department of Horticulture of the State Experiment Station at Geneva, N. Y., in this project.

[2] A. B. Stout, "A New Hardy Seedless Grape," *Jour. Heredity*, 19: 316–323, 1928.

[3] T. H. Goodspeed, Paper presented in Section G, 73rd meeting A. A. A. S., December 28, 1920.

[4] T. Susa, "Sterility in Certain Grapes," Mem. Hort. Soc. N. Y. 3: 223–232, 1927.

[5] Helen Pearson, "Parthenocarpy and Seedlessness in *Vitis vinifera*," Science, 76: 594, 1932.

zygous for certain of the complementary factors involved.

A preliminary study of the seed-like structures in the mature fruits of these new seedless grapes shows several degrees of development. In a few cases there are only tiny rudiments of seeds, quite as exist in the fruits of the Sultanina grape. But in most cases there is some development of the tissues of the seed coats, but the structures, even when their size approaches that of a seed, are either without embryo and endosperm or with only traces of them and are so soft and pulpy that they are not noticed when the fruits are masticated in eating. It appears that the type of seedlessness in these plants corresponds to that of the pollen parent, but that the inhibition in the development of the seeds which results in their abortion is less complete in most of them.

The seedless plants already obtained are being utilized as pollen parents in crosses with sister plants that have seeds. The latter are being selfed and crossed to obtain a second generation and they are being used in back crosses with the seedless parents. The results should give further data on hereditary behavior, and, it is hoped, provide more of the seedless grapes.

Several of the seedlings which bear seedless or near-seedless fruits possess considerable merit. For these the clusters are well filled and of good size or even large. In size the berries range from larger than Delaware fruits to nearly the size of Concord. The colors include green, amber, red, mottled red and shades of black. In quality there is considerable variation, but the best are vinous, sweet and meaty. Several ripen early. The most promising of these grapes are being propagated for trial under cultural conditions.

A. B. STOUT

NEW YORK BOTANICAL GARDEN

## THE OCCURRENCE OF ROTENONE AND RELATED COMPOUNDS IN THE ROOTS OF CRACCA VIRGINIANA[1]

CRACCA VIRGINIANA, the most abundant species of the genus Cracca indigenous to the United States, has recently been reported as possessing insecticidal properties.[2] This, together with the fact that other species of Cracca, namely, *C. toxicaria* from South America and *C. vogelii* from Africa, have yielded substances related to the rotenone group of fish poisons,[3] has made a chemical study of the American species interesting and desirable. Such an investigation has been in progress and to date the following results have been obtained:

Ether extraction of the roots of the plant yielded from 4 to 6 per cent. of resinous materials having a pleasant characteristic odor. The extract, when tested as a fish poison, showed essentially the same toxicity as pure rotenone. It contained 9 per cent. methoxyl[4] and in many ways resembled the non-crystallizable extractives from derris and cubé roots.[5] Attempts to obtain individual major constituents by distillation, crystallization or the formation of derivatives were for the most part unsuccessful, although four substances were obtained in small quantities. These were rotenone, dehydrorotenone, tephrosin and a colorless crystalline material, $C_{22}H_{24}O_4$, whose M.P. is 131°.

The rotenone was obtained by dissolving one part of the resin in an equal part of *n*-butyl ether and allowing the solution to crystallize for from two to three weeks. The yield was usually about 5 per cent. of the weight of the resin, but apparently much more rotenone was present which did not crystallize because of the complex nature of the mixture. This was shown by the fact that a slightly more dilute solution failed entirely to crystallize or at most gave only traces of crystals, and also by the fact that solutions of the resin in other solvents, from which rotenone readily crystallizes from very dilute solutions, would not crystallize.

Dehydrorotenone was obtained from the resin in approximately 2 per cent. yield by treating the material in a methanolic solution with alkali (50 gm. resin, 200 cc. methanol and 0.5 gm. potassium hydroxide). Sometimes crystallization occurred in a short time, and again a month or more was required for the process to take place. The dehydrorotenone was frequently contaminated with material which appeared to be a dehydro derivative of a somewhat higher molecular weight. The first specimen obtained, for example, melted sharply at 217°. It gave analytical values approximately half-way between that required for dehydrorotenone and dehydrotoxicarol and could not be further purified. Hydrolysis with alcoholic alkali, however, gave a fair yield of derrisic acid, and examination by the optical immersion method[6] showed that much of the material was dehydrorotenone. This particular phenomenon is the same as was recently reported for certain naturally occurring mixtures of dehydrodeguelin and dehydrotoxicarol.[7] Other specimens of the dehydro

[1] From the Insecticide Division of the Bureau of Chemistry and Soils, United States Department of Agriculture, Washington, D. C.

[2] Little, SCIENCE, 73, 315 (1931); *Jour. Econ. Ent.*, 24: 743 (1931).

[3] Clark, *Jour. Am. Chem. Soc.*, 52, 2461 (1930); 53, 729 (1931).

[4] A ligroin (B.P. 40–60°) extract was employed for this purpose.

[5] Clark, SCIENCE, 71: 396. 1930.

[6] The optical identifications involved in this communication were performed by George L. Keenan, of the Food and Drug Administration, U. S. Department of Agriculture.

[7] Clark and Keenan, *Jour. Am. Chem. Soc.*, 55, 422, 1933.

derivative from the same or other samples of resin were easily purified and identified by melting-point, mixed melting-point and optical properties.

Tephrosin was obtained by removing the methanol from the dehydrorotenone mother liquors, dissolving the residue in approximately an equal volume of *n*-butanol and allowing the solution to crystallize over a period of several weeks. The material was purified and identified by melting-point, mixed melting-point and optical properties.

The fourth substance, $C_{22}H_{24}O_4$, sometimes crystallized in small amounts from the alkaline methanolic solutions upon standing. A small quantity could always be obtained by adding approximately 5 per cent. of water to the alkaline alcoholic solution and allowing the turbid liquid to stand until it cleared. Crystallization usually occurred. If this did not take place, the oily insoluble layer in the bottom of the flask was dissolved in boiling petroleum ether and concentrated to about one fifth of its volume. Upon standing the solution crystallized. The material was purified by recrystallization from petroleum ether. It consisted of colorless rods which melted at 131° and gave in alcoholic solution a greenish purple color with ferric chloride, but it did not dissolve in aqueous alkali. Analysis for carbon and hydrogen and molecular weight determinations showed it to have the formula $C_{22}H_{24}O_4$. The material reacted with hydriodic acid in a Zeisel apparatus, giving an alkyl iodide, but the results were of such a character as to show that probably neither methoxyl nor ethoxyl groups were present. The material in a concentration of 1–100,000 when tested for toxicity, employing goldfish as test animals, was inert.

The yields of tephrosin and the $C_{22}$ compound were small and variable, but, as with rotenone, there were ample indications that much more material than was obtained was present in the resin. In all probability the complex character of the extractives inhibited the crystallization of the individual constituents.

While the results here recorded account for only a small portion of the extractives of *Cracca virginiana*, it is interesting that this is the first native plant of the United States in which members of the rotenone group of fish poisons have been found.

E. P. CLARK

## EFFECT OF TEMPERATURE ON EVERSPORTING EYE COLOR IN DROSOPHILA MELANOGASTER[1]

OUR x-ray experiments have produced three mottled-eyed stocks.[2] All are caused by some change in the normal allelomorph at the white locus of the x-rayed wild type sex chromosome. Regular males receiving a treated X-chromosome, and regular females heterozygous for a treated X and for white eye color, have mottled eyes.

Since the mutation rate varies directly with temperature in *Drosophila melanogaster*,[3] it might be expected that temperature would influence such conditions of genetic instability. Similar cases of eversporting in other forms have been tested for effect of temperature. Eyster[4] found that strains of maize with variegated pericarp color raised in Arizona showed less extreme variegation patterns than the same strains raised in a cooler climate in California. Demerec,[5] on the other hand, found that a difference of 10° C did not affect mutable miniature in *Drosophila virilis*.

Preliminary tests at 29°, 24° and 18° C show that the cooler the temperature at which the flies are raised the larger the light areas of mottled eyes in our stocks. Temperature affects viability as well as eye color. Mottled-2 is almost completely lethal to males at 18° and 24°, but at 29° a fair proportion of the expected males survive, demonstrating that genetic constitution may be a factor in determining the survival value of an organism in an unfavorable environment.

This temperature effect offers a means of determining the larval stage at which mottling occurs, which may furnish a clue as to the mechanism involved. Eyster's work and ours both indicate that the incidence of eversporting varies inversely with temperature, which seems to imply that something other than regular gene mutation is responsible for these cases of unstable genetic constitution.

JOHN W. GOWEN
E. H. GAY

[1] From the Rockefeller Institute for Medical Research, Department of Animal and Plant Pathology, Princeton, N. J.; and the Department of Biology, School of Hygiene and Public Health, Johns Hopkins University, Baltimore, Md.

[2] J. W. Gowen and E. H. Gay. "Eversporting as a Function of the Y-chromosome in *Drosophila melanogaster*," *Proc. N. A. S.*, 19: 122–126. 1933.

[3] H. J. Muller. "The Measurement of Gene Mutation Rate in Drosophila, its High Variability, and its Dependence upon Temperature." *Genetics*, 13: 279–357. 1928.

[4] W. H. Eyster. "The Effect of Environment on Variegation Patterns in Maize Pericarp." *Genetics*, 11: 372–386. 1926.

[5] M. Demerec. "Effect of Temperature on the Rate of Change of the Unstable Miniature –3–γ Gene of *Drosophila virilis*." *Proc. N. A. S.*, 18: 430–434. 1932.

## BOOKS RECEIVED

COUDERC, PAUL. *Discussion sur l'Evolution de l'Univers.* Pp. xii + 67. Gauthier-Villars et Cie, Paris. 15 fr.

HALDANE, J. B. S. *Science and Human Life.* Pp. vii + 287. Harper. $2.50.

PLANCK, MAX. *Wege zur Physikalischen Erkenntnis.* Pp. 280. S. Hirzel, Leipzig. 8. RM.

WHEELER, WILLIAM M. *Colony-Founding Among Ants.* Pp. viii + 179. 23 figures. Harvard University Press. $2.00.

# SCIENCE

VOL. 77 — FRIDAY, MARCH 31, 1933 — No. 1996

*Thermodynamics and Relativity. II:* PROFESSOR RICHARD C. TOLMAN ..... 313

*Active Iron:* DR. OSKAR BAUDISCH ..... 317

*Scientific Events:*
*The Junior Science Clubs of the American Institute; The Sixth Annual Summer Symposium in Theoretical Physics at the University of Michigan; Conferences on Recent Developments in Chemistry at the Johns Hopkins University; In Honor of Dr. Elihu Thomson* ..... 319

*Scientific Notes and News* ..... 321

*Discussion:*
*Patents are Ethical:* DR. YANDELL HENDERSON. *University Patents:* DR. ABRAHAM FLEXNER. *Maturation Divisions in Tradescantia, Rheo and Oenothera:* PROFESSOR E. C. JEFFREY. *Local Electric Anesthesia:* DR. FREDERICK PETERSON. *Self-sterility in Nemesia:* DR. HERBERT PARKES RILEY. *A New Vascular Fusarium Disease of Peas:* DR. WILLIAM C. SNYDER ..... 324

*Special Correspondence:*
*The Ella Sachs Plotz Foundation for the Advancement of Scientific Investigation* ..... 328

*Societies and Meetings:*
*The Colorado-Wyoming Academy of Science:* PROFESSOR R. J. GILMORE. *The Alabama Academy of Science:* PROFESSOR EMMETT B. CARMICHAEL ..... 329

*Scientific Apparatus and Laboratory Methods:*
*Ammoniation of Peat for Fertilizers:* DR. R. O. E. DAVIS and WALTER SCHOLL. *An Accurate Method for Measuring New-born Mice:* DR. ARTHUR SVIHLA. *A New Source of Working Current for Potentiometers:* LESTER F. BOSS ..... 330

*Special Articles:*
*The Effect of Galactose Feeding upon Depancreatized Dogs:* PROFESSOR J. H. ROE and RUSSELL F. CAHOON. *The Incidence of Color Blindness among Races:* DR. THOMAS R. GARTH 331

*Science News* ..... 5

SCIENCE: A Weekly Journal devoted to the Advancement of Science, edited by J. MCKEEN CATTELL and published every Friday by

THE SCIENCE PRESS

New York City: Grand Central Terminal

Lancaster, Pa. — Garrison, N. Y.

Annual Subscription, $6.00 — Single Copies, 15 Cts.

SCIENCE is the official organ of the American Association for the Advancement of Science. Information regarding membership in the Association may be secured from the office of the permanent secretary, in the Smithsonian Institution Building, Washington, D. C.

# THERMODYNAMICS AND RELATIVITY. II

By PROFESSOR RICHARD C. TOLMAN

CALIFORNIA INSTITUTE OF TECHNOLOGY

(5) CONSEQUENCES OF RELATIVISTIC THERMODYNAMICS

To complete our discussion, we must now consider the possible consequences of relativistic thermodynamics. The technical modifications in thermodynamic theory needed to secure its extension to relativity may have seemed too trivial and obvious to warrant the expectation that these consequences could be very novel or interesting. Nevertheless, the actual effect of replacing classical ideas as to the nature of space and time by relativistic ideas is so fundamental as to lead to important differences between the results of classical and relativistic thermodynamics. Three examples may now be given to illustrate both the essential novelty and the inherent rationality of the consequences of relativistic thermodynamics.

(*a*) *Temperature Gradient in Gravitational Field.* In the classical thermodynamics we have become accustomed to the conclusion that a system which is in thermal equilibrium will necessarily have uniform temperature throughout. As a result of relativistic thermodynamics, however, it is found that this conclusion must be modified in the presence of appreciable gravitational fields. Thus if we consider a spherical distribution of material held together in static equilibrium by its own gravitational forces, corresponding to the line element,

$$ds^2 = -e^{\mu}\,(dr^2 + r^2 d\,\theta^2 + r^2 \sin^2\theta\, d\,\phi^2) + e^{\nu} dt^2 \qquad (23)$$

where $\mu$ and $\nu$ are functions of r alone, it can be shown[8] that the condition for thermal equilibrium is given by

$$\frac{d \log T_o}{dr} = -\tfrac{1}{2}\frac{d\nu}{dr} \qquad (24)$$

where $T_o$ the proper temperature as measured by a local observer decreases as we go outward instead of remaining constant. And for the more general static case of a system, not necessarily having spherical

[8] Tolman, *Phys. Rev.*, 35: 906, 1930.

symmetry, but corresponding to the more general line element

$$ds^2 = g_{ij}\,dx^i dx^j + g_{44}dt^2 \qquad (i, j = 1, 2, 3) \qquad (25)$$

where $g_{ij}$ and $g_{44}$ are independent of t, it has been shown by Professor Ehrenfest and myself[9] that the condition for thermal equilibrium would be given by a constant value throughout the system for the product

$$T_o \sqrt{g_{44}} = \text{const} \qquad (26)$$

rather than for the proper temperature $T_o$ itself.

From an observational point of view, this new conclusion may not be very important, since the change in temperature with position would only be

$$\frac{d \log T}{dr} = 10^{-17}\ \text{cm}^{-1} \qquad (27)$$

in a gravitational field having the intensity of that at the earth's surface. From a theoretical point of view it is of interest, however, in leading to a modification of one of the most cherished results of the classical thermodynamics.

It should be emphasized, nevertheless, that this modification is entirely reasonable from the point of view of relativity. In accordance with that theory all forms of energy have mass and weight, and it is hence indeed not surprising that a temperature gradient is necessary to prevent the flow of heat from regions of higher to those of lower gravitational potential when thermal equilibrium has been reached. Furthermore, since the pressure of black-body radiation in equilibrium with a thermal system would evidently have to increase as we go to lower gravitational levels, in order to support the weight of radiation above, we can also see from purely mechanical considerations that temperature must increase with depth.

(*b*) *Possibility for Reversible Processes at a Finite Rate.* To turn to a second example, we have long been accustomed to believe as a result of the classical theory that *reversible* thermodynamic processes taking place at a *finite rate* could never occur in nature, since a finite rate of change would make it impossible to achieve that maximum efficiency which would permit a restoration both of the system and its surroundings to their original states.

To illustrate this we may consider a fluid contained in a cylinder with non-conducting walls and provided with a piston as shown in Fig. 1. The *reversible* expansion of this fluid with the piston moving out at a *finite rate* would evidently be impossible, in the first place since there would be friction between the piston and the walls, and in the second place since the fluid in flowing in behind the moving piston would not be able to maintain as high a pressure and hence do as much external work as at an infinitesimal rate of expansion. It has hence been concluded in the past that the reversible expansion of a fluid at a finite rate would under all circumstances be impossible.

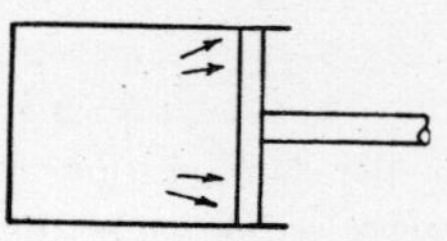

Fig. 1. Classical cylinder

[9] Tolman and Ehrenfest, *Phys. Rev.*, 36: 1791, 1930.

In relativistic thermodynamics, nevertheless, this situation is altered in an important manner by new possibilities for changes to take place in the proper volume of an element of fluid, because of changes in the gravitational potentials which were neglected in the older theory. To illustrate this, Fig. 2 attempts

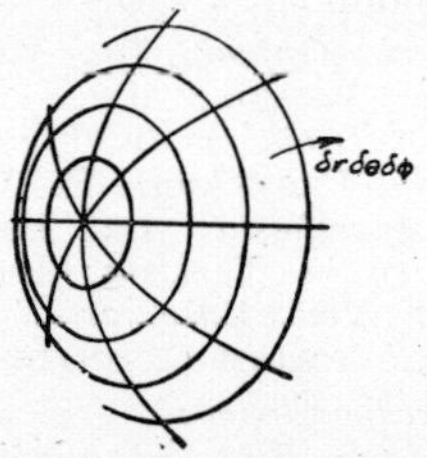


Fig. 2. Relativistic non-static universe

to give a symbolic two-dimensional representation of the space-like coordinates, corresponding to the line element

$$ds^2 = -\frac{e^{g(t)}}{\left[1+\frac{r^2}{4R^2}\right]^2}(dr^2 + r^2\,d\,\theta^2 + r^2 \sin\theta\, d\,\phi^2) + dt^2 \qquad (28)$$

which characterizes the homogeneous distribution of fluid, that we usually call a non-static model of the universe. These coordinates are so selected that any element of fluid lying in a given coordinate range $\delta r\ \ \delta\theta\ \ \delta\phi$ will remain permanently therein. The proper volume of such an element of the fluid as measured by a local observer will then be

$$\delta V_o = \frac{e^{\frac{3}{2}g(t)}}{\left[1+\frac{r^2}{4R^2}\right]^3} r^2 \sin\theta\, \delta r\, \delta\theta\, \delta\phi \qquad (29)$$

and this will change with the time t at a finite rate on account of the occurrence of the function g(t) in the gravitational potentials and hence also in the expression for proper volume.

These changes in proper volume take place, however, in the first place quite obviously without any friction of moving parts, and in the second place with a perfect balance between internal and external pressures owing to the uniformity of conditions throughout the fluid. Thus the two sources of irreversibility in the previous classical illustration are completely eliminated. Furthermore, there can be no irreversible heat flow in the model under consideration, again owing to the uniform conditions throughout the fluid and the possibility of irreversible processes within each element of the fluid can be eliminated by the choice of a sufficiently simple substance. As a consequence it has proved possible to construct conceptual models of this kind[10] which can expand or contract at a finite rate, and nevertheless satisfy the relativistic condition for reversibility by maintaining the sign of equality instead of inequality in the simple expression

$$\frac{d}{dt}(\phi_o \, \delta V_o) \geqq 0 \qquad (30)$$

which results from the application of the general form of the relativistic second law (19) to the present case.

This possibility for reversible thermodynamic processes taking place at a finite rate seems very strange from the point of view of the classical thermodynamics. Nevertheless, from the relativistic point of view the result seems both rational and, indeed, perhaps inevitable, when we recall that the principles of *relativistic mechanics* alone, without bothering about thermodynamics, have been found sufficient to show[11] the possibility of constructing models of the kind in question, which—when filled with such simple fluids as a perfect monatomic gas or black-body radiation—would expand at a finite rate to an upper limit and then precisely retrace their steps to their original density, pressure and temperature.

(*c*) *Possibility for Irreversible Processes without Reaching a Final State of Maximum Entropy.* As a final example of the differences between classical and relativistic thermodynamics, let us now turn to the classical conclusion that the ultimate result of irreversible processes taking place in a system having no interaction with its surroundings would necessarily be a state of maximum entropy where further change would be impossible.

To illustrate the classical reasons for belief in this principle, let us consider a simple homogeneous system consisting of a gas of uniform pressure, temperature, and composition throughout. The state of such a system can be specified by its energy E, volume v, and the number of mols $N_1$, $N_2$, etc., of the different chemical substances which it contains, and in accordance with a fundamental expression, provided by the work of Gibbs himself,[12] its entropy can then be determined with the help of the general equation

$$dS = \frac{dE}{T} + \frac{p}{T}dv + \left(\frac{\partial S}{\partial N_1}\right) dN_1 + \left(\frac{\partial S}{\partial N_2}\right) dN_2 + \ldots \qquad (31)$$

[10] Tolman, *Phys. Rev.*, 37: 1639, 1931; *ibid.*, 38: 797, 1931.

[11] Einstein, Berl. Ber. (1931) p. 235; Tolman, *Phys. Rev.*, 38: 1758, 1931.

[12] Allowing for the difference in notation and form, equation (31) is equivalent to the fundamental equation (12) given in the "Collected Works of Gibbs." Vol. I, p. 63. Longmans, Green and Company, 1928.

In applying this expression, however, to the special case of a system having no interaction with its surroundings, it was necessary in the classical thermodynamics to take the energy change dE equal to zero to agree with the classical principle of energy conservation. It was also necessary, for a system having no interaction with its surroundings, to take either the volume-change dv equal to zero or the pressure p itself equal to zero to prevent the performance of work on the surroundings. In both cases the only chance for entropy increase and hence for change would then lie in the readjustment of chemical composition. At constant energy and volume, moreover, this would have to cease when the entropy reached the maximum possible value compatible with the fixed value of energy and volume; while at constant energy and zero pressure the gas would be infinitely dilute and a final state of maximum entropy would be reached when all the molecules of gas had disassociated into their atoms.

In the relativistic treatment of this problem, nevertheless, the application of relativistic mechanics alone is sufficient to show a very different state of affairs. In the relativistic treatment, the analogue of the preceding homogeneous isolated system will evidently be a non-static model of the universe, since the line element for these models corresponds to a completely homogeneous distribution of fluid with no interaction with anything outside the system itself. By the application of relativistic mechanics, however, it has been shown by the work of Professor Ward and myself,[13] that there is a great class of such models, obtained by taking the cosmological constant $\Lambda$ equal to zero or less, which could apparently undergo a continued succession of expansions and contractions without ever coming to rest. To be sure, the equations that we now have available for our highly idealized models are only sufficient to describe the expansion of the models to their upper limit and return, and not sufficient to describe their passage through the exceptional point at their lower limit of volume. Nevertheless, on physical grounds we must be inclined to assume that contraction to the lower limit of volume would be followed by renewed expansion.

It is to be specially noted now, however, that our conclusion as to the possibility of such behavior is based solely on mechanical equations alone and is quite independent of assumptions as to the reversibility or irreversibility of any thermodynamic processes that may take place in the fluid, although in the case of irreversible processes it can be shown that successive expansions have a tendency to go to larger and larger volumes before returning. The possibility thus

[13] Tolman, *Phys. Rev.*, 39: 320, 1932; Tolman and Ward, *ibid.*, 39: 835, 1932.

provided for an unending succession of irreversible expansions and contractions seems very strange from the point of view of classical thermodynamics, but can nevertheless be shown to be reasonable from the point of view of relativistic thermodynamics.

The application of the relativistic second law to these non-static models leads to the general result

$$\frac{d}{dt_o}(\phi_o\,\delta V_o) \geqq 0 \qquad (32)$$

which states that the proper entropy of each element of the fluid as measured by a local observer can only remain constant or increase with local time. With a fluid of composition simple enough to eliminate the possibility for changes other than in density, we obtain the conditions necessary for constant entropy, and are led to the reversible expansions and contractions at a finite rate previously considered. With a slightly more complicated fluid, such as a gas which tends to disassociate as the density is lowered, we can obtain the irreversible increases in entropy in which we are now interested, since the composition of the fluid will then lag behind the changes in volume, and the processes of disassociation and recombination will always take place in the direction of an equilibrium which has not been attained.

From a classical point of view, such a continuous irreversible increase in entropy in an isolated system which undergoes a never-ending succession of expansions and recontractions to an earlier volume might seem impossible, since the energy of the isolated system would have to remain constant, and with a given value of energy and volume there would be a definite, maximum possible value of entropy.

From the relativistic point of view, nevertheless, it is easy to see that this continued increase in entropy could be made possible by the failure in relativistic mechanics of the ordinary principle of energy conservation. Indeed the application of relativistic mechanics to the models in question leads to the result

$$\frac{d}{dt_o}(\rho_{oo}\,\delta V_o) + p_o\frac{d}{dt_o}(\delta V_o) = 0 \qquad (33)$$

which shows that the proper energy ($\rho_{00}\,\delta V_0$) of each element of fluid in the model will decrease as the model expands and increase as it contracts, and since the general effect of irreversibility would be to give higher pressures during compression than during the preceding expansion, we are thus provided with the needed mechanism for a gradual increase in proper energy and hence also in the proper entropy of the elements of fluid.

The difference between the classical and relativistic points of view can also be illustrated in a somewhat different manner, if we return to the classical cylinder and relativistic model of the universe given by Figs. 1 and 2, and consider a continued succession of expansions and contractions, in both cases providing for irreversibility by again introducing for example a gas which tends to disassociate when the pressure is lowered.

The classical man who is engaged in moving the piston of his cylinder successively in and out reports that the entropy inside the cylinder is all the time getting greater and greater, because the gas can not disassociate fast enough on the way out nor recombine fast enough on the way in to maintain equilibrium. He also reports, however, that the energy inside his cylinder—which is now no longer an isolated system—is also getting greater and greater, since the pressure has a tendency to be too high to correspond to equilibrium on compression and too low on expansion, so that he does more work on the way in than he gets back on the way out. He then finally remarks that this continued increase in energy indeed provides in the case of this non-isolated system an opportunity for the entropy to go on increasing forever, but that he personally is getting very tired of the silly experiment, and is going to have to stop:—not now because the irreversible processes will ever lead to an unsurpassable maximum of entropy but because he actually won't have the necessary energy to push in the piston one time more.

How different the remarks of the relativistic man as he sits calmly by and—in his mind's eye—watches his conceptual model expand and contract. "Yes," he says, "I notice that the proper entropy of each element of fluid is all the time increasing owing to successive processes of disassociation and recombination under conditions that do not correspond to equilibrium." "I do not worry, however, since I also notice that the proper energy of each element of fluid is also increased after a succession of expansions and contractions sufficiently to allow for this increase in entropy, and I know that the principles of relativistic mechanics not only permit such increases in proper energy, but indicate—without reference to reversibility or irreversibility—the continued succession of expansions and contractions that I observe."

This completes the discussion of examples illustrating the kind of conclusions that we may expect from the extension of thermodynamics to general relativity.

## (6) Conclusion

Much remains to be done in the further application and development of relativistic thermodynamics. The application to systems in which heat flow is taking place from one portion of the fluid to another has not yet been undertaken and might lead to interesting results. It could be of special importance when we have made more progress in the treatment of nonhomogeneous models of the universe which may well be necessary for a better understanding of the actual universe. The development of relativistic thermodynamics to include an appropriate treatment of fluctuations might also be attempted with the help of the statistical methods introduced by Gibbs himself. The effect of fluctuations on the behavior of cosmological models might be specially important at certain stages of their history.

In trying to estimate the significance of the applications of relativistic thermodynamics that have already been made, we must not misjudge the nature of the two applications to cosmological models that were described in the foregoing. It should be emphasized that the homogeneous cosmological models which we now consider are not only very highly simplified and idealized, but at best are constructed to agree throughout their entire extent with that small sample of the actual universe which lies within the range of some $10^8$ light years. Furthermore, it must be remembered that among the different possible kinds of homogeneous cosmological model, there is a class which would expand never to return as well as the class that could undergo an unending succession of expansions and contractions; and we do not now have sufficient data so that we could assign the actual universe to either class. Hence we must be very careful, in extrapolating to the actual universe any conclusions that we may draw as to the behavior of our conceptual models.

The dangers of long-range extrapolation were specially emphasized to you by Professor Bridgman in his beautiful Gibbs memorial lecture of last year, and these dangers, as we see, are specially present in cosmological speculations, based on the observation of a small fragment of the total universe for an inappreciable time span. Nevertheless, it certainly seems significant that conceptual models of the universe can be constructed, which are permitted by the principles of relativistic thermodynamics to exhibit behavior in serious conflict with the classical conclusions, that reversible processes could never take place at a finite rate, and that the end result of irreversible processes would necessarily be a stationary condition of maximum entropy. Hence at the very least it would now seem desirable to extrapolate to a cautious position, in which we no longer dogmatically assert that the principles of thermodynamics necessarily require a universe created at a finite time in the past and fated for stagnation and death in the future. Indeed, the chief duty and glory of theoretical science is certainly, not merely to describe in complicated language those facts that are already known, but to extrapolate—as cautiously and wisely as may be—into regions yet unexplored but pregnant with human interest.

# ACTIVE IRON

By Dr. OSKAR BAUDISCH

DEPARTMENT OF CHEMISTRY, YALE UNIVERSITY

IN the year 1806 the Bergrat Johann Georg Lenz named a natural iron oxide hydrate "goethite," in honor of the celebrated naturalist and poet, Johann Wolfgang von Goethe. This mineral had already been known in the literature previously under the name ruby mica (Rubinglimmer).[1] Although comparatively rare, it is found in good crystalline form in Siegen, in Westphalia. The splendid crystals, one to two millimeters long, indeed resemble rubies in their beautiful color and luster. The crystals or powder made from them are non-magnetic, but if one dehydrates the powder by heating it a magnetic iron oxide, $Fe_2O_3$, is obtained. This interesting observation was described as early as 1838 in the book "Grundzüge der Mineralogie" by Franz von Kobel (published in Nürnberg in 1838). The names ruby mica and goethite are used interchangeably for this macro-crystalline brown iron ore in the "Manual of Mineralogy" by Robert Allan (Edinburgh, 1834). It is seen, therefore, that historically the names ruby mica and goethite properly apply to the natural iron oxide hydrate which becomes magnetic on heating.

In the year 1848, Plücker made a magnetic study of the natural and artificial iron oxides and oxide hydrates, and observed that an iron oxide hydrate prepared in a certain way gave a magnetic iron oxide on dehydration. He found it almost a hundred times stronger magnetically than the original hydrate from which it was prepared, and remarked that the powdered material could be picked up by even a small horseshoe magnet. Robbins mentioned a magnetic iron oxide in *Chemical News* in the year 1859.

Malaguti in 1863 (*Compte Rendus*) published more exact chemical and physical data on the properties of magnetic iron oxide. He obtained the oxide in various ways, as, for example, by explosion of magnetite with potassium chlorate and by heating ferrous salts of organic acids in the air. In France the magnetic iron oxide is also known under the name Malaguti-oxide.

1 J. F. L. Hausman, ''Handbuch der Mineralogie,'' Göttingen, 1813.

The fact that this magnetic iron oxide contained iron only in its completely oxidized state (ferric), was definitely established by Hilpert in 1909. Until this time all samples had contained varying amounts of incompletely oxidized iron (ferrous).

To turn again to the iron oxide hydrates, it must be noted that our view-points on these important iron compounds, which occur so abundantly in nature, have been fundamentally changed. Formerly on a basis of chemical analysis and superficial characterization, the natural iron oxide hydrates were classified as to water content. Thus, iron oxides combined with 3, 2, 1½, 1, ¾ and ½ molecules of water were classed as separate species. These distinctions did not recognize the fact that part of the total water present is chemically linked and part only absorbed. Consequently, the majority of the older chemical formulas assigned to iron oxide hydrates are meaningless.

More exact studies, in particular x-ray analyses, have proved that there is only one definite chemical combination between iron oxide and water, namely, the monohydrate, $Fe_2O_3 \cdot H_2O$. This is known to exist in two different modifications, both of which exist in nature and may be prepared synthetically. Since the oxides prepared by dehydration of the two monohydrates are genetically related to the natural dimorphous aluminum oxides, diaspore and bauxite, according to a proposal of Haber (*Naturwissenschaften,* 1925) they were named α and γ hydrates and oxides. This designation has been adopted not only by chemists and physicists but by mineralogists as well.

There are two common differences between the α and γ hydrates. Each has a distinct x-ray spectrum. Also they may be more easily distinguished by their magnetic properties. The α hydrates on dehydration yield a non-magnetic α oxide (hematite), while the γ hydrates yield a strongly magnetic (ferromagnetic) γ oxide. Since goethite, as we have seen, becomes ferromagnetic on dehydration it belongs to the γ hydrate class.

The various natural iron oxide hydrates formerly mentioned are merely micro-crystalline aggregates of α $Fe_2O_3 \cdot H_2O$ (Böhm, 1928; Albrecht, 1929). The differences depend partly on a chemical reaction (polymerization) of the molecules, and partly on the difference in the arrangement, form and size of the crystallites (clusters of sub-microscopic crystals). The different shades of color depend mainly on the particle size.

For the more detailed study of the structure (fine and hyper-fine structure) which remains to be carried out, it is necessary first of all to have pure materials. It is important to prepare iron oxide hydrates and iron oxides which are free from electrolytes, since such impurities may greatly influence the magnetic and surface properties. This we have succeeded in doing, through the use of organic bases, for example, pyridine and aniline. The purest obtainable iron, that prepared from iron pentacarbonyl, serves as starting material. It is dissolved in hydrochloric acid and autoxidized in the presence of pyridine to a very pure γ iron oxide hydrate, with the study of which we are now concerned. This γ hydrate gives on dehydration a ferromagnetic ferric oxide which is free from all impurities of electrolytes.

There now remains only to report briefly of the progress that has been made with γ oxide since the work of Hilpert, and how our study in this field has brought us to designate the concept "active iron."

The fundamental discovery which led to the introduction of the concept "active iron" into biology was that of Welo and Baudisch[2] concerning the interesting and peculiar behavior of ferromagnetic ferric oxide. We found that the lattice of ferromagnetic ferric oxide, $Fe_2O_3$, is cubic, whereas hematite, $Fe_2O_3$, is rhombohedral, as was already known. The paramagnetic modification corresponding to hematite is stable, while the ferromagnetic modification is unstable and can pass over, with loss of energy and loss of ferromagnetism, into the stable form. The surprising observation that magnetite retains its spinel crystal structure on oxidation and first passes to the rhombohedral hematite structure on strong heating led us to designate the ferromagnetic gamma oxide as "active" in contrast to the inactive form corresponding to hematite. The strikingly different physical and physico-chemical behaviors of these chemically identical iron oxides led us to compare their biological actions. The experiments of Webster and Baudisch showed, in fact, that the two oxides had different biological effects. The designation "active iron" therefore assumed biological significance.

Since, in the medical literature, the term "active iron" has often been completely distorted and confused in relation to and in comparison with the sense in which we use it, it seems necessary to include a further discussion of the development of the problem. The original identification of the two forms of ferric oxide (alpha and gamma), became, one might say, only an introduction to further study and further knowledge of the topochemistry and the magnetic properties of iron oxides. The designations "active" and "inactive" had, later, to be expanded and developed.

It has been mentioned that by x-ray analysis one can determine only the type of arrangement, while by magnetic measurements one can at least detect

[2] SCIENCE, 62: 1605, 311–312. 1925.

finer structural anomalies and consequent surface irregularities. We therefore made detailed magnetic studies of magnetite and several ferromagnetic iron oxides prepared in different ways. This was done, as is usual in the study of ferromagnetic materials, by taking the magnetization curves for increasing and decreasing magnetizing fields; that is, we determined the hysteresis loops. The four constants characteristic of ferromagnetic materials may be obtained from these curves. They are: the permeability (simply related to susceptibility), which is a measure of the magnetization; the hysteresis loss, which is a measure of the resistance to orientation of the elementary magnets and hence appears as a transformation of electromagnetic energy into heat; the remanence, which is the residual magnetization after the field is removed, since orientation, when once attained, may persist in varying degree; and finally, the coercive force, which is the field that must be applied in the opposite direction to demagnetize the substance. Both remanence and coercive force are secondary features of the hysteresis phenomenon. If the hysteresis loss is large, both the remanence and the coercive force are large. For example, in steel hysteresis loss, remanence and coercive force are large, while in soft iron all three of these quantities are relatively small.

The result of these studies was that while the several oxides differed somewhat as to permeability, they differed enormously as to the constants associated with hysteresis. But after the several differently prepared oxides had been annealed at high temperatures they gave nearly the same values for the hysteresis loss, remanence and coercive force. It is this fact which is the basis for our conclusion that it is the crystal quality (lattice perfection and absence of atomic deformation) which is markedly affected by changing the method of preparation. The magnetic investigation, therefore, gave us a means of tracing the finer structural features which occur in regions of too small dimensions or are for other reasons not accessible to x-ray analysis. In other words, while we can establish the fine structure of ferromagnetic iron oxides by the x-ray, it becomes possible by magnetic analysis to establish the existence of a still finer one—a hyperfine structure.

To these exact physical methods of investigation the biological methods joined themselves naturally and it was found that the latter were not less but rather more sensitive than the magnetic methods to hyperfine structural differences. By combination of these methods one can gain an insight into biological phenomena that would otherwise be quite impossible.

Our investigations, as they have been briefly described in the foregoing, have given rise to a whole array of researches in the field of the metal oxides, especially those of iron. Chemists, physicists, engineers, mineralogists, geologists, pharmacologists and medical men have repeated the experiments and supplemented them in various directions, according to their particular fields of interest.

# SCIENTIFIC EVENTS

## THE JUNIOR SCIENCE CLUBS OF THE AMERICAN INSTITUTE

THE Junior Science Clubs of the American Institute were the guests, on the morning of March 25, of the Museum of Science and Industry and the American Museum of Natural History.

Museum Day was planned by the American Institute as a new departure in its program of science educational projects for children. Recently the institute, a century old organization, has associated hundreds of science clubs made up of young people all over the city into its new branch, the Junior Science Clubs. The members of these clubs represent some seven or eight thousand children, all under eighteen years of age.

The meeting at the Museum of Science and Industry was open to all member Physical Science Clubs. The group was divided into two sections, one going directly to the main exhibit hall and one to the museum theater. In the main exhibit hall, Robert P. Shaw, of the Museum of Science and Industry, spoke on "The Story of Electricity." The hall was darkened and a spotlight was thrown on the various exhibits as they illustrated Mr. Shaw's talk. In the museum theater, the second group was shown the following series of science motion pictures: "The Romance of Power"; "Dynamic America"; "A. B. C. of Electricity," and "Finding His Voice." The groups then changed places and the program was repeated.

To the American Museum of Natural History meeting members of the Biological Science Clubs were invited.

At the meeting at the museum Paul B. Mann, chairman of the department of biology of Evander Childs High School, spoke on "The Museum's Part in Exploration," illustrated with motion pictures taken by Roy Chapman Andrews.

The group was then broken up into five sections, each of which visited one of the various museum trails. Members of the museum's staff were stationed in the different halls, where they gave short talks on the contents of each. The children then, under the guidance of these staff members, spent the rest of the morning inspecting the Darwin Hall, Insect Hall, Mammal Hall, Bird Hall and Fish Hall.

## THE SIXTH ANNUAL SUMMER SYMPOSIUM IN THEORETICAL PHYSICS AT THE UNIVERSITY OF MICHIGAN

IN the summer of 1923, the University of Michigan invited Professor Karl T. Compton of Princeton University and Professor F. A. Saunders of Harvard University to give special lectures during the summer session. These lectures initiated a policy which has been maintained ever since. For the first five years the subjects covered by the lecturers were primarily in the field of experimental physics, but beginning with the session of 1928, a symposium in theoretical physics was inaugurated, and since that date the visiting lecturers have treated theoretical subjects exclusively. An examination of the list of lecturers discloses the fact that many of the foremost physicists of America and Europe have appeared on these summer programs. Particularly in recent years these meetings have attracted not only advanced students but also members of other university and college faculties, and research physicists from governmental and industrial laboratories. The summer is apparently the only time that such men can attend, and the course of eight weeks is sufficiently long to give a very adequate treatment either of an introductory course in modern theoretical physics or of a very advanced one covering perhaps material receiving its first public presentation. In addition to the regular lecture courses there are numerous informal meetings of groups limited to those interested in special problems.

The sixth symposium will be held between the dates June 26 and August 18. In the first or second week of this period Professor Niels Bohr of Copenhagen will give several lectures on "The Foundations of Atomic Mechanics." Professor Enrico Fermi of Rome will lecture throughout the eight weeks of the session on "The Structure of the Atomic Nucleus." Following Professor Bohr's lectures Professor J. H. Van Vleck of Wisconsin will lecture for four weeks on "The Recent Developments in the Theory of Magnetism." Professor G. E. Uhlenbeck of Michigan will give a course on "Quantum Mechanics" and Professor D. M. Dennison of Michigan a course on "The Theory of Band Spectra." Both of these last courses will be given throughout the summer. The informal seminars which meet several times weekly will be under the general supervision of Professors Fermi and Van Vleck. Holders of doctors degrees may attend all lectures, courses and seminars as guests of the university.

In addition to the symposium lectures the department of physics offers its regular advanced courses. Facilities for experimental research are available, particularly in spectroscopy in the fields of x-rays, ultra violet, visible, near and far infra-red, in sound, in electronics and in vacuum tube phenomena.

## CONFERENCE ON RECENT DEVELOPMENTS IN CHEMISTRY AT THE JOHNS HOPKINS UNIVERSITY

THE Johns Hopkins University will this summer conduct a second conference on recent developments in chemistry in conjunction with the regular summer session at the institution.

The conference will be divided into five consecutive sessions of one week each. Each week will be devoted to one phase of chemical progress, and will include lectures by men known in that particular field.

"Organic Chemistry Related to Medicine" will be the subject of discussion during the week of June 26, and speakers from the Johns Hopkins School of Medicine and from outside institutions will present various phases of the work. E. Emmet Reid and G. H. Corwin will have charge of the week's program. On June 26, Hugh Young, Justina Hill, Fitzgerald Dunning, Edwin C. White and W. C. Harden will deal with the general subject of "Antiseptics." On June 27, "Oxidation and Reduction" will be discussed by E. Emmet Reid, Leslie Hellerman and G. H. Corwin.

Gordon M. Dean and Hans Jensen will be the speakers on June 28, presenting phases of the topic, "Insulin and Proteins." A sound film, "Some Biochemical, Pharmacological and Medical Experiences as Told to Chemists," by Dr. John J. Abel, will be shown in the evening of that day. On June 29 Joseph C. Bloodgood will preside over a program devoted to "Chemistry and Physics in Cancer." The speakers will include Dr. Bloodgood, Charles F. Geschickter, E. A. Peterson, Dudley Jackson, Curtis Burnam, M. A. Tuve, Carl Voegtlin, Warren H. Lewis, Margaret Lewis and George Otto Gey. Motion pictures related to the subject of cancer will be presented in the evening. June 30 will be devoted to "Chemotherapy," aspects of which will be discussed by Hugh Young, Justina Hill and David I. Macht.

During the week of July 3, Joseph E. Mayer will preside over a program devoted to "Physical Treatment of Molecular Binding." The speakers for the week, in the order in which they will present their discusisons, are Dr. Mayer, Maurice L. Huggins, Hugh M. Smallwood, Henry Eyring and Saul Dushman. "X-rays and Structure of Matter" will be the general topic for the week of July 10. Emil Ott will preside, and speakers for the week will include Ralph W. G. Wyckoff, Maurice L. Huggins and Dr. Ott. For the week of July 17, a topic of especial interest to physicists has been selected. "The Application of Optical Methods and Instruments to Chemical Research" will be discussed, A. Herman Pfund presiding over the week's program. The speakers will be Dr. Pfund, George F. A. Stutz, H. E. Merwin and Ralph H. Muller.

The final week will be devoted to the subject of "Catalysis." J. C. W. Frazer will be chairman of the program for the week of July 24, and the speakers for the conference will include Paul Hugh Emmett, Dr. Frazer, Arthur F. Benton, J. A. Becker and Herbert G. Tanner.

Those interested in the conferences may register for the full five weeks, or for any part of the program that attracts them. Cottages on the shore of the Chesapeake Bay, within commuting distance of the university, are available for those who wish to combine a summer vacation with scientific study and discussion.

### IN HONOR OF DR. ELIHU THOMSON

ACCORDING to the final plans for the dinner held at the Massachusetts Institute of Technology on March 29, leaders in science, engineering and education paid tribute to Dr. Elihu Thomson, dean of electrical engineers and inventor, on his eightieth birthday.

A correspondent writes: "Within the span of four score years Dr. Thomson, a pioneer in electrical science, has witnessed and played an important part in the development of the country's great electrical industry. He is the last of the magnificent 'big four,' Thomas A. Edison, Charles F. Brush and James J. Wood. Three of them gave the people electric lighting systems, Edison invented the incandescent lamp. To-day Dr. Thomson is the 'last of the first,' with more than seven hundred United States patents to his credit. From 1920 to 1922 Dr. Thomson was acting president of the Massachusetts Institute of Technology. He is a life member of its corporation and a non-resident professor of applied electricity."

On the afternoon of Dr. Thomson's birthday there was a conference at which brief lectures on the historical development of the applications of electricity, modern theories and the present trends of research were presented. According to the program, President Karl T. Compton, of the Massachusetts Institute of Technology, discussed the historical aspects of electricity with particular reference to Dr. Thomson's achievements in this field. Dr. John C. Slater, head of the institute's department of physics, discussed modern theories of electricity, and Dr. K. K. Darrow, research physicist at the Bell Telephone Laboratories, spoke on the trends of modern research.

As part of this celebration, many models and some of the originals of Dr. Thomson's most significant inventions were on exhibition. This exhibition was open to guests on Wednesday, continuing for the public from Thursday to Sunday, from 2 to 5 P. M. The models included the frictional electrical machine made from a discarded wine bottle by Dr. Thomson when he was eleven years old, and a dynamo invented in 1878, which has all the essentials of the great modern generators. Many early types of the arc lamps designed by Dr. Thomson and his colleague, Professor E. J. Houston, are shown. One of the most significant exhibits was the Thomson recording wattmeter, forerunner of the 30,000,000 meters now installed in homes, factories and stores to record the amount of energy consumed. There were shown early types of lightning arresters, as well as Dr. Thomson's first electrical resistance welding transformer, a method which is now universally used in almost every branch of manufacturing.

It was expected that President Karl T. Compton would preside at the dinner, at which Governor Joseph B. Ely, of Massachusetts, would voice the tribute of the people of Massachusetts to Dr. Thomson. George B. Cortelyou, president of the Consolidated Gas Company of New York, was expected to speak for the electrical industries and Dr. Harry P. Charlesworth, president of the American Institute of Electrical Engineers, in the name of the engineering societies, to pay honor to the inventor. The tribute of educational institutions, many of which had bestowed upon Dr. Thomson their highest academic honors, was to be given by Dr. Vannevar Bush, vice-president of the institute and dean of engineering. Other speakers announced were Dr. Harvey Cushing, of Harvard University, who represented professions other than engineering, and Mr. E. W. Rice, Jr., honorary chairman of the board of the General Electric Company, its former president, and one of Dr. Thomson's earliest associates in the electrical industry in Lynn, for his friends and colleagues.

## SCIENTIFIC NOTES AND NEWS

DR. WILLIAM H. WELCH, whose eighty-third birthday occurred on April 8, has been confined to the Brady Clinic of the Johns Hopkins Hospital since February 1. It is announced that there is a slow improvement in his condition.

DR. THEOBALD SMITH, of the department of animal pathology, Rockefeller Institute for Medical Research, Princeton, New Jersey, will deliver the Thayer Lectures at the Johns Hopkins Medical School on April 5, 6 and 7.

PROFESSOR ARTHUR H. COMPTON, of the University of Chicago, will direct courses in "Electricity and Magnetism" and on "X-Rays and Electrons" during the summer session of Columbia University.

AT a dinner in celebration of the seventy-fifth anniversary of the Pathological Society of Philadelphia on March 9, honorary membership was conferred on Drs. Harvey Cushing and Frank B. Mallory, of the Harvard Medical School; on Dr. James Ewing, of Memorial Hospital, New York, and Dr. Karl Landsteiner, of the Rockefeller Institute. Dr. Fielding H. Garrison, of the Johns Hopkins University, and Dr. David Riesman, of the University of Pennsylvania, were the principal speakers.

DR. FRITZ VON WETTSTEIN, professor of botany at Munich, has been elected a member of the Bavarian Academy of Sciences. Corresponding members have been elected as follows: Dr. Franz Meyer, professor of mathematics at Königsberg; Dr. Kurt Hensel, professor of mathematics at Marburg; Dr. Paul Guthnick, professor of astronomy at Berlin, and Professor Hans Ludendorff, director of the Astrophysical Observatory at Potsdam.

THE Royal Aeronautical Society has awarded its gold medal to Sir Richard Glazebrook, from 1899 to 1919 director of the British National Physical Laboratory. This medal has been awarded six times previously: to the Wright brothers, Octave Chanute, Professor Bryan, E. T. Busk, Professor Lanchester and Professor L. Prandtl. Sir Richard Glazebrook has been chairman of the Aeronautical Research Committee since its formation as the Advisory Committee for Aeronautics in 1909. He is retiring from the position next month.

AT the fifty-fifth annual general meeting of the Institute of Chemistry, held in London on March 1, the Meldola Medal was presented to Dr. Leslie Ernest Sutton, of Oxford, and the Sir Edward Frankland Medal and Prize to Dr. Leslie Young, of the Royal College of Science. Dr. Jocelyn Field Thorpe, professor of organic chemistry in the Imperial College of Science and Technology, London, was elected president in succession to Dr. G. C. Clayton, director of Imperial Chemical Industries.

DR. WILLIAM BOWIE, chief of the divison of geodesy, U. S. Coast and Geodetic Survey, was reelected honorary president of the Pan-American Institute of Geography and History at the congress held last December in Rio de Janeiro, Brazil.

THE officers of the Harvey Society for 1933–34 are as follows: *President,* Alfred F. Hess; *Vice-president,* R. Keith Cannan; *Treasurer,* T. M. Rivers; *Secretary,* Edgar Stillman; *Council,* S. R. Benedict, Robert F. Loeb and Wade H. Brown.

DR. ARTHUR B. LAMB, president of the American Chemical Society, was the speaker at a luncheon meeting of the writers of abstracts and the assistant editors of *Chemical Abstracts* on March 28. Dr. Charles E. Munroe, who was honorary chairman of the Washington meeting of the American Chemical Society and who has served as an assistant editor of *Chemical Abstracts* since its beginning in 1907, was also a guest of honor.

DR. CHARLES FREDERICK ROOS, formerly assistant professor of mathematics at Cornell University and later permanent secretary of the American Association for the Advancement of Science, has been awarded a Guggenheim fellowship. He plans to write a book on dynamical economics in consultation with European scholars.

DR. A. R. MOORE, research professor of general physiology, University of Oregon, sailed from San Francisco for Japan on March 24, to spend a year as visiting professor of biology in the Tohoku Imperial University at Sendai. He will be in the Biological Institute of the university, the director of which is Professor Shinkishi Hatai. The visiting professorship is maintained by the Rockefeller Foundation.

PROFESSOR J. PROUDMAN has been appointed to the chair of oceanography at the University of Liverpool, vacant through the death of Professor J. Johnstone.

HERBERT L. DAVIS, for the past four years a Heckscher research assistant to Professor W. D. Bancroft at Cornell University, has been appointed assistant professor of chemistry at Westminster College, New Wilmington, Pennsylvania.

DR. CORNELIA T. SNELL has left the Fifth Avenue Hospital to take a position at the College of Physicians and Surgeons of Columbia University. She will work with Drs. T. F. Zucker and Benjamin Berg in connection with their studies of diabetes.

PROFESSOR RALPH J. FOGG, formerly head of the department of civil engineering at Lehigh University, is serving as a technical expert under the National Transportation Committee.

DR. OTTO APPEL, director of the Federal Biological Experiment Station at Berlin, Germany, will visit the Wisconsin potato sections this summer following his visit to the Century of Progress Exposition in Chicago.

DR. R. E. COKER, professor of zoology at the University of North Carolina, who is on leave of absence from the university on the Kenan Foundation during 1932–33, is working at the University of Paris.

A PAPER by Dr. M. A. Tuve and L. R. Hafstad on "Atomic Nuclear Studies at the Department of Terrestrial Magnetism," was presented before the Philosophical Society of Washington on March 25.

Mr. John Ruel Manning, in charge of technological investigations, Bureau of Fisheries, Washington, addressed the Alpha Mu chapter of Tri Beta at Western Maryland College on March 21, on "The Nutritional Value of Marine Products."

Professor James Westfall Thompson addressed the History of Science Club at the University of California in Berkeley on March 3 on German science in the fourteenth and fifteenth centuries, giving a presentation of the mathematical achievements and the interconnections of Jordanus Nemorarius, Georg Purbach, Regiomontanus and Cardinal Nicholas of Cusa.

The Bruce-Preller lecture of the Royal Society of Edinburgh will be delivered by Professor C. H. Lander, on October 23. His subject will be "The Utilization of Coal."

A symposium on the utilization of coal, arranged by the British Science Guild, was held on March 27 at the Royal Institution under the chairmanship of Mr. H. T. Tizard. The speakers included Captain B. Acworth, S. Lacey, Eng.-Rear-Admiral W. Scott Hill and A. C. Hardy. The discussion was opened by Dr. O. M. W. Sprague.

During February and March the following visitors gave clinics at the Duke Hospital of the Duke University School of Medicine: Dr. Addison G. Brenizer, of Charlotte, on "The Evolution of Thyroidectomy"; Dr. Hugh Trout, of the Jefferson Hospital, Roanoke, on "The Surgical Treatment of Pulmonary Tuberculosis"; Dr. W. W. S. Butler, Jr., of the Jefferson Hospital, Roanoke, on "Transurethral Resection of Prostate"; Dr. Thomas M. Rivers, of the Hospital of the Rockefeller Institute, on "Filterable Viruses in Relation to the Practise of Medicine"; Dr. B. C. Willis, of the Boyce-Willis Clinic, Rocky Mount, North Carolina, on "Perforated Wounds of the Abdomen."

The fifth lecture to the faculty and students of the School of Medicine, the George Washington University, on the Smith-Reed-Russell Society series was given on March 16 by Dr. Maurice C. Hall, chief of the Zoological Division of the Bureau of Animal Industry, U. S. Department of Agriculture. Dr. Hall's subject was "Drama Anthelmintica." The next lecture in this series, to be given on April 6, by Dr. William H. Howell, chairman of the National Research Council, is entitled "Recollections of a Physiologist during the Past Half Century." The regular faculty seminar for March was given by Professor Charles S. White, of the department of surgery, who spoke on "Chronic Peptic Ulcer in Childhood."

Dr. Bronislaw Malinowski, professor of anthropology in the School of Economics of the University of London, gave a series of lectures on the Messenger Foundation at Cornell University during March on "The Development of Culture: an Enquiry into the Function, Origins and Evolution of Human Beliefs, Customs and Social Organization." The Messenger lectures on the evolution of civilization were inaugurated in 1925, the first lecturer being Professor James H. Breasted, whose subject was the origins of civilization. Other lecturers have been Robert A. Millikan, H. J. C. Grierson, Thomas F. Tout, Edward L. Thorndike, Roscoe Pound, Thomas H. Morgan and Frank Jewett Mather, Jr.

The Rutgers University chapter of Sigma Xi adopted last year the plan of having monthly lectures, sometimes by members of the university faculty, describing their own research work, and sometimes by visitors. The same plan has been in effect this year, and the complete program is as follows: October, Dr. S. A. Waksman, New Jersey Agricultural Experiment Station, "Humus"; November, Dr. Hugh S. Taylor, Princeton University, "The Concept of Speed in Chemical Reactions"; December, Dr. T. C. Nelson, Rutgers University, "A Comparative Study of the Feeding Mechanism of American and European Oysters"; January, Dr. J. W. Shive, New Jersey Agricultural Experiment Station, "The Rôle of Iron in Plants"; February, Dr. C. G. Abbot, Smithsonian Institution, "The Sun"; March, Dr. T. J. Headlee, Rutgers University, "Some Effects of High Frequency Electrostatic Fields on Insects"; April, Dr. Homer W. Smith, New York University Hospital, "The Physiological Evolution of the Kidney."

Public lectures to be given on Saturday at 3:30 p. m. at the New York Botanical Garden are as follows: "Spring Wild Flowers," Dr. John Hendley Barnhart, bibliographer and administrative assistant; "Floral and Scenic Features of the Bahamas," Dr. Marshall A. Howe, assistant director; "Minute Marvels of Aquatic Life," Mr. Robert Hagelstein, honorary curator of Myxomycetes; "Sex in the Fungi," Dr. B. O. Dodge, plant pathologist; "Variegated Plants," Dr. A. B. Stout, director of the laboratories; "Floral and Scenic Features of Porto Rico," Dr. H. A. Gleason, head curator; "Travels through the Mountains of Colorado, Wyoming and South Dakota," Dr. Fred J. Seaver, curator; "A Trip to the Philippines," Dr. Elmer D. Merrill, director-in-chief; "Mushrooms," Dr. William S. Thomas, physician.

The one hundred eighty-fourth regular meeting of the American Physical Society will be held in Washington on April 27, 28 and 29. The Thursday and Friday sessions will be held at the Bureau of Standards and the Saturday sessions at the National Academy

Building. Subsequent meetings are: Salt Lake City, June 15–16, 1933, Pacific Coast; Chicago, June 19–24, 1933, a joint meeting with the American Association for the Advancement of Science; Cincinnati, December 1 and 2, 1933; December, 1933, Pacific Coast, time and place to be announced later; annual meeting, December, 1933, Boston.

THE Canadian Institute of Mining and Metallurgy will meet at Toronto on April 4, 5 and 6. The program calls for some forty addresses by authorities on various phases of mining. For the first time, the Institute of Mining and Metallurgy of London will send its president, Dr. Sydney W. Smith, to confer with the Canadian Association. R. B. Bennett, prime minister, will be the chief speaker at the annual dinner. Other speakers will be Robert C. Stanley, president of the International Nickel Company; Wesley Gordon, federal minister of mines; Charles McCrea, minister of mines for Ontario, and Dr. Smith.

ARRANGEMENTS are being completed for the holding of the 1933 meeting of the Canadian Phytopathological Society at Regina, Saskatchewan, in July. A committee under the chairmanship of Dr. P. M. Simmonds, Saskatoon, has been appointed to look after local arrangements.

THE International Museums Office, on the invitation of the Spanish government, has called a conference to be held in October at Madrid for the study of museum problems.

THOSE interested in forming a Society for Research on Meteorites, whose purpose shall be to promote the discovery, collection, investigation and preservation of meteorites and to advance the science of meteoritics and related sciences through the increase and diffusion of knowledge concerning meteorites, are invited to communicate with the acting secretary of the preliminary organization, Professor H. H. Nininger, director, The Nininger Laboratory, 1955 Fairfax St., Denver, Colorado, or with Frederick C. Leonard, acting president, Department of Astronomy, University of California at Los Angeles, California.

THE following message was sent by President Roosevelt to the fourth congress of the Pan-American Medical Association, which opened at Dallas, Texas, on March 21: "I extend to you and your fellow members of the Pan-American Medical Congress, on behalf of the government, cordial greetings on the opening of the fourth congress, the first to be held in an English-speaking country. The medical profession is deeply interested in the accomplishment of this meeting, which means so much to the health and welfare of the nation, to say nothing of the promotion of friendly relations and mutual understanding between the United States and her sister republics of Latin-America. I am confident that you will find a most hearty welcome by the medical profession and an earnest desire to cooperate with you in every way in furthering the high object of the congress. I wish the members of the fourth congress every success in their great undertaking."

THE Marqués Sanchez Dalp, of Seville, has presented to the Institute of Agrarian Reform his large estates on the banks of the Guadalquivir, covering nearly 10,000 acres and containing 200,000 olive trees and several model farms linked by 56 miles of roads. The Marqués has improved his lands for 40 years and they are now valued at 30,000,000 pesetas (about £700,000). The object of the gift is to help the Spanish government with its schemes of agrarian reform, the intention being that the estates with all the installations on them, such as olive-oil factories and maize and bean sorting and packing machinery, should be used as a school for agriculture.

# DISCUSSION

## PATENTS ARE ETHICAL

THERE has recently been considerable discussion of the propriety of members of a university faculty taking out patents based on their discoveries. Such comments as I have seen have tended to the view that, if patents are obtained, they should ethically be transferred to the university.

With this view I very decidedly disagree; and my opinion is based, not on theory, but on extensive practical experience.

In the first place very few inventions are financially remunerative. If the university is to take the profit, it should also pay the expenses; and if it did pay the expenses, it would generally have a net loss. If an occasional patent does return more than the fees to the U. S. Patent Office and lawyers, the inventor is not thereby tempted to an enervating luxury. As a member of a university faculty, he generally needs an increase of income over and above his university salary. A good invention is as proper a source of income as the authorship of a good book. If the holder of the patent is freed to some extent from financial stringency and care, he will be the better able to devote himself to further scientific discoveries and useful inventions. Bread, or even a little butter on the bread, for a man and his family is one of the prime requisites for research, although this nutritional feature of productive scholarship is often overlooked.

But there are even better reasons for patenting new ideas whenever possible, and for the discoverer or inventor holding the patent himself. He can push it with more knowledge and energy, and can control it for the general welfare more effectively, than can the financial officers of a university. There is an opinion imputed to Emerson to the effect that the inventor of even a better mouse trap, although he hide in a cabin deep in the forest, will find that the world will beat a wide path to his door. I understand that it is doubtful whether Emerson ever said or wrote anything of the sort. He was a sensible man of considerable experience with new ideas; and certainly this statement is utterly contrary, in the large majority of cases, to actual experience. Inventions, like all other new ideas, have generally to be forced on conservative mankind. It would be easy to point to many inventions and other applications of discovery now saving large numbers of lives that would not yet be in use without advertising and the efforts of salesmen. Without commercialization a large part of all the scientific ideas that are now in constant and active use in our daily lives would be locked in books on the dusty shelves of university libraries. It is properly the business of the creative scholar to see to it that, if possible, his ideas serve mankind in his own generation.

But an even stronger duty rests on a discoverer or inventor. He should see to it that his idea or invention is not misused. He should control it. He should find one or more high-grade concerns to develop it. He should afford them at least such little protection as a patent gives against cut-throat competition, after they have spent money to put the invention into practical form and have made a market for it. Without some assurance of such protection it is difficult to get an idea developed and commercialized. The inventor should so far as possible prevent the sale of inferior or harmful imitations.

Often the investigator or inventor will be unable to accomplish all this. But at least he can do it better than the financial officers of a university. Their responsibilities and duties are sufficiently trying just now without this addition.

In this matter, as in all the other relations of scholars to their universities, it should always be assumed that members of university faculties are men of the highest character. Any new practise, rule or regulation that involves even the smallest imputation to the contrary, or that in any way impairs scholarly freedom, will tend rather to diminish than to insure the maintenance of scholarly ethics and faculty morale. Regulations impair ethics.

YANDELL HENDERSON

YALE UNIVERSITY

## UNIVERSITY PATENTS

DR. ALAN GREGG has done a notable service not only to research in medicine but to scientific research in general. John Maynard Keynes has recently said that nothing is more important than that we should get rid of the profit spirit in modern life. His opinion applies more definitely to research than to any other social or human activity. As a matter of history, the scientific discoveries that have ultimately inured to the benefit of society either financially or socially have been made by men like Faraday and Clerk Maxwell who never gave a thought to the possible financial profit of their work. They were driven on by the spirit of curiosity, and that alone should animate workers in scientific laboratories. The moment that research is utilized as a source of profit, its spirit is debased. The state's and the individual's interest in its support is necessarily weakened, and the most glorious characteristic of modern science is debased. There may be a few who will think that Dr. Gregg is treading on their toes. If so, let the "galled jade wince."

ABRAHAM FLEXNER

## MATURATION DIVISIONS IN TRADESCANTIA, RHEO AND OENOTHERA

IN a recent communication Dr. Belling,[1] whose sudden and untimely death is a great loss to biology, has made comments on my recent short article in SCIENCE for January 13, 1933 (pp. 49–50). His courteous criticisms seem to turn on the definition of a univalent chromosome. This may conveniently be described as a single (that is not paired with another) chromosome of the first meiotic division. Consequently neither the so-called bivalents nor their constituents can logically be called univalents. According to the results of a number of investigators, in *Tradescantia virginica,* there are found two kinds of chromosome pairs (the so-called synaptic mates), namely, ring pairs, which resemble those generally seen in meiosis in favorable objects, such as Allium, Lilium, etc., and by contrast a varying number of so-called rod pairs. The ring couples are regarded as parasynaptically mated side by side, while the rod bivalents are believed to represent chromosomes paired telosynaptically end to end. We have thus the truly remarkable paradox of the chromosomes of the same species in the identical meiotic division, conducting themselves in fundamentally different fashions. The conception of telosynapsis or end-to-end pairing has long been in growing disrepute, particularly among geneticists. Favorable material seems to show clearly that the meiotic so-called bivalents are primitively always in relation side by side. My extended and somewhat

[1] SCIENCE, 77, p. 260, March 10, 1933.

comprehensive investigations, covering a wide range of both plants and animals, appear to make it clear that the side-by-side pairs are invariably present in the primary meiotic division. *Tradescantia virginica* presents no exception in this respect. Although the profile view of the metaphase seems to show the contrasting ring and rod bivalents, the polar aspect, which appears to have been neglected by other investigators, makes it clear that the two are identical and only represent the face and lateral views of identical structures.

Further, in *T. virginica,* the so-called zygotene or zygonema phase can always be seen at the appropriate stage. Since this stage is properly regarded as the precursor of the side-by-side bivalents (the so-called parasynaptic mates), its presence automatically excludes the possibility of end-to-end pairs of chromosomes (telosynaptic mates). There is thus an additional reason for regarding all the chromosome pairs of *T. virginica* as side-by-side mates and *none* of them as end-to-end mates. Following a sound practise in cytology and transferring these results to the interpretation of the less clear conditions presented by the genus Rheo and certain species of Oenothera, it becomes obvious that the pairs of consecutive homologous segments present in the persistent spireme in these cases in reality represent so-called parasynaptic bivalents, strung out in a longitudinal series. Thus, if we were to arrange the vertically elongated bivalents found at metaphase in Allium or Lilium end to end they would accurately correspond to the strings of chromosomes found in the three genera as discussed in the present connection.

E. C. JEFFREY

## LOCAL ELECTRIC ANESTHESIA

IN the issue of SCIENCE for February 24, 1933, is an interesting article, "A Method of Outlining Cutaneous Nerve Areas," by Professor Thompson and Dr. Inman, of the University of California, in which an important use of anesthesia from an alternating current is described and discussed.

During the summer of 1892 I worked with A. E. Kennelly, chief electrician of the Edison Laboratory at Orange (later professor of electrodynamics at Harvard), studying the effects of alternating currents and the huge magnets there upon the human body. Professor Kennelly and I published a paper on "Some Physiological Experiments with Magnets at the Edison Laboratory."[1]

We noted that summer that anesthesia and analgesia could be produced by alternating currents above 2,000 vibrations, though this was not alluded to in the paper mentioned.

[1] *New York Medical Journal,* lxi: 729–732. 1892.

However, in an article[2] of mine in the *American Medical and Surgical Bulletin* appeared the following paragraphs, which I have just copied from the *Bulletin* at the Academy of Medicine Library:

> Several years ago Mr. Kennelly and I experimented at the Edison Laboratory with the sinusoidal current. The results of these experiments have never been made public, for lack of time, until the present moment. We established one singular and interesting fact, which is of therapeutic value, and which I will detail here. The experiments were tried upon Mr. Kennelly, Dr. Charles E. Atwood, one of the assistants at the Vanderbilt Clinic, who kindly aided me, and upon myself. The same results were obtained in each of us. Applying one pole to a nerve trunk, say at the wrist, and another at an indifferent point, there were no perceptible effects as long as the vibrations were below 2000 per second. When we reached that point the parts supplied by the nerve beneath the pole became anaesthetic, so that pricking with a needle or knife, or touching the part, was not perceived. Both the anaesthesia and analgesia were so marked that an incision might have been made without the consciousness of the individual operated upon. The higher the rate of vibration the more noteworthy was this effect. Our apparatus did not permit of our going beyond 3000 vibrations per second. * * * The return of sensibility was instantaneous on interruption of the electric current. Doubtless small operations might be performed by this new method of local anaesthesia. As yet the procedure is in its infancy.

In the autumn of 1892 after this summer work at Orange I asked the surgeons in the surgical department of the Vanderbilt Clinic to be on the lookout for some simple case on which the newly found electric anesthesia could be tested. I was testing it out for various nervous disorders in the Nervous Department of the Vanderbilt Clinic, where I was chief of clinic, with Professor Allen Starr. In a few days Dr. Percy Turnure brought in a young woman with a painful felon of the left forefinger which was exactly suitable for the purpose. The electric anesthesia was quickly produced and Dr. Turnure lanced the finger tip. The operation was apparently painless, though as soon as the current was removed sensation returned, with of course such pain as would be natural after any similar incision.

So far as I know this was the first operation under that type of local anesthesia.

About 1902 Leduc in France began writing articles on electrical anesthesia.

FREDERICK PETERSON

NEW YORK, N. Y.

## SELF-STERILITY IN NEMESIA

SEVERAL years ago, working in the greenhouse at Princeton University, I undertook to study the genetic

[2] *Am. Med. and Surg. Bull.* ix: 765–808. 1896.

factors which control flower color in plants of the genus Nemesia. A packet of seeds, labeled "Nemesia —Newton's Glories Mixed," was obtained from Peter Henderson and Co. in New York City, and sixteen plants were raised. Comparison with the description of this genus in the Flora Capensis seemed to indicate that these plants belonged to the species *N. strumosa.*

It was desired to obtain seed from self-pollinations for the next generation, but every flower which was selfed set no seed whatever, and as many as fifteen flowers were pollinated on some plants. Some crosses between these plants, made at the same time as the selfings, were fertile, proving that both the pollen and ovules were functional and that the failure to set seed was due to physiological incompatibility, commonly called self-sterility. Two families studied in the succeeding generation gave the same results, although few intra-family crosses were made.

In the third generation, three families were studied more intensively. In one, ten plants were selfed and all proved self-sterile, although one plant exhibited a slight tendency to be pseudo-fertile. Seventy-four of the ninety possible crosses were made and showed that two and only two intra-sterile, inter-fertile groups were present, of which one consisted of seven and the other of three plants. Ten plants of a second family were completely self-sterile when as many as ten flowers on a plant were self-pollinated. Fifty-nine crosses were made within this family and again two groups were found to be present. All crosses behaved regularly. In the third family, six plants belonged to one intra-sterile, inter-fertile class and six to another and all twelve were self-sterile. Only one cross exhibited behavior not in accordance with the general trend. Inter-family crosses between the two latter families showed that no group was common to both. A similar result was noted for the first and third families but, unfortunately, I did not cross the first two.

This study is being continued this year to learn whether Nemesia behaves like Nicotiana and most other plants which have been studied with respect to self-sterility.

HERBERT PARKES RILEY

BUSSEY INSTITUTION
HARVARD UNIVERSITY

## A NEW VASCULAR FUSARIUM DISEASE OF PEAS

DURING the course of an investigation of pea diseases, particularly of Fusarium wilt, carried on under the direction of Dr. J. C. Walker, of the Department of Plant Pathology, University of Wisconsin, a wilt disease possessing many of the characteristic symptoms of Fusarium wilt, caused by *F. orthoceras* v. *pisi* but produced by another species of Fusarium, has been repeatedly separated from the pea disease complex. This disease was first seen in Wisconsin in 1931, and was encountered frequently and found to be wide-spread in Wisconsin, Maryland and Delaware during the 1932 season. Specimens were also received from New Hampshire, Massachusetts, Idaho and Montana.

The new disease is tentatively referred to as "near-wilt" because of its close resemblance to the wilt disease previously described by Linford.[1] As they occur in the field and upon plants grown in artificially infested soil, the symptoms of the two diseases are so similar that it is practically impossible to differentiate them by this means. Typically the foliage takes on a yellowish cast, the leaflets and stipules become recurved and the stunted plant dies prematurely. Usually the vascular elements become brightly stained an orange or reddish color some distance up the stem.

One of the significant features of the new disease is that it occurs upon varieties known to be 100 per cent. resistant to *F. orthoceras* v. *pisi.* This is of great importance to both growers and seedsmen, for it means that certain seed stocks sold as resistant to the wilt caused by *F. orthoceras* v. *pisi* may wilt in the field because of another fungus.

Satisfactory diagnoses of these two diseases can only be made by culturing the causal fungi. The purple pigmentation of the near-wilt Fusarium upon certain media is useful in distinguishing it from the wilt pathogen. Although there is a wide range of pigmentation exhibited by the various strains of *F. orthoceras* v. *pisi* this purple type seldom is approached. An additional aid in distinguishing them is the abundance of spores, including macroconidia, produced by the near-wilt Fusarium, inasmuch as *F. orthoceras* v. *pisi* produces but few spores in culture and these few are microconidia, with infrequent exceptions.

The new disease may be distinguished from Fusarium rootrot, caused by *F. martii* v. *pisi,* since in rootrot a cortical decay of the underground stem conspicuously precedes the invasion of the stele, while both near-wilt and wilt are primarily diseases of the xylem tissue and not of the cortex. Under field conditions diseased plants frequently show both cortical and vascular invasion, and culturing must be used to identify the fungi present. *F. martii* v. *pisi* is easily distinguished in culture from the two vascular Fusaria by its masses of blue green spores.

WILLIAM C. SNYDER

DIVISION OF PLANT PATHOLOGY,
UNIVERSITY OF CALIFORNIA, BERKELEY

[1] M. B. Linford, "A Fusarium Wilt of Pea in Wisconsin," Wis. Agr. Exp. Sta. Res. Bul. 85, 44 pp. illus. 1928.

# SPECIAL CORRESPONDENCE

## THE ELLA SACHS PLOTZ FOUNDATION FOR THE ADVANCEMENT OF SCIENTIFIC INVESTIGATION

DURING the ninth year of the Ella Sachs Plotz Foundation for the Advancement of Scientific Investigation, ninety applications for grants were received by the trustees, sixty-five of which came from sixteen different countries in Europe, Asia, South and North America and Australia, the remaining twenty-five coming from the United States. The total number of grants made during this year was thirty-three, one of these being a continued annual grant. Eighteen of the new grants were made to scientists in countries outside of the United States.

In the nine years of its existence the foundation has made 179 grants, and investigators have been aided in Argentina, Austria, Belgium, Chile, China, Czechoslovakia, Esthonia, Estland, France, Germany, Great Britain, Hungary, Italy, Latvia, Netherlands, Palestine, Poland, Portugal, South Africa, Sweden, Switzerland, Syria and the United States.

The list of investigators and the purpose of their researches aided in the current year is as follows:

Dr. Z. M. Bacq, Brussels, Belgium, $300 for research on problems in relation to the physiology of the sympathetic nervous system.

Dr. E. T. Bell, University of Minnesota, $500 for continuation of kidney studies.

Dr. R. Bossert, Munich, Germany, $400 for continuation of work on cholesterol-ergosterol metabolism.

Dr. Henry Chabanier, Paris, France, $400 for researches to determine the iso-electric points of blood proteins and to do ultrafiltrations of blood.

Professor Robert Chambers, New York University, $500 for work on problems in kidney secretion.

Professor Alfred Chanutin, University of Virginia, $300 for chemical analysis of blood and tissues in his partially nephrectomized rats fed on a variety of diets.

Dr. Erwin Chargaff, Berlin, Germany, $400 for investigations dealing with the chemistry of pathogenic bacteria, especially lipoids and carbohydrates of acid-fast group and of diphtheria bacteria.

Professor Dr. Herbert Elias, Vienna, Austria, $200 for continuation of investigations on the globulin and albumin contents in sera of patients with nervous diseases.

Professor Dr. Philipp Ellinger, Düsseldorf, Germany, $300 for continuation of work on physiology, pathology and pharmacology of the kidney.

Professor Boris Ephrussi, Paris, France, $400 for a new method for the measurement of respiratory exchanges in tissue-culture cells.

Dr. Emil Epstein, Vienna, Austria, $300 for study of the Neiman-Pick disease and amaurotic idiocy and the lipoids of the brain.

Dr. G. Favilli, Florence, Italy, $300 for continuation of research on the relation between undulant fever and epizootic abortion.

Professor Dr. Alfred Fleisch, Tartu-Dorpat, Estland, $200 for investigations concerning the adequate stimulus for dilatation of the arterioles during work.

Professor E. Gellhorn, University of Oregon, $300 for continuation of work on the influence of internal secretions on permeability.

Dr. R. W. Gerard, University of Chicago, $300 for work on the chemical and physical changes in nervous tissue during rest and activity.

Dr. David Glusker, Jewish Hospital of Brooklyn, $400 for study of blood lipids in children.

Professor Allen D. Keller, University of Alabama, $250 for continuation of research on brain-stem function.

Dr. Walter P. Kennedy, Edinburgh, Scotland, $300 for investigation on "The Reproductive Endocrine Balance in the Human Female."

Dr. Th. Konschegg, Graz, Austria, $400 for research on the relationship of the glandula suprarenals, adrenalin and blood pressure.

Dr. H. A. Krebs, Freiburg, Germany, $350 for continuation of studies on the breakdown of protein in animals and on the metabolism involved in the action of insulin.

Professor William deB. MacNider, University of North Carolina, $175 for work on nephritis.

Dr. F. Mainzer, Rostock, Germany, $300 for studies of excreted albumin to clear up the physico-chemical forerunners of albuminuria.

Dr. David Marine, Montefiore Hospital, New York City, $300 for continuation of an attempt to separate the powerful goitrogenic agent present in cabbage.

Professor C. A. Mills, University of Cincinnati, $200 for continuation of metabolic experiments.

Professor H. O. Mosenthal, New York Post-Graduate School, $350 for research on the result of continuous infusions of small doses of adrenalin on kidney, blood pressure, and peripheral blood vessels as measured by temperature.

Dr. Louis A. Rapkine, Paris, France, $350 for research on cell division.

Dr. William T. Salter, Huntington Memorial Hospital, Boston, $500 for work on the metabolic changes in animals, particularly with regard to the enzymes concerned with protein metabolism and with oxidation.

Dr. Gordon H. Scott, Washington University School of Medicine, St. Louis, $300 for study of the mineral constituents of the walls of the blood vessels.

Dr. E. A. Spiegel, Temple University, $300 for continuation of experiments on epilepsy and on the vegetative nervous system.

Thorndike Memorial Laboratory, Boston City Hospital (Prof. George R. Minot, Director), $500 a year (continued since 1927) in recognition of Dr. Francis W. Peabody's services.

Dr. C. Van Caulaert, Strasbourg, France, $400 for biological work on nephritis.

Professor René Wurmser, Paris, France, $500 for continuation of studies of oxidation-reduction phenomena in cells.

Professor Edgard Zunz, Brussels, Belgium, $100 for studies of pancreatic secretion.

Applications for grants to be held during the year 1933–1934 should be in the hands of the executive committee before May 1, 1933. They should be sent to Dr. Joseph C. Aub, Collis P. Huntington Memorial Hospital, 695 Huntington Avenue, Boston, Massachusetts.

# SOCIETIES AND MEETINGS

## THE COLORADO-WYOMING ACADEMY OF SCIENCE

THE sixth annual meeting of the Colorado-Wyoming Academy of Science was held on November 25 and 26, 1932, at the Colorado Agricultural College, Fort Collins.

Friday and Saturday mornings were given over to the reading of papers in section meetings. One hundred thirty-six papers were presented, These were distributed as follows: Chemistry, 12; education, 13; geology and geography, 10; physics, 15; plant science, 25; psychology, 16; social science, 16, and zoology 29.

About 175 members were present. The attendance of the public and college students was unusually large.

A new feature of the program was the display of exhibits of the scientific work carried on by members of the academy. Sixty exhibits were presented. These included teaching devices, demonstrations of collections of animals and plants, rare scientific books, chemical and physical apparatus, experiments in physics and chemistry, cooking devices, historical manuscripts, charts for psychology and education, experiments in hydraulics, plant breeding, plant pathology, models of ecological situations, etc. These were on display during the entire session. The enthusiastic interest shown by academy members, students and the visiting public insured the continuance of this feature.

At the academy dinner on Friday evening, A. S. Adams, of the Colorado School of Mines, spoke on "A Defense of Mass Production."

The following officers were elected: *President:* F. C. Jean, Colorado State Teachers College; *Vice-President:* S. H. Knight, University of Wyoming; *Secretary:* R. J. Gilmore, Colorado College; *Treasurer:* O. M. Dickerson, Colorado State Teachers College.

C. H. Hutchinson, University of Colorado, was appointed chairman of the program and publications committee.

F. E. E. Germann, University of Colorado, was appointed representative to the conference of state academies.

Members of the executive committee are: O. A. Beath, University of Wyoming; F. F. Coen, Colorado Agricultural College; F. F. Ramaley, University of Colorado; A. S. Adams, Colorado School of Mines; T. R. Garth, University of Denver; F. P. Goeder, Colorado Agricultural College; R. G. Gustavson, University of Denver.

The 1933 meeting will be held at the University of Wyoming, Laramie, on December 1 and 2, 1933.

R. J. GILMORE,
*Secretary*

## THE ALABAMA ACADEMY OF SCIENCE

THE tenth annual meeting of the Alabama Academy of Science was held at Birmingham-Southern College, Birmingham, Alabama, on March 10 and 11. The attendance was better than at any previous meeting.

The presiding officer was Professor J. F. Duggar, Alabama Polytechnic Institute. There were two general sessions and sectional meetings were held by the following sections: biology, chemistry, physics and mathematics, industry and medicine. A fifth section was organized at the meeting, which will cover the following subjects: anthropology, archeology and geology.

The internal organization of the academy was changed at this meeting. The plan adopted is in some respects similar to that of the American Association for the Advancement of Science; that is, sectional chairmen are automatically vice-presidents of the academy. The offices of first vice-president and second vice-president were discontinued.

The officers elected for 1933–34 are as follows:

*President:* James L. Brakefield, Howard College, Birmingham, Alabama.

*General Secretary:* W. A. Whiting, Birmingham-Southern College, Alabama.

*Treasurer:* A. G. Overton, Alabama By-Products Corporation, Tarrant.

*Councilor to the American Association for the Advancement of Science:* Emmett B. Carmichael, University of Alabama.

*Editor of the Journal:* E. V. Jones, Birmingham-Southern College.

The following were elected as chairmen and secretaries of the various sections:

*Anthropology, Archeology and Geology:*

*Chairman:* R. S. Poor, Birmingham-Southern College.
*Secretary:* G. Andrews, University of Alabama.

*Biology:*

*Chairman:* Septima Smith, University of Alabama.
*Secretary:* Thera Towery, Howard College.

*Chemistry, Physics and Mathematics:*

*Chairman:* Roger W. Allen, Alabama Polytechnic Institute.
*Secretary:* W. N. Arnquist, Alabama Polytechnic Institute.

*Industry:*

*Chairman:* E. A. Hawk, Birmingham, Alabama.
*Secretary:* T. N. McVay, University of Alabama.

*Medicine:*

*Chairman:* Franklin S. DuBois, University of Alabama.
*Secretary:* G. D. Matthews, Birmingham.

Representatives from eleven high schools met with the academy on Saturday morning, March 11, and organized the Junior Academy of Science of Alabama. Each high school had one exhibit and one member to give a paper. There were more than a hundred in attendance at the high school program. Officers of the Junior Academy are:

*President:* Winthrop R. Hubler, Ensley High School.
*Vice-president:* R. E. Chambers, Woodlawn High School.
*Secretary:* Martha Bray, Ramsay Technical High School.

EMMETT B. CARMICHAEL,
*Vice-president of the Academy Conference*

# SCIENTIFIC APPARATUS AND LABORATORY METHODS

## AMMONIATION OF PEAT FOR FERTILIZERS

FOR several years much of the higher grade organic fertilizer materials, such as cottonseed meal and animal tankage, has been diverted into feedstuffs. To use such material in fertilizer mixtures it was necessary to compete with their valuation on a protein basis in feeds. Under such competition the price paid for nitrogen of this sort was considerably greater than nitrogen contained in inorganic fertilizer materials. While in the last few years the price differential has not been so great, due to the low price of feeds from grain products, it still exists and the demand for organic nitrogenous materials in fertilizers has held this price higher than that of the inorganic materials. The desirability of utilizing some abundant organic substance as a carrier of the cheap nitrogen derived from synthetic ammonia led to the investigation by the Fixed Nitrogen Research Laboratory of peat as a possibility in this direction. It is well known that peat occurs in large quantities and in commercially workable beds at widely distributed points throughout the eastern part of the United States. Such deposits may be found from Minnesota to Maine, from Maine to Florida, and along the coast of the Gulf of Mexico.

Experiments have been carried out by the authors to utilize peat as a nitrogen carrier by treating the air-dried material with anhydrous ammonia. Four types of peat have been used and the conditions of treatment have been varied to study the effect of time of treatment, concentration of ammonia and temperature. A quantity of the ground peat passing a 14-mesh screen was loaded into a steel bomb and anhydrous ammonia added in excess. The closed bomb was placed in an electric oven at the temperature under which the experiment was carried out. The temperature used varied from room temperature to 300° and the pressure developed was that obtained under conditions necessary to retain the ammonia in the bomb varying from 100 to 300 atmospheres. The four types of peat investigated yielded products of a nitrogen content of 4 to 6 per cent. at 50°, 10.5 to 13 per cent. at 180°, and 14 to 21 per cent. at 300° C. It was found that treatment after 20 hours had very little effect in adding more nitrogen. Increasing amounts of moisture tended to lower the content of nitrogen in the product, but did not decrease it very sharply. From these results it appears that the temperature variation affects the amount of nitrogen more than any of the other conditions and that by controlling the temperature and water content of the material practically any nitrogen content up to 20 per cent. is obtainable, depending somewhat upon the character of the peat used.

The original peats contained from 1 to 3 per cent. of nitrogen, which is very slowly available as plant food, but under the conditions of treatment here described, this nitrogen becomes a part of the total nitrogen, practically all of which is available according to chemical tests. Analyses have shown that the nitrogen contained in the ammoniated peat is partly water-soluble and partly water-insoluble, although the water-insoluble part is roughly about two thirds of the total. The ammoniated material is considerably darker than the untreated peat, ranging from dark brown to almost black in color. It is slightly more dense than the original peat and decidedly more easily wetted on coming in contact with water.

The product is of such physical condition as to be well suited for use as a conditioner in mixed fertilizer or for direct application. It promises to be of great importance in offering a cheap nitrogen carrier which, used in mixed fertilizer, will prevent caking of the mixture and keep it in condition suitable for easy distribution. The condition of the nitrogen being partly water-soluble and partly water-insoluble makes it of essential value where danger of leaching or loss through drainage is encountered. Substitution of this material for part of the inorganic materials in the fertilizer mixtures will also be of value in diminishing the burning effect of highly concentrated mixtures, as the amount of water-soluble nitrogen would be reduced thereby.

The advantages of ammoniated peat from the standpoint of fertilizer use are numerous and apparently convincing, and in addition both peat and ammonia from which it is made are cheap and abundant. There are estimated to be 14 billion tons of peat covering 110 million acres in the United States, and ammonia as produced from nitrogen fixation processes is one of the cheapest forms of nitrogen. While the process of manufacture has not yet been worked out, indications are that it will be relatively simple and cheap. Investigations on the details of the technical problems involved are being actively prosecuted.

In the soils unit of this bureau, H. G. Byers and I. C. Fenstal, while engaged on a study of the decomposition of peat, on heating it with aqueous ammonia in a closed vessel obtained a peat product with an increased nitrogen content.

R. O. E. DAVIS,
WALTER SCHOLL
BUREAU OF CHEMISTRY AND SOILS
U. S. DEPARTMENT OF AGRICULTURE

## AN ACCURATE METHOD FOR MEASURING NEW-BORN MICE

WHILE carrying on growth studies of the mice of the genus *Peromyscus*, it became necessary to devise some method for the accurate measurement of new-born and very young mice. For the first two or three days after birth, these mice are so small, squirmy and curled in posture that it is almost impossible to take accurate measurements of the total length, tail length and hind foot by the usual hand methods.

The idea was therefore conceived of taking pictures of each litter with a Leica camera. A metric scale was pictured at the same exposure so that the mice were all taken at a fourth natural size. The negatives were then projected upon a screen by means of an ordinary lantern slide projector at forty times the negative size or ten times natural size. The measurements were then taken from the screen picture and divided by ten. The curved areas, such as the total length, were measured with a pair of dividers. The cost per picture is nominal where a Leica camera and a projecting apparatus are available, and the accuracy of this method fully compensates for the small amount of time and labor involved. It is suggested that this method may also prove efficient in measuring other small animals.

ARTHUR SVIHLA
STATE COLLEGE OF WASHINGTON

## A NEW SOURCE OF WORKING CURRENT FOR POTENTIOMETERS

THE writer has observed that a two-volt primary battery on the market, known as an "air-cell" battery,[1] has characteristics which make it an almost ideal source of working current for a potentiometer.

This battery has a rated capacity of 600 ampere hours and a flat voltage discharge curve if the current drain does not exceed the specified 650 milliamperes. This is ample capacity for a potentiometer for many months' use.

The writer has used such a battery in place of a storage battery and has found that when protected against changes of temperature the working current will remain constant for hours and in some cases an entire working day without adjustment.

The above features, together with its cheapness and continuity of service, make it a very desirable source of current. The potential of a storage battery drops steadily until it reaches a point where it must be replaced and recharged.

LESTER F. BOSS
MARINE BIOLOGICAL LABORATORY
WOODS HOLE, MASS.

[1] Eveready Air-Cell "A" Battery, manufactured by the National Carbon Company.

# SPECIAL ARTICLES

## THE EFFECT OF GALACTOSE FEEDING UPON DEPANCREATIZED DOGS

THE studies of Roe and Schwartzman,[1] in which it was shown that diabetic subjects have practically as good a tolerance for galactose as normal subjects, suggested that it would be of interest to study the influence of pancreatectomy upon the metabolism of galactose. We have therefore undertaken an investigation of the metabolism of galactose in depancreatized dogs,

[1] J. H. Roe and A. S. Schwartzban, *Jour. Biol. Chem.*, 96: 717, 1932.

and wish to make a brief preliminary report at this time.

Dogs were placed in metabolism cages and water was allowed *ad libitum.* Twenty-four hour samples of urine were collected under toluene. The principal chemical data obtained were determinations of the fasting blood sugar and of the amounts of galactose, glucose and nitrogen of the urine, and the D : N ratio. After obtaining control data the dogs were totally depancreatized under ether anesthesia. Our usual procedure was to determine the D : N ratio of the urine upon the second and sometimes third days after pancreatectomy under fasting conditions, and the dogs were then fed galactose in water in amounts varying from 1 to 6 grams per kilo per day for periods varying from 4 to 9 days. During the period of galactose feeding the amounts of galactose, glucose and nitrogen in the 24-hour samples of urine were determined and the D : N ratio was calculated. The fasting blood sugar was also determined each day upon samples of blood collected in the morning before galactose was fed. Following these studies the surviving animals were given food mixed with galactose, and observations, together with irregular chemical studies, were made until the animals died.

In control studies the dogs were found to excrete in the urine 17 to 30 per cent. of the ingested galactose. Following pancreatectomy the urinary excretion increased to quantities ranging from 32 to 57 per cent. of the ingested galactose.

After pancreatectomy the D : N ratio of the urine

TABLE I

COMPARISON OF GALACTOSE AND GLUCOSE TOLERANCE OF DEPANCREATIZED DOGS

| Dog | Days after Pancreatectomy | Feeding | 24-Hour Urine: Galactose Gms. | Glucose Gms. | Nitrogen Gms. | D : N |
|---|---|---|---|---|---|---|
| 1 | 21 | 18 gm. galactose | 8.84 | 4.69 | 2.43 | 1.9 |
| | 22 | 18 gm. glucose | ......... | 17.50 | 2.26 | 7.7 |
| 2 | 7 | 18 gm. galactose | 7.29 | 7.28 | 2.95 | 2.4 |
| | 8 | 18 gm. glucose | ......... | 15.35 | 1.89 | 8.1 |
| 3 | 8 | 30 gm. glucose | ......... | 26.23 | 4.56 | 5.8 |
| | 9 | 30 gm. galactose | 9.95 | 15.16 | 4.30 | 3.5 |
| 4 | 6 | 32 gm. galactose | 13.20 | 10.58 | 3.21 | 3.3 |
| | 7 | 32 gm. glucose | ......... | 27.60 | 2.96 | 9.3 |
| | 8 | 32 gm. galactose | 13.44 | 5.41 | 2.11 | 2.5 |
| 5 | 8 | 21 gm. galactose | 7.25 | 4.00 | ......... | ....... |
| | 9 | 21 gm. glucose | ......... | 15.50 | ......... | ....... |

during galactose feeding either kept at essentially the same value as obtained in the control studies before galactose feeding or in some cases decreased considerably. This finding shows that the galactose was not converted into glucose by the depancreatized animals, and since only 32 to 57 per cent. of the ingested galactose was excreted in the urine, the evidence indicates that about one half of the galactose fed to the depancreatized dogs was retained in their tissues and apparently was utilized.

In Table I are shown comparative studies of galactose and glucose feeding to depancreatized dogs upon consecutive days. When glucose was fed there was a much greater excretion of glucose in the urine than when galactose was fed and the D : N ratio was approximately 2 to 4 times as great. Even if one totals the amounts of galactose and glucose that were excreted in the 24-hour period of galactose feeding (a procedure that is unwarranted because the normal dog excretes galactose in the urine) it will be found that there was less total sugar excreted upon galactose feeding than upon glucose feeding. These data show that there is a preferential utilization of galactose as compared with glucose by the depancreatized dog.

The fasting blood sugar of 5 depancreatized dogs ranged from 221 to 350 mg per cent. during the period when galactose only was fed. While receiving galactose the fasting blood sugar of one dog increased from 261 to 304 mg per cent. and that of the others either remained at essentially the same level or diminished, the greatest decrease being from 350 to 252 mg per cent. in 3 days of galactose feeding.

By galactose feeding we were able to prevent or suppress some of the sequelae of pancreatectomy. Vomiting was either suppressed or prevented in the dogs receiving galactose by mouth or intravenously. Apparently there is no other conclusion than that the galactose was responsible for this favorable result. As a result of the prevention of vomiting, the dogs were able to take water and did not become dehydrated. Ketone body formation and acidosis developed in our animals, but most of them survived the acute period of ketonuria, during which galactose only was administered in some instances, while in other instances sodium bicarbonate was administered in addition to galactose.

The survival periods of the depancreatized dogs, which did not receive insulin and to which we administered galactose, are as follows: One dog lived 5 days; 2 dogs 6 days; 1 dog 7 days; 1 dog 12 days; 1 dog 14 days; 1 dog 19 days; 1 dog 30 days; and 1 dog was sacrificed 41 days after pancreatectomy. There is no record in the literature of survival periods of totally depancreatized dogs not receiving insulin through the post-operative period that are as long as some of those obtained by us with galactose feeding.

The influence of galactose feeding with respect to healing of the dog's operative wound is apparently of significance. It is very well known that the abdominal incision of the depancreatized dog becomes infected and does not heal. We obtained complete healing of the mid-line incision of the dogs which lived 30 and 41 days, and in the other dogs, which lived 10 days or more, there was more or less healing. Apparently there is no other conclusion than that galactose feeding had some influence in bringing about these favorable results.

Grateful appreciation is expressed to Smith, Kline, and French, Inc., Philadelphia, Pa., for donations of galactose.

Joseph H. Roe

Department of Biochemistry
George Washington University
Medical School

Russell F. Cahoon

Department of Physiology
Georgetown University
Medical School

## THE INCIDENCE OF COLOR BLINDNESS AMONG RACES[1]

In Science in 1930,[2] the writer announced the beginning of an experimental study of the incidence of color blindness among Indians. Since then there have been, under his direction, expeditions to test various races in America by trained investigators, *i.e.*, four expeditions to test Indians—at Santa Fé and Albuquerque, New Mexico; Holy Rosary and St. Francis Missions in South Dakota; Haskell Institute at Lawrence, Kansas; in Colorado and New Mexico at various points, where we tested Utes, Apaches and Navajo; three expeditions to test Mexicans, the native-born (Spanish-Americans) and another to test immigrant Mexicans in Colorado, and still another to test the natives of Old Mexico in Mexico City; three expeditions to test Negroes, one in Tennessee, one in North Carolina and still another in Colorado. The unselected whites and Jews were tested in and around Denver.

The first three Indian expeditions were made possible by a joint grant between the National Research Council and the University of Denver. All the other expeditions were financed by the university.

The test used in the present investigation was the Ishihara Color Blindness Test, which has been used rather extensively in this country, particularly by Miles, Haupt and Clement. Our procedure was to test one eye at a time, but followed the general directions of the author of the test. By means of automobile goggles, with the glasses punched out and exchangeable blinds, one eye was tested at a time. It should be said that no case of monocular color blindness was discovered by the investigator. No case of total blindness was brought to light; consequently these results are for complete and incomplete red-green blindness. With results from the same test Miles[3] has reported for various groups of white males

[1] Paper read before the Colorado-Wyoming Academy of Sciences on November 25, 1932.

[2] T. R. Garth, "The Color Blindness of Indians," Science, 71: 468, 1930.

[3] W. R. Miles, "One Hundred Cases Color Blindness

TABLE I

The Incidence of Color-Blindness Among Races Obtained with the Ishihara Color-Blindness Test by Garth *et al.*

| Racial group | Males | | | Females | | |
|---|---|---|---|---|---|---|
| | Number tested | Color-Blind No. | Color-Blind Per cent. | Number tested | Color-Blind No. | Color-Blind Per cent. |
| Whites, unselected | 795 | 67 | 8.4 | 232 | 3 | 1.3 |
| " Jews | 200 | 8 | 4.0 | 175 | 0 | 0 |
| Indians, F. B. var. tribes | 562 | 14 | 2.5 | 337 | 0 | 0 |
| " " " Navajo | 535 | 6 | 1.1 | 456 | 3 | 0.7 |
| " mixed bloods | 480 | 25 | 5.2 | 523 | 4 | 0.8 |
| Mexicans, Old Mexico | 571 | 13 | 2.3 | 494 | 3 | 0.6 |
| " immigrants | 523 | 13 | 2.5 | 469 | 4 | 0.9 |
| Spanish-Americans | 346 | 13 | 3.8 | 390 | 3 | 0.8 |
| Negroes, Southern | 538 | 21 | 3.9 | 496 | 4 | 0.8 |
| " Northern | 254 | 7 | 2.8 | 165 | 0 | 0 |

an average incidence of 8.2 per cent. and around 1 per cent. for white females; Haupt's report[4] indicates incidence of 7.8 per cent. for white males; and Clement[5] certain incidences given below for Indians, full bloods, mixed bloods of the southwest, and northern Negroes of Connecticut. His Indians numbered 392 full bloods, 232 mixed bloods, his Negroes 323.

The Indians of the present study represent practically the whole of the United States—for instance, one mixed blood from New York City, seven full bloods from North Carolina, seven from California. The various Indian tribes are well represented, though most of the Indians are Pueblos, Navajos and Sioux.

In Table I is given a preliminary report of the results of the investigation to determine the incidence of color blindness among races with the Ishihara test. It is our intention to continue carrying on the investigation, particularly in America and in the countries of Turkey and India.

Upon examination of Table I, it will be seen that the result of testing unselected whites in Colorado agrees well with results gotten by Miles in California and Haupt in Baltimore, *i.e.*, for white males an incidence of about 8.0 per cent. and females 1.0 per cent. Full-blood Indians and Negroes agree fairly well with results gotten by Clement, but our percentage results for mixed-blood Indians do not agree with Clement's results. He obtained for full bloods 2.0 per cent.—mixed bloods 1.2 per cent., and Negroes 3.4 per cent. The Navajos tested by us show a great departure from Indians of other tribes, since they have for males an incidence of 1.1 per cent. This is the first report of testing Mexicans with any color blindness test, though it is not the first time they have been tested. Information has come direct to the author of the testing by Dr. Luis Serrano with the *Mosaics Serrano*—a test derived from the Stilling test—of an incidence of 2.3 per cent. for males and 0.0 per cent for females, the numbers tested being respectively 609 and 415.

It will be seen upon examining Table I that according to the Ishihara test unselected white males are afflicted with the defect of color blindness more than any one of the others of the racial groups. In fact, when we treat the data with a view to determining whether or not the differences in the proportions are real, we find they are so between unselected white males and the males of any of the other racial groups, full-blood Indians, Negroes and Mexicans, excepting in the case of the mixed-blood Indians, with an approximation to a difference (2:75) in the case of the Jews. When a real difference between the percentages is indicated $D/\sigma_{\text{diff.}}$ should be 3 and more.[6] We may say, then, that a real difference or a close approximation to it is indicated between unselected whites and the other racial groups here represented, excepting the mixed-blood Indians, and even between them and Mexicans.

As to differences in percentages between the remaining groups, these are not indicated, excepting in the case of full-blood Navajos and the mixed-blood Indians, where there is a close approximation to a difference (the figure is 2.9), between Navajos and Southern Negroes. It is interesting to note that neither the Jewish groups, the Mexican groups, the Negro groups nor the full-blood Indian groups differ among themselves when classified geographically, nor do they differ when classified superficially racially, with the exception mentioned, Navajos and Southern Negroes.

The investigator is not disposed to call the indicated differences racial differences, since they do not hold to racial lines, but he is disposed to think they may be due to some selective factor.

THOMAS R. GARTH
UNIVERSITY OF DENVER

Detected with the Ishihara Test,'' *Jour. of Gen. Psy.*, 2, 535–543, 1929.

[4] I. Haupt, ''The Nela Test for Color Blindness Applied to School Children,'' *Jour. Comp. Psychol.*, 7: 179–184, 1922.

[5] Forest Clement, ''Comparative Racial Differences in Color Blindness,'' SCIENCE, 72: 203–204, 1930.

[6] K. J. Holzinger, ''Statistical Methods for Students of Education.'' Ginn and Company, pp. 248f. 1928.

## BOOKS RECEIVED

*Annual Report of the General Education Board, 1931–32.* Pp. xv + 79. General Education Board, New York.

COLE, L. HEBER and R. A. ROGERS. *Anhydrite in Canada.* Pp. v + 89. Illustrated. Department of Mines, Canada.

DAVIS, HAROLD T. *Philosophy and Modern Science.* Pp. xiv + 335. Illustrated. Principia Press.

EGLOFF, GUSTAV. *Earth Oil.* Pp. xi + 158. 41 figures. Williams & Wilkins. $1.00.

LIDDLE, CARL and DAVID THIBAULT. *Tunchi.* Pp. v + 312. Century. $2.00.

*Memoirs of the Indian Museum.* Vol. X: *The Copepoda of Indian Seas; Calanoida.* By R. B. Seymour Sewell. Pp. 223–407. Illustrated. Vol. XII, No. 1: *Annelida Polychaeta of the Indian Museum, Calcutta.* By Pierre Fauvel. Pp. 262. 40 figures. 9 plates. Zoological Survey of India, Calcutta.

MOTT-SMITH, MORTON. *Heat and Its Workings.* Pp. x + 238. 50 figures. Appleton. $2.00.

*Records of the Indian Museum.* Vol. XXXIII, Part II, June, 1931: Pp. 71–210. Vol. XXXIII, Part IV, December, 1931: Pp. 328–516. Vol. XXXIV, Part I, March, 1932: Pp. 79. Vol. XXXIV, Part II, June, 1932: Pp. 81–228. Vol. XXXIV, Part III, September, 1932: Pp. 229–356. Illustrated. Zoological Survey of India, Calcutta.

*Report of the Department of Scientific and Industrial Research, 1931–32.* Pp. 193. His Majesty's Stationery Office, London. 3s.

THOMSON, SIR J. J. and G. P. THOMSON. *Conduction of Electricity Through Gases.* Third edition. Vol. II: Ionisation by Collision and the Gaseous Discharge. Pp. viii + 608. 231 figures. Macmillan. $6.50.

WIENER, NORBERT. *The Fourier Integral and Certain of Its Applications.* Pp. xi + 201. Macmillan. $3.25.

WILLIAMS, JOSEPH J., S.J. Voodoos and Obeahs. Pp. xix + 257. Dial Press. $3.00.

WOLTERECK, RICHARD. *Grundzüge einer allgemeinen Biologie.* Pp. xvi + 629. 271 figures. Ferdinand Enke, Stuttgart. RM 43.

# SCIENCE

Vol. 77 — Friday, April 7, 1933 — No. 1997

*Tendencies in the Logic of Mathematics:* Professor E. R. Hedrick ... 335

*Obituary:*
*Edward Bruce Williamson:* Professor Fernandus Payne. *Recent Deaths* ... 344

*Scientific Events:*
*International Standard for the Ovarian Follicular Hormone; The Eleventh International Symposium on Physics at the University of Michigan; Geology and Geography at the Chicago Meeting of the American Association; Award to Professor H. C. Sherman; Professor Einstein and the Prussian Academy* ... 344

*Scientific Notes and News* ... 346

*Discussion:*
*Naming the Grand Canyon:* Dr. Frederick S Dellenbaugh. *The Reaction of Individual Bacteria to Irradiation with Ultra-violet Light:* Dr. Frederick L. Gates. *Lactobacilli in Frozen Pack Peas:* James Alex. Berry. *Vitamin A in the Pimiento Pepper:* Dr. Leah Ascham. *Earthquakes in the Holy Land:* Professor Bailey Willis. *A Rare Publication:* Wm. J. Fox ... 349

*Scientific Apparatus and Laboratory Methods:*
*Double Staining by the Cajal-Brožek Method:* Dr. K. Hruby. *A New Paraffin Embedding Mixture:* Dr. Robert T. Hance ... 352

*Special Articles:*
*Photoperiodism as a Cause of the Rest Period in Strawberries:* Dr. George M. Darrow and George F. Waldo. *A "Scurvy-like" Disease in Chicks:* Dr. Walther F. Holst and Everett R. Halbrook ... 353

*Science News* ... 8

SCIENCE: A Weekly Journal devoted to the Advancement of Science, edited by J. McKeen Cattell and published every Friday by

THE SCIENCE PRESS

New York City: Grand Central Terminal
Lancaster, Pa. — Garrison, N. Y.

Annual Subscription, $6.00 — Single Copies, 15 Cts.

SCIENCE is the official organ of the American Association for the Advancement of Science. Information regarding membership in the Association may be secured from the office of the permanent secretary, in the Smithsonian Institution Building, Washington, D. C.

# TENDENCIES IN THE LOGIC OF MATHEMATICS[1]

By Professor E. R. HEDRICK

UNIVERSITY OF CALIFORNIA, LOS ANGELES

## 1. Introduction

I approach this subject which I have announced for to-day, "Tendencies in the Logic of Mathematics," with some trepidation, with many misgivings, and, I trust, with due humility. To many, the logic of mathematics is old, fixed, immutable. To shake faith in it, even to express a doubt concerning it, is to these nothing short of heresy. As Professor C. I. Lewis, of Harvard University, says in the October issue of *The Monist:* "From Aristotle down, the laws of logic have been regarded as fixed and archetypal; and as such that they admit of no conceivable alternatives. Often they have been attributed to the structure of the Universe or to the nature of human reason; and in general they have been regarded as providing an Archimedean fixed point in the realm of thought."

Yet long ago, as I shall indicate, doubts appeared; and within my own lifetime definite and undeniable difficulties have arisen which leave no room for a complacent acceptance of the logic of the ancients in unchanged form. I shall attempt to-day to state some of the difficulties and some of the proposed remedies. We shall see that there is to-day, if not universal agreement on the details of new systems, at least essential agreement that fundamental changes are necessary. As Lewis remarks in the article quoted: "There are no laws of logic which can be attributed to the universe or to human reason in the traditional form." Acceptance of such doctrine, however, like acceptance of other revolutionary changes in the history of human thought, of which the most recent is the theory of relativity, comes slowly; always men's minds revert to older ways of thought, always the interpretations placed upon the newer statements may be mistaken, always there is need for slow and detailed statement

[1] Address of the retiring chairman and vice-president of Section A—Mathematics, American Association for the Advancement of Science, Atlantic City, December 28, 1932.

of the essential grounds on which the need for changes rests.

If, then, I seem to some of you present, who know full well all—or well-nigh all—that I shall say, to go too slowly over the familiar grounds, I beg you to bear with me, since there is real need for patient and repeated statement of these things. I address myself to-day essentially to those to whom the reasons for change are not thoroughly known. To them, and to others who may later read these lines, I wish to make clear in not too lengthy form the larger outlines, with some details.

I am saved the necessity of a long introduction, recounting the slow growth of mathematical rigor, by the fact of easy access by all of you to two reports essentially on the same field: the Gibbs Lecture, by Professor James Pierpont, presented at the Nashville meeting of these organizations in 1927, and the invited address by Professor Arnold Dresden, presented at the same meeting, both of which were printed in Volume 34 (1928) of the *Bulletin of the American Mathematical Society*.

Pierpont gave a general résumé, going back at least to the beginnings of the Calculus, and coming down the centuries from Newton and Leibnitz through Euler and Lagrange and Cauchy to the days of Weierstrass and Kronecker and Cantor and Poincaré, and thence to our own generation and the present decade, with sketches of the three chief movements of this period, which are associated in men's minds most vividly with the names of Whitehead and Russell, Hilbert, and Brouwer, respectively. These remain the three chief directions of research in this field, and it is to them that I shall give particular attention in what follows. By name, these three schools of thought, or methods of procedure, are most often called the logistic, the postulational or formalistic, and the intuitional schools or methods, respectively. While my own sympathies will doubtless appear, I will attempt to give an impartial account of the progress in these fields, in grand outlines, and their present states.

Dresden, in his address, states what appear to him to be the underlying philosophical aspects. Both here, and in a former report published in Volume 30 (1924) of the *Bulletin,* he gives special attention to the work of Brouwer and to its underlying philosophy, but he does so with great impartiality, and his views on the doctrines which underlie mathematics and mathematical logic are still worthy of careful study. These two reports by Dresden were preceded by a translation by him of an article by Brouwer, published in the *Bulletin* in 1913. The two papers in 1913 and 1924 deal primarily with Brouwer's work; with the present article, they span two decades, and it may be of interest to observe by a comparison with them the slow but certain progress of the principal ideas during these two decades.

## 2. Introduction of Infinities

In a large sense, though with certain notable exceptions, such as the controversies over the parallel postulate, the origin of logical difficulties appears to lie in the introduction of infinities into mathematics. Even in the case of the parallel postulate, the rôle of infinity is clearly apparent, and might be held to be the paramount difficulty. With the advent of the Calculus, at any rate, with its troublesome concepts of infinitesimal and of limit, the effect of infinities upon mathematics and mathematical reasoning becomes striking and undebatable. It is with these difficulties that Pierpont begins in his address.

That essentially the same difficulties had arisen in the old Greek paradoxes is now clear to us; but such paradoxes were regarded mainly as philosophical playthings, and the mathematical controversies in the same field awaited the important development of the Calculus. At one other point, however, an objection had been raised before that time; and it is so important for our more recent studies that I wish to emphasize it, particularly because it is not mentioned in the addresses quoted above. Isaac Barrow, who was one of Newton's teachers, and one to whom Newton owed much, had objected, before the Calculus controversy, to the development of the theory of proportion in the Fifth Book of Euclid. He pointed out that Euclid's argument, and in particular his definition of the sense of inequalities for what we should now call irrational numbers, requires, for a determinate answer, the use of an infinite number of steps. This objection, which Barrow stated in clear language, makes him the forerunner of such modern scholars as Kronecker, Poincaré, Brouwer, Weyl and E. T. Bell, all of whom have reiterated this objection. In it, the notion of infinity enters in mathematical reasoning again, in a very different, and in a very disturbing fashion.

The position of Kronecker is stated in some detail by Pierpont. In his *Festschrift,*[2] Kronecker attacked particularly the definition of reducibility of a polynomial, which is ordinarily stated by saying that a polynomial is reducible, or not, according as it has, or has not, a rational factor. Without means for decision, and faced with a possible infinite number of trials, Kronecker declares such a definition not only unusable, but meaningless. For the same reasons, he attacked bitterly the whole theory of irrational numbers, and the entire structure of the Weierstrass theory of functions. To this day, these objections

[2] *Zeitschr. für Math.*, Vol. 92. 1882.

stand. They have been voiced again and again, most strenuously, perhaps, by Brouwer, which may be a misfortune. To many other great mathematicians, however, including Poincaré and Weyl, objections of this character, involving both definitions and existence proofs, have seemed weighty and soberly ominous. It is indeed surprising that so little heed has been paid to the reasonable warning given time and again by men of the first rank, from Barrow to Poincaré; and it must be admitted that every such definition, every such existence proof, which does not contain in itself an explicit means for setting up the concept discussed in a finite number of steps, is open to question, and can not be said to be established with logical rigor.

That insistence upon such a point would destroy much of mathematical literature, as has been urged by such equally great figures as Weierstrass and Hilbert, seems to me to be as much beside the point as is that argument for immortality which depends upon our displeasure at mortality. If there be no better argument, we may as well begin at once some effort toward reconstructing those parts of mathematics that depend on such debatable procedures.

In one instance, this has already happened. In 1897, Burali-Forti[3] published his now famous paradox on transfinite numbers. As a result, that theory is now quite re-formed, and parts of it are no longer used, while some theorems, such as the theorem that every closed set consists of a countable set together with a perfect set, once proved by means of that theory, is now commonly proved otherwise. Possibly due to this very paradox, and surely due to some similar considerations, Poincaré showed a most interesting change of attitude—a volte-face, indeed—from the Paris Congress in 1900, where he said, "One may say to-day that absolute rigor has been attained," to the Rome Congress in 1908, where he said, "Later generations will regard the Mengenlehre as a disease from which one has recovered." His other writings from that time on betray his lack of faith in that rigor which he had called "final" in 1900.

Such objections are climaxed and most vociferously proclaimed by Brouwer, as I have stated above, but he is by no means alone.[4] These objections, however, should be differentiated from what is the central part of Brouwer's thesis, the so-called intuitionism. It is by no means necessary to become an adept of intuitionism in order to adopt the objections of Kronecker and Poincaré, which Brouwer also advocates. Nor is Brouwer's objection to the Law of the Excluded Middle an integral part of intuitionism. One may, and, as I shall point out, one now must, admit that the Law of the Excluded Middle is not a necessary part of logic, whether one is an intuitionist or not. All these objections are advocated strongly—perhaps too strongly—by Brouwer, and his adherents as well as he will justly claim them as an integral part of his whole thinking and of his works. This I will not deny. What I wish to emphasize is that neither the objection to an infinite number of steps in an argument or definition or existence theorem, nor the objection to the Law of the Excluded Middle as a fixed principle, is so tied to intuitionism that one must accept it in order to accept these others. I believe that the general impression that these ideas can not be accepted without acceptance of all that is associated with Brouwer's name is one of the reasons why the mathematical world has so long delayed acceptance of them, and action based upon them.

### 3. Brouwer's Position. Excluded Middle

In what precedes, I have dwelt upon one objection voiced by Brouwer, but also by many great scholars before him. His objection to the Law of the Excluded Middle is, as I have remarked, also independent of the method or school called intuitionism. Leaving that method for later discussion, I wish to call attention now to his position, and the position of others, regarding the Law of the Excluded Middle. His own statements sometimes lack complete clarity, and even the expositions of Dresden mentioned above may not be wholly obvious. Certainly the attitude of Brouwer was not clear to many of his opponents. Thus Barzin and Errera obviously misunderstood him, as they themselves state in a later article.[5]

That Brouwer rejects the law is quite obvious. His reasons also seem not hard to find for one who wills, and they certainly appear in the examples which he cites.[6] One such example is to know whether there exists a number k which expresses the number of digits in the number $\pi$ at which, for the first time, the sequence 0123456789 begins in the decimal representation of $\pi$. It is not provable at present that k exists, for such a sequence does not occur in the decimal representation of $\pi$ as far as its expression has been calculated.

It is then obvious that Brouwer is thinking, as others are thinking, that it may not be possible to arrive at a demonstration of a proposition p, or of its denial p′, by a finite sequence of syllogisms, without the use of the law mentioned. If not, there may be a proposition not provable, whose denial (p′) is also not provable. This may even be the case if argu-

[3] *Rend. Circ. Mat. de Palermo,* 11: 154–164. 1897.

[4] See Brouwer (trans. by Dresden), *Bull. Amer. Math. Soc.,* 20: 81 *ff.* (1913); Brouwer, *Jahresbericht D. M. V.,* 28: 203; 1920); Brouwer, *Zeitschr. für Math.,* 154: 1 (1925); Pierpont, *Bull. Amer. Math. Soc.* 34: 23–53 (1928); Dresden, *Bull. Amer. Math. Soc.,* 30: 31–40 (1924) and 34: 438–452 (1928).

[5] *Acad. de Belgique, Classe des Sciences,* 13: 56–71 (1927); *Arch. Soc. Belge Philos.,* pp. 3–26. 1928–29.

[6] *Zeitschr. für Math.,* 154: 1. 1925.

ments that are equivalent to the use of an infinite number of steps are allowed. Such propositions need not be *absurd,* as some have claimed: the preceding example does not introduce any new concepts, and is within what is sometimes called the "universe of discourse"; the question involved can not be called absurd, or rejected; indeed, it is entirely thinkable that the question can be answered.

The immediate reply of many persons is that the proposition that k exists must either be true or else false, on the basis of "ultimate" truth. This is, indeed, precisely the Law of the Excluded Middle. If the topics discussed form a part of the concrete universe, thought of as externally real, such a position would be justified. In how far such a position is tenable will be discussed in the next section. The belief in a real external existence of the objects and relationships under discussion is undoubtedly the basis for the law, as it is, no doubt, the basis for all logic. Again, as Dresden has remarked[7] in his discussion of Brouwer's position, the law would be granted if the proposition dealt with a finite system. That Brouwer's own statements are not particularly clear on these matters will appear from the quotations which Dresden makes in the article just cited, and from Dresden's own comments.

## 4. Reality. The External World

As I have just stated, a crucial element in any such discussion is the meaning of the words "true" and "false," and the associated question of the conceived real existence of the concepts and relationships under discussion in the real external world. It may be as well to grant at once that the law hold in an *a priori* sense in such an *a priori* system.

On the other hand, so far as I know, no modern school of mathematical thought, least of all the postulational or formalistic school, would accept such a tenet. Beginning with the discussions of the parallel axiom of Euclid, the whole course of mathematical logic has tended strongly toward the abandonment of the claim that an axiom or a postulate necessarily represents the realities of the external universe. Thus every present school of mathematical thought, in so far as I know, would accept either Euclidean geometry or any one of the non-Euclidean geometries, with no claim that one of them more than any other represents the realities. Thus, while I have not yet discussed the different schools nor the differences that exist in their fundamental thinking, I may assume that no one of these schools would attempt to base its systems on a claim of reality. The nearest approach to such a claim would be the school associated with Brouwer himself, but since he freely accepts the different geometries mentioned above as equally valid, for example, it is clear that any claim of the intuitionists for the reality of their systems would be quite limited; to this I shall return.

If the claim for reality, the claim that the objects and the relationships under discussion form a part of an existent external world, disappears, then the *a priori* nature of "truth" and "falsity" of propositions also disappears, and with it disappears also the *a priori* assumption that any proposition is either true or else false, that is, the Law of the Excluded Middle. To reestablish it, we need at the least a clear agreement on the meaning of the words "true" and "false"; and we need new assurance of the validity of the law.

That a confusion of thought arises continually from the tendency of the human mind to revert to the primeval definitions or *a priori* conceptions of "true" and "false" appears very frequently in the literature. Thus, such a careful thinker as Church,[8] in his keen criticism of Barzin and Errera, says of the Brouwer position: "The latter point" (a statement essentially quoted from Brouwer) "depends, of course, on identifying the truth of a proposition with the possibility of proving the proposition. But it seems more in accord with our usual ideas to think of truth as a property independent of our ability to prove it. Consequently we prefer to take the truth of a proposition merely as an undefined term subject to certain postulates, among them, if we choose to include it, the law of the excluded middle." While I must admit at once that Church's position is entirely tenable and logically sound, and while it is only just to Church to admit that he says elsewhere that one may also choose to deny the law, his position seems to be to avoid trying to define "true" and "false" in order to save the Law of the Excluded Middle. One must admit the correctness (logically) of his statement, since what he proposes is precisely what is done in the system of Principia, as we shall see. To admit that such a system is a possible system of logic, however, is far from admitting that it is the only system of logic; and to assert that such a system (*e.g.,* Principia) is "more in accord with our usual ideas," that is, with the *a priori* conception of "true" and "false" in an external world of realities, seems strange to one to whom the rudiments of the Principia are known.

Still closer to the *a priori* conception of "truth" is the position taken by Barzin and Errera. In the second article just cited, they criticize the definition given by Levy, which we shall mention in a moment. They say (page 5): "M. Levy . . . defines a truth or falsity which he calls *brouwerian,*" and they speak of the "usual" sense of truth and falsity, without further comment.

[7] Dresden, *Bull. Amer. Math. Soc.,* 30: 39. 1924.

[8] Church, *Bull. Amer. Math. Soc.,* 34: 75–78. 1928.

The definition given by Levy[9] deserves attention. Although he calls it "brouwerian," he has stated also that it does not agree precisely with Brouwer's own view. Levy says that a proposition is "true" if it is possible to demonstrate it (obviously without the use of L. E. M.), and "false" if it is possible to prove its denial p′. I myself had used essentially these same definitions[10] in a paper presented to this society, and I have been told by Weyl, in conversation, that this is probably Brouwer's point of view, though I am not aware that he has stated it distinctly and clearly.

The effect of such a definition upon the law (L. E. M.) is clear enough. If a proposition p is not "true," does it follow that it is "false"? This now has a distinct meaning, at least. It means: if p can not be proved (in a finite number of steps and without L. E. M.) then p′ can be proved. Of this there is no present guarantee. Hence the law (L. E. M.) has no present validity. What further effects such a position may have upon (say) the mathematics of a postulational system, and in how far the validity of the law (L. E. M.) may be secured in such a system, will be discussed later.

As a result of the present discussion, it is sufficient to point out that a crucial element in any treatment of these matters is to determine what the author means by "truth," that is, whether he reverts to the *a priori* concept based on a claim of reality; or assumes, with Church, what is essentially the Principia position, that "truth" is an undefined property; or uses what I shall call, with Levy, the "brouwerian" definition of "truth"; or gives some other definition of the term. Clearly, the law (L. E. M.) has totally different significances in these various cases.

### 5. The Formalistic or Postulational Method

It is probable that the postulational or formalistic view-point is the one most familiar to my audience, but a precise statement of it is not easy to give. A clear statement is given by Bernstein,[11] and I will not repeat it. Many other authors have given clear descriptions. One given with a clear consciousness of the existence of Brouwer's ideas is that of Dresden,[12] which is nevertheless, in its essence, a description of the postulational view-point.

I wish to refer hurriedly to some of the fundamental ideas present in modern discussions of any postulational system, but I shall assume that you are familiar with them. It is usual to prove that the postulates stated are *independent,* that is, that no one can be deduced from the others; that they are *consistent,* that is, that they contain no hidden contradiction, which is done (ordinarily) by exhibiting a set of objects and operations or relations whose existence is supposed known and which satisfy all the postulates. It is desired also to show that the system of postulates is *complete,* that is, that no new postulate may be added to the set without the introduction of a new undefined concept; and that they are *categorical,* that is, that two systems that satisfy the postulates can be made to correspond isomorphically.

The present status of this school of thought is also known to you perhaps better than is that of any other school. Its results have been quite successful in many fields of mathematical thought, and the extent to which such examination of systems of postulates has been carried surely exceeds any estimate which might have been made, say, in 1900. One serious bar remains. In general, the proofs of consistency have been made on the assumption of the soundness of the postulates of arithmetic. These postulates themselves have been discussed extensively, and most strenuous efforts have been made to prove that they themselves are consistent. Hilbert and his followers have been most hopeful that final success would be achieved, and a partial success has been attained by Hilbert himself,[13] von Neumann[14] and others. The means employed by Hilbert and others, however, particularly the employment of arbitrary marks, seem of doubtful validity to many, and one must hesitate to announce that a final success has been attained.

The present status, then, remains that we must assume the validity of the postulates of arithmetic, in some form. We need, indeed, thus much of assumed *reality,* or at least assumed *consistency.* If it be an assumption of *reality,* then the L. E. M. would have a certain *a priori* validity based on that assumption; but even that would not of itself carry through to other sets of postulates based upon this one, since a proof of consistency by no means demonstrates reality.

As for "truth," we may assume, with Church, that it is an undefined property, and we may adjoin (see Bernstein, *loc. cit.*) some such set of postulates for logic as that of the Principia. To do so, however, is clearly an act of *choice,* not of necessity; and this Church clearly indicates.

On the other hand, it would appear more in keeping to call these things "true," just as we call the postulates themselves "true," not because of an instinctive belief in their ultimate reality in an external world, but simply because they follow from the postulates.

[9] *Acad. de Belgique Classe des Sciences,* 13: 256–266. 1927.

[10] *Bull. Amer. Math. Soc.,* 34: 436. 1928.

[11] *Bull. Amer. Math. Soc.,* 37: 484. 1931.

[12] *Bull. Amer. Math. Soc.,* 34: 442. 1928.

[13] Hilbert, *Jahresbericht D. M. V.,* 8: 1900; *Math. Annalen,* 78: 405. 1918; *Abh. Hamburg Univ.,* 1: 157. 1922; *Math. Annalen,* 88: 151. 1922–23, and 95: 161. 1926. Also references given by Dresden, *Bull. Amer. Math. Soc.,* 34: 440. 1928.

[14] v. Neumann, *Math. Zeitschrift,* 26: 1 (1927), and *Math. Annalen,* 154: 219. 1925.

This is indeed no other than the position that I myself have taken, that Levy took, and that I have called, with Levy, "brouwerian." It seems to me, however, not primarily brouwerian; rather, it seems to me very decidedly in accord with the very spirit of the postulational school. In that case, however, some support would have to be given to establish the validity of the L. E. M., since it ceases to be obviously true.

If we could prove the set of postulates have the property that any proposition p can be proved, or else its denial p′ can be proved, from the set of postulates, we should have turned the trick. If we can not do this, then of what avail is it to have adopted rules of logic which essentially beg the question? Such rules of logic *do* essentially beg the question, for, after all, what we want to know is precisely whether or not we can prove p or else p′. To assume that we can always do one or the other of these things, or, what amounts to the same thing, to say (in no matter how disguised a form) that p is to be called "true" not only when we can give a direct proof of it, but also whenever we can not prove p′, seems strangely out of accord with the spirit of the postulational method. It is, however, logically possible to do this.

A dilemma to which we are led if we take this position has been stated by Church in his discussion of the Zermelo postulate.[15] Here he himself is dealing with a possible *addition* to the laws of logic, and, since alternatives present themselves, it is obvious that we can not decide all questions until some such additional law has been assumed. Realizing the relation of this question to the L. E. M., Church states (p. 186) that the fact that we might be led, after assuming one or the other of two additional postulates, to different conclusions regarding the same proposition, he concludes that we should then have not a violation of the L. E. M. but rather two universes of thought, each self-consistent, proceeding forever side-by-side, perhaps after the manner of the two universes of thought contained in Euclidean geometry and one non-Euclidean geometry. It seems obvious, however, that *just before* the additional postulate is chosen, we should certainly be in possession of a consistent set of postulates for which the L. E. M. does not hold. Nor is it clear how one may know when this situation exists. For example, before the explicit statement of the Zermelo postulate, would it have been clear that the L. E. M. did *not* then apply to the system as it was? Let me say distinctly, however, that the remark of Church seems to me to be sound in so far as it goes.

### 6. The Intuitional School

I have discussed already two phases of the work of Brouwer, namely, his attitude toward the L. E. M. and his attitude toward proofs or definitions that are based effectively upon the use of an infinite number of steps. Neither of these has a specific relation, however, to the intuitional method, in the sense that one may adhere to either or both of these other principles without attaching himself thereby to the intuitional school; indeed, as I have pointed out, many mathematicians of note have done so, without participating thereby in the intuitional movement.

Brouwer has stated his position on intuitionalism as the proper basis for mathematical work in numerous articles cited above. Two quotations from him that are given by Dresden[16] seem to give in brief space something of his view. "This intiution," says Dresden, "upon which not only mathematical thinking, but all intellectual activity is held to be based, is found in the abstract substratum of all observation of change, 'a fusion of continuous and discrete, a possibility of conceiving simultaneously several units, connected by a *between* that can not be exhausted by the interpolation of new units.'" And again: "It [the fundamental intuitive concept of mathematics] manifests itself in the intuition of time, which makes possible 'repetition, as being object in time, and again object.'"

Without pretending that this represents the whole of the point of view of the intuitionists, I may say that one concept which seems to stand out clearly is the acceptance on the basis of intuition, of some essential properties of *time*. In particular, the indefinite divisibility of it, the occurrence of a time between any two other times, appears; and the idea of *unit* is emphasized. These are indeed fundamental properties of pure number, as it is conceived in arithmetic. The recognition of *time* as a primordial prototype is not at all novel: Hamilton defined *mathematics* as "the science of pure time," and many another has done his fundamental *intuitional* thinking (which we may grant all mathematicians *must* do in some way) in terms of *time*.

While I reiterate that this does not exhaust the views of Brouwer on this field of thought, it does appear to me that there is here a common ground which I have not seen emphasized, as between intuitional and postulational thinking: it is that in both, if I have not too much distorted the facts, the essential properties of *time* (that is, of *real number*), are at present assumed to be valid upon the basis of our intuition, for I have pointed out that the present state of the postulational school is essentially just this.

At at least one other point, however, the two schools of thought part company in a more decisive manner. Brouwer contends that logic is not a sure guide toward the building-up of mathematical thought, and that the existence of a variety of possible logical sys-

[15] *Trans. Amer. Math. Soc.*, 29: 178–208. 1927.

[16] *Bull. Amer. Math. Soc.*, 30: 32. 1924.

tems leads one to feel that results obtained by one such system may not be wholly convincing. This position has been clearly stated by Boutroux.[17] It is admirably demonstrated, in fact, by the results which have been obtained by the use of the Zermelo postulate, as contrasted with results obtainable with no such postulate, or with a different one. I think that Brouwer would hold that the intuition must be called upon to decide when such a situation arises. That few of us would be able to do this with any degree of confidence, is, perhaps, not a valid objection. Certainly the formalistic or postulational school would not agree to such a procedure, except, perhaps, in an extremely restricted and narrow form. To what extent the modern developments of logic tend to confirm Brouwer's views, we shall see presently.

I have referred in what precedes chiefly to the Zermelo postulate because it is in some senses the best known case of an addition to the preceding logical system. There are others, however, which are nearly if not quite as prominent in the minds of mathematicians. Among these, I may mention the proposed postulate of Russell[18] that "whatever involves all of a collection must not be one of the collection," and the proposed postulate of Hilbert[19] to sanction the use of complete induction in the transfinite case. These notable instances of additions to the logical system, and their possible alternatives illustrate in themselves the possible variety of logical systems of which Boutroux speaks.

While I make no claim to have exhausted the views of intuitionists, I have presented some which seem to have their support. It is to be noted that the advances in logical theory tend rather to support them than otherwise, but perhaps not in precisely the manner that was intended by their originators.

## 7. LOGISTICS. THE PRINCIPIA

The logistic school has attempted to introduce a symbolism to replace ordinary language, in order to avoid the errors traceable to the ambiguities of ordinary language, and to express mathematics essentially as a part of logic by means of this symbolism. A first comprehensive attempt was begun by Peano in the "Formulaire de Mathématique" (Vol. 1, 1895), which was extended and completed in four volumes during the years 1895–1903 by Peano and several other Italian mathematicians. A still more comprehensive and exhaustive treatment began with a paper by Russell in the *American Journal* in 1908, and led to the monumental work "Principia Mathematica," by Whitehead and Russell (2d ed., 1925–27), to which reference has been made above. It was thought by the authors and by many followers that the procedure followed was subject to no errors, and that the resulting system was indeed final. Many mathematicians, however, including most German mathematicians, remained skeptical, and it is true that the authors felt obliged to introduce fundamental changes in the second edition, largely due to the work of H. M. Sheffer. A brief statement of the essential purposes and methods of the "Principia" is given by Bernstein,[20] and I may refer any who are not familiar with its nature to that article In his review of "Principia,." Bernstein pointed out certain difficulties of interpretation, and he has insisted upon these difficulties in his later articles[20] A simple instance is that the symbol "p" is often read "p is true," in spite of a warning by the authors of "Principia" against doing so. There are also certain "informal" statements in the "Principia" which were intended to clarify the more formal ones; but it appears that there are real differences between the "formal" and the "informal" systems, so that it may be said that the "Principia" consists of two different systems conducted simultaneously.

The definition of *implication* is stated essentially in the form: "p implies q if it is true that either not-p is true or else q is true." This definition is entirely sound, but it departs fundamentally from the Aristotelian system. Thus a false proposition implies any proposition whatever; and a true proposition implies any other true proposition. For this reason, the authors of the "Principia" took the position that the usual concepts of *independence* and of *consistency* do not apply to their own system, since any (true) postulate must imply any other (true) postulate. Bernstein has shown that this is not the case, however, by reducing the "Principia" assumptions to the form of postulates for a Boolean Algebra, since the definition of implication stated above essentially divides all propositions into two classes, which may be identified with the symbols 1 and 0 of a Boolean Algebra, for which postulates paralleling those of the "Principia" are then stated. These postulates are subject to examination for independence and for consistency, so that the original "Principia" postulates are also. It also proves possible to state the entire system in terms that make it a strict mathematical science in the sense of the postulational method. Another comprehensive survey of the situation is in type and will be published in the January, 1933, issue of the Transactions of the American Mathematical Society by E. V. Huntington. His system differs from that of Bernstein chiefly in the introduction, not only of the class K of all propo-

[17] Boutroux, ''L'Idéal des Mathématiciens.'' 1908.

[18] *Amer. Jour. Math.* 30: 225 (1908); Whitehead and Russell, ''Principia Mathematica'' (2nd ed., 1925), p. 58.

[19] Hilbert, *Math. Annalen,* 88: 151. 1922–23.

[20] Bernstein, *Bull. Amer. Math. Soc.,* 32: 711–713 (1926); 37: 480–488 (1931); 38: 388–390 (1932); 38: 589–593 (1932).

sitions, but also of another class T of propositions, a subclass of K, in terms of which the postulates are stated. The independence and consistency of these postulates are examined with great care. It is shown that the resulting system is equivalent to the "informal" "Principia" system, but the inherent difficulty of deriving it from the "formal" "Principia" system again manifests itself. Quite informally, one may think of T as the subclass of *true* propositions.

In either Bernstein's or Huntington's systems, and therefore in the "informal" "Principia" system, the L. E. M. follows from the postulates, though this is not the case for the "formal" "Principia" system. However, no immediate conclusion as to the universal validity of that law can be said to follow, since it is here simply postulated. The only conclusion is that the "informal" "Principia" is a dichotomy; that is, it is a two-valued system. This does not show that every mathematical system must also be dichotomous; it shows only that the "informal" "Principia" system is not applicable to a mathematical system unless that system is shown to be a dichotomy. This is quite a different statement.

### 8. OTHER LOGICAL SYSTEMS. ABANDONMENT OF L. E. M.

Despite the monumental nature of the "Principia," it follows from what precedes that we must again face the question as to whether or not the L. E. M. is of universal application. The recent work of Bernstein, Huntington and others have not altered the inherent nature of the "Principia"; they have simply refined it, and have transformed it into a mathematical system, freed from essential disagreements between "informal" and "formal" system.

Attempts have been made to demonstrate the law. I have referred to the attempt of Barzin and Errera. Many replies were made to this attempt, of which two that are noteworthy are the papers of Church and Levy, in which the difficulties of the attempted argument are clearly established. Indeed, if the L. E. M. could be proved from the remaining standard laws of classical logic, it would follow, of course, that there would be no necessity of stating it. In a sense, therefore, any such attempt was predestined to fail, if any statement of the law is needed.

In 1930, however, a very definite settlement of all such controversy was given by Lukasiewicz and Tarski,[21] who actually set up a trichotomy which satisfies every requirement of implication, and which possesses a strict table of implications, including a *middle,* which I may call "uncertainty," as well as the customary "true" and "false." An excellent account has been given by C. I. Lewis in *The Monist* for October, 1932. It appears from their work, and from some later papers, that it is perfectly possible to set up and to operate perfectly sound systems which have just as definite "implication" systems as that of the "Principia," which have any desired number of intermediate "truth-values." One such which has been worked out with care is a quadruple system whose "truth-values" I may call "true," "probable," "improbable" and "false." Indeed the resulting system bears at least as close a relation to the popular interpretation of these four concepts as does the "Principia" to the popular interpretations of "true" and "false."

[21] *Comptes Rendus Soc. de Varsovie,* 23, III: 51–77. 1930.

We are then obliged to conclude, with Lewis, that the L. E. M. is not "writ in the heavens," that it is not a law of universal application in logic. Rather it "reflects our stubborn adherence to the simplest of all possible modes of division, and our predominant interest in concrete objects as opposed to abstract concepts." These words of Lewis should have strong import to mathematicians, for in mathematics we deal habitually with just such abstract concepts.

### 9. EXAMPLES. THEORY OF PROBABILITY

Lewis, in the paper cited above, and Lewis and Langford, in their "Symbolic Logic" use the phrases "certainly true," "certainly false," "doubtful" as names for the "truth-values" of a trichotomy. I have insisted above upon such situations as actually existent, useful and commonly employed for practical ends, with at least as close adherence to the theoretical systems as obtains in the dichotomy "true" and "false" in the logic of ordinary reasoning.

It would seem that any desired scheme of "truth-values," however numerous, would find again a parallel in human thinking. The quadruple system "true," "probable," "improbable," "false," mentioned above, is such a case; though again I must insist that the precise rules for implication would be followed no more than in the case of ordinary reasoning. To obtain a similar parallel to any number of "truth-values," it is only necessary to appeal more openly to the theory of probabilities, and to assign to definite degrees of probability from 0 to 1 various "truth-values," that is, various gradations of certainty. I am attempting only to point out that such systems are by no means bizarre systems (or at least no more bizarre than is the "Principia" system), for something much akin to them is actually present in our minds, and forms habitually a basis for a great part of our actual thinking.

Nor is the limiting case of all this at all bizarre. It is quite legitimate to set up a scale of probabilities, and we do commonly do so, in which each rational proper fraction expresses a degree of probability, with the extreme limits 0 and 1, which express impossibility and certainty. The parallel logical system with an infinite number of graduations in "truth-values" from "false" to "true" appears to be just as feasible. Finally, a continuous scale might be established in either the popular sense of the theory of probability, or in the exact "implication" sense of a strict logical system. That the theory of probabilities may be thought of, at least informally, as constituting in itself a scheme of logical thinking in which there are many gradations of "truth-values" may form a clue toward rational appreciation of logical systems in which the L. E. M. is violated. It is unnecessary, however, to pretend to precise correspondence in this case, any more than there is precise correspondence between the "Principia" system and ordinary reasoning, for in each case independent and satisfactory proof exists that the logical system in question is legitimate.

## 10. Conclusions

I have attempted to outline in its major details the development of the logic of mathematics in recent years. If it appear to any that the acceptance of such ideas will destroy mathematics or parts of it, I would point out that a certain amount of discarding of what has been is necessary in order to assure progress. If we are to deny new developments whenever they require relinquishment of the ideas of the past, we shall be serving not truth but only our vanity.

It is indeed true that many famous mathematicians have given up in despair. Cantor, Dedekind, Frege, all consciously accepted defeat, and bitterly. I have mentioned the protest in a former generation of Weierstrass; in our generation, of Hilbert; these great men cry out that great portions of mathematics will fall if such ideas prevail. True, but that is no reason why they must not prevail if they be correct.

Nor is despair the note of all scholars. Brouwer, Weyl, Poincaré, show no sign of pessimism. They, and many lesser men, feel only that we may go on to new conquests of truth. New minds will arise who will carry mathematical truth in the next generation not to destruction, but to yet greater heights, to new and higher ideals of rigor.

For young men, there is a challenge in all this. Not that we can presume that Rome can be rebuilt after the conflagration in a single day. For a long time we must proceed as we now seem to be: asserting that our results are valid if we postulate the L. E. M. along with our other postulates. While this is a fundamentally weak situation, in view of our inability to show that our postulates are categorical, it is at worst defensible in the present state of our knowledge. We must proceed slowly. A vast amount of work that should and must be done lies in exploring the whole of mathematical literature to determine which theorems in a given field require the use of the L. E. M. for their demonstration, in the form in which we now do demonstrate them. Next, we may find out how to give better proofs, in which that law is not assumed, at least in some cases. On the basis of any philosophy, such discoveries would be valuable. For a reconstruction of mathematics they are quite necessary.

Can definitions and existence theorems be revised in every field, at least in some cases, so that the concepts discussed can be actually arrived at in a finite number of steps?

Such reconstructions are in fact already in progress. Not only Brouwer, but many others who have seen the need for such investigation, irrespective of an ultimate acceptance of all that now appears to be true, have been working toward these very goals. One need by no means accept the intuitionist point of view to see the value of such reconstruction. If it be only partial in our time, we should not fear the ultimate future. Generations yet unborn will doubtless face still some of our doubts, some of our problems.

There is, no doubt, some sense of tragedy in this, as in every previous instance of advancing ideals of logical exactness. We too lay down our task, unfinished. I shall only paraphrase the sentiments of great mathematicians of the past who have seen their labors end incompleted, if I quote to you some of the lines of a poem of Kipling which I treasure deeply, "The Palace"; in it, the master builder, after years of proud effort, lays down his task at last, saying:

When I was a King and a Mason,
In the open noon of my pride,
They sent me word from the Darkness,
They whispered and called me aside;
They said: "The *end* is forbidden."
They said: "Thy use is fulfilled;
"Thy Palace shall stand as that other's,
"The Spoil of a King who shall build."

I called my men from my trenches,
My quarries, my wharves, and my shears,
All I had wrought I abandoned
To the Faith of the faithless years.
Only I cut on each timber,—
Only I carved on each stone:
"After me cometh a builder;
"Tell him I too have known."

# OBITUARY

## EDWARD BRUCE WILLIAMSON

EDWARD BRUCE WILLIAMSON, entomologist and naturalist, died at Ann Arbor, Michigan, on February 28, 1933, at the age of fifty-five. His boyhood days were spent on a farm near Bluffton, Indiana. After graduating from Ohio State University in 1898, he was assistant curator at the Carnegie Museum, 1898–99, and a fellow at Vanderbilt University, 1900–01. From 1905 to 1930 he served as president of the Wells County Bank at Bluffton, and since 1930, as research associate at the Museum of Zoology, University of Michigan.

His first paper on the *Odonata* appeared in 1897 and in the interval between then and his death he published more than 65 papers on this group of insects. Much of the work was done before and after banking hours. While the papers were mainly of a systematic nature, they also contain much data of a general biological nature observed during his extensive collecting trips in the United States, Central and South America. The value of these contributions is attested by the high esteem in which he was held by entomologists the world over. In addition to his work as an entomologist he was one of the pioneer breeders of iris. He developed and placed on the market many of the best varieties and his interest in this field was maintained until the end. His interests, however, were not limited to these two fields. In his earlier years he had collected birds' eggs and during his boyhood days he was much interested in pets. In fact, he was interested in all living things, a naturalist in the true sense of the word.

The things which have been said, however, give to the stranger no real concept of Bruce Williamson. One had to know him personally in order to appreciate him. He was a rare personality; an amateur in spirit and enthusiasm, energetic, stimulating alike to the non-scientist as well as the scientist. So contagious was his enthusiasm for natural phenomena that he was able to interest either children or adults in the things he was doing. It was literally impossible to be around him without getting an insect net to chase dragon-flies or without planning an iris garden. One could not remain static in his presence, because of his seemingly inexhaustible supply of energy. Perhaps, because of the use of so much energy, his death came somewhat prematurely, but who can say that he did not live more richly and abundantly than those of us who creep at a slower pace. We who had the privilege of knowing him intimately prized his friendship in a way difficult to express in words, and hence his loss to us is the greater. The world would be richer if we had more naturalists like him.

FERNANDUS PAYNE

## RECENT DEATHS

THE death is announced of Dr. Frank Mann Life, physicist, dean of the College of Letters, Arts and Sciences at the University of Arizona. He was in his sixty-third year.

JOHN LEMUEL STONE, emeritus professor of farm practise at the New York State College of Agriculture at Cornell University, died on March 8. He was in his eightieth year.

CHARLES E. EVELETH, a vice-president of the General Electric Company and formerly manager of the Schenectady plant, died on March 25, at the age of fifty-seven years.

DR. ROYAL EDGAR JEFFS, associate professor of botany in the University of Oklahoma, died on February 17, at the age of fifty-three years.

ARTHUR BLISS SEYMOUR, since 1886 assistant in the cryptogamic herbarium at Harvard University, died on March 29, at the age of seventy-four years.

DR. FERNANDO WOOD MARTIN, formerly vice-president of Randolph-Macon Woman's College and for thirty-six years head of its department of chemistry, died on March 22, at the age of sixty-nine years. He retired in 1929 as emeritus professor.

THE REV. FREDERICK L. ODENBACH, S.J., for the past forty years meteorologist and seismologist at John Carroll University, Cleveland, Ohio, died on March 15, at the age of seventy-five years. It was through Father Odenbach's influence and initiative that seismographic equipment was installed and stations were organized at fifteen Jesuit colleges and universities in the United States and Canada during the years 1909 to 1912.

DR. WILLIAM HENRY PORTER, professor emeritus of pathology and internal medicine at the New York Post-Graduate Medical School, died on March 27. He was in his eightieth year.

DR. JOHN MILLAR THOMSON, emeritus professor of chemistry at King's College, London, died on March 22, at the age of eighty years.

# SCIENTIFIC EVENTS

## INTERNATIONAL STANDARD FOR THE OVARIAN FOLLICULAR HORMONE

DURING the past summer the Health Organization of the League of Nations held a meeting on the standardization of the estrus-producing hormone. Sir Henry Dale presided over the conference, which was composed of A. Butenandt, E. A. Doisy, E. Laqueur, G. F. Marrian and A. S. Parkes. In an abbreviated form the most important points of the agreement were:

(1) That a material standard preparation should be preserved as a central standard of reference.

(2) That this material standard should consist of the hydroxy-ketonic form of the hormone.

(3) That the various countries will be invited to contribute samples which will be combined to form the standard preparation.

(4) That the unit will be the specific estrus-producing activity contained in 0.1 gamma of the standard preparation.

(5) That by the term "estrus-producing activity" is to be understood the power of producing in an adult female animal completely deprived of its ovaries an accurately recognizable degree of the changes characteristic of normal estrus, *i.e.*, the changes in cellular contents of the vaginal secretion of the rat or mouse.

(6) That the comparison of an unknown preparation with the standard can only be accurately made if the conditions of administration and interpretation of results are identical.

(7) That a bio-assay procedure, which has been proved to be capable of determining the equality of activity with an error not greater than plus or minus 20 per cent., should be used in comparing a preparation with the international standard.

(8) That proper precautions will be observed in the preparation and storage of the international standard. The international standard will be kept at the National Institute for Medical Research in London, but a portion will be available for distribution in each country.

The adoption of an international standard should solve many of the vexing problems of bio-assay of the estrus-producing hormone. In the past, many modifications of the original Allen-Doisy bio-assay procedure have been introduced. This has led to a great many different units, since so many different factors alter the absolute weight of the hormone required to produce estrus. The result was that no investigator could compare his results with those of another investigator with any feeling of assurance of accuracy. With the establishment of an international standard it is hoped that investigators will make use of this standard preparation and that pharmaceutical houses will also label their products in terms of the international unit.

E. A. D.

## THE ELEVENTH INTERNATIONAL SYMPOSIUM ON PHYSICS AT THE UNIVERSITY OF MICHIGAN

THE eleventh International Symposium on Physics at the summer session of the University of Michigan will be held as usual. Owing to reduced university appropriations its support has been provided for from private sources.

The foreign lecturers this year will be Professor Niels Bohr, of the University of Copenhagen, Nobel laureate, the founder of modern atomic physics, and Professor Enrico Fermi, of the Royal University at Rome, authority on quantum theory. Professor John H. Van Vleck, of the University of Wisconsin, specialist in the theory of magnetism, will also lecture, as will Professors Ernest F. Barker, David M. Dennison and George E. Uhlenbeck, of the university.

Dr. Edward H. Kraus, dean of the summer session, states that the symposium brings together annually leading native and foreign authorities who conduct classes and meet together with their students in give and take discussions of both the theoretical and experimental aspects of the laws of the atom, infra-red rays, the revelations of the spectroscope and like problems.

In recent years physicists from outside the United States who have attended the symposium include Professors Erhenfest, of Leiden; Heisenberg, of Leipzig; Sommerfeld, of Munich; Pauli, of Zurich, and Kramers, of Utrecht, as well as Brillouin, of Paris; Dirac, of Cambridge, and Milne, of Oxford.

## GEOLOGY AND GEOGRAPHY AT THE CHICAGO MEETING OF THE AMERICAN ASSOCIATION

SECTION E of the American Association for the Advancement of Science will meet in Chicago on Tuesday, Wednesday and Thursday, June 20, 21 and 22 in conjunction with members of the Geological Society of America, the Geographical Society of Chicago and other affiliated organizations. The Hotel Southmoor at Sixty-seventh Street and Stony Island, will serve as headquarters. An informal dinner will be held on Tuesday evening at the University of Chicago and will be followed by a lecture on "Variation and Evolution in Earth History" by Professor Albrecht Penck, Berlin, who with Professor J. J. Sederholm, Helsingfors, Finland, is among the foreign guests who will address the members of this section and their friends. The meetings will be held at the University of Chicago and at the Field Museum of Natural History.

The Tuesday morning session will be devoted to papers on general geology and, if necessary, the reading of papers will be continued on Tuesday afternoon. On Wednesday afternoon there will be a joint session with the physicists, chemists and astronomers, devoted to a symposium on "The Measurement of Geologic Time." Among those who will participate in this symposium are: A. F. Kovarik, A. C. Lane, H. Schlundt, A. V. Grosse and W. D. Urry. For the Thursday session, which will be held jointly with the Geographical Society of Chicago, a program of papers on geography is being arranged by Professor Charles C. Colby, of the University of Chicago.

Local arrangements are in charge of Professor D. Jerome Fisher, of the University of Chicago. Hotel reservations should be made directly with the Hotel Southmoor. Titles and abstracts of papers for the program on geology should be submitted to Professor Kirtley F. Mather, Harvard University, Cambridge, Massachusetts, prior to May 10.

### AWARD TO PROFESSOR H. C. SHERMAN

THE medal of The American Institute of Chemists, presented annually for outstanding service to chemistry in America, has been awarded this year to Dr. H. C. Sherman, head of the department of chemistry at Columbia University, according to an announcement made by President Henry G. Knight from the office of the institute. The award is made in recognition of Dr. Sherman's food researches, and his services to the profession through the training of chemists.

One of the pioneers in food chemistry from the time he first began to teach at Columbia in 1898, Dr. Sherman has been prominent most recently for his studies of the effect of diet on longevity, carried out in collaboration with the Carnegie Institution of Washington. He was the first to insist on quantitative analysis of iron and other minerals in foods; and he has also carried out research on enzymes and on the vitamin values of foods and the significance of vitamins in nutrition.

Dr. Sherman's work for fifteen years with the food supply committee of the New York Association for Improving the Condition of the Poor has resulted in a marked improvement in the food and nutrition conditions of the average New York family.

Describing Dr. Sherman's work as "use-research," Dr. Knight called for increased scientific efforts to teach people how to live intelligently. "Industry can always afford to pay for the discovery of products it can sell," Dr. Knight said, "but only educational institutions, subsidized foundations and state and national governments can improve living conditions by showing people how to use the things they already have. The individual can not pay for his own nutrition research. Instead, he pays for medicine and doctors, after he has guessed wrong."

Last year's medalist of the American Institute of Chemists was Dr. Charles H. Herty, whose newly discovered process for making paper from the Southern slash pine has just turned out its first mill run of newsprint. Other past medalists include Andrew W. Mellon and Richard B. Mellon, honored for establishing the Mellon Institute for Industrial Research; the late George Eastman, who made fine organic chemicals available to the chemists of the country, and Mr. and Mrs. Francis P. Garvan, who established the Chemical Foundation.

The medal will be presented to Dr. Sherman at the annual meeting of the American Institute of Chemists, to be held in New York in May.

### PROFESSOR EINSTEIN AND THE PRUSSIAN ACADEMY

ACCORDING to a special cable to the *New York Times*, the Prussian Academy of Science accepted on April 1 the resignation of Professor Einstein and announced that he was renouncing the Prussian citizenship conferred on him in 1913 on his admission to membership. He was born in Ulm, Germany, but subsequently his family moved to Switzerland and he became a Swiss citizen.

Professor Einstein has also withdrawn from the management of the Kaiser Wilhelm Institute, which recently appealed in the United States for funds for the construction of a new physical laboratory.

The Prussian Academy, its statement declares, "learned with indignation of Professor Einstein's participation in atrocity propaganda in America and France" and immediately demanded an explanation. His reply, it is stated, was that he "could no longer serve the state under the present government."

"The Prussian Academy," the announcement continued, "deplores Professor Einstein's propagandist activity abroad the more since, of old, the academy and its members have felt themselves intimately conjoined with the Prussian State and for all the strict reserve they have maintained respecting political questions, have always emphasized and preserved the idea of nationality. The academy, therefore, has no reason to regret Professor Einstein's retirement."

It is further reported that funds and securities in a Berlin bank have been seized by the Nazi Government "to prevent their use for treasonable purposes."

Professor and Mrs. Albert Einstein arrived at Antwerp aboard the liner *Belgenland* on March 28. Mayor Camille Huysmans went aboard to welcome them. Professor de Groodt, who lives near Antwerp, will be their host for several days. They plan to remain in Belgium four or five months, taking a cottage at Coq-sur-Mer near Ostend. Professor Meyer, his assistant, will join him.

## SCIENTIFIC NOTES AND NEWS

ANNOUNCEMENT of the establishment of the Elihu Thomson Professorship of Electrical Engineering at the Massachusetts Institute of Technology was made on March 29 by President Karl T. Compton, at the dinner given at the institute to Professor Thomson in honor of the eightieth anniversary of his birthday.

In announcing the plan, Dr. Compton said that the institute's executive committee had voted to establish the professorship "under terms which may be expected continually to draw as the incumbent a man of such qualifications for teaching and research as shall fittingly and permanently carry forward those high ideals of creative scholarship and productive service as have so distinguished the man whose name this professorship will bear."

DR. LYMAN J. BRIGGS has been nominated by President Roosevelt to be director of the National Bureau of Standards. Dr. Briggs, who had been acting director since the death of Dr. C. K. Burgess, had been previously nominated for the position by President Hoover, but the appointment had not been confirmed by the Senate.

DR. WILLIAM I. MYERS, professor of farm management at the New York State College of Agriculture at Cornell University, has been appointed assistant secretary to Henry Morgenthau, Jr., chairman of the Federal Farm Board. Dr. Myers has been given leave of absence from the university until October.

DR. S. H. KNIGHT, professor of geology at the University of Wyoming, has been appointed state geologist, as the office of state geologist at the State Capitol, Cheyenne, has been abolished. The Legislature has provided for the creation of the Geological Survey of Wyoming, to function under the department of geology of the University of Wyoming.

DR. LYMAN J. BRIGGS, Walter S. Gifford, Admiral William V. Pratt and Dr. Alexander Wetmore have been elected trustees of the National Geographic Society. They will fill vacancies caused by the deaths of former President Coolidge, Dr. George K. Burgess, Rear Admiral Colby K. Chester and O. P. Austin. George W. Hutchinson has been elected secretary of the society.

DR. J. T. DUNN has been elected president of the British Society of Chemical Industry for the year 1933–34 in succession to Dr. R. H. Pickard. Dr. Dunn is the public analyst of Northumberland and represents the Fuel Research Board on the North Eastern Coalfields Survey.

DR. HARVEY CUSHING, Moseley professor of surgery, emeritus, at the Harvard Medical School, has been appointed an associate fellow of Trumbull College, one of the new colleges in Yale University.

THE Langmuir Award of the American Chemical Society for chemical research has been conferred this year on Dr. Frank Harold Spedding, of the University of California. The award, which carries a prize of $1,000, is for Dr. Spedding's study of the atom by spectrographic methods.

DR. CHARLES A. MOSS and Herbert D. Brown, of the General Electric Company, recently received Charles A. Coffin Foundation awards from the company. Dr. Moss was cited for his design of the centrifugal supercharger or "tamed torpedo" which reinforces airplane engines, and Mr. Brown received the award because of his work in the development of the mercury-arc rectifier. These awards, established in memory of Charles A. Coffin, first president of the General Electric Company, are granted each year for outstanding service in advancing electrical industry.

DR. DICKINSON W. RICHARDS, JR., assistant professor of medicine in the Columbia University School of Medicine, has received the Walter Belknap James Fellowship for 1933–34, in recognition of his research on "Blood Flow in Cardiac Disease."

DR. ROYD R. SAYERS, of the U. S. Public Health Service, who has been assigned to the U. S. Bureau of Mines for the past sixteen years, has been transferred back to the service to take charge of the division of industrial hygiene and sanitation. Dr. Albert Eugene Russell will succeed Dr. Sayers.

*The American Physics Teacher,* the initial number of which appeared in March, is a new quarterly journal sponsored by the American Association of Physics Teachers. It is an addition to the list of seven periodicals which the American Institute of Physics now publishes. Devoted to the interests of teachers of physics, the journal will feature articles on the teaching of physics and related problems, and will have departments devoted to discussion, laboratory and demonstration apparatus and abstracts. The editor is Dr. Duane Roller, associate professor of physics at the University of Oklahoma. Associate editors are: Dr. A. A. Knowlton, Reed College; Dr. C. J. Lapp, University of Iowa; Dr. Louise S. McDowell, Wellesley College; Dr. F. K. Richtmyer, Cornell University; Dr. L. W. Taylor, Oberlin College, and Dr. David L. Webster, Stanford University.

*Nature* writes: "With the close of 1932, Mr. T. Sheppard retired from the editorship of the *Naturalist,* having served it as editor for thirty years. As an illustrated monthly journal, designed for readers within the domain of the Yorkshire Naturalists' Union, the *Naturalist* has maintained a high standard, and in its comments and reviews it conveyed a touch of the editor's vitality and boisterousness. The occasion of his retirement was made an opportunity of presenting Mr. Sheppard with his portrait in oils by Mr. Vincent Galloway."

DR. DONALD A. LAIRD, director of the psychological laboratory of Colgate University, has been appointed to supervise the exhibit on sleep and fatigue for the

Century of Progress Exposition. The exhibit, which is being supported by the Master Bedding Makers of America, will feature the actual use of apparatus used on recent studies of sleep and fatigue at several universities, giving visitors an opportunity to take some of the tests.

THE Committee on Scientific Research of the American Medical Association has made grants to Dr. James L. O'Leary, of the department of anatomy of Washington University Medical School, St. Louis, to aid his work on the nervous mechanisms controlling blood pressure, and to Dr. Helen C. Coombs, of the department of physiology of the New York Homeopathic Medical College, for an investigation of the effects of bromides on experimentally induced convulsions.

DR. PAUL BARTSCH, Smithsonian Institution biologist, who led the Johnson-Smithsonian Deep-Sea Expedition to investigate the Puerto Rico Deep, has returned to Washington. Some of the specimens obtained by the expedition at depths extending to 3,200 feet are believed to be new. The expedition was made possible through the generosity of Mr. Eldridge R. Johnson, of Philadelphia, who placed at the disposal of the Smithsonian Institution his motor yacht *Caroline,* and who himself accompanied the expedition. Much of the scientific work was made possible by the gyro-stabilizer equipment of the yacht, which eliminated rolling.

DR. WALTER HOUGH, of the U. S. National Museum, who has been conducting field-work in southern Arizona for the past two months, was expected to return to Washington at the end of March.

F. TRUBEE DAVISON, president of the American Museum of Natural History and until recently Assistant Secretary of War for Aviation, and Mrs. Davison, will leave in June for a two months' exploration of the Kenya jungles of East Africa. They will join Mr. and Mrs. Martin Johnson on their trips, and will live at their home at Nairobi, on Lake Rudolf.

PROFESSOR H. J. MULLER, of the University of Texas, is spending the year abroad as fellow of the Guggenheim Foundation and has been working at the Kaiser Wilhelm Institute for the Study of the Brain at Berlin-Buch. He delivered a lecture at the institute on March 9. His subject was "Studies on Mutation."

THE subjects of the Dohme lectures to be given on April 20, 21 and 22 by Sir Henry Dale at The Johns Hopkins University under the general title of "Progress in Autopharmacology" are: "The Action of Histamine, and the Evidence Restricting its Probable Significance. Evidence for Other Natural Vasodilators." "Acetylcholine; its Natural Occurrence and Probable Function. Adenosine and its Derivatives." "Kallikrein. Vasodilators from Blood-vessels, Blood, Intestine and Brain. A General Survey of the Possible Functions of Such Constituents of the Tissues, in Relation to Those of Nerves and Specific Hormones."

PROFESSOR OTTO HAHN, director of the Kaiser Wilhelm Institute for Chemistry at Berlin, lectured on April 6 and 7, under the auspices of the Carnegie Institute of Technology at Pittsburgh on "Radioactive Elements and their Use in Chemical Research" and on "Gaseous Radio-elements and their Applications." Under the auspices of the Royal Canadian Institute, he lectured at Toronto on April 8, discussing in a popular manner progress "From the Ponderable to the Imponderable" in chemical work. Professor Hahn is the George Fisher Baker non-resident lecturer in chemistry at Cornell University during the spring semester, where he is lecturing on "Applied Radiochemistry."

PROFESSOR WILLIAM D. HARKINS, of the University of Chicago, gave on March 21 the last of a series of lectures on "The Neutron and Modern Alchemy." These lectures were presented at the University of Michigan, Princeton University, University of Kansas, University of Iowa, University of Chicago, Iowa State College, Kansas State College, University of Missouri, University of Indiana, and to sections of the American Chemical Society at Kansas City, Omaha, Chicago, Indiana, Wilmington, Philadelphia, and at the Research Laboratory of the Corning Glass Company.

THE Iowa Academy of Science will hold its forty-seventh annual meeting at Coe College, Cedar Rapids, Iowa, on April 21 and 22. Professor H. J. Gilkey, head of theoretical and applied mechanics at the Iowa State College, will be the speaker at that meeting. His subject will be "The Hoover Dam." Mr. Gilkey is a member of the board of consulting engineers on concrete problems for the Hoover Dam.

THE department of geology and geography of Northwestern University announces the institution of an exchange of lectures with Washington University, St. Louis. Under this arrangement Chester K. Wentworth, associate professor in the department of geology and geography, gave five lectures at Northwestern University, and Dr. Charles H. Behre, Jr., associate professor of economic geology, gave a similar series of lectures at Washington University. Professor Behre's lectures dealt principally with the geology of central Colorado and with various phases of economic geology, and those given by Professor Wentworth with problems of sedimentation and glaciation. Professor Wentworth also spoke before the Society of the Sigma

Xi of Northwestern University on "Power Sites in the Missouri River Basin."

Under a plan of exchange speakers the Iowa and Missouri Chapters of the Society of Sigma Xi have cooperated this winter. Professor A. G. Hogan, of the University of Missouri, addressed the Iowa Chapter at its first soirée on December 14, discussing "Nutritional Deficiency Diseases." On March 31, Dean George F. Kay, of the University of Iowa, addressed the Missouri Chapter on "Glaciation: the Background of Mississippi Valley Development." At the annual election of the Iowa Chapter of the Society of Sigma Xi new officers for the 1933–1934 period were named. Professor Henry A. Mattil succeeds Professor J. H. Bodine as president; Professor Norman C. Meier succeeds Professor John A. Eldridge as vice-president; Professor E. P. Tyndall succeeds Professor A. C. Tester as secretary; Professor Roscoe Woods completes a two-year term as treasurer. The society has sponsored a program of exchange speakers and soirées conducted by the College of Medicine, the College of Engineering, the department of mathematics, and the department of geology. Professor J Harlen Bretz addressed the society on February 15, on "The Grand Coulee," at the soirée conducted by the department of geology.

Announcement is made that Sir Henry Dale, director of the National Institute for Medical Research of England and a leading authority on pharmacology, will be the principal speaker at the dedication of the new Merck Research Laboratory, to take place at Rahway, New Jersey, on April 25. Dr. Dale will be welcomed by the following guests of honor, who have accepted invitations to be present on the occasion of the formal dedication: Representing chemistry and the chemical industry, Lammot du Pont, president of E. I. du Pont de Nemours and Co., Inc., chairman of the Board of General Motors, Inc., president of the Manufacturing Chemists' Association; representing pharmacy and the pharmaceutical industry, J. K. Lilly, chairman of Eli Lilly and Company; representing medicine and the Public Health Service, Surgeon General Hugh S. Cumming, of the United States Public Health Service. The State of New Jersey will be represented by Governor A. Harry Moore. Over three hundred leaders in medicine and chemistry of the country will be present at the dedication.

*The Johns Hopkins Alumni Magazine* reports that a gift of $6,000 for the continuation of Dr. J. J. Abel's work on the pharmacology and chemistry of insulin has been received from the Commonwealth Fund.

*Museum News* states that the University of Richmond, Richmond, Virginia, will open a museum of biology in April. The museum will be housed in the new biology building of the university. It will occupy a room 34 by 40 feet with high windows so that 7-foot cases can stand beneath them, a room equipped with steel herbarium cases, and a room with 150 glass top insect cases in special cabinets and display cases. The case equipment is of bronze and plate glass by Russell. In addition, display cases will be set up in the halls and in each of the laboratories, and there will be a room with 24 cages for live animals, 22 aquaria of 12 to 200 gallons capacity, and a greenhouse on the roof. Other material besides the biological exhibits will also be shown in the museum. The building in which the museum is housed is three stories high, of brick and concrete, and includes lecture rooms, store rooms and the library of the department of biology with 500 feet of book-shelf space. Dr. John Wendell Bailey, professor of biology, is in charge.

# DISCUSSION

## NAMING THE GRAND CANYON

There seems to be some uncertainty in the public mind as to when the Grand Canyon was named and who named it. The first Spaniards to see it were members of a scouting party of the Coronado expedition in 1540 under Don Garcia Lopez de Cardenas, but, so far as the available records go, no name was then given to the great chasm. It was more than three centuries after this discovery by Cardenas that the canyon came into common knowledge though still with no name.

At last, in 1858, Lieutenant Ives and Professor Newberry wrote of it as the "Big Cañon" and the "Great Cañon." Then came Major Powell, in 1869, who was the first to explore its depths by descending through it in rowboats and he called it the "Grand Cañon."

In 1871 and 1872 Major Powell made a second descent of the Green and Colorado rivers. His report, published after this, spoke of it as the Grand Cañon (the Englished spelling "Canyon" was adopted later). The name was not recorded on any map till his topographers (of whom I was one) produced the first preliminary map of the region in the winter of 1872–73 in a tent in Southern Utah.

On Powell's first (1869) trip through the Grand Canyon it was not yet definitely named by him. John C. Sumner, one of his most active and intelligent men, says in a narrative he later wrote:

About fifteen miles below the Little Colorado the first bad rapid occurs in what I wanted to name Coronado Canyon. Major Powell told me it should bear my name if he got through and ever had the opportunity to place it on the Government map. Well, he got through all right, but forgot his vows and named it Grand Canyon.

There is no doubt whatever that the Grand Canyon was named by Major Powell not long after he came out of it on his 1869 trip.

FREDERICK S. DELLENBAUGH

NEW YORK

## THE REACTION OF INDIVIDUAL BACTERIA TO IRRADIATION WITH ULTRA-VIOLET LIGHT

STUDENTS of the effect of ultra-violet light on bacteria have commonly accepted absence of multiplication, tested by clouding of broth or by colony formation, as the criterion of bactericidal action. This is a convenient but arbitrary endpoint, for "death" is not necessarily coincident with failure to multiply.

Observations on single organisms (*B. coli communis*) in the first hours after irradiation with measured monochromatic light, λ 2377 to 3022, show that there is a wide reaction zone between the behavior of cells which are not visibly affected and those which seem to be killed outright by the exposure. Single organisms which apparently have been unaffected grow and divide regularly on the surface of nutrient agar, producing typical colonies of normal-looking bacteria that ultimately coalesce into a confluent growth. Organisms which are exposed to quickly lethal doses show no increase in size and no cell division, but soon lose their high refractility, become beaded or irregularly refractile and degenerate into ghosts or shadows which are undoubtedly dead. In the intermediate zone between these two extremes the irradiated organisms present a remarkable picture. They increase in size, especially in length, without apparent inhibition, but do not divide when the normal adult stage is reached; so that long filaments of clear, highly refractile protoplasm are formed that look like spaghetti and may attain measured lengths of 50 to 150 microns. The transverse diameter is 1 to 3 times that of normal bacteria. These long forms are actively motile in a fluid medium, progressing with a sinuous motion, or drilling back and forth like spirochaetes. In 2 to 4 hours at 37.5° C the cells reach a limit of individual growth, forming long rafts of parallel filaments on an agar surface. Then cell division or degenerative changes begin. (1) The long cells may undergo a gradual degeneration, with loss of hyaline refractility, beading and ghost formation. (2) They may divide by cross fission into a number of large or small units, which then degenerate without further growth. (3) One or more normal-looking daughter cells may pinch off at one end and multiply rapidly to colony formation. The rest of the filament follows courses 1 or 2 above. Daughter cells have not been observed to form filaments; the reaction is limited to cells directly exposed to ultra-violet light.

Here is an apparent separation of two coordinate functions commonly essential to life. Cell division is regulated by a mechanism which is much more sensitive to wave-lengths below 3,000 than is the concomitant function of growth. By appropriate exposures the one can be temporarily or permanently suppressed, while the other proceeds for hours without hindrance. Ultimately, however, a limit is reached, and unless the division mechanism is restored the cell degenerates. A further study of this cell reaction is in progress.

FREDERICK L. GATES

HARVARD UNIVERSITY

## LACTOBACILLI IN FROZEN PACK PEAS

MICROBIOLOGICAL analyses of frozen pack peas held in storage from 1 to 26 months show that lactic acid bacteria tolerate well cold storage temperatures. The peas under consideration, representing several batches, were packed in a variety of ways—blanched and unblanched, dry and in brine, in 1 pound paper containers, and in No. 2 tin cans both vacuumized and unvacuumized. The storage temperature in most cases was 15° F., though some containers of the current year's pack were held at minus 5° F.

Some 40 samples from the different packs have been studied from the spoilage view-point alone, the containers being held at ordinary room temperature for 2 to 7 days, at the end of which time the contents were analyzed bacteriologically. Without exception the peas presented a bleached appearance and had a sour odor. Those in tin had developed more or less pressure in the container. The clouded liquors gave positive ferric chloride tests for lactic acid. Acidities of 1.0 to 1.3 per cent., calculated as lactic acid, were found, and the pH values ranged between 4.2 and 4.6. Direct microscopic examination invariably showed gram-positive rods, and medium-sized gram-negative rods were often present, but in smaller numbers. Appropriate cultural technique yielded the *Aerobacter aerogenes* ("colon") type and lactobacilli.

Study of 15 cultures of the lactobacilli isolated places the majority with the *Lactobacillus cucumeris* type, since they ferment arabinose and trehalose in addition to sucrose, dextrose and maltose. Inoculation of pure cultures of these into sterile peas yielded products entirely similar to the fermented frozen pack peas as regarded appearance, sauerkraut-like odor and acidity.

Organisms of this type are widely distributed and occur commonly on vegetables, and their presence on shelled peas is to be expected. Since they are not spore formers, it is noteworthy that they withstand a temperature of 15° F. for over 2 years. While no peas stored at minus 5° F. for more than a month have to date been analyzed, the lactobacilli in all probability would persist at this temperature, for experience has shown that micro-organisms generally tolerate zero Fahrenheit as well as or better than higher freezing temperatures.

James Alex. Berry
U. S. Bureau of Plant Industry
Seattle, Washington

## VITAMIN A IN THE PIMIENTO PEPPER

The pimiento pepper is utilized in the culinary art chiefly as a condiment. This rather limited use in the diet may perhaps be an explanation for the relative paucity of research concerning its food value.

MacLeod and Booher[1] report that the vitamin C content of the canned product is equivalent to that of fresh grapefruit, and analyses have determined its chemical composition.[2] Capsanthin, or an allied pigment so masks any other color present in the pepper that it seems expedient at this time to call attention to its high carotene content.

In the biological study the Sherman technique was followed. Rats varying from 40 to 50 grams at weaning were put upon his vitamin A-free diet until symptoms of depletion were manifest, *i.e.*, signs of ophthalmia and stationary or slightly declining weight. Fresh, commercially canned and dried pepper were each then fed upon three different levels with an average of eighteen animals in the several groups.

This preliminary investigation has shown that, computed upon the dry basis, four milligrams of pepper induced a growth response above that of the Sherman unit. Further, a chemical assay has indicated from 200 to 300 mg of carotene per kilogram of the dried material. Work is in progress to establish the unit level for the pimiento pepper and to ascertain its carotene value.

Leah Ascham
Georgia Experiment Station

## EARTHQUAKES IN THE HOLY LAND: A CORRECTION

In an article on earthquakes in the Holy Land[1] there is given a list of 207 shocks, of which there is record, between the years 1606 B. C. and 1927 A. D. Among these are 27 dates from an Arabian authority, As-Soyuti, whose work appears in translation in the *Journal of the Asiatic Society of Bengal.* In transcribing these dates I failed to observe that they were stated as A. H., *i.e., Anno Hejira,* instead of *Anno Domini.* They are, therefore, as quoted in my list something over six centuries too early. The corrected dates are as follows:

| A.H. | A.D. | A.H. | A.D. | A.H. | A.D. |
|---|---|---|---|---|---|
| 94 | 712 | 434 | 1042 | 552 | 1157 |
| 98 | 716 | 455 | 1063 | 565 | 1169 |
| 130 | 747 | 460 | 1067 | 575 | 1179 |
| 220 | 835 | 462 | 1069 | 578 | 1182 |
| 233 | 847 | 479 | 1086 | 597 | 1200 |
| 242 | 856 | 484 | 1091 | 600 | 1203 |
| 245 | 859 | 532 | 1137 | 702 | 1302 |
| 393 | 1002 | 538 | 1143 | 791 | 1388 |
| 425 | 1033 | 551 | 1156 | 889 | 1484 |

Inasmuch as the Hejira dates from July, 622 A. D., and there are adjustments of the calendar dates for fractions, these figures may be off one year. It is also probable that the original dates are approximate. Hence where As-Soyuti differs by a year from others given in the list as published, one shock only is presumably meant.

In this connection I would call attention to a very ancient, yet definite observation regarding the now well-known earthquake fault that traverses the eastern slope of the Mount of Olives:

> And His feet shall stand upon the Mount of Olives which in that day is before Jerusalem on the east; and the Mount of Olives shall be cleft in the midst thereof toward the east and toward the west, and there shall be a very great valley; and half of the mountain shall remove toward the north and half of it toward the south.[2]

Activity on this fault was the occasion of destructive tremors in 1927. That it was the scene of more obvious displacement some 2,500 years earlier we can not doubt in view of the graphic description of the Old Testament writer, although his identity and the exact date of his prophecy are matters of uncertainty, especially with reference to this particular passage.

Bailey Willis
Stanford University

## A RARE PUBLICATION

The library of the Academy of Natural Sciences of Philadelphia recently acquired from a dealer in second-hand books a copy of Volume 1, 1892–94 (1895) of the Transactions of the Natural History Society of Queensland. The fact that this is not listed in the Union List of Serials and that the natural

[1] Grace MacLeod and Lela Booher, "The Antiscorbutic Vitamin Content of Some Preserved Foods," *Jour. Home Econ.*, 22: 588. 1930.

[2] J. G. Woodroof and J. E. Bailey, "Pimiento Peppers," *Ga. Exp. Sta. Bull.*, 150. 1929.

[1] *Bull. Seismol. Soc. Amer.*, Vol 18, 1928.

[2] The Old Testament, Zechariah, 14, 4–6, 520 B. C.

history library of the British Museum and that of the Linnean Society of London, when their library catalogues were issued a few years back did not have this volume, would indicate that this is a rare work. The library of the Zoological Society of London lists the work in its catalogue, although the new species described in the "Transactions" are not noted in the *Zoological Record*. There are but two articles of taxonomic interest in the volume, one by C. J. Wild, describing *Dendroceros subtropicus*, a new species of moss (pp. 49–50); and "Australian Lepidoptera: Thirty New Species," by Thomas P. Lucas, entirely moths (pp. 101–116).

WM. J. FOX

ACADEMY OF NATURAL SCIENCES OF PHILADELPHIA

# SCIENTIFIC APPARATUS AND LABORATORY METHODS

## DOUBLE STAINING BY THE CAJAL–BROŽEK METHOD

WHEN making durable microscopic slides, many different ways of dyeing are in use, of which some are of chief importance in cytological work. But the double staining is such that only quite definite parts of the cells, *e.g.*, chromosomes or nucleoles are stained by one color; whereas the other color stains another part, *e.g.*, cytoplasm. The method, which the author of this account wishes to describe briefly, has been worked out with a few alterations, by Ramon y Cajal. It has been used from time to time and still is used in zoological work, but only for the last three years in botanical studies, where it has been introduced by Professor Arthur Brožek with considerable success, in a modified form.

It is a cytological method, which stains the chromosomes splendidly, and when compared with Heidenhain's iron-hematoxylin method, so much used nowadays, has certain advantages, which will be pointed out below. By our method, the chromosomes are stained a bright red with magenta—which is basic fuchsin, while the nucleole and the other parts are stained sky-blue with picro-indigo-carmine. Picro-indigo-carmine is a mixture of 2 parts saturated aqueous solution of indigo-carmine and one part of picric acid. Both the magenta and picro-indigo-carmine are used in concentrated solutions.

The process of staining is quite simple and short. The preparation—paraffin sections mounted on supporting glass—is freed from paraffin by xylol and brought through a mixture of alcohol-xylol and then through a series of alcohol baths to water; after which the object is placed for 3 to 5 minutes in concentrated magenta. The exact time must be found out for various objects, although the preparation always appears quite right, if treated for the length of time mentioned above. At the expiration of this time, the object is rinsed in distilled water and immediately placed in picro-indigo-carmine, where it is left for 10 to 15 minutes. It is better to find out the precise time for various objects by experiment. Then the object is placed in very slightly acid water for about one minute, into a beaker of distilled water with 1 to 2 minims acetic acid, after which an automatic differentiation is made with 80 per cent. alcohol. The slip is simply rinsed from the acid water, allowed to drain and plunged directly into 80 per cent. alcohol, where it remains until the red stain from the section remains, which can easily be seen with the naked eye. The time for differentiation is one half to one minute. Then the object is brought into 96 per cent. alcohol, 100 per cent. alcohol and a mixture of alcohol-xylol to xylol, and then mounted in Canada balsam. The whole process, from the placing in xylol to the mounting in Canada balsam, does not last more than 40 to 45 minutes. This is a great advantage when compared with Heidenhain's method, in which the procedure in the best case lasts for eight hours, and with careful working may even last for two and a half days. Another advantage is that the chromosomes stained with magenta can be distinguished from one another, even when they lie close to each other, or actually on each other. Such a method with hematoxylin is quite impossible on account of the covering color. A certain disadvantage of the method is that it can only be used successfully after sufficient acid fixing. It is best to use Nawashin's method, which is at the same time the most perfect, after fixing—15 parts 1 per cent. chromic acid, four parts formol and 1.5 parts glacial acetic acid. This method has been tried with success after fixing in highly diluted $HNO_3$. After using Němec fixing solution I., color tends to disappear—100 ccm 1 per cent. chromic acid and 8 ccm formol—but no change is apparent after using Němec II—50 ccm 1 per cent. chromic acid, 50 ccm 3 per cent. bichromate of potash, and 8 ccm formol; or after Regaud's method—80 parts 3 per cent. bichromate of potash and 20 parts formol. It proceeds badly after alcohol or formol fixing, but quite well after sublimate with acetic acid. There is no need to mention other fixing methods, which are for the greater part special. It is important that our method works excellently after Nawashin's fixing, which is most used to-day in plant-cytology. This method can be recommended, as it furnishes beautiful slides in a relatively short time, which can be studied in all their details, drawn and excellently photographed with a green filter.

K. Hruby
Charles University
Prague, Czechoslovakia, Europe

## A NEW PARAFFIN EMBEDDING MIXTURE

Difficulty in obtaining a paraffin of satisfactory consistency in which to embed and section biological material led to the development of the following formula. The use of neither of the substances added to the common paraffin is original with the writer (having been in fairly common use fifteen to twenty years ago) although the proportions and combinations may be.

A stock solution of crude rubber in paraffin is first made. Crude rubber is available in thin sheets, either smoked or unsmoked. Both kinds work equally well. The sheets of crude rubber are chopped up with a scissors and dropped in melted Parawax or any similar common paraffin. The paraffin should be smoking hot and the mixture should be stirred occasionally. Three to four hours are required to completely melt the rubber. About 20 grams of rubber can be dissolved in 100 grams of paraffin.

Embedding Mixture

| | |
|---|---|
| Parawax | 100 grams |
| Rubber-paraffin mixture | 4–5 grams |
| Beeswax | 1 gram |

Filter through paper (paper towels serve this purpose excellently).

This mixture is pale yellow in color, does not crystallize readily, and is of a waxy consistency that sections unusually well. It has been in use in this laboratory for the past three years and has materially increased the success of large classes in micrology.

Robert T. Hance
University of Pittsburgh

# SPECIAL ARTICLES

## PHOTOPERIODISM AS A CAUSE OF THE REST PERIOD IN STRAWBERRIES

Experiments made by the authors on the light requirements of strawberries have suggested an explanation of the cause of the rest period in this plant. The strawberry plant in northeastern United States becomes more or less dormant with the onset of low temperatures in the fall. Low temperatures alone are not responsible for dormancy, for many varieties remain dormant even when taken into a warm greenhouse in late fall. However, if plants are first given a low temperature rest period until about January 1, when brought into a warm greenhouse, all varieties grow vigorously, even though the days are still short. After the rest period has been broken, leaf growth and flower production is rapid. Plants covered with boxes in the field in January, so placed as to exclude all light, blossomed at about the same time as those in the open. Temperature and not light was the controlling factor after the rest period was broken.

If plants in the greenhouse are given additional light for several hours each night, beginning in November before they have had a low-temperature rest period, many but not all varieties grow vigorously. Each variety and species shows a characteristic response to the length of the daily light period at this time. If, however, the daily light period is lengthened beginning in early fall (September 1) before the days become short, the plants of all varieties we have tested make a vigorous vegetative growth throughout the entire winter and do not require a low-temperature rest period. Some varieties under such increased light periods produce some flower clusters, depending on their particular daily light period response. In contrast, plants not given additional light start fruit bud formation with the onset of short days, and if the temperature is above 60° F., plants of many kinds go into the rest period.

In one test, plants of some 51 varieties were given electric light until 10:00 each night to supplement daylight, beginning September 1. Until February their growth was almost entirely vegetative. They produced an average of 0.7 flower clusters per plant by that time, while control plants under normal light but similar temperatures had averaged 3.8 clusters. By June 9, the control plants had averaged 20.2 clusters, while the plants under the lights had averaged 4.8 clusters each. Continued growth seems to be correlated with relatively constant exposure to the photoperiodic requirements of the particular variety. Growth in some form apparently can continue over a fairly wide range of light exposures. For ordinary varieties very short daily light periods initiate a rest period, short light periods result in continuous fruiting and longer periods in vegetative growth only. Rest periods then seem to result from nutritional conditions following exposures to short daily light periods. *Fragaria virginiana* and varieties adapted to the Northern and Eastern states require a rest period after exposure to days as short as 12 hours daily light. *F. chiloensis,* varieties of the Northwest derived in part from it recently, and Southern varieties do not need a rest period until the days are much less than 12 hours. In fact, after exposure to days as short as 9 hours at the relatively low temperatures used they still grew freely.

Strawberries are grown commercially from regions having several weeks of continuous light in midsummer, such as Alaska, to regions of successively shorter daylight periods southward to Ecuador having 12 hours of daylight, and in winter, in Florida in days with less than 11 hours of daylight. Varieties that succeed in subtropical climates do not require a rest period, at least when grown under the day lengths in the subtropics. Although there is evidence that better growth may sometimes be obtained on such varieties after exposure to low temperatures for a time, they do not require a rest period under light conditions that prevail at Washington, D. C.

A study of the responses to light and rest periods seems to show that the strawberry varieties now grown in regions of short and of long days have actually though unconsciously been selected for adaptation to the light and rest period conditions of those regions. Varieties grown in subtropical regions are sufficiently adaptable to grow continuously under light periods of less than eleven to more than thirteen hours, and in these regions do not require a dormant period. Varieties adapted to Northern United States do not grow well under the short days of Southern states, and soon die out, while southern varieties make too vigorous a growth under the long days of summer in the North.

The strawberry is an evergreen, and upon exposure to suitable light periods some varieties after becoming dormant resume growth. In others apparently nutritional conditions have progressed to a point where light alone as we have used it is insufficient to cause renewal of growth. If the rest period in some other plants, especially in the deciduous ones, is due to similar causes, attempts to produce continued growth or to break the rest period by the use of lights should start before the leaves have fallen, or in some cases even as early as the end of June when the days are longest or even earlier to prove successful

GEORGE M. DARROW
GEORGE F. WALDO

BUREAU OF PLANT INDUSTRY
U. S. DEPARTMENT OF AGRICULTURE

## A "SCURVY-LIKE" DISEASE IN CHICKS

IN the course of nutritional studies we have observed the development of a scurvy-like disease in baby chicks. The first external symptoms are usually observed about the third week. They are nervousness and lameness, which is apparently due to stiffness of the hock joints. These symptoms are followed by bleeding from pin feathers on the neck, wings or thighs. About the same time blood clots appear beneath the skin and in the muscle of the thigh, around the hock joint and at the base of the wings. Closely following these abnormalities are frequent hemorrhages around the head, neck, back, ribs, breast and keel. Abdominal hemorrhages and small hemorrhagic spots in the muscle of the intestinal wall are common. The most frequent symptom is that of dark erosion spots on the gizzard lining[1] similar to the condition described by McFarlane, *et al.*[2] In these experiments approximately 95 per cent. of the chicks had erosions on the gizzard lining, while over 70 per cent. were affected with external or internal hemorrhages. In chicks suffering from the disease the bones were often brittle and the bone marrow dry and colorless. The blood showed an extremely low hemoglobin content (as low as one gram per hundred cubic centimeters of blood) and the blood picture microscopically resembled that described by Hess[3] for human scurvy. There further seemed to be an association between the symptoms described and growth in that the more rapid the growth the earlier the symptoms occurred and the more severe they were.

The symptoms described were produced by feeding a ration composed of fish meal, ground yellow corn, yeast, ground oyster shell and sardine oil or cod-liver oil to chicks confined in battery brooders. Rations in which the yeast was omitted produced the symptoms to a lesser extent. The substitution of 10 per cent. of dried skim-milk for the yeast and a portion of the fish meal produced about normal chicks. However, a few cases of eroded gizzard lining and small hemorrhages were observed, even when the milk was included in the diet. Five grams of cabbage per bird fed to affected individuals during the fifth and sixth weeks resulted in a complete recovery at the end of this period.

In view of the symptoms described, the diets used in order to produce the disease and the fact that cabbage in small quantities brought about a cure, we believe that, contrary to previous reports, growing chicks may suffer from scurvy due to an absence of vitamin C in the diet. We further believe that they are either unable to synthesize vitamin C or under certain conditions they are unable to synthesize this vitamin in sufficient amounts to meet their requirements.

A more detailed report of these investigations is being prepared for publication.

WALTHER F. HOLST
EVERETT R. HALBROOK

UNIVERSITY OF CALIFORNIA

1 Similar gizzard affections have been observed in baby chicks as early as the seventeenth day of incubation.

2 W. D. McFarlane, W. R. Graham, Jr., and G. E. Hall, *The Journal of Nutrition*, 1931, Vol. IV, 331.

3 Alfred F. Hess, "Scurvy, Past and Present," Philadelphia, 1920.

# SCIENCE

VOL. 77 — FRIDAY, APRIL 14, 1933 — No. 1998

*A History of the National Research Council, 1919–1933:*
*Foreword:* DR. W. H. HOWELL ... 355
*General Organization and Activities:* DR. ALBERT L. BARROWS ... 356
*Division of Physical Sciences:* PROFESSOR F. K. RICHTMYER ... 358
*Obituary:*
*Memorials; Recent Deaths* ... 360
*Scientific Events:*
*Proposed Planetarium for the American Museum of Natural History; Weather Station on Mt. Wachusett; Annual Report of the Brooklyn Botanic Garden; Fellowships of the Charles Lathrop Pack Forest Education Board* ... 361
*Scientific Notes and News* ... 363
*Discussion:*
*A Civilization without Native Mathematics:* PROFESSOR G. A. MILLER. *Theories of Cortico-adrenal Function:* PROFESSOR S. W. BRITTON and H. SILVETTE. *The "Spread" or "Scatter" of the Influence from a Reward, in Relation to Gestalt Doctrines:* DR. EDWARD L. THORNDIKE. *Stratigraphic Nomenclature:* DR. F. X. SCHAFFER. *Frequency of Vertebrate Fossils in River Deposits:* DR. ELLIS W. SHULER ... 366
*Scientific Apparatus and Laboratory Methods:*
*Apparatus for Slide Technique:* EMORY S. JAMES. *A Simple Device for the Perfusion of the Mammalian Heart:* PROFESSOR J. W. WILSON and J. M. DARLINGTON ... 369
*Special Articles:*
*The Perihelion of Mercury:* DR. THADDEUS MERRIMAN. *Some Factors Influencing the Susceptibility of Albino Rats to Injections of Sodium Amytal:* DONALD H. BARRON. *Sibling Resemblance and its Relation to Age Interval:* DR. F. H. FINCH ... 371
*Science News* ... 8

SCIENCE: A Weekly Journal devoted to the Advancement of Science, edited by J. MCKEEN CATTELL and published every Friday by

THE SCIENCE PRESS

New York City: Grand Central Terminal
Lancaster, Pa. — Garrison, N. Y.

Annual Subscription, $6.00 — Single Copies, 15 Cts.

SCIENCE is the official organ of the American Association for the Advancement of Science. Information regarding membership in the Association may be secured from the office of the permanent secretary, in the Smithsonian Institution Building, Washington, D. C.

# A HISTORY OF THE NATIONAL RESEARCH COUNCIL 1919—1933

## FOREWORD

DURING the year 1932 the Committee on Policies of the National Research Council was directed by the Executive Board to make a survey of the organization of the Council and to present recommendations in regard to needed changes. As a preparation for their labors they called upon the officers of the Council and the chairmen of the several divisions for a report upon the activities of the Council since its organization upon a peace-time basis in 1919.

The Council has felt that it is desirable to bring the substance of this report to the attention of the scientific workers of the country, since what it has been able to accomplish has depended so largely upon their interest and cooperation. Accordingly, a summary of the report will be published in SCIENCE, through the courtesy of the editor, as a series of short articles prepared under the supervision of Dr. Fernandus Payne, Chairman of the Division of Biology and Agriculture, and Dr. A. T. Poffenberger, chairman of the Division of Anthropology and Psychology.

The first of this series of ten articles follows, describing briefly the organization of the council and its general activities. Subsequent articles of the series will be published in later issues of SCIENCE.

W. H. HOWELL,
*Chairman, National Research Council*

## I. GENERAL ORGANIZATION AND ACTIVITIES

By Dr. ALBERT L. BARROWS
ASSISTANT SECRETARY

THE origin of the National Research Council lies in an offer which the National Academy of Sciences made of its services to President Wilson following the spring meeting of the Academy in 1916, when it was seen that the United States would probably become involved in the world war. The services offered by the Academy were for the coordination of the non-governmental scientific and technical resources of the country with the military and naval agencies of the Government, in the interests of national security and preparedness for the emergency which this country was then facing. A similar crisis had, in fact, brought about the organization of the National Academy for the assistance of the Government in 1863.

President Wilson at once accepted this offer, and at his request the Academy organized a central committee which it called the "National Research Council." This committee set up a number of special technical committees on various problems involved in the mobilization of the scientific and technical resources of the country. During the ensuing two years the National Research Council was engaged largely in the service of the Federal Government, acting as the Department of Science and Research of the Council of National Defense, and also as the Science and Research Division of the Signal Corps of the Army, and in cooperative relationship with other branches of the Government to meet its military and naval needs.

By the close of the war the recognition of the valuable services which such an organization might continuously render to the country under peace conditions had become apparent. This was particularly appreciated in view of the "new and important possibilities . . . opened through the heavy demands upon science and research which had arisen through the exceptional necessities brought about by the war." Accordingly, President Wilson issued an executive order on May 18, 1918, requesting the National Academy to perpetuate the National Research Council. The purpose of the Council is expressed in its Articles of Organization as follows:

> It shall be the purpose of the National Research Council to promote research in the mathematical, physical, and biological sciences, and in the application of these sciences to engineering, agriculture, medicine, and other useful arts, with the object of increasing knowledge, of strengthening the national defense, and of contributing in other ways to the public welfare, as expressed in the Executive Order of May 11, 1918.

During the early part of 1919 the Research Council was reorganized by the Academy on a permanent basis centering around an executive board of some 44 members as a central governing body, with certain additional general committees called divisions, representing the major fields of interest of the Council. The number of these divisions is now eleven, four of them representing general relationships of the Council with the Federal Government, with international scientific organizations, with educational institutions and with scientific agencies of the state governments. The divisions of science and technology number seven, including the physical sciences, engineering and industrial research, chemistry and chemical technology, geology and geography, the medical sciences, biology and agriculture, and anthropology and psychology. The membership of these several divisions ranges in number from 18 to 44. The Council also maintains a research information service for the organization of general data and for assistance in locating sources of information.

The reorganization of the National Research Council in 1919 further provided for the enlistment of the cooperation of research men throughout the country, by inviting the national technical and scientific societies of the United States to designate representatives in the membership of the Council. In the seven divisions of science and technology these society representatives constitute the majority of the divisional membership. Each division also contains in addition a limited number of members-at-large, selected by the division. At present 79 societies are affiliated with the National Research Council in this way. The total number of members of the Council in its executive board and in its divisions is this year 285. The administrative and technical committees through which the Council conducts most of its operations number 135, and include 888 members in addition to the officers and members of the Council, making a body of 1,173 scientific men directly related to the Council, besides a large number of other collaborators in its various undertakings.

The chairmen of the Council and the chairmen of its executive board, since the inception of the Council, have been:

| | |
|---|---|
| George E. Hale, | 1916–1919 |
| John J. Carty, | 1916–1918 |
| James R. Angell, | 1919–1920 |
| H. A. Bumstead, | 1920 |
| John C. Merriam, | 1921–1923 |
| Gano Dunn, | 1923–1928 |
| George K. Burgess, | 1928–1932 |
| William H. Howell, | 1932–1933 |

The office of secretary, executive secretary or permanent secretary of the Council during this period has been filled by:

| | |
|---|---|
| Cary D. Hutchinson, | 1916–1918 |
| John Johnston, | 1918–1919 |
| A. O. Leuschner, | 1919 |
| Vernon Kellogg, | 1919–1931 |

In addition to relating the National Research Council to the national research societies of the country, the reorganization of the Council in 1919 provided in each of its divisions of science and technology for an active leader as the chairman of the division. Each division chairman during his term of office has given his major attention to the promotion of the projects sponsored by his division, with the constant assistance of an executive committee which has met with him at stated intervals. This leadership, supported by the extensive relationships afforded through the membership of the divisions and by other facilities offered by the Council, has been the unique feature in its organization.

During the past year the Research Council has been giving particular study to the problem of its organization and relationships in the light of its experience in the past thirteen years. Certain changes, principally in the direction of economy of organization, which are to be put into effect next year, will, it is hoped, result in a simplification of its administration and in an increased effectiveness.

The financial resources of the Council came from various sources during the war years, but largely from the Engineering Foundation and from the Federal Government. Subsequently, the Council has been supported in its general administration wholly from private sources and mainly on the income from an endowment provided by the Carnegie Corporation of New York. Of the original gift of $5,000,000 from the Carnegie Corporation, about one third was taken for the erection of a building in Washington, D. C., to service as headquarters for the National Academy of Sciences and for the National Research Council.

In addition to its income from endowment, which is used mainly for administrative expenses, the Council among its other activities administers funds placed in its hands for special research purposes. These funds in recent years have totalled about $800,000 annually. The purposes for which they have been used include (1) the maintenance of research fellowships, (2) the support of coordinated programs of cooperative research through the allotment of grants to collaborators in these projects, (3) the awarding of individual grants in support of research, and (4) the administration of the funds of independent scientific bodies without the assumption, however, of responsibility for their work.

One of the most important of the undertakings of the Council has been the administration of three series of post-doctorate fellowships in physics, chemistry and mathematics, in the medical sciences and in the biological sciences, including anthropology and psychology and the fundamental aspects of forestry and agriculture. These fellowships are supported on funds furnished by the Rockefeller Foundation, and, in the earlier years of the series of medical fellowships, by the General Education Board also. The purpose of these fellowships is to give promising investigators at the beginning of their careers additional years of training and experience in research. At present about 140 appointments are made annually at basic stipends of from $1,600 to $1,800 per year, with additional allowances for dependents. Some of these fellows are appointed to study abroad. Altogether about 850 fellows have been appointed, about one third of the total number of applications. Of the 700 or more past fellows approximately four fifths now hold positions in educational institutions.

For the past three years the Council has also had the administration of a research aid fund for the assistance mainly of individual research. During this time 375 grants have been made to individuals and 19 grants for conferences and other general research purposes. The total amounts thus granted is $250,-775.01.

Among other general undertakings the Council has sponsored the publication of the "International Critical Tables of Numerical Data of Physics, Chemistry and Technology," in seven volumes, with a comprehensive index now in the course of preparation. The Council has also given its assistance to the collection of funds in this country for the publication in Paris of the "Annual Tables of Numerical Data of Chemistry, Physics, Biology and Technology." At the request of the trustees of the Chicago "Century of Progress" Exposition, the Council organized a group of committees in 1929 and 1930 to advise the trustees in regard to certain aspects of the plans for the scientific exhibits at this exposition. The Council has acted as the fiscal agent for the Tropical Plant Research Foundation, for the Crop Protection Institute and for the Commission on Standardization of Biological Stains in the early years of these organizations, and still administers the editorial funds for the "Biological Abstracts." The Council has also supported the work of the American Geophysical Union, which is the principal coordinating agency in the United States for research in geodesy, oceanography and related subjects.

In addition to the material support of research, represented by the research funds administered by the Council, largely through committees of the divisions of the Council, other special committees of the divisions have sponsored a wide variety of enterprises which require not so much funds as other forms of assistance. These enterprises have included the encouragement of research through the coordination of investigations in certain fields, the preparation of surveys of the conditions of research in special subjects, and the holding of conferences for the discussion of the current status of research in problems of large scope. The chairmen of divisions have themselves undertaken special studies of conditions affecting the course of research in their respective fields. A long series of publications has been issued in a *Bulletin* and a *Reprint and Circular Series,* consisting of reports of committees of the Council and the reissue of timely articles in various fields of scientific research. Several books have been prepared under auspices of committees of the Council and have been issued through commercial publishers.

"The primary function of the Council is the promotion of research in the United States; . . . it justifies its existence not through the maintenance of an organization but solely through the definite projects which that organization is maintaining and promoting." With this object in view the Council has functioned as an agency through which many cooperative undertakings have been initiated. It has furnished auspices under which scientific men have acted by a wide variety of means for the encouragement of research. By virtue of its organization and its affiliations it has been in position, also, in many cases, to bring together the workers and the benefactors of science in a common endeavor to promote the advancement of knowledge. Whatever has been accomplished, however, in the support of research has been possible mainly because of the personal contributions of the large body of American scientific men associated with the Council, who have collaborated in these enterprises and have given generously to them of their time and effort. The Council relies upon this cooperation from the scientific men of the country for the successful operation of the mechanism which has been set up.

## II. DIVISION OF PHYSICAL SCIENCES[1]

By Professor F. K. RICHTMYER

CHAIRMAN

THE Division of Physical Sciences of the National Research Council, formally organized May 1, 1919, was the natural outgrowth of the activities of the Physics Committee and later the Division of Physics, Mathematics, Astronomy and Geophysics of the Council, and also of the Science and Research Division of the Signal Corps, which rendered important research services during the war. For perhaps the first time, it was realized that, in addition to direct results, the indirect benefits of directed cooperative effort among scientists was very great. The men who sponsored the Division of Physical Sciences had all seen war service in one way or another, but the organization of the division which they set up and the program of activities which they initiated were directed toward the peace-time development of the sciences of physics, mathematics and astronomy. Accordingly, "the primary object of the Division is to stimulate and to facilitate research in the various related sciences grouped in the Division."

Two methods were adopted to accomplish this purpose. First, the Division was so organized as to bring together in its organization men in the different sciences and geographically separated—it being believed that such association would promote better acquaintance and would pave the way for spontaneous cooperation. Second, the policy was adopted of setting up research committees to survey and summarize research in various fields and to prepare short monographs which should be "distributed to all scientists in the group . . . to put the readers *au courant* with the present state of the science as regards the subject of the monograph." A third method was soon added. The Rockefeller Foundation generously provided support for the now well-known National Research Fellowships in physics (including astronomy), chemistry and mathematics. And the Division of Physical Sciences was asked to organize and to sponsor a fellowship board to administer these fellowships.

The organization of the division provided for a chairman, vice-chairman, members-at-large and representatives from each of the several national societies in the fields of science included within the division. During the past several years the division has contained twenty-one members, of which three are members-at-large and seventeen represent the following societies: American Astronomical Society, Acoustical Society of America, American Mathematical Society, American Physical Society, Mathematical Association of America and the Optical Society of America. Meetings of the division are held annually to discuss matters of general policy, work of the preceding year and plans for future activities.

It will be not without interest to record the names

[1] This is the second of a series of ten articles prepared to describe briefly the nature of the activities with which the National Research Council has been engaged during the past fourteen years.

of those who have served as chairmen of the division since its organization:

1918–1919—R. A. Millikan
1919–1920—C. E. Mendenhall
1920–1921—Augustus Trowbridge
1921–1922—Henry G. Gale
1922–1923—William Duane
1923–1924—Oswald Veblen
1924–1927—Joseph S. Ames
1927–1930—Dayton C. Miller
1930–1933—F. K. Richtmyer

Since 1919, there have been associated with the division as officers, or members, or as members of research committees, altogether some 355 *different* persons. Many of these persons, through their connection with the division in one way or another, have become mindful of the value of cooperative support of research, as well as of the latent possibilities of the service which such an organization as the National Research Council can render. These contacts have tended to emphasize the community of interest which scientists have in the promotion and general well-being of science as a whole.

Recognizing the importance of these indirect influences, the division has not thought it wise to undertake a great variety of activities in the promotion of research in physics, mathematics and astronomy. Rather, the efforts of the division have been concentrated on the formation of various research committees to survey and to report upon timely research topics, whenever such a survey would seem to serve a useful purpose.

Since the organization of the division in 1919 there have been appointed a total of thirty-eight research committees in such subjects as: Acoustics, Algebraic Numbers, Analysis Situs, Atomic Structure, Celestial Mechanics, Electrodynamics of Moving Media, Hydrodynamics, Line Spectra of the Elements, Luminescence, Numerical Integration, Photo-Electricity, Physics of the Earth with various subsidiary committees, Quantum Theory, Radiation in Gases, Theories of Magnetism, X-rays and Radioactivity, X-ray Spectra and many others. Of these committees, seven are still active. A large proportion of the remainder, having completed the reports for the preparation of which they were appointed, has been discontinued.

In addition to numerous articles in current scientific periodicals, reports to the number of thirty-three prepared by these committees have been published or are in press as bulletins of the National Research Council. These bulletins have ranged from pamphlets of forty or fifty pages up to large volumes of several hundred pages. They are sold at cost of manufacture. The subjects covered are varied; to mention only a few: The Quantum Theory (1920); Problems of X-ray Emission (1920); The Present Status of the Atomic Problem (1921); Certain Problems of Acoustics (1922); The Present Status of Visual Science (1922); Algebraic Numbers (1923); Critical Potentials (1924); Radioactivity (1925), reprinted (1929); Quantum Principles of Line Spectra (1926), reprinted (1928); Molecular Spectra in Gases (1926), reprinted (1930); Hydrodynamics (1932).

As illustrative of the service which the division is rendering in the preparation of these monographs, special mention should be made of the Committee on the Physics of the Earth, organized by Dr. Joseph S. Ames during his term as chairman. This committee, with a total membership of approximately 100 physicists, chemists, geologists, geophysicists and others, is divided into nine subcommittees as follows: The Figure of the Earth; Age of the Earth; Meteorology; Oceanography, Volcanology; Seismology; Internal Constitution of the Earth; Terrestrial Magnetism and Electricity; and Field Methods for Detecting Unhomogeneities in the Earth's Crust. The first six of these subcommittees have completed their reports, and they have been published in the Bulletin Series of the National Research Council. Reports from the remainder are nearing completion. This group of bulletins is a noteworthy contribution to the literature of this important subject. Although intended to stimulate research in the general field of earth physics, the bulletins are nevertheless of particular interest to the general scientific reader, since for the most part they are written in non-technical language.

It is the purpose of the division to form new committees whenever work in any field of research would be furthered thereby. It has been felt that the research bulletins have been of special service to investigators in providing up-to-date surveys not otherwise available; and in suggesting new problems and lines of attack. Research, particularly in pure science, is most effectively carried on as a result of individual initiative, rather than by the organized parcelling out of problems. The division has never attempted to "organize" research.

In 1920 and 1922, the division received from the National Research Council a sum of $1,500 to initiate a revolving fund for the publication of mathematical books. It was the purpose of this fund to underwrite the publication of important mathematical books which could not find publication through commercial channels. To date three such books have been published by and from this fund. Royalties received have slightly exceeded expenditures.

In 1926 and 1928, the division received from the International Education Board a total sum of $20,000 in support of astronomical research surveys under the direction of Professor A. O. Leuschner.

As was mentioned above, the Fellowship Board in

Physics, Chemistry and Mathematics—the first of the three National Research Council Fellowship Boards now operative—was organized under the auspices of the division in 1919. The administration of these fellowships has been one of the chief activities, as well as one of the major accomplishments, of the division. The chairman of the division serves, *ex officio,* as the secretary of the board, which in addition to its chairman and secretary consists of ten members—three in physics, three in mathematics and four in chemistry, the last named including, *ex officio,* the chairman of the Division of Chemistry and Chemical Technology. The board meets once each year, in April, for the appointment of fellows for the ensuing year.

Appointments are for one year, and are offered only to those who have the Ph.D. or who have had equivalent training. A limited number of appointments are made for work abroad, but for the most part fellows work at the various universities and other research institutions in the United States and Canada. Appointments are frequently renewed for one year.

Since 1919 the Fellowship Board in Physics, Chemistry and Mathematics has considered upwards of 1,000 applications. In that period nearly 400 appointments have been made, over fifty of which have been for work abroad. At present there are sixty fellows active, of whom six are working abroad. In this period nearly $1,300,000 has been paid to fellows in stipends.

About 39 per cent. of appointments have been in chemistry, 39 per cent. in physics, and the remainder in mathematics.

Fellows have been appointed from (that is, have taken their respective Ph.D's in) some thirty-five different universities in America. While the larger proportion of fellows have come from the larger universities, a study of the distribution shows that the relative number of appointees from the several universities is roughly proportional to the number of Ph.D's conferred by each.

There is an equally wide distribution of institutions in which fellows have worked. Some thirty-two American and twenty-five foreign universities and research institutions have cooperated with the National Research Council in offering facilities to fellows to carry on research. In the aggregate this service which the various institutions have thereby rendered is very great indeed.

It was the original purpose of those who sponsored the fellowship program to provide the more able young scientists with opportunities to acquire "momentum" in research, before settling down to permanent positions. That this objective is being realized is at once evident from a consideration of the present location and activities of past fellows. Nearly 80 per cent. of past fellows hold positions in educational and similar research institutions, where not only are they continuing their researches, but they are in many cases leaders in promoting the research program of the institution. The remainder are connected with industrial or governmental institutions. *With very few exceptions, all past fellows are entering upon active research careers.* There are many who would heartily endorse the statement that had the National Research Council engaged in no activity other than the promotion and administration of the National Research Fellowships, its existence would have been justified.

The services of the Division of Physical Sciences have been utilized in providing a sponsorship for the American sections of several international unions. At present there are organized under the auspices of the division the American sections of, respectively, The International Astronomical Union, The International Scientific Radio Union and the International Union of Pure and Applied Physics.

Each of the several divisions of the National Research Council can be of most effective service by organizing and by engaging in activities so as most adequately to meet the needs of the particular group of sciences concerned, due regard being had for other agencies in the field, such as societies, research institutes, academies and the like. In common with other divisions, it is the policy of the Division of Physical Sciences to stand ready to be of service wherever and whenever such service can be best rendered, and to cooperate to the fullest extent with other agencies so as to avoid needless duplication of effort.

# OBITUARY

## MEMORIALS

A BRONZE tablet in memory of Josiah Royce was placed on April 9 by the Harvard Club of San Francisco in the library of his native city, Grass Valley. At the ceremony Rudolph Altrocchi, professor of Italian and chairman of the department of Italian, and now president of the Harvard Club of San Francisco, presided. A paper on Josiah Royce was read by Jacob Loewenberg, vice-president of the club and professor of philosophy in the University of California. Dr. Royce was professor of philosophy at Harvard University from 1882 until his death in 1916.

A BRONZE bust of Ernest Haeckel, the German naturalist, was unveiled at the Cincinnati Society of Natural History on January 18.

SIR HARRY GOSCHEN, chairman of the board of the London School of Hygiene and Tropical Medicine, has received from Mr. Robert Holland Martin and the committee of the Avebury Memorial Fund a sum of £2,000 for the establishment in the school of a fund in memory of Lord Avebury, to be applied to the advancement of study and research in entomology.

SIR F. GOWLAND HOPKINS has unveiled a plaque which has been placed in the Halliburton laboratory of physiology at King's College, London, in memory of Professor W. D. Halliburton, who was professor of physiology at the College from 1890 until 1923. *Nature* writes: "When Professor Halliburton was appointed, the laboratory was on the Embankment in small and badly lit rooms where Ferrier and Lister had worked. Yet, by his enthusiasm, he managed to attract many young physiologists to the college. The present laboratory is the result of his great efforts during his tenure of office as professor of physiology." Professor Halliburton was elected a fellow of the Royal Society in 1891 and died on May 21, 1931, aged seventy years.

A CORRESPONDENT of the London *Times* writes from Bournemouth recently that the evidence supplied by an inscription on a gravestone in the parish churchyard of the village of Worth Matravers, near Swanage, Dorset, shows that Edward Jenner, who discovered inoculation by cowpox, or vaccination, as a preventive of smallpox, was forestalled by two years by Benjamin Jesty, a Dorset farmer. The facts are known to the medical profession, but not generally. Edward Jenner's first inoculation by cowpox is recorded as having been made on a boy in May, 1776. Jesty's gravestone inscription shows that he inoculated his wife and two sons with cowpox in 1774. The gravestone was noticed recently by a medical man now practising in Bournemouth, who was walking through Worth Matravers. The inscription relates that Benjamin Jesty "was an upright honest Man: particularly noted for having been the first Person known that introduced the Cow Pox by Inoculation, and who from his great strength of mind made the Experiment from the Cow on his Wife and two Sons in the year 1774." Adjoining Benjamin Jesty's grave is that of his wife, and the fact that she died at the age of 84 in 1824, 50 years after the experiment, proves fairly conclusively that the experiment made on her by her "strong-minded" husband did not affect her health.

## RECENT DEATHS

FREDERICK E. BEACH, assistant professor of physics at Yale University, from 1895 to 1931, died in his seventieth year on April 6.

LUTHER MARION DEFOE, emeritus professor of mechanics at the University of Missouri, died on April 3, in his seventy-third year.

DR. CLARENCE ALBERT SHORE, for twenty-five years director of the North Carolina State Laboratory of Hygiene, died on February 10, at the age of sixty years.

DR. JOHN MILLAR THOMSON, emeritus professor of chemistry at King's College, London, died on March 22, at the age of eighty-four years.

WALTER EDMUND ROTH, anthropologist and curator of the British Guiana Museum, died on April 6. He was seventy-two years old.

THE death is announced of Dr. Friedrich Rinne, professor of mineralogy and petrography at Leipzig.

# SCIENTIFIC EVENTS

## PROPOSED PLANETARIUM FOR THE AMERICAN MUSEUM OF NATURAL HISTORY

F. TRUBEE DAVISON, president of the American Museum of Natural History, and George McAneny, president of the Regional Plan Association, recently discussed with Mayor O'Brien, of New York City, plans for the creation of a Planetarium Authority. Mr. Davison has also discussed the plan with Governor Lehman. The proposal has been under consideration for several years, but the plans were postponed because of lack of funds.

At a recent luncheon at the Museum, Mr. Davison explained that it was hoped to obtain state legislation that would permit the creation of a Planetarium Authority similar to the New York Port Authority, with power to issue bonds. The measure would also enable the city to transfer to the authority, for a time, some of the city-owned museum land, just north of the African Hall.

Mr. Davis said in part:

The bill is purely a permissive measure. It does not bind the museum to take any action toward the planetarium project and it does not commit the city to endorse the project unless it is in whole-hearted accord with the museum's attitude.

The reason for the measure is that we hope to borrow the money from the Reconstruction Finance Corporation, provided we are satisfied that the planetarium will be self-supporting; in other words, the planetarium, through admission fees, must not alone pay its own way with respect to maintenance and so on, but must also yield enough income to retire any bonded indebtedness incurred in connection with its construction.

The reason we ask for legislation now is because it is needed in the event we determine to put the completed project before the city for further action.

Tentative plans call for a planetarium similar to the Adler Planetarium in Chicago. It would seat 600 persons. Though admission would be charged until the bonds have been paid, school children would be admitted free at specified times, when they attended as part of their classroom work.

## WEATHER STATION ON MT. WACHUSETT

ON this isolated peak in central Massachusetts, 2,018 feet above sea-level, a new meteorological station has been established under the auspices of Blue Hill Observatory, Harvard University, in connection with the work of the International Polar Year. Unlike the Mt. Washington Observatory, however, there will not be resident observers. A meteorograph, designed and built by Professor S. P. Fergusson to run two or three months without attention, is keeping the record of wind direction and velocity, atmospheric pressure, temperature and humidity.

According to a news release of Science Service, permission to install the apparatus in the fire lookout's tower on the top of the hotel on Mt. Wachusett was granted by Everett W. Needham, superintendent of the Wachusett State Reservation. The meteorograph and the exposed elements were prepared and adapted by F. B. Towle and his son, Philip, of Holden, Massachusetts, who will also look after the station weekly.

The wind vane and three-cup anemometer, loaned by the U. S. Weather Bureau, are exposed a few feet above the top of the tower and are connected to the pens which record the wind direction and velocity on the large drum of the meteorograph in the fire-lookout room. Under the eaves of the summit-house tower, the temperature and humidity elements are exposed in a louvered box to protect them from the full force of the gales that beset this summit. A coil of brass and steel is indicating the temperature, while a bundle of 150 strands of child's hair, prepared by Clifford L. Davis, of Worcester, operates the humidity recorder. The motion of these elements is transmitted several feet to the pens on the recorder by means of 100-year-old light wooden connecting rods from an old church organ which are hung on sewing machine needles.

Mt. Wachusett stands alone and is exposed to more or less frequent high winds. Mt. Washington, 127 miles away, is sometimes visible in extremely clear weather, and Blue Hill, 45 miles distant, is also in sight. Ice storms occur quite often. At the beginning of this month, the east side of the hotel was plastered with almost solid ice, two to three inches thick.

Mt. Wachusett is characterized by a strong edition of the typical ever-changing New England weather. It is intermediate between the arctic character of Mt. Washington and the more temperate weather of Blue Hill, where are the other two mountain and hill top stations of New England. These three stations will help to show how sudden weather changes progress over New England.

## ANNUAL REPORT OF THE BROOKLYN BOTANIC GARDEN

THE twenty-second Annual Report of the Brooklyn Botanic Garden records the facts that the garden closed the year without a deficit and with more than $11,400 added to its permanent endowment fund and with the 1933 budget balanced. The director points out that this accomplishment has been made possible only by the most rigid economies.

During 1932, there was a registered attendance of 1,307,964, which was an increase of more than 200,925 over the preceding year. The registered attendance for May (232,737) was nearly half the attendance for the entire year of 1924. The week-end attendance of May 14 and 15 was 38,804.

4,555 packets of seeds of American wild flowers were supplied to more than 120 gardens in more than 20 foreign countries. The request for these packets of seeds was about 500 in excess of the garden's ability to respond.

During the year, lectures, addresses, informal talks and class exercises reached a total number of 1,762. 780 adults were enrolled in classes and 597 children. Teachers from the public schools brought more than 41,000 pupils to the garden for instruction, and 6,105 teachers were supplied with living plant material and sterilized agar for class work for the instruction of 257,527 pupils. 740 potted plants were placed in the classrooms of public schools and more than 670,000 packets of seeds were supplied to pupils for planting in school and home gardens. The school service of the Brooklyn Garden now extends to all five boroughs of Greater New York.

Progress in the research program of the garden is also recorded covering the subjects of plant pathology, genetics and plant breeding, forest pathology, ecology and systematic botany. Eight research students were registered during the year. Progress in the development and beautifying of the grounds is also recorded.

The library of the garden now has more than 17,450 volumes and more than 30,900 bound pamphlets. The library of the American Fern Society is now deposited there. In contrast to the experience of many organizations and many institutions, the garden reports an increase of new members for 1932 of 97, or 9.3 per cent.

The report includes an urgent plea for an addition of not less than one million dollars to the endowment of the garden in order to care for the increased service which it is being called upon to render to the general public and to botanical science and education.

## FELLOWSHIPS OF THE CHARLES LATHROP PACK FOREST EDUCATION BOARD

MAKING its fourth annual award of fellowships for training leaders in forestry, the Charles Lathrop Pack Forest Education Board announces its selection of three American and two Canadian fellows for the year 1933. The fellowships were established to encourage men to obtain advanced training to better qualify them for leadership in forestry and in the forest industries. The successful candidates are:

Walter U. Garstka, instructor in forestry, Penn State Forest School. To make organic analysis of leaf litter, immediately after its fall in the autumn, collected from forests growing on podzolized and brown-earth soils.

Harold R. Hay, graduate student, University of Wisconsin. To make a study of changes in the physical properties and chemical constituency of wood subjected to steam treatments.

John Edward Liersch, junior forester, British Columbia Forest Service. To continue a demonstration begun under Charles Lathrop Pack Fellowship awarded in 1932 regarding the practicability of economic selection in the Douglas fir region.

Nicholas T. Mirov, graduate student, University of California. To make a study of transpiration by different forest cover species with reference to precipitation and to moisture content of the soil.

Louis René Scheult, graduate student, University of Toronto, Toronto. To make a regional study of forest development.

This is the fourth award of fellowships by the board. They are available to Americans and Canadians for further training in the general practise of forestry, in the forest industries, in the teaching of forestry, in forest research, or in the development of public forest policy.

The directors of the board are: Henry S. Graves, dean, Yale Forest School; Samuel T. Dana, dean, School of Forestry and Conservation, University of Michigan; John Foley, forester, Pennsylvania Railroad; William B. Greeley, secretary-manager, West Coast Lumbermen's Association; Arthur Newton Pack, director, Charles Lathrop Pack Forestry Trust; E. O. Siecke, director, Texas Forest Service; Ellwood Wilson, acting professor of silviculture, New York State College of Agriculture; Hugo Winkenwerder, dean, College of Forestry, University of Washington, and Raphael Zon, director, Lake States Forest Experiment Station.

The offices of the board are at 1214 Sixteenth Street, N.W., Washington, D. C., and correspondence should be addressed to Tom Gill, secretary.

# SCIENTIFIC NOTES AND NEWS

DR. HENRY NORRIS RUSSELL, research professor of astronomy and director of the observatory at Princeton University, president this year of the American Association for the Advancement of Science, will deliver the Halley Lecture at the University of Oxford on June 1. His subject will be "The Composition of the Stars."

DR. ROBERT A. MILLIKAN, of the California Institute of Technology, has accepted the invitation of Oberlin College to deliver the Centennial Commencement address on June 20. Dr. Millikan was recently reelected alumni trustee for a term of six years; he has served on the Board of Trustees since 1918.

DR. IRVING LANGMUIR, of the General Electric Company, Schenectady, New York, will be made an honorary member of the School of Engineering Alumni Association of Columbia University at the annual dinner on April 26. Dr. Langmuir and Dr. Michael I. Pupin will be the principal speakers.

DR. WALDEMAR LINDGREN, Rogers professor of economic geology and head of the department of geology at the Massachusetts Institute of Technology, will retire at the end of the academic year.

THE Paris faculty of medicine has conferred the degree of doctor, *honoris causa,* on Professor Sanarelli, director of the Hygienic Institute of the University of Rome.

THE Bessemer Gold Medal of the British Iron and Steel Institute has been awarded to Dr. W. H. Hatfield, director of research in the firm of Messrs. Thos. Firth and John Brown, Ltd., in recognition of his distinguished services in the advancement of metallurgical science.

THE Gold Medal of the British Institution of Mining and Metallurgy, the highest distinction in its power to confer, has been awarded to Sir John Cadman in recognition of his work in the advancement of technical education and the development of the mineral industries, and of his distinguished public services. The following awards have also been made: The Consolidated Gold Fields of South Africa Gold Medal to Mr. Charles Arthur Banks for his paper on

"Air Transportation of Gold Dredges in New Guinea"; and the premium of 40 guineas conjointly to Mr. J. L. Francis and Mr. John C. Allan for their paper on "Driving a Mines Drainage Tunnel in North Wales"; the William Frecheville Student's Prize of ten guineas to Mr. Gordon J. Williams for his paper on "The Genesis of the Perrunal-La Zarza Pyritic Ore-body, Spain."

*Nature* reports that the prize of the Institute of Physics for the best paper published in the *Journal of Scientific Instruments* during the year 1932 has been awarded to Mr. E. Lancaster-Jones, of the Science Museum, for his paper on "The Principles and Practice of the Gravity Gradiometer," and the prize for the best contribution to the Laboratory and Workshop Notes in the *Journal* has been awarded to Dr. J. L. Miller and Mr. J. E. L. Robinson, of Messrs. Ferranti, Ltd., for their joint note entitled "A Three-Dimensional Adjustment of an Electrode in Vacuo."

SIR RONALD GRAHAM, the British Ambassador at Rome, presented Signor Mussolini on March 24 with the silver medal of merit conferred upon him by the Royal Society for the Prevention of Cruelty to Animals—the highest award in the gift of the society—in recognition of his recent action in making the Island of Capri a bird sanctuary.

OFFICERS of the New York Branch of the American Psychological Association were elected at the recent New Haven meeting as follows: *Honorary President,* Dr. J. McKeen Cattell; *Directors,* Dr. H. E. Garrett, Columbia University, and Dr. H. S. Langfeld, Princeton University.

OFFICERS of the Ray Society, London, were elected at the annual meeting held on March 22, as follows: *President,* Sir Sidney Harmer; *Treasurer,* Sir David Prain, and Dr. W. T. Calman, *Secretary.*

AT the annual meeting of the Physical Society, London, the following officers were elected: *President,* Professor A. O. Rankine; *Vice-president,* Professor W. Wilson; *Secretaries,* Dr. Allan Ferguson, Dr. Ezer Griffiths; *Foreign Secretary,* Professor O. W. Richardson; *Treasurer,* Mr. R. S. Whipple; *Librarian,* Dr. J. H. Brinkworth; new members of council, Professor E. V. Appleton, Dr. L. F. Bates and Dr. L. Hartshorn.

DR. PHILIP BARD, assistant professor of physiology at the Harvard Medical School, has been appointed professor of physiology at the School of Medicine of the Johns Hopkins University.

DR. ROBERT B. MACLEOD, formerly an honor student in psychology and philosophy at McGill University and winner in 1927 of the Moyse Traveling Scholarship in the Classics, has been appointed an assistant professor in psychology at Swarthmore College.

IN the Bell Telephone Laboratories, Vice-president H. P. Charlesworth has resigned to accept the position of assistant chief engineer of the American Telephone and Telegraph Company. Dr. E. H. Colpitts, who has been appointed to succeed him, is assistant vice-president of the American Telephone and Telegraph Company in charge of the Development and Research Department under Dr. F. B. Jewett, vice-president.

SENATORS Kendrick, Hayden, McNary and Carey are urging the retention of Dr. Elwood Mead as commissioner of reclamation under the new administration. The recommendation is based on Commissioner Mead's long service in various government departments in the interest of irrigation and drainage works. He has devoted nearly forty years to reclamation projects in the West. In 1924 he was appointed commissioner of the Reclamation Service by President Coolidge. Secretary of the Interior Harold L. Ickes is reported to have said that he would give the recommendation every consideration.

DR. EDWARD H. GRAHAM, assistant curator of botany at the Carnegie Museum, Pittsburgh, and Mrs. Graham, will leave on April 15 on a botanical collecting expedition of several months to the southeastern Uinta Mountains in the vicinity of Vernal, Utah, in order to obtain representatives of the spring flora and thus augment the collections made by the same party in the summer and fall of 1931.

DR. JOHN C. MERRIAM, president of the Carnegie Institution of Washington, was the chief speaker at the Jefferson Day exercises at the University of Virginia on April 13.

DR. A. V. KIDDER, chairman of the division of historical research of the Carnegie Institution of Washington, will give a lecture at the annual meeting of the American Philosophical Society on Friday evening, April 21, on "Mayan Explorations and Their Results."

DR. HARRY BOYER WEISER, professor of chemistry at the Rice Institute, gave the annual lecture of the Sigma Xi Club of the University of Alabama on March 30. His subject was "Colloidal Phenomena in the Formation of Gallstones."

THE Cutter Lectures on preventive medicine at the Harvard Medical School will be delivered on April 17 and 18, at 5 P. M., by Dr. Eugene L. Opie, professor of pathology in the Cornell University Medical College, on "The Epidemiology of Tuberculosis."

ROBERT FECHNER, vice-president of the International Association of Machinists and a lecturer on labor questions at Harvard University and Dartmouth College, has been appointed by President Roosevelt to be director under the unemployment reforestation act. Those present at the conference following which the appointment was made were Horace Albright, director of the National Park Service; John D. Coffman, fire control expert of the National Park Service; William G. Howard, director of lands and forests of the New York Conservation Department; R. Y. Stuart, chief United States forester; C. H. Granger, assistant chief forester; Colonel Duncan K. Major, Jr., of the general staff of the War Department, and W. Frank Parsons, of Chicago. This committee will direct the preliminary work and will have offices in the Interior Department.

THE Committee on Scientific Research of the American Medical Association has granted to Professor Ludwig A. Emge, associate professor at Stanford University, and his associates a grant to be used toward a study of the effect of pregnancy on tumor growth. This study forms part of a more extensive study on the behavior of benign tumor growth, which is now in its fifth year. A grant has also been made to Dr. Arthur Grollman, associate professor of pharmacology and experimental therapeutics at the Johns Hopkins University, to aid in work on the hormone of the adrenal cortex.

DR. T. WAYLAND VAUGHAN, director of the Scripps Institution of Oceanography of the University of California at La Jolla, and Mrs. Vaughan, have returned from a journey around the world, which started last August and has taken them as visitors to the principal oceanographic stations.

THE April lecture to the faculty and students of the School of Medicine, the George Washington University, on the Smith-Reed-Russell Society series was given by Dr. William H. Howell, chairman of the National Research Council. He spoke on the "Recollections of a Physiologist during the Past Half Century." The regular faculty seminar for April was given by Professor George B. Roth, of the department of pharmacology, who spoke on "The Arsphenamines; their Nature and Behavior."

THE scientific session of the American Heart Association will be held on Tuesday, June 13, from 9:30 A. M. to 5:30 P. M., in the Knickerbocker Hotel, Milwaukee, Wisconsin.

THE fourth annual Connecticut Valley Student Scientific Conference is meeting at Wesleyan University on Saturday, April 15. The conference is modeled after the meetings of the American Association for the Advancement of Science. The colleges represented are Amherst, Dartmouth, Mt. Holyoke, Smith, Massachusetts State, Connecticut State, Springfield, Trinity, Connecticut and Wesleyan. About seventy-five titles of papers or demonstrations appear on the program. It is expected that about three hundred students will attend. The conference is organized entirely by the graduate students and undergraduates of the colleges concerned.

APPLICATIONS for grants from the Cyrus M. Warren Fund of the American Academy of Arts and Sciences should be in the hands of the chairman of the committee, Professor James F. Norris, Massachusetts Institute of Technology, Cambridge, Mass., not later than May 15.

A DAVID ANDERSON-BERRY GOLD MEDAL, together with a sum of money amounting to about £100, will be awarded in July, 1935, by the Royal Society of Edinburgh to the person, who, in the opinion of the council, has recently produced the best work on the nature of x-rays in their therapeutical effect on human diseases.

ANNOUNCEMENT is made of a fellowship for graduate study at the medical faculty of the University of Geneva providing for tuition and a stipend of 3,000 Swiss francs (about $600) for the academic year, 1933–34. To be eligible, a candidate must be an American citizen, a graduate of an approved American medical school or the holder of a master's or doctor's degree in a science related to the medical field and must have a thorough knowledge of the French language. The fellowship will be administered by the Swiss American Student Exchange under the auspices of the Institute of International Education.

A HISTORICAL exhibit of maps, arranged by Dr. Erwin J. Raisz, is being shown at the Institute of Geographical Exploration, Harvard University. Many of the maps are originals, and come from the collections of Widener Library and Dr. Hamilton Rice. In addition to the maps, there are shown a number of old instruments connected with navigation and surveying, loaned by the Peabody Museum of Salem. The exhibit, open from 9:30 to 4:30 o'clock every day except Saturday and Sunday, will continue until May 1.

FREDERICK S. DELLENBAUGH, who was artist and one of the topographers with Major Powell in his second descent through the canyons of Green River and the Colorado, in 1871 and 1872, has presented the flag of Major Powell's boat, the *Emma Dean,* to the National Museum in Washington. The flag was made in Salt Lake City in 1871 by Major Powell's sister, Mrs. Ellen Powell Thompson. Major Powell's boat was named after his wife. There were two other boats, the *Nellie Powell,* named after Mrs. Thompson, and the *Cañonita.*

THE Bureau of Ethnology has received the first report of the field activities of the party undertaking archeological reconnaissance in the eastern section of Honduras, made up of Dr. W. D. Strong, of the bureau staff, Alan W. Payne, and Norman Haskell. The report states that on February 10 the party left Puerto Castilla, proceeded to the mouth of the Patuca River, and went upstream. Studies were undertaken on the Guampu and Cuyamel Rivers, tributary to the Patuca. Two archeological sites marked by the presence of earth mounds were studied and excavated. The few remaining Sumu Indians were encountered, and a brief study was made of them. The conclusion was reached that the Maya culture did not extend that far to the eastward, as nothing indicative of this culture was found. The party learned that several hundred Sumus had been living on the river until four years ago, when an epidemic of smallpox swept them away. The next trip to be made will be from the westward of the Patuca Valley overland *via* muleback into the mountain region.

# DISCUSSION

## A CIVILIZATION WITHOUT NATIVE MATHEMATICS

IN a recent number of the historical periodical entitled "Quellen und Studien zur Geschichte der Mathematik, Astronomie und Physik," volume 2 (1932), page 255, there appears an article by P. L. van Hee, in which it is stated that if the Chinese mathematical books of every epoch would disappear science would suffer no loss as regards mathematics. It is claimed here that China has contributed nothing towards raising the edifice of modern mathematics, but that the mathematics which appears now in the Chinese literature is due to other nations and was often credited by Chinese writers to natives of their own country. Among the recent writers who are said to have been misled by these false claims is Y. Mikami, whose work entitled "The Development of Mathematics in China and Japan," 1913, is widely known and has been frequently referred to as an authority.

There is a remarkable contrast between the recent historical developments relating to China and those relating to Egypt and Babylonia. In the former case these developments seem to tend to show that their early mathematical attainments were overestimated, while in the latter they were underestimated, especially as regards Babylonia. In particular, the issue of the periodical noted above contains also the remarkable announcement that the ancient Babylonians had a rule equivalent to a general formula for the sum of the squares of the first $n$ natural numbers. It was formerly supposed that the first discovery of such a rule was due to the ancient Greek mathematicians. A few years ago it was announced that the ancient Egyptians had a rule which is equivalent to our modern formula for the area of a sphere, but this seems now to be incorrect, having been due to a mistranslation.

The chief interest in the article to which we referred at the beginning of this note is due to the fact that it exhibits a lack of mathematical initiative on the part of the Chinese extending over a long period of time. When mathematics was introduced from other countries it received considerable attention and some of it was permanently retained, but no definite evidences of native advances seem as yet to have been established. The exaggerated claims made by some of the Chinese writers have really been harmful to the reputation of their country and they have made it difficult to form a correct judgment as regards their possible contributions It seems clear, however, that from the standpoint of mathematics ancient China was far behind ancient Egypt and ancient Babylonia. Their ancient as well as their modern civilization exhibits unusual mathematical weakness and many of the references to their achievements along this line are untrustworthy according to some of the most recent investigations.

G. A. MILLER
UNIVERSITY OF ILLINOIS

## THEORIES OF CORTICO-ADRENAL FUNCTION

WITHIN the past year three theories of cortico-adrenal function have been advanced. They postulate that the adrenal cortex (1) prepotently regulates carbohydrate metabolism,[1] (2) produces a general tissue hormone,[2] (3) controls the circulating blood volume.[3] The first appeared about a year ago, the second shortly after, and the third in January of this year.

In presenting their theory of blood-volume regulation and the relation of the adrenals to shock, Swingle and his associates ride rough-shod over other hypotheses. "None," they state, "have materially advanced (*sic*) the problem of cortical function." Not even a foot-line was given to bibliographic mention of the earlier theories mentioned above.

It is not *in justitia scientiae* merely that mention should be made of the praiseworthy contributions of

[1] S. W. Britton and H. Silvette, *Amer. Jour. Physiol.,* 100: 701, 1932.

[2] F. A. Hartman, K. A. Brownell and J. E. Lockwood, *Endocrinology,* 16: 521, 1932; *Amer. Jour. Physiol.,* 101: 50, 1932.

[3] W. W. Swingle, *et al.,* SCIENCE, 77: 58, 1933.

Hartman and his colleagues toward the elucidation of cortico-adrenal problems. Contemporaneously with, if not prior to Swingle and Pfiffner, the Buffalo investigators produced a potent extract of the adrenal cortex, and they have published extensively on its effects. Furthermore, they have formulated a theory of cortico-adrenal function as noted above, and supported it with considerable experimental evidence.

That the adrenals are of importance in maintaining a normal circulation has been known for many decades, and the ideas of Swingle and his associates are not at all novel. In a small section of a review a few years ago, one of us (Britton)[4] drew attention to more than a score of observations on the subject. Antedating by two years the recent report of Swingle *et al.*, there appeared a comprehensive experimental study by Wyman and Suden on "The blood volume in suprarenal insufficiency, anaphylactic shock and histamine shock."[5]

Our own observations lead us to conclude that changes in blood pressure and in the amount of circulating blood are indirect and illustrative only of the general effects of adrenalectomy throughout the body. We have sought an understanding of the *underlying* chemical changes and conditions in adrenal insufficiency which are antecedent to, or take precedence over, because of their critical nature, the altered permeability relationships in the body.

Breakdown to the point of utter collapse of the normal carbo-metabolic processes appears to us still to constitute the primary critical contingency in adrenal insufficiency. The adrenalectomized animal suffers from glucose and glycogen lack, which becomes progressively more severe after the operation, and parallels the development of symptoms. All the symptoms, too, are compellingly suggestive of severe hypoglycemia. We have never observed such profoundly critical glucose and glycogen disturbances in any other cachexic status which involves carbohydrate metabolism—*e.g.,* the cachexia following hepatectomy or pancreatectomy or heavy insulin dosage. Cortico-adrenal extract appears to have a primary effect, moreover, in restoring promptly the normal carbohydrate levels.

Animals dying of adrenal insufficiency show convulsive seizures some hours before death which are identical in type with those observed in insulin hypoglycemia. By contrast we have never observed such convulsions in animals in which the circulating blood volume has been markedly reduced by hemorrhage and other operative procedures.

It may be that carbohydrate deficiencies do not explain the whole problem of adrenal insufficiency. Glucose does not prolong the lives of adrenalectomized animals many days. Similarly, carbohydrate injections only slightly extend the survival of hepatectomized animals. In a number of cases we have observed, too, that glucose does not restore severely insulinized animals. Many substances are furthermore known to reduce the blood sugar in diabetes, but that without remedy. It is to be emphasized in this connection that we have been concerned for the present simply with *the first crucial signs of failure* in the adrenalectomized animal. That there occurs primarily and fundamentally a failure in glycotaxis in the body appears as best fitting the mass of evidence at hand.

Swingle and his colleagues state that in cases of adrenal insufficiency blood dilution "never occurs . . . unless the hormone is injected." In our experiments we have observed that restoration of the normal blood volume of adrenalectomized animals may readily be brought about by saline injections. The symptoms of insufficiency are not at all ameliorated by such restoration, however, nor is life even slightly prolonged. In contrast, augmentation of the blood sugar by glucose injections alleviates the symptoms very rapidly, and lengthens significantly the survival period.

We have observed that the adrenalectomized animal is somewhat hydrated, rather than dehydrated.[6] Increased amounts of water are held in the hepatic and muscular tissues. The blood plasma and total blood volume are in contrast reduced, but not until symptoms are developed are these reductions noteworthy. Fluid accumulations in the liver and muscle in adrenal insufficiency more than balance the loss of fluid by the blood.

We gain the impression from our data that water is more necessary for the maintenance of normality conditions in the liver and muscle than for any of the demands of the circulation, important though the latter may be. Furthermore, one of the earliest and most striking effects of cortico-adrenal extract which we have observed is the *elimination* of fluid by the production of a striking diuresis. Space limits can not be imposed on for further considerations here.

The most critical emergency in the career of the adrenalectomized animal results from virtually complete disappearance of liver glycogen, and concomitantly profound reduction of blood sugar, as well as muscle glycogen. Thus, severe hypoglycemic convulsions supervene, and death results during the convulsive seizures. Our data compel adherence to our first-proposed theory of the prepotent function of the adrenal cortex—that of the regulation, in cooperation

[4] S. W. Britton, *Physiol. Rev.*, 10: 617, 1930.

[5] L. C. Wyman and C. tum Suden, *Amer. Jour. Physiol.*, 94: 579, 1930.

[6] H. Silvette and S. W. Britton, *Amer. Jour. Physiol.*, (in press), 1933.

with other tissues or secretions, of carbohydrate metabolism in the organism.

S. W. BRITTON
H. SILVETTE
UNIVERSITY OF VIRGINIA

## THE "SPREAD" OR "SCATTER" OF THE INFLUENCE FROM A REWARD, IN RELATION TO GESTALT DOCTRINES

IN SCIENCE of February 10, I reported the discovery of the "spread" or "scatter" of the influence of a reward, and especially the significance of the phenomenon as an independent proof of the so-called law of effect. Circumstances prevented a prompt reply to Ogden's criticisms (SCIENCE, March 3) and the need has perhaps vanished as a result of Boring's ingenious *modus vivendi* for Gestaltists and connectionists (SCIENCE, March 24). But I venture to note the following:

The "whole process" in my experiments consists of 40 words chosen at random said by the experimenter, to each of which the subject responds by a number from 1 to 10, or of equally arbitrary multiple choices. An announcement of "Right" after one of the 40 word-number units in the experiments certainly does not strengthen or confirm the whole process equally. An announcement of "Wrong" seems to the observers to be as "final" or as "consummatory" of, the connection it follows as an announcement of "Right." Certainly any difference in this respect is very small, but the difference in strengthening of the connection is enormous. And this enormous difference uniformly goes with the satisfyingness of the after-effect.

My note in SCIENCE presented evidence for these conclusions: (1) The strengthening of the connection which the reward immediately follows and to which it belongs does not occur indirectly by reason of repetitions or rehearsals of the connection or by way of memories that such and such a number was right, or successful, or rewarded for such and such a word, because the announcements of "Wrong" have no negative influence comparable to the positive influence of the announcement of "Right."

(2) The reward does not have to search out the "right" or "successful" act by any mysterious power and attach itself to it, as Peterson has objected. It strengthens whatever its physiological equivalent influences in the neurones.

(3) The reward strengthens chiefly the connection which immediately precedes it and of which it is (by sophisticated humans) felt to be the after-effect. But it also strengthens the connections one and two steps further back or forward, though these were definitely punished and most emphatically did *not* belong to the reward in the Gestalt's meaning of "belong" if I understand them. Each belongs to its punishment. Nothing happening to the subject equally near the time of the reward could belong to it much less in the sense of forming with it a "perfectly integrated unit."

In the very different sense in which I use the word, the reward may belong to these preceding and succeeding connections, though rather tenuously and indirectly, as neighboring tasks related only by the conditions of the experiment.

I can guarantee this. Let any Gestaltist choose a hundred multiple-choice tasks as "discrete and independent" one from another as he can find or make, each composed of a situation and *n* responses from which choice is to be made such that the situation and the responses are as "discrete and independent" from each other as he can find or make, and let him choose rewards and punishments as "discrete and independent" from anything in the tasks as he can find and make. Then the situation-response connection which has a reward attached to it utterly arbitrarily by the experimenter will be strengthened thereby, so long as it is a satisfying after-effect of that connection to the learner. And the influence of the reward may, and often will, spread or scatter so as to strengthen other connections in the physiological neighborhood.

EDWARD L. THORNDIKE
TEACHERS COLLEGE
COLUMBIA UNIVERSITY

## STRATIGRAPHIC NOMENCLATURE

IN SCIENCE (Vol. 76, p. 489) Professor G. D. Harris, of the Paleontological Laboratory, Cornell University, writes: "Perhaps others as well as the writer have often been at a loss for a concise, logical and self-explanatory term for indicating all that portion of the geologic sequence (or geologic time) below or antedating the Cambrian system (or time). Strangely enough, the embarrassment becomes more acute if one searches for a term to include the Paleozoic, Mesozoic and Cenozoic."

I want to make the statement, that in my "Textbook of Geology" (*Lehrbuch der Geologie*, Wien, 1924) I introduced the term "Euzoische Schichtfolge" (Euzoic sequence), which includes the Paleozoic, Mesozoic and Cenozoic.

F. X. SCHAFFER
NATURHISTORISCHES STAATSMUSEUM
WIEN

## FREQUENCY OF VERTEBRATE FOSSILS IN RIVER DEPOSITS

THE following observation, dated "Monday 17, 1805," taken from "History of the Expedition of Captains Lewis and Clark,"[1] is of more than usual interest

[1] Vol. I, p. 352, New Amsterdam Book Company, New York.

to vertebrate paleontologists. The scene was at the great Falls of the Missouri.

There are vast quantities of buffalo feeding on the plains or watering in the river, which is also strewed with the floating carcases and limbs of these animals. They go in large herds to water about the falls, and as all the passages to the river near that place are narrow and steep, the foremost are pressed into the river by the impatience of those behind. In this way we have seen ten or a dozen disappear over the falls in a few minutes. They afford excellent food for the wolves, bears, and birds of prey; and this circumstance may account for the reluctance of the bears to yield their dominion over the neighborhood.

Ellis W. Shuler
Southern Methodist University

# SCIENTIFIC APPARATUS AND LABORATORY METHODS

## APPARATUS FOR SLIDE TECHNIQUE

The apparatus illustrated in the following figures has been found very practical and a great time-saver in the preparation of slides. The small cost of materials and time required for construction are negligible, compared with the efficient service they render.

### Warming Plate for Spreading Paraffin Sections

The warming plate shown in Fig. A is practically

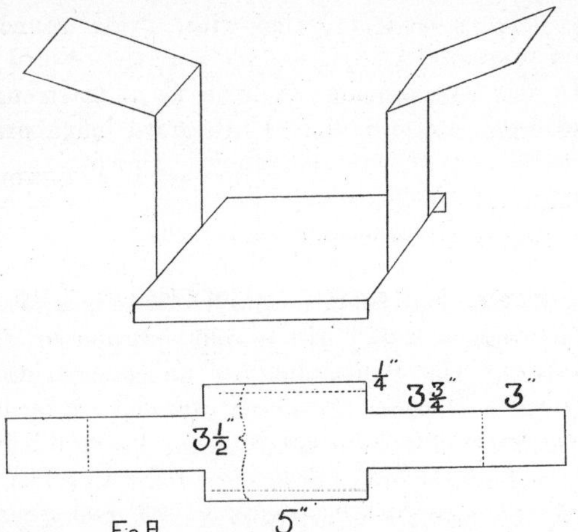


Fig A.

self-explanatory for its use in spreading paraffin sections. It is made from a single sheet of thin copper and heated by conduction from alcohol flames under the wing tips. By placing bits of paraffin, having the same melting point as that used in preparing the tissue, on the ends of the stage, the best working temperature can be determined and controlled by moving the flames closer to or farther away from the wing tips. The small diagram gives the dimensions and shows the shape of the sheet before being bent. The height of the wings could be changed to compensate for the lamp to be used.

### Slide Drying Cabinet

In preparing a large number of slides for study, it is advantageous to hasten the drying of the balsam after the covers are in place. The slide drying cabinet in Fig. B is a very efficient piece of apparatus for

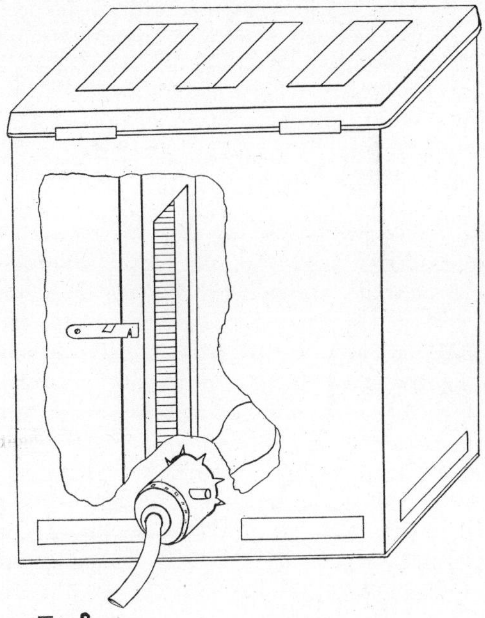

Fig B.

this purpose. It was made from a cracker can, two slide boxes, a small sheet of copper and a light socket with several feet of cord.

The light socket was placed in the rear wall so that the bulb would just clear the bottom and give room for a slide box to stand on end on either side. A 25 watt clear bulb furnishes sufficient heat for good circulation of air without having a temperature over 50° C. The air enters through the openings at the bottom, passes over the slides and goes out through the openings in the lid. A copper slide, supported beneath the lid, makes it possible to close the openings if a higher temperature is desired.

Through the opening in the back of the cabinet a slide box can be seen in position. The lids and bottoms were cut out, leaving just enough edge to hold the slides. Catches on the sides hold the lids firmly in place. After 48 hours in the drying cabinet slides are ready for their final cleaning and polishing.

Emory S. James
Ohio Wesleyan University

## A SIMPLE DEVICE FOR THE PERFUSION OF THE MAMMALIAN HEART

IN the course of some experiments in which we used the heart-beat to test the properties of some balanced salt solutions, the apparatus here described was devised. Most devices for the perfusion of the mammalian heart[1,2,3] are elaborate and present considerable difficulties in manipulation. While this is undoubtedly necessary in experimentation on some physiological function of the heart we found the simplified apparatus here presented adequate to our purpose. We are presenting it with the expectation that a device so easily assembled might be found useful in lecture demonstrations or classroom experiments.

There are three factors, the control of which presents the greatest difficulty in the perfusion of the mammalian heart: (1) Temperature of the fluid; (2) Pressure of the fluid; (3) Oxygenation.

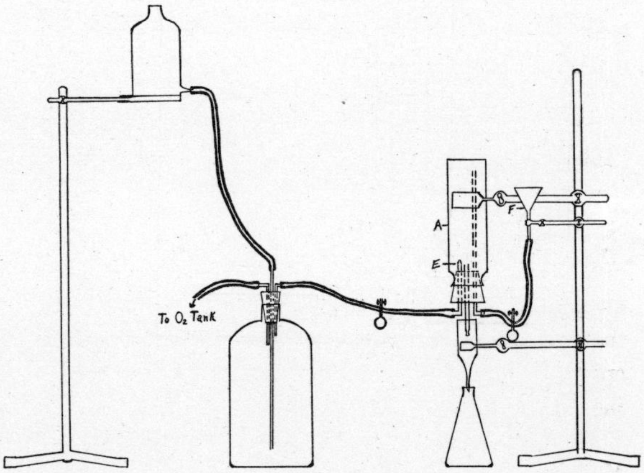


FIG. 1.

As far as the temperature is concerned it is merely necessary to control it within a degree or a degree and a half. This is readily accomplished by means of the vacuum flask (A). The cannula to which the heart is attached is inserted in rubber tubing which is attached to a piece of glass tubing inserted in the rubber stopper of the flask. The cannula and tubes are all as short as possible to avoid cooling of the fluid. The heart is suspended in a filter tube the mouth of which can be closed by a wad of moist cotton. The temperature of the heart is maintained by the passage of the perfusion fluid through it. Unless the room is very warm it is desirable to warm the filter tube by an electric lamp suspended near it. However crude this temperature control may seem to the physiologist who is accustomed to working with apparatus capable of control to a tenth or even a hundredth of a degree C., we have found it quite sufficient to keep the heart beating vigorously 6 to 8 hours.

Pressure and oxygenation are controlled by a single apparatus. Medical oxygen is released from a cylinder into a gasometer consisting of two bottles at different levels, connected by a rubber tube, the lower partly filled with water. As pressure is increased water is displaced within the lower bottle and rises in the upper. Pressure is controlled by the difference in the level of the bottles. The oxygen is conducted from the gasometer through a tube drawn out into a capillary (E) inserted in the rubber stopper of the flask, where it bubbles through the perfusion fluid. This gas is then allowed to escape through the trap (F) consisting of a funnel on a rubber tube, filled with water to counterbalance the pressure in the gasometer. This funnel may be raised and lowered to keep the pressure constant as the fluid within the flask is used. By this device the perfusion fluid is very readily kept saturated with oxygen at any desired pressure.

In our experiments we have used hearts of rat, guinea-pig and rabbit. Of these we have had the greatest success with the rabbit. The rat heart and frequently that of the guinea-pig stopped beating during the manipulation in attaching it to the apparatus. If it resumed beating at all the beat was irregular and of short duration. This is apparently the phenomenon of fibrillation or delirium cordis.[4]

Our procedure in setting up an experiment is as follows: The flask, previously warmed by the introduction of water heated to 37.5° C, is filled with perfusion fluid also warmed to 37.5° C. The fluid, preparatory to the beginning of the experiment, is saturated by a lively stream of oxygen. The animal is killed by a blow on the head and bled quickly from the carotid artery. The heart is immediately removed, taking particular care to leave the systemic aorta sufficiently long to accommodate the tip of the cannula. The heart is then placed in a small dish of warm perfusion fluid and permitted to beat in it, under the slight pressure of the finger, to clear itself of blood. The aorta is carefully dissected away from the surrounding tissue to make sure that none of the nerves will be tied in the ligature. The cannula, already attached to the flask, has now a slow stream of perfusion fluid, controlled by a clamp on the rubber tube (C), passing through it. The heart is lifted by the aorta, and the aorta is drawn over the tip of the cannula. The aorta is held in position so that the cannula does not protrude beyond the semi-

[1] Knowlton and Starling, *Journ. of Phys.*, 44: 206. 1912.

[2] Anrep and Hausler, *Journ. of Phys.*, 65: 357. 1928.

[3] Gunn, *Journ. of Phys.*, 46: 506. 1913.

[4] Starling, "Human Physiology," p. 758. Philadelphia. 1926.

lunar valves and in this position is firmly tied. The clamp on the rubber tube is then completely opened. The filter tube is raised to enclose the heart and its top closed with moist cotton.

For perfusion simply to maintain the heart-beat as long as possible we have had the greatest success with Locke's fluid as given by Baylis,[5] with the difference that it was buffered with 100 mg of sodium bicarbonate and 50 mg of primary sodium phosphate per liter.

We have found that the size and shape of the cannula and the care with which it was tied in the proper position in the aorta were very important in the success of the experiment. The cannula must be sufficiently large to permit the fluid expelled by the beating heart to flow rapidly back through it. The tip of the cannula must be above the semi-lunar valves so that at the beginning of the beat the full pressure of the perfusion fluid is not exerted on the wall of the ventricle. A complete relaxation of the ventricles is necessary to insure a proper perfusion of the coronary vessels. This will not be possible if the cannula projects beyond the semi-lunar valves into the left ventricle and maintains a constant distention of the ventricle. Even when the cannula is correctly inserted a certain amount of fluid accumulates in the ventricles. This may come from leakage past the valves or from the Thebesian vessels. It is for the rapid release of the pressure of this fluid as the heart contracts that it is necessary to make the aperture of the perfusion cannula as large as possible. If, in spite of all precautions, a distention of the ventricle does develop during the experiment it may be relieved by inserting a cannula through the pulmonary vein and the mitral valves into the ventricle. It is obviously necessary to be certain that the tip of the perfusion cannula does not project so far into the aorta that its wall occludes the opening into the coronary arteries.

As the perfusion continues, the pressure in the gasometer is maintained at a constant level by admitting oxygen from the tank as necessary. Oxygen is permitted to bubble slowly through the perfusion fluid by adjusting the level of the funnel of the trap. If the fluid in the flask becomes exhausted it is merely necessary to fill another flask and replace the one originally used.

J. W. WILSON
J. M. DARLINGTON
BROWN UNIVERSITY

# SPECIAL ARTICLES

## THE PERIHELION OF MERCURY

THE law of Newton states that every particle of matter in the universe attracts every other particle with a force that varies directly as the product of the masses and inversely as the square of the distance. For two bodies this law gives accurate results (a), as they are very far apart and (b), as their dimensions are small in relation to the distance between them but, when two bodies of substantial size are near together and when a small body is near to a large one, there is ground for doubting its precision.

Let the formula for the force of gravitation F, be written,

$$F = G\frac{M_1}{d} \times \frac{M_2}{d}$$

G being the gravitational constant, $M_1$ and $M_2$ the individual masses of two bodies and $d$ the distance between their centers. From this it may be inferred that gravitation is the resultant of two forces each varying directly as the mass which produces it and inversely as the distance from the other. These forces are directed toward each other. Each acts at the distance $d$ from the other and their product is the resultant which is called Gravitation.

If the above proposition be true, then the actual attraction between two spheres can not be the same as that which is computed on the supposition that the entire mass of each is concentrated at its center as on the basis of the inverse square.

In Fig. 1, $M_1$ and $M_2$ are homogeneous spheres, $M_2$ being very small, and $M_1M_2 = d$. The inner circle

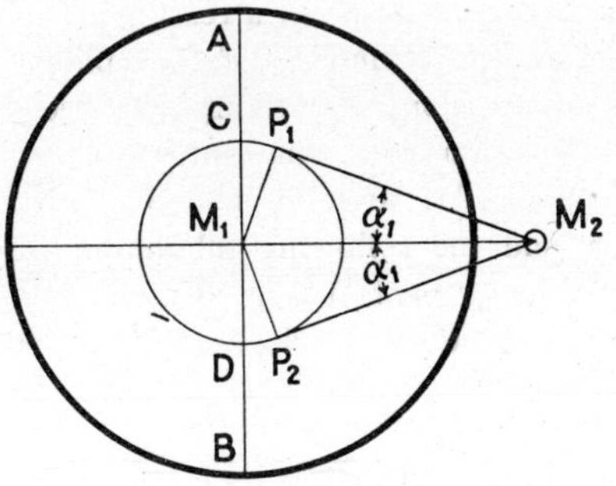


FIG. 1

$CP_1P_2$ DC is drawn so that $M_1C = 0.4244 M_1A$ and it is, therefore, the locus of the centers of gravity of all the halves of the circle AB which is a diametral section of $M_1$; $M_2P_1$ and $M_2P_2$ are tangents to this circle and $P_1$ and $P_2$ are the points at which the resultant attractions on $M_2$ of the upper and lower semi-circles of $M_1$ may be considered as concentrated. The value of the attraction of each of the semi-circles, if $a$ rep-

[5] Baylis, "Principles of General Physiology," p. 211. London. 1927.

resent its area, is proportional to $a \cos\alpha_1$, where $\alpha_1$ is the angle $P_1M_2M_1$ and, as the attraction varies inversely with the distance, the attractive force exerted by each semi-circle on $M_2$ is, if $g$ is a constant and since $P_1M_2$, the distance at which this force acts is $d \cos\alpha_1$,

$$\frac{\text{ga} \cos\alpha_1}{\text{d} \cos\alpha_1} = \frac{\text{ga}}{\text{d}}$$

The attractive force of the upper semi-circle is exerted on $M_2$ in the direction $M_2P_1$ and its component along $M_2M_1$ is ga $\cos\alpha_1/d$ while, for the entire circle, the attraction is $g\ 2a \cos\alpha_1/d = g\ A \cos\alpha_1/d$. If now, the circle AB is rotated through 180° it will generate the sphere AB and what is true for each of its sections will be true for its mass. The attraction of $M_1$ for $M_2$ therefore is, $gM_1\cos\alpha_1/d$ and, in an exactly similar manner, the attraction of $M_2$ for $M_1$ is $gM_2\cos\alpha_2/d$. The total force of attraction F, which is that of Gravitation, between the two spheres is, then, the product of the individual forces, thus,

$$F = \frac{g\, M_1 \cos\alpha_1}{d} \times \frac{g\, M_2 \cos\alpha_2}{d} = g^2 \frac{M_1 \cos\alpha_1 \times M_2 \cos\alpha_2}{d^2} \quad (1)$$

and this, when G is written for $g^2$, is an advanced statement of the law of gravitation.

The relative acceleration $f$ of the spheres $M_1$ and $M_2$ therefore is,

$$f = G \frac{M_1 \cos\alpha_1 + M_2 \cos\alpha_2}{d^2} \quad (2)$$

In nearly all cases $\cos\alpha_1$ and $\cos\alpha_2$ are so close to unity that no practical difference between the above formula and that of Newton can be detected. However, the value of $\cos\alpha$ for the Sun, at the distance of Mercury, is such as to point a reason for the observed "advance" of the perihelion of that planet. To this end the acceleration of Mercury has been computed for three positions with the center of gravity of the Sun's semi-circular area at 0.28 of its radius from its center and the following tabulation presents the values of the exponent of $d$ in Newton's law which are necessary to produce the accelerations given by formula (2) above.

| Position of Mercury | Necessary exponent of $d$ in Newton's Law |
|---|---|
| Aphelion | 2.00000013 |
| Mean | 2.00000019 |
| Perihelion | 2.00000031 |

Allowing for the longer time spent by Mercury in the outer portion of its orbit, the mean value of the exponent of $d$ necessary to conform the law of Newton with formula (2) is 2.000000192 and this is comparable with the value of 2.000000161 which was suggested[1] in order to account for the then known advance of 42″ per century in the position of the perihelion point. Now, if the exponent 2.000000161 accounts for an advance of 42″, then the exponent 2.000000192 represents an advance of 50.″1 per century, which value compares with the recent determination[2] by Morgan of 50.″9.

The quantitative agreement which has been shown between the observed and the computed values for the advance of Mercury's perihelion is of especial interest and the principles on which this finding is based extend into many fields. The placing of the center of gravity of the sun's semi-circular section at the 0.28 point of its radius is merely a recognition that the density of the sun increases toward its center. In a homogeneous sun this ratio would be 0.4244.

A detailed outline of the studies on which the conclusions herein presented are founded is being prepared.

THADDEUS MERRIMAN
NEW YORK CITY
December 14, 1932

## SOME FACTORS INFLUENCING THE SUSCEPTIBILITY OF ALBINO RATS TO INJECTIONS OF SODIUM AMYTAL[1]

IN an earlier account[2] of the use of sodium amytal (Lilly) as an anesthetic for albino rats a sex difference in the reaction to the drug was noted. The concentration of the solution in which the anesthetic was given was found to have a marked effect upon its efficacy. These two facts have been investigated in an attempt to analyze further the action of the anesthetic.

A record has been kept of the amount of sodium amytal in a 10 per cent. solution required to produce anesthesia in male animals of weights ranging between thirty and four hundred grams. These animals have been anesthetized in experiments of various types during the past year and a half. From these individual records Fig. 1 has been composed. A total of over one thousand observations have been made on animals of varying weights.

In the graph the weight of the animals has been plotted against the milligrams of sodium amytal in a 10 per cent. solution necessary to produce a deep anesthesia from which the animal will recover. This extends the observations on the dosage required for

1 Simon Newcomb, article, "Gravitation." Encyclopaedia Britannica, 9th Edition.

2 H. R. Morgan, *Jour. Optical Society of America*, Vol. 20, p. 228.

1 The sodium amytal used in these experiments was generously furnished by Eli Lilly and Company.

2 J. S. Nicholas and D. H. Barron, *Jour. of Pharmacol. and Exper. Therapeut.*, 46: pp. 125–130, 1932.

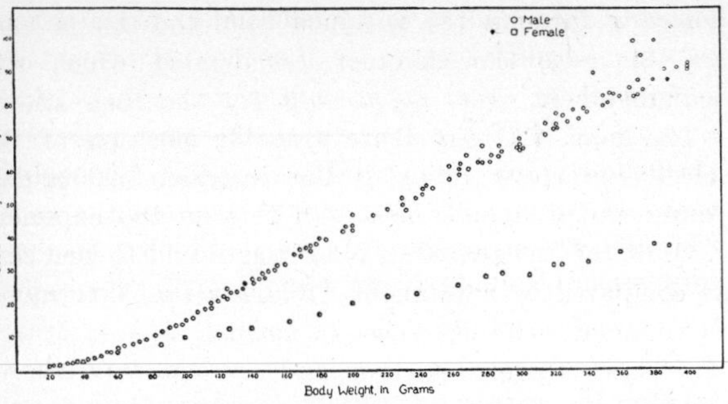


Fig. 1. A graph illustrating the relation between the body weights of albino rats and the amount of sodium amytal in milligrams necessary to produce deep anesthesia.

male rats which in a previous report were obtained only upon males ranging between one hundred and twenty-five and two hundred and fifty grams in weight. For comparison, the dosage for females of a corresponding range of weights has also been plotted. The graph therefore demonstrates the sex difference in the reaction to sodium amytal and defines clearly the weight at which this sex difference appears.

To determine whether or not the greater resistance of the male rats was to be associated with the presence of the gonads, ten adult male rats weighing about one hundred and seventy-five grams each were castrated. Six weeks later these animals were weighed and given the male dose normal for their weight. None of the animals survived. A second group of five adult animals about two hundreds grams in weight were castrated and anesthetized at the end of six weeks. These animals were more resistant to sodium amytal than females but were markedly less resistant than normal males.

A third series of ten young males about thirty grams each were castrated. Each week following castration the animals were anesthetized. The normal male dose for their weight was invariably necessary to produce deep anesthesia. These animals were castrated before they had developed the sex difference in their reaction to sodium amytal; nevertheless they retained the resistance normal to uncastrated males throughout their growth and development. The resistance of males castrated before the sex difference has appeared, therefore, is unaltered, but males castrated when adults become definitely more susceptible.

Although not more than suggestive, it is interesting to note that the weight at which the sex difference appears—between fifty and sixty grams—is also the weight at which the differential growth relation of both the hypophysis and the suprarenals first appear between the males and females.[3] The female rat has the heavier hypophysis and suprarenal glands.

The effect of the dilution of the solution of sodium amytal with which anesthesia is produced has been discussed earlier. The animals were much more resistant to equal quantities of the drug if administered in more dilute solutions. This fact suggested that injections of mammalian Ringer's into the blood stream of an over-anesthetized animal might reduce the effectiveness of the original dose and aid in the recovery of the animal.

Both males and females were injected with one and a half times the normal dose for their weight. After the animal was well under the anesthetic the femoral vein was exposed and eight cubic centimeters of mammalian Ringer's—either warm or cold—was injected into the blood stream. The controls were anesthetized in the same way but were not injected with Ringer's. All the animals that received the injection of Ringer's solution (ten) recovered from the anesthetic. The ten control animals, however, all died from respiratory failure typical of over-anesthetized animals. This method of reducing the effectiveness of the drug by injections of Ringer's into the blood stream has proved of value in saving an occasional animal which is more susceptible to sodium amytal than the normal.

These facts appear to be directly related to the action of sodium amytal, for rats demonstrate no sex difference to nembutal. The dose for both males and females is the same as the male dose of sodium amytal in a ten per cent. solution. The injection of Ringer's into the blood stream of rats over-anesthetized with nembutal is not effective.

The injection and dilution experiments indicate that resistance to sodium amytal is in some way related to the water metabolism of the animal. This is further supported by the correlation between the time of the development of the sex difference in rats and the differential growth rate of the hypophysis and the suprarenal glands. The castration experiments then imply that in the adult the testes influence the water metabolism control, although when removed before this function is developed, other factors within the body compensate for their loss.

Donald H. Barron
Osborn Zoological Laboratory
Yale University

## SIBLING RESEMBLANCE AND ITS RELATION TO AGE INTERVAL

Stocks[1] has recently published an investigation in which the resemblance of siblings in a number of

[3] H. H. Donaldson, "The Rat: Data and Reference Tables." Memoirs of the Wistar Institute of Anat. and Biol., No. 6, Philadelphia, pp. 469, 1924.

[1] Percy Stocks, "A Biometric Investigation of Twins and Their Brothers and Sisters," *Annals of Eugenics*, 4: 49–108. 1930.

physical and physiological traits has been examined to determine whether the interval between births of children of the same parents is related to degrees of resemblance. His results furnish no definite evidence that the interval between births has any influence on degree of resemblance in the traits studied. To date there has been published no direct attack of a similar nature upon the question of resemblance in mental traits.

For the past two years the author has been collecting data from intelligence tests administered to two or more members of a family with the idea of trying to reveal any relationship existing between age interval and degree of resemblance of siblings in mental capacity (within the limits to which paper and pencil tests measure mental capacity). The present results are based on the records of 1,012 pairs of native-born white siblings, representing 614 families and having age differences ranging between one and eleven years. Three groups, including superior, average and inferior ability, respectively, were obtained by drawing upon schools enrolling children from widely different socio-economic strata.

In all cases the two members of a pair were tested with the same tests and under similar conditions, in so far as this was possible. For example, children from any one school were all tested when they had progressed to a given grade level, so that the average age at test was approximately equal for the older and younger members of all pairs.

The principal method of analysis employed to discover any possible relationship existing between age interval and difference in intelligence was that of product-moment correlation. For each group of data this relationship was computed by entering the difference of a pair in I. Q. on the x axis, and their difference in age on the y axis. The obtained correlations, as will be seen from Table 1, indicate no tendency for children within a family, far apart in age, to resemble each other less than children born near together.

TABLE 1

RELATION BETWEEN I. Q. DIFFERENCE AND AGE INTERVAL OF SIBLINGS

X = I. Q. difference
Y = Age difference in months

| Group | $r_{xy}$ | P.E.* | $M_x$ | $M_y$ | $\sigma_x$ | $\sigma_y$ | N* |
|---|---|---|---|---|---|---|---|
| I | −.001 | .036 | 10.59 | 41.04 | 7.83 | 23.70 | 359 |
| II | −.006 | .049 | 11.55 | 32.34 | 8.04 | 15.78 | 188 |
| III | +.058 | .032 | 10.86 | 43.20 | 8.10 | 25.26 | 465 |

* The values of N given here, and employed in computing the values of P. E. here reported, are in each case the number of pairs, and, since some individuals entered more than one pair, are greater than the actual number of cases involved. These P. E. values are therefore slightly below the true probable errors.

The data of Group I are probably most free from selective factors favoring the inclusion of bright young and dull older sibs. In this group the mean I. Q. of the 359 paired as older was found to be 117.6 as compared to a mean of 118.0 for the 359 paired as younger. The difference in mean I. Q. (.4) is less than its own probable error, and gives no evidence of superiority of later over earlier born members of a family. It may also be pointed out that the degree of sibling resemblance has been computed for each group of data. This has been done by entering the I. Q. of the older member of each pair on the x axis, and the I. Q. of the younger on the y axis. The resulting values for r were .49, .52 and .34, respectively. The first two of these are probably fairly accurate measures of the degree of sibling resemblance in representative groups; the latter is lower than the true degree of resemblance because of a marked restriction of range in the data employed.

F. H. FINCH

UNIVERSITY OF MINNESOTA

## BOOKS RECEIVED

FALK, I. S., C. RUFUS ROREM and MARTHA D. RING. *The Costs of Medical Care.* Pp. xviii + 623. University of Chicago Press. $4.00.

FALK, I. S., MARGARET C. KLEM and NATHAN SINAI. *The Incidence of Illness and the Receipt and Costs of Medical Care Among Representative Family Groups.* Pp. xii + 327. University of Chicago Press. $3.00.

KLÜVER, HEINRICH. *Behavior Mechanisms in Monkeys.* Pp. xvii + 387. 52 figures. University of Chicago Press. $4.00.

PLANCK, MAX. *Introduction to Theoretical Physics.* Translated by Henry L. Brose. Vol. I: *General Mechanics.* Pp. vii + 272. $2.50. Vol. II: *The Mechanics of Deformable Bodies.* Pp. 234. $2.50. Vol. III: *Theory of Electricity and Magnetism.* Pp. viii + 247. $2.50. Vol. IV: *Theory of Light.* Pp. vi + 213. $2.50. Vol. V: *Theory of Heat.* Pp. viii + 301. $2.75. Macmillan.

REED, LOUIS. *The Ability to Pay for Medical Care.* Pp. x + 107. University of Chicago Press. $2.00.

ARKELL, W. J. *The Jurassic System in Great Britain.* Pp. xii + 681. 97 figures. 41 plates. Oxford University Press. $7.75.

COLLINS, A. FREDERICK. *Experimental Optics.* Pp. xiv + 318. 174 figures. Appleton. $2.00.

MCALPINE, ROY K. and BYRON A. SOULE. *Qualitative Chemical Analysis.* Pp. xii + 697. Van Nostrand. $4.50.

MOORE, R. L. *Foundations of Point Set Theory.* Colloquium Publications, Vol. XII. Pp. vii + 487. American Mathematical Society.

RITT, JOSEPH F. *Differential Equations from the Algebraic Standpoint.* Pp. x + 173. American Mathematical Society.

STONE, MARSHALL H. *Linear Transformations in Hilbert Space and Their Applications to Analysis.* Pp. viii + 623. American Mathematical Society.

# SCIENCE

VOL. 77 FRIDAY, APRIL 21, 1933 No. 1999

*The American Association for the Advancement of Science:*

*Solar Eclipse Problems:* DR. J. H. MOORE ... 375

*Obituary:*

*Achilles de Khotinsky:* DR. PAUL E. KLOPSTEG. *Recent Deaths* ... 382

*Scientific Events:*

*The Eightieth Anniversary of the Founding of the California Academy of Sciences; The New Commissioner of Indian Affairs; In Honor of Charles E. Munroe; The Award of the Willard Gibbs Medal to Dr. Richard Willstaetter* ... 383

*Scientific Notes and News* ... 386

*Discussion:*

*Zoological Nomenclature:* DR. J. BROOKES KNIGHT. *The Involved Genetics of Fish:* PROFESSOR A. BRAZIER HOWELL. *Note on the Life-cycle of Ectocarpus siliculosus Dillw.:* GEORGE F. PAPENFUSS. *On the Scientific Name of the Webbing Clothes Moth:* PROFESSOR GLENN W. HERRICK and DR. GRACE H. GRISWOLD. *Human Necrobacillosis:* DR. FREDERICK W. SHAW ... 389

*Scientific Apparatus and Laboratory Methods:*

*A Method and the Apparatus for the Study of Permeability of Gases through the Bird's Eggshell:* DR. ALEXIS L. ROMANOFF. *A Method for the Preparation of Fossils:* DR. G. ARTHUR COOPER 393

*Special Articles:*

*The Utilization of Adsorbed Ions by Plants:* DR. HANS JENNY and E. W. COWAN. *Observations on Early Developmental Processes in the Living Egg of Drosophila:* GEORGE P. CHILD and PROFESSOR RUTH B. HOWLAND ... 394

*Science News* ... 6

SCIENCE: A Weekly Journal devoted to the Advancement of Science, edited by J. MCKEEN CATTELL and published every Friday by

THE SCIENCE PRESS

New York City: Grand Central Terminal

Lancaster, Pa. Garrison, N. Y.

Annual Subscription, $6.00 Single Copies, 15 Cts.

SCIENCE is the official organ of the American Association for the Advancement of Science. Information regarding membership in the Association may be secured from the office of the permanent secretary, in the Smithsonian Institution Building, Washington, D. C.

# SOLAR ECLIPSE PROBLEMS[1]

By Dr. J. H. MOORE

ASTRONOMER IN THE LICK OBSERVATORY

A TOTAL solar eclipse affords an opportunity to study the faint outer portions of the sun, invisible under ordinary conditions. Several serious attempts have been made to observe the solar corona without an eclipse, and although partial success has recently attended certain observations of this character we still are confined to the fleeting moments of totality for a study of its detailed structure. Moreover, at the time of a solar eclipse we are able to investigate most efficiently the spectrum of the chromosphere, and from such studies to obtain important information, not only concerning the distribution of the elements within the sun's atmosphere, but also of the physical conditions that obtain there. These two fields of research in solar physics may be regarded as preeminent among those associated with a total eclipse of the sun, and it is to certain of the problems related to the constitution of the chromosphere and the corona that I wish to direct your attention, stressing the observational more than the theoretical aspect.

[1] Address of the retiring vice-president and chairman of Section D—Astronomy, American Association for the Advancement of Science, Atlantic City, December, 1932.

### THE CHROMOSPHERE

Immediately preceding and following totality when the glaring photosphere is hidden behind the moon's limb, the outer portion of the solar atmosphere appears as a narrow brilliant scarlet-colored crescent. To this envelope of the sun, Lockyer gave the name of chromosphere. Its spectrum was first observed at the eclipse of 1870 by Young, who found it to consist of bright lines on a dark background, which flash out as the photosphere is hidden, and remain for a few seconds, until covered by the advancing moon. This "flash spectrum" was regarded by Young as a reversal of the Fraunhofer lines whose origin was ascribed to the "reversing layer," a shell of comparatively shallow depth, as shown by the brief duration of the flash.

Although numerous attempts were made to observe the spectrum of the chromosphere visually at succeeding eclipses, it was not until 1893 that the first photographs of the flash spectrum were secured by Fowler in West Africa and by Shackleton in Brazil. These observers employed prismatic cameras, a type of instrument admirably adapted to this particular problem, since the chromospheric crescent is so narrow that the slit of the spectrograph may be dispensed with. The spectrum recorded on the photographic plate consists of monochromatic images of the crescent in the different wave-lengths emitted by the chromosphere. Spectrographs of this form have generally been used in photographing the spectrum of the chromosphere at subsequent eclipses. Prism systems, of one, two or three prisms, or plane gratings, have been employed with camera lenses of various focal lengths, depending upon the region to be studied and the dispersion desired. Some observers have obtained beautiful flash spectra with the concave grating spectrograph in its slitless form. Photographs made in quick succession with an instrument of this type will record the changing spectrum at the sun's limb, Fraunhofer, flash and prominence spectra.

At the moment when the last vestige of the photosphere has disappeared the dark lines of the ordinary solar spectrum are replaced by the bright lines of the chromosphere, the lengths of the arcs being obviously an indication of the heights to which the various emissions can be traced. The majority of the lines are found at low levels and disappear at heights of only a few hundred kilometers, while a few, like those of helium, hydrogen and ionized calcium, ascend to heights of from 7,500 to 14,000 km.

While the procedure of recording the chromospheric spectrum, outlined above, appears to be quite simple, in practise it encounters certain difficulties. Aside from those common to most eclipse observations of adjusting and operating apparatus under trying conditions, there is the serious one of making the exposure at the proper time to obtain the fainter lines, which are visible for only about a second. This difficulty is obviated by the method devised by Campbell, in which the changing spectrum in a short central section of the crescent is recorded on a moving plate. The procedure consists in placing immediately in front of the plate a narrow slit parallel to the length of the spectrum, so that only a very short section of the crescent falls upon the sensitive film. The plate is then moved at a uniform rate behind the slit in a direction perpendicular to its length. By starting the exposure 25 or 30 seconds before second or third contact and continuing it for as many seconds after, a continuous record is obtained of the changing spectrum at the sun's limb from the Fraunhofer to the emission lines. The method was successfully employed by Campbell at the eclipses of 1898, 1900, 1905 and 1908. One of the chief difficulties he encountered with it was in obtaining a uniform motion of the photographic plate with the mechanical devices then available. Trouble from this source has been overcome at recent eclipses by driving the plate carriage by an electric motor of constant speed.

Spectrograms taken on the moving plate furnish a continuous record of the changes that take place in the spectral lines at only one point on the sun's limb as different levels of the solar atmosphere are covered or uncovered by the moon. On such photographs we note again the great heights shown by the lines of ionized calcium, hydrogen, helium, ionized strontium, the intermediate heights given by the lines of other atoms, generally in the ionized state, and the great number of the lines in the lower levels given for the most part by neutral atoms. One is impressed with the fact that while the spectrum of the chromosphere appears to be a reversal of the Fraunhofer spectrum, there are marked differences between the intensities of corresponding lines in the two spectra. The most pronounced dissimilarities are found in the enhanced lines or those that are given by ionized atoms, such lines being especially prominent in the chromosphere. Certain radiations appear in the flash spectrum that are not represented in the solar spectrum, while to some strong Fraunhofer lines there correspond only weak lines in the spectrum of the chromosphere. Most of these peculiarities that were once so puzzling, are now explained in a beautiful manner by the theory of ionization, first stated by Saha and developed in further detail by the contributions of Milne, Russell, R. H. Fowler, Eddington, and others.

Since the intensity of a spectral line depends upon the number of atoms acting in a given time to produce it, the relative number of atoms that are in the neutral and ionized states becomes a question of considerable importance in the interpretation of spectra. On the assumption that the general laws of thermodynamics apply equally well to electrons and molecules, Saha was able to calculate the degree of ionization that takes place in gases under different conditions of temperature and pressure. It was found that ionization is favored by increase in temperature or decrease in density of the gas, and that for different elements at the same temperature and pressure the degree of ionization is less for the one of greater ionization potential.

At the higher levels in the chromosphere the density must be much less than in those near its base, consequently the ionization is increased in spite of the somewhat lower temperature. The extension of the enhanced lines to heights greater than those of the neutral atom and the strength of these lines in the flash spectrum is thus seen to be the result of decreased density within the chromosphere. The familiar lines of calcium furnish an interesting illustration of the point in question. The ultimate line of the neutral atom, g, or λ 4227, extends to a height of about 5,000 kilometers, while the H and K lines given by the ionized atom are visible to a height of 14,000 kilometers. Above 5,000 kilometers practically all the calcium atoms are ionized, leaving none to emit the lines of the neutral atoms, while the lines of the ionized atom appear as far up as the level where the chromosphere thins out entirely. Similar differences are found between the enhanced lines and those of the neutral atoms of strontium, scandium, titanium and other elements.

One might expect that the relative heights of the lines would correspond to the atomic weights of the elements, the greater heights being associated with elements of lower atomic weights. Calcium, however, with an atomic weight nearly twice that of sodium, can be traced to a greater height than either hydrogen or helium. This puzzling fact may be explained as the selective effect of radiation pressure. Above 1,500 km the sodium atoms are completely ionized, and the lines of ionized sodium lie in the far ultraviolet, where they are not observable. Ionized calcium, on the other hand, has strong ultimate lines in the visible region and so ascends to great heights.

Not only do the lines of greatest intesity, in general, reach the highest levels, but it is found that for any element the lines of greatest intensity and extending to the greatest heights in the chromosphere arise from multiplets of the lowest excitation potential. An interesting example of the relation of intensity and excitation potential is shown by the two pairs of Fe lines given by the neutral atom at λλ 3887.0 and 3886.3, and λλ 3878.0 and 3878.6. Though of comparable intensity in the sun, the second line of each pair is stronger in the flash, and arises from the lowest energy level in the atom, while the first ones come from the next higher level, with an excitation potential greater by only one volt.

This qualitative study of flash spectra has called attention to the fact that the heights to which the individual lines can be traced depends largely upon their intensities, which in turn are functions of abundance, atomic weight, ionization potential, excitation potential, etc.

A quantitative investigation of such spectrograms involves the determination of the wave-lengths, intensities and heights of the various spectral lines and is obviously a work of considerable magnitude. Studies of this character have been made by several investigators. Two of these have been published within the last two years, the one by S. A. Mitchell and the other by D. H. Menzel. Since they are the most extensive and thorough investigations of the flash spectrum that have been made, they merit our special attention at this time.

Mitchell's discussion is based largely upon his flash spectra obtained at the eclipses of 1905, 1925 and 1930, and includes the region from λ 3066 to λ 7065. His spectra were taken on a stationary plate, with a concave-grating spectrograph used in its slitless form. Menzel's results were derived from the Lick spectrograms taken without slit, the dispersion being given by prisms of flint or ultra-violet glass. These were supplemented by data obtained from spectra secured at the 1905 eclipse on fixed plates. The region of spectrum investigated by him was from λ 3229 to λ 5328.

Intensities of the chromospheric lines were estimated on the Rowland scale and for these the two observers are in satisfactory agreement. Their values for the relative heights of the high and low level lines, however, exhibit marked disagreement. Several explanations for this have been offered. The heights of the chromospheric vapors are derived from the angular length of the cusps on the stationary plate, while on the moving plate these heights are measured from a zero level somewhat arbitrarily chosen as the point where the continuous background seems to fade out. Moreover, these heights would be expected to be different, since they depend in part upon the speed of the spectrograph and of the photographic plate used. Differences arising from the choice of zero level, or from the speed of the recording apparatus, should not affect materially the relative heights of high and low level lines. The presence of a valley or mountain on the moon at the point of contact or near the ends of the cusps may readily give erroneous values of relative heights determined on the stationary plate, while lack of uniformity in the motion of the moving plate will produce similar errors. In order to check the uniformity in motion of the plate the second-breaks of a chronometer have been recorded on spectrograms secured by the method of the moving plate at recent eclipses. This is not the place to discuss the relative merits of the two methods of observing the flash spectrum; each has its own advantages and disadvantages. The record obtained by the one method offers a valuable check upon that of the other, and both were used by the Lick Observatory expedition at the eclipse of last August, as well as in 1905.

From the preceding discussion it will be evident that great caution should be exercised in drawing conclusions concerning apparent variations in the depth of the chromosphere from observations made at different eclipses. Both Mitchell and Menzel have found evidence of such changes in chromospheric structure. On Mitchell's spectrograms of the 1905 and 1925 eclipses, taken with the same instrument, the lines of intermediate level are noticeably higher in 1925 than 1905, although no systematic difference is shown for the high level lines. Menzel's heights for the 1908 eclipse are uniformly lower than those derived from the 1905 plate. After careful consideration of all possible contributory factors, he is led to the conclusion that his observations indicate a real difference of height in the chromosphere at the two dates. In each case the greater heights were obtained at the time of greater solar activity, which is in harmony with what we should be led to expect from our present views of the structure of the chromosphere. More data, however, are needed before a variation of the character suggested can be considered as established.

Data of intensities and heights determined from flash spectra enable us to derive the distribution of the atoms at different levels, or the density gradient in the chromosphere. There are two independent methods by which this may be accomplished: (1) from the line intensities measured at different levels; (2) from the relation of the theoretical intensities of the members of multiplets to the heights of the corresponding lines. Menzel determined the relative intensities at six different levels in the chromospheric spectrum from microphotometer measures of the 1905 spectrogram. Laboring under the severe handicap of not having the characteristics of his plate defined by standard squares, he was forced to check his material from the interagreement of the data for different lines. The method of employing intensities at different heights along the spectral line, although apparently the most direct one for determining the density distribution, is complicated by the fact that the energy at a given level is the integrated light of this and the higher levels. It also becomes necessary to correct the observed intensity for the effect of self-reversal.

Both Mitchell and Menzel have used the second method of deriving the density gradient in the chromosphere up to a height of 2,500 km. The intensities of the members of a multiplet may be computed from the formulae relating the transition probabilities to the energy emitted by the different lines. It is then possible to derive a simple expression for the number of atoms per unit volume that are involved in the emission of a line of given intensity. From a knowledge of the heights to which the different lines of the multiplet extend in the chromosphere and the relative number of atoms concerned in the production of the lines, the relative concentration of the atoms at different levels may readily be obtained. In Menzel's discussion, all elements were grouped together, while Mitchell discussed the elements separately. Their results are in good agreement and show that the density gradient for the lower chromosphere is much less than would be expected in an isothermal atmosphere. It corresponds closely to that which would be given by an atmosphere of hydrogen in gravitational equilibrium, while at higher levels the chromosphere is even more distended. It is of interest to note in this connection that Menzel found the electron pressure at the base of the chromosphere to be about $10^{-7}$ atmospheres or about 500 times smaller than Russell's value for the pressure at the base of the reversing layer.

One of the most important fields of spectroscopic investigation is the determination of the energy emitted by a spectral line or the absolute intensity of the line. The problem on the experimental side is an extremely difficult one. Some progress, however, has been made by Unsöld and others for the strong resonance lines in the solar spectrum. Pannekoek and Minneart have attempted a similar investigation for the lines of the flash spectrum, utilizing for this purpose their high dispersion spectrograms secured at the eclipse of 1927. After calibration of the spectra through comparison with standard sources and elimination of the effects of instrumental and atmospheric absorption they were able to determine the absolute surface intensity of the chromosphere. The observed intensities for lines in well-known multiplets were compared with their theoretical intensities and found to increase more slowly than the latter. They interpret this as indicating an appreciable amount of self-absorption in the chromospheric layer when viewed tangentially. The density gradient for hydrogen deduced by them shows characteristics similar to those noted above.

The intensity of a spectral line, whether emission or absorption, is a function of the abundance of the element producing it. For an assembly of atoms in thermodynamic equilibrium the relation may be easily derived. Russell has, after making allowance for departure from thermodynamic equilibrium, utilized this relation in a most skilful investigation of the abundance of the various elements in the solar atmosphere, on the basis of the lines in the Fraunhofer spectrum. Since the intensities in the solar spectrum are estimated on an arbitrary scale, that of Rowland, it is necessary to reduce these to the scale based on theoretical intensities, before they can be used for determining the relative number of atoms engaged in the production of different lines. The calibration of Rowland's scale was obtained by comparison of the estimated and theoretical intensities of multiplets. Following Russell's procedure, both Mitchell and

Menzel have determined the abundance of the various elements in the chromosphere. The results show that for all the elements investigated, there appears to be little difference, except for hydrogen, between the relative abundance derived from Fraunhofer and flash spectra. Hydrogen seems to be considerably more abundant in the chromosphere than in the reversing layer.

By plotting the ratio of the number of atoms giving rise to multiplets in the reversing layer and chromosphere against the excitation potential of these lines Menzel finds evidence that the number of highly excited atoms in the chromosphere is greater than that predicted by the Boltzmann law. This excess, which increases with the excitation potential, is closely allied with the effect found by Russell and Adams from stellar spectra and generally known as the deviation of stellar atmospheres from thermodynamic equilibrium. In the chromosphere, however, it seems to be greatly intensified.

Determination of the temperature gradient in the chromosphere from the intensities and heights of the flash lines meets with certain difficulties, chiefly for the reason that the procedure of referring the observed intensities to the theoretical ones automatically corrects for possible temperature gradient. The observations afford some evidence that the mean temperature of the chromosphere is about 1,000 degrees lower than that of the reversing layer, and that the temperature gradient is low.

It appears then that the observed chromosphere lies above the layers that contribute the major portion of the absorption in the wings of the Fraunhofer lines, and that the chromospheric absorption accounts only for the central dark cores of some of the strongest lines. To this extent alone is the chromosphere the seat of Fraunhofer absorption.

The need for more observations of the flash spectrum is apparent. Spectrograms should be secured with both stationary and moving plates with as high dispersion as feasible and should be provided with photometric standards to permit of accurate calibration. The region of the infra-red is still a virgin field. The study of prominence spectra is also an important and closely related field of investigation which has been cultivated but slightly. A further investigation of the relation of the structure of the chromosphere to the cycle of solar activity is worthy of attention. Advantage should be taken of the excellent opportunity for securing spectrograms of the flash at a partial eclipse.

On the theoretical side important contributions to the problem of the structure of the chromosphere have been made by a number of investigators in an attempt to explain the small density gradient and the great heights to which the chromosphere extends. Milne has developel a beautiful theory of the equilibrium of an atmosphere of ionized calcium atoms supported by radiation pressure. It accounts for the high levels at which ionized calcium is found, and certain other phenomena of the chromosphere, but does not give the observed density gradient or emission of sufficient intensity. Moreover a chromosphere of the quiescent type postulated by the theory does not exist. McCrea and Rosseland have called attention to the effect of turbulence in the sun's atmosphere as an efficient aid in the support of the chromosphere. Pannekoek has shown that the electrons in an atmosphere, owing to their small atomic weight, would rise to great heights if they were not kept down by the attraction of the positively charged ions. This attraction, on the other hand, aids in keeping the ionized atoms at high levels. Menzel has made a careful discussion of the various theories and concludes that an extension of McCrea's theory to include the effects of self-reversal and Pannekoek's and Stewart's theories of electrostatic levitation gives a fair representation of the observed density gradient in the chromosphere and of the general featurs of the flash spectrum.

### THE CORONA

From the brief review of the present status of certain problems relating to the structure of the chromosphere, it will be seen that real progress has been made toward a solution of at least a few of them. The situation with reference to the problems of the corona is less encouraging. Important facts concerning it have been established, but they are more or less isolated and in general their relations to each other are unknown. The paucity of results obtained thus far is due, primarily, to the unique condition that the opportunities for observing the corona are few and the time available for its study, at any one eclipse, is at best of but a few minutes' duration. Fortunate indeed would be the observer who could obtain an hour of totality with clear skies, in his entire lifetime.

Photography of the corona has comprised a part of the work of most expeditions that have observed total eclipses of the past fifty years. One of the most extensive series of coronal photographs is that obtained by eclipse expeditions of the Lick Observatory. These photographs were secured with cameras of various focal lengths, but since 1892 the more important observations of this character have been made with a form of photographic telescope designed by J. M. Schaeberle and used by him at that time in Chile. In this instrument the lens, of 5 inches aperture, remains stationary and the diurnal travel of the sun is allowed for by moving the photographic plate in the focal plane of the lens. The photographs secured with it have generally been of excellent quality and reveal the intricate detail of structure, as well as the faint outer portions of the corona. The obvious advantages of large scale photographs of the corona have led other observers to employ cameras of even greater focal lengths.

At the eclipse of August 31, 1932, the responsibility for this part of the Lick Observatory program was undertaken by W. H. Wright. After careful consideration of the most advantageous form of instrument for coronal photography, he abandoned the 40-foot camera of the Schaeberle type for two photographic telescopes of 5 inches aperture and 15 feet focal length, rigidly mounted on a polar axis. The lenses are of excellent quality and are estimated to have about five times the speed of the 40-foot camera. This arrangement proved to be a very fortunate one at an eclipse where clouds were present, since it was possible to secure a greater number of photographs and to obtain a few of exceptionally long effective exposures. The superior quality of Wright's photographs fully supports the wisdom of his choice of instruments. When enlarged to the scale of those taken with the 40-foot camera they are equal, if not superior, in the excellence of their definition and in the delineation of coronal detail.

Photographs of the corona secured in this manner, although subject to the limitations of a composite picture of structural detail at different positions along the line of sight, afford a basis for study of the general form and structure of the corona.

It has long been known that the shape of the corona near the time of maximum in the sun-spot cycle is different from that near minimum sun-spots. The type of corona associated with sun-spot maximum is approximately circular in form, while that near minimum is roughly rectangular with the polar brushes and wing-like extensions at lower latitudes in which the sun-spots and prominences are found. Ludendorff has devised a simple method of representing more precisely the form of the corona through the ellipticity of lines of equal intensity drawn on coronal photographs. Studies made by him in this way, of the coronas from thirteen eclipses secured at different phases in the sun-spot cycle, reveal a closer relation between the coronal shape and the actual number of spots visible for a few days preceding and following the date, than with the phase in the solar cycle. From a study of the coronas observed since 1860, Lockyer has found a close correlation between the shape of the corona and the position of the prominences, the maximum type occurring when prominences are near the polar region.

Examination of the individual details in the corona has revealed a connection in some cases between the long streamers and prominences visible at the limb. The structure of the inner corona is affected to a marked extent in the neighborhood of prominences. On the other hand, in only a few instances has it been possible to trace a direct connection between disturbed areas in the corona and large spots, or groups of spots, visible near the sun's limb. "Arches," "hoods" or "striated cones" are marked features of the inner and middle corona and are especially conspicuous near sun-spot maximum. In most instances, they are found to be erected over a large prominence and their forms suggest that the coronal materials are being driven outward from the prominence. That such is the case was found by Miller, who compared large scale photographs of the corona in 1918, taken at three separate stations, those of the Lick, Lowell and Sproul expeditions. Measures were made on three arches surrounding three conspicuous prominences. These gave fairly accordant results and indicated that in the twenty-six minutes that elapsed between the times of the Lick and Sproul photographs the arches had receded from the sun, with an average speed of about ten miles per second. Other attempts to detect motion of the coronal details on direct photographs taken at one station or by comparing those from widely separated stations have yielded little more than the result that, for the most part, the motion is small.

Progress in acquiring information about the spectrum of the corona has been painfully slow. The reasons are not far to seek. The coronal spectrum is very weak and the opportunities for observing it are few. The inner corona, up to about ten minutes of arc from the sun's limb, gives a continuous spectrum upon which are superimposed a number of bright lines extending to distances of from 5′ to 10′ from the sun. With the possible exception of the strong red line at $\lambda$ 6374, none of these have been observed in laboratory spectra or in those of the stars or nebulae. About 42 coronal emission lines in the region $\lambda$ 3164 to $\lambda$ 6800 have been reported by various observers but in the case of half of these it is extremely doubtful whether they are of coronal origin. The strongest lines are the well known one in the green, $\lambda$ 5303, and the ultra-violet line, $\lambda$ 3888. Next in intensity are $\lambda\lambda$ 6374, 3601, 4231, etc. The wave-lengths of but a few are known to a tenth of an angstrom, those of $\lambda$ 5303 and $\lambda$ 6374 being the most accurately determined.

Although the slit spectrograph is superior to the slitless form for wave-length determinations, spectrograms obtained with the latter instrument yield information of the greatest value concerning the distribution of intensities in the coronal emissions. The radiation in a single line is found to have very different intensities in different parts of the inner corona. The coronal ring exhibited by λ 5303, for example, is very faint in the polar regions and even at lower latitudes shows a marked variation in intensity. At the eclipse of 1918, this radiation was strengthened near the bases of the prominences and had its greatest intensity near the eruptive prominence at the southwest limb of the sun. Similar effects are to be seen in the green coronal ring obtained at the eclipse of last August, its greatest strength being shown near the two prominences on the west limb, while it was extremely faint over the whole east limb. On the same spectrogram the coronal ring in λ 6374 shows a more uniform distribution than λ 5303, although it, too, is weak in the polar regions and of greatest strength near the prominence on the southwest limb. In other details the distribution in the two radiations shows great dissimilarity. This difference, noted also by other observers, indicates that the two radiations can not take their origin in the the same atom in the same state of ionization.

Studies of the distribution of the intensities exhibited by the different coronal radiations enable us to group together lines of like behavior and should prove an important aid in the identification of the atom, or atoms, responsible for these emissions. Some of the stronger coronal lines have been so grouped by several observers, but there is a manifest disagreement in their opinions in this matter. At present, there seems to be reliable evidence that λ 3601 and λ 4086 belong together and that λ 5303 and λ 3388 form a pair, but the data for the others are not sufficient to permit their classification.

The great variation in intensity of the emission in different parts of the corona obviously limits the value of line intensities derived from spectra secured with a slit spectrograph and also accounts to a large extent for the failure to observe certain lines at one eclipse, which were obtained in good strength at another. To this cause may be ascribed some of the observed variation in the green line shown by comparing slit spectrograms of different eclipses, although there seems to be some evidence that this line is stronger near sun-spot maximum than near the minimum in the cycle. One of the most fruitful fields of coronal spectroscopy is undoubtedly that of the investigation of the forms, intensities and structural details in the coronal rings obtained with slitless spectrographs of fairly high dispersion.

Several observers have attempted to study the green line with an interferometer of the Fabry and Perot type, but without success. At the eclipse of last August, Shane made use of a slit spectrograph provided with an etalon of 2.5 mm separation and obtained very weak interference fringes in the green line. The observation is of importance not only because it explains the failure of previous attempts in which higher orders of interference were used, but also because it gives definite indication as to the width of the line. This, Shane estimates to be of the order of one third of an angstrom. The observed width of the line is probably due to the effect of turbulence in the inner corona.

A number of suggestions have been made as to the atom giving the coronal emissions. Pannekoek once suggested that they were due to doubly ionized calcium. Freeman, from coincidences in wave-length, attributed them to argon, while Rosenthal attempted to identify them with radiations of the helium atom in a special state. None of these identifications are entitled to any weight. Recently Hopfield has called attention to an unclassified line in the spectrum of oxygen, having wave-length 6374.29 A. and in close agreement with that of the red coronal line 6374.28 A. de Bruin has calculated three additional lines in the spectrum of neutral oxygen which he identifies with λ 5303, λ 6704 and λ 6775, but here again the identification appears to be open to serious criticism, so that the great mystery of the coronal lines still remains unsolved.

Many attempts have been made to study the corona without an eclipse, but until recently all have ended in failure. One of the most important advances in the investigation of the inner corona made in recent years is that due to Bernard Lyot, who, in full sunlight, obtained the red and green lines with his spectrograph and determined their wave-lengths. Moreover, with a spectroheliograph he photographed the inner corona in light of these two radiations. It is well known that the great obstacle standing in the way of observations of this character is that of the light scattered by the atmosphere and by the image-forming lens. By working at the observatory of Pic du Midi at an altitude of 2,870 meters, he reduced to a minimum the scattering of light by particles suspended in the air. A carefully ground simple lens was used to obtain the image, the light scattered by it being excluded through use of properly arranged diaphragms. Only by careful attention to the elimination of every possible source of scattered light in his instrument was success finally attained. The possibilities offered by this method to astronomers at mountain observatories for studies of coronal radiation, without the necessity of waiting for a total eclipse, are certainly alluring.

The spectrum of the corona beyond 8′ to 10′ from the sun's limb exhibits the Fraunhofer lines of the solar spectrum. The relative intensities of the coronal lines seem to be quite similar to those of the sun's spectrum. They have, however, a hazy appearance which is doubtless due to the fact that they record light scattered by different portions of the corona in the line of sight. That the Fraunhofer spectrum of the corona is caused by the scattering of sunlight by coronal material in a finely divided state is substantiated by the fact that the light of the corona is polarized. Measures by R. K. Young of the photographs obtained with polarigraphs by Lick observers show that the polarization is radial and that the percentage of polarized light increases rapidly from the sun's limb, reaching a maximum of 37 per cent. at a distance of 5′, and then diminishes slowly as the distance from the limb increases.

On the spectrograms secured in 1922, I measured the positions of the Fraunhofer lines in the coronal spectrum at points east and west of the sun and found that these were displaced toward the red with reference to the ordinary solar lines. The displacements, interpreted as a Doppler-effect, indicate radial motion of the coronal particles at points 20′ east and west of the sun's limb of about 12 or 15 miles per second, a speed of the same order as that found by Miller. These results are subject to considerable uncertainty on account of the character of the spectra measured. For this reason an attempt was made to repeat the observations at the eclipse of last August, with spectrographs especially designed for this particular problem. Unfortunately, the value of the spectrograms secured is somewhat impaired by the effect of scattered light from the clouds covering the sun during totality. Preliminary measures of these plates indicate the presence of small displacements in the Fraunhofer lines of the corona east and west of the sun, corresponding to a velocity of recession of about ten miles per second. At present we have no reliable information concerning the rotation of the corona.

Our knowledge of the total light of the corona and the distribution of its intensity with distance from the sun is still in an unsatisfactory state. The most reliable information we have at present, concerning the total brightness of the corona is to the effect that it is about 0.50 that of the full moon, although it probably varies with the cycle of solar activity. Observations of this character are beset with numerous difficulties but those made by recent investigators give evidence that many of them have been overcome. A most thorough investigation of the distribution of coronal intensity with distance from the sun was made by Bergstrand, who brought to this problem many years of experience in the methods of photographic photometry. He found that the intensity of coronal light in the photographic region varies inversely as the square of the distance from the sun's surface. Other observers have derived the law of variation to be according to the fourth, sixth, seventh and eighth powers.

Of coronal theories there is a sufficient number to permit of choice according to the particular phase of coronal studies in which one happens to be interested. Mechanical, electric, magnetic and other theories have been suggested, but in the present state of our knowledge with respect to the phenomena of the corona, it would not be profitable to give serious consideration to any of them. A corona composed of electrons and ions will account for many of the phenomena, especially those associated with its radiation. While there is much to commend the theory, it too meets with its share of difficulties.

The problems of the structure of the chromosphere and the corona are many and the solutions for a number of them are still to be given. Most encouraging progress has been made in unraveling the structure of the chromosphere, largely through the aid of the recent developments in our ideas of the behavior of the atom under different conditions and the manner in which it radiates energy. Regarding the corona our knowledge is in a less advanced state, but the time is not far distant, in my opinion, when many of its complex phenomena will receive a satisfactory interpretation.

# OBITUARY

## ACHILLES DE KHOTINSKY

ON March 28, 1933, occurred the death, in Pentwater, Michigan, of Captain Achilles de Khotinsky, who, through his genius in invention, design and construction, leaves a permanent impression on physics and chemistry in America. Captain de Khotinsky was born on January 6, 1850, in St. Petersburg, Russia. Having completed the course in the Imperial Naval Academy, he spent the next 13 years in the Russian navy, in which he attained the rank of captain. It was during this period, in 1878, that he first saw America, while on commission to supervise the construction of three battle cruisers for the imperial navy. In the late seventies he obtained European patents on incandescent lamps which he manufactured on a large scale in Russia, Germany, Austria, England, France and Holland. He also held a basic French patent on the pasted storage battery plate. While in England, he developed the widely used de Khotinsky cement, known to every research physicist as indispensable in investigations involving vacuum technique.

Returning to America in 1891, he established an incandescent lamp factory in Massachusetts. As a result of patent difficulties, the plant was closed after about a year of operation. Deprived of practically all he possessed, he came west, spending about a year at Purdue University. In the middle nineties he located at Chicago. During the next twenty years he was associated with various firms and institutions, among them the Western Electric Company, Wm. Gaertner and Company, Armour Institute of Technology and the University of Chicago. Many physicists and chemists who obtained their degrees from Chicago will affectionately recall "the Captain," as he was always known to his associates and acquaintances. He spent eight years with Professor Michelson at Ryerson Laboratory, designing and constructing research apparatus and ruling diffraction gratings, after which he spent some years in Kent Laboratory as research mechanician. In 1916 he joined the development staff of Central Scientific Company, where he remained until 1922. Here he developed miscellaneous constant temperature devices, including ovens, water baths and thermoregulators. His contributions to design and production methods of military instruments which the company manufactured for the government during the war were numerous.

In 1922 Professor Randall, of the University of Michigan, asked the writer to suggest some one who might undertake the design and construction of a dividing engine for ruling special diffraction gratings, to be used in researches in the region of the longer wave-lengths. No one seemed better qualified than Captain de Khotinsky. Although 72 years old at that time, he was happy for the opportunity of spending the next few years in the kind of work he loved and in most congenial and pleasant surroundings. In three years the ruling machine was completed and in operation. Not the smallest part of his achievement was the method of shaping the diamond ruling points to produce grooves of predetermined shape, by means of which intense spectra in selected wave-length regions could be obtained.

In 1926 Captain de Khotinsky retired to Pentwater, to spend his declining years.

His achievements are numerous. In engineering he has to his credit many inventions and patents on incandescent lamps, storage battery plates, and automatic gun-firing devices. He devised the first switchboard signal lamp. In physics he is best known for his de Khotinsky cement and his work in the production of diffraction gratings, while chemists and bacteriologists will remember him for his laboratory devices for the maintenance of constant temperatures.

Paul E. Klopsteg

## RECENT DEATHS

Dr. Jermain Gildersleeve Porter, professor of astronomy at the University of Cincinnati and director of the Cincinnati Observatory from 1884 to 1931, died on April 15 at the age of eighty-one years.

Mrs. Zelia Nuttall, honorary special assistant at the Peabody Museum of Harvard University and honorary professor of archeology at the National Museum of Mexico, died at her home in Mexico City on April 12, in her seventy-fifth year.

The death is announced of Dr. Ernst Grossmann, professor of astronomy at Munich.

The Duke of the Abruzzi, who conducted explorations in Africa, India and the far north, died on March 18, aged sixty years.

Jules Piccard, for forty years professor of chemistry at Basle, died on April 11. Dr. Piccard was the father of Dr. Auguste Piccard, professor of physics and physical measurements and director of the laboratory of physics at the University of Brussels, who is now visiting the United States.

# SCIENTIFIC EVENTS

## THE EIGHTIETH ANNIVERSARY OF THE FOUNDING OF THE CALIFORNIA ACADEMY OF SCIENCES

On April 4, the eightieth anniversary of its founding was celebrated by the California Academy of Sciences in its Simson African Hall, where a preview was arranged of the installations of habitat groups of African mammals which are now in a stage of particular interest. At this function, there was a brief address of welcome by Mr. William H. Crocker, the president of the Board of Trustees, who has held this position since 1897. Dr. C. E. Grunsky, president of the academy for over twenty-one years, referred briefly to the history of the academy as a scientific research and educational institution, whose activities since its inception have been made possible by generous contributions and endowments from private individuals, outstanding among which is that of James Lick some sixty years ago. The Lick endowment placed the academy in unrestricted ownership of downtown property in San Francisco, the improvements on which, made with borrowed money, yield most of the income which makes its activities possible.

When Mr. Leslie Simson some years ago made his offer to furnish to the academy, free of cost, specimens of African mammals which would be needed for an African hall of habitat groups, provided that a house for the collection were provided, it was hoped that some one might come forward with an endowment for much needed new buildings. But this did not happen. Mr. Simson then offered to the academy property worth $150,000, but with the condition that income therefrom should be his during life. His proposition was accepted and the academy borrowed $255,000 and erected a new unit to its museum buildings in Golden Gate Park in which it has provided space for the departments of entomology and ichthyology, for the administrative offices, and for the Simson African Hall.

In this hall, under the direction and general planning of Mr. Frank Tose, the chief of exhibits, the habitat groups are being installed. There will be ten large groups, thirteen intermediate small size groups and one very large waterhole group at the end of the hall. Of these groups, only one is now under glass. The backgrounds of three small groups have been painted and the backgrounds of five other large groups are nearing completion. The lighting of the habitat groups will all be artificial. Their backgrounds are domed so that all structural work is concealed. The observer gets no impression of a painted wall. Glass fronts will be inclined so that reflections of opposite light areas will be thrown well up above the horizon where they will interfere least with a view of the mounted specimens. In the lion group, the preparator of which throughout is Mr. Tose, sunlight effect by a transparency behind a rugged foreground is startling and exceptionally realistic, made to merge perfectly into the surrounding well-lighted surface painting.

It is notable in connection with this installation that there are no lighting fixtures in the hall. Abundant indirect light radiates from the habitat groups, all of which are artificially illuminated.

The hope was expressed that sponsors would be found for the individual habitat groups, as has been the case in the academy's hall of California wild life.

## THE NEW COMMISSIONER OF INDIAN AFFAIRS

JOHN COLLIER has been nominated by President Roosevelt to succeed Charles J. Rhoads as Commissioner of Indian Affairs. In making the announcement Harold L. Ickes, Secretary of the Interior, made the following statement:

John Collier will bring to the administration of the Bureau of Indian Affairs a wide knowledge of the subject based upon personal contacts and intensive study during the past several years. In my judgment, he is the best equipped man who has ever occupied that office.

Drafted by the government four years ago, Mr. Charles J. Rhoads has served as Commissioner of Indian Affairs with great distinction. His uprightness of character, his ability and his single-hearted desire to serve have impressed all who have known him and realized the difficult task he undertook. It has been my pleasure to know Mr. Rhoads and the fine work he has done. Respecting his repeated request to be permitted to retire to private life, a conscientious effort has been made to find an outstanding and experienced man to take over his burdensome duties. Such a man I believe Mr. Collier to be.

I am deeply concerned about the welfare of the American Indians. I am persuaded that they are entitled to every consideration that the government can give them. The Commissioner of Indian Affairs ought to be the representative of the Indians themselves in the Department of the Interior. He should be their advocate, fighting for their interests and pleading their cause. Those who seek to encroach upon the rights and privileges of these original Americans are amply able to look out for themselves. Unless the government selects the right kind of a man as Commissioner of Indian Affairs, the Indians themselves are, in effect, without a friend at court when substantial rights and interests of theirs are up for adjudication.

I have known John Collier for a number of years, and I have had opportunity to acquaint myself at first hand with the soundness of his views and his attitude toward the Indian question. In addition to safeguarding the property rights of the Indians, he will help them to help themselves toward a fuller and happier life. He will respect their customs, encourage them in their arts and assist them to maintain their rich and unique culture. He will try to interpret them sympathetically to their white fellow Americans. He realizes that on the purely material side, our American Indians possess possibilities in which the white people themselves may share, if those possibilities are realized and cultivated.

## IN HONOR OF CHARLES E. MUNROE

AT the subscription dinner at the recent Washington meeting of the American Chemical Society Dr. Charles E. Munroe, past president of the society and its only surviving charter member, was the guest of honor. In testimony of the esteem of the society, Dr. Munroe was presented with a jeweled emblem of the society and a purse. In presenting these tokens, Dr. Arthur B. Lamb, professor of chemistry and director of the laboratory at Harvard University, president of the society, said, in part:

The American Chemical Society was definitely organized on April 20, 1876, in New York City. Of the one hundred and thirty-three charter members at that time the sole survivor to-day is Charles Edward Munroe.

The first general meeting of the society was held in Newport, Rhode Island, on August 6 and 7, 1890, at the suggestion and under the chairmanship of Dr. Munroe, who was at that time a member of the technical staff of the United States Navy Torpedo Station at that city. Dr. Munroe was president of the society in 1898 to 1899 and is honorary chairman of this, the eighty-fifth general meeting of the American Chemical Society. He is with us here to-night, as keen of wit and as full of energy, optimism, kindness and good will as when he assisted in the establishment of our society fifty-seven years ago!

Dr. Munroe was born in Cambridge, Massachusetts, in 1849. He graduated from the Lawrence Scientific School at Harvard in 1871 and stayed on as instructor in quantitative analysis in the chemical department of the university until 1874.

From Harvard, Dr. Munroe went as professor of chemistry to the Naval Academy at Annapolis. After twelve years there he became chemist to the Torpedo Corps, United States Naval Station, and War College, and to other bureaus of the Federal Government; and thereafter, professor of chemistry and dean of the graduate faculty of George Washington University. He is the inventor of smokeless powder, discoverer of the ''Munroe Effect,'' and author of a hundred or more articles and books on chemistry and explosion.

But as Dr. Wiley has said, Dr. Munroe's greatest works are not found in the scientific papers that he has published nor in the dangerous researches that he has made, but in the hearts and lives of the thousands he has taught.

Dr. Munroe, as I have said, was born in 1849. Gold was discovered that year in Cambridge as well as in California—for Dr. Munroe's heart is made exclusively of that noble metal!

It is then with the greatest pleasure and satisfaction that I hand to you, Dr. Charles Edwin Munroe, first, this gold pin carrying the emblem of our society, and secondly, these gold certificates of the United States Treasury, as tokens of our respect, our admiration and our affection.

## THE AWARD OF THE WILLARD GIBBS MEDAL TO DR. RICHARD WILLSTAETTER

DR. RICHARD WILLSTAETTER, of Munich, who received the Nobel Prize in 1915, has been awarded the Willard Gibbs Medal of the Chicago Section of the American Chemical Society.

The award is made for Dr. Willstaetter's work in chemistry, especially in the chemistry of chlorophyll. His name is added to the list of twenty-one other Willard Gibbs medalists "whose work in either pure or applied science has received world-wide recognition." The jury which voted the medal consisted of twelve American leaders representing every branch of chemistry.

The medal will be conferred on Dr. Willstaetter in Chicago on September 13 during the eighty-sixth meeting of the American Chemical Society, which will be held in connection with the Century of Progress Exposition. A distinguished group of scientists from Europe and America will witness the ceremony.

A statement from the American Chemical Society says:

Dr. Willstaetter is known for his researches in organic chemistry, particularly in biochemistry. The chronicle of his career in science is the record of a great mind successfully attacking, in logical sequence, some of the most difficult problems in organic and bio chemistry.

The greatness of Dr. Willstaetter as a chemist lies not only in his signal accomplishments, but in his ability to perpetuate his influence by opening the way for the work of others. He has conquered barren wildernesses of ignorance and left them fertile fields where others as well as himself might gain rich reward.

Honored by scientific societies all over the world for his contributions to the field of organic chemistry, Dr. Willstaetter last year was awarded the Davy Medal of the Royal Society in London. His sixtieth birthday last August was widely celebrated in Germany.

One of the best known of all European chemists, Dr. Willstaetter's first great independent research was with the cocaine alkaloids, the result of which ''set the field in order'' and culminated in the synthesis of cocaine. Next he attacked the quinines and quininoid substances, and discovered ortho-quinine and proof of the structure of aniline black.

Work on the cyclic hydrocarbons, important in the oil industry, was the next step in Dr. Willstaetter's scientific career, the most notable achievement in this field being the synthesis of cyclo-octatetrene, a cyclic substance having alternating single and double bonds, but not aromatic in nature.

An outstanding chapter in Dr. Willstaetter's studies was his investigation on the structure of chlorophyll, the green coloring matter of leaves which is present in all growing vegetable cells, and the assimilation of carbon dioxide by plants. He proved the identity of chlorophyll from many plants, demonstrated the existence of two chlorophylls, and their close association with the carotinoids, a widely distributed plant pigment.

From products derived after breaking down chlorophyll, Dr. Willstaetter disclosed most of the secrets of its structure, thus contributing greatly to science's knowledge of the vegetable kingdom. His researches with the anthocyanins, flower pigments, demonstrated the close relationship of this varied-hued substance to chlorophyll, and the simple means by which nature changes the blue of the cornflower to the red of the rose or the purple of the grape. This study of plant pigments was crowned in 1915 by the award of the Nobel Prize for outstanding chemical research.

Dr. Willstaetter next considered the related field of the enzymes, chemical compounds of vegetable or animal origin that cause chemical transformation. By developing new methods and by insisting upon checking each procedure through quantitative analysis, he revolutionized research in this field.

Valuable contributions on many other subjects, such as hydrogenation with platinum and the hydrates of metals, have been made by Dr. Willstaetter, in addition to his major researches. In most cases these lesser studies grew out of the need for information to assist some principal experimental procedure. These investigations have been found to be so numerous that there is "scarcely a phase of organic chemistry in which one can read far without encountering Willstaetter's name."

Dr. Willstaetter's work with the cocaine alkaloids made possible the commercial synthesis of local anesthetics. His studies in chlorophyll paved the way for the triumphs of Professor Hans Fischer, at Munich, and Professor James Bryant Conant, at Harvard, in this field.

Dr. Willstaetter's experiments with the carotinoids have made possible the separation of the individual components of this group and their relation to Vitamin A, while his researches in the enzymes "lifted the veil that obscured the complex processes of protein hydrolysis."

# SCIENTIFIC NOTES AND NEWS

ACCORDING to press dispatches, Dr. Albert Einstein has accepted "with the greatest pleasure and gratitude" a professorship in the University of Paris. It is said that the professorship is at the Sorbonne, but it is also reported that the French government has proposed to establish a chair of mathematical physics for him in the Collège de France. It is understood that this new appointment will not interfere with Dr. Einstein's professorship in the University of Madrid or with appointments that he has accepted in Brussels and Glasgow. Dr. Einstein will return to the United States in the autumn to occupy for part of the year the chair of mathematical physics in the Institute for Advanced Study at Princeton.

THE Trustees of Princeton University announce the retirement of Dr. Edwin Grant Conklin, professor of zoology; of Dr. Charles F. W. McClure, professor of comparative anatomy, and of W. B. Harris, professor of geodesy. They will continue their connection with the university as lecturers. The resignation of Professor Augustus Trowbridge, dean of the graduate school, on account of ill health, is also announced. Professor Edmund Newton Harvey, professor of physiology, has been assigned to succeed Dr. Conklin in the Henry Fairfield Osborn professorship of biology, and Professor Wilbur Willis Swingle has been appointed to the Edwin Grant Conklin professorship of biology.

DR. MORTIMER E. COOLEY, dean emeritus of the College of Engineering and Architecture of the University of Michigan, celebrated his seventy-eighth birthday on March 28. During the day Dr. Cooley received his colleagues and friends in his room at the Engineering Building.

DR. FRANK A. HARTMAN, professor of physiology at the University of Buffalo, has been awarded the Schoellkopf Medal for 1933, for his work on cortin. This medal is bestowed annually by the western New York section of the American Chemical Society for outstanding achievement in science.

THE Joseph A. Capps Prize for 1932 of the Institute of Medicine of Chicago has been awarded to Eugene L. Walsh, Northwestern University Medical School, 1931, for his "Studies on the Etiology of Gallstones." Dr. Walsh holds the George W. Belcher fellowship in urology at the Cleveland Clinic Foundation. Honorable mention was given to Edward E. P. Seidmon, University of Illinois College of Medicine, 1932, for his paper on "Influence of Vitamin Deficient Diets upon Intestinal Acid-base Equilibrium." The Joseph A. Capps Prize of $500 is awarded annually for meritorious medical research by a graduate of a medical school in Chicago completed within two years after graduation.

DR. THEODOR WIEGAND, Berlin, president of the Imperial Archeological Institute, has been made an honorary doctor of the medical faculty of the University of Berlin.

DR. VICTOR GOLDSCHMIDT, of Heidelberg, has been elected an honorary member of the German Mineralogical Society.

THE Makdougall-Brisbane Prize of the Royal Society of Edinburgh for 1930–32 has been awarded to Dr. A. C. Aitken, of the University of Edinburgh, for contributions to mathematics published in the *Proceedings* of the society, and the Gunning Victoria Jubilee Prize for 1928–32 to Sir James Walker, for work in physical and general chemistry.

THE *Journal* of the American Medical Association reports that three hundred and seventy-five friends of Dr. Howard A. Kelly, Baltimore, gathered at a dinner on February 20, in celebration of his seventy-fifth birthday. Dr. Thomas S. Cullen, Baltimore, was toastmaster, and speakers included Dr. Walter W. Chipman, emeritus professor of obstetrics and gynecology, McGill University, and Dr. Abraham Flexner, director of the Institute for Advanced Study, Princeton. A special tribute was sent to Dr. Kelly by Dr. William H. Welch, emeritus professor of the history of medicine at the Johns Hopkins University School of Medicine, who, since February 1, has been a patient in the Brady Clinic, Johns Hopkins Hospital. Dr. Kelly, who is known as the "father of gynecology," is professor emeritus of gynecology at Johns Hopkins, with which he has been associated since 1889, retiring from active work at the school in 1919.

DR. WILLIAM H. PARK, general director of the Bureau of Laboratories of the Department of Health of

New York City, professor of bacteriology and hygiene at New York University and professor of preventive medicine at Bellevue Hospital Medical College, was the guest of honor at a dinner given at the Biltmore on April 19 by his friends and associates. The date was the fortieth anniversary of Dr. Park's founding in New York of the first public bacteriological laboratory in the world. Dr. Linsly R. Williams, director of the New York Academy of Medicine, was chairman of the dinner committee and Dr. Shirley W. Wynne, Health Commissioner, was toastmaster. The speakers included, in addition to Dr. Williams, Dr. Matthias Nicoll, Homer Folks and Dr. C.-E. A. Winslow.

WE learn from *Nature* that at the annual general meeting of the Institute of Metals, the following officers were elected for the year 1933–34: *President,* Sir Henry Fowler; *Vice-presidents,* Professor C. H. Desch and Professor R. S. Hutton; *Members of Council,* Eng. Vice-Admiral Sir Robert Dixon, Mr. Wesley Lambert, Mr. H. C. Lancaster, Mr. A. H. Mundey, Mr. A. J. G. Smout, Mr. F. Tomlinson. The silver jubilee meeting of the institute will be held in Birmingham from September 18 to 21. It was in Birmingham that the first general meeting of the institute was held in the autumn of 1908, under the presidency of the late Sir William White.

DR. HARRY A. CHARIPPER, assistant professor of biology at the Washington Square College of New York University, has been appointed head of the department.

MARGARET M. FULFORD, of the department of botany of the University of Cincinnati, has been appointed curator of hepatics and a member of the advisory board of the Sullivant Moss Society.

WORK at the new Leonard Wood Laboratory for the Eradication of Leprosy on Culion Island, the Philippines, is planned by Dr. Malcolm H. Soule, University of Michigan; Dr. E. B. McKinley, George Washington University; Dr. E. W. Goodpasture, Vanderbilt University; Dr. E. R. Long, University of Pennsylvania; Dr. T. M. Rivers, Rockefeller Institute, and Dr. Hans Zinsser, Harvard University. A correspondent writes: "Recently Drs. Soule and McKinley succeeded in isolating the leprosy bacillus, or germ, outside the human body. Monkeys inoculated with the bacillus developed conditions suggestive of the human disease, but soon recovered. Other laboratory animals failed to show any signs of the disease. Drs. Soule and McKinley have been granted leave of absence from June next to February, 1934. They will be the first of the group who within the next few years will endeavor to work out preventive treatment and, if possible, a cure for the disease."

DR. SVEIN ROSSELAND, director of the observatory at Oslo, has arrived at the Massachusetts Institute of Technology to make an intensive study of the differential analyzer designed by Dr. Vannevar Bush, vice-president of the institute and professor of electrical power transmission.

PROFESSOR OTTO HAHN, director of the Kaiser Wilhelm Institute in Berlin, non-resident Baker lecturer at Cornell University, will deliver the second John Howard Appleton Lecture at Brown University on April 28. His subject will be "The Radioactive Elements and their Application in Chemical Research."

DR. OTTO LOEWI, professor of pharmacology at Graz, will deliver at 5 o'clock on May 4 and 11 the Edward K. Dunham Lectures for the promotion of the medical sciences at Harvard University. The subjects of the lectures are "Humoral Transmission of the Nerve Impulse" and "Regulation and Adaptation."

DR. FELIX BERNSTEIN, director of the Institute of Mathematical Statistics of the University of Göttingen, spoke before the Sigma Xi Chapter of the University of Cincinnati on April 10 on "Solution of Mathematical Problems in Physics and Engineering by New Mechanical Means."

PROFESSOR H. J. MULLER, of the University of Texas, lectured at the University of Stockholm on April 4 on "Evolution in the Light of the Modern Mutation Theory." On April 6 he lectured at the University of Oslo, on April 8 before the Mendelian Society of Lund and on April 11 at the University of Copenhagen. He is to address the Genetical Society of London on April 27.

PROFESSOR A. E. KENNELLY spoke on April 11 on "Experiences during the Development of Electrical Engineering since the Year 1875," before a joint meeting at Harvard University of the Boston Section of the American Institute of Electrical Engineers with the Student Branches of Harvard University, Massachusetts Institute of Technology, Northeastern University and Tufts College.

THE program of illustrated lectures arranged by the California Academy of Sciences during April and May, at San Francisco, under an endowment by an unnamed friend, is announced as follows: "Natural and Cultural Pearls," Dr. Charles A. Kofoid, professor of zoology, University of California; "Explorations in Plant Life," Arthur C. Pillsbury; "Crystals and Crystallization," Dr. Austin F. Rogers, professor of mineralogy, Stanford University, and "Some Protozoa and Causes of Disease in Animals and Man," Dr. Charles A. Kofoid, professor of zoology, University of California. These lectures are free to the public.

THE Pennsylvania Topographic and Geologic Survey has recently moved its offices from the Claster Building on Market Street in Harrisburg, Pennsylvania, to the sixth floor of the South Office Building of the Capitol group. The scientific staff and its special interests now is as follows: George H. Ashley, state geologist, coal; Ralph W. Stone, assistant state geologist, structural materials; Stanley H. Cathcart, associate geologist, oil and gas; Bradford Willard, associate geologist, paleontology; Charles K. Graeber, associate geologist, mineralogy and areal geology; Forrest T. Moyer, assistant geologist, areal geology; W. O. Hickok, 4th, assistant geologist, areal geology and metals; M. N. Shaffner, technical assistant.

*Industrial and Engineering Chemistry* writes that at the Tenth Conference of the International Union of Chemistry, held at Liége in September, 1930, the committee on thermochemical data, formed in 1925 for a limited time, was replaced by the standing committee on thermochemistry, which includes the following: L. Keffler, Great Britain; C. Matignon, France; W. A. Roth, Germany; F. Swarts, Belgium; W. Swietoslawski, chairman, Poland; P. E. Verkade, Holland, and E. W. Washburn, United States. One of the main functions of that committee consists in the preparation of an International Table of Thermochemical Data, to be published under the patronage of the International Union of Chemistry under the same conditions as the International Tables of Atomic Weights. Authors of papers connected with thermochemistry and published within the last five years are requested to send two copies to the secretary of the committee, L. Keffler, Thermochemical Laboratory, University of Liverpool.

A DISPATCH to *The New York Times* from Paris reports that a decree creating the Superior Council for Scientific Research was signed by President Lebrun on April 14. The council will resemble France's Superior Council of Public Instruction and will coordinate scientific organizations and facilitate research in pure science. It will have eight divisions covering mathematical, mechanical, statistical, astronomical, physical, chemical, biological, natural, historical, philosophical and social sciences.

As a result of its recent petition the council of the Institute of Marine Engineers have received official information that King George has approved the grant of a charter to the institute. The attainment of this distinction follows closely on the forty-fourth anniversary of the foundation of the institute, in 1889. To-day the membership amounts to 3,550, including over 2,800 corporate members, among whom are many of the foremost marine engineers in Great Britain and the Dominions. The King became patron of the institute in 1918. The grant of the Royal Charter signifies recognition of the institute's record of work and achievement and affirms its status as the representative organization of the marine engineering profession.

THE Yosemite School of Field Natural History will be held in the Yosemite National Park from June 26 to August 11. The headquarters of the school are at the Yosemite Museum, but the greater part of the time will be spent in field work.

THE new Saguaro National Monument in Arizona comprises about 60,000 acres, mainly within the Coronado National Forest, on the slopes of the Santa Catalina mountains about 25 miles northeast of Tucson. It was created a National Monument by proclamation of President Hoover on March 1. Administration of the area will be in the hands of the Forest Service. The land will be protected from any use that would interfere with the preservation of the native flora, which is considered of great educational and scientific interest. Some of the specimens of the Giant Cactus on the area are believed to be more than 100 years old. Examples of European and American Indian and European archeological handiwork have been placed on display for the first time in Denver by the department of anthropology of the University of Denver. Pieces of Continental Paleolithic and Neolithic implements of the early man are arranged in the collection. Many of the specimens have been gathered personally by Dr. E. B. Renaud, head of the department of anthropology, during his archeological work in Spain and France. The greater portion of the exhibition is devoted, however, to the display of Indian native art and craftsmanship.

ACCORDING to the *Journal* of the American Medical Association, the Deutsche Gesellschaft für Kinderheilkunde, at its meeting in Dresden in September, 1931, expressed in a proclamation the fear that the long-continued economic crisis might cause a general weakening of resistance to disease in the oncoming generation. Observations made during the war show that children suffer the most from inadequate nutrition. For that reason, Drs. Gottlieb and Stransky, of the Vienna Public Health Service, examined 800 young children, establishing the weight of each child. They report in an article in the *Klinische Wochenschrift* that the number of underweight children in families that had been at least a year without a definite source of income was considerably higher than the number of children showing overweight. Among the children of employed parents, however, the number showing overweight was more than twice as large as the number presenting underweight. The children of the unemployed, ranging between 2 and 4 years of age, show an especially large number who are underweight. In children 5 and 6 years old, the differences are not so marked.

*Nature* reports that at a recent meeting of the Industrial Advisory Committee of the Ross Institute, London, reports were received of the over-seas activities of the institute. Seven research centers in Assam and northern Bengal have been opened, and anti-malarial work and the testing of new drugs for the treatment of malaria have been pursued there and in Rhodesia and East and South Africa. In the Assam tea gardens, anti-malarial work has resulted in much improved health, for in 1930 among a population of 13,248 the admissions to hospital were 23,226, but in 1932 with a slightly larger population the admissions were reduced to 15,141. A standard oil mixture for killing mosquito larvae has been devised in conjunction with the Burma-Shell group. The health among lead miners in Yugoslavia was investigated and a health scheme was formulated and is now in operation. At the conclusion of the proceedings, Mr. Still and Sir Malcolm Watson addressed the meeting on the subject of yellow fever. Now that travel by aeroplane is so rapid, the grave danger that infection may be carried from the yellow fever zone in West Africa to East Africa and Asia, which would be followed with disastrous consequences, was emphasized.

# DISCUSSION

## ZOOLOGICAL NOMENCLATURE

PROFESSOR A. S. PEARSE, of Duke University, has recently contributed to SCIENCE[1] a number of thought-provoking reviews of recent text-books of zoology.

Professor Pearse makes, rather dogmatically, two statements in his reviews that to the taxonomist stand out as though they were printed in red ink and, though they are of distinctly minor importance, are as startlingly incongruent with the established formalities of nomenclature as red ink would be on a page of SCIENCE.

Professor Pearse makes the statement that "the scientific name of an animal consists of the genus, species *and the name of the author.*"[2] (The italics are Professor Pearse's). Had Professor Pearse said that the name of the author should be *appended* to the scientific name of an animal at least once in the publication using the name, one could agree with him, and might even walk with the International Commission on Zoological Nomenclature and add that the date of the proposal or some other clue to the original use of the name might also appear to advantage.[3]

Article 2 of the International Rules of Zoological Nomenclature states that "the scientific designation of animals is uninomial for subgenera and all higher groups, binomial for species, and trinomial for subspecies." Article 22 reads in part as follows (there is no need of quoting it in full): "If it is desired to cite the author's name, this should follow the scientific name without interposition of any mark of punctuation;—"[4] If the author's name is a *part* of the scientific name, as Professor Pearse contends, how is it possible for it to *follow* the scientific name? How can the part follow the whole?

Professor Pearse at another place[5] makes the following comment: "Evidently the writer disapproves of the modern tendency to begin even generic names with small letters, —" Let us refer to the Code. Article 8 reads: "A generic name must consist of a single word, simple or compound, written with a capital initial letter—."

Of course, a word may be used in more than one sense. The word felis, for instance, may be used as a formal scientific name, in which case it is properly capitalized. Also it may be used as a common noun, just as is its English equivalent, cat. In the latter usage it is not capitalized. Can it be this that Professor Pearse means? If so, he fails to make himself clear and has no need to appeal to a non-existent "modern tendency" for support of what has always been good usage.

Any tendency, however trivial, to flout the International Rules, the only hope we have for ultimate stability in zoological nomenclature, should bring a vigorous protest, even though the protestee is one as eminent and respected as Professor Pearse. Indeed, the more eminent the offender, the more necessary the protest.

J. BROOKES KNIGHT

YALE UNIVERSITY

[1] SCIENCE, n. s., 77: 169–172.

[2] *Loc. cit.*, p. 170, first paragraph.

[3] See resolution of the International Commission on Zoological Nomenclature at Budapest, 1927, as published in U. S. Public Health Service, Public Health Reports, Oct. 28, 1927, pp. 2639–2640.

[4] International Rules of Zoological Nomenclature; Proc. Biological Society of Washington, volume 39, pp. 75–104.

[5] *Loc. cit.*, p. 170, second column, first paragraph.

## THE INVOLVED GENETICS OF FISH

THE recent paper by Hubbs and Hubbs on "Apparent Parthenogenesis in Nature, in a Form of Fish of Hybrid Origin"[1] is of great interest to any one concerned with the extremely puzzling phenomena of ichthyological genetics. The matter is puzzling for the reason that although some crosses behave in normal Mendelian fashion, other crosses, like those

[1] SCIENCE, n. s., 76: 628. 1932.

recorded by Hubbs and Hubbs, refuse to conform to anything that the geneticist seems able to explain in the light of his studies with fruit-flies, birds or mammals.

For years the writer has bred tropical fish as a hobby and now has aquaria and indoor heated pools totaling 2,500 gallons capacity, with a number of sorts of hybrids under observation. Some of the facts connected therewith are worth recording.

First it should be stated that the commonest cross attempted in domestication is that of a male platy (*Platypoecilus*) of one or another of the developed color phases, with a female swordtail (*Xiphophorus helleri*). In the absence of live food, at least, the young hybrids are not produced as freely as those of pure lineage, but the former are all different from either parent, with size of mother and with color approaching or surpassing that of the father. These hybrids are known as "black helleris," "red helleris" or similarly according to color. At least when a female black helleri is mated to a pure male swordtail, approximately three quarters of the resultant young will be colorless like the father and one quarter black like the hybrid mother. The genetics of some of these various hybrids are extremely difficult to investigate, for many of them are sterile, and it is even claimed that males of some of the crosses are always so.

Hubbs and Hubbs found that when males of either *Mollienisia latipinna* or *M. sphenops* are mated with females of a hybrid between the two, which is a form currently known as *M. formosa,* all the offspring are always *formosa* in type. In other words, the hybrid characters are inherited by the young from the mother in a block, without respect to dissimilar paternity. And the offspring are invariably female. In this connection, however, the authors state that "the consistent and abundant production of purely matroclinous and constantly female offspring by this hybrid form of fish finds its most plausible explanation as parthenogenesis. It is apparently not a spontaneous parthenogenesis, since many controls, unmated, have shown no indication of becoming pregnant. We provisionally assume that we are probably dealing with a case of gynogenesis . . . a condition recorded as naturally occurring among certain invertebrates." Comment upon the above may be divided into three headings as follows:

(a) It is unwise to intrude the suggestion of parthenogenesis, even of a modified sort, into vertebrate literature. The phenomenon is so at variance with what is known and believed about vertebrate development that I am sure no vertebrate morphologist would admit for a moment that the natural development from egg to sexual maturity of an individual vertebrate without direct inclusion of the male element is within the realms of probability. Certainly extremely convincing cytological evidence would be necessary and the experiments verified several times.

(b) The fact that all the hybrids of *Mollienisia* produced were female appears to be ascribable in this instance, perhaps, to a sex-linked lethal factor acting on male eggs, or possibly to some type of non-disjunction. In this connection it may be mentioned that a yellow (mutant ?) strain of *Xiphophorus,* developed in domestication and known as the golden swordtail, consistently produces two or three times as many females as males, and the case of the *Mollienisia* may be an instance of this factor carried to an extreme.

(c) The matroclinous character of the offspring can involve no argument in favor of parthenogenesis, for I can cite reverse evidence, of a patroclinous nature, as follows: I have a strain of hybrids produced by crossing a male black platy (*Platypoecilus*) with a female of the golden swordtail strain of *Xiphophorus,* which are large, spectacular fish, mostly black but with many spots and blotches of green and orange. Apparently all individuals of this hybrid or at least a large proportion of them, are fertile, and when bred to one another they behave as a true species. In other words all the young of the second generation resemble their parents rather than either of the grandparents. So far so good, with nothing very remarkable. But when a male of this hybrid strain is mated with a female of pure strain green swordtail (*Xiphophorus helleri*), none of the young will be of dull color like the mother but all blackish like the hybrid father. This patroclinous inheritance has been tested in a number of individuals and litters. I have no doubt that it will hold throughout successive generations, but for proof or disproof of this assumption sufficient time has not yet elapsed.

A. BRAZIER HOWELL
JOHNS HOPKINS UNIVERSITY

## NOTE ON THE LIFE-CYCLE OF ECTOCARPUS SILICULOSUS DILLW.

THE generally accepted view that the plurilocular sporangia of *Ectocarpus siliculosus* produce gametes is based primarily on the classical work of Berthold[1] at Naples. His results have been confirmed by Oltmanns, Hartman, and, more recently, by Knight.[2] Knight demonstrated also that all the plants of this species that she found at Naples had a haploid soma.

[1] G. Berthold, "Die geschlechtliche Fortpflanzung der eigentlichen Phaeosporen," *Mitt. a. d. Zool. Stat. z. Neapel,* II. 1881.

[2] M. Knight, "Studies in the Ectocarpaceae. II. The Life-History and Cytology of Ectocarpus siliculosus, Dillw." *Trans. of the Royal Society of Edinburgh,* Vol. LVI. 1929.

Knight, on the other hand, found that all the plants of *E. siliculosus* studied by her at the Port Erin Biological Station have a diploid soma and bear both plurilocular and unilocular sporangia on the same plant. The plurilocular sporangia in this locality produce diploid zoospores. In the unilocular sporangium, however, the first nuclear division is a reduction division, and the haploid zoids from this structure are gametes which fuse in pairs. At Port Erin, she states, no alternation of generations occurs, and the diploid phase is the only one in the life-cycle.

The fact that zoids from plurilocular sporangia may at times act like zoospores has long been known; and the work of Knight suggests that in such cases they came from diploid plants. The zoids from unilocular sporangia have always been regarded as zoospores; and Knight is the only author who has found them sometimes behaving like gametes.

From aquarium cultures made at Naples, Berthold obtained plantlets that bore both plurilocular and unilocular sporangia on the same plant. The precise origin of the young plants in question was not determined. Berthold suggested that they may have come from zygotes. Since, however, unfertilized gametes, which he had already found to be capable of parthenogenetic development, were present in these aquaria we must keep in mind also the possibility that these in reality may have given rise to the small plants. Berthold also did not learn the function of the zoids from these cultured plants. Although he raised plants with unilocular sporangia in culture, he makes no mention in the text of finding these in the sea at Naples. (The plant shown in his Fig. 8 is referred to as having been found in the open). Knight states positively that she was unable to find unilocular sporangia there after careful search. The part that is played by unilocular sporangia in the normal life-history of this species at Naples therefore remained quite problematical.

It was apparent that further research on Ectocarpus was very essential. The facts that were known suggested the occurrence of an alternation of generations in this plant, but the evidence was far from adequate to substantiate this. It was also important to know whether the plants whose unilocular sporangia produce zoospores were diploid or whether unilocular sporangia may sometimes arise on haploid plants and give rise to zoospores which serve to multiply this generation.

This paper is a preliminary report of the results of an attempt to determine the course of the life-cycle of *Ectocarpus siliculosus* on the Atlantic coast of North America. The aim was to learn whether both haploid and diploid plants occur here and, if so, the rôle played by each in the life-cycle.

The material for this study was collected about Woods Hole, Massachusetts, during the summers of 1931 and 1932. All plants at Woods Hole itself were like those studied by Knight at Port Erin, since they were diploid and bore both kinds of sporangia. It was found, however, that the presumably haploid zoids of the unilocular sporangia as well as the diploid zoids of the plurilocular sporangia invariably germinate directly. That is, the zoids of the unilocular sporangia of these plants do not act like gametes, as Knight reported for the plants at Port Erin. Sexual plants as well as the asexual ones were found at Penikese, an island twenty miles from Woods Hole. The sexual plants are haploid and bear only plurilocular sporangia; their zoids serve as gametes, and they are distinctly dioecious. These sexual plants are therefore like those found at Naples. Parthenogenetic development of both male and female gametes occurs.

The cytological studies thus far made indicate that the number of chromosomes in asexual plants, with both kinds of sporangia, is twice as large as that found in the sexual plants, which bear plurilocular sporangia only.

The life-cycle of *E. siliculosus* near Woods Hole therefore exhibits a definite alternation of generations. Diploid asexual plants with both unilocular and plurilocular sporangia produce, in the plurilocular sporangia, diploid zoids which develop directly into other diploid plants. The first division of the nucleus in the unilocular sporangium is presumably a reduction division such as Knight found. The haploid zoids produced in this structure germinate to form haploid sexual plants. The haploid sexual plants are dioecious and produce gametes in plurilocular sporangia. After the fusion of these gametes in pairs the zygotes develop into diploid asexual plants and thus complete the cycle. The haploid sexual generation propagates itself by the parthenogenetic development of unfertilized gametes.

George F. Papenfuss
The Johns Hopkins University

## ON THE SCIENTIFIC NAME OF THE WEBBING CLOTHES MOTH

The webbing or common clothes moth, *Tineola bisselliella,* was first described by Hummel in 1823 (Essais Entomologiques 3: 13). In spite of the fact that the specific name was spelled with two s's in the original description, only one s is used by most writers at the present time. This is true of authors in Europe as well as of those in this country. Dyar[1] and Walsingham,[2] however, both spell the name with two s's.

The mistake in spelling is probably due to the fact that few writers have had an opportunity to see Hum-

[1] *U. S. Nat. Mus. Bul.,* 52: 570, 1902.
[2] *Zool. Soc. London, Proc.,* 1907, p. 1026, 1908.

mel's original description. The publication, "Essais Entomologiques," Nos. 1 to 7, was printed in St. Petersburg and was evidently issued in installments from 1822 to 1829. According to the Union list of serials in libraries of the United States and Canada, only three institutions have copies, and none of them owns the complete work. The Museum of Comparative Zoology (Cambridge) is listed as having Nos. 4 and 6; the Academy of Natural Sciences (Philadelphia) Nos. 4 to 7; and the American Philosophical Society (Philadelphia) No. 6.

The department of entomology at Cornell University has the good fortune to own all seven numbers of these interesting essays. On the inside of the front cover appears the following statement: "A very rare work. This copy contains No. VII, of which Hagen observed, "so excessively rare as scarcely to be known." " In Hagen's "Bibliotheca Entomologica" (1862, Vol. 1, p. 391) under the title, "Essais Entomologiques" he says, "Die Essais sind nicht häufig; No. 7 sogar äusserst selten und kaum gekannt."

Hummel's original description of the webbing clothes moth, in this rare and interesting publication, is written in Latin and is followed by a brief statement in French regarding the habits of the insect. Suggestions are also given for controlling the pest, especially in furniture. Preceding the description is the scientific name, *Tinea bissellìella,* followed by an asterisk which refers to a footnote at the bottom of the page. The footnote reads, "Du mot latin 'bissellium,' canapé." But Hummel may not have been as well versed in the classics as he was in entomology, for his spelling of the Latin word is incorrect. The word "bisellium" has but one s. A Latin lexicon gives the following definition: "Bisellium, a splendid ornamental seat of honor (so called because there was room for two persons upon it, although only one sat thereon). . . ."

When Zeller[3] wrote a more extensive description of this insect he dropped the second s in *bissellìella.* Perhaps Zeller was a better student of the classics than Hummel. In 1853 Herrich-Schäffer placed the species in the genus *Tineola* and he also used one s. Walsingham[2] criticizes Zeller's spelling and calls attention to the fact that Hummel used two s's.

According to the rules of priority, a name must stand as published in the original description. Therefore, although the Latin word was misspelled by Hummel, the mistake must stand and the specific name of the webbing clothes moth must remain *bissellìella.*

GLENN W. HERRICK
GRACE H. GRISWOLD

CORNELL UNIVERSITY

[3] *Linnaea Entomologica,* 6: 166, 1852.
[4] *Syst. Bearb. Schmett. Eur.,* 5: 81, 1853.

## HUMAN NECROBACILLOSIS

NECROBACILLOSIS is an acute infectious disease due to *Actinomyces necrophorus* Löffler. This condition was probably first noticed by Dammann, in 1870, in diphtheritic infections in calves. Schmorl (1891) reported a fatal enzootic occurring the previous year among his laboratory rabbits. *A. necrophorus* was isolated from the caseonecrotic lesions. Schmorl and one of his assistants each had a small abscess on one finger from handling these rabbits. Stained smears of the pus showed the characteristic gram-negative, beaded bacillus. In 1910, the writer isolated *A. necrophorus* from the lesions on the hand of a veterinary inspector.

Following the above reports of human necrobacillosis, the literature contains cases of pseudodiphtheria, infections of the arm, abscesses and necrosis of the tissues of the hip joint, retropharyngeal abscess with gangrene and extension into the perithracheal and subcutaneous tissue and mediastinum. Two deaths occurred in the series. Recently the writer isolated *A. necrophorus* from a lung abscess of man.

Among the principal pathologic conditions (other than man) in which *A. necrophorus* is found may be mentioned lip and leg ulceration of sheep, gangrenous dermatitis of horses and mules, necrotic stomatitis in cattle and multiple necrotic foci in the livers of cattle and hogs. Spontaneous necrobacillosis has been observed in nineteen different species of animals.

*A. necrophorus* is a pleomorphic anaerobe. It may vary from cocci to long filaments, and from solid stained rods to filaments with granules. Spores are not formed. It is gram-negative.

Several mediums have been used for the growth of *A. necrophorus,* but a medium of veal infusion, peptone and cystine is very satisfactory. For primary isolation serum should be added.

To obtain the woolly colonies in agar stab cultures, one must not use too stiff an agar, 0.3 per cent. being satisfactory for the demonstration.

As *A. necrophorus* does not produce group agglutinins the agglutination reaction can not be used for the differentiation of this organism.

Hemolysis is another property that is variable; some authors state that necrophorus is strongly hemolytic, while others state that it is non-hemolytic.

The fermentation of carbohydrates is, likewise, at variance.

Subcutaneous injection of the microorganism into the rabbit produces an area of necrosis and, after a time, invasion of the internal organs, although some strains do not produce anything beyond the local lesion, which heals.

The difficulty of isolation of anaerobes in general, and of *A. necrophorus* in particular, is probably responsible for the low record of human cases of necrobacillosis. Material containing a pleomorphic bacillus with beaded threads should be grown under anaerobic conditions, in or on mediums containing serum. Anaerobic cultures of the blood should be made in all cases of infectious jaundice. Some of the tubercular hips are, in all probability, necrophorus infections.

FREDERICK W. SHAW

MEDICAL COLLEGE OF VIRGINIA
RICHMOND

# SCIENTIFIC APPARATUS AND LABORATORY METHODS

## A METHOD AND THE APPARATUS FOR THE STUDY OF PERMEABILITY OF GASES THROUGH THE BIRD'S EGG-SHELL

OUR previous study[1] of such physical factors of the eggshell as breaking strength, thickness, and relative number and size of pores (observed microscopically) convinced us that the eggshell has definite characteristics peculiar to the species of bird, the flock of birds of the same species, the birds of the same flock, and in a less degree to the eggs laid by the same individual.

Yet the structural and physical properties of the eggshell are found to be very important in regard to the storage and preservation of eggs for future use. For example, an egg with a thin or very porous eggshell would likely more rapidly evaporate or lose moisture, more readily absorb outside odors and gases, and allow more easy penetration by micro-organisms. All these conditions eventually would lead to some changes in physical state and possibly in chemical composition of the egg-contents and thus soon to a decrease in the nutritive value of the eggs.

Furthermore, the structural and physical properties of the eggshell have their biological significance. There is a constant loss of moisture and interchange of respiratory gases through the eggshell during the incubation. This rate of interchange of gases, or absorption of oxygen and elimination of carbon dioxide, is gradually increasing in volume per time with the embryonic growth and development. On the other hand, the eggshell furnishes the largest portion of the calcium needed for the building up of the skeleton of the developing embryo, thus leading to some changes in its physical properties. An egg with extremely thin or thick shell may therefore present an important biological problem in relation to the developing embryo.

It is evident, however, that from both the economic and biological points of view a reliable quantitative direct method of measuring the quality of a bird's eggshell would be very desirable.

In view of the above facts, during the past three years, our laboratory of experimental embryology has developed and improved primarily for scientific use a special electric apparatus for the direct and accurate measurement of the permeability of the bird's eggshell to various gases.

The apparatus, as shown diagrammatically in the accompanying Fig. 1, operates on the principle of

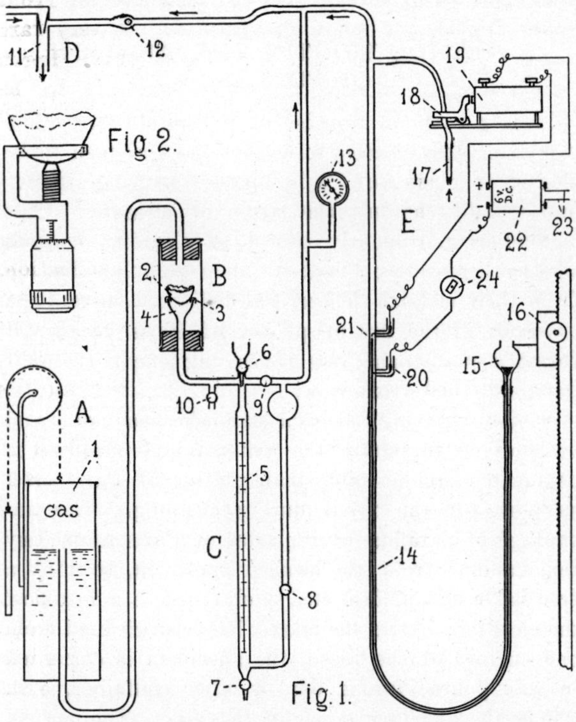


FIG. 1. A diagram of the apparatus for measurement of the permeability of a gas through the bird's eggshell. A, gas holder (1) with a gas; B, eggshell chamber, shown with eggshell (2), rubber gasket (3), and funnel (4) of one-inch inside diameter; C, micro-gas meter, consisting of a 50-cc. burette (5) funnel with glass stopper (6) for refilling of the burette (5) with water, drain stopcock (7), control stopcock (8), set up stopcock (9), vacuum relief stopcock (10); D, vacuum pump, including water suction pump (11) and back pressure valve (12); E, automatic vacuum controlling mechanism, consisting of vacuum gauge (13), adjustable monometer (14) with level bulb (15) and slide with screw (16), capillary tube (17), lever (18), induction coil (19), fixed contact point of the monometer (20), break point of the monometer (21), rectifying transformer (22), line of alternating current (23), and switch for the vacuum-controlling mechanism (24).

FIG. 2. A micrometric spherometer shown with a portion of eggshell, the surface of which is to be measured.

[1] A. L. Romanoff, "Study of the Physical Properties of the Hen's Eggshell in Relation to the Function of Shell-secretory Glands," *Biol. Bull.*, 56: 351–356, 1929.

suction of the gas in question through the portion of the eggshell (B-2). The passing gas is measured in an especially designed micro-gas meter (C) and a constant predetermined vacuum is maintained by an adjustable self-controlled monometer (E), operated automatically by electricity.

The volume of gas which passes through the portion of eggshell is read in cc./min./sq. cm. The data are obtained from the table of calculated and corrected values obtained after measurement of the curvature of eggshell by a special micrometric spherometer (Fig. 2).

ALEXIS L. ROMANOFF

CORNELL UNIVERSITY

## A METHOD FOR THE PREPARATION OF FOSSILS

IT is a common practise of paleontologists, when preparing fossil shells, to cement the specimen to be cleaned in plaster of Paris, thereby insuring rigidity and stability against the strain of cleaning. This method is particularly useful in cleaning delicate shells otherwise too fragile to allow complete freeing from their matrix. There is a distinct disadvantage, however, in the use of plaster of Paris because it forms a permanent base concealing one surface of the fossil shell from view.

While preparing Paleozoic star-fishes, echinoids and brachiopods for study, the writer found paraffine to be much more desirable than plaster of Paris as a support for the fossil during cleaning. The advantage of paraffine over plaster of Paris is its easy removability from the cleaned specimen, so that a free valve or star-fish, etc., is obtained as a result of the cleaning. After the matrix has been cleaned from one surface of the fossil, the specimen is cemented in wax poured into a box or other container, with the cleaned surface down in the wax. The matrix is then worked off the opposite surface, leaving a completely cleaned specimen embedded in the wax. For greater rigidity, the specimen and its paraffine base can be cemented in plaster. After cleaning, the plaster is broken away from the wax base and the paraffine dissolved away by xylol or cotton soaked in xylol for very delicate shells. In this way a number of Paleozoic star-fishes of all sizes have been freed completely from their matrix, and many rare and new brachiopod shells have been cleaned internally and externally.

The method has proved useful in preparing such delicate structures as the loops of the Terebratulidae. The loop is exposed on one side, then wax is poured on this exposed surface of the loop. This gives a rigid base which will allow working the matrix away from the loop from the other side. Dissolving the paraffine leaves a free loop.

In order to prevent the paraffine from softening during the cleaning, which is commonly carried out near a strong, hot light under a binocular microscope, it is frequently necessary to plunge the embedded specimen into cold water. As long as the wax is kept cool and stiff it is quite as safe a bedding medium as plaster of Paris. It is sometimes desirable to perform the entire cleaning process under water. Besides keeping the wax stiff, this has the advantage of making a strong contrast between shell and matrix.

By the above method it is possible to secure the interior of either valve of brachiopods in which both valves are in conjunction. The particular valve desired is cemented in the paraffine base. Then the valve whose interior is not wanted is ground away and cleaning of the desired valve progresses.

In making preparations such as those described above, the dental engine is very useful, but for the most delicate work against the shell, needles sharpened to a chisel edge are the best tools.

G. ARTHUR COOPER

UNITED STATES NATIONAL MUSEUM

# SPECIAL ARTICLES

## THE UTILIZATION OF ADSORBED IONS BY PLANTS[1]

RESTRICTED Brownian movement of ions is one of the great differences between a nutrient solution and a natural soil. In culture solutions the nutrient ions are free to move (diffusible), while in soils they are "adsorbed" on colloidal particles, fixed in crystals and thus exist under conditions of constraint.

In the study of the liberation of adsorbed ions by the plant itself it is necessary that at the outset the nutrient ions be present in adsorbed form only. Otherwise the free ions in the liquid phase could replace the adsorbed elements (ionic exchange)[2] and the problem would approach a mere nutrient solution experiment. Soybean plants were grown in systems containing but *one nutrient ion* (calcium), which for purposes of comparison was either free in solution or adsorbed on colloids or fixed in the interior of crystals.

### EXPERIMENTAL METHOD

(a) *Free calcium ions in the soil solution.* Ca-acetate and $CaCl_2$ are very soluble. $CaCO_3$ furnishes Ca ions according to the $CO_2$ content of the system.

(b) *Adsorbed Ca ions on colloids.* Prolonged electrodialyses of soil colloids removes all free and adsorbed

[1] Missouri Agricultural Experiment Station, Journal Series No. 329.

[2] H. Jenny, *Jour. Phys. Chem.*, 36: 2217–2258, 1932.

ions and the resulting H-systems can be transformed into pure Ca-colloids by addition of $Ca(OH)_2$. These adsorbed Ca ions are all exchangeable. Putnam clay and colloidal bentonite were thus treated. Artificial zeolite (permutite) was prepared as described previously.[3]

(c) *Non-exchangeable Ca ions in the interior of close packed crystal lattices.* Anorthite, a Ca-alumino silicate, was ground in a mortar and—as all the other dried colloids—passed through a 100 mesh sieve. Only those Ca ions seated in the outer surface of the mineral particles are exchangeable.

Soybean seedlings were put into nursery bottles (four plants) containing a uniform mixture of 300 grams of purified quartz sand and various amounts of the above Ca-compounds. All systems had an initial pH of 7. The water content was adjusted twice daily to 20 per cent. of the weight.

### COMPARISON BETWEEN ADSORBED IONS AND NON-EXCHANGEABLE IONS

Fig. 1 (solid lines) shows that the soybean plant can live and do well in media which contain mainly

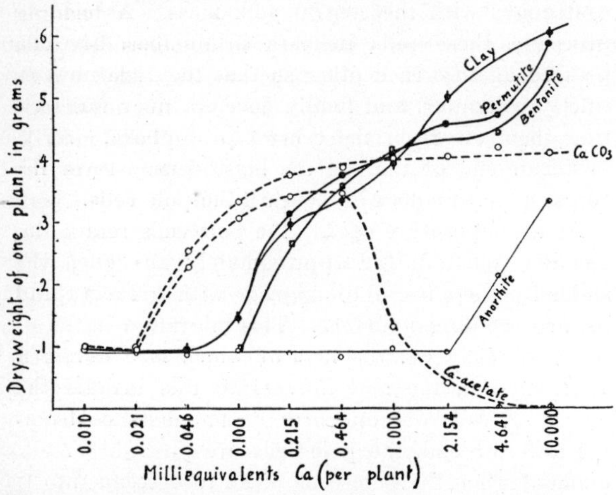


FIG. 1. Growth of soybean plants as a function of amount and form of calcium in the medium.

adsorbed Ca ions. This holds true even for sterile systems, in absence of microorganisms. On the other hand, Ca ions in the interior of crystal lattices can not be utilized or only with difficulty. The growth observed on anorthite at very high calcium concentrations is very likely due to exchangeable surface cations resulting from the grinding process of the mineral.

### COMPARISON BETWEEN ADSORBED IONS AND FREE IONS

Under low calcium concentrations the plant yields are much higher for the "free Ca" system than for the "adsorbed" one, indicating that the plant encounters considerable difficulty in obtaining the adsorbed ions. The situation becomes entirely reversed at higher Ca concentrations where, most strikingly, the plants grow best on adsorbed ions, surpassing even the $CaCO_3$ system. This indicates a specific behavior of adsorbed ions in regard to plant growth.

[3] H. Jenny, *Kolloid. chem. Beih.* 23: 428–472, 1927.

### THE MECHANISM OF LIBERATION OF ADSORBED IONS BY PLANTS

Fig. 1 demonstrates that plants are able to free adsorbed ions. This is by no means a simple process. The Ca-colloids used form no true solutions, and the concept of the solubility product can not be applied. In a strictly physico-chemical sense, the Ca-colloids are practically insoluble.

One might conceive the picture that the plant simply removes the adsorbed Ca, attracts it, pulls it away, so to speak. But in this case free electric charges would be left on the particle, leading to enormous potential differences in the electric double layer. It would be difficult to reconcile such a mechanism with the known laws of electrostatics.

It is possible, however, to have a liberation of adsorbed Ca by means of ionic exchange. In such a case—where hydrolysis is negligible—the plant would have to excrete cations other than Ca and these ions would replace the adsorbed calcium. The excreted cations should be found on the colloid. The following experiment is interesting in this respect.

Thirty soybean seedlings were transplanted into 100 cc of 2.50 per cent. pure Ca-clay suspension having a pH of 6.30 and containing 1.500 milliequivalents of adsorbed Ca ions. The plants were harvested 35 days later and after subtracting the original Ca content of the sprouted beans (0.0280 minus 0.0076g. Ca) it appeared *that the plants had removed from the clay 1.020 milliequivalents Ca.* The reaction of the sol had dropped from pH 6.30 to 4.32. Evidently the colloidal particles contained now numerous H ions. These were determined by titration with $Ca(OH)_2$ and it was found that *the clay carried 0.948 milliequivalents H ions which it did not possess at the beginning of the experiment.* In other words, it appears that an exchange has taken place which is stoichiometrical (93 per cent.) within the limits of the present technique. These data and other unpublished trials suggest that *the plant has excreted H ions which have replaced the Ca ions on the clay enabling them to enter the plant.* For every Ca ion that went into the plant, two hydrogen ions are found on the colloidal particles.

### PRACTICAL CONCLUSIONS

(1) It has been demonstrated quantitatively that total analysis of the soil is a poor indicator of soil fertility because the determination does not differentiate between adsorbed and non-exchangeable lattice ions.

(2) Since the plant can feed successfully on adsorbed ions, it appears that the significance of the "soil solution" has been overestimated.

(3) The solubility concept is not adequate enough to account for plant growth in soils of humid regions. Ionic exchange must be taken into consideration.

(4) The study of the adsorbed (exchangeable) ions in the soil offers great possibilities for a better understanding of many soil-plant relationships and soil fertility problems (*e.g.*, utilization of fertilizers, distribution of pasture vegetation, soil acidity, activity of soil microorganisms).

HANS JENNY
E. W. COWAN

DEPARTMENT OF SOILS
COLUMBIA, MISSOURI

## OBSERVATIONS ON EARLY DEVELOPMENTAL PROCESSES IN THE LIVING EGG OF DROSOPHILA

DUE to the fact that the egg of Drosophila is covered by a semi-opaque chorionic membrane, our knowledge of the course and rate of early developmental processes has, up to the present time, been gained only by a study of preserved material, prepared by means of the usual cytological technique. Such a study has not only been a laborious one because of the inherent limitations of a method requiring the reconstruction of a three-dimensional object from serial sections, but it has also been open to error because of the uncertainty as to the age of an egg at the time of deposition. This latter source of difficulty has heretofore been overcome to a large extent by keeping under observation a laying female, rejecting the first eggs laid, and carefully timing eggs laid subsequently. Under suitable conditions, fertilized eggs are not retained by the female for more than twenty minutes.

During the past summer, we found a simple and satisfactory method for observing early embryonic development in the living egg. An egg, firmly imbedded in the agar in which it has been laid, or fastened to a glass slide by a film of Ambroid cement, may be dechorionated with fine, sharp needles under a binocular microscope. It is then mounted in water, and a thin coverslip, supported by bits of glass, placed over it. As the inner membranes are transparent, developmental changes may be followed under high powers, though the definition of the earliest cleavage figures is somewhat obscured by the overlying yolk granules. While under observation, the egg can be rolled about by pushing the coverlip slightly from side to side.

In the early egg, the protoplasmic islands around the first cleavage nuclei appear as lighter spherical regions well marked off from the dense surrounding yolk. As cleavage proceeds, these islands increase in number and decrease in size, giving the egg a "dappled" appearance. Soon a lighter grayish cap arises at the posterior end, presaging the formation of the pole or germ-tract cells. These are pushed out as large buds, which then constrict off from the underlying ooplasm with great rapidity, forming a conspicuous layer; this is separated from the adjacent ooplasm by a clear fluid-filled space. At a temperature of 22° the pole cell formation is approximately complete within 20 to 30 minutes after the first bud forms. Protoplasmic islands containing the yolk nuclei now remain in the center, while the cleavage nuclei migrate to the periphery of the egg to form the blastoderm. Here they push out bud-like prominences over the entire surface, except in the region of the pole cells. This gives the cleaving egg a morula-like appearance, which is most pronounced at the anterior end. Dividing walls can now be seen growing inward and enclosing each blastodermic nucleus in a cubical protoplasmic area which is still continuous with the central yolk mass. As cleavage proceeds, these cells increase in number, are compressed against each other so that they are now distinctly columnar, and finally develop inner walls cutting them off from the central protoplasm. At the posterior end of the egg the blastodermic layer next forms a continuous wall beneath the pole cells.

At a temperature of 22° the pole cells retain their terminal position for approximately an hour, when suddenly they begin to migrate with great rapidity toward the dorsal surface. This migration initiates a series of changes: the first of which is a dorsal invagination in the mid line. Into this invagination, which arises about one fifth of the distance toward the anterior end, the pole cells are pushed.[1] At the moment when the pole cells begin to descend into the cup-like invagination, the cells along the entire dorsal surface begin to group themselves into metameres. These are pronounced by the time the pole cells disappear within the dorsal invagination. At 22° C. the entire series of growth changes, including migration, invagination and metamere formation, occurs within the brief period of 10 to 15 minutes.

Cinematographic records of the processes described above as well as of subsequent embryological changes are now being made, and will serve as the basis for a more extensive report to be given later.

GEORGE P. CHILD
RUTH B. HOWLAND

WASHINGTON SQUARE COLLEGE
NEW YORK UNIVERSITY

[1] The force exerted seems to be due to a rapid upward growth of the ventral blastoderm. This point, however, needs further careful study.

# SCIENCE

VOL. 77 FRIDAY, APRIL 28, 1933 No. 2000

*From the Ponderable to the Imponderable:* PROFESSOR OTTO HAHN 397

*Scientific Events:*
*Human Remains Discovered by the British East African Expedition; The Morris Arboretum of the University of Pennsylvania; Dedication of the George Eastman Research Laboratories of the Massachusetts Institute of Technology; The Minnesota Academy of Science; The Salt Lake City Meeting of the Pacific Division of the American Association for the Advancement of Science* 404

*Scientific Notes and News* 406

*Discussion:*
*The High Cost of German Medical and Scientific Periodicals:* EILEEN R. CUNNINGHAM. *Is Longevity Compatible with Optimum Growth?:* DR. C. M. MCCAY. *Soluble Sesquioxides and Organic Matter from Alkali Treatments on Soils:* G. T. SHAW and DR. R. R. MCKIBBIN. *The Attraction of Spheres:* HENRY NORRIS RUSSELL 409

*Scientific Apparatus and Laboratory Methods:*
*A Two-field Stroboscope:* PROFESSOR PAUL F. GAEHR. *Regulating the Air Supply of Micro Burners:* CORNELIUS A. DALY 412

*Special Articles:*
*Accelerated, Experimental Poliomyelitis in Nasally Instilled Monkeys:* DR. SIMON FLEXNER 413

*Science News* 8

SCIENCE: A Weekly Journal devoted to the Advancement of Science, edited by J. MCKEEN CATTELL and published every Friday by

THE SCIENCE PRESS

New York City: Grand Central Terminal
Lancaster, Pa. Garrison, N. Y.

Annual Subscription, $6.00 Single Copies, 15 Cts.

SCIENCE is the official organ of the American Association for the Advancement of Science. Information regarding membership in the Association may be secured from the office of the permanent secretary, in the Smithsonian Institution Building, Washington, D. C.

# FROM THE PONDERABLE TO THE IMPONDERABLE[1]

By Professor OTTO HAHN

DIRECTOR KAISER WILHELM INSTITUTE FOR CHEMISTRY, BERLIN-DAHLEM, NON-RESIDENT LECTURER IN CHEMISTRY AT CORNELL UNIVERSITY ON THE GEORGE FISHER BAKER FOUNDATION

CHEMISTRY has for its purpose the study of the composition of our material world. Its first task is to determine the simple basic substances—the chemical elements—out of which all other substances are made, and artificially to produce new kinds of substances from these same elements. After its problem had been thus recognized and defined, thanks chiefly to Robert Boyle, chemistry could be spoken of as a "science," striving, in contrast to the direction of earlier efforts, towards an ideal objective through unprejudiced researches. The prerequisite for these researches was the recognition of the fact that the weight of a chemical compound is equal to the sum of the weights of its constituents. We owe to the French chemist Lavoisier the recognition of the full significance and the ingenious application of this law. We have him to thank for introducing the well-known balance as a reliable guide in chemical work, whereby Lavoisier became the true founder of modern chemistry whose victorious march began in the nineteenth century and has continued at a steadily increasing tempo.

To be sure, Lavoisier's immortal services were poorly rewarded by his contemporaries; in 1794, during the confusion of the French Revolution, the Revolutionary Tribunal sent him to the guillotine.

My topic is "From the Ponderable to the Imponderable" in chemistry, in physics, and I might also add, in biology. How far can we extend the limits of our qualitative and quantitative tests of chemical compounds? Are there methods of investigation that are reliable at and beyond the present limits of our balances? What are the lower limits?

As a science develops, its methods are improved and its aids become more and more refined. The

[1] Introductory public lecture.

quantitative analytical balance of the time of Lavoisier certainly differed very considerably from the balances used in chemical laboratories to-day by every young student of chemistry. But even along this line development has not yet ceased. As it becomes possible to work with smaller and still smaller quantities of material, to that same degree we refine our analytical methods and the delicacy of our tests. The methods of "microchemistry" have now been added to those of ordinary or "macro" chemistry.

The usual modern analytical balance permits a mass of a few hundred grams to be weighed accurately to within one ten-thousandth of a gram. About thirty years ago Nernst devised the micro-balance that bears his name, which weighs a few milligrams of material to within a few millionths of a gram. This device was followed by the Kuhlmann balance—now widely used in microchemistry—which weighs amounts of even twenty grams to within a millionth of a gram. This was a tremendous advance, but the end was not yet; special methods enable us to weigh smaller amounts of material with very much greater accuracy.

In such direct weighings the material is always still available in masses that are fractions of grams; by other methods it is possible to make qualitative and quantitative determinations of chemical compounds in masses whose lower limit is finally determined by their visibility under the microscope. It may be stated as a quite general truth that whenever, for any reason, it seems necessary positively to determine minute amounts of material, there will be found means and ways for doing so. This statement may be explained by a few examples.

When the world war was over and the victors imposed upon Germany the task of finding enormous sums for "reparations," Fritz Haber proposed to himself the most interesting scheme of extracting gold from the inexhaustible reservoir of the oceans. Previous determinations by other investigators had placed the gold content of sea water at five to ten milligrams of gold per metric ton (one thousand kilograms) of water. The gold ores of South Africa contain about one thousand times more gold per ton than does sea water, but the greater ease of working water, as compared with rigid rock, made the task seem very promising. If it succeeded it would open up an inexhaustible source of gold, for Arrhenius had estimated that, with a richness of six milligrams of gold per ton of water, the total content of all the seas amounted to eight billions of tons of gold.

The plan itself—to secure gold in this way—did not succeed and could not succeed. Instead of the assumed gold-content of five to ten milligrams per ton, Haber's numerous experiments showed only about one thousandth as much. But they accomplished a great advance in the analytical methods for separating out minute amounts of material. Microscopic measurement of the tiny gold spherules obtained from the precipitation enables one to determine with certainty one ten-millionth of a gram or less. This determination of microscopic traces of gold was successfully employed in explaining and combating experiments that in their day caused great excitement because they seemed to indicate the supposed transmutation of mercury into gold.

Mercury furnishes another illustration in this connection. While Alfred Stock was working in Berlin he became a victim of the injurious effects of small amounts of mercury. He combined his great educational campaign regarding the deleterious nature of the cheaper amalgam dental fillings, with the development of a demonstration of the presence of very small amounts of mercury in the saliva, in urine, and in exhaled air. As a result it is possible to demonstrate the presence of a hundred millionth of a gram of mercury in the form of tiny crystals of mercury iodide, so minute as to be barely visible under the microscope.

Many other chemical elements and compounds might be cited, that have been identified in such amounts by weight as would never have been possible without the aid of the increasingly important methods of microchemistry.

It will now be asked whether there is really any good reason for such extraordinary refinement in our experimental aids for recognizing and quantitatively determining such small amounts. It is by no means a matter of indifference whether we can prove the presence somewhere of a minute amount of a metal or of a chemical compound as an impurity of other metals or compounds. Modern research has demonstrated the great influence exerted upon the hardness, ductility and durability of metals by very small additions of other substances to them. Again, in all the life processes of plants as well as of animals, substances present in minutest amounts often play a much greater rôle than do those substances occurring in easily determinable quantities. Mere mention of enzymes, hormones, vitamins, is sufficient to point out such substances to you; we shall return later to their consideration.

In order to understand how it is that the smallest amount of a substance can so often produce such great effects, it must be remembered that even the smallest of the weights mentioned above, *viz.*, one one-hundred-millionth of a gram consists nevertheless of a very large number of those minute particles that we call atoms or molecules.

As to the number of molecules obtained in a given weight of a chemical compound, this can be accurately determined if we know its molecular weight, as it is called; and the latter can almost always be readily ascertained. The atomic or molecular weight in grams of a substance contains the inconceivably large number of $6 \times 10^{23}$ atoms or molecules. Some interesting computations by the English physicist Aston[2] enable one to form some conception of their quantity. Suppose we have an absolutely evacuated incandescent lamp bulb of the usual size, and make an opening into it so fine that one million molecules of air enter in one second. Then one hundred million years must elapse before the bulb will fill with air to atmospheric pressure.

Again, suppose that in some way each of the molecules in the two hundred grams of water contained in an ordinary glass of water could be made visible, could be labeled or tagged. If this glassful of water were then poured into the ocean at any point—Australia, the Gulf of Mexico, some Russian river—then after a very long time the two hundred grams would be uniformly distributed throughout the oceans of the globe. Now if a glass of water were dipped up at random from the ocean at any point, whether from the surface or from a depth of six thousand meters, there would be found more than two thousand of those tagged molecules in this glass of sea water.

Finally, take an example from my own particular field of radioactivity. Through atomic disintegration the element uranium gradually changes into the element lead, in fact during every second ten thousand atoms are converted per gram of uranium. But seventy-one million years must elapse before this single gram of uranium has formed one hundredth of a gram of lead.

Returning to the tiny amounts of gold and of mercury mentioned above, it is easily computed that there must be millions of millions of atoms or of molecules in the microscopic particle of gold or of the mercury salt referred to. It is justifiable to inquire whether there are methods by which one can recognize amounts even smaller than those considered above—quantities lying beyond the limits of direct weighing or of direct vision. This question is answerable distinctly in the affirmative, and we shall now consider a series of such methods.

First in interest among these methods is that of spectrum analysis, devised by Bunsen and Kirchhoff, which reveals the chemical composition of a substance by the spectral lines that its vapor emits under appropriate excitation. You all know that this method has revealed to us the chemical composition of the heavenly bodies, and proved that they consist of precisely the same elements as does our earth. Bunsen and Kirchhoff sought to determine the smallest amount by weight that was recognizable by their method, and they found that in the case of sodium as little as $3 \times 10^{-10}$ gram could be detected spectroscopically. To be sure, the practical execution of their experiments required considerably larger amounts (practical *vs* theoretical sensitivity). Many gaseous elements have a much higher spectroscopic sensitivity than do the solid metals like sodium. Paneth's researches in particular should be mentioned in this connection. He has been able to identify the noble gas helium in amounts as small as $2 \times 10^{-14}$ gram, and to make quantitative determinations of as little as $2 \times 10^{-11}$ gram, employing Otto Stern's later refinements of Pirani's method. Here again is illustrated the fact—so gratifying for the progress of science—that when a new task is set the means and methods for accomplishing it are also often discovered. Paneth and his coworkers employed his refined spectroscopic method in their quantitative determinations of the minute helium content of a large number of iron meteorites, and thereby determined the age of these heavenly bodies. Paneth came to the remarkable conclusion that meteorites probably originated within our solar system and not—as was previously assumed—from fixed stars outside that system.

Spectrum analysis has recently found an extraordinarily fruitful field in applied qualitative and quantitative chemical analysis. The demonstration by spectrum analysis of the "ultimate lines" of the elements now enters into an ideal contest with former micro-analytical methods, "spot" analysis and potentiometric titration in the determination of the least traces of impurities in metals, forensic preparations, and other substances (Gerlach and his coworkers).

Of late years x-ray spectroscopy also has developed as a powerful tool for chemical research, making possible the discovery of new elements at their lowest concentration, and the determination of impurities in metals that would certainly have escaped detection by ordinary chemical analysis.

To consider this broad and fruitful field of study in more detail would take us far beyond the limits of a one-hour address. A single method of optical identification may briefly be considered, however, since it served in its day to solve a problem that was of interest to the non-technical world. Organic chemistry knows of dyes whose aqueous solutions have very intense coloring powers; infinitely minute amounts of these dyes can be detected even at extraordinary degrees of dilution. Among these coloring substances is fluorescein, discovered by A. von Baeyer. At the suggestion of von Baeyer this property of fluorescein was employed in 1877 to determine a supposed subterranean connection between the Danube and the Rhine rivers. A solution of ten kilograms of fluorescein was sunk in the Danube near

[2] F. W. Aston, *Nature*, 110: 702, 1922.

its head springs. After an interval of about sixty hours the characteristic fluorescence of the dye appeared in a little river which empties into Lake Constance and thence into the Rhine, but has no visible connection with the Danube. The coloration lasted for about thirty-six hours. The supposed connection between the two rivers has been proven experimentally.

Turning from these optical methods that impress the vision, to methods working through other senses, our attention is held above all by such substances as appeal to the sense of smell. Here it is found that through this sense one can recognize substances present in quantities that are far below the limits of the chemical balance.

As early as 1887 a classical investigation in this field was carried out jointly by Emil Fischer and E. Penzoldt. Up to that time the sense of smell was thought to be most sensitive toward the odor of attar of roses. The presence of an unbelievably small trace of this perfume can be detected in this manner. But these two investigators found that even smaller amounts of a derivative of hydrogen sulfide, mercaptan, could readily be recognized through its powerful and highly disgusting odor. When the air of the room contained by volume one part of mercaptan in three hundred million parts of air, the stench was so penetrating that "the odor passed off only gradually even after opening four windows, two doors, and setting up a strong draft." Fischer and Penzoldt found that as minute an amount as one part in fifty thousand million of air could thus be recognized. On the assumption that about fifty cubic centimeters of air must flow past the olfactory nerves of the nasal passages to make an odor noticeable, the amount of mercaptan that can be recognized by its stench is one four hundred and sixty thousand millionth of a gram, an absolutely unweighable quantity.

In the course of time the limits of detection by smell were determined for many other agreeable and evil smelling substances, and a great many of them were found to be as potent as is mercaptan. Among the fragrant substances are ionon (the essence of the violet) and vanillin (the fragrant substance in vanilla). Among the evil-smelling bodies may be mentioned butyric acid, whence comes the stench of rancid butter. The enjoyment of sweet butter is spoiled for us by absolutely unweighable amounts of that compound.

A computation of the number of molecules of these substances detectable by smell always shows that many million molecules of the substance are involved per cubic centimeter of air. There is no great wonder, then, that certain animals seem to be able to recognize a very much smaller amount of disagreeable and of fragrant substances. The dog's and the insect's sense of smell are good examples, and particularly that of butterflies—whose scenting powers actually border on the marvelous. The Swiss naturalists Fabre and Forel report the following experiment: The caterpillar of a butterfly was raised in the city of Zurich, spun its cocoon and emerged the following spring as a female butterfly. This female was imprisoned in a room with windows open, but within two days more than one hundred males of the same species had gathered in the room; they had traveled a number of kilometers from the forests in the environs of Zurich. Such statements might be relegated to the realm of fable had they not been adequately confirmed.

We turn now to another field. The preceding methods for identifying minute amounts of material have in common the feature that the substance is always recognized by some one of its specific characters. But there is an almost boundless number of phenomena in which the presence or absence of minute amounts of substances is detected, not directly, but through the effects they produce. Among these the most important are the effects upon life processes.

Thus, many metals and chemical compounds exert a poisoning influence on the lower organisms. Disinfection and antiseptic methods are based upon this fact. A couple of pictures showed how small the amount may be and yet produce an evident effect.

The first slide showed a group of houses in a small town of southern Germany. These houses are roofed with a flaggy limestone from the Jura, and in the course of time the growth of a great variety of mosses and lichens has given these slabs a beautiful dark patina. The picture showed that some of these house roofs are crossed by a pair of parallel white streaks. There the growth of moss and lichens is absent. The reason for this is that two naked copper wires pass above these houses, the rain dissolves traces of copper, the extremely dilute copper solution drips on the roofs, and in these areas the plant growth is interrupted.

This poisoning effect upon the lower organisms of minute amounts of metal was clearly shown in the next slide. A nutrient agar-agar preparation was inoculated with a culture of *Staphylococcus*, and a silver coin was laid upon it.[3] The dish was kept in the dark and at a low temperature for several days. Under these conditions the bacteria do not multiply, but traces of the silver can nevertheless diffuse through the nutrient. Later the dish was placed in a warm incubator, whereupon a luxuriant growth of bacteria developed. Around the coin, however, there was a space free from bacteria, where the dissolved metal had prevented their growth. In such a case it certainly would be very difficult to prove the presence

[3] H. Beehold, *Kolloid-Z.*, 25: 158, 1919.

of silver by one of the usual chemical methods, for the silver content per cubic centimeter of nutrient solution could have been only a few hundred-millionths of a gram.

Recently the katadyne process had made extensive use of this so-called "oligodynamic" effect. The very large number of papers and patents relating to the sterilization of water, milk, and other substances, testify to the steadily increasing significance of this process. It is interesting to find that the ancient Egyptians employed this disinfecting action of minute amounts of dissolved metal. Open wounds healed better and more rapidly if they were covered with silver plates. The traces of dissolved silver prevented infection. Bone fractures repaired with silver wire show a greatly reduced tendency to infection.

In the cases here mentioned these infinitesimal amounts of material acted as poisons toward low forms of life. Much more important for all life-processes are those cases where the presence of a very small amount of substance is essential for life-processes, where lack of it produces deficiency phenomena and can mean illness and death.

This brings us to the supremely important field of the enzymes, vitamins and hormones. The catalytic enzyme or ferment reactions that are so determinative of organic phenomena find their inorganic, model-like counterpart in the catalytic decomposition of hydrogen peroxide into water and oxygen by minute traces of the noble metals present in the most finely divided state. Many years ago Bredig found that three millionths of a gram of colloidal platinum per liter of water produced a marked acceleration in the decomposition of hydrogen peroxide. Conversely, the slightest trace of "catalytic poisons" suffices to hinder this action by platinum; scarcely more than one millionth of a gram of hydrocyanic acid per liter of water was found to produce such a "poisoning."

The living cell shows corresponding catalytic reactions. The respiratory ferment, which is indispensable for cell growth, and which has been studied in detail by Otto Warburg, contains minute traces of iron—the so-called "enzyme iron." Only very delicate qualitative reactions can prove the presence of this iron. Nevertheless, the cell's life is extinguished if the iron is removed or its action is chemically prevented. As in the catalysis of hydrogen peroxide by platinum, very minute amounts of hydrocyanic acid put an end to the catalytic action, "poison" the respiratory ferment, and the respiratory activity ceases.

Less understood, as yet, than these enzyme reactions is the mechanism of the effects observed in connection with the "hormones." A few illustrations may be given. The human thyroid gland secretes thyroxine, an organic compound containing iodine, whose absence can induce severe metabolic diseases; in the lower animals a hereditary lack of this compound causes extraordinary effects. An American species of salamander, the Axolotl, often fails to complete its metamorphosis—particularly when in captivity—from the aquatic, gill-breathing larval stage to the fully developed terrestrial, lung-breathing animal. A single abdominal injection of a hundred thousandth of a gram of thyroxine suffices to produce promptly and positively the otherwise suspended metamorphosis.

A tadpole that develops very slowly if at all in water wholly freed of iodine, accomplishes its metamorphosis in a thyroxine solution of one part thyroxine to five thousand million parts water, and more rapidly than it would in an otherwise normal environment.

In these cases minute amounts of organically combined iodine have released vitally important functions, and in other cases minute amounts of other chemical elements have produced corresponding phenomena. During the past year Schmucker[4] in Göttingen has strikingly demonstrated the extraordinary and specific physiological activity of a minimum concentration of boric acid. He experimented with the pollen grains of tropical water lilies whose natural nutrient liquid contains small amounts of boric acid. If this boric acid is removed development ceases; if it is added in amounts of a hundred thousandth to a millionth, normal development is resumed. In this case the boric acid may actually be described as an "inorganic hormone."

Special interest attaches to the growth-producing substance "auxin" recently investigated by the Dutch botanist Went,[5] and prepared in the pure state by the German chemist Kögl.[6] The growth of plants requires extremely slight amounts of this hormone-like compound, in addition to the other materials belonging to plant structures. When an oat-sprout is "topped" to remove the tip, the growth of the sprout is stopped. If a trace of the "auxin" preparation—which can be extracted from the cut-off tip—is applied to the truncated end, growth is revived. An application of the "auxin" to one side of the sprout's end revives the growth on that side only; the sprout therefore curves toward the opposite side. The unit amount of "auxin," that which suffices to cause a curvature of about 10°, has been called the "avena unit." Kögl has now successfully prepared the pure crystallized growth-producing substance "auxin," and it has been found that the growth-unit just defined is produced by the fifty-millionth part of a milligram, that is, $2 \times 10^{-11}$ gram of "auxin." In the first attempts to secure this very interesting substance maize

[4] Schmucker, *Naturwissenschaften*, 20: 839, 1932.
[5] Went, *Naturwissenschaften*, 20: 596, 1932.
[6] Kögl, *Chem. Weekblad*, 29: 21, 1932.

and oat sprouts were used; but even one hundred thousand maize tips contain only very small amounts of "auxin." Its best source was finally found to be human urine, which is a source of many highly important physiological substances. It has been found that every human being, regardless of age or sex, secretes on the average two milligrams of auxin daily.

The foregoing expositions have shown that there are many ways, some direct and some indirect, for proving the presence of substances and determining their exact amounts when the latter are beyond the scope of the chemical balance. At the same time, however, it has been found that even the least of the amounts we have considered consists of a very large number of molecules. Is there, then, no bridge leading from these relatively gross quantities to the individual atoms?

In the closing years of the last century there were discovered the radioactive substances, and these actually do furnish the key that has, at one turn, opened the gate to this field formerly regarded as closed to exploration. The final section of this lecture will therefore be devoted to a consideration of these radioactive substances.

Radioactive elements are those which are subject to spontaneous intra-atomic disintegration. The discharge of small fragments of atoms—the so-called "radioactive rays"—gives rise to new elements possessing new chemical and physical properties. The radiant particles emitted during the disintegration are characterized by an enormous initial velocity and it is because of their high velocity that the particles, in spite of their merely atomic magnitude, reveal their presence in the most varying ways through the effects they produce. These effects of the radiation constitute the fundamental difference between the long-known chemical and the new radioactive methods of investigation. In the former case ordinary stable atoms are used for investigation, and all that has been said shows that many millions of atoms or of molecules are required for such work. In the case of the radioactive substances one measures at the instant of emission the rays coming from the disintegrating atoms. Thus it is not the absolute number of atoms present, but the number of atoms disintegrating during the period of measurement that is of importance. By studying this radiation-intensity it is possible to investigate a whole series of different radioactive atoms (chemical elements) in masses that are far below the limits of chemical identification. By means of their radiations invisible and unweighable masses can be recognized as present, and they can also be accurately analyzed and determined quantitatively. The broad field of applied radiochemistry employs these properties of radioactive substances to study the behavior of imponderable amounts in the presence or the absence of inactive accompanying substances; it puts into our hands the means for attacking and solving chemical and physico-chemical problems unanswerable by other methods.

There is not time to discuss this matter now in any detail and a few brief references must suffice. In connection with spectrum analysis it was mentioned that optical methods enabled us to demonstrate the presence of traces of impurities in metals and chemical compounds. Radioactive methods enable us to go yet further and to study the laws according to which unweighable amounts of foreign materials are taken up by their carriers.

The next photograph showed two crystals of different salts. One was a natural crystal, gypsum, which after irradiation had the striking property of phosphorescence along certain of its crystalline surfaces.[7] There is hardly any doubt but that this selective phosphorescence was due to minute amounts of impurities deposited regularly on the crystal as it was growing. The probable correctness of this explanation was shown by the second crystal, rubidium sulphate, which we made artificially and which contained less than one billionth of a gram of a radioactive substance (lead). This crystal was placed in the dark upon a photographic plate, and the latter was developed after a short exposure. The picture showed plainly that these absolutely imponderable amounts of radioactive material here also were deposited in a regular manner. The remarkable character of this distribution could not possibly be determined by other than radioactive methods, because the infinitesimal amounts involved in these inclusions can not be detected by analytical chemical methods.

When the radioactive substance is not embedded in a crystal, as in the case just considered, but is adsorbed by minute particles in a liquid or a gas, it is possible to determine directly the nature of the radioactive element emitting the rays, from their effects on a photographic plate. The next illustration showed how this is possible.[8]

One could notice that there were a number of dark circular figures of various diameters; the diameters of these circles are quite definitely characteristic of certain radioactive substances. Were other substances of this kind present, the circles or zones would have a different radius. This makes it possible to identify a chemical element in this way when perhaps a thousand or less atoms are present, and there is nothing to prevent the detection of a still smaller number of atoms.

These circles, called "radioactive zones," produced here artificially upon the photographic plate, occur naturally in many minerals and are of prime significance in problems on the history of our earth. In

[7] *Handbuch der Experimentalphysik*, Band XXIII, 2 (Tomaschek).

[8] See Mlle. C. Chamié, *Comptes rendus*, 1929–1931.

the pleochroic halos, so-called, one has to do with very small, circular images; they are found in particularly beautiful development in a fluorite from southern Germany. The colored medium in this case is the decidedly less sensitive rock in place of the highly sensitive photographic plate. Our next slide showed photographs of such zones or halos.[9] They appear as a large number of concentric circles, each circle corresponding to a particular one of such radioactive decomposition-products as are found in uranium or thorium minerals. The interruption of the circular area by brighter annular bands results because the rays are most effective at the respective limits of their so-called "range." Minute traces of radioactive minerals are embedded in the inactive fluorite, and have sent their rays into the surrounding mineral which they have colored.

Experimental determinations of the number of rays necessary to produce these zones and the microscopical measurement of the volume of the radioactive dust particles that caused the halo, enabled Rutherford and Joly to figure out that in many cases several hundreds of millions of years were required to produce such halos. This demonstrates the tremendous age of the solid crust of the earth. The study of these pleochroic halos reveals the almost overwhelming fact that it is possible in this way to demonstrate atomic transformations in which, every few years, one single atom breaks down with the emission of a radiant particle. Compare with this the fact that in one milligram of radium, seventeen million atoms disintegrate every second, and yet thousands of years must elapse before this minute mass of radium has been completely transformed.

Radioactive phenomena, in fact, now offer us the possibility of determining and studying the behavior of substances consisting of only single atoms. The so-called "Wilson cloud-chamber" carries out such work in an especially intensive manner, and in conclusion some slides were presented demonstrating the principle of this method and pointing out what it can accomplish.

When the alpha rays of radioactive substances traverse the air it is well known that they produce positively or negatively charged air particles—the so-called "ions." If this air is saturated with water vapor and then rapidly cooled, the cooling causes the vapor to condense in cloud droplets where these ions are present. Under suitable illumination, the mist in the air chamber is plainly seen to be divided into sharp lines, and these lines correspond to the paths of the ions from the alpha rays. The length of the path represents the range of the alpha rays in air.

Each of the many straight lines corresponds to a radiant particle and therefore to a disintegrated atom. In a case illustrated, the disintegration of two different substances was involved, therefore there were noted two different groups of rays, one having a greater and the other a lesser field of action. Clearly a much smaller number of rays than that shown can be recognized in this way.

The next figure showed something else. In addition to the brush of numerous normal alpha rays, there appeared in one place a longer and much thinner ray.[10] This was a hydrogen ray that had been set in rapid motion by an alpha ray, a rather unusual phenomenon. These fog-tracks aid in the photographic recording of such rare atomic processes. The modern terms atomic disintegration, atomic structure, neutrons, indicate how extraordinarily fruitful for the modern physics of the atom is this method of photographing fog-tracks.

The Wilson photographs clearly demonstrate our ability to detect extremely minute amounts of material, but an even more striking illustration of the sensitivity of this method was furnished by an occurrence in the speaker's laboratory in the Kaiser Wilhelm Institute in Dahlem.

While Wilson photographs were being made in Professor Lise Meitner's room in the physics section of the institute, one of the speaker's collaborators opened, in the distant chemistry section, a vial containing a solution of a few milligrams of radium. A fraction of the radium emanation, not more than about one one-hundred-millionth of a gram, escaped into the laboratory. Thence a smaller fraction escaped into the corridor, and thus an infinitesimally small quantity entered the room where the Wilson photographs were being made. The result was recorded on the photograph shown in the last view. One could see a multitude of Wilson-paths running crisscross through the photographing chamber; these had been made by emanation atoms that had entered the Wilson-chamber, and, at the moment of exposure, had been disintegrated by ray emission. These minute traces of emanation "infected" the apparatus, and perfect records could not be made again until the last trace of emanation had been removed from the chamber, or had disintegrated.

We may esteem ourselves fortunate that the detection of non-radioactive substances is less sensitive than those that have been described. If we could see how many nuclei of dirt, dust, and disease are contained in the air we constantly inhale, we might be terrified and hardly dare to breath. Nature in her wisdom has arranged matters so that in the course from the ponderable to the imponderable the limits of visibility coincide approximately with the limits of weighability. Let us be thankful that it does not reach down to the individual atoms!

[9] Gudden, *Z. Physik*, 26, 110, 1924.

[10] For these Wilson-photographs the speaker was indebted to Professor Lise Meitner.

# SCIENTIFIC EVENTS

## HUMAN REMAINS DISCOVERED BY THE BRITISH EAST AFRICAN EXPEDITION

A CONFERENCE was called by the Royal Anthropological Institute on March 18 and 19 to discuss the early human remains recently discovered by the East African Expedition of Dr. L. S. B. Leakey, and to examine the material which is now assembled in Cambridge. *Nature* reports that after hearing Dr. Leakey's exposition of his discoveries, and a general discussion of questions arising therefrom, the conference appointed committees to report, respectively, on the geological, paleontological, anatomical and archeological evidence.

The committee on paleontology reported that Kanam East and Kanam West exhibit differences only in the relative numbers of the fossils of different groups. With the human jaw at Kanam West were found close relatives of the two types of rhinoceros still living in the region, a small hippopotamus, a pig, an antelope, fragments of mastodon, two teeth of a very large deinotherium and remains of *Trionyx*. In Kanam East the collection consists chiefly of mastodon with a primitive elephant, deinotherium, and a few specimens of hippopotamus, rhinoceros, horse and a young monkey.

The fossils from Kanjera have a later aspect. One elephant has dental plates as deep as those of *E. antiquus,* and all the remains of elephant are of Asiatic or European type. At least two antelopes, *Hylæochœrus, Phacochœrus,* and a large pig distinct from that of Kanam West, have a very modern appearance. A baboon is remarkable for its comparatively short face. One equine upper molar approaches *Hipparion,* if it does not actually belong to that genus. Typical *Equus* also occurs. Fragments of mastodon, rhinoceros, a giraffoid, hippopotamus and a carnivore have also been found.

The committee thinks that the Kanam deposit should be referred to the Lower Pleistocene, in which the deinotherium and mastodon are survivals from the Upper Pliocene. It also thinks that the Kanjera fauna can not be later than the Middle Pleistocene.

The conference, according to *Nature,* after detailed discussion and after receiving supplementary information furnished by Dr. Leakey and Mr. McInnes as to the circumstances of their discoveries, accepted the reports; congratulated Dr. Leakey on the exceptional significance of his discoveries, and expressed the hope that he may be enabled to undertake further researches, seeing that there is no field of archeological inquiry which offers greater prospects for the future. It especially urged the early organization of another expedition. The following were present and concurred in the above conclusions: Sir Arthur Smith Woodward (*chairman*), A. L. Armstrong, H. Balfour, Miss D. M. A. Bate, P. G. H. Boswell, M. C. Burkitt, V. G. Childe, L. C. G. Clarke, W. L. H. Duckworth, H. J. Fleure, C. Forster Cooper, V. E. Fuchs, A. C. Haddon, A. T. Hopwood, O. T. Jones, Sir Albert Kitson, L. S. B. Leakey, D. McInnes, E. H. Minns, J. Reid Moir, J. L. Myres, T. G. Mollison, F. Oswald, K. S. Sandford, R. A. Smith, W. J. Sollas, J. D. Solomon, Miss M. L. Tildesley and D. M. S. Watson.

## THE MORRIS ARBORETUM OF THE UNIVERSITY OF PENNSYLVANIA

THE Morris Arboretum of the University of Pennsylvania will share in a collection of more than 30,000 mounted botanical specimens from eastern Asia as a result of its participation in a botanical expedition which has been at work there under the direction of Dr. Joseph F. Rock, of the U. S. Department of Agriculture.

According to Dr. Rodney H. True, professor of botany at the university and director of the arboretum, in addition, the seed of several hundred varieties of Oriental plants, many of which offer possibilities of reproduction in this country, will also come to the arboretum from the Rock expedition.

Of the collection made by Dr. Rock, who has been agricultural explorer in the office of foreign plant introduction of the Department of Agriculture since 1920, only about one third has thus far been classified.

These classified specimens, which include more than five hundred rhododendrons, one hundred and fifty primulas, and many varieties of lilies, magnolias and the poppy-like mecanopsis, were found near the headwaters of the Irrawaddy River, in the province of Tsurong west of the Kaaker range, along the upper Salween River, and in other districts chiefly in southeastern Tibet. The remaining two thirds of the specimens, as yet unclassified, have been collected in a wide area which includes in general the region between the Yangtze and Mekong Rivers and a section north of Muli. This latter section hitherto had been untouched in botanical explorations.

In addition to the Morris Arboretum, the shareholders in Dr. Rock's expedition include the Arnold Arboretum, of Boston; the New York Botanical Garden; the Edinburgh Botanical Garden; H. D. MacLaren, of Bodnant, Wales; the Morton Arboretum, Lisle, Illinois, and the University of California.

The material collected is being sent to the University of California where it is being assembled and classified for future distribution to all the shareholders in the expedition.

According to Dr. True, the participation of the Morris Arboretum in the Rock expedition marks the first step in the arboretum's program for the collection of rare botanical specimens from all parts of the world. Although the arboretum already has a wide representation of Oriental plants, its herbarium will be greatly enriched by the mounted specimens from Tibet. It is expected that the seeds from the Rock expedition will enable the arboretum to grow many varieties of Oriental plants.

## DEDICATION OF THE GEORGE EASTMAN RESEARCH LABORATORIES OF THE MASSACHUSETTS INSTITUTE OF TECHNOLOGY

The George Eastman Research Laboratories of the Massachusetts Institute of Technology will be dedicated on Monday, May 1.

The new building, which takes its place in the main educational group, will be devoted to advanced training and research in physics and chemistry, and many former students and members of the faculty in these fields will return for the dedication. It was built from a fund originally provided by the late George Eastman for new buildings, and was completed last autumn. The laboratory offers the most advanced facilities for fundamental study and teaching.

The ceremonies will open with a meeting in the large lecture room of the laboratories in the morning, when the guests and official delegates will be welcomed in an address by President Karl T. Compton. Dr. Harry M. Goodwin, dean of the Graduate School, will speak on "The Graduate School," and Professor Frederick G. Keyes, head of the department of chemistry, will discuss "Chemistry at the Massachusetts Institute of Technology," tracing the development of advances in this field at the institute since its beginning. "Physics at the Massachusetts Institute of Technology" will be the subject of an address by Professor John C. Slater, head of the department of physics. The meeting will be followed by an inspection of the laboratories and special exhibits.

After a buffet luncheon in the Walker Memorial Building, the delegates will attend a meeting at which Dr. Arthur H. Compton, of the University of Chicago, will contribute a paper entitled "Cosmic Rays," and Professor Charles A. Kraus, of Brown University, will speak on "Thirty Years of Physical Chemistry."

After the meeting, the inspection of laboratories and exhibits will be resumed, to be followed by a tea in the Forris Jewett Moore Room late in the afternoon. At 6:30 in the evening the delegates will attend a dinner in Walker Memorial. The ceremonies will close with a reception by President Compton and the staff of the George Eastman Research Laboratories.

As a preliminary to the dedication of the new building, the Northeastern Section of the American Chemical Society, with members of various other New England sections as its guests, will meet in the new building on Saturday afternoon and evening, April 29. Dr. Gilbert N. Lewis, dean of the College of Chemistry at the University of California, a former member of the faculty, will make an address at the afternoon meeting on "The Preparation and Properties of Pure Hydrogen Isotope." At the dinner in the evening, Professor Ernest H. Huntress, of the department of chemistry, will perform a number of unusual experiments in chemistry.

## THE MINNESOTA ACADEMY OF SCIENCE

Last October there were held in the Twin Cities several meetings with a view to organizing a Minnesota Academy of Science. Formal organization was finally completed at a meeting held on November 18. The officers elected and appointed were:

*President,* Wm. A. Riley, University of Minnesota, St. Paul.
*Vice-president,* H. E. Stork, Carleton College, Northfield.
*Secretary-Treasurer,* D. E. Minnich, University of Minnesota.
*Councilors,* George Friedrichs, State Teachers College, St. Cloud; Richard U. Jones, Macalester College, St. Paul; Reverend Wendel Luetmer, St. John's University, Collegeville; E. T. Tufte, St. Olaf College, Northfield.

On April 15, the first annual meeting of the academy was held in the Zoology Building at the University of Minnesota. At a morning and an afternoon session eighteen papers were read. The papers covered a wide variety of fields, including biology, chemistry, geology and astronomy. The noonday luncheon was the occasion of two addresses: one by Dr. L. M. Gould, of Carleton College, on "Antarctic Glaciation," and one by Dr. A. E. Jenks, University of Minnesota, on "Anthropologic Problems of Special Interest in Minnesota." Forty-nine new active members and five new associate members were elected to the academy.

The following officers were elected for the coming year:

*President,* H. E. Stork, Carleton College, Northfield.
*Vice-president,* T. B. Magath, Mayo Clinic, Rochester, Minnesota.
*Secretary-Treasurer,* H. K. Wilson, University of Minnesota, St. Paul.
*Councilors,* George Friedrichs, State Teachers College, St. Cloud; Richard U. Jones, Macalester College, St.

Paul; Wendel Luetmer, St. John's University, Collegeville; E. T. Tufte, St. Olaf College, Northfield.

## THE SALT LAKE CITY MEETING OF THE PACIFIC DIVISION OF THE AMERICAN ASSOCIATION FOR THE ADVANCEMENT OF SCIENCE

BY invitation of the University of Utah, the Pacific Division of the American Association for the Advancement of Science and associated societies will hold their seventeenth annual meeting at Salt Lake City. Unusually attractive rates have been offered by the railways for members proposing to attend the meeting.

The sessions will commence on Monday, June 12. In the afternoon a series of reviews pertaining to the progress of scientific research will be presented. The subjects and authors are: Meteorology, H. H. Kimball, Harvard University; Geology and Seismology, Eliot Blackwelder, Stanford University; Astronomy and Astrophysics, R. G. Aitken, Lick Observatory; Chemistry in Relation to Medicine, Chauncey D. Leake, University of California.

Problems of major interest and the most noteworthy accomplishments in each of these fields will receive attention.

The morning of Tuesday, June 13, is to be devoted to a symposium on "Scientific Problems of the Great Salt Lake." The subjects selected for consideration will be presented as follows:

"The Ancestry of Great Salt Lake," F. J. Pack, professor of geology, University of Utah.

"Climatological and Hydrological Problems," T. C. Adams, associate professor of civil engineering, University of Utah.

"Chemical Deposits and Problems," T. B. Brighton, professor of metallurgy, University of Utah.

"Animal Life and Relations," R. V. Chamberlin, professor of zoology, University of Utah.

"Observations on Artemia," E. G. Martin, professor of physiology, Stanford University.

"Plant Life and Relations," W. P. Cottam, professor of botany, University of Utah.

The general addresses to be delivered before the division at large are scheduled for the evenings of June 12, 13 and 14. The first will be by Dr. W. F. Durand, president of the Pacific Division, on "The Development of our Knowledge of the Laws of Fluid Mechanics"; that of Tuesday evening will be given by Dr. H. H. Kimball, of the Blue Hill Observatory, Harvard University, on "Meteorology—Ancient and Modern; its Development and Applications," and that of Wednesday evening, June 14, by Professor Bailey Willis on "Earthquake Habits of Many Lands."

June 15 will be the closing date for all the organizations participating in the meeting, except the American Physical Society and the Astronomical Society of the Pacific, whose programs extend over June 16.

Members of associated societies are reminded that the titles of papers to be presented at the meeting must be submitted as soon as possible for inclusion in the program.

# SCIENTIFIC NOTES AND NEWS

WILLIAM HENRY HOLMES, chief of the Bureau of American Ethnology from 1902 to 1910, who retired last June as director of the National Gallery of Art, died on April 20 at the age of eighty-six years.

AT the meeting of the American Philosophical Society held in Philadelphia on April 21, the following members were elected. *Members resident of the United States:* Donald H. Andrews, Baltimore; William Bell Dinsmoor, New York; Edward Vermilye Huntington, Cambridge; B. E. Livingston, Baltimore; Edward Martin, Media; Marshall S. Morgan, Philadelphia; G. Kingsley Noble, New York; Francis Randolph Packard, Philadelphia; Samuel Price Wetherill, Jr., Haverford; Westel Woodbury Willoughby, Baltimore, and James Thomas Young, Philadelphia. *Foreign residents,* James Colquhoun Irvine, St. Andrews, Scotland, and Max Planck, Berlin, Germany.

AT the recent charter day exercises of the University of California, the doctorate of laws was conferred on Dr. William E. Ritter, emeritus professor of zoology at the university, emeritus director of the Scripps Institution of Oceanography and honorary president of Science Service.

THE honorary degree of LL.D. was conferred at the graduation ceremony on March 29 of the University of Aberdeen on Dr. D'Arcy Wentworth Thompson, professor of natural history at the University of St. Andrews, "in recognition of the fact that he had played a leading part in guiding the scientific investigation of an industry of immense importance to the city of Aberdeen, since the time when, in 1897, as a British delegate, he had attended the Behring Seas Fisheries Conference."

THE University of St. Andrews will confer on June 30 the honorary doctorate of laws on Professor Carl Neuberg, director of the Kaiser Wilhelm Institute for Biochemistry, Berlin, and editor of the *Biochemische Zeitschrift,* and on R. S. Pearson, director of the Forest Products Research Laboratory, Princes Risborough.

ROYAL MEDALS of the Royal Geographical Society have been awarded as follows: The Founder's Medal to Mr. J. M. Wordie, for the work he has done in polar exploration from the voyage of the *Endurance* in the Weddell Sea in 1914–17 to the present day, and the Patron's Medal to Professor Erich von Drygalski, for his researches in glaciology, both in the Arctic and the Antarctic regions. The Murchison Grant has been awarded to Dr. Noël Humphreys, for his expeditions in Ruwenzori; the Back Grant to Miss Freya Stark, for her journeys in Luristan; the Cuthbert Peek Grant to Dr. L. S. B. Leakey, for his studies on climatic changes in East Africa; and the Gill Memorial to Khan Sahib Afraz Gul Khan, Survey of India, for his frontier and trans-frontier explorations and surveys.

Dr. Wilhelm His, professor of internal medicine at Berlin, has been awarded the silver Carl Ludwig Medal for 1933, which is given every year for outstanding services in research on the circulation.

Dr. Roscoe W. Thatcher, who resigned as president of the Massachusetts State College on account of ill health in September, 1932, and has since been on leave of absence in Florida, expects shortly to return to the college where he has been appointed to a research professorship.

Dr. Carl Einar Hille, associate professor of mathematics at Princeton University, has been appointed professor of mathematics at Yale University. Dr. Hille is a fellow of the American Academy of Arts and Sciences and managing editor of the *Annals of Mathematics.*

At Harvard University, Dr. William Caspar Graustein has been promoted to a professorship and Dr. Marshall Harvey Stone, of Yale University, has been appointed associate professor of mathematics and tutor in the division. Dr. George Bogdan Kistiakowsky has been promoted to an associate professorship of chemistry, and Dr. Bartholomeus Jan Bok, Willson teaching fellow, has been made assistant professor and tutor in the division of the physical sciences.

Dr. Lawrence R. Blinks, of the Rockefeller Institute for Medical Research, has been appointed associate professor of plant physiology in the department of botany of Stanford University.

Dr. Hervey W. Shimer, professor of paleontology at the Massachusetts Institute of Technology, has been made acting head of the department of geology to succeed Dr. Waldemar Lindgren, whose retirement was recently announced.

The nomination of Commander R. S. Patton as head of the U. S. Coast and Geodetic Survey has been sent to the Senate by President Roosevelt. Commander Patton has been connected with the survey since 1904 and became director under the Hoover administration in 1929.

According to an Associated Press dispatch Professor James Franck, who, jointly with Gustav Hertz, was awarded the Nobel Prize in physics in 1925, presented his resignation from the University of Göttingen to the German Ministry of Education on April 18. He is reported to have said: "I have requested my superior authorities to release me from office but will endeavor to continue scientific work in Germany."

A wireless dispatch to *The New York Times* reports that the supervising board of the German Bureau of Standards, of which Professor Albert Einstein long has been a member, has expelled him on the ground that the "attitude he has taken toward the national renaissance of Germany has made his remaining a member impossible."

An Associated Press dispatch from Berlin dated April 21 states that the German Government has appointed Gottfried Feder as president of the Reich's Technical Society, giving him control of the eighty professional scientific organizations which it represents.

Dr. Vern O. Knudsen, associate professor of physics at the University of California at Los Angeles, has been nominated for president of the Acoustical Society of America. The annual meeting of the society will be held in Washington on May 1 and 2.

The following officers of the Society for Experimental Biology and Medicine have been elected for the ensuing year: *President,* A. R. Dochez; *Vice-president,* E. L. Opie; *Secretary-treasurer,* A. J. Goldforb; *Additional Councilors,* C. R. Stockard and G. B. Wallace; *Nominating Committee,* F. R. Sabin, *chairman,* T. Addis, W. R. Bloor, R. Chambers, W. T. Longcope, D. Marine, A. N. Richards, C. R. Stockard, C. J. Wiggers.

Officers of the American Society of Biological Chemists for 1933–34 have been elected as follows: *President,* William M. Clark, the Johns Hopkins University; *Vice-president,* Howard B. Lewis, the University of Michigan; *Secretary,* Henry A. Mattill, the State University of Iowa; *Treasurer,* Cyrus H. Fiske, Harvard Medical School; *Councilors,* Harold C. Bradley, University of Wisconsin; Paul E. Howe, U. S. Department of Agriculture; William C. Rose, University of Illinois.

Dr. A. O. Rankine, professor of physics at the Imperial College of Science and Technology, was elected president of the Physical Society, London, at the annual meeting on March 17. Dr. William Wilson,

Hildred Carlile professor of physics in the University of London, was elected vice-president.

AT the recent annual meeting of the Geological Society of London, Sir Thomas Holland was elected president and Professor E. J. Garwood, J. F. N. Green, W. Campbell Smith and Professor W. W. Watts were elected vice-presidents.

RECENT awards from the Elizabeth Thompson Science Fund have been made to Dr. S. W. Britton, University of Virginia, $150 additional, to be used for the purchase of chemicals and other supplies necessary in his study of the function of the adrenal glands, and to Dr. Erwin Chargaff, Hygienische Institut, University of Berlin, $100, for aid in his investigations dealing with the chemistry of pathogenic bacteria, especially with the lipoids and carbohydrates of the acid-fast group. The trustees of the Elizabeth Thompson Science Fund meet ordinarily during the last ten days of the months of February, May and November. Applications for grants should be sent well in advance of the meeting to the secretary of the fund, Dr. Alfred C. Redfield, the Biological Institute, Divinity Avenue, Cambridge, Massachusetts.

EIGHTEEN fellowships in medicine, including two renewals, for study in the United States and Europe during 1933–1934, were awarded at the spring meeting of the Medical Fellowship Board of the National Research Council, Washington, D. C., of which Dr. G. Carl Huber, dean of the Graduate School, University of Michigan, is the chairman. A list of the successful candidates follows: Caroline C. Bedell, Maurice Brodie, James K. W. Ferguson, Earl W. Flosdorf, Louis S. Goodman, William G. Gordon, Arthur T. Hertig, Joseph Hughes (renewal), Thomas H. Jukes, James M. Orten, Alwin M. Pappenheimer, Wesley T. Pommerenke, Clarence F. Schmidt, Jr. (renewal), Henry G. Schwartz, Randall L. Thompson, William McC. Tuttle, Arthur J. Vorwald and Samuel J. Weinberg. The 1933 fall meeting of the board will be held in September and applications to be considered at that time should be filed with the Washington office of the Medical Fellowship Board on or before August 1.

AN award of the Charles A. Coffin Foundation was recently made to Dr. Sanford A. Moss, of the General Electric Company, not Dr. Charles A. Moss, as recently reported in SCIENCE.

PROFESSOR RAYMOND L. WILDER, of the department of mathematics of the University of Michigan, has leave of absence during the next academic year to enable him to continue his special work for a year at the Institute for Advanced Study at Princeton.

DR. LEROY ABRAMS, professor of botany and director of the Dudley Herbarium at Stanford University, sailed recently from San Francisco. He expects to study during the summer in London, Paris and Geneva.

LEAVE of absence for the next academic year has been granted by Princeton University to Professor Howard Crosby Warren, of the department of psychology, and to Professor Warner Fite, of the department of philosophy, and for the first term to Professor Raymond S. Dugan, of the department of astronomy.

THE Edgar Fahs Smith Memorial Lecture will be delivered at the University of Pennsylvania on the evening of May 8 at 8:15, by Dr. James B. Conant, professor of chemistry at Harvard University. The title of his lecture will be "A Study of Extremely Weak Acids and Bases."

THE Faraday Lecture of the Chemical Society was delivered at the Royal Institution on March 29 by Professor Peter Debye, of the University of Leipzig. He took as his subject "The Relations between Stereochemistry and Physics."

PROFESSOR H. E. ARMSTRONG will deliver the Huxley Memorial Lecture at the Imperial College of Science and Technology, South Kensington, on May 4. His subject will be "Our Need to Honor Huxley's Will."

ON the occasion of the visit of Professor N. Bohr, of Copenhagen, to Pasadena for two weeks beginning on May 15, the staff of the Norman Bridge Laboratory of Physics of the California Institute of Technology plans to conduct a symposium on the general subject of the physics of nuclei and high energy transformations. Professor Bohr will deliver four lectures on the foundations of atomic mechanics, and Professor E. O. Lawrence, of the University of California, will speak on the artificial disintegration of nuclei. Other phases of recent work in this field will be discussed by various members of the staff, including Professor P. S. Epstein, Professor C. C. Lauritsen, Professor J. R. Oppenheimer, Dr. C. D. Anderson, Dr. H. V. Neher and Dr. R. M. Langer. It is planned to have lectures at 4:30 P. M. five days weekly. Professor Bohr probably will speak on Wednesdays and Fridays. A cordial invitation is extended to all who may be interested to attend and to take part in the discussions.

THE North Dakota Chapter of Sigma Xi, University of North Dakota, on March 30, had as their guest speaker Dr. G. W. Stewart, of the University of Iowa. He delivered three addresses. In the forenoon his convocation topic was "Ordinary Made Extraordinary"; at the noon luncheon he made a plea for better teaching of college subjects, and at the dinner meeting, he discussed what civilization may expect from science in the future.

THE New England Association of Chemistry Teachers and the Eastern Association of Physics Teachers held a joint meeting on April 8 in the new Thompson Science Building of the Phillips Exeter Academy, Exeter, New Hampshire. This new building, the gift of the late Colonel William Boyce Thompson, of Yonkers, New York, and a graduate of the academy in the class of 1890, embodies the latest equipment and facilities for teaching chemistry and physics.

THE sixth annual scientific meeting, and twenty-seventh annual South African Medical Congress, will be held in Capetown from September 25 to 30, under the presidency of Mr. E. Barnard Fuller. The work of the congress will be divided among five sections as follows: medicine, surgery, gynecology and obstetrics, public health and special subjects (six subsections). At the three plenary sessions the topics for general discussion are: diet in relation to health in South Africa; prevention of maternal mortality in urban and rural areas in South Africa, and medico-legal problems of general practise. An exhibition of specimens of medical interest from a historical point of view is being arranged in conjunction with the trades exhibition.

# DISCUSSION

## THE HIGH COST OF GERMAN MEDICAL AND SCIENTIFIC PERIODICALS

THE financial problem of literature in the scientific fields, especially those of medicine and the biological sciences, has for some time been a matter of concern to those interested in educational institutions and in providing facilities for investigators engaged in scientific work. Fortunately, in most countries this type of literature has not been extensively commercialized. Wise editorial policies and economical management have prevented prices from becoming exorbitant. This has not, however, been equally true of all countries, notably Germany. Much of the German scientific literature appears in periodicals which, while containing excellent work, are since the war published at absolutely prohibitive prices. The high prices of German periodicals have affected all scientific libraries, and especially medical libraries, since the increase in prices has been the largest in the field of medicine, biology and chemistry. The Medical Library Association has been concerned for some time over this situation, which has been growing progressively worse until the subscription rates for some of these journals have now reached $90.00 to $173.00 a year.

Several interesting articles on this subject have appeared. Dr. Raymond Pearl,[1] of Johns Hopkins University, Mr. Charles H. Brown,[2] of Iowa State College Library, Colonel Fielding H. Garrison,[3] of the Welch Medical Library, Mr. Alfred L. Robert and Mr. Hans Schaltenbrand,[4] of the College of Physicians and Surgeons in New York, Dr. Wilfrid Bonser,[5] Librarian of the University of Birmingham, England, and others[6] have made excellent studies regarding the cost of scientific periodicals, and the dangers inherent in some of the present policies.

The Medical Library Association appointed a committee, consisting of Colonel Fielding H. Garrison, Mr. Alfred L. Robert and Mrs. Eileen R. Cunningham, to investigate the high cost of German medical periodicals, and see what might be done to alleviate this situation. This study has brought out several interesting facts. It is evident that in a large or medium-sized medical library in this country, two thirds or even more of the total annual appropriation for current periodicals is expended on German periodicals, issued chiefly by one or two firms, leaving less than one third of the funds available to be used for the scientific output of all other nations, including the United States and many of the more reasonably priced German publications. This is obviously an absurd situation. Appeals to these German publishers have been met with promises to reduce the volume output, but so far prices have increased and nothing constructive has been accomplished.

The fact that German scientific publications do not usually receive financial aid from foundations and scientific societies undoubtedly renders it more difficult for publication cost to be as low as in other countries, but there seems to be no justification for prices which vary from five to eight, or more, times as much as those of any other nation. It seems difficult to explain these publishers' prices on a cost plus basis. No definite yearly subscription price is announced;

1 Raymond Pearl, "Cost of Biological Books in 1928." *Quarterly Review of Biology*, 3: 600–603, 1928.

2 Charles H. Brown, "A Hazard to Research," *Journal of Higher Education*, 2: 420–426, 1931.

3 Fielding H. Garrison, "Dangers Besetting the Literature of Recent Medicine." Festschrift zur Feier des 60. Geburtstages Max Neuburger, Wien, 1928. "The High Cost of Current Medical Periodicals." *Bulletin of the Medical Library Association*, n. s., 20: 165–169, 1932.

4 Alfred L. Robert and Hans Schaltenbrand, "The Comparative Cost of Medical Journals." *Bulletin of the Medical Library Association*, 20: 140–155, 1932.

5 Wilfrid Bonser, "The Cost of German Biological Publications." *Library Association Record*, n. s. 6: 252–256, 1928.

6 "The Cost of German Medical Journals." Editorial, *Canadian Medical Association Journal*, 27: 63–64, 1932.

one number of a journal may cost $5, while the next may cost $10, and yet only perhaps thirty to forty more pages are included, and the plates, curves and charts do not seem essentially different from those of the less expensive number.

We are also convinced that if the editors and publishers of these expensive journals would really cooperate in an earnest effort to bring down prices, something could be accomplished. The chief responsibility rests with the publishers, however, for in Germany they control the medical publications, employ the editors and pay for the papers printed in the journals. Lately, in every commercial undertaking, prices have been scaled to meet changed economic conditions, and the publishing business should be no exception to this rule.

These German publishers have cautioned libraries against cancellation, as they say that a decrease in the number of subscriptions would lead to an increase of prices for the remaining subscribers. Many American libraries are facing reduction of income, and every means possible is being considered whereby economies can be effected. Therefore, it is obviously impossible for many of them to continue subscriptions to these high priced journals. Many European libraries and individual subscribers, even in Germany, have been forced to cancel their subscriptions, and unless there is evidence of a change in policy on the part of the German publishers, it will not be long before there will be wide-spread cancellation of these high-priced journals by American libraries, who are at present among the most extensive subscribers. If this is to be met by further increase in prices, still further cancellations will result, and a vicious cycle established which would certainly be unfortunate for all concerned.

The Medical Library Association therefore decided to issue an appeal to the German scientific and medical societies and to editors of German medical journals. The American College of Physicians joined the Medical Library Association in this appeal, which was issued in January 1933.[7] This letter summarized the situation and urged German scientists to use their influence and cooperation wherever possible to bring about a decrease in the cost of these journals before wide-spread cancellation had become inevitable.

A few suggestions were made as to possibilities in accomplishing this objective: (1) Decrease in the size and number of the volumes, through briefer articles and careful editorial selection; (2) fixed annual subscription prices for the journals; (3) statements in advance of the approximate number of volumes to appear each year.

That the present situation is considered unfortunate by many Germans is indicated by several articles which have appeared lately in the German journals,[8, 9] showing that the subject is being given consideration there as well as elsewhere.

The situation is a serious one, and those interested in medical education, scientists and investigators, especially in the fields of medicine and the biological sciences, should use any influence they may have with German colleagues to urge their cooperation in reducing the prices of these scientific journals. It is also of the utmost importance for such individuals to study the situation in regard to the particular library from which their reference material is drawn.

In view of present economic conditions, it is likely that the next few years will see the cancellation of large numbers of these expensive German journals, until they will be available only in the large cities, and in libraries with large endowments. This means that investigators working at a distance from such centers will be at a disadvantage as compared with other colleagues; but unless within the next few months marked cooperation is shown on the part of the editors and publishers of these high-priced German journals, the unfortunate results outlined above will inevitably take place.

That we, in this country, can continue indefinitely to expend 70 per cent. of our current periodical budgets for perhaps forty or fifty journals published by a few German firms is extremely unlikely; especially when there are three to five hundred journals necessary for a good medical library, many of which certainly contain material as valuable as that appearing in the journals which are so excessively high priced.

EILEEN R. CUNNINGHAM,
*Chairman, Committee on Cost of Current Medical Periodicals, Medical Library Association*

VANDERBILT UNIVERSITY
SCHOOL OF MEDICINE

[7] This letter was published in full in the *Bulletin of the Medical Library Association*, n. s., 21: 90–91, 1933. Reprints can be obtained by those interested on application to the Chairman of the Committee on Cost of Current Medical Periodicals.

## IS LONGEVITY COMPATIBLE WITH OPTIMUM GROWTH?

MODERN nutrition is governed by the philosophy that a diet which produces optimum growth in the young animal is the ideal. This carries with it the assumption that optimum growth means optimum health. When experimental findings are applied to

[8] Georg Leyh, Address delivered before the Vereins Deutscher Bibliothekare und des Verbandes Deutscher Volksbibliothekare in Jena am 18. u. 19. Mai 1932. *Zentralblatt für Bibliothekswesen* 49, Heft 8, 1932.

[9] H. Morstatt, "Über die Notwendigkeit, den Umfang der wissenschaftlichen Veröffentlichungen einzuschränken." *Die Naturwissenschaften*, 19: 968, 1931.

man, they usually imply the additional assumption that optimum growth leads also to long duration of life, commonly termed longevity. There is no doubt that the nutrition of animals that are to be slaughtered for meat shortly after they mature should be considered from the point of view of rapid growth, since that implies efficient feed conversion. On the other hand at the present time it is the general practise of those who are concerned with child nutrition to attempt to attain the maximum growth of the child without regard to the possible interrelationship between such growth and a short life span. The same philosophy dominates the practises of rearing dairy calves and horses to maturity as rapidly as possible although it is desirable that they have a long productive life span.

In 1912 Slonaker[1] reared three male rats upon an omnivorous diet. Their mean length of life was 1,222 days, but it required 391 days for these rats to attain their maximum weight. A study of Slonaker's growth data indicates that these rats really grew very slowly to maturity and that they did not grow rapidly and then merely fatten to a maximum weight as middle age approached. I have disregarded Slonaker's data upon exercised rats, because there is nothing in the literature for comparison. I have not cited his data upon the vegetarian groups because they died relatively young and need not be considered in a discussion of longevity.

In a report concerning the rat diet that has proved satisfactory as far as reproduction and growth in our colony is concerned, Maynard[2] showed most of the growth of the male rat takes place before the sixteenth week with a gradual weight increase until the twenty-eighth week. During the past four years we fed a group of seventy-five male rats upon this diet until they died. Their mean age at death was $503 \pm 12$ days. Only 1 of these rats lived for more than 900 days.

Although Slonaker's data are very limited they indicate that our rats upon the stock diet are dying in middle age. Our rats matured rapidly, those of Slonaker slowly.

In our studies upon brook trout we have reported experiments twice in which trout that failed to grow lived much longer than those that grew upon similar diets.[3, 4] This first called our attention to the possible relationship between the rate of growth and the span of life within a given species. A relationship between rate of attaining maturity and life span between various species is frequently mentioned by early biologists, however Zabinski[5] from his studies with insects has noted the possibility of prolonging life by retarding the growth rate. Osborne and Mendel[6] suggested the same possibility from their studies with rats.

Miss Campbell[7] found she could extend the mean length of life as well as the growth of rats slightly by increasing the milk in the diet. In the light of Slonaker's data, these findings have only negative bearing upon the problem of longevity because even her group that lived the longer died in approximately middle life at a mean age of 664 days. All her many hundreds of rats died without any attaining the mean age of Slonaker's three males and her value for mean age disregards early deaths. Therefore her data indicate nothing concerning the interrelationship of growth and longevity. Her findings also confirm those of others that the female rat grows more slowly and outlives the male.

We may then have diets that are entirely satisfactory for growth and reproduction and these same diets may be unsatisfactory for longevity. It is known from many experiments that we may have a slow growth rate and a short life span upon a deficient diet. No one has ever found it possible, however, to have both rapid growth with early attainment of maturity, and longevity. It is possible that longevity and rapid growth are incompatible and that the best chance for an abnormally long life span belongs to the animal that has grown slowly and attained a late maturity.

C. M. McCAY

CORNELL UNIVERSITY

## SOLUBLE SESQUIOXIDES AND ORGANIC MATTER FROM ALKALI TREATMENTS ON SOILS

ALKALI treatments, equivalent to one ton per acre, on Appalachian upland podzol soils of Quebec have been studied in percolators in an attempt to break down the relatively large amount of organic matter and to decrease the acidity (pH about 5.0, "lime requirement" 3 tons CaO per acre). The results found differ from those reported by Meyer[1] based on the effects of calcium carbonate applied to Caddo silt loam of pH 4.8. Liming podzol soils has not produced the large increases in soluble iron and organic matter found in the case of the acid Louisiana soils. On the other hand, equivalent treatments with sodium hydroxide and sodium carbonate on these podzol soils give marked increase of soluble organic matter in

[1] J. R. Slonaker, Leland Stanford Jr. Univ. Publications (1912).

[2] L. A. Maynard, SCIENCE, lxxi: 192. 1930.

[3] J. W. Titcomb, *et al.*, *Trans. Am. Fish. Soc.*, 58: 205. 1928.

[4] C. M. McCay, *et al.*, *Trans. Am. Fish. Soc.*, 61: 58. 1931.

[5] J. Zabinski, *Jour. Exp. Biol.*, vi: 360. 1929.

[6] T. B. Osborne, *et al.*, SCIENCE, xlv, 294. 1917.

[7] H. Louise Campbell, Thesis, Columbia Univ. (1928).

[1] A. H. Meyer, "Iron Toxicity from Liming," SCIENCE, 76: 56. 1932.

colloidal suspension in the soil solution. In addition, iron and aluminum are found adsorbed by this organic material to the extent of about 40 p.p.m. and 20 p.p.m. of the soil, respectively. These soils and soil solutions with this treatment remain acid between values of pH 6.1 and 6.7.

Iron toxicity, due to increase in soluble iron after liming, has been claimed for the Louisiana soils, but the evidence that we possess indicates that the presence of the soluble sesquioxides in small amounts after sodium alkali treatment does not inhibit production from these Quebec soils but permits positive increases.

G. T. SHAW
R. R. MCKIBBIN

MACDONALD COLLEGE

## THE ATTRACTION OF SPHERES

IT is appropriate that some warning should be given the inexperienced reader of Mr. Thaddeus Merriman's article in SCIENCE for April 14 (p. 371). His method of calculating the attraction of a homogeneous sphere upon a neighboring body involves assumptions inconsistent with the generally accepted methods of the integral calculus, as well as with the Newtonian law of gravitation. Newton's beautiful geometrical proof that the net attraction of such a sphere is exactly the same as if all the mass was concentrated at its center is, of course, fully confirmed by the rigorous analytical discussion which may be found in any standard treatise on mechanics, and so need not be reproduced here.

Mr. Merriman's proposed substitute law is inconsistent not only with theory but with the fact. For a small sphere near the earth's surface, it reduces to $F = G\,\frac{M, \cos \alpha}{d^2}$, when M is the earth's mass, d its radius, and $\alpha$ the angle between a line drawn to the earth's center and one tangent to a circle of radius 0.424 times the earth's. The factor $\cos \alpha$, which is omitted in Newton's equation, has the value 0.911 for a point on the earth's surface. Without it the attraction at the surface is known to be in complete agreement with that inferred from the orbital motion of the moon. To introduce it destroys the agreement, which provided Newton with the first conclusive test of his theory.

HENRY NORRIS RUSSELL

PRINCETON
APRIL 21, 1933

# SCIENTIFIC APPARATUS AND LABORATORY METHODS

## A TWO-FIELD STROBOSCOPE

IN stroboscopic observation of vibrating strings for measurement of frequency, no use seems to have been made of a two-field illumination. The two fields are contiguous and are alternately illuminated. The two-field method removes some ambiguities of the one-field method. But more important is the fact that a feeble resonance of the string to a tuning-fork or other source is more easily detected.

For the laboratory, the simplest device is the type of Neon bulb built for a. c. lighting circuits and having semi-cylindrical electrodes. Such a bulb can be held behind a string in such a manner that half of each electrode is visible. The two electrodes light up in alternation, the flash frequency of either side being equal to the frequency of the current.

For lecture demonstration, one can take a siren disk with an even number of holes. Alternate holes are half covered on the half nearest the center of the disk; the remaining holes are half covered on the side next the edge of the disk. The disk is set as closely as possible to the string, with the center of the disk level with the string. When a hole is level with the string, a strong beam of light is made convergent by means of a condenser, and is arranged to just cover either type of hole. On the other side, an objective focusses the string on a screen. When the disk is rotated and the string made to vibrate, a two-field stroboscopic view of the string is obtained. (Many other methods may be used.)

To understand the patterns seen, the procedure is to construct in advance the patterns to be expected. To do this, imagine a stroboscope disk with a single spot; rotate this at S revolutions per second, S being the string frequency; and illuminate the disk by F flashes per second. When the pattern has been worked out, project the spots of the pattern on a vertical line in the plane of the disk. Then repeat the process for a series of flashes beginning one half flash-period later. The projections of this second pattern gives the string pattern in the other field. The figure herewith illustrates the case when the flash frequency is 3/5 of the string frequency. Small circles give the first disk pattern, and crosses give the second.

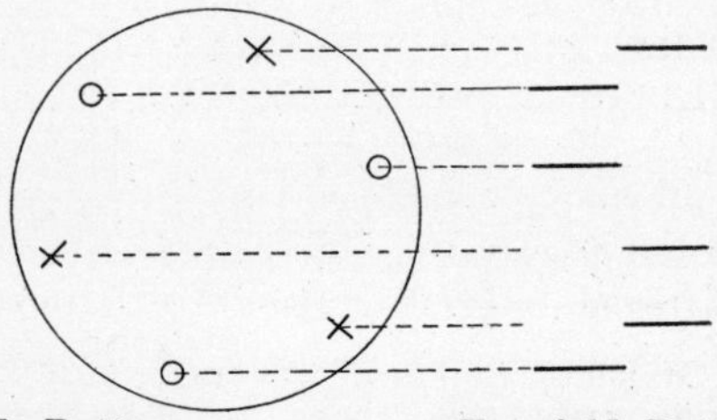

Disk Pattern Two-field Pattern

Figure illustrating the construction of the two-field pattern for $F = S.3/5$.

A few simple rules may be given here. Assume that F = S.f/s.

*For the disk patterns:*

(1) Sf/s flashes per second produce a pattern of f spots, independently of the value of s.

(2) If s is even, the crosses coincide with the circles.

(3) If s is odd, the crosses alternate with the circles.

*For the two-field string patterns:*

(1) The number of lines seen in either field is equal to f; when two lines merge into one, that line must be counted twice.

(2) If s is even, the two fields are identical, and appear as a single field.

(3) If s is odd, the two fields are similar but not identical.

It is rarely the case that f/s is a simple ratio. Then, as in Lissajou curves, one sees changing patterns. These can be worked out by shifting the initial position of the disk in the construction shown above. It is just this fact that makes the two-field method so convenient. Assume that a string has been tuned to the frequency F, for which we obtain just one line in either field. If the string starts to resonate to some source, one can usually observe two lines moving in opposite directions. The writer has used a ×25 microscope to observe such resonances.

The changing patterns just mentioned can be worked out by a slow rotation of the disk patterns, as stated. From this it will be understood that a complete cycle of change means that the disk has moved by an angle equal to the angle between two spots of the same set. Or in the two-field patterns, we have made a complete cycle of changes when we return to some pattern in the same way. Then, if the pattern corresponds to a ratio f/s, and there are R complete repetitions per second,

$$\frac{F}{f} - \frac{S}{s} = \frac{\pm R}{fs}$$

Although, for simplicity, we have spoken of strings, the two-field method is adaptable in many ways to the observation of other bodies, *e.g.*, the writer used a Neon bulb in the selection of steel springs which were to vibrate at a frequency of 240.

PAUL F. GAEHR

WELLS COLLEGE

## REGULATING THE AIR SUPPLY OF MICRO BURNERS

MOST of the micro burners obtainable from supply houses have an inflexible and very often an inefficient adjustment of the gas-air mixture. The usual practise with laboratory workers has been to test a number of burners and then select the best of the lot, without attempting adjustment. Obviously, this is an awkward and somewhat unsatisfactory solution of the problem.

A method, almost as convenient as that used for the Bunsen burner, has been found for regulating the air supply of micro burners. The small burner is connected to the gas line and lit. While the flame is burning, twist with a pair of pliers the metal gas connection which projects from the base, loosening or tightening until the proper type of flame is obtained.

Occasionally a burner will be found which requires further treatment. In these cases the gas connection is unscrewed and, using a small three-cornered file, two flat channels about 5 mm wide and 6 or 8 mm long are filed on each side of the tube. These shallow channels start from the middle of the tube and slant upward, meeting at the pin hole gas outlet on top. The connection is replaced frequently while filing and the gas-air mixture tested as described above, in order to prevent spoiling the burner by too much filing. If necessary, the small gas outlet can be made larger by reaming with a pin. However, it is usually found that the opening is already too large. This can be remedied by filing the sides of the hole rather thin and then pressing the edges inward until the desired opening is obtained.

CORNELIUS A. DALY

MEDICAL DEPARTMENT, UNION UNIVERSITY
ALBANY MEDICAL COLLEGE

# SPECIAL ARTICLES

## ACCELERATED, EXPERIMENTAL POLIOMYELITIS IN NASALLY INSTILLED MONKEYS

IN a previous communication,[1] attention was directed to the accelerating effect of a second virus injection, after an interval of from 7 to 10 days, in provoking experimental poliomyelitis in *Macacus rhesus.* The earlier report dealt with the phenomenon from the point of view of establishing human strains of virus in monkeys. Since that report was made, additional studies of the subject of accelerated infection have been undertaken.

The first test, made by injecting the human virus intracerebrally and intraperitoneally, were soon followed by the injection of sub-infective doses of monkey virus intracerebrally alone. The results showed that acceleration does not depend on the

[1] S. Flexner, "Accelerated Infection in Experimental Poliomyelitis," SCIENCE, 1931: 74, 520.

presence of foreign (human) nervous tissues along with the virus, and probably is not simply a summation effect of the two virus injections.

The events following the second or accelerating injection of virus are characterized by an abrupt rise in temperature (105° to 106° + F.) and the onset of paralysis, often rapid, which may progress quickly to prostration and death. The accelerating action has now been shown to apply also to monkeys receiving the virus by instillation into the nasal cavities. Since the natural infection in man takes place through these cavities, this observation may prove to have practical import. The virus, in suspension, is dropped into the nares on two successive days; and if infection does not manifest itself in from 7 to 10 days, the instillations are repeated. After one or two such instillations, symptoms, consisting of fever and paralysis, may manifest themselves promptly, as in the instances of intracerebral inoculation.

The sudden onset of severe symptoms following the second nasal instillations has suggested not only relationship with the phenomenon in children described by Draper[2] under the term "dromedary" type of poliomyelitis, but has also supplied a possible explanation of its nature. According to this provisional explanation, the "dromedary" effect is a result of reinfection, arising either from the patient himself (autochthonous infection) or from a new exposure to the virus.

The path of the virus introduced into the nares—ascending by way of olfactory nerve cells in the mucous membrane to the olfactory lobes of the brain, and then to other parts of the nervous system in regular sequence—has become more firmly established as the experimental study of poliomyelitis has progressed.[3] The part taken by the meningeal choroid plexus complex in the extension of the virus has been little studied.[4] Upon examining, on successive days, the cerebrospinal fluid withdrawn by lumbar puncture after the first and second sets of nasal instillations of virus, it was found that the number of mononuclear cells in the fluid increases considerably, even before the appearance of any symptoms of infection, except sometimes fever (105° F.), and that the occurrence of fever, increased cells and the presence of globulin in the fluid may be the only detectable pathological effects of the instillations. However, the second instillations are succeeded, but not invariably, by a further rise in cells and by the appearance of paralysis, which may extend rapidly, leading to death; or the paralysis may be partial, become arrested and terminate in recovery. It remains to be determined whether monkeys which develop the cerebrospinal fluid changes only, exhibit later a heightened resistance (immunity) to the virus injected intracerebrally, and whether the blood serum has acquired antiviral properties. The occurrence of these mild effects from the instillations may profitably be compared to the alterations in the cerebrospinal fluid observed during epidemics of poliomyelitis in certain children who develop no detectable paralytic symptoms whatever.

The acceleration procedure has been employed advantageously in still other ways: (1) To determine the neutralizing action of blood sera in respect to strains of virus differing qualitatively and quantitatively from one another; and (2) to throw light on the degree and duration of active immunity in monkeys that have recovered from an acute attack of experimental poliomyelitis, or have been rendered immune by the intradermal injection of virus. In the first instance, intracerebral, and in the second, intranasal inoculation is performed. A greater degree of regularity and accuracy has been introduced into these difficult tests by the use of the acceleration method in the experimental study of poliomyelitis.

SIMON FLEXNER
LABORATORIES, THE ROCKEFELLER INSTITUTE
FOR MEDICAL RESEARCH, NEW YORK

[2] G. Draper, "Acute Poliomyelitis," p. 40. P. Blakiston Son and Co., Philadelphia, 1917.

[3] S. Flexner and P. F. Clark, "A Note on the Mode of Infection in Epidemic Poliomyelitis," *Proc. Soc. Exper. Biol. and Med.*, 10: 1, 1912.

[4] S. Flexner and H. L. Amoss, "The Relation of the Meninges and Choroid Plexus to Poliomyelitic Infection," *Jour. Exper. Med.*, 25: 525, 1917. "Mechanisms that Defend the Body from Poliomyelitic Infection, (a) External or Extra-nervous, (b) Internal or Nervous," *Proc. Nat. Acad. Sciences*, 3: 416, 1917.

## BOOKS RECEIVED

BOAS, GEORGE. *The Happy Beast in French Thought of the Seventeenth Century.* Pp. vii + 157. Johns Hopkins Press. $2.00.

BROWN, W. NORMAN. *The Story of Kalaka.* Pp. 149. Illustrated. Smithsonian Institution.

ESCLANGON, ERNEST. *Dix Leçons D'Astronomie.* Pp. 108. Illustrated. Gauthier-Villars, Paris. 25 fr.

FREUDENBERG, K., Editor. *Stereochemie.* 8. Lieferung. Pp. 1117–1276. Franz Deuticke, Leipzig.

FOLDES, EUGENE. *A New Approach to Dietetic Therapy.* Pp. xii + 434. Badger.

FUTCHER, PALMER H. *Giants and Dwarfs: A Study of the Anterior Lobe of the Hypophysis.* Pp. 80. Illustrated. Harvard University Press.

GREY, ROBERT M. and F. TRACY HUBBARD. *List of Plants Growing in the Botanical Garden of the Atkins Institution of the Arnold Arboretum, Cuba.* Pp. 245. Harvard University Press.

HARNWELL, G. P. and J. J. LIVINGOOD. *Experimental Atomic Physics.* Pp. xiii + 472. Illustrated. McGraw-Hill. $5.00.

MAXIM, HIRAM P. *Life's Place in the Cosmos.* Pp. xii + 176. Illustrated. $2.50.

PIEPER, CHARLES J. and WILBUR L. BEAUCHAMP. *Everyday Problems in Science.* Revised edition. Pp. xxxiv + 734. 546 figures. Scott, Foresman. $1.60.

ROBACK, A. A. *Self-Conciousness and Its Treatment.* Pp. 122. Sci-Art Publishers. $1.50.

# SCIENCE

VOL. 77 FRIDAY, MAY 5, 1933 No. 2001

*The Significance of Professor Thomson's Work in the Development of Electrical Engineering:* DR. KARL T. COMPTON 415

*In Honor of Professor Elihu Thomson:* DR. VANNEVAR BUSH 418

*Scientific Events:*
*Industrial Research Laboratories; The Field Museum of Natural History; Centenary of the British Entomological Society; Award of the Loubat Prizes; The National Academy of Sciences* 420

*Scientific Notes and News* 423

*Discussion:*
*The Crisis in Scientific Research and the Way out:* PROFESSOR DR. SERGEI TSCHACHOTIN. *A Compendium of Culture Methods for Invertebrate Animals:* PROFESSOR JAMES G. NEEDHAM. *Reversal of the Pinhole Image:* PROFESSOR ERNEST C. BRYANT. *The Adrenal Glands in an Editor's Office:* DR. J. MCKEEN CATTELL 426

*Scientific Apparatus and Laboratory Methods:*
*A New Form of Centrifuge-Microscope for Simultaneous Observation of Control and Experimental Material:* PROFESSOR E. NEWTON HARVEY. *The Agitation of Material in Aerated Water:* PROFESSOR H. B. SIFTON 430

*Special Articles:*
*The Atomic Weight of Lead from Katanga Pitchblende:* PROFESSOR G. P. BAXTER and C. M. ALTER. *Free Positive Electrons Resulting from the Impact upon Atomic Nuclei of the Photons from Th C″:* DR. CARL D. ANDERSON. *Method of Extraction of Suprarenal Cortical Hormone-like Substance from Urine:* DR. DAVID PERLA and DR. J. MARMORSTON 431

*Science News* 8

SCIENCE: A Weekly Journal devoted to the Advancement of Science, edited by J. MCKEEN CATTELL and published every Friday by

THE SCIENCE PRESS

New York City: Grand Central Terminal

Lancaster, Pa. Garrison, N. Y.

Annual Subscription, $6.00 Single Copies, 15 Cts.

SCIENCE is the official organ of the American Association for the Advancement of Science. Information regarding membership in the Association may be secured from the office of the permanent secretary, in the Smithsonian Institution Building, Washington, D. C.

# THE SIGNIFICANCE OF PROFESSOR THOMSON'S WORK IN THE DEVELOPMENT OF ELECTRICAL ENGINEERING[1]

By Dr. KARL T. COMPTON

PRESIDENT OF THE MASSACHUSETTS INSTITUTE OF TECHNOLOGY

ANY one with the misapprehension that engineering practise consists in following a set of fixed formulas, rules and specifications will do well to consider that electrical engineering and the art of useful application of electricity has developed almost entirely during the lifetime of Professor Elihu Thomson. The basic scientific discoveries of electromagnetic induction by Faraday and Henry had been made during the decade just preceding his birth, as had the first crude form of telegraph. But generators, motors, transformers, transmission lines, electric meters and regulators, electric lights, telephones, x-rays, electric discharges through high or partial vacuum, lightning protectors, converters, rectifiers, electrical insulators, wireless, radio and all the theory and practise of electrical networks are the product of science and invention since Thomson's birth on March 29, 1853. These things, and the economic problems associated with them, constitute the field of electrical engineering. Some of them Professor Thomson has himself invented, a majority of them owe much of their development to him, and there is scarcely a one on which he has not left his imprint in one way or another. Yet I suspect that he himself would be the first to maintain that we are as yet only at the threshold of the possibilities which are inherent in electricity for the services of man, and that no one would more stoutly advocate the continued endeavor to discover these possibilities and make them effective.

Granted this, it must nevertheless have been a particularly thrilling experience to be connected with the early engineering and industrial developments of electricity, in the early 1880's, when it first became evident that in electricity lay a mighty force whose

[1] Address given on the occasion of the eightieth birthday of Professor Elihu Thomson at the Massachusetts Institute of Technology, March 29, 1933.

potentialities were as yet but dimly imagined, yet which opened up in new directions, week by week, to the eager and talented young men, Edison, Thomson, Rice, Brush, Edgar, and the others.

Inspired by the possibilities which he had come to realize while experimenting with electricity as professor in the Boys' Central High School of Philadelphia, Professor Thomson and his colleague, Professor Houston, formed the Thomson-Houston Company in 1882, at the age of 29. With the able assistance of his pupil, Edwin W. Rice, he then began his long career of industrial and scientific research and its commercial development.

Perhaps Professor Thomson's first great contribution to electrical engineering was his invention in about 1879 of the three-coil dynamo with its automatic regulator and other features, which formed the basis of the first successful electric lighting system. This was put out by the Thomson-Houston Company in the early 1880's, and quickly found its place not only in this country but also in the leading countries of Europe. The machine was entirely automatic in its operation and so adjusted that it could maintain constant regulation in a system of many electric arcs, no difference how many of these arcs might be turned off or on. The need for such a regulator and its general nature were suggested to him by his earliest serious electrical studies, which were on the relation between the current and voltage in an electric arc, and which led him to the discovery that as the current increases the voltage falls—a relation which accounted for the instability of an arc, and pointed out characteristics which an arc dynamo should have.

It is interesting to note that this three-coil dynamo was a direct-current machine provided with a commutator, since in those days direct currents were more readily handled than were alternating currents and had certain advantages for arc-lighting purposes. However, exactly the same machine, simply with different connections, constitutes the three-phase generator which is so important in present-day electric power and was so represented by Professor Thomson in his original patent application. This is one of many cases in which Professor Thomson's ideas were years in advance of the world's readiness for their acceptance and utilization.

About two years later (1881) there was another great invention, that of a magnetically operated lightning arrester. Although this was designed for the particular purpose of protecting his arc-light systems from lightning, it was the invention of a fundamental method of breaking electric circuits, which has found very numerous applications, one of the most important of which was by Professor Thomson himself in the control of electric cars and trains.

The fundamental idea of this was again based upon an accurate knowledge and study of scientific phenomena involved in the discharge of electricity through gases. A transmission line, of course, has to be insulated from the earth by insulators adequate to prevent spark-over at the voltages used. If, however, the line is struck by lightning or an abnormally large electric surge passes through it, a spark may pass around the insulation, and it is a peculiarity of sparks through air that when once the insulation of the air is broken down by a spark there is literally no limit to the amount of current which can flow. Thus these sparks frequently cause serious short circuits.

Professor Thomson's discovery consisted in placing the insulator between the poles of a magnet, with the result that the spark or arc which might be produced was acted on by electrical forces in such a way as to elongate it in the form of a bow which became more and more extended until it finally became so long that it went out. This principle is of just as great importance to-day as ever, and is the foundation of many recently improved schemes for the switching of very large currents.

Again in these very early days and long before the importance of it was realized, Thomson invented the now universally used method of transmitting electric power, stepping it down from a high tension with the aid of a local transformer for consumption. This was set up as a working model at the Franklin Institute in Philadelphia in 1879, a patent was applied for in 1885, and after an unusually strenuous history in the patent office, the fundamental patent for multiple-arc distribution systems with transformers was granted in 1902. During this same time and as an additional safety device for high voltage operation, Thomson patented the procedure of earthing the secondary coil of the transformer, a practise which has now become universal. In passing, I should note here, as an illustration of a notable characteristic of Professor Thomson, that this patent on his advice was dedicated by the General Electric Company to the public from a feeling that no patent or invention which has to do with public safety should in any way be restricted or made unavailable to the people.

In the further development of alternating-current machinery, he invented the constant-current transformer and the inductive regulator in which a movable secondary or primary coil could be adjusted automatically to give constant-current output. Again in the direction of increasing the power capacity of transformers, in 1887–89 he first proposed the use of oil for cooling and for insulation purposes in transformers, and furthermore called attention to the great and deleterious effect of moisture in the oil, an effect whose full significance students of insulators are only now beginning adequately to realize.

I pass now to two of the most important and characteristic of Professor Thomson's discoveries. The first of these is that process of electrical welding whereby the welded surfaces were fused and united by the heat developed on account of the resistance in the contact between them. This method of welding has come into enormous use in industry and the indications are that it will be even more used in the near future. As examples in widely different fields may be mentioned the welding of seamless metal tubing, the attachment of filaments and other electrodes in incandescent lamps and vacuum tubes, and the fastening together of most of the parts of the new Ford automobile. In the former of these applications, it may be interesting to know that a single manufacturer has manufactured in a single year enough bedstead tubing to reach around the earth.

Professor Thomson was not the first to utilize an arc in welding. The Demeritens patent, which was fundamental, was bought on advice of Professor Thomson by the Thomson Electric Welding Company in the early days, and, had arc welding developed within the life of the patent, that company would have controlled the arc as well as the electric resistance welding art.

Again, one of Professor Thomson's most fundamental discoveries was the principle of dynamical repulsion between a primary and secondary coil. This can be demonstrated by a variety of interesting lecture experiments, most of which were suggested and shown first by Professor Thomson himself. For example, a vertical iron core was wound with a coil through which an alternating current could be passed. The core projected above the coil into a jar of water. Fitting loosely around the core was a second small coil, free to slip up and down the core in the water, and supporting by its terminals an incandescent lamp. When an alternating current was sent through the primary coil, a current was induced in the movable secondary coil which lighted the lamp and at the same time raised the coil, against the force of gravity, high up in the jar of water. This scientific observation was developed by Professor Thomson into an alternating current repulsion motor which is nothing more nor less than our ordinary induction motor, which is in almost universal use for small single-phase motors.

In connection with this discovery you will be interested in the following quotation from the *Electrical World* of May 28, 1887, commenting upon this work.

> It is, as yet, too early to assign to its proper place and limit the part which the alternating current will take in the electric arts. It has started on its career with most rapid strides, and it now only remains to devise means for its accurate measurement, regulation and distribution. Certain it is that Professor Thomson's brilliant paper can not fail to act as a powerful stimulus to those whose attention is now absorbed in the direction indicated, and the fruits of which will soon be noted. We hope that at a later meeting of the Institute Professor Thomson will give to the world his practical results, which he has only hinted at in the present paper.

Professor Thomson was then 34 years of age. These practical results are now seen, for example, in probably a million induction motors in daily use.

During the years 1885–1895 Professor Thomson was busily engaged with the development of electric meters, especially recording watt meters, of which more than 4,000,000 are now in operation, and for this invention Professor Thomson was awarded the Paris Meter Prize of 1890 at a competition held after the exposition of 1889.

As early as 1890 and continued intensively for half a dozen years thereafter were a series of brilliant experiments on high-frequency alternating currents, paving the way for many of the developments in wireless and other high-frequency applications which are being so actively applied at the present time. He constructed the first high-frequency dynamo, operating at frequencies of 30 to 40 times as great as any previously designed, and in connection with experiments with this type of electric power, he designed also the first special high-frequency transformers. While working in this field, he discovered a method of producing still higher frequency alternating current from a direct-current arc, by shunting the arc with inductance and capacitance, thus discovering the method which played such an important rôle in wireless transmission up until its virtual replacement by electronic tube devices only within the past few years. This interesting method of producing alternating currents was actually applied to wireless telegraphy by Poulsen, and is therefore generally known as the Poulsen arc. Also in connection with these high-frequency investigations, he made the important discovery that the insulating power of oils at these high frequencies is very much greater than at the ordinary low commercial frequencies, if this insulating power is measured in terms of the path at which a spark will pass. Just one other item can be mentioned in connection with his high-frequency work, namely, the fact that he discovered and was the first to use the method of tuning electric circuits, which is, of course, absolutely fundamental to modern electrical communication systems. This was done very early in his career while he was still a professor at Boys' Central High School in Philadelphia, and was done in connection with experiments on wireless signaling which antedate the famous experiments of Hertz by about a dozen years, and, as far as I have been able to ascertain, constitute the first experiments on the propagation of electric waves and wireless signaling, with the sole exception of some experiments conducted still a dozen years previous to his by Joseph Henry in Princeton. These earlier experiments of Henry's were apparently never published.

Immediately upon the announcement of the discovery of Röntgen rays, Professor Thomson began a series of interesting experiments and valuable developments in connection with the x-ray art. The foundation for this work had been laid by previous experiments on electric discharge through gases at low pressures, and led to the first application of stereoscopic methods in Röntgenology only one year after the publication of the Röntgen rays themselves had been announced, and led also to various practical improvements in the design of x-ray tubes, as, for example, the double-focus x-ray tube and a cooled-target tube within less than a year after the discovery of Röntgen rays. In connection with these experiments Professor Thomson also took a lively interest in the physiological effects of x-rays, including x-ray burns, and in the laws governing diffusion of x-ray matter, subjects which have been developed on the one hand to exceedingly important applications in medical therapy, and on the other hand to give some of the most intimate knowledge which we possess of the internal constitution of matter, such as the arrangement of atoms in crystals and molecules, and the arrangement of electrons in atoms.

Things like these, and many more of them, constitute the tangible contributions of Professor Thomson to electrical engineering. His intangible contributions are less easy to talk about, but are none the less real and important. I can not close without mentioning a few of them.

Still quite tangible are his services to engineering education. From his earliest work as a teacher of science in the Boys' High School of Philadelphia, to his many years of service to the Massachusetts Institute of Technology as member of its corporation and executive committee, its acting president during a critical period, a frequent member of the visiting committee of its department of electrical engineering and non-resident professor in that department, he has been a continual inspiration and source of help to students and colleagues.

Rather less tangible is his influence in the many professoinal engineering and scientific bodies of which he is a member. Not only have his scholarly contributions been many and important, but he has consistently been an ideal connecting link between the practical and the theoretical, the commercial and the academic, by his example keeping them from being too narrow and maintaining a generous spirit of mutual appreciation and cooperation.

Still less tangible, but perhaps most important of all have been his inspiration to his thousands of business and research colleagues, his example of enthusiasm, perseverance, ingenuity, unselfishness, love of truth, generosity and broadmindedness.

As I have come to know it, the electrical engineering profession is on a remarkably high plane, both technically and also in general attitude. I believe its debt to men like Professor Thomson for making it a good profession in which to work is at least as important as its debt to him for so much of its basic technical development.

# IN HONOR OF PROFESSOR ELIHU THOMSON[1]

By Dr. VANNEVAR BUSH

DEAN OF ENGINEERING AND VICE-PRESIDENT OF THE MASSACHUSETTS INSTITUTE OF TECHNOLOGY

THERE are many titles which I might use in presenting to you these greetings on the occasion of your birthday; but I feel sure that that of "Professor" is most welcome to you. It emphasizes an aspect of your accomplishments which I know is close to your heart. Great material changes have followed upon your scientific and engineering accomplishments, and these are visible to all of us in our daily lives. More subtle but none the less lasting is the influence of your many contacts with academic affairs. You have touched and moulded many institutions which are dedicated to the education of youth, and I bring you the felicitations of your colleagues everywhere.

Sixty-three years ago you were a professor in Philadelphia. We take great pride that you are still, and we hope will long be, professor of applied electricity at the Massachusetts Institute of Technology. Through these years your interest in collegiate affairs has been continuous. I need recite but a few instances. In 1890, just as I was born, and when you were thirty-seven, Yale recognized you as a master of arts. Tufts has the distinction of having conferred upon you your first doctorate, that of philosophy. Harvard made you doctor of science, and the University of Pennsyl-

[1] Address given at the dinner to mark the eightieth birthday of Professor Elihu Thomson, March 29, 1933.

vania, doctor of laws. Victoria University reached across the ocean to confer the degree of doctor of science.

Your contacts with educational institutions have been much more than occasional, however. They were bound to be, for your interest in their affairs has always been constructive. I find you, very early, organizing a scientific society, lecturing to audiences in an artisan's night school, at the Franklin Institute, and at many other places. And in later years, you have served on the visiting committees of this institution and of several departments of Harvard University.

Your contacts with the Massachusetts Institute of Technology have been particularly close. It was a fortunate thing for us when your acquaintance with Professor Cross brought you to lecture here fifty years ago on electrical machinery. Since that time we have always felt your presence. For thirty-five years a member of the corporation, and for twenty years on its executive committee, you have guided our steps. One of the most helpful things you have ever done for us was when you were highly instrumental in bringing to the institute the president we all so deeply honor, Dr. Maclaurin. Another act, a small one this time, but one that reminds me of you every time I look out of my window, was when you classified for him the names that appear graven on our buildings. And finally, when he died, you became for two years our acting president and gave of your time and effort to steady us on our feet as we staggered from that blow. And now you are still "Professor" and our colleague.

There has long been, on the part of the layman, an inclination to associate the title "professor" with the pedantic and the cloistered. To fully earn the title it is sometimes popularly supposed that one must cultivate an intense absent-mindedness and a lack of knowledge of the every-day affairs of the world. You have certainly done much to dissipate this idea, and your colleagues rise and call you blessed. That there exist professors who can put up a window-shade while conversing in ordinary language, or who can set the timing of an automobile as a form of recreation, is a fact of the modern world which is still incredible to the laity. That there is one who has hundreds of patents to his name for all sorts of things which very practical men have been very glad to use has given the title a significance which is well added to its dignity. I hope that every farmer who uses a cream separator will realize that it was invented by a professor, for it will do much to counter that persistent fallacy that those who think deeply are necessarily beings apart.

The world progresses only so fast as it learns to pass on its accomplishments from one generation to the next. The material things, those that are of direct utility, machines and structures, can hardly be passed on at all to-day, for obsolescence is much more rapid than deterioration. The written word, the recorded science of yesterday, is here to-day, and we may delve and explore for the thoughts of the pioneer in order that the gains made by those who blaze the path may not be lost to those who follow. But there is a means of transfer of accomplishment which transcends either of these, just as the speed of thought is greater than the working of tools or the reading of words. It is the direct contact between the alert mind of youth and the seasoned and inspiring mind of experience. This is education in its essence. All the paraphernalia of the college, the faculties and curricula, the tall towers and the basement laboratories, have but one purpose, to bring together in an atmosphere of progress the youth and his teacher, and to make it possible for them to work.

It is not by chance that you, who have been scientist, inventor, organizer, engineer, man of business, have been for sixty-odd years professor. It is because that profession holds for you, as it does for us your colleagues, the key to an accomplishment that is more truly satisfying even than the pushing back of the boundaries of science or the application of the fruits thereof to the material benefit of man. There must have been a glorious feeling of triumph when you first watched an electric arc stream out and attenuate in a magnetic field. The satisfaction of electrically making one piece of metal where there were two before was intensified by the realization of what the process would mean in the comforts of life to all. But I venture the thought that these were not as stimulating or as lasting as the satisfaction which was yours when you first caught in the eyes of a youngster that gleam of fire which told you that a spark of your own wisdom had transferred to another mind. The joy of teaching is deep seated in our primary instincts, and there is an immortality more specific than fame.

You have taught us many things of less tangible nature than how to make a transformer yield constant current. You have showed us that a man may be truly a professor and at the same time very practical. And one thing more which I wish to emphasize. You have shown us that a scientist or engineer may be, even in this complex modern world, versatile and yet not superficial. I recall that you were first a professor of chemistry and of mechanics, and you are now professor of applied electricity, and you have been organizer, inventor, man of business, engineer, astronomer, executive, philosopher. In these days, when there is a tendency to specialize so closely, it is well for us to be reminded that the possibilities of being at once broad and deep did not pass with Leonardo da Vinci or even with Benjamin Franklin. Men of our profession—we teachers—are bound to be impressed with the tendency of youths of strikingly capable minds to become interested in one small corner of science and uninterested in the rest of the world. We can pass by those who, through mental laziness, prefer to be superficially and casually interested in everything. But it is unfortunate when a brilliant and creative mind insists upon living in a modern monastic cell. We feel the results of this tendency keenly, as we find men of affairs wholly untouched by the culture of modern science, and scientists without the leavening of the humanities. One most unfortunate product is the type of engineer who does not realize that, in order to apply the fruits of science for the benefit of mankind, he must not only grasp the principles of science, but must also know the needs and aspirations, the possibilities and the frailties, of those whom he would serve. There are students who may realize this fallacy only when it is too late. To those we would say: "There is one of your professors to whom we would call your attention. He exemplifies that combination of breadth with a definiteness of grasp of the affairs of this world to which we may humbly aspire. He has made significant advances in many diverse branches of engineering, represented by many inventions relating to such things as the uniflow steam engine, the lightning arrester, the cream separator, the electric meter, the resistance welder, x-rays, the automobile muffler, the use of helium in diving, the heat treatment of steels and various chemical processes. He has written of such matters as the nature of comets, the light of the firefly and the aurora. He has organized and guided business and one of the great electrical companies of the world bore his name. He has many, many friends. May some of you follow in his distinguished footsteps that the world may be brighter and more replete with the opportunity which comes with material advance! May you make many friends, as he has, that those who inherit these benefits may know and understand each other better. May you grasp his kindly philosophy, that you may be happy as you create."

I bring you, sir, not only the salutations of your colleagues, but also their heartfelt gratitude that you have dignified and enriched the title of professor, and that we may hail you as friend and colleague.

# SCIENTIFIC EVENTS

## INDUSTRIAL RESEARCH LABORATORIES

WE learn from Science Service that while over 55 per cent. of the research laboratories serving America's industries have either maintained their staffs of investigators at the same level or actually increased their workers, there has been a decrease of over 12,000 in the staffs of other industrial laboratories in the past three years. However, at least 90 per cent. of the concerns reporting have maintained at least a skeleton research organization. This is shown in a survey just completed by Dr. C. J. West and Miss Callie Hull, of the Research Information Service of the National Research Council.

This year 1,467 laboratories reported 21,464 scientists on their staffs, while in 1930 there were 33,596 scientists on the staffs of 1,420 laboratories. This is taken to mean that at least 10,000 highly trained industrial research scientists are not engaged in scientific research due to the economic depression. The potential value of the lost services of these scientists must run into millions of dollars annually. Some of these scientifically trained workers have been transferred to plant and sales jobs, it is believed.

The 500 laboratories that reported decreases in staff employed 23,783 in 1930 and now have at work only 9,686. The 628 laboratories that reported no change employ 5,268 investigators. In 186 laboratories the staffs were increased from 3,768 in 1930 to 5,338 in 1933. The number of laboratories discontinued during the three-year period between the National Research Council surveys numbered 106 and they employed 775 scientists in 1930. In the course of the survey 153 laboratories now employing 1,172 scientists were included in the survey for the first time. Some of these may be new laboratories, but most are small research organizations that were not discovered in the course of the 1930 survey.

## THE FIELD MUSEUM OF NATURAL HISTORY

THE annual report of the director of Field Museum of Natural History to the board of trustees, a book of 141 pages with nine photogravure illustrations, has been published by the Field Museum Press. In this book Director Stephen C. Simms outlines the activities of the museum during the year 1932.

The fact is emphasized that the museum has been able to continue its full service to the public, and has even extended its educational influence to a greater number of persons (attendance in 1932 having been 1,824,202) than in any previous year, despite having, like other endowed institutions, suffered a heavy decline in revenue. With income in 1932 $267,000 less than that in 1931, the museum reduced its expenses by $273,000 through calling expeditions home, making payroll adjustments, and putting economies in force throughout the institution.

Among contributions to the museum during the year were the following: from Marshall Field, a trustee of the museum, $96,000; from Stanley Field, president of the museum, $35,788; from Mrs. E. Marshall Field, $50,000; from Mrs. Charles H. Schweppe, $18,000; from Mrs. James Nelson Raymond, $3,000; from Frederick H. Rawson, $3,000; from the American Friends of China, Chicago, $1,075; and various sums from Leon Mandel II, Fred Mandel, Jr., William J. Chalmers and Arthur M. Barnhart.

The report gives a full account of the work of the various scientific departments; the educational activities of the James Nelson and Anna Louise Raymond Foundation and the N. W. Harris Public School Extension, which are units of the museum organization for cooperative work with the schools of Chicago; a résumé of new exhibits; of gifts of material received for the collections, lists of the several thousand members of the museum, and other data on the institution's activities.

## CENTENARY OF THE BRITISH ENTOMOLOGICAL SOCIETY

The Entomological Society of London celebrated the centenary of its foundation at meetings held on May 3 and 4 in the rooms of J. G. Children, of the British Museum. According to the London *Times*, the society received a Royal Charter in 1885, and the King became patron of the society in 1914.

On May 3 a general meeting of the society was held in the rooms of the Royal Geographical Society, Kensington Gore, at which delegates from other learned bodies at home and abroad were received and presented addresses. A scientific conversazione was held in the evening in the house at 41, Queen's Gate, which the Entomological Society now shares with the Imperial Institute of Entomology, and fellows brought with them exhibits.

The following day an afternoon conversazione took place for the delegates at the British Museum (Natural History), and an evening reception at Lancaster House was given by the Government, the guests being received by Major Walter Elliot, minister of agriculture. The delegates from abroad were invited to spend the two following days visiting collections and entomological laboratories in the country, including in their tour Whipsnade and Lord Rothschild's collection at Tring.

Professor E. B. Poulton, who was president in 1903–04 and in 1925–26, has been elected president for the centenary year, while the vice-presidents are Dr. H. Eltringham, Dr. K. Jordan and Mr. R. W. Lloyd. Dr. S. A. Neave, assistant director of the Imperial Institute of Entomology, is the honorary secretary. In addition to fellows of the society (now numbering nearly 700) delegates from about 140 learned institutions, universities and museums at home and abroad accepted invitations to be present.

Minute-books in the possession of the society show that an almost continuous history links the present Entomological Society of London with predecessors as far back as 1745, when the Aurelian Society held meetings at the Swan Tavern, 'Change Alley. The present Entomological Society of London occupied rooms in turn at 17, Old Bond Street, at 12, Bedford Row, and as tenants of the Medical Society of London at 11, Chandos Street. The move to 41, Queen's Gate, took place in 1920, and a meeting-room of great beauty, with panelling and decoration copied from the Bromley Room in the Victoria and Albert Museum, was subsequently constructed through the generosity of Mr. R. W. Lloyd and opened in May, 1930, by Dr. Addison.

## AWARD OF THE LOUBAT PRIZES

Award of the Loubat prize of $1,000 to Dr. Charles O. Paullin, of Washington, D. C., and Dr. John Kirtland Wright, of New York, author and editor, respectively, of the "Atlas of the Historical Geography of the United States," has been announced. The second prize of $400 was awarded to Professor Walter Prescott Webb, of the University of Texas, for "The Great Plains."

The Loubat prizes, instituted in 1893 by a grant of Joseph Florimond, Duc de Loubat, are conferred at the end of every succeeding five-year period for "the best work printed and published in the English language on the history, geography, ethnology, philology or numismatics of North America."

The work of Dr. Paullin and Dr. Wright, issued jointly by the Carnegie Institution and the National Geographic Society in 1932, is described by the Jury of Award as "the first major historical atlas of the United States and probably the most comprehensive study of its kind that has yet been published for any country." The purpose of the atlas is to illustrate cartographically the essential facts of geography and history that "condition and explain" the development of the United States. Presentation will be made formally at Columbia University on Commencement Day, June 6.

Dr. Paullin, formerly a member of the faculties of Johns Hopkins and George Washington Universities, was born at Jamestown, Ohio. He received his bachelor of science degree from Union Christian College, Merom, Indiana, in 1893, and pursued graduate studies at Johns Hopkins University until 1895. The doctor of philosophy degree was conferred on him by the University of Chicago in 1904. After lecturing on diplomatic history at the Johns Hopkins University, and on naval history at George Washington University, Dr. Paullin joined the research staff of the Carnegie Institution, Washington.

Dr. Wright, librarian of the American Geographical Society, was born at Cambridge, Massachusetts, and is a graduate of Harvard University, having received his bachelor of arts degree in 1913, his master's in 1914, and his Ph.D. in 1922. He was an instructor in history at Harvard in 1916 and 1917, and assumed his present position in 1920.

The prize-winning work of Professor Webb, issued in 1932 by Ginn and Company, is declared by the jury of award to be an accurate study of what happened in American civilization when, in its westward progress, it emerged from the woods and "essayed life on the Plains." Professor Webb's answer, the jury continued, "explores all the shaping influences of land, climate and rainfall and displays in fascinating detail the innovations forced upon the pioneers of the Great Plains—innovations in weapons, in agricultural methods and utensils, in fencing, in water supply, in law and custom."

Members of the Loubat jury were Dr. Isaiah Bowman, director of the American Geographical Society, chairman; Dr. Arthur M. Schlesinger, professor of history in Harvard University, and Dr. Carl Russell Fish, professor of American history in the University of Wisconsin.

## THE NATIONAL ACADEMY OF SCIENCES

AT the closing session of the meeting of the National Academy of Sciences held in Washington on April 24, 25 and 26, the following scientific men were elected to membership: Dr. Oswald Theodore Avery, member, Rockefeller Institute for Medical Research, bacteriology; Harold Delos Babcock, physicist at the Mount Wilson Observatory, physics; Dr. Thomas Barbour, director of the Museum of Comparative Zoology, Harvard University, zoology; Dr. Alphonse Raymond Dochez, professor of medicine, Columbia University, medicine; Dr. Bernard O. Dodge, plant pathologist at the New York Botanical Garden, botany; Dr. Eugene F. DuBois, professor of medicine, Cornell University Medical College, pathological physiology; Dr. Griffith C. Evans, professor of pure mathematics, Rice Institute, mathematics; Bancroft Gherardi, vice-president of the American Telephone and Telegraph Company, New York City, engineering; Dr. Herbert Eugene Ives, physicist, Bell Telephone Laboratories, physics; Dr. W. R. Miles, professor of psychology, Yale University, psychology; Samuel Alfred Mitchell, director of the Leander McCormick Observatory, University of Virginia, astronomy; Dr. Linus Pauling, professor of chemistry, California Institute of Technology, chemistry; Dr. J. F. Ritt, professor of mathematics, Columbia University, mathematics; Dr. H. C. Sherman, Mitchill professor of chemistry, Columbia University, chemistry.

At the same session, Dr. Arthur L. Day, director of the Geophysical Laboratory of the Carnegie Institution of Washington, was elected vice-president, succeeding Dr. David White, of the U. S. Geological Survey, resigned. Dr. J. McKeen Cattell, editor of SCIENCE, and Dr. Karl T. Compton, president of the Massachusetts Institute of Technology, were reelected to membership in the governing council of the academy.

At the dinner given on the evening of April 25 medals were presented to five scientific men for distinguished work:

The Alexander Agassiz Medal for Oceanography was given to Dr. Albert Defant, of the Institute for Oceanography, Berlin, for his studies on atmospheric and oceanic circulation and his notable contributions to theoretical oceanography. The address was made by Dr. Henry B. Bigelow, of Harvard University, director of the Woods Hole Oceanographic Institution, and the medal was received by the German ambassador.

The Public Welfare Medal was awarded to Dr. William H. Park, of New York, for his work as head of the research laboratories of the New York City Department of Health as a pioneer and leader both in research and in the application of scientific discovery to the prevention of disease. The address was made by Dr. Simon Flexner, director of the Rockefeller Institute for Medical Research.

The John J. Carty Medal and Award for the Advancement of Science was awarded before his death to Dr. Carty, in whose honor the medal was established, for his distinguished accomplishments in the field of electrical engineering. Dr. Frank B. Jewett, president of the Bell Telephone Laboratories, a colleague of Dr. Carty, made the address, and the medal was received by his son, Dr. John Russell Carty.

The Henry Draper Medal was presented to Dr. V. M. Slipher, astronomer of the Lowell Observatory, Flagstaff, Arizona, in recognition of his spectroscopic researches. The address was made by Dr. Henry Norris Russell, research professor of astronomy and director of the Princeton University observatory.

The Mary Clark Thompson Medal was given to Dr. Francis Arthur Bather, of Wimbledon, England, for his distinguished services in the fields of paleontology and geology. The British ambassador having been detained by the political situation, the medal was received by Ralph Howard Fowler, of the University of Cambridge.

# SCIENTIFIC NOTES AND NEWS

DR. ROSS G. HARRISON, Sterling professor of biology at Yale University, has accepted the invitation of the Royal Society of London to give the Croonian Lecture on June 29.

PROFESSOR NIELS BOHR, of the University of Copenhagen, will give the Graduate School Convocation address at Brown University on June 17, his title being "Explanation in Natural Science."

THE John Fritz Gold Medal, which was awarded last November to Daniel Cowan Jackling, of San Francisco, for "notable industrial achievement in initiating mass production of copper from low-grade ores, through the application of engineering principles," was presented to him at a recent meeting in New York of the American Institute of Mining and Metallurgical Engineers. Dr. Geo. Otis Smith, chairman of the Federal Power Commission, made the principal address.

THE gold medal of the National Institute of Social Sciences will be presented to Clifford W. Beers, who initiated the movement for mental hygiene which led to the establishment of the National Committee for Mental Hygiene, the twenty-fifth anniversary of which will be celebrated in New Haven on May 6. Mr. Beers will also be the guest of honor at a meeting to be held on May 10 at the Twentieth Century Club, Boston, to commemorate the twentieth anniversary of the establishment of the Massachusetts Society for Mental Hygiene and the twenty-fifth anniversary of the movement.

FRANK A. PERRET, director of the new volcanological station at the foot of Mt. Pelée, St. Pierre, Martinique, has been appointed Chevalier de la Légion d'honneur by the French Government.

A CORRESPONDENT of the *Journal* of the American Medical Association states that at a recent meeting of the All-Russian Central Executive Committee the degree of honorary science-worker was awarded to the following physicians: Professors Alexis I. Abrikosov, of the First Moscow Medical Institute, for his scientific work in the field of pathology; Professor Nicolas N. Bourdenko, for his scientific work in neuropathology and medical education; Professor Wladimir I. Wojachek, of the Military Medical Academy, for his studies in otolaryngology; Professor Ivan I. Grekov, of the Second Leningrad Medical Institute, who instructed many scientific workers in the field of surgery; Professor Alexis W. Martynov, of the Moscow First Medical Institute, for his surgical work and teaching, and Professor Basil B. Cramer, for his scientific work in the field of neuropathology.

BY an order of the Committee of Privy Council of Great Britain made after consultation with the Medical Research Council and with the president of the Royal Society, Sir Thomas Lewis, director of the department of clinical research in University College Hospital, London, has been appointed a member of the council in succession to Professor J. J. R. Macleod, of the University of Aberdeen.

LORD DAWSON of Penn was reelected on April 10 as president of the Royal College of Physicians, London.

AT the annual election of the Pennsylvania Academy of Sciences Dr. John C. Johnson, State Teachers College, West Chester, was elected *president;* Dr. S. H. Derickson, Lebanon Valley College, Annville, *vice-president;* Dr. H. W. Thurston, Pennsylvania State College, *treasurer;* Dr. T. L. Guyton, Pennsylvania Department of Agriculture, Harrisburg, *secretary;* Dr. V. Earl Light, Lebanon Valley College, *assistant secretary,* and R. W. Stone, Geological Survey, Harrisburg, *editor.* The annual summer meeting will be held in August at Ohio Pyle. The place of meeting for the tenth annual meeting has not been selected.

THE officers elected for a three-year term by the Wisconsin Academy of Sciences, Arts and Letters at the annual meeting held at Madison, April 7 to 8, include: *President,* Rufus M. Bagg, Lawrence College, Appleton; *Vice-president for the Division of Sciences,* Storrs B. Barrett, Yerkes Observatory; *Vice-presidents—for the Division of Arts,* Anselm M. Keefe, St. Norbert College, West De Pere, *for the Division of Letters,* A. R. Hohlfeld, University of Wisconsin; *Secretary-Treasurer,* H. A. Schuette, University of Wisconsin; *Librarian,* W. M. Smith, University of Wisconsin; *Curator,* C. E. Brown, State Historical Museum.

THE council of the University of Bristol has accepted with regret the resignation as from July 31 of Professor A. J. Sutton Pippard from the chair of civil engineering on his appointment to the London University chair of civil engineering at Imperial College. Professor Pippard is a graduate of the university and returned to fill the chair vacated by Professor Ferrier in 1928.

IN recognition of the work of Dr. Evans in metallurgy, the General Board of the University of Oxford has appointed him assistant director of research in metallurgy, without stipend from the university, for the period during which he holds the Royal Society Armourers' and Brasiers' research fellowship in metallurgy.

LAWRENCE MCHUEY, curator of birds and mammals at the Natural History Museum at San Diego, California, has been appointed federal inspector of exotic birds and mammals entering the port of San Diego.

THE J. T. Baker Chemical Company Eastern Analytical Research Fellowship for 1933–34 has been awarded to Mr. G. W. Low, Jr., graduate of Princeton University, 1931. Mr. Low will engage in analytical investigations at Princeton.

GERALD ASHLEY WARING, geologist in the U. S. Geological Survey, has returned to Washington after two years spent on a detailed survey of the coal deposits of Alaska.

DR. FORREST SHREVE and Dr. T. D. Mallery, of the Desert Laboratory of the Carnegie Institution, and Dr. Ira L. Wiggins, of Stanford University, recently returned from an expedition to the valleys of the Yaqui and Mayo Rivers in southern Sonora. The transition from desert to thorn-forest was studied, some physiological work was done on *Larrea* and *Encelia,* and nearly 400 plants were collected.

SIR HUBERT WILKINS has sailed on the *Bremen* to take part in the proposed Antarctic flight of Lincoln Ellsworth and Bernt Balchen. Sir Hubert is *en route* to Germany, where he will make preparations for the flight before going on to Cape Town and then to New Zealand, where he will meet the Ellsworth-Balchen expedition.

DR. W. F. G. SWANN, director of the Bartol Research Laboratories of the Franklin Institute at Swarthmore, addressed the institute on April 19, on "The Work of the Bartol Research Foundation."

DR. HENRY E. SIGERIST, formerly director of the Institute of Medicine at the University of Leipzig, who succeeded Dr. William H. Welch as director of the Institute of the History of Medicine of the Johns Hopkins University, delivered an illustrated lecture before the Washington Academy of Sciences on April 20. His subject was "Medicine of the Renaissance."

DR. FLORENCE R. SABIN, member of the Rockefeller Institute for Medical Research, gave on May 2 the first lecture on the foundation established at Goucher College by the Baltimore Association for the Promotion of the University Education of Women. The subject of the lecture was "Cells in Relation to Tuberculosis."

DR. WILLIAM BEEBE, director of the department of tropical research at the New York Zoological Park, will address the Phi Beta Kappa Alumni in New York at the annual meeting on May 10. The title of his lecture will be "Four Hundred Fathoms Down."

MARKUS RENIER, visiting research professor of Lafayette College, an engineer of the Department of Public Works of the British government in Palestine, is giving a series of lectures on mathematical rheology at the John C. Green School of Engineering, Princeton University.

DR. MILTON J. ROSENAU, professor of preventive medicine and hygiene, Harvard Medical School, will give two courses at the summer session of the University of California. One course will deal with epidemiology, the other with public health.

THE eleventh Colloid Symposium, which was scheduled to be held at the University of Wisconsin on June 15, 16 and 17, has been postponed for one year.

THE twenty-first annual meeting of the Eugenics Research Association will be held on June 3 at the American Museum of Natural History, New York City.

THE annual spring meeting of the Association of Consulting Psychologists will be held on May 6 at the University of Pennsylvania.

THE third annual meeting of the Field Conference of Pennsylvania Geologists is to be held at Harrisburg, Pennsylvania, on May 27, 28 and 29 at the invitation of the Pennsylvania Topographic and Geologic Survey. Field trips will include Cornwall Mines, the Triassic and the Paleozoic sections of south-central Pennsylvania.

THE ninth annual field conference of the New York State Geological Association will be held in the New York City region on May 12 and 13. The association will convene at Newburgh, New York, on the morning of Friday, May 12, and will proceed by car through Peekskill to northern New York City; stops will be made at localities displaying the overthrusting of the crystalline rocks of the Highlands northwestward on the younger Paleozoic rocks, and the metasediments of northern New York City will be examined. An evening session will be held at Columbia University. Saturday, May 13, will be devoted to a study of the Triassic rocks west of the Hudson River, and of the glacial features and the serpentine on Staten Island. Further information may be obtained from the secretary, Dr. G. Marshall Kay, Columbia University.

*Museum News* reports that at the meeting of the American Association which will be held in Chicago in June the dates will articulate with those of other conventions which are attended by museum workers: June 8–10, American Federation of Arts; June 12–14, American Association of Museums; June 14–15, Association of Art Museum Directors; June 15–17, College Art Association; June 19–30, American Association for the Advancement of Science. The sections and chairmen are as follows: Art, Walter H. Siple, Cincinnati; History, Robert W. Bingham, Buffalo;

Science, Charles C. Adams, Albany; Art Technique, Edward W. Forbes, Cambridge; Technical (Science technique), E. L. Judah, Montreal; Superintendents, J. Francis McCabe, Chicago; Education, Mrs. Grace Fisher Ramsey, New York; Public Relations, I. T. Frary, Cleveland; Radio, Chauncey J. Hamlin, Buffalo; College, Carl E. Guthe, Ann Arbor.

THE American Mining Congress will be held in Pittsburgh from May 8 to 12. Discussions will be centered about present problems of the coal industry, these including management, mining methods, safety program, mechanical production, haulage, and coal analyses. A large exhibit will be installed in the William Penn Hotel in Pittsburgh, where most of the manufacturers will display products used by the coal mining industry. J. B. Warriner, president of the American Mining Congress, will lead the sessions held in Pittsburgh, with subchairmen in charge of divisional activities. The Pittsburgh committee is headed by Dr. L. E. Young, vice-president of the Pittsburgh Coal Company.

THE ninety-third annual meeting of the German Society of Naturalists and Physicians will be held in Hannover in 1934. There will be no meeting during the present year.

FOLLOWING the resignation of Dr. James Franck, professor of physics at the University of Göttingen and member of the Kaiser Wilhelm Institute of Physical Chemistry and Electrochemistry at Berlin, the resignations have been received, according to press reports, of Professor Herbert Freundlich, distinguished for his work in colloid chemistry, and of Dr. Michael Polanyi, physicist, vice-directors of the institute. An Associated Press dispatch, dated April 28, states that Professor Hermann Jacobsohn, of the University of Marburg, has committed suicide by throwing himself before a train. It is also reported that Dr. Bernhard Zondek, who has been forced from his professorship of gynecology in the University of Berlin, may be given a position in the University of Stockholm. Dr. Gustav Bucky, for three years director of the Central Röntgen Institute and the cancer department at the Rudolf Virchow Hospital, who was reported early this month to be "on vacation," has also resigned and is now in New York. Dr. Bucky is an American citizen of German-Jewish birth.

IN regard to dismissals of German professors, a correspondent of *The New York Times* writes: "Twenty-six Jewish professors were dismissed from the faculties of the leading Prussian universities on April 25 by Bernhard Rust, Nazi Minister of Culture for that state. This makes a total of forty-two Jewish or Republican savants who have lost their teaching posts at Prussian universities within the month, but it is announced officially that these removals constitute only a first instalment in a general house-cleaning of the German academic groves from what is known, in Nazi parlance, as "alien influence." No fewer than eighteen among the Jewish professors who lost their positions belonged to the faculty of the University of Frankfort-am-Main, while seven were dropped from the University of Göttingen and one from the University of Marburg."

THE seventy-eighth annual exhibition of the Royal Photographic Society of Great Britain is to be held in London from September 9 to October 7, inclusive. It is requested that all entries for the technical section from residents of the United States be sent to Dr. Walter Clark, Eastman Kodak Research Laboratories, Rochester, New York. Exhibits should be mounted but not framed, and should reach Dr. Clark not later than June 20. Exhibits for Section III may consist of photographs or transparencies related to the following subjects: natural history, photomicrography, radiography, astronomical and aerial photography, stereoscopy, survey and record work, press and theatrical photography, meteorological, geological and metallurgical applications of photography and useful photographic devices. It is hoped that a generous contribution will be made in order to maintain the high standard set by American contributors to the technical section in previous years. Entry forms may be obtained on application to Dr. Clark. There is no fee.

DURING the past fall and winter the Bacteriological Laboratories at the Pennsylvania State College have been entirely remodeled and reequipped and have been used during the first semester. Specially designed laboratory desks have been installed. Rolling doors make it possible to divide the larger laboratory with ample accommodations for a section of fifty students into two laboratories for smaller groups when desirable. An important item of new equipment is the constant temperature room (37° C.) which affords sufficient space for incubation of class cultures. The facilities now provide excellent working conditions for 280 students registered in the division of bacteriology.

IN connection with the commemoration of the one hundred and ninetieth birthday of Thomas Jefferson, founder of the University of Virginia, presentation to the university was made of a ten-inch photographic telescope of 45-inch focal length from Mount Wilson Observatory. The telescope is to be used by Dr. S. A. Mitchell, director of the McCormick Observatory, in photographing 18,000 stars to determine their proper motions. Funds to provide a complete new mounting have been provided by the Carnegie Institution of Washington.

FRANK A. WARDLAW and his son, Frank A. Wardlaw, Jr., have recently presented to the U. S. National Museum the only cast now known to exist from a life mask of Thomas A. Edison. The mask was made in 1878, the year of the invention of the phonograph and the year before the invention of the incandescent lamp. As this was the only mask of Edison ever made, it will be of value as a record. The same donors presented original Edison lamps of the first types of paper filament and bamboo filament lamps, a galvanometer used by Joseph Henry, and several models of locomotives and marine engines.

THE executive committee of the sixth International Congress for Industrial Diseases and Accidents, held at Geneva last year, has instituted a prize of 1,000 Swiss francs for the best essay on the estimation of the consequences of an industrial accident. The typescript of the essay, which may be written in English, French, German or Italian, should be sent to the general secretary of the congress, Geneva, before December 31, 1934.

AT a recent meeting of the American Institute of Nutrition—Dr. H. C. Sherman, president, and Dr. John R. Murlin, secretary-treasurer—*The Journal of Nutrition,* owned by the American Institute of Nutrition, was transferred to The Wistar Institute. Beginning in January, 1934, this journal will be published by the institute under the same editorial management. Announcement of an increase in the number of yearly issues will be made later. The acquisition of *The Journal of Nutrition* is the first step in the creation of a department of nutrition at The Wistar Institute.

THE return of a permanent American delegate to the International Institute of Agriculture at Rome is probable as the result of action by the Senate Foreign Relations Committee, which has approved a bill by Senator Hiram Johnson, of California, to finance representation at a cost of $48,500 a year. The institute is the nucleus for world planning in crop production. Seventy-four nations participate and America had a permanent delegate at the institute up until four years ago.

THE New York Botanical Garden is now conducting a school for gardeners modeled on those of Kew and Edinburgh. In the past the gardening profession in the United States has been recruited almost entirely from Europe. Student-gardeners are temporary employees remaining at the garden for two years. During the day-time they perform the duties of gardener, being moved as opportunity permits from one department to another to broaden their experience. They attend a two-year course of evening lectures, including such subjects as general and systematic botany, physics and chemistry, soils and fertilizers, plant pathology, entomology, genetics and plant breeding. They also attend demonstrations by the staff and visit other gardens. On satisfactory completion of the two years course a certificate is awarded, also a year's extension of employment at the garden during which time the student is expected to seek employment elsewhere. Appointment as student-gardener is limited to those prepared to do the work without remuneration. The New York Botanical Garden, in cooperation with the Horticultural Society of New York and the National Association of Gardeners, is also conducting a course for professional gardeners in the basic sciences underlying gardening practise.

# DISCUSSION

## THE CRISIS IN SCIENTIFIC RESEARCH AND THE WAY OUT

WE find ourselves, to-day, faced with a crisis in scientific research, especially in biology and medicine. Professor Krogh has already referred to it at the Thirteenth International Congress of Physiology, held at Boston in 1929.

The causes of this difficulty would seem to lie in a discrepancy between the efforts and the results of research work. The effects of collective scientific endeavor are to-day quantitatively so vast that the possibility of surveying and applying them with complete assurance and certainty becomes ever more remote. From this results a constant increase in specialization; one perceives the various connections less and less clearly, the great clear directing lines and historical points of view tending to disappear. Or, one is obliged to undertake a quite incredible amount of labor, in fact, to devote one's entire life, so to speak, to the subject, without even being certain that the results will prove worth the trouble.

This often only half perceived, almost unconsciously felt, recognition discourages many young scientists so that they turn more willingly towards those forms of activity which promise more practical results, and this constitutes the chief danger to scientific research and its traditions.

The principal cause of all this lies, in my opinion, in the fact that in the technique of publication and survey of scientific results, in the method of mental and scientific synthesis, the old established customs still hold sway, but these are no longer suited to the pace and necessities of our time. We are, to-day, accustomed to the scientific organization of work in every sphere of industry, commerce and administration, one may even say in politics and political propaganda. Only in the realm of science one fails to trace any kind of scientific organization worthy of the importance of science; and in this way much time, energy and economy of means is wasted.

This is especially conspicuous in the production of scientific literature. Science, whilst it is one and international, appears in publications in more than twenty languages, in hundreds of magazines, in thousands, even tens of thousands of pamphlets, in a year. The themes of research work are left mostly to chance, thousands of problems are worked up without any logical discrimination, without intrinsic power, often occasioned by purely external circumstances, for reasons which have nothing to do with the research itself. And these millions of pages are poured out over us like a flood, they cover and swamp us, they inundate us so that we stand continually in a despairing struggle to keep our heads above this sea of papers.

The way out of this chaos is the same as that taken by economics and by the state, namely, rationalization or so-called scientific management. One need not think that through rationalization intuition, the creative faculty, will be suppressed; on the contrary, it will then first obtain a real facility for its awakening, and will then first be able to develop itself satisfactorily. The less energy required to be expended on overcoming difficulties, the more there will be for creation, for invention, and the higher will be the quality of its output.

I have tried for some years to apply to the realm of science the principles of scientific management in industry, administration and politics, and have worked out a system for the means of rationalizing the scientific institutes for research activities and for the collective scientific institutions.

The whole refers to the following system of subjects:

I. Scientific laboratory management:
   (1) Administration of scientific institutes.
   (2) Application of specific scientific activities:
      Practical arrangements.
      Economy of time.

II. Work of research-workers:
   (1) Physical and psychic hygiene of mental work.
   (2) Systematic method in research, especially time- and plan-schedules.
   (3) Application of the card system for collecting scientific data and ideas.

III. Collective scientific activities:
   (1) Congresses—their organization and general plan of research.
   (2) Scientific literature—systematization of periodicals, libraries, reports, scientific treatises, schedules and card indices.
   (3) Scientific language and standardization of expert expressions.

I suggest that an International Committee might consider these problems systematically and make definite propositions.

SERGEI TSCHACHOTIN

KAISER WILHELM INSTITUT FÜR MEDIZINISCHE FORSCHUNG
HEIDELBERG

## COOPERATION AMONG AMERICAN ZOOLOGISTS TOWARD A COMPENDIUM OF CULTURE METHODS FOR INVERTEBRATE ANIMALS

AT the Atlantic City meeting of the American Association for the Advancement of Science, this matter again came up. Vice-president Zeleny, chairman of Section F—Zoology, appointed as a committee to consider it Dr. Frank E. Lutz, of the American Museum of Natural History, Dr. Paul S. Welch, of the University of Michigan, and Dr. J. G. Needham, of Cornell University.

At the present time there is difficulty in finding information about culture methods. Much more experience has been gained by individuals than has ever been made available through publication. Much also undoubtedly exists in papers whose titles give no clue of its presence. Such information if gathered together and made available to the many whose work nowadays demands the use of living materials in continuous supply would be a great aid to biological research.

The committee has found a very general feeling of need for such a compendium and is proceeding with plans for it. Its plans are as yet wholly tentative. A book is contemplated, to contain the information that is needed by the one who is trying to rear and maintain cultures. It is proposed to have a short introductory chapter on general principles of management, with the main body of the book made up of signed articles, volunteered by individual workers and based on their own practical experience.

It is hoped that for at least one species of each considerable group of invertebrates there may be included a fairly complete account of maintenance requirements, covering collecting methods and devices, cages and breeding quarters, plans for feeding and watering, cleaning and aerating quarters, breeding management, and all else that enters into the maintenance of the species through successive generations. Such full accounts, however, will be few, and less comprehensive items will be welcome.

The committee reserves the right to condense and to combine where necessary to avoid duplication. An effort will be made to include bibliographical references to all the more important relevant published material; also summaries and cross-references to aid in finding things.

The scope proposed is North American invertebrates. It goes without saying that Apis and Bombyx are not to be discussed beyond laboratory usages, since their culture has long passed the stage of pioneering that we are to record.

This call goes out to all American zoologists. Let any one who has tested out a reliable method of culture maintenance, or any device that he has found to be particularly useful to that end, write it up and submit it for a place in this book to any member of the committee.

JAMES G. NEEDHAM,
*Chairman*

CORNELL UNIVERSITY

## REVERSAL OF THE PINHOLE IMAGE

IT was my good fortune to be associated with Dr. Oliver J. Lee, director of Dearborn Observatory, in a problem he investigated at the time of the solar eclipse in August, 1932. He wished to obtain information regarding temperature changes produced by the moon's shadow at various altitudes. For elevations of 700, 3,000 and 10,000 feet, this information was furnished by recording meteorographs carried by airplanes, which cruised at constant altitudes in circles about a mile in radius. Lieutenant Baker and I were in the highest plane, which stayed at 10,400 feet most of the time, but rose to 15,000 feet for a while. The report of the observations which I made to Dr. Lee that evening included one phenomenon which I have not seen described by any of the observers who were in airplanes during the eclipse.

For about fifteen minutes preceding totality, while the solar crescent was very narrow, whenever I looked where the shadow of the airplane would have been cast on the clouds more than a mile below, I saw a halo about five degrees in diameter, red on the outside, yellowish on the inner side, with a dark, shadow-like crescent at its center. The angular diameter of the shadow crescent was the same as that of the solar crescent. The thickness at the middle was somewhat greater. What attracted my attention particularly was the fact that the cusps of this shadow crescent pointed eastward, while those of the solar crescent pointed westward. After totality the whole appearance was repeated, except that the cusps of both crescents were reversed in direction.

It was a phenomenon similar to that seen by Edwin Edser in England during the partial eclipse of 1912 and described by him in *Nature* for May 2 of that year. It was the reverse of the familiar pinhole image. A huge screen with a relatively small hole at the position of the airplane would have caused a bright, inverted crescent against a dark background on the clouds, crescent image and solar crescent having the same angular dimensions as seen from the screen. Interchanging screen and hole would interchange image and background, giving the dark crescent which I saw on the bright clouds.

I have repeated, with some modifications, the experiment Edser described. A piece of ground glass close to the condenser of a stereopticon was nearly covered with a circular disk of black paper, leaving only a bright, narrow crescent exposed. The objective of the lantern was removed. A screen with a small hole placed ten feet from the lantern produced a pinhole image on the crescent on the wall an equal distance from the screen. Then a brass ball about the size of the hole was used in place of the screen and a dark, shadow-like crescent appeared on the wall, corresponding exactly to what I saw on the clouds. A small square of black paper substituted for the ball gave the same dark crescent. A little airplane made of black paper also produced the same result. The shadow crescent was independent of the shape of the obstacle, as a pinhole image is independent of the shape of the pinhole, provided obstacle or hole is small enough in comparison with the object. As stated by Edser, in order to obtain the shadow image, the screen must be beyond the apex of the umbra of the shadow cast by the obstacle.

ERNEST C. BRYANT

MIDDLEBURY COLLEGE

## THE ADRENAL GLANDS IN AN EDITOR'S OFFICE

A DISTINGUISHED physiologist wrote to the editor of SCIENCE on April 14:

At the recent meetings of the American Physiological Society in Cincinnati Dr. Britton of the University of Virginia made the statement in open meeting that SCIENCE had published an article on the adrenals by Professor Swingle of Princeton University, the publication of which was paid for by Professor Swingle, and that the pages of SCIENCE have been subsequently closed to Professor Britton and possibly others on the subject of Professor Swingle's original paper or article. If true, this appears to me both a curious and serious situation. I had the understanding that SCIENCE was an organ of the American Association for the Advancement of Science. If scientific articles published in SCIENCE are paid for by authors, that fact should be stated, it seems to me, in connection with the article as it appears in SCIENCE, because otherwise we appear to be in danger of under-cover paid propaganda.

A distinguished physicist wrote on April 19:

From a number of influential and reputable sources, I have run into a considerable amount of irritation over the article by Swingle, Pfiffner, Vars, Bott, and Parkins in SCIENCE for January 13. This irritation is on the following grounds: First, that the article implies that the discoveries there reported were made by the authors; second, that the material was rushed to publication through a subsidiary of [subsidy to] SCIENCE; and third, that replies to this article by recognized leaders in the field have either not been accepted or have not been acknowledged.

I admit that the field is entirely outside my own knowledge. Nevertheless, I am assured by men who are the leaders of similar work at the Harvard Medical School and in Massachusetts hospitals that every one of the 12 points published by Swingle, et al, had been published by others, as indicated in part in the enclosed bibliography. I am further informed that this is not the first instance in which Swingle has been in a similar position.

Under these circumstances, therefore, I can not but feel that this incident has reacted unfavorably to the Association and in particular, will be a handicap to the cooperation which we hoped to secure next winter.

The letter from the physiologist was sent to Professor Britton with the following request:

Please be so kind as to let me know whether Professor ——— reports correctly what you said at the meeting of the American Physiological Society. In case he does not state correctly what you said, please let me know what this was.

In his reply Professor Britton wrote:

In prefacing my paper at Cincinnati, since Swingle coming just before me had again neglected to recognize the earlier work of others, I remarked that a recent situation which had come up in connection with the adrenal controversy should perhaps be aired at that time; that Swingle and his associates had recently published an article on a circulatory theory of cortico-adrenal function in which they had stated that all other theories were practically valueless, and gave no reference at all to the previous theories of others, although the paper had been greatly extended over several pages; that the article had been paid for apparently out of special research funds as stated in their foot-note; that other workers in the field (excepting Freeman's partial reply, of course) wishing to reply to the article found that publication could not be secured; that we ourselves could not at first get a reply published on offering to pay for it, but that eventually a short article had been accepted by the journal; and further, that subsidizing or paying for research publications set up a very unfortunate precedent, to say the least. Later, in question time, I asked Swingle if he would mind telling *why* he found it necessary to pay for science publications, and he declined to answer. To my knowledge, this is all I said on the subject.

The facts of the case are these. Professor E. G. Conklin, of Princeton University, wrote (he permits the quotation) on December 22:

I am sending you herewith a manuscript by Professor Swingle and his associates on the physiological activity of the adrenal cortex. I think that this is an extraordinarily important discovery, comparable in many ways to the discovery of insulin, and likely to be of very great service in medicine and surgery.

Professor Swingle had written:

The contents of this paper should be placed before biologists and medical men at the earliest opportunity since there can be no question but that the adrenal cortical hormone is specific in the treatment of surgical and traumatic shock. This form of shock costs the lives of thousands of people yearly and now that the cortical hormone is available for use, it seems a pity that the facts should not be made known and lives saved as speedily as possible.

To Professor Conklin the editor of SCIENCE replied:

I am pleased to learn of the important work of Professor Swingle and also that you and he regard SCIENCE as the best place of publication. As you know, we can not under ordinary circumstances print longer research articles in SCIENCE. . . . The Physical Society has adopted a plan, which is also used in connection with other journals and will I dare say become general in the future, of making the cost of publication part of the cost of the research. . . . If SCIENCE could be enlarged to the extent of the length of the paper it could be printed at once, it being stated that the cost of printing had been defrayed by the institution from which it came. However, this is something that has never been done and I suppose that it is not worth while to take up the possibility at the present time.

After conversation with Professor Conklin at the Atlantic City meeting of the American Association, the editor wrote to him on January 7 as follows:

I have been a good deal bothered about Professor Swingle's article. The journals that I edit have not charged for illustrations, tables or proof alterations, and it is a very considerable departure from long usage to enlarge the journal and charge the cost to the author or institution. Scientific journals, however, seem to be coming to this policy, even when the journal is not enlarged for the purpose of prompt publication, and I expect that it will be generally adopted.

In the case of Professor Swingle's article, it is not only the question of the cost, though under existing conditions that is somewhat serious, but of giving precedence to a long article over the other articles that we have been compelled to hold for a considerable time and especially over the addresses and other material presented at Atlantic City to which we aim in January and February to give most of the space in SCIENCE.

The situation could be explained by a footnote to the effect that SCIENCE had been enlarged to publish this article, the cost having been defrayed by the Macy Foundation or the Princeton Laboratory, as the case may be. On the whole, therefore, though not without reluctance, I shall accept Professor Swingle's offer.

After the publication of Professor Swingle's article three criticisms were received. One of them, abusive and probably libelous, was returned; one by Dr. Norman E. Freeman was promptly printed; the third, by Dr. Britton, was too long for publication in SCIENCE, but a shorter reply was published. After this had been accepted Professor Britton wrote: "Let me again assure you of my gratitude in granting this privilege of reply in your much-esteemed journal." A counter reply by Professor Swingle containing new data was not accepted, though he was informed that a short reply would be.

Professor Britton has published within the last two years five articles in SCIENCE. Indeed the adrenal glands and the whole field of chemical physiology have received, not more attention than their importance deserves, but more space than has been given to other subjects equally important. Now it is necessary to print more words (it costs three cents each to print a word in SCIENCE) on the adrenals; but that and the troubles of an editor are obviously small matters compared with the saving of thousands of lives (see above).

J. MCKEEN CATTELL

# SCIENTIFIC APPARATUS AND LABORATORY METHODS

## A NEW FORM OF CENTRIFUGE-MICROSCOPE FOR SIMULTANEOUS OBSERVATION OF CONTROL AND EXPERIMENTAL MATERIAL

IN centrifuge studies on the effect of substances on the viscosity or the tension at the surface of living cells, comparison of experimental conditions with control conditions is a necessity. This can be accomplished by a slight modification of the centrifuge-microscopes[1] previously described, which very greatly adds to the convenience and usefulness of the instruments. In the same field of view a perfect image of control and experimental material side by side can be obtained for any power of the microscopes (except oil immersion objectives) and for any rate of rotation that will not shatter the materials of which the instrument is made. Adaptation to the Beams air turbine is possible.[2]

As illustrated in Fig. 1 the device is a special head in the form of a bar, fitting on the ½ inch shaft (A) of a high speed electric motor. At the two ends of the bar are depressions for the special slides S, S¹, which hold the living cells, two microscope objective systems mounted horizontally, and small right angle reflecting prisms to reflect the images to the axis of rotation. Here two ½ inch right angle prisms ¼ inch wide are mounted facing in opposite directions, so as to reflect from both ends of the bar vertically to the stationary ocular (Oc.).

If the lights (L, L′) are incandescent filaments whose images are thrown on the slides parallel to a radius of rotation, the distance of S and S′ to the axis of rotation must differ by 3 to 5 mm, so that S will not be illuminated by L′ and *vice versa*. Since

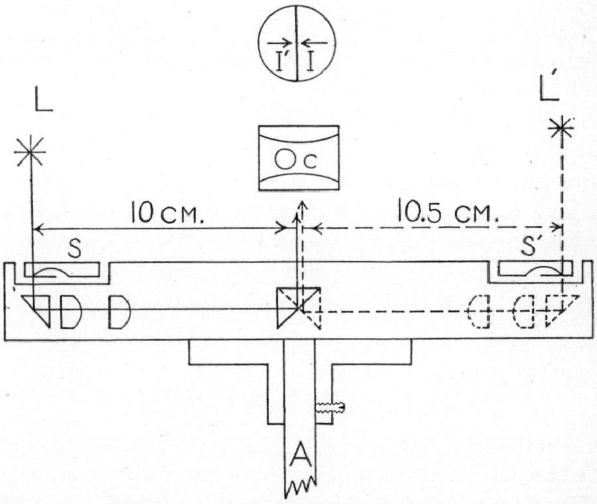


FIG. 1. Diagram of centrifuge-microscope for simultaneous observation of control and experimental material.

the radius of rotation may be 100 mm, this makes a difference of only 3 to 5 per cent. in the centrifugal force on the two slides. The image of material in S′ appears in the left field of the ocular, I′, and the image of material in S appears in the right field, I, the direction of the centrifugal force being indicated by arrows. For successive observation of S and S′, only one light need be used, say L. It is moved 5 mm further from the axis for observation of S′ and back again for observation of S.

If a high voltage condenser discharge in Hg. vapor is used as the source of illumination, L and L′, the distance of S and S′ from the axis may be exactly the same, but the contact surfaces which set off the lamps are arranged at different radial distances from the axis, so that lamp L discharges only when over S and lamp L′ only when over S′. The mercury discharge lamp gives a clearer image over the whole field of view, but necessitates a more complicated accessory mechanism.

[1] E. N. Harvey and A. L. Loomis, SCIENCE, 72: 42, 1930; E. N. Harvey, *Jour. Franklin Inst.*, 214: 1, 1932. I express my sincere thanks to Mr. Alfred L. Loomis for the generous hospitality of his laboratory at Tuxedo Park, N. Y., where the new head was made. The Bausch and Lomb Optical Company will place the standard centrifuge-microscope on the market.

[2] J. W. Beams, SCIENCE, 74: 44, 1931; E. N. Harvey, SCIENCE, 75: 267, 1932.

In this manner the remarkable difference in behavior under the influence of centrifugal force of unfertilized and just fertilized sea-urchin eggs can be observed, and quantitative comparison made of the effect of any substance on the viscosity or form of living cells.

E. NEWTON HARVEY

BIOLOGY DEPARTMENT
PRINCETON UNIVERSITY

### THE AGITATION OF MATERIAL IN AERATED WATER

IN a recent issue,[1] McCutcheon described an apparatus for circulating and aerating material. The purpose of this note is to describe an arrangement that has been found particularly useful for difficult material, and is successful in a number of cases where other methods have not been entirely satisfactory.

It consists of a circular flat-sided flask (a standard Kolle culture flask serves admirably) filled with water, into which is inserted a glass tube bent and connected with a compressed air outlet.

The bubbles of air, rising at one side of the flask, set up a circular motion in the water, the rapidity of which can be adjusted at will by controlling the stream of air, so as to keep the material continuously circulating.

The apparatus is especially useful when the shape or size of the objects circulated renders them likely to become tangled or lodged against obstructions in their path. The smooth, circular motion, with a minimum of subsidiary vortices makes for a very efficient utilization of the air current. A relatively small amount of air is sufficient to keep light objects submerged and circulating, and objects with a specific gravity considerably greater than water circulate freely.

The use of a filter pump to supply the air current is feasible if the joints of the apparatus be made airtight.

The addition of two siphons, with their outer ends immersed below water surfaces of properly adjusted height, will provide for a gradual change of water in the flask, and convert it into an efficient washing apparatus.

H. B. SIFTON

UNIVERSITY OF TORONTO

[1] SCIENCE, November 4, 1932.

# SPECIAL ARTICLES

### THE ATOMIC WEIGHT OF LEAD FROM KATANGA PITCHBLENDE

THROUGH Professor A. C. Lane, chairman of the Committee of the National Research Council on the Measurement of Geologic Time, we have recently received a fine specimen of Katanga pitchblende, a gift from Radium Belge. Petrographic examination by Professors Lindgren and Newhouse, of the Massachusetts Institute of Technology, showed the black base to be permeated with microscopic veins of yellow material which Davis has already found to be readily soluble in dilute hydrochloric acid. Extraction of the very finely powdered material with dilute hydrochloric acid removed 22.8 per cent. of the original. Approximate analysis of the residual black pitchblende and of the extract yielded the following percentages of uranium and lead. Other analysts have found similar material to be nearly if not quite free from thorium.

| | Per cent. U | Per cent. Pb | Pb/U |
|---|---|---|---|
| Pitchblende | 74.9 | 6.7 | 0.089 |
| Extract | 58.5 | 8.4 | 0.144 |
| Whole | 71.2 | 7.1 | 0.100 |

Lead was extracted from both portions and was purified chiefly by many crystallizations as nitrate in quartz and as chloride in quartz and platinum. Next it was twice distilled in dry hydrogen chloride, and finally it was fused in nitrogen containing hydrogen chloride in a weighed quartz boat.

Analysis of the chloride was effected by solution and comparison with a solution of nearly equivalent quantity of pure silver. The end point of the comparison was found by the equal opalescence method with the aid of hundredth normal silver and chloride solutions and a nephelometer. For comparison, samples of chloride similarly purified were prepared from common lead (Coeur d'Alene) and from Bedford cyrtolite[1] and analyzed.

The result for common lead agrees closely with that commonly accepted (207.22) and that from Bedford cyrtolite with the value previously found by ourselves (205.92). The varieties from Katanga pitchblende both apparently possess atomic weights appreciably lower than that found by Hönigschmid and Birckenbach,[2] 206.05, with lead extracted from secondary minerals associated with Katanga pitchblende. If the original untreated pitchblende is considered as a whole the average atomic weight of the lead is 205.99. Aston[3] has found Katanga lead to be com-

[1] See Baxter and Alter, SCIENCE, 76: 524, 1932.
[2] Ber. 56: 1837, 1923.
[3] *Nature*, 129: 649, 1932.

THE ATOMIC WEIGHT OF LEAD

*Katanga Pitchblende*

| Wt. of $PbCl_2$ in vacuum g. | Wt. of Ag in vacuum g. | Ratio $PbCl_2$ : 2Ag | At. wt. of Pb. |
|---|---|---|---|
| 4.57229 | 3.56261 | 1.28341 | 206.00 |
| 6.20083 | 4.83143 | 1.28344 | 206.00 |
| 4.45462 | 3.47094 | 1.28340 | 205.99 |
| | Average | 1.28342 | 206.00 |
| | *Katanga Pitchblende Extract* | | |
| 2.62575 | 2.04615 | 1.28326 | 205.96 |
| 3.75342 | 2.92474 | 1.28333 | 205.98 |
| 3.28347 | 2.55867 | 1.28327 | 205.96 |
| 3.19222 | 2.48745 | 1.28333 | 205.98 |
| | Average | 1.28330 | 205.97 |
| | *Bedford Cyrtolite* | | |
| 0.59044 | 0.46015 | 1.28315 | 205.94 |
| | *Common Lead* | | |
| 2.56818 | 1.99234 | 1.28903 | 207.21 |
| 4.34481 | 3.37050 | 1.28907 | 207.22 |
| | Average | 1.28905 | 207.21 |

posed of the isotopes $Pb^{206}$ and $Pb^{207}$ in the proportions of 14 to 1. From this evidence the isotopic weight of $Pb^{206}$ would seem to have the surprisingly low value 205.90–205.93.

It is difficult to explain the difference in the atomic weights of the lead from the black and yellow portions of the original mineral. If the veins were formed by infiltration, an external source of lead of atomic weight 205.97 is required. If, as seems more probable to us, the yellow material is an alteration product, it might indicate a different rate of decay of uranium isotopes, as v. Grosse has recently proposed.[4] But since then the yellow material must contain on an average older lead than the black, this hypothesis would require a higher rate of decay for $U^{238}$ than for $U^{239}$, a conclusion which is contrary to v. Grosse's.

G. P. BAXTER
C. M. ALTER

T. JEFFERSON COOLIDGE, JR.,
MEMORIAL LABORATORY OF
HARVARD UNIVERSITY

[4] *Phys. Rev.*, 42: 565, 1932.

## FREE POSITIVE ELECTRONS RESULTING FROM THE IMPACT UPON ATOMIC NUCLEI OF THE PHOTONS FROM TH C″

THE discovery of the fact that free positive electrons are present among the secondary particles resulting from the disruption of nuclei by the cosmic radiation,[1] together with various kinds of evidence that the primary cosmic radiation at sea-level consists largely of photons, made it appear of value to study the hard γ-rays of natural radioactive substances for similar effects. Experiments have been carried out which gave conclusive evidence that positrons[2] are ejected from lead by the γ-radiation of Th C″.

Near the bottom of a vertical Wilson cloud-chamber operating in a magnetic field of about 400 gauss a plate of lead was placed through which a collimated pencil of γ-rays from Th C″ was allowed to pass. About 5 cms above the lead was inserted an aluminum plate of 0.5 mm thickness for the purpose of differentiating between particles of positive and negative charge, a method previously used by the author and later by Blackett and Ochialini for the same purpose.

Out of 1,500 exposures three photographs were obtained, each one of which showed a positron ejected from the lead, the direction of ejection being nearly in the direction of the incident γ-ray beam. The positrons penetrate the aluminum plate and emerge with an appreciably lower energy; in all three photographs the tracks cross practically the whole chamber, and their curvatures are readily measurable and of the right order of magnitude. The general indications are that the positrons are not very rare among the electrons ejected from the lead.

These photographs offer unambiguous evidence that photons when absorbed by nuclei do eject both positive and negative electrons quite in accordance with the evidence which has appeared in cosmic-ray studies. Further, many of the tracks which we have obtained from the γ-rays of Th C″ resemble the showers such as those obtained by us[3] and particularly emphasized in the photographs of Blackett and Ochialini.[4]

I wish to express my gratitude to Mr. Seth H. Neddermeyer, for his assistance and to the Carnegie Corporation for their support of this whole program.

CARL D. ANDERSON

CALIFORNIA INSTITUTE
OF TECHNOLOGY

[1] SCIENCE, 76: 238, 1932.

[2] The contraction positron is here used to denote the free positive electron.

[3] C. D. Anderson, "Cosmic-Ray Bursts," *Phys. Rev.*, 43: 5, 368, March 1, 1933.

[4] *Proc. Roy. Soc.*, 139, 699, 1933.

## METHOD OF EXTRACTION OF SUPRARENAL CORTICAL HORMONE-LIKE SUBSTANCE FROM URINE

IN view of the physiological significance of the possible presence of a substance in the urine that raises the resistance of suprarenalectomized rats to histamine poisoning,[1] the exact method of extraction of this substance is given below:

[1] D. Perla and J. Marmorston-Gottesman, *Proc. Soc. Exp. Biol. Med.*, 28: 1024, 1931.

The urine of young adult males and females is collected during the evening and night in large amber-colored bottles, packed in ice and containing a small cube of $CO_2$ snow; 50 cc of benzene is added to each bottle. A large funnel is inserted through an opening in the cork of the bottle, and the stem of the funnel is closed by a cork attached to a long glass rod. When in use this cork is removed and urine passed into the funnel. The cork is then immediately replaced. This method of collection results in a minimal amount of decomposition of the urine and keeps the freshly voided urine cold in an atmosphere saturated with $CO_2$ and under a layer of benzene. The following morning the bottles are removed to a dark room and the urine extracted with 50 cc of benzene for each liter of urine. An electrical mechanical mixer with a small fan-shaped stirring rod is used for agitation and extraction. The extraction with benzene is continued for from 10 to 15 minutes, and repeated with fresh benzene. The benzene is separated, and the fractions pooled and evaporated at 40° in vacuo to dryness. The residue is taken up in ether, the ether evaporated and the ether residue is shaken with the desired amount of physiological saline. The final aqueous product is colorless, has no odor of urine, turns faintly pink in 20 hours, and is non-irritating to rats when injected subcutaneously or intraperitoneally. The final product is made so that 1 cc of the extractive is equivalent to 300 cc of urine. The potency of such extracts will vary with the concentration of the original urine. The precautions employed in the collection of the urine minimize the effect of light and oxidation of the substance in the urine.

Although the substance obtained by the above method from urine raises the resistance of suprarenalectomized rats to histamine poisoning, as also does the life-prolonging hormone of the suprarenal cortex, proof is lacking that it is identical with the life-prolonging hormone.

DAVID PERLA
J. MARMORSTON

## PRELIMINARY REPORT ON REDUCING TRANSPIRATION OF TRANSPLANTED EVERGREENS

IN the semi-arid Great Plains Region, coniferous evergreens are the most desirable shelterbelt trees and are the most permanent when once established. Unfortunately, their mortality in transplanting is particularly high, losses of 50 to 100 per cent. being not uncommon on prairie farms. Probable factors responsible for this loss are: (1) Climatic conditions favoring a high transpiration rate; (2) necessity of moving evergreens in full foliage; (3) slow rate of regeneration of roots destroyed in digging and resetting.

Since the fall of 1931 the Cheyenne Horticultural Field Station has been investigating means of reducing the transpiration rate of transplanted conifers. Through the work of Neilson[1,2] and others[3,4,5] the coating of dormant deciduous nursery stock for protection in storage, shipment and transplanting is being used to some extent in horticultural practise. Following the work of these investigators, various materials have been applied to the above-ground parts of dormant conifers in an attempt to cut down excessive transpiration of transplants until the damaged root systems can develop sufficiently to again support the trees.

Many materials have been tested, consisting chiefly of waxes, gums, resins, oils and asphaltic compounds, alone, and in various mixtures. Proprietary preparations employed included a rubber compound, a special petroleum wax, a Duco formula, a paraffin emulsion and four commercial nursery waxes. Early in the trials it was found that waxy materials which gave thick and nearly complete coverage of coniferous needles reduced transpiration almost to nothing; however, such heavy coatings caused severe injury to the plants. The temperatures at which materials can safely be applied to dormant evergreens is much lower than for dormant deciduous trees, but varies somewhat with different species, *e.g.*, Colorado blue spruce (*Picea pungens*) can not safely be treated with materials above 65° C., while yellow pine (*Pinus ponderosa*) can stand 5 to 10 degrees higher. Difficulty of securing thin coatings of waxy materials at these temperatures led to the use of pure oils and emulsions of oils and waxes which can be applied with a sprayer. Of the many oils tested, castor oil and corn oil were the only ones that did not injure the conifer needles when applied in pure form. Emulsifying some of the injurious oils greatly reduced or entirely removed their toxicity.

The non-toxic oils and several emulsions of oils and waxes have been tested on different typyes of conifers

1 J. A. Neilson, "Paraffine Wax—an Aid to Growth in Transplanted Trees and Shrubs," *North. Nut Grow. Ass'n. Proc.*, 19: 44–51. 1928.

2 J. A. Neilson, "Reducing Storage and Transplanting Losses in Nursery Stock" *Flor. Exch. and Hort. Trade World*, 78: (No. 5) 27, 35. 1931.

3 C. N. Pillsbury, "The Use of Rubber in the Propagation, and for the Protection of Nursery Stock," *Flor. Exch. and Hort. Trade World*, 77: No. 17, 28–29, 41. 1931.

4 H. B. Tukey and Karl Brase, "The Effect of Paraffining, Pruning and Other Storage Treatments upon the Growth of Roses and Cherry Trees, *Am. Soc. Hort. Sci. Proc.*, 28: 489–495. 1931.

5 T. J. Maney, "An Apparatus for Spraying Plants with Melted Paraffin or Other Waxes," *Am. Soc. Hort. Sci. Proc.*, 28: 496–497. 1931.

without injury, and the efficacy of these coatings in reducing transpiration has been determined. The table shows a comparison of a few materials sprayed on uniform lots of five-year-old dormant pines.

PINE (PINUS AUSTRIACA)

| | *Daily loss before treatment | †Daily loss after treatment |
|---|---|---|
| Corn oil | 20.7 gms | 2.4 gms |
| (1) Sulphonated linseed oil emulsion 33⅓ per cent. | 20.8 | 8.4 |
| (2) Crystal No-Dri 50 per cent. solution | 20.7 | 18.0 |
| Beeswax emulsion | 20.9 | 18.3 |
| Untreated (control) | 20.3 | 26.3 |

* Averages for 8 days.
† Averages for 7 days.
(1) Prepared by heating 9 parts boiled linseed oil to 470° F. and adding 1 part flowers of sulfur to the hot oil. Emulsified by mixing with laundry soap and water.
(2) Manufactured and sold by the Crystal Soap and Chemical Co., Inc., Philadelphia.

The trees had been grown in pots long enough to be thoroughly established and to ensure that all were living. The pots were sealed in metal cans and the trees exposed to outdoor conditions. Trees were grouped into five lots of four trees each and transpiration (loss of weight) was determined every two days, water being added after each weighing to make good the loss. After a period of eight days during which the comparative transpiration rates of the five lots were determined, different treatments were applied to each lot and the loss in weight determined for seven more days, water loss being replaced as before. It will be noted that in the period before treatment the groups were selected so that their average daily transpiration rates were practically equal. After treatment the groups showed wide variation in water loss. The data show that all coatings reduced transpiration as compared with the untreated control, pure corn oil in this instance, causing a reduction of 88.4 per cent. Whether such a great reduction in transpiration is necessary or even desirable is not yet known, although no detrimental effects were noticeable after several months. Further investigations are under way to determine the ultimate effect of these coatings on the tree's metabolism.

In actual practise the materials are best applied by spraying seed beds or nursery rows before digging. Thousands of conifer seedlings and transplants have been treated this year with oils and emulsions, apparently with good results. It is believed that these coatings may also prove useful in protecting coniferous seed beds from excessive drying out over winter. In this connection the efficiency of the sulphonated oil is of interest, as this material is also a repellent for rodents that attack nursery beds.

A complete report of these investigations will appear in a later publication.

J. L. EMERSON
A. C. HILDRETH
CHEYENNE HORTICULTURAL FIELD STATION
U. S. DEPARTMENT OF AGRICULTURE

## BOOKS RECEIVED

ANTEV, ERNST. *Alpine Zone of Mt. Washington Range.* Pp. viii + 118. 38 figures. Merrill and Webber.

BAILEY, L. H. *The Cultivated Conifers.* Pp. ix + 404. 114 figures. Macmillan. $7.50.

BOYNTON, PAUL L. *Intelligence: Its Manifestations and Measurement.* Pp. xi + 466. Appleton. $2.50.

*Bulletin of the Academy of Sciences of the United Provinces of Agra and Oudh, Allahabad, India.* Volume I, 1931–32. Pp. 150 + 49. Illustrated. The Academy.

*Bulletin of the Association of Field Engineers, June, 1932.* Pp. 128. Illustrated. U. S. Coast and Geodetic Survey.

*Contributions to the Calculus of Variations,* 1931–32. Theses Submitted to the Department of Mathematics of the University of Chicago. University of Chicago Press. $3.00.

CRUM, ROY W., Editor. *Proceedings of the Eleventh Annual Meeting of the Highway Research Board, December, 1931.* Part I: *Reports of Research Committees and Papers.* Pp. 443. Illustrated. National Research Council, Washington.

FAIRCHILD, HERMAN L. *A Chapter in Earth Science History.* Pp. xvii + 232. Illustrated. The Geological Society of America. $2.50.

GALT, WILLIAM. *Phyloanalysis.* Pp. 151. Kegan Paul, Trench, Trubner & Co., London. 2/6.

GOWANLOCH, JAMES N. *Fishes and Fishing in Louisiana.* Pp. 638. Illustrated. Bulletin No. 23, Department of Conservation, State of Louisiana.

GRAY, LEWIS C. *History of Agriculture in the Southern United States.* Pp. xix + 567. Carnegie Institution of Washington.

HEGNER, ROBERT W. *Invertebrate Zoology.* Pp. xiii + 570. 403 figures. Macmillan. $3.75.

LASLEY, JOHN W. and EDWARD T. BROWNE. *Introductory Mathematics.* Pp. xvi + 439. McGraw-Hill. $2.75.

LINDSEY, ARTHUR W. *A Textbook of Genetics.* Pp. xvi + 354. 128 figures. Macmillan. $2.75.

LINGEL, ROBERT. *Educational Broadcasting, a Bibliography.* Pp. x + 162. University of Chicago Press. $1.50.

LINTON, RALPH. *The Tanala: A Hill Tribe of Madagascar.* Pp. 334. 35 figures. Field Museum of Natural History. $2.25.

MILLER, CASPER O. *The Ether in its Relation to the Structure of Matter and the Transmission of Force.* Pp. 442. 45 figures. Henkel Press.

MOSELEY, EDWIN L. *Other Worlds.* Pp. xi + 231. 55 figures. Appleton. $2.00.

*Recent Social Trends in the United States:* Report of the President's Research Committee on Social Trends. Vol. I: Pp. xcv + 750. Illustrated. Vol. II: Pp. vi + 751–1568. McGraw-Hill. $10.00.

ROQUETTE-PINTO, E. *Boletim do Museu Nacional.* Vol. III. No. 3. Pp. 133–256. Illustrated. Museu Nacional, Rio de Janeiro.

TYSON, LEVERING, Editor. *Radio and Education.* Pp. viii + 298. University of Chicago Press. $3.00.

WOODS, ALAN C. *Allergy and Immunity in Opthalmology.* Pp. xiv + 176. Johns Hopkins Press. $2.25.

# SCIENCE

VOL. 77 — FRIDAY, MAY 12, 1933 — No. 2002

*Perfect Quality and Auditory Perspective in the Transmission and Reproduction of Music:* DR. FRANK B. JEWETT ... 435

*Obituary:*
*Arthur Hollick:* PROFESSOR E. C. JEFFREY. *Memorials. Recent Deaths* ... 440

*Scientific Events:*
*Representation of Museums at the Century of Progress Exposition; Deaths from Asphyxiation; The Dedication of the George Eastman Laboratories at the Massachusetts Institute of Technology; Professor Einstein* ... 442

*Scientific Notes and News* ... 444

*Discussion:*
*Destruction of Mooring Ropes by Teredo:* PROFESSOR W. R. COE. *The Effects of Media on Bacterial Filtrability:* JEROME ALEXANDER. *A Test for the Presence of Novocaine in Nervous Tissue:* PROFESSOR MANUEL GRODINSKY, DR. MEYER BEBER and CHARLES P. BAKER. *Sponge Spicules from the Lower Ordovician of Wisconsin:* PROFESSOR C. E. NEEDHAM. *The Water Content of Medusae:* J. B. BATEMAN ... 447

*Quotations:*
*Medical Patents* ... 451

*The American Association for the Advancement of Science:*
*Spring Meeting of the Executive Committee:* PROFESSOR HENRY B. WARD. *Hotel Headquarters for the Chicago Meeting* ... 452

*The National Academy of Sciences:*
*Abstracts of Papers Presented at the Washington Meeting* ... 454

*Science News* ... 8

SCIENCE: A Weekly Journal devoted to the Advancement of Science, edited by J. MCKEEN CATTELL and published every Friday by

THE SCIENCE PRESS

New York City: Grand Central Terminal
Lancaster, Pa. — Garrison, N. Y.

Annual Subscription, $6.00 — Single Copies, 15 Cts.

SCIENCE is the official organ of the American Association for the Advancement of Science. Information regarding membership in the Association may be secured from the office of the permanent secretary, in the Smithsonian Institution Building, Washington, D. C.

# PERFECT QUALITY AND AUDITORY PERSPECTIVE IN THE TRANSMISSION AND REPRODUCTION OF MUSIC[1]

By Dr. FRANK B. JEWETT

BELL TELEPHONE LABORATORIES

IT is quite impossible in the short space of the fifteen or twenty minutes allotted to me to attempt anything in the way of detail, either in the matter of the scientific principles involved in the apparatus and equipment of this particular system of music transmission or in the elaborate arrangement of parts involved in the demonstration to be given in Constitution Hall next Thursday evening. As a matter of fact, all the scientific material has been or will be incorporated in various technical papers. Further, the demonstrations which Dr. Harvey Fletcher is proposing to give at the time of the Thursday demonstration will be more illuminating than anything which I could hope to reproduce here.

All that I propose to do, therefore, is to outline briefly the fundamentals of the problem, the extent to which we have succeeded in solving them, and the general arrangement of parts which will be employed in the transmission and reproduction of a complete symphonic concert from the stage of the Academy of Music in Philadelphia to the stage of Constitution Hall in Washington.

For the perfect pick-up, transmission and reproduction of orchestral music a system is needed, such that the sound reproduced in the ears of the listener is the same as that which would be produced in his ears if he were listening to the orchestra directly. In other words, the frequency, intensity and phase relations of the sound in each ear must be accurately reproduced in order best to convey the frequency and intensity range of the sounds and the spatial relations of the instruments. So far as we now know, this can be done

[1] Presented to the annual meeting of the National Academy of Sciences, Washington, D. C., April 25.

only by means of a binaural telephone system, using two head receivers for each listener. In other words, to obtain what might be called an acoustic facsimile, a separate telephone system must be used for each ear of the listener. Such an arrangement was necessarily employed in working out the arrangements which have been developed, although for obvious reasons it was never contemplated that such a system could ever be used for a general audience.

Although such a facsimile can not be produced by means of loud-speaking telephones, it is possible by their means to reproduce music which has auditory perspective, and which in many ways gives just as pleasing an effect as though it were a perfect facsimile. As an illustration of how this might be accomplished, it is possible to imagine a system of microphones and sound projectors which will approach facsimile reproduction as follows.

Suppose the stage of the music hall is acoustically insulated so that the only sound reaching the audience is that coming through the opening occupied by the curtain when it is lowered. If now a large number of microphones are distributed over the plane occupied by the curtain when it is lowered and each microphone is connected to a loud speaker similarly placed before the audience where the music is to be reproduced, then if the microphones, the loud speakers and the connecting lines have the right characteristics, the audience should receive sound which is a very close approximation to the original. In such a system the microphones must be so small as not to interfere with the free passage of the sound waves and must produce an electrical facsimile of the sound waves in front of them. Similarly, each of the connecting lines must be distortionless. The loud speakers must be very small and must produce an acoustic facsimile of the electrical waves. At the present time, we do not know how to produce loud speakers of this character. Even if we did know how to produce them, the expense involved would be prohibitive on account of the amount and complexity of apparatus required and of the cost of the multi-channel connecting lines. Fortunately, however, experience has shown that a very close approximation to complete facsimile reproduction can be obtained by using a three-channel system. With such a system the auditory illusion is substantially complete except for those persons sitting very near to the stage.

Broadly speaking, the frequency range which is needed to secure perfect reproduction is the entire frequency range that is audible to the human ear. However, tests with reproduced orchestral music have shown that the elimination of the frequency range below 30 or 40 cycles per second and that above 15,000 cycles per second is hardly detectable. These eliminated frequencies are very close to the audible limits for the average person.

A full-sized symphonic orchestra is capable of producing sound through an intensity range of about 65 or 70 db. For perfect reproduction any electrical system to be satisfactory must be capable of handling an intensity range of at least this amount. The range that a system can handle is determined by the difference between the noise level and the overload level. When a system capable of handling a greater intensity range than that ordinarily produced by an orchestra was finally developed musicians were quick to take advantage of it as a means of increasing the sound intensity during crescendo passages above normal and in decreasing the intensity during very soft passages below normal. This indicates apparently that the intensity range, which an ideal system should be capable of handling, is set by the range between the loudest sounds that a listener can hear comfortably and the faintest sounds that he can hear in a quiet audience. This range is somewhere between 80 and 100 db, depending upon the character of the music. Roughly, such an ideal system will produce maximum sounds in crescendo periods about ten times as loud as those which a one hundred piece orchestra is capable of producing directly.

### Characteristics of the Pick-up Microphones Employed and Their Location

The characteristics of the microphones which have been developed for this reproducing system are described in two papers entitled, "Moving-Coil Telephone Receivers and Microphones," by Wente and Thuras, and "A Sensitive Moving-Coil Microphone of High Quality," by Thuras.

### Characteristics of Loud Speakers Employed and Their Location

Each loud speaker assembly employed in reproducing transmitted music consists of three units. One of these units is of large dimensions and is designed for the perfect reproduction of frequencies below 300 cycles per second. The remaining two units, which are small and alike, are designed for the perfect reproduction of all frequencies above 300 cycles per second. These two small units are mounted on top of the low frequency unit and the combination of the three units is so designed and arranged that the entire frequency band of sound is distributed uniformly throughout the hall.

### Characteristics of Power Amplifiers

Time does not permit any detailed description of the power amplifiers which it is necessary to employ in order to obtain the requisite amount of energy. Suffice to say, these amplifiers must have substantially flat amplification characteristics for all frequencies at all intensity levels and must be capable not only of maintaining continuously these characteristics for the normal sound range of the orchestra, but must also be capable of handling for short periods and without distortion the greatly increased sound range in crescendo passages.

### QUASI-BINAURAL ARRANGEMENT EMPLOYED

As is shown in Fig. 1, three complete channels are used. Each channel consists of a microphone, amplifier, volume control, connecting line and loud speaker. Hall. The volume control which Dr. Stokowski will use permits of changing the three channels simultaneously as a group or of changing each individually as he may elect in order to obtain any desired tonal coloring.

The response characteristic of the overall system is obviously dependent upon the acoustic properties of the rooms in which the sounds are picked up and reproduced. In order to obtain a proper overall characteristic, the loud speakers were put on the stage at the Academy of Music and connected to an electrical oscillator. The pick-up microphones were hung in their proper positions in front of the stage. The electrical power developed by the transmitters was compared with the electrical power supplied to the loud speakers for sinusoidal waves in the frequency range 40 to 15,000 cycles per second. The system was then equalized so that the power ratio was a constant over the entire frequency range. Since each channel of the system is capable of furnishing a steady acoustic power of at least 35 watts at any frequency in the entire range, the three channels together are capable of furnishing at least 100 watts of power. In the middle of the frequency range several times this amount of power can be produced without distortion. When the energy frequency distribution of orchestral music is taken into account, it turns out, as was indicated earlier, that the system is capable of magnifying the total sound output of a one hundred piece orchestra about tenfold.

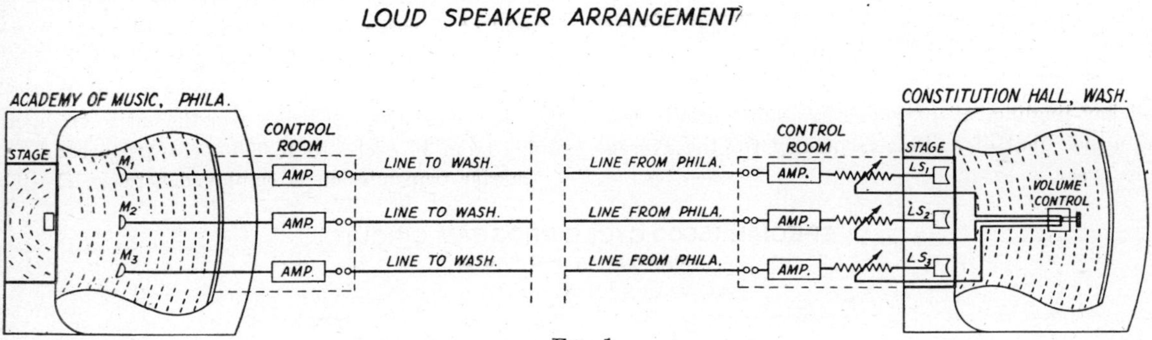


FIG. 1

In the Academy of Music in Philadelphia, the microphones are placed about ten feet in front of the stage and ten or twelve feet above the floor. These microphones are connected to loud speakers in corresponding positions on the stage of Constitution Hall, *i.e.,* the microphone at the left of the Philadelphia stage connects to a loud speaker at the left of the Washington stage, etc. Thus, the three channels, left, center and right, reproduce the sounds arising in corresponding positions on the Philadelphia stage.

### METHOD OF VOLUME CONTROL WHICH DR. STOKOWSKI WILL EMPLOY

In the system to be demonstrated in Constitution Hall Thursday evening, provision is made for Dr. Stokowski to control the volume of sound from the loud speakers on the stage of Constitution Hall while seated at a monitoring position in the audience at Constitution Hall. He will also have facilities for communicating directly with the orchestra on the stage at the Academy of Music in Philadelphia. The general features of the plan for the demonstration are to transmit without change the program to Washington as it is picked up at Philadelphia. The unchanged program coming to Washington may then be changed at will by means of the volume control before reaching the loud speakers on the stage of Constitution

### AUDIBLE FREQUENCY RANGE FOR MUSIC, SPEECH AND NOISE

As a matter of passing interest, Fig. 2 shows the audible frequency range for speech and for various kinds of noises and musical instruments which the system is capable of reproducing without noticeable distortion. As will be seen, these frequencies extend from the deep low notes of the bass viol and bass tuba to the high frequencies emanating from the snare drum, cymbals, violin, oboe, footsteps, hand-clapping

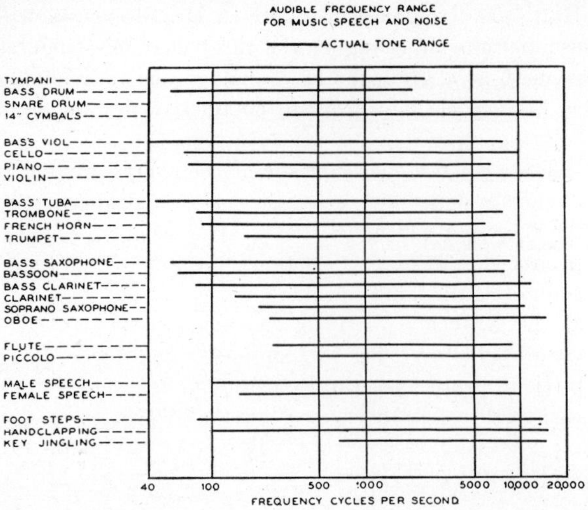


Fig. 2

and key-jingling, all of which are substantially near the upper limit of audible frequency for the average human ear.

### Transmission Lines

The general route of the transmission lines, together with the location of the repeater or amplifier stations, is shown on Fig. 3. The distance between Philadelphia and Washington is approximately 140 miles and the transmission circuits are in lead-covered underground cable.

This figure also shows in schematic form the three separate channels required for the system just described. It also shows in rough schematic the energy level variations along the line. As will be seen, the energy amplification at each repeater station is about 50 db. In other words, at each repeater station the gradually weakened currents are enormously magnified to the end that the level of energy, as it is delivered at Constitution Hall, will be substantially the same as that at the Academy of Music.

The transmission lines themselves have substantially flat characteristics (± 1 db) over the entire frequency range from 40 cycles to 15,000 cycles per second.

Carrier transmission is employed between the tele-

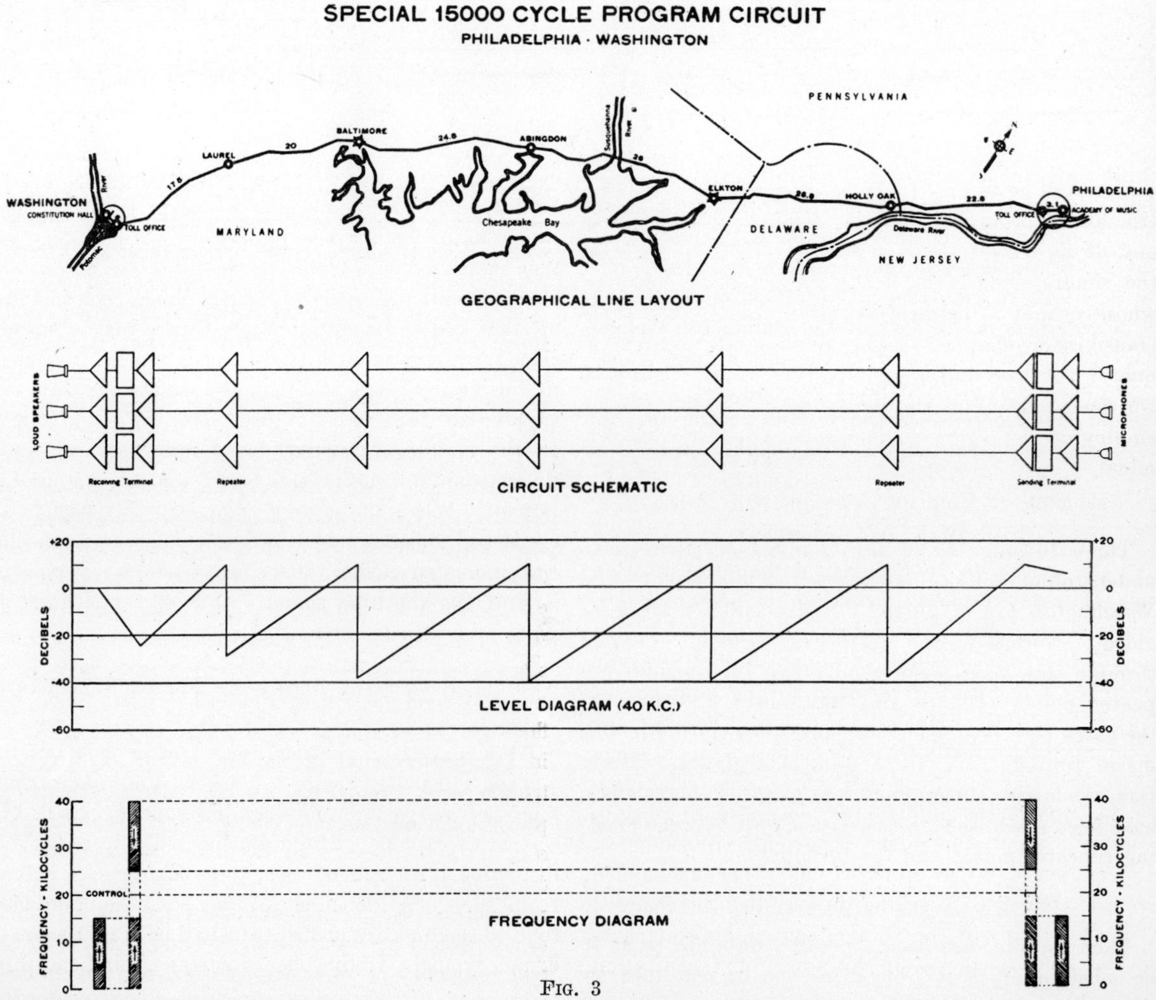


Fig. 3

phone toll offices in Philadelphia and Washington, a distance of approximately 140 miles. The carrier band lies in the frequency range between 25,000 and 40,000 cycles per second.

Fig. 4 shows a schematic of the special program circuit employed. As will be seen in this schematic and very stable with respect to wide power variations. The gain at each repeater is about 50 db. An important feature at each repeater point are the equalizers to adjust the degree of amplification proportional to the line loss for the different frequencies. This is essential since, as is well known, the higher frequen-

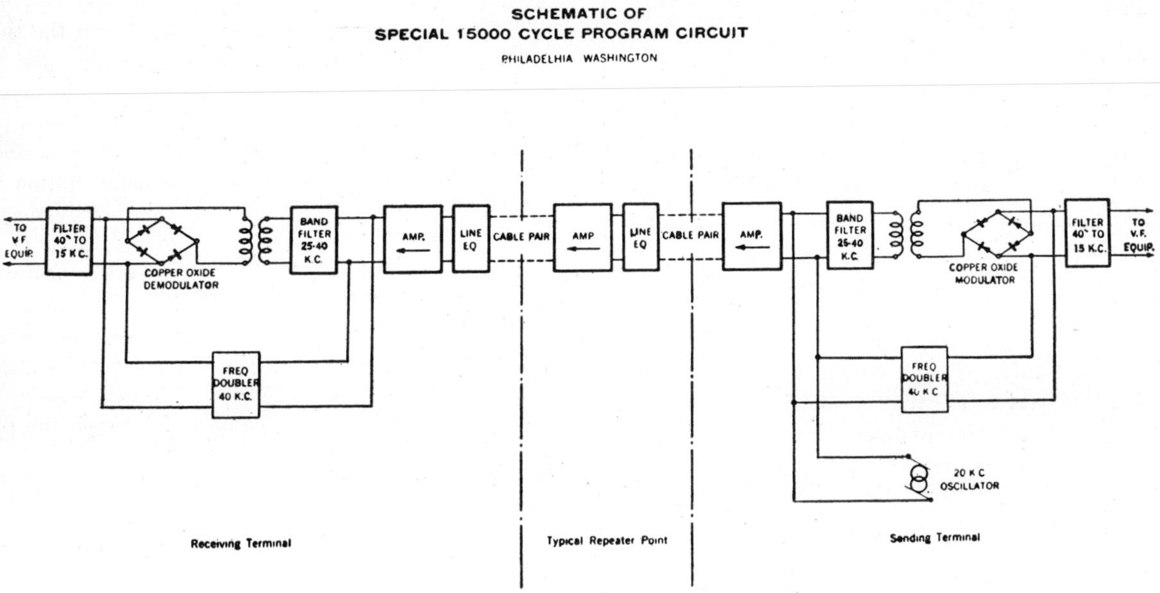


FIG. 4

and as will be referred to in a moment, accurate control of frequency and phase throughout the system and at its terminations is obtained by employing at the sending end a 20 kilocycle oscillator, part of whose output is transmitted over each of the three transmission channels. The 40 kilocycle carrier required for modulating at the transmitting end and for demodulating at the receiving end is obtained by employing a frequency doubling device at each terminal.

### LINE LAYOUT

Three 16-gauge (1.29 mm) non-loaded pairs in an underground toll cable between Philadelphia and Washington are employed. Spare circuits are provided. Normally, the telephone circuits operated through this cable require only two intermediate repeater points (Elkton and Baltimore). Because of the extra high frequency transmission required in this music reproduction, three additional points (Holly Oak, Delaware, Abingdon and Laurel, Maryland), have been established, located as shown between existing repeater points and the terminals.

### REPEATERS OR AMPLIFIERS

Each repeater has been especially designed so as to be substantially free from distortion or non-linearity cies suffer a much greater attenuation during transmission over a cable circuit than do the lower frequencies. Without these equalizers enormous distortion would result.

One new repeater point (Holly Oak) is established in an existing telephone office. At two other points (Abingdon and Laurel) temporary huts have been erected to house the demonstration repeaters.

### CARRIER APPARATUS

The carrier system employed is single sideband with the carrier frequency at 40 kilocycles and lower sideband transmission. In order, however, to obtain satisfactory transmission of the very low musical frequencies, what is known as "vestigial" sideband transmission is employed. This means that the unwanted (*i.e.*, upper) sideband is not entirely suppressed in the neighborhood of the carrier but is allowed to pass through the circuit to some extent so as to help out in the preservation of the low notes. This type of transmission circuit requires very careful attention to phase relations in filter design and accurate phase control of the carrier current which is supplied to the demodulator circuit in respect to that supplied to the modulator. As has already been mentioned, this is accomplished by transmitting some of the special control frequency of 20 kilocycles over each transmission line, together with the music band. This transmitted 20 kilocycle control current is used at the receiving end by a frequency doubling device to supply the accurately phased carrier needed for demodulation.

### Noise

As has been referred to earlier, noise entering the transmission system is a limiting factor in determining the extent to which low level sounds can be transmitted and reproduced. Noise can reach a cable circuit in either of two ways. (a) It may enter the cable through the sheath from radio or power fields through which the cable passes, or (b) it may enter the cable at the ends or intermediate points along other circuits in the cable which are operating in a lower frequency range.

So far as (a) is concerned at the frequencies employed and for the transmission levels used, this particular Philadelphia-Washington cable is quiet and was found to require no special arrangements.

With respect to (b) the repeater layout is such that it was not necessary to take special steps, except at Baltimore. Here the volume levels from the north were sufficiently low so that high frequency noises produced in the office as a by-product chiefly of telegraph and switching operations passed into the cable over working circuits and cross-talked into the pairs used for the special broad band transmission. To prevent this the cable north was "isolated" from the office by putting choke coils in every pair in the cable. These choke coils are non-inductive to ordinary telephone or telegraph currents. They are inductive, however, to currents flowing over any of the conductor systems to ground.

### Local Circuits

The carrier apparatus is located in the toll terminal offices at Philadelphia and Washington. Small gauge equalized underground cable circuits are used between the Academy of Music and the telephone office in Philadelphia and similarly at Washington between the telephone office and Constitution Hall.

### Auxiliary Features

As has been previously mentioned, spare circuits are available in the cable to substitute in the event of any breakdown of the regularly assigned carrier pairs. Secondary spares of slightly lower frequency range capacity have also been provided in another cable to be available in the remote possibility of something happening to completely disrupt the cable carrying the regular circuits.

### Summary

In conclusion, all that need be pointed out is that the system just described is one designed for the reproduction in auditory perspective of symphonic or other music to an audience. Because of its multichannel character and its wide range of frequency and energy capacity, it is not readily adaptable for use in small rooms. While theoretically susceptible of employing any set of transmission channels capable of handling the desired frequency and volume range, it is at least in the present state of the art restricted essentially to wire transmission systems. This restriction arises from three main sources: (1) The ability to free the system against extraneous electrical or noise disturbances which at times so frequently mar radio transmission. (2) The uniformity with which transmission characteristics can be maintained and the relative ease with which the effects of attenuation can be overcome by intermediate repeaters. (3) The fact that under existing statutory regulation of radio it is impossible to secure clear channels of a frequency band requisite for the complete transmission of all the fundamental and overtone frequencies produced throughout the full range of musical instruments and the human voice.

Whether for local or distance use, the easily controlled and very tremendous volume ranges which the apparatus is capable of handling without distortion have placed in the hands of the musical director an implement for tonal effects not hitherto attainable. What the future use of the system in all its parts is likely to be will depend in large measure not only on the extent to which it is desirable to produce perfect music in auditory perspective at a distance remote from the source but likewise on the extent to which musical composers and directors find it effective in producing artistic effects beyond the capacity of the largest orchestras or choruses.

# OBITUARY

## ARTHUR HOLLICK

1857–1933

Dr. (Charles) Arthur Hollick was born in 1857, the son of Frederick and Eleanor Eliza (Bailey) Hollick. He graduated from the Columbia School of Mines, 1879, and from the George Washington University in 1897 with the doctor's degree. He married Adeline Augusta Talkington in 1881. Although scientifically he was a paleobotanist of distinction, he filled many public offices, since he was a man of wide human interests. He was a member of the City of New York Board of Health from 1883 to 1893, a member of the New York State Board of Education from 1907 to 1910, and of many local public services during the whole course of his life.

His academic positions were as follows: Tutor and fellow of Columbia University in geology, 1890–1900; curator of fossil botany, Columbia University, 1900–13; honorary curator, 1914–21; paleobotanist, New York Botanical Garden, 1921 to the time of his death; geologist to the United States Geological Survey; director of the Board of Education of New York City, 1907–10. He belonged to a large number of scientific organizations, including the New York Academy of Sciences, the Torrey Botanical Club, the Staten Island Institute of Arts and Sciences, the Geological Society of America, the Paleobotanical Society of America, the Botanical Society of America, etc.

His main scientific activities were in connection with fossil plants, and his first contribution was the editing of "The Later Extinct Floras of North America," left in form of notes by J. S. Newberry. He published during his active years a large number of papers on paleobotany, covering the Mesozoic and later floras. His most notable contributions were on the Cretaceous floras of New England, which were summarized as an important Memoir of the United States Geological Survey. Another extremely important and indeed classic contribution was on "The Fossil Flora of Alaska," which appeared a short time before his death. Not only was he the author of innumerable papers on fossil plants, but he acted officially in the paleobotanical publications of Puerto Rico, Louisiana, Maryland, New Jersey, New York State Museum and the Dominion of Canada. He was likewise a contributor to several general works, including the articles on paleobotany and fossil plants in the new International Cyclopaedia and also the Encyclopaedia Americana.

Hollick was a singularly lovable man and it was a great pleasure to make visits to the field in his company. The present writer recalls the happy days spent in this way on Staten Island, Long Island, Martha's Vineyard, the coast of New Jersey, etc. He was an indefatigable collector and was physically almost tireless. He would walk for hours through mud and rain and other discomforts in search of new discoveries in his favorite field. A not infrequent experience in paleobotanical excursions is dirt and discomfort (including parasites). These he endured most philosophically and the tedium which invariably arose at times was relieved from the rich store of his experiences. His last excursion was in Cuba, where he rode many hundreds of miles on horseback in the company of a good Spanish officer of the Church, who was at the same time a geologist. He returned from this last excursion apparently in the best of health, but unfortunately soon developed a malignant malady which was unsuccessfully operated on, and he passed away with traumatic pneumonia.

Dr. Hollick has left an enduring mark on American paleobotany, and particularly his works on the fossil floras of New England and Alaska will long stand as classic contributions to the subject. It has been for years a deplorable fact that too little interest has been devoted to the important subject of fossil plants in the United States. The older generation was passing and there were almost no promising successors. Fortunately at the present time this tendency has been corrected, and now a considerable number of young men of ability are taking up the study of extinct plants. In spite of the prevailing mechanistic tendencies of the hour, it is indubitable that paleontology occupies the same position on the intellectual side of biology that the ancient classics do in literature. There seems to be no doubt that the depth and background furnished by the study of extinct forms is an invaluable preparation for biological studies of any kind.

E. C. Jeffrey

## MEMORIALS

A friend of the late Olive M. Lammert, formerly professor of chemistry at Vassar College, has given $4,000 to establish the Olive M. Lammert fund to further the work in physical chemistry, and $1,000 for additional equipment in the precision laboratory, in which this work is carried on. The rooms in the Sanders Laboratory set aside for this field of study will be designated the Olive M. Lammert Laboratories.

At a memorial meeting for the late Professor William Henry Holmes, held in the National Museum on April 22, the following resolution was passed:

Whereas: Notice of the passing of our colleague and friend, Professor William Henry Holmes, which occurred at Royal Oak, Michigan, on April 20, 1933, has been received with deep sorrow by members of the Smithsonian Institution and his other associates and friends; be it

*Resolved:* That we, assembled here to do honor to him, offer our tributes to this eminent man of science in whom the various phases of both art and science were fused to a degree seldom given in one man. Art, science and technic were the agencies he applied to the elucidation of his favorite science, anthropology. His passion for pure art is seen in his paintings which are poetical transcriptions of nature, not only portraying nature but revealing his inmost soul;

That his scientific writings and explorations form permanent contributions to the sum of human knowledge;

That we here record our sense of loss at the passing of Professor Holmes and extend to his family our sympathy in their sorrow.

According to the London *Times* the hundredth anniversary of the death of Richard Trevithick, the pioneer of the steam locomotive, on April 22, 1833, was celebrated on that day by a demonstration in Camborne, Cornwall. On April 23 a memorial service took place at 11 A.M. in the parish church of Dartford, Kent, where Trevithick died. The service was conducted by the vicar, the Rev. Elliott Mitchell, and the preacher was the Bishop of Rochester. An address on "The Life and Work of Richard Trevithick" was given by L. St. L. Pendred, past president of the Institution of Mechanical Engineers, and a chaplet was deposited at the foot of the Trevithick Memorial Tablet. At a service in Westminster Abbey special mention of the great engineer was made by the Archdeacon of Westminster in his sermon and a chaplet was placed below the Trevithick Memorial Window in the North Aisle. A memorial service was also held at Tregajorran Methodist Chapel, near Carn Brea, Cornwall. The chapel is on the site of Trevithick's birthplace. On April 24 a memorial lecture was delivered at the Institution of Civil Engineers by Professor C. E. Inglis. Sir Murdock MacDonald, president of the institution and chairman of the executive committee of the commemoration, presided.

### RECENT DEATHS

DR. WILLIAM OPHÜLS, professor of pathology and dean of the Stanford University Medical School, died on April 27. He was sixty-one years of age.

DR. HENRY SMITH MUNROE, formerly a professor of mining at Columbia University, from 1877 until he became emeritus in 1915, died on May 4. He was eighty-three years old.

DR. JERE WILLIAMS LORD, for thirty-one years clinical professor of dermatology at the Johns Hopkins Medical School and consulting dermatologist at the time of his death, has died at the age of sixty-nine years.

PROFESSOR ERNEST WILLIAM HOBSON, formerly Sadleirian professor of pure mathematics in the University of Cambridge, died on April 18, at the age of seventy-six years.

DR. GEORGE HERBERT PALMER, professor of philosophy at Harvard University from 1873 until he became professor emeritus in 1913, died in Cambridge on May 8, at the age of ninety-one years.

## SCIENTIFIC EVENTS

### REPRESENTATION OF MUSEUMS AT THE CENTURY OF PROGRESS EXPOSITION

MUSEUMS from coast to coast and in Canada are arranging, as reported in *Museum News,* to send representatives to the Chicago meeting of the American Association of Museums, June 12 to 14. Some museums at a distance which can not pay the traveling expenses for members of their staffs are granting a week's extra vacation with pay for attendance at the meeting; and one museum is allowing this extra week and a week of the regular vacation to be taken consecutively. From hotel headquarters comes a renewal of notice that reservations should be made before May 15 in order to secure the best rates.

Railroads are making special rates for visitors to Chicago and there are indications that still further inducements to the World's Fair will be available to travelers from certain quarters. Prospective delegates should make inquiry of local railroad agents. Under some circumstances round trips to Chicago may be made for only ten per cent. more than one way fares.

The program of the meeting, including the programs of ten sections, will occupy three days and will include sessions at the Chicago Historical Society, the Art Institute of Chicago, the Field Museum of Natural History and the Chicago Academy of Sciences. Most of those attending will spend some days before or after the meeting in visiting the other museums of Chicago and the World's Fair. There is the Adler Planetarium and Astronomical Museum and the Shedd Aquarium, both with new buildings near the entrance to the exposition. *Museum News* calls attention to the fact that at the other end of the fair grounds is the new Chicago Museum of Science and Industry which will have in operation a coal mine in which 5,000 people daily may witness an unparalleled venture in realistic museum exhibition, including the illusion of a drop down a shaft and miles of travel underground past moving curtains. There is also the Oriental Institute Museum with its new building. The Century of Progress Exposition will have museum features—in its science building and elsewhere—which will be worth observing also.

Probably the greatest loan exhibition of art ever shown in America will be on display at the Art Institute of Chicago, which has been commissioned to assemble the official art exhibition of the World's Fair. The Art Institute is preparing a 300-page catalogue of the exhibition.

### DEATHS FROM ASPHYXIATION

As a first step in a nation-wide educational program designed to reduce the number of avoidable deaths from the various forms of asphyxiation, an all-day state conference on the problem will be held on May 24, at the New York Academy of Medicine. Dr. Chevalier Jackson is chairman of the medical advisory board of the Society for the Prevention of Asphyxial Death, which is calling the conference. The meeting will be held under the auspices of the public health relations committee of the New York Academy of Medicine.

The morning session will include an address by Dr. Shirley W. Wynne, commissioner of health of the City of New York, on vital statistics relating to asphyxia, with Dr. Haven Emerson, of Columbia University, opening the discussion; Dr. Harrison P. Martland, medical examiner of Essex County, New Jersey, will present medical examiners' findings in asphyxial cases, with discussion opened by Dr. Thomas A. Gonzales, deputy chief medical examiner of New York City; Albert W. Whitney, associate general manager of the National Bureau of Casualty and Surety Underwriters, will speak on the economic aspects of asphyxial mortality, with discussion by Leon Senior, manager of the Compensation Insurance Rating Board; Chief Surgeon Daniel J. Donovan, of the New York City Police Department, will explain through motion pictures the first-aid resuscitation methods used by the department.

Dr. Chevalier Jackson, of Philadelphia, will open the afternoon session with a paper on the fundamentals of laryngoscopy as applied in resuscitation, with discussion led by Dr. Charles J. Imperatori, professor of laryngology at the New York Post-Graduate Medical School and Hospital; Dr. Yandell Henderson, professor of applied physiology at Yale University, will present the fundamentals of gas therapy as related to the use of oxygen and carbon dioxide in resuscitation, with discussion opened by Dr. Dayton J. Edwards, associate professor of physiology at Cornell Medical College.

Dr. Edmund B. Piper, professor of obstetrics, University of Pennsylvania Medical School, will show the practical application of laryngoscopy and gas therapy in the treatment of the asphyxiated, with discussion led by Dr. H. J. Stander, professor of obstetrics and gynecology at the Cornell Medical College; Dr. Pol. N. Coryllos, professor of clinical surgery at Cornell Medical College, will give the principles and practise of the negative pressure cabinet in the treatment of asphyxia; Dr. John F. McGrath, vice-president of the Society for the Prevention of Asphyxial Death, will suggest ways and means of applying the improved resuscitation principles to medical and hospital practise.

A report preliminary to the conference has been issued by the Society for the Prevention of Asphyxial Death, of which the directors are: Dr. Paluel J. Flagg, president; Dr. Cornelius J. Tyson, medical director, St. Vincent's Hospital; Dr. Joseph D. Kelley; Dr. John F. McGrath, of the New York Hospital-Cornell Medical Center, and Dr. George W. Cumbler, of the Neurological Institute of the Presbyterian Hospital-Columbia Medical Center.

The report calls attention to the "alarming and needless loss of life through neglect and improper treatment of asphyxial cases." More than 50,000 deaths from asphyxia, many of which are preventable, occur annually in the United States, with approximately 2,800 deaths occurring each year in New York City alone. The death rate from this cause in New York City is twice that from automobile accidents, eighteen times that from diphtheria and nearly forty times that from typhoid. Of the total of 5,579 infants stillborn in New York City in 1931, approximately one fourth may be classed as having been capable of response to resuscitation properly applied.

## THE DEDICATION OF THE GEORGE EASTMAN LABORATORIES AT THE MASSACHUSETTS INSTITUTE OF TECHNOLOGY

CHEMISTS and physicists gathered at the Massachusetts Institute of Technology on May 1 for the dedication of the great George Eastman Research Laboratories. President Karl T. Compton, of the institute, made the address of welcome to a large gathering of official delegates from scientific and engineering organizations and various educational institutions in this country and abroad.

In an address on "Science at the Massachusetts Institute of Technology," Dr. Samuel C. Prescott, dean of science, reviewed the contributions of the institute to the progress of science and commented upon its present status and prospects for the future.

Dr. Harry M. Goodwin, dean of the Graduate School, discussed the field of advanced education at the institute, while Dr. Frederick G. Keyes, head of the department of chemistry, discussed the significance of chemistry. The address of Dr. John C. Slater, head of the department of physics, described education and research in physics.

Following the morning meeting, which was held in the main lecture hall of the new building, there was an inspection of the various laboratories of physics and chemistry, followed by a luncheon.

The exercises included the dedication of a tablet at the entrance to the present Rogers Laboratory of Physics, commemorating the establishment in 1869 by William Barton Rogers, founder of the institute, of the first physical laboratory for purposes of instruction.

Many of the official delegates to the dedication, representing scientific societies and educational institutions, attended a reunion dinner of the Research Laboratory of Physical Chemistry in the Forris Jewett Moore Room. The dinner was given in honor of Dr.

Arthur A. Noyes, founder of the laboratory and acting president of the institute from 1907 to 1909, now director of the Gates Chemical Laboratory at the California Institute of Technology.

The program in the afternoon included a meeting at which Dr. Arthur H. Compton, of the University of Chicago, described the latest work on the origin and nature of the cosmic rays. At this meeting Dr. Charles A. Kraus, professor of chemistry at Brown University, made an address on "Thirty Years of Physical Chemistry."

At the conclusion of the afternoon meeting the inspection of laboratories was resumed, after which the visitors attended a tea in the Forris Jewett Moore Room. In the evening they were the guests at a private dinner in Walker Memorial, and later attended a reception by President Compton and members of the staff of the new laboratories.

### PROFESSOR EINSTEIN

As SCIENCE has reported, the French Government has offered its hospitality to Professor Einstein, and for this purpose has created a chair of mathematical physics at the College of France. This has been offered to Professor Einstein, who has accepted the call.

The London *Times* states that the creation of this new chair required legislation, and a bill was hastily prepared by the Ministry of Education. It was introduced into the Chamber by M. de Monzie, the responsible minister, and was rapidly passed through all the necessary stages before the deputies separated for the recess.

In the preamble to the bill M. de Monzie recalled as a precedent the action of the French Government in 1840 in creating a Chair of Slavonic Literature for the Polish poet Adam Mieckiewicz, then in exile, and declared that the Third Republic should show itself to be at least as liberal as the July Monarchy. The chair was destined for the occupation of a foreign *savant* who would find in the foundation of Francis I. the spiritual liberty and serenity necessary to his labors and the welcome due to his genius.

At the close of a brief discussion of the measure in the Chamber M. Daladier asked the deputies to associate themselves with the government in passing the bill and thus honor not only a man of genius but a man of courage. The measure was unanimously adopted.

Professor Einstein has addressed the following open letter to the Prussian Academy of Sciences, from which he recently resigned:

I have received from absolutely reliable sources the report that the Academy of Sciences, in an official declaration, spoke of the "participation of Albert Einstein in the atrocity campaign in America and France."

I hereby declare that I have never taken part in any atrocity campaign, and I must add that I have seen nothing whatsoever of such a campaign. In the vast majority of cases people contented themselves with repeating and commenting upon official declarations and decrees of responsible persons in the German Government as well as the program for the economic destruction of the German Jews.

The information I have given to the press was that I would resign my position in the academy and surrender my rights of German citizenship; I gave as my reason the fact that I did not want to live in a country where equality before the law and freedom of speech and of teaching were not granted to the individual.

In addition I explained the state of present-day Germany as one of psychic illness in the masses and said something about the causes. In an article which I gave for circulation purposes to the International League for Combating Anti-Semitism, and which was in no way intended for the press, I further summoned all thoughtful people who remain true to the ideals of a threatened civilization to do everything possible to prevent this mass psychosis, which had manifested itself in such an appalling way in Germany, from spreading further.

It would not have been difficult for the academy to have acquired a proper text of my statements before talking about me in the way it has done. The German press has misrepresented my statements in a tendentious manner, as is only to be expected in view of the present gagging of the press.

I stand by every word I have uttered. But I expect in return that the academy—particularly as it has contributed to my defamation before the German public—should put this statement of mine before its members and the German public before whom I was calumniated.

## SCIENTIFIC NOTES AND NEWS

DR. JAMES B. CONANT, Sheldon Emery professor of organic chemistry, was on May 8 elected president of Harvard University by the corporation to succeed Dr. A. Lawrence Lowell.

AT a meeting of the board of trustees of the American Museum of Natural History on May 1, a resolution was adopted directing that the hall which houses the collection of the Pleistocene period be known as the "Osborn Hall of the Age of Man," in recognition of Dr. Osborn's "untiring devotion to vertebrate paleontology." At this meeting a portrait of Dr. Osborn by Mr. Julian Lamar was presented to the museum by the trustees.

DR. MAX PLANCK, professor of physics in the University of Berlin, celebrated his seventy-fifth birthday on April 23.

Professor D'Arsonval recently retired from the chair of physiology at the Collège de France on the occasion of his eighty-first birthday.

The Berlin correspondent of the *Journal* of the American Medical Association writes: "The recognized leader among German pharmacists, Professor Hans Horst Meyer, of Vienna, celebrated his eightieth birthday, March 17. At the age of twenty-nine he held the chair of pharmacology at the University of Dorpat, Estonia. From Dorpat he was called to Marburg; in 1904 he was given the chair of pharmacology at Vienna, and, refusing a call to Berlin, he held this position until he reached the age of enforced retirement. On his seventieth birthday, the Vienna Academy of Sciences established the Hans Horst Meyer prize, which is bestowed every five years for the best research in the German language in the field of experimental medicine."

On the occasion of the celebration of a half-century of progress in dentistry at the University of Pennsylvania on May 8 the honorary degree of doctor of science was conferred on Dr. Herbert S. Jennings, director of the zoological laboratory of the Johns Hopkins University; Dr. Milo Hellman, professor of orthodontia at Columbia University and research associate of the American Museum of Natural History; Dr. Leroy Matthew Simpson Miner, dean of the Harvard Lental School, and Dr. Charles Root Turner, dean of the Dental School of the University of Pennsylvania. The doctorate of laws was conferred on Dr. Samuel P. Capen, chancellor of the University of Buffalo. Addresses were made by Professor Herbert S. Jennings on "The Biologist's Outlook on the World" and by Surgeon-General Hugh S. Cumming, U. S. Public Health Service, on "The Relationship of Dentistry to Public Health." At the annual dinner addresses were made on "The Field of Dentistry," by Dr. Leroy M. S. Miner; on "Dental Education," by Dr. Samuel P. Capen, and on "The Dental School in the University," by Dr. Thomas S. Gates, president of the University of Pennsylvania.

The Mendel Medal, awarded annually by Villanova College to "a Catholic who has achieved distinction in the advancement of the sciences," was presented on May 4 to Dr. Hugh S. Taylor, David B. Jones professor of chemistry and chairman of the department of chemistry at Princeton University. Rev. Edward V. Stanford, president of the college, made the presentation.

Felix M. Warburg has resigned as a member of the board of trustees of the American Museum of Natural History after a membership of twenty-three years. The vacancy has been filled by the election of Mr. Warburg's son, Frederick M. Warburg. John D. Rockefeller, 3rd, has been elected to succeed Frederick E. Brewster, who resigned in January after serving for twenty years.

Professor J. T. J. Morrison, on his retirement from the chair of forensic medicine and toxicology at the University of Birmingham, has been elected by the Court of Governors emeritus professor and a life governor of the university.

Dr. Benno E. Lischer, professor of orthodontics in the University of California, has been appointed dean of the School of Dentistry, Washington University, St. Louis.

Dr. Solomon Lefschetz, professor of mathematics at Princeton University, has been appointed to the Henry Burchard Fine chair of mathematics to succeed Professor Oswald Veblen, now a member of the faculty of the Institute for Advanced Study.

Dr. Henry McE. Knower, research fellow in the Osborn Zoological Laboratory at Yale University, has been appointed research associate in biology with the rank of associate professor.

Dr. S. F. Hildebrand, senior ichthyologist of the U. S. Bureau of Fisheries, has been "loaned" to Mississippi to make investigations on which to base a scientific program for fish conservation and propagation in Mississippi, following representations to the bureau from the State Fish and Game Commission and the congressional delegation of that state asking for assistance in securing information on spawning seasons of the various fish.

Dr. George M. Sutton, curator of birds at Cornell University, has left for the Chisos Mountains in the Big Bend Region of Texas, on a joint Cornell-Carnegie Institution bird-hunting expedition.

New officers of the Western Reserve University Chapter of Sigma Xi include: Dr. Harold S. Booth, associate professor of chemistry, *president;* Dr. James Angus Doull, professor of public health, *vice-president;* Dr. Wilton Marion Krogman, associate professor of physical anthropology, *secretary;* Dr. Amos Henry Hersh, assistant professor of biology, *treasurer;* Dr. Webster G. Simon, professor of mathematics, and Dr. Bradley M. Patten, associate professor of histology and embryology, *members of the nominating committee.*

At the annual meeting of the Boston Society of Natural History, held on May 3, the following officers were elected for 1933–1934: *President,* Charles H. Taylor; *Vice-presidents,* Nathaniel T. Kidder, Glover M. Allen, William M. Wheeler; *Secretary,* Clinton V. MacCoy; *Treasurer,* Augustus P. Loring, Jr.; *Trustees,* Thomas Barbour, John A. Blanchard, William

L. W. Field, Ralph Hornblower, Frederic H. Kennard, John C. Phillips. At the same meeting the annual Walker Prizes in Natural History, offered this year for the best memoir on any subject in the field of botany, were awarded to Lyman B. Smith, of Harvard University, for his paper on "Evolutionary Lines in the Bromeliaceae," and to George Hume Smith, of Indianapolis, for his paper on the "Anatomy of the Embryonic Leaf." Alice A. Mackenzie, of Pittsburgh, Pennsylvania, received honorable mention for her paper entitled "A Few Observations on Adaptations for Support Exhibited by Plants."

THE Board of Directors of the Bache Fund, composed of Professors E. B. Wilson, W. J. V. Osterhout and Heber D. Curtis, chairman, at their meeting in Washington on April 26, made grants as follows: To Miss Cecilia H. Payne, Harvard College Observatory, Cambridge, Mass., for the determination of photographic magnitudes of southern stars; to Robert R. McMath, McMath-Hulbert Observatory, for motion picture researches on the solar prominences; to Dr. Graham Edwards, School of Medicine, University of Buffalo, for renal researches; to Dr. O. J. Lee, Dearborn Observatory, for investigation of the spectra of faint stars; to Dr. J. Elery Becker, Iowa State College, for researches on the protozoal parasites of ground squirrels; to Dr. Michael Heidelberger, Presbyterian Hospital, New York, for the purchase of an interferometer for the study of precipitin reactions.

DR. JOYCE CLENNAM STEARNS, professor of physics and mathematics at the University of Denver, has been given a grant of $300 from the Carnegie Institution and another for the same amount from the Rumford Committee, which he will use for further study of the cosmic ray.

THE Secretary of Agriculture, Henry A. Wallace, spoke before the Franklin Institute, Philadelphia, on May 9, the title of his address being "Agriculture and Science." He described the present situation of the scientific departments of the government, as well as the relationship of science to agriculture.

DR. JOHN CAMPBELL MERRIAM, president of the Carnegie Institution, delivered a James Arthur Foundation lecture on May 4, entitled "Time and Change in History."

DR. GEORGE W. MCCOY, director of the National Institute of Health of the United States Public Health Service, delivered a public address on April 27, under the auspices of the Lehigh University Chapter of Sigma Xi, on "Our National Defense against Disease."

DEAN GEORGE F. KAY, head of the department of geology at the State University of Iowa, and state geologist of Iowa, lectured recently at the University of Rochester, Cornell University and Vassar College, on "Glaciation: the Background of Mississippi Valley Development."

DR. E. W. GOODPASTURE, professor of pathology, Vanderbilt University School of Medicine, gave the annual address of the LaFayette Guild chapter of the Gorgas Medical Society at the University of Alabama, on April 28. The subject of his address was "A Medical Pageant." Following the address, Dr. Goodpasture was made an honorary fellow of the Gorgas Medical Society.

DR. ALEXANDER PRIMROSE, formerly dean and professor of clinical surgery, University of Toronto Faculty of Medicine, Toronto, delivered the seventh annual Donald C. Balfour Lecture in Surgery at the university on April 5. Dr. Primrose's subject was "The Interrelation of Anatomy and Surgery." The day was the one hundred and sixth anniversary of the birth of Lister.

SIR FRANK DYSON, formerly astronomer royal of Great Britain, who has arrived at Capetown on a holiday in South Africa, addressed a meeting of the Astronomical Society of South Africa, giving a critical summary of the work of his predecessors at Greenwich.

ALL works of Dr. Franz Boas, professor of anthropology in Columbia University, have been removed from the library of the University of Kiel. The writings of Professor Boas are particularly distasteful to the Nazi, because of his opposition to the theory of "Nordic" or "Aryan" racial superiority which forms the basis of the National Socialist social philosophy. Professor Boas received the doctorate degree from Kiel in 1881 and was last year given an honorary degree by the university.

AFTER a period of inactivity since 1918 the Arkansas Academy of Sciences held its annual meeting in Little Rock on April 14 and 15. The academy was organized and chartered by the state in 1917 and was active into 1918, but because of the war, activities were suspended until last fall when the organization was revived. The following officers were elected: *President,* D. M. Moore, University of Arkansas; *Vice-president,* C. F. Allen, Little Rock; *Treasurer,* H. H. Schwardt, University of Arkansas; *Permanent Secretary,* L. M. Turner, University of Arkansas.

A GROUP of fifty-seven advanced and graduate students of the department of chemical engineering of the Ohio State University left Columbus on May 1, on the twenty-seventh Annual Chemical Engineering (Eastern) Inspection Trip under the direction of Dr. James R. Withrow, chairman of the department, and Assistant Professor Joseph H. Koffolt. They planned to visit plants in Rittman, Barberton, Akron, Cleveland, Niagara Falls, N. Y., Rochester, New York City, Grasselli, New Jersey, Wilmington, Delaware, Baltimore, Maryland, and Pittsburgh, Pennsylvania. The industries visited included the paper board industry, rubber industry, chemical stoneware, dirigible fabrication, paints, varnishes, insulators, high tension problems, manufacture of tungsten filaments, glass bulb blowing, hydroelectric power development, carborundum, petroleum refining, heavy chemical manufacture, manufacture of graphite, rayon, electrolytic caustic soda, chlorine, glass-lined equipment, silver salts, photographic films, sugar refining, dyes, chemicals and intermediates, industrial alcohol, alcohol chemicals, the U. S. Bureau of Mines, Pittsburgh, and the Fuel Testing Laboratory of the Carnegie Institute of Technology, Pittsburgh.

GIFTS to the National Research Council since last October include three new appropriations from the Rockefeller Foundation: (*a*) A fund of $50,000 for the continuation of the general research aid fund which has been administered by the council since 1929, making a total of $320,000 provided by the foundation for this purpose. (*b*) A fund of $75,000 for the support of the program of research in problems of sex which has been directed by the council since 1922, with the aid of grants from the foundation now amounting to $735,000. (*c*) A further appropriation of $75,000 has been made by the foundation to *Biological Abstracts* for the expense of the editorial work of this journal. This fund will be administered through the National Research Council. Altogether a total of $793,000 has been provided by the foundation toward the support of the *Abstracts* since the establishment of the journal, which began publication in 1926. The firm of E. R. Squibb and Sons has given the sum of $1,400 for the support of two fellows working in cooperation with the Committee on Drug Addiction, one with the group engaged upon chemical investigations for the committee at the University of Virginia, and one with the group at the University of Michigan, which has charge of the physiological investigations of the committee.

THE late Dr. Alexander S. Monro, Vancouver, B. C., former president of the Canadian Medical Association, who died on August 12, 1932, bequeathed to the University of British Columbia a fund of $80,000 for medical research. The bequest will become available after the death of all beneficiaries of the will.

ACCORDING to the London *Times,* an official decree issued by the commissarial burgomaster of Munich, Herr Fiehler, restricts all Jewish doctors in the Munich municipal hospitals (including most of the university institutions) to Jewish bodies in their dissection work, and bans all Jewish medical students from these hospitals.

THE transmission of weather maps by teletype, over a mileage of airways which already amounts to about 13,000 miles, is a new feature introduced in the weather service in the United States through a cooperative arrangement made between the Weather Bureau of this department and the Department of Commerce. Such transmission is a valuable improvement in the efficiency of weather service for air traffic of all kinds, says the Weather Bureau. For the purpose of the teletype distributing system the country is divided into three regions, for which Cleveland, Kansas City and Oakland, Calif., serve as distributing centers. At these centers Weather Bureau personnel prepare base weather maps every four hours for the respective regions. These base maps are then given to teletype operators of the Department of Commerce, who place them in a teletypewriter and type on them symbols representing ceiling, visibility, lines of equal barometric pressure, etc. The maps are sent over a number of electric circuits simultaneously by use of an automatic perforator and perforated tape. With the use of the perforated tape the map is duplicated at all teletype-equipped points in the circuits. After a map has been transmitted to the circuits in its own region it is then relayed to circuits in other regions.

# DISCUSSION

## DESTRUCTION OF MOORING ROPES BY TEREDO; GROWTH AND HABITS IN AN UNUSUAL ENVIRONMENT

IN the summer and autumn of 1930 a species of *Teredo* appeared in Long Island Sound in unprecedented numbers. Instead of confining their borings exclusively to piles and other submerged pieces of wood, as is usually the case, the young mollusks also attacked the ropes which held buoys and mooring floats at anchor. In a number of cases the ropes were entirely severed and the boats set adrift. The greatest damage seems to have occurred in New Haven Harbor, but similar trouble was reported from near New York. Mr. Raymond E. Miskelly, of the Plymouth Cordage Company, who first called my attention to this attack on rope, informs me that injuries of this nature were more or less general along the coast south of Cape Cod, as well as in Long Island Sound, during the same months.

The species responsible for this aberrant behavior

was identified by Dr. Paul Bartsch as *T. morsei* Bartsch,[1] which is always found in submerged timbers in these localities and which has been usually considered merely a local variety of the widely distributed *T. navalis* Linn. Although all the individuals in the ropes were young, the variations in structure of shell and shape of pallets fall within the limits found by Miller[2] to occur in *T. navalis* under various environmental conditions.

Only ropes that had been continuously submerged for several weeks were seriously damaged and these mainly at the lower ends near the attachments to the anchors, corresponding with the usual preference of teredos for wood placed within about a meter above the surface of the mud.[3,4] In the rope, however, the damage usually extends for two meters or more, due to the slack which falls to the bottom at low tide.

The habits of the young mollusks in the rope are somewhat different from those of other individuals when boring in wood. The fibers of the rope are all twisted into close spirals in the yarns of which the rope is composed and the yarns are again twisted spirally into the cords which are themselves twisted into the finished rope. The *Teredo* in boring tends to penetrate at right angles to the surface, but, due to the twist of the fibers, the tunnel actually cuts obliquely across the yarn. The diameter of the yarn is frequently between 2 and 4 mm and as soon as the tunnel approximates this diameter the yarn is completely severed. The individual fibers of the rope are thus cut into bits, ranging from a few millimeters to a few inches in length, according to the distance between adjacent borings. When the borings are close together the affected portion of the rope falls into shreds. The parting of the fibers leads to the death of all the borers, which drop out into the water.

It has been observed[3] that the *Teredo* seldom passes from one piece of wood to another closely applied, but in the rope many of the tunnels lead from one yarn to the next.

The young mollusks had evidently found the ropes less suitable than wood for normal growth, for many of them were approaching sexual maturity when only 10 to 12 mm in length. In wood the size at sexual maturity may reach 40 to 50 mm if conditions are favorable; otherwise growth may be retarded while the development of sexual products continues, but more slowly than in individuals growing in a more favorable environment.

Examination of the gonads of many of these young teredos shows that in this unusual situation there is a strong tendency toward protandric bisexuality. In approximately half the sexually differentiated individuals studied the gonads consisted of a cortical layer of yolk-forming ovocytes, with spermatogenic cells filling the lumen of each follicle. There was a fairly close correlation between the size of the ovocytes and the abundance of spermatozoa already formed, indicating a typical protandric condition. In a few individuals most of the spermatozoa had been previously discharged and in these the ova were fully mature. Some evidence of protandry has been reported for another species of the genus.[5]

In addition to the protandric females other individuals were presumably exclusively male, the cells of the cortical layer remaining small and apparently undifferentiated. Others had only a few scattered ovocytes in the cortical layer of an otherwise typical spermary. Thus all individuals first function as males, at least in this unusual environment.

The fibers of the rope are devoured and partially digested, as is normally the case with wood,[6] but the animals remain stunted and produce but few gametes as compared with the vast numbers formed by normal individuals.

Even if a certain amount of reproduction does occur by the teredos living in the rope, this material is highly unsuitable for long survival, and the mortality before reaching the reproductive period must be very great. If the borers are numerous the cut fibers of the rope separate or the entire rope parts; in either case the adjacent borers perish by being dropped out into the water.

While the damage reported in 1930 was unusually serious, these are not the only records of teredos boring in rope or in plant structures other than wood. Lobstermen state that they experience trouble of this nature from time to time, as the borers attack not only the wooden trap but the adjacent part of the buoy rope as well. The unprecedented abundance of this mollusk in that year is thought to have resulted from unusually favorable conditions for the survival of the larvae, which float for two to three weeks[3,4] near the surface of the water before settling upon the objects in which they bore and mature. The free-swimming stage is always precarious and most of the larvae die without completing metamorphosis. Their potential numbers are exceedingly large, however, for a single female may produce more than a million larvae in one season.[3,4] The conditions for survival were evidently better in 1930 than in any other recent year and this is true not only for the teredo but for

[1] Paul Bartsch, *Bull. 122, U. S. Nat. Mus.*, 1922.

[2] R. C. Miller, *Univ. Calif. Publ. Zool.*, 22: 292–328; 401–414, 1922–23.

[3] H. B. Grave, *Biol. Bull.*, 55: 260–282, 1928.

[4] C. A. Kofoid and R. C. Miller, *Final Rept. San Francisco Bay Marine Piling Comm.*, 188–343, 1927.

[5] C. M. Yonge, *Quart. Jour. Mic. Sci.*, 70: 391–394, 1926.

[6] C. M. Yonge, *Trans. Roy. Soc. Edinburgh*, 54: 703–718, 1926.

other mollusks, such as the oyster and clams, which have similar free-swimming larvae, for these survived in unusual numbers the same year.

The presence of even a few adult teredos in piling or in other submerged wooden structures may thus lead to a repetition of this unusual behavior whenever the environmental conditions are such as to favor the survival of their innumerable progeny, provided there is not sufficient wood in the areas to which the pelagic larvae are carried by the currents in the water.

W. R. Coe

Osborn Zoological Laboratory
Yale University

## THE EFFECTS OF MEDIA ON BACTERIAL FILTRABILITY

The fact that Seastone and Lawrence[1] were unable to duplicate Kendall's filtration experiments on the Rawlins strain of *B. typhosus*, even with "K" medium made from "K" powder supplied by him, indicates the probable existence, in this work, of one or more neglected but variable factors. This is further evidenced by the statement of Seastone and Lawrence that their "K" medium showed no uniformity of pH from tube to tube, and also that it occasionally developed a spontaneous turbidity without inoculation.

I query whether bacteriologists, in carrying out filtration experiments, consider or give due weight to the following physico-chemical or colloid factors operative in their media, even when using identical filters; for variations in the filters themselves involve a series of additional factors, based on the specific attractions between filter constituents, bacteria and media constituents:

(1) Colloids may favor the passage of fine particles through filters.
(2) Variation in bacterial deformability may affect filtrability.
(3) The flocculative or deflocculative power of the medium, at the time of filtration, must be considered.

At a symposium on filtration held by the American Society of Bacteriologists at Philadelphia in December, 1926, I heard no reference to factors (1) and (2), and felt constrained to draw attention to them in the open discussion and later on in Science for February 25, 1927.

Factor (1) was dealt with by R. Zsigmondy ("Colloids and the Uultramicroscope" [1909], Chapter 14 on Filtration Experiments), and the fact that moistening the gut with bile increases its permeability to some products of digestion is known to physiologists. Factor (2) was pointed out by Bechhold and Neuschloss,[2] in connection with work on lecithin emulsions where the individual droplets, several μ in diameter, under a pressure above 150 g./cm$^2$, passed through an ultrafilter which completely retained hemoglobin, and whose pores were less than 30 mμ in diameter. Bechhold's explanation is that the lecithin passes the filter-pores in filiform fashion, and reforms droplets after its exit.[3] Apart from the stage of growth of the inoculum, and the relative growth-producing quality of the medium for the bacteria, both of which affect bacterial size, it is not impossible that changes in the medium (and pH is only one factor) may affect the *turgidity* of the bacteria present, and therefore their filtrability under constant pressure.

As to factor (3), the protective or coagulative action of any medium is the summation of various factors, including the specific colloids present. Filtration conditions are affected by pH, salts, temperature, cumulative protective relations, etc. There is an extensive literature on the wide variation in the protective action of colloids, especially of albumins, albumoses and their fractions, toward colloidal gold ("gold number"). Some fractions, instead of being protectors, are active coagulators.[4]

On first reading of Kendall's results,[5] it seemed possible that they might, in part, be accounted for by some or all of the factors above stated. Through the kindness of Dr. L. W. Famulener and his staff at the Pathological Laboratory of St. Luke's Hospital (New York), I was able to have made some preliminary tests on the relative protective behavior of three bacterial media, obtained through courtesy of the New York City Board of Health.

On March 24, 1932, samples of beef broth, veal broth and "K" medium were subjected to the "colloidal gold reaction," according to the technique described by Karl M. Vogel.[6]

The results were:

| | | | | | | | | | | |
|---|---|---|---|---|---|---|---|---|---|---|
| Beef broth | 5 | 5 | 0 | 0 | 0 | 0 | 0 | 0 | 0 | 0 |
| Veal broth | 0 | 0 | 0 | 0 | 0 | 0 | 0 | 0 | 0 | 0 |
| "K" medium | 0 | 0 | 0 | 0 | 0 | ½ | 1 | 2 | 2 | 1 |

Here 0 represents satisfactory protection, 5 represents complete coagulation and precipitation of the gold, and the intermediate numbers represent varying degrees of aggregation of the gold ultramicrons. The figures in the first column are for the original concentrations; those in subsequent columns are the results for progressively doubled dilutions.

1 Science, 77: 259, 1933.

2 *Kolloid Zeitschrift*, 1921.

3 H. Bechhold, "Colloids in Biology and Medicine," 1920.

4 Zsigmondy, *lib. cit.*, pp. 79–89.

5 Science, 75: 295–301, 1932.

6 *Arch. Int. Med.*, 22: 496–516, 1918.

While these results are no criterion for the protective action of media wherein bacteria have grown, towards these same bacteria, they do indicate that media may exhibit wide differences in "gold number," which often parallels protective and deflocculative action, as well as the ability to aid the passage of particles through filters. Thus, Hans Zinsser[7] reported that Ward and Tang, in his laboratory, found that the agents of vaccine and herpes would pass through a filter more readily when suspended in certain types of broth than when suspended in isotonic salt solutions, irrespective of pH; further, that Grinnell found that *B. prodigiosus* passed through all their "V" Berkefeld and Mandler filters, and through most of grade "N," if taken from old cultures and suspended in hormone broth of about pH 7.8.

Speaking of filtrable viruses, T. M. Rivers stated:[8] "Methods of filtration are crude and inaccurate, and the most any one can say concerning viruses is that under given experimental conditions they either pass or do not pass through certain filters. The failure to pass through a filter, however, is certainly not determined in every instance by the size of the virus."[8]

There are, no doubt, many other factors to be considered, besides the three above suggested. Thus, discrete particles in the medium might adsorb otherwise filtrable particles; or oppositely charged particles might form with bacteria a non-filtrable coagulum or union. As pointed out by May Annetts,[9] changes in conductivity, pH and stability may be expected to accompany the filtration of suspensoid sols. Filters described as "certain" may prove to be very uncertain, under special conditions. There is a wide call for bacteriologists, suitably equipped, to give proper recognition and evaluation to all these physicochemical factors, while attempting to establish exact technique for reproducible filtration experiments.

JEROME ALEXANDER
NEW YORK, N. Y.

## A TEST FOR THE PRESENCE OF NOVOCAINE IN NERVOUS TISSUE

DURING the course of some research work upon spinal anesthesia, it became desirable to determine the degree of penetration of novocaine solution into the substance of the spinal nerve roots, spinal cord and medulla, when injected into the subarachnoid space of live animals. At first we attempted to follow the course of the novocaine by adding a dye (methylene blue) to the novocaine solution and checking the distribution of the color post-mortem. The dye was effective in coloring the surface of the nervous tissue and membranes but, on section, none was found within the substance of the nervous tissue. If the extension of the dye were an indication of the extension of the novocaine itself, the failure of the color to penetrate the nervous substance was not in accord with the production of anesthesia and, in some cases, the death of the animal. That the novocaine penetrated further into the nervous tissue than the dye with which it was in solution was the inevitable conclusion. To obtain direct evidence of this as well as to determine the exact distribution within the nervous tissue, a method of recognizing novocaine within the substance of the latter was sought. It occurred to one of us (Beber) that the novocaine might be diazotized, and a color reaction obtained with beta naphthol.

The method evolved is briefly as follows: The nervous tissue to be tested is placed in a beaker of cold 5 per cent. sodium nitrite solution. After a few minutes hydrochloric acid (1:10) is added in the proportion of one of the latter to five of the former solution. This liberates nitrous acid, which in turn diazotizes the novocaine. It is essential that the solution be kept cold for this reaction. After five minutes, the specimens are washed in distilled water and transferred to a 5 per cent. alcoholic solution of beta naphthol. The tissue containing novocaine takes on an orange red color which is greatly intensified by transferring to a weak solution (2 per cent.) of sodium hydroxide. The color fades if placed in water or carried through the usual solutions used in preparing paraffin sections. For section work it is found best after bringing out the color reaction to fix the tissue in 10 to 20 per cent. formalin for fifteen to twenty minutes, freeze and cut thick (fifty $\mu$).

Control experiments, in which the nervous tissue was either treated with distilled water instead of novocaine or not treated at all, failed to produce a similar color reaction when subjected to the same process.

MANUEL GRODINSKY
MEYER BEBER
CHARLES P. BAKER
COLLEGE OF MEDICINE
UNIVERSITY OF NEBRASKA

## SPONGE SPICULES FROM THE LOWER ORDOVICIAN OF WISCONSIN

WHILE examining insoluble residues from the Oneota dolomite (Lower Ordovician) of Wisconsin the writer came upon numerous detached sponge spicules from one locality. The location in question is on U. S. Highway 12, about three or four miles south of Springfield Corners, Wisconsin. Although the writer has examined several hundred samples of the Oneota from numerous localities in the Upper

[7] SCIENCE, 75: 257, 1932.

[8] Jordan and Falk, "The Newer Knowledge in Bacteriology and Immunology" (1927), p. 519; see also S. P. Kraemer, *ibid.*, 557.

[9] *Phys. Chem.*, 36: 2939, 1932.

Mississippi Valley, no sponge remains have been observed elsewhere.

The Oneota near Springfield Corners is a medium to thick bedded dolomite, having a gray or flesh color and carrying a few lenses and thin beds of chert. The sample yielding the spicules is from a pure, non-cherty bed, the insoluble residue consisting of a minute quantity of very fine sand, silt and sponge spicules.

Under the microscope the spicules are seen to be composed of amorphous silica, with considerable amounts of crystalline silica. In form they are uniaxial needles, sharpened at each end, and show no evidence of having been fused in the organism. The longest one observed measures 0.41 mm in length and 0.02 mm in diameter. Axial canals in the spicules can not be plainly seen, but there is a suggestion that they were present in life. It is believed, therefore, that the spicules are to be classified as Silicispongia, order Monactinellida Zittel.

The fauna of the Oneota is a meager one, and nearly all the forms found have been in the chert nodules. These sponge spicules may be the first sponge remains reported from the Oneota formation, as the writer has found no mention of them in the available literature describing these rocks. It is stated by Zittel[1] and Berry[2] that Monactinellid spicules are known from rocks as old as Silurian. No mention is made of their occurrence below the Silurian. If the writer's identification is correct, the spicules from southern Wisconsin may be the oldest Monactinellid spicules thus far discovered.

C. E. NEEDHAM
NEW MEXICO SCHOOL OF MINES

### THE WATER CONTENT OF MEDUSAE

DR. GORTNER'S faith[1] in a marine jelly-fish which is more than 99 per cent. water obviously can not be "flatly contradicted," but there are plenty of data which show his belief to be unfounded in the case of the commoner genera, and which justify skepticism.

In my paper I did not present new data because there was nothing to add to the old; but Dr. Gortner must have observed that the calculation of the "bound water" results in Table 3 necessitated routine determinations of total water. The total solid of *Cyanea* varied from 4.7 to 5.9 per cent., and that of *Aurelia* was always within the range given by Krukenberg. With Gortner's statement that the fraction of *organic* matter may be less than 1 per cent. I have no quarrel; indeed I once crudely estimated it by keeping a dead *Cyanea* in running tap water for 3 days and then drying it. The dry weight was 0.9 per cent. of the wet weight. The effect of the salts is clearly shown, also, by comparing the dry weight data of Krukenberg, whose jelly-fish came from the Gulf of Trieste, with those of Moebius, from the dilute sea water of Kiel Bay. The mean values for *Aurelia* were 4.88 and 2.08 per cent., respectively.

HEIDELBERG J. B. BATEMAN

# QUOTATIONS

## MEDICAL PATENTS

CEREMONIOUS opening of the new laboratories of an important drug manufacturing company is not an occasion on which we expect to hear plain speaking of the kind in which Sir Henry H. Dale indulged at Rahway, on the danger of being too practical in medical research, and of keeping a too eager eye on profits to be derived from the patenting of medical discoveries. The laboratories in question will undoubtedly develop many a useful remedy which will become the subject of a patent monopoly. Sir Henry spoke with authority. Once upon a time he was the director of just such a laboratory. Does not his own career argue against his contention that the pursuit of the practical is incompatible with the pursuit of pure science? He owes his present position of director of Great Britain's National Institute of Medical Research to the distinguished work that he managed to do as a chemist employed by a drug company whose patents are probably its most valuable assets.

There certainly has been no worshiping of false gods in the laboratories of the great German and American industrial organizations. Such Nobel Prize winners as Langmuir, Bosch and Bergius won their laurels as the employees of wealthy corporations. Indeed, certain kinds of research can apparently be conducted most effectively only with the financial aid and equipment of an industrial laboratory. If we want to learn anything about low-pressure chemistry, we must go to the General Electric Company; the best information on speech and hearing is likely to be obtained from the Bell Telephone Laboratories; the Eastman Kodak Laboratories are the recognized authorities on photochemistry. The larger and more liberal corporations have learned to leave their research staffs alone. Even pure science can not help making discoveries that yield a profit when exploited with the aid of patents.

Yet physicians as a class will endorse Sir Henry's warning. Deep down in all of us there is a repug-

[1] Karl A. von Zittel, ''Text-Book of Paleontology,'' Eastman translation, p. 51, Macmillan Company, 1927.

[2] E. W. Berry, ''Paleontology,'' p. 29, McGraw-Hill Company, 1929.

[1] SCIENCE, March 17, 1933.

nance to making money out of human suffering. Even the men in university laboratories who patent their medical discoveries share it. They apply at least part of their royalties to conducting fresh research. But it is a question whether royalties do not quench the disinterestedness that is the very essence of pure research. A patented drug becomes the object of jealous concern. Is it likely that the merits of a competitive product will be objectively appraised and conceded? Questions such as these were probably uppermost in Sir Henry's mind. No doubt the men who have given us patented insulin, patented liver extract and patented ergosterol can be trusted to observe the medical tradition. Yet there is a clear need for some method which will enable a researcher to obtain the money that he needs and yet pursue his studies with a serenity that knows nothing of profits.
—*The New York Times.*

# THE AMERICAN ASSOCIATION FOR THE ADVANCEMENT OF SCIENCE

## SPRING MEETING OF THE EXECUTIVE COMMITTEE

The spring meeting of the executive committee of the council of the American Association for the Advancement of Science was held at the Hotel Stevens in Chicago on March 24 and 25.

Dr. Fox, as executive secretary of the Committee on Foreign Guests for the Chicago meeting, reported regarding the acceptance of invitations issued jointly by the Century of Progress Exposition and the association, and also on the assignment of guests to sectional and society programs.

Dr. Fox stated that he had sent out communications from his office to colleges and universities in order to provide opportunities for such guests as desired invitations to lecture at various points. Different foundations in the United States have been cooperating with Dr. Fox in furnishing information concerning other foreign scientists whom they might have in this country about the time of the Chicago meeting. The executive committee voted that distinguished foreigners who expect to be in the country at the time of the meeting should be invited to participate as honorary foreign guests and members of the association for the Chicago meeting.

The permanent secretary laid before the executive committee the record of receipts and expenditures at the Atlantic City meeting and a summary of the condition of the various funds of the association up to February 28, 1933. From these data it appeared that the balances available were narrow and care must be exercised in making further appropriations. The paid-up membership had fallen off slightly but was still at an encouragingly high level. Some items regarding succeeding meetings were reported and especially the plans for the Boston meeting, which, due to a highly efficient local committee, had already reached a well-advanced stage.

The permanent secretary reported that since Dr. A. F. Woods had been elected a member of the executive committee at the Atlantic City meeting a vacancy in the council was created. Dr. W. W. Cort, of the School of Hygiene and Public Health of the Johns Hopkins University, was elected to fill the vacancy. Dr. Cort's term will expire at the close of the Pittsburgh meeting, in December, 1934.

Certain members, on the basis of credentials duly presented, were elected as fellows of the association.

The question of branch registration offices for the Chicago meeting was discussed. In view of the widely separated locations fixed upon by affiliated societies and sections and of the complexity of the program, the permanent secretary's office was instructed to arrange for branch registration at a limited series of places. This arrangement was approved for the Chicago meeting only.

The presentation of the financial report led to a discussion regarding miscellaneous expenses. The permanent secretary was requested to prepare a communication to section secretaries, urging the need of economy and pointing out the necessary limitations in incurring expenses in connection with the work of the section. It was voted that other items of expense than those regularly included under the regulations of the association be paid only provided that approval was secured from the office of the permanent secretary before the expense had been incurred.

The permanent secretary was asked to revise the general statement for travel and per diem allowances of executive committee members and section secretaries so as to provide for pro-rated distribution of expense whenever travel is undertaken for purposes other than those of the meeting.

In view of general economic conditions and of the two meetings held this year it was voted that section secretaries in attendance at the Chicago meeting be allowed actual minimum railroad fare plus pullman charges and a room at the headquarters hotel as regularly arranged for by the permanent secretary's office for a period not to exceed one week. The per diem allowance was discontinued for the Chicago meeting.

In view of the special circumstances surrounding the summer meeting, the permanent secretary's office was authorized to extend invitations to persons living within a radius of three hundred miles from Chicago to join the association until July 15, 1933, without making payment of the usual entrance fee.

Information was presented to the executive committee that a volume containing papers delivered at the symposium on "The Stabilization of Employment," held in connection with the Atlantic City meeting, had been printed by the Principia Press. The volume was edited by Dr. Charles F. Roos, former permanent secretary. The Principia Press and the Far-Reaching Foundation of Denver proposed to distribute a special edition of the volume to the president, members of Congress and other national officers. The permanent secretary was authorized to prepare and approve the use of a statement to accompany each volume to indicate the part of the association in the undertaking.

The payment of life membership fees in instalments as approved by the council in the Atlantic City meeting was further considered by the executive committee and it was voted that such payment be approved in instalments of not less than $20 in each of five successive years. Such periodic payments would include the annual dues for each year during this period. The permanent secretary was requested to formulate the exact conditions of the plan and present the same for record and approval at the next meeting of the executive committee.

Dr. Henry Norris Russell, president of the association, was delegated as its representative for the meeting of the British Association for the Advancement of Science to be held in Leicester, from September 6 to 13, 1933.

Correspondence from the general secretary of Phi Beta Kappa was presented to the committee, and the permanent secretary was asked to invite that organization to arrange for an address at the Boston meeting, the address to be given by a leading scholar.

Various communications concerning the great increase in the cost of German scientific publications were read to the committee and discussed at considerable length. The possible complications as affecting intimate contacts and proper exchange of information between scientific men were pointed out. In view of the opportunity for misinterpreting definite action, the matter was laid aside for the present.

The proposal to select from the fellows in membership in the association a certain number to be designated as research fellows was presented and after much consideration was on recommendation of the chairman made a special order of business for the June meeting.

The finance committee presented a report regarding defaulted interest payments on mortgages held in the endowment funds, and it was voted that collection of interest should not be pressed during present conditions.

The committee was entertained at luncheon Saturday noon at the Administration Building of the Century of Progress Exposition. Following the luncheon there was a joint meeting with some of the officers of the Century of Progress and with the local committee for the Chicago meeting. Opportunity was afforded for seeing plans of the exposition, learning of the progress made on the installation of scientific features of the same and the general outlook for the exposition. Reports were made by members of the local committee representing individual sections and affiliated societies. They showed that the plans had been adequately worked out, that the work was well advanced towards completion, and that the exhibits, facilities and programs assured not only satisfactory conditions for the summer meeting but a scientific gathering of unusual extent and significance.

HENRY B. WARD,
*Permanent Secretary*

## HOTEL HEADQUARTERS FOR THE CHICAGO MEETING

THE local committee has arranged for the Chicago meeting, the hotel headquarters of the association and its sections as follows:

General Headquarters: Stevens Hotel, Michigan Avenue at 7th Street.

Section A (Mathematics): Judson Court, University of Chicago.

" B (Physics): Windermere Hotel, 1642 E. 56th Street.

" C (Chemistry): Hotel Sherman, 106 W. Randolph Street.

" D (Astronomy): Hotel Stevens, Michigan Avenue at 7th Street.

" E (Geology): Southmoor Hotel, 67th at Stony Island Avenue.

" F (Zoology): Hotel Stevens, Michigan Avenue at 7th Street.

" G (Botany): Hotel Stevens, Michigan Avenue at 7th Street.

" H (Anthropology): Bismarck Hotel, 175 W. Randolph Street.

" I (Psychology): Great Northern Hotel, 237 S. Dearborn Street.

" K (Social and Economic Sciences): Hotel Stevens, Michigan Avenue at 7th Street.

" L (Historical and Philological Sciences): Drake Hotel, Lake Shore Drive and Michigan Avenue.

" M (Engineering): Palmer House, 15 East Monroe Street.

Section N (Medical Sciences): Knickerbocker Hotel, 163 E. Walton Place.
" O (Agriculture): Morrison Hotel, Madison and Clark Streets.
" Q (Education): Drake Hotel, Lake Shore Drive and Michigan Avenue.

The affiliated societies are in general housed in hotels of the section to which they are related. The engineering societies, however, are distributed as follows:

Palmer House: American Society of Civil Engineers; American Society of Mechanical Engineers.
Edgewater Beach: American Institute of Electrical Engineers.
Stevens Hotel: American Institute of Mining and Metallurgical Engineers; American Society for Testing Materials; Society of Industrial Engineers; American Ceramic Society; Society for the Promotion of Engineering Education; National Council of State Boards of Engineering Examiners; American Foundrymen's Association.
Hotel Sherman: Institute of Radio Engineers.

For those who may be coming to Chicago by car and may be interested in automobile camps, the following operated by the Century Cabins, Inc., 7 South Dearborn Street, have been approved by the Century of Progress:

Desplaines Avenue where crossed by Chicago Rapid Transit Line, Forest Park, Illinois. On World's Fair marking—Illumination Route—U. S. 330—Lincoln Highway.

Milwaukee Avenue and Oakton Street, Park Ridge, Illinois. On World's Fair marking—Radio Route—Illinois Route No. 21—Milwaukee Avenue.

22nd and Manheim Road, Westchester, Illinois. On World's Fair marking—Illumination Route—U. S. 330—Lincoln Highway.

Other camps are no doubt available, information concerning which can be obtained from automobile associations and clubs.

Correspondence regarding reservations should be sent directly to the appropriate hotel. Members are advised to make early application for rooms and to specify their connection with the association. It is important to have a definite understanding regarding space and rates.

# THE NATIONAL ACADEMY OF SCIENCES

## ABSTRACTS OF PAPERS PRESENTED AT THE WASHINGTON MEETING

AT the annual meeting of the National Academy of Sciences, held in Washington, D. C., on April 24 and 25, the following papers were presented:

*Geometry of the Laplace equation:* EDWARD KASNER. The Laplace differential equation, $\frac{\partial^2\varphi}{\partial x^2}+\frac{\partial^2\varphi}{\partial y^2}=0$, has its origin in the theory of gravitation, $\varphi$ being the potential; but of course it is of importance in many other branches of physics and in the theory of functions of a complex variable. The curves $\varphi(x, y) =$ constant constitute an isothermal family, so called because they are the curves of equal temperature in a steady flow of heat. The author finds purely geometric properties of such families. We state seven of these properties as follows, each one being completely characteristic: (1) If we construct the osculating circles at any point P of the curve of the given isothermal family and the orthogonal trajectory, these circles meet at another point $P_1$, and the transformation T from P to $P_1$ is conformal. (2) A related transformation is of the Darboux type. (3) If we construct all the $\infty^2$ isogonal trajectories these form a natural family of the kind arising in optics and in the dynamics of conservative forces. (See Kasner's Princeton Colloquium Lectures.) (4) Of all the isogonal trajectories at any point P, two will admit circles of curvature of higher than second order contact, and these two will be orthogonal. (5) The isogonal trajectories form a linear family (as proved by the writer in *Math. Annalen,* 1904), and therefore we can form a Desargues configuration. This gives a characteristic construction in finite form. (6) Any isothermal family and the two families of minimal straight lines form a Blaschke hexagonal web. (7) Any isothermal net may be regarded as the orthogonal projection of the asymptotic lines of some surface. In conclusion, various geometric operations are described by means of which given isothermal families yield new isothermal families. The generalization to the Laplace equation in three dimensions is not direct and will be studied in another paper.

*The geometry of spinors:* OSWALD VEBLEN.

*Finding the velocities of the spiral nebulae:* V. M. SLIPHER. This paper gives a brief account of the velocity studies of the spiral nebulae made at the Lowell Observatory, where work in this field was begun. It touches on the development of the efficiency of the instruments for the work and gives results. There are mentioned the early tests and the reasons stated in support of the velocities being real in spite of their most extraordinary magnitudes. Examples of nebulae in rapid rotation are cited, and objects are referred to which are of exceptional interest because of their speeds of translation or rotation or because of their exceptional spectra.

*Absorption and space reddening in the galaxy from the colors of B-stars:* JOEL STEBBINS and C. M. HUFFER. The stars of spectrum class B, with intrinsic luminosities ranging from a hundred to several thousand times that of the sun, furnish an excellent means for testing the presence of dark matter in space. With a photo-electric cell attached to a 15-inch telescope, the brightness and colors of some seven hundred B-stars have been determined at the Washburn Observatory of the University of Wisconsin. This survey of such objects in the northern sky, complete down to visual magnitude 7.5, has been supplemented by measures of fainter stars and clusters with the large reflectors at Mount Wilson. The observations confirm the existence of a layer of absorbing material in our stellar system, extending along the central plane of the Milky Way. For distances of the first few hundred light-years the effect of this dark gas or dust is inappreciable, but from five hundred to five thousand light-years from the sun the absorption and space reddening become increasingly evident. The present results are in striking agreement with distribution of extra-galactic nebulae determined by Hubble at Mount Wilson. Where the nebulae appear in great numbers the stars are normal in color, but in obscured regions, where the nebulae can not be photographed through the veil in the foreground, the stars show a pronounced effect of coloration. Due to the eccentric position of the sun in the galaxy, stars in the outer regions, like those of the constellation of Orion, are less affected than objects in the opposite direction toward the center of the galaxy, where the loss from absorption amounts to at least three fifths of the visual or five sixths of the photographic light. The growing evidence from B-stars, globular clusters and nebulae supports the conclusion that we do not see out as far as the galactic center, and that objects hitherto supposed to be beyond the nucleus are really on this side of the center of the system. The scale of stellar distances must be revised with allowance for the effect of absorption. Finally, because of the general amount and extent of the obscuration, it is shown that the dark matter in space, counting only that which has so far been detected, may well be greater in total mass than the luminous material which we see in the form of shining stars.

*Luminosity curves and average density of matter in twenty-five groups of galaxies:* HARLOW SHAPLEY. Preliminary calculations at Mount Wilson and at Harvard have indicated that the average density of matter in intergalactic space is of the order of $10^{-30}$ grams per cubic centimeter. Throughout large volumes of space, however, the density is much higher and its evaluation is of significance in consideration of the evolution of the Metagalactic System. The luminosity curves of the galaxies in twenty-five groups, differing in richness, angular extent and volume, have been found from Harvard observations, with appropriate corrections for the random galaxies of the general metagalactic field. The luminosity data permit estimates of distance and mean density. The number of galaxies per cubic megaparsec in the groups varies from ten times to more than a thousand times the average number for metagalactic space. These groups of galaxies (super-galaxies) occur occasionally in pairs, the boundaries of the component groups separated apparently by less than the diameter of either.

*On the masses of binary stars:* HENRY NORRIS RUSSELL and CHARLOTTE E. MOORE. The dynamical parallaxes computed by the writers have been revised by the inclusion of new material for many stars, and compared with determinations from other sources. We are indebted to Dr. Schlesinger for access to the Yale card catalogue of trigonometric parallaxes, to Dr. Adams for unpublished spectroscopic parallaxes from Mt. Wilson, and to Dr. Aitken for valuable double star measures. These comparisons indicate a close agreement with Eddington's mass-luminosity relation, for giants and dwarfs alike, with the well-known exception of the white dwarfs. The total number of stars available for investigation of mass is approximately five hundred and sixty.

*The absolute motion of the solar system and the orbital motion of the earth, determined by the ether-drift experiment:* DAYTON C. MILLER.

*Solar variations and atmospheric pressure:* H. H. CLAYTON (introduced by C. G. Abbot).

*Long-range forecasting:* C. G. ABBOT. There is presented with verification a two-year forecast of the variation of the sun made in November, 1930, and published in February, 1931. The average deviation of observed from predicted monthly mean values is 0.3 per cent. The analysis of solar variation from January, 1924, to September, 1932, and its exhibition as the summation of seven regular periodicities of 6–2/3, 8, 11, 21, 25, 45, and 68 months, respectively is presented. The average deviation of this summation from observed monthly mean values, is 0.15 per cent. The author ventures a detailed forecast of solar variation to December, 1934. Expected values generally below normal, with strong minima June, 1933, and July, 1934. The author presents the analysis of the departures from normal temperature of Bismarck, North Dakota, from 1875 to 1925. In addition to the seven periodicities found in solar variation, he finds others of 9–1/2, 12–3/4, 18 and 135 months, respectively. All these periodicities continue over the 50-year period from 1875 to 1925, but with fluctuations of amplitude, phase and form. He attempts to determine empirical relations governing these fluctuations. Employing the preferred adjustments of this kind, he compares the summation of adjusted periodicities with the actual departures from normal temperature, 1875 to 1925. Finally, he compares his forecast for 1925 to 1932 with observed departures of that interval.

*The phosphorescence of solid nitrogen and its relation to crystal structure:* L. VEGARD.

*Forbidden lines in astrophysical forces:* JOSEPH C. BOYCE, DONALD H. MENZEL and CECILIA H. PAYNE (introduced by Harlow Shapley).

*The physical state of Novae:* DONALD H. MENZEL and CECILIA H. PAYNE (introduced by Harlow Shapley).

*The action of the parenteral administration of sugars in the hydrogen-ion concentration of normal and malignant tissues in living animals:* CARL VOEGTLIN, H. KAHLER and R. H. FITCH (introduced by C. S. Hudson). [To be printed in SCIENCE.]

*Crystalline pepsin and trypsin:* JOHN H. NORTHROP (introduced by Simon Flexner). A crystalline protein (pepsin) which digested other proteins in acid solution with great rapidity was isolated three years ago from commercial pepsin preparations. More recently another crystalline protein (trypsin) which digests other proteins in slightly alkaline solution has been isolated from pancreas. These proteins behave like pure substances in that the chemical and physical properties, including enzymatic activity, are the same in a number of different preparations and are not changed by repeated fractional crystallization. Partial destruction of the protein by heat, acid, gamma rays or ultra-violet light, results in a corresponding loss in activity. The inactivation by heat is partly reversible. These results confirm the conclusion that the enzymatic activity is a property of the protein molecule. A number of physical and chemical properties of the proteins have been determined.

*Gluconeogenesis from Fat:* JOHN R. MURLIN (introduced by Lafayette B. Mendel). There has been much theorizing but little convincing evidence in favor of the conversion of fatty acids to glucose in the animal body. It is certain that the reaction at best is difficult and probably takes place very little at a time, if at all. Studied by the method of respiratory metabolism the conversion should give a low R.Q., but if it were followed immediately by combustion of the sugar the low R.Q. would blend with a high R.Q. and the evidence consequently would be obscured. With the castor bean it has been possible to separate the two reactions clearly. Conversion of fatty acids to cane sugar takes place in the endosperm and its oxidation in the young plant. With the help of Drs. R. G. Daggs and H. B. Pierce we now have the evidence complete, (1) by the R.Q., (2) by combustion in a modified oxycalorimeter, and (3) by chemical analysis. With the assistance of Drs. Estelle E. Hawley and Carroll W. Johnston, an attempt has been made to devise conditions for the human subject, which would possibly separate conversion from combustion. Deprived of glycogen the tissues, offered sugar, prefer to restore the glycogen rather than burn the sugar. If under these conditions easily assimilable fat were offered and if any glucose were formed, it would be converted to glycogen and retained, thereby disclosing low R.Q.s. Later it would be oxidized, giving a special sequence of quotients following a high-fat meal, namely, first low, then medium, then high. Seven subjects have been used, and rich cream (approximately 40 per cent. fat) furnished the sole diet for several days. Thereby glycogen was reduced and a flood of fatty acids became available suddenly to supply materials for replacement. The special sequence of quotients predicted was obtained several times especially at an early test for each subject. Later the phenomenon of adaptation or increased tolerance for fat supervened to obliterate this sequence. Many very low R.Q.'s were obtained, however, outside the predicted sequence. There are three other known ways of explaining low R.Q.s, aside from the conversion of fatty acids to glucose: (1) Formation of sugar from protein; (2) formation of sugar from glycerol; (3) production of the acetone bodies. Consideration of these several reactions under the conditions of the experiments described proves that none or all of them combined can explain the lowest R.Q.s obtained. The latter undoubtedly are correct, for they have been duplicated many times by both the Benedict and the Tissot-Haldane techniques. It seems clearly possible, therefore, that we have here a method of demonstrating gluconeogenesis from fat. To make it perfectly convincing we should be able, as in the castor bean, to find the sugar. That has not yet been accomplished.

*Origin of bioelectric potentials:* W. J. V. OSTERHOUT. In *Nitella* (as in muscle and in nerve) we find an outwardly directed potential on which the current of action and the current of injury depend. Our experiments on *Nitella* indicate that this may be largely due to the diffusion potential of potassium salts which exist inside at a higher concentration than outside (the mobility of the potassium ion in the protoplasmic surface is apparently very high). This has a paradoxical look because the potassium must penetrate from the outside and thus diffuse inward against an electrical gradient created by itself. It is therefore of considerable interest to find that suitable models can do this very thing and can imitate in many other ways the behavior of the living cell. The apparent paradox is explained by the fact that potassium penetrates in one form and goes out in another and that it sets up less diffusion potential in entering than in leaving the cell. In the model, as in the living cell, a non-aqueous layer lies between two aqueous phases and more potential is produced in this layer by potassium than by sodium. But if certain substances be removed from the non-aqueous layer potassium produces no more effect than sodium. Experiments in collaboration with S. E. Hill show that a similar change is brought about by treating the living cell with suitable solutions. The cell is then in a state of anesthesia: it is no longer excitable by ordinary electrical stimuli. The process is perfectly reversible. This suggests that anesthesia is due to the removal of certain substances from the cell.

*The precocious development of sexual characters in the fowl by daily injections of hebin:* L. V. DOMM and H. B. VAN DYKE (introduced by F. R. Lillie). Brown Leghorn cockerels ranging from 1 to 47 days in age received daily subcutaneous injections of hebin. The quantities administered ranged from 4 to 32 rat units in single daily injections. The duration of the experiments varied from 14 to 36 days. The first effect noticed was a pronounced stimulation of head furnishings. This could be definitely noted, in some instances, as early as 48 hours after injections began. The comb revealed steady growth throughout and at the conclusion of experiments was usually considerably larger than controls. Precocious sexual behavior was noted. Young males were found crowing when 9 days old and to reveal the initial treading reactions at 13 days. Post-mortem revealed hypertrophy of testes. These were usually larger and heavier than controls. Thyroids were likewise larger and heavier in treated birds. The spleen, liver and heart did not seem to show significant changes in weight though experimental spleens were fairly consistently somewhat lighter than controls. The ductus deferens revealed hypertrophy. In the cases studied histologically tubules of control testes were distinctly juvenile showing primordial germ cells, whereas those in treated testes revealed spermatogenesis. Thyroids from treated individuals revealed larger vesicles. In a second series of experiments brown Leghorn females received daily subcutaneous injections of hebin. Concentrations injected, age range, and duration of experiments were identical with the experiments on cockerels. Here also the first effect noticed was a striking growth of head furnishings. This was definitely noticeable within 48 hours in individuals receiving higher concentrations. In such experiments head furnishings revealed a continuous high growth rate throughout becoming masculine in character. The comb became stout of blade and erect whereas that of similar size in normals, only found in much older females, shows a thin loppy blade. Plumage and behavior were apparently unaffected. Post-mortem revealed considerable hypertrophy of ovaries. These were larger and heavier than controls but showed no indications of ovulation. The surface of more advanced ovaries had a mulberry appearance indicating follicular development. The more advanced oviducts showed astonishing hypertrophy comparable to that normally preceding ovulation. The weight of these frequently exceeded 15 times that of controls. Thyroids were larger and heavier than controls. Differences in weights of liver, spleen and heart were probably not significant though experimental spleens were usually heavier. Histologically experimental ovaries showed larger follicles. Sections of normal oviducts showed low mucous folds devoid of tubular glands and conspicuous muscle layer, whereas experimentals showed high mucous folds, well-developed tubular glands and conspicuous peripheral muscle layer. Experimental thyroids showed larger vesicles. Effects were in general proportional to concentrations injected. The results generally confirm the earlier experiments of Domm ('31) following daily hypophyseal implants on juvenile males and females.

*The anterior hypophyseal substance which synergizes with prolan:* HERBERT M. EVANS, MIRIAM E. SIMPSON and PAUL R. AUSTIN. In 1931 Evans, Meyer and Simpson[1] discovered that the gonadotropic effect of the substance found in the urine of pregnant women (prolan) is greatly increased if certain extracts of the anterior hypophysis, themselves of low gonadotropic potency, are added to prolan. The phenomenon has been recently confirmed by Leonard,[2] similar synergistic effects with prolan having been secured by him through the employment of extracts high in gonadotropic potency. Our earlier experiments led to the suggestion of the growth hormone as the synergistic substance, while the Leonard series provoked his hypothesis that the gonadotropic hormone itself was involved. Continued study of the phenomenon has shown that the anterior hypophyseal substance which increases the gonadotropic effects of prolan (when mixed *in vitro* with prolan) is neither the gonadotropic nor growth hormone. The new substance does not possess either growth- or gonad-stimulating properties, and is characterized by physical and chemical traits which clearly distinguish it from the hormones in question.

[1] H. M. Evans, K. Meyer and M. E. Simpson, "The Relation of Prolan to the Anterior Hypophyseal Hormones," *Proc. Soc. Exp. Biol. and Med.*, 28: 845, 1931.

[2] S. L. Leonard, "Increased Stimulation of Immature Rat Ovaries by Combined Injections of Prolan and Hypophyseal Sex Hormone, *Proc. Soc. Exp. Biol. and Med.*, 30: 665, 1933.

*The effects of deprivation of magnesium in the animal body:* E. V. MCCOLLUM, H. D. KRUSE and ELSA R. ORENT. When young rats are deprived of magnesium but are given adequate amounts of other dietary essentials, they show a spectacular series of symptoms denoting a condition that is short and abruptly fatal in its course. Successively they pass through stages of vasodilatation and hyperirritability of the nervous system before succumbing in tonic-clonic convulsions. This syndrome fits into the category of tetany, when the term is used in its broadest sense. It has, however, characteristic features that differentiate it from all other forms of tetany. The chemical changes in the blood serve as further evidence to the distinctiveness of magnesium tetany, since magnesium is the only inorganic ion undergoing alteration. Adult males, restricted to the magnesium-deficient ration, suffer damage of the reproductive system, resulting in sterility. A study of females as yet is incomplete. In addition to these effects on the nervous and reproductive systems which may be designated as local effects, adult animals show constitutional changes in the form of nutritive failure, which is reflected in loss of body weight. Again, chemical examination of the blood offers an explanation of the nutritive failure, since it reveals an unusual disturbance in lipid metabolism unlike that seen hitherto in any other disease. It has been asserted that the mechanism of failure in fasting and deficiency diseases is identical; the blood picture in magnesium deficiency indicates that the mode of failure is entirely different in the two conditions. Studies of inorganic metabolism in animals deprived of magnesium reveal that while the animal runs a negative magnesium balance it retains calcium in the earlier stages to an extent far in excess of control animals. If the animal has a long survival, period, however, this retention of calcium is broken. The retention of calcium is reflected in the calcification of the long bones, analyses of which show a higher content of calcium.

*Rate of development of primate embryos:* G. L. STREETER. Being able to study macaque embryos of known age throws light on the rate of development during the first few embryonic weeks concerning which in human specimens only inadequate clinical data have thus far been available. The two genera differ in minor details of form and in rate of differentiation but these differences become progressively less in the early stages. The close morphological parallelism between embryos of monkey and man will be shown and a comparison will be made between some of the well-known human specimens and similar monkey specimens of known ages.

*Morphine and the cat:* Wilder D. Bancroft, Robert S. Gutsell and John E. Rutzler, Jr. It is usually stated that the action of morphine on the cat is fundamentally different from its action on man or on the dog, the cat becoming violently excited. We have tested six cats with varying amounts of morphine—five to twenty milligrams per kilogram—injected subcutaneously and intramuscularly. While the cats showed a slight excitement, there was nothing approaching mania, and it is not certain that the effect is anything more than the irritability corresponding to sub-anaesthetic doses. Oral administration of sodium rhodanate decreases the excitement produced in cats by morphine. Toxic, but not lethal, doses destroy the excitement almost completely. In the presence of histamine, an agglomerating agent, the effect of morphine lasts almost twice as long. Morphine caused dilatation of the pupils and a doubling under of the hind quarters in all six cats. Sodium rhodanate eliminated the doubling under but had no appreciable effect on the dilatation. A few men and more women are said to become violently excited under morphine and this is said to be true of all human beings in the manic state. There is therefore no fundamental difference in the action of morphine on men and on cats though the relative incidence of the drug is undoubtedly different. It is possible that a greater percentage of cats than of men become violently excited by morphine; but there is no real evidence either way.

*The isotopic fractionation of water:* Edward W. Washburn, Edgar R. Smith and Mikkel Frandsen. When water is subjected to electrolysis an isotopic fractionation occurs.[1] It has been found that the heavier isotope of hydrogen and the heavier isotopes of oxygen are concentrated in the residual water. The specific gravity of the residual water rises continuously as the electrolysis proceeds. The rise in specific gravity is accompanied by a rise in the freezing point and in the boiling point and by a decrease in the refractive index. No indication of approach to an electrolysis equilibrium has been found, and there is every reason to hope that it will be possible to obtain the various isotopes of hydrogen and oxygen in a pure state, certainly in highly concentrated form. If the oxygen from the electrolysis of normal water is combined with normal hydrogen, the water produced has a lower specific gravity than normal water. If this water be again partially electrolyzed and the oxygen combined again with normal hydrogen, a further drop in the specific gravity of the water occurs. It will consequently be possible to prepare isotopically pure water of the composition $H^1O^{16}H^1$ and hence to determine very accurately the atomic weight of normal oxygen on the $O^{16} = 16$ scale. With the different isotopes of hydrogen and oxygen available in pure form, a new field of chemistry and possibly also of biology will be opened up, since the different isotopes of hydrogen, at least, may be expected to exhibit pronounced differences in chemical behavior. A survey is being made of water from different natural sources to find out whether differences in isotopic composition occur in nature.

*Neutrons and atomic nuclei:* William D. Harkins. The neutron is an electrically neutral nuclear particle of about $10^{-13}$ cm diameter and of about the mass of a hydrogen atom. The existence of neutrons in the radiations from beryllium, when a piece of this material is bombarded by fast $\alpha$-particles, was recognized by Chadwick in 1932. That the nucleus of the beryllium atom contains a neutron was assumed in 1915 by Harkins and Wilson, and the characteristics of free neutrons were given in 1920 by the writer and by Rutherford. Photographs of the disintegration of nitrogen nuclei by fast neutrons from beryllium have been obtained by Gans, Newson and the writer. One of these photographs shows the effect of a neutron of extremely high energy, which amounts to 15 million electron volts or a velocity of about 33 thousand miles per second. This is by far the fastest neutron thus far detected. The work of Feather in Cambridge, together with that of this laboratory, indicates that in disintegrations of nuclei by neutrons kinetic energy is either conserved or disappears and is converted into gamma rays. The energy found to disappear in the reaction—Nitrogen 14 + Neutron 1 = Boron 11 + Helium 4—is represented by only a few definite energy values, so it seems probable that definite energy levels exist in some of the nuclei involved, in that of boron of mass 11. A neutron plus a proton may be assumed to form a hemi-alpha particle or nucleus of a hydrogen atom of mass 2. Certain interesting relations are found if it is assumed that atomic nuclei consist of alpha particles, neutrons and hemi-alpha particles. These will be discussed in connection with the Harkins-Masson nuclear formula $(np)_Z n_I$, or $\left(\frac{\alpha}{2}\right)_Z n_I$, in which Z is the atomic and I the isotopic number; n, a neutron; p, a proton; and $\alpha$ represents an $\alpha$-particle of group. The completion of an $\alpha$-particle in a nucleus by the addition of a hemi-$\alpha$-particle gives an extremely large amount of energy: 20 million electron volts or more. It is found that neon gives the smallest and nitrogen the largest number of nuclear disintegrations from bombardment by neutrons of the three gases thus far tested—nitrogen, oxygen and neon. Experiments with other gases, such as ethylene, are in progress.

*A possible alternative formula for sucrose:* C. S. Hudson and C. B. Purves. In an attempt to prepare a methyl fructoside possessing the same ringed structure as that depicted for the fructose residue in the generally accepted formula for sucrose, cane sugar was dissolved at room temperature in methyl alcohol containing hydrogen chloride. The reaction was found to proceed with remarkable rapidity and to give rise initially to glucose in a reducing condition and to a mixture of methyl fructosides of a gamma type. On the basis of the usual structure for sucrose, stable alpha methyl glucoside and an individual beta methyl gamma fructoside had been expected as the sole initial products of the reaction. This unforeseen result induced the authors to review the experimental evidence upon which the chemical constitution of sucrose is at present based and they point out that the

[1] Washburn and Urey, *Proc. Nat. Acad. Sci.*, 18: 496, 1932.

whole of these experimental data can be equally well satisfied by an alternative structure for the disaccharide. In the possible alternative structure sucrose is regarded not as a glucosido gamma fructoside but as a dicyclic acetal condensation product of open chain glucose and open chain fructose.

*The widths of the K absorption limits in x-ray spectra:* F. K. RICHTMYER and S. W. BARNES. By means of a two-crystal spectrometer the widths of the following elements have been studied: Mo(42), Ag(47), In(49), Sn(50) and W(74). Except in the case of Sn(50) none of the limits showed any trace of fine structure. After making an approximate correction for the width of the rocking curves of the pair of crystals used, the widths of the several limits in volts are as follows: Mo(42), 18 volts; Ag(47), 28 volts; In(49), 31 volts; W(74), 133 volts; Au(79), 160 volts. Within experimental error there seems to be no difference between the limit of Ag(50) in the metal and in the oxide. The absorption limit of Sn(50) seems to show a structure which perhaps may be associated with the fact that Sn has a large number of isotopes, in contrast with Ag, which has two, and In, which has only one constituent.

*New optical properties of the alkali metals:* R. W. WOOD. Continuing an investigation made over fifteen years ago, on the remarkable transparency of films of sodium and potassium to ultra-violet light, and their opacity and high reflecting power in the visible region, it has now been found that there is a fairly sharp transition point in the spectrum at which an alkali metal ceases to exhibit the properties of a metal and assumes those of a dielectric. A potassium film, through which the sun's disc is invisible, transmits 25 per cent. of the energy in the region between 3,000 and 1,860. For this spectral range it gives plane polarization by reflection of unpolarized light, having a Brewsterian angle of about 37°. The spectrum of a light source giving a continuous spectrum, reflected from a film of the metal several wavelengths in thickness, shows interference maxima and minima the fifth order or higher being recorded. The transition point, at which the properties change, descends in the spectrum, with decreasing atomic number being at about 4,000 for caesium and 2,000 for lithium. The use of the films as ray filters for spectroscopic work will be discussed.

*Application of the three-color principle to oil painting:* HERBERT E. IVES. The experimentally well-established fact that all colors may be matched by the mixture of three properly selected primaries has been extensively used in color photography and typographic printing. It has not, however, been heretofore successfully used in painting. The usual artist's palette consists of a dozen or more pigments, with the result that the number of ways of making desired colors by mixture is very large and quite unamenable to systematization. Learning how to use these numerous pigments is a matter of long experience. The simplification indicated by the three-color principle has been retarded in realization largely owing to the mistaken but widely held belief, that the primary pigment colors are red, yellow and blue. Actually the pigment primaries, which act by subtraction or absorption of light from white, should be complementary in hue to the red, green and blue, which are the primaries for mixing light by addition. Those colors are a minus red (spectrum minus red) or turquoise, a minus green, or crimson, a minus blue, or yellow, each having wide overlapping spectral reflection bands. Pigments of these colors, of proper spectral characteristics, are capable of mixing in pairs to make red, green and blue, and all three together to make black. When mixed with white all variations of saturation and hue are obtained. The practical problem consists in procuring pigments possessing the indicated spectral reflectivities and having satisfactory chemical properties, such as freedom from reaction with the oil or other medium, and satisfactory permanence. Due to the very great advances which have been made in the dye industry to meet recent demands for permanent colors for automobiles and outdoor signs, it is now possible to select pigments nearly enough meeting the scientific requirements to test the practicability of the principle. This has been done with success, and pictures so painted are exhibited in connection with the presentation of this paper.

*On supraconductivity and the Hall effect:* EDWIN H. HALL. The experiments of Onnes from which he concluded that the Hall effect does not exist in the supraconductive state of metals are inconclusive. These experiments were of two kinds. In one the metal under examination was tested in the usual direct method which reveals the effect in the ordinary conductive state. In the other a metal spherical shell, in which persistent (self-sustaining) currents had been set up, was subjected to a magnetic field which, in the opinion of the experimenter, tended to swing the currents into new orbits within the metal. Failure to discover such a deflection led Onnes to infer the non-existence of a Hall effect. There is reason to doubt whether in either of these methods of experimentation the magnetic lines of force penetrated the metal to any appreciable degree. A different procedure for testing the question at issue is proposed.

*The Pleistocene diversion of the Mississippi River across Crowley's Ridge, southeastern Missouri:* F. E. MATTHES. The lower Mississippi Valley throughout its upper half is divided longitudinally into two parallel lowlands by a narrow strip of hilly upland, 100 to 250 feet high, known as Crowley's Ridge. Originally the Mississippi followed the lowland on the west side of this ridge, but now the river cuts across it at Thebes, Illinois, in spite of the fact that the ridge there is seven miles broad and composed in part of hard limestone. In consequence of this remarkable change in course the Mississippi now joins the Ohio 200 miles north of its original point of confluence with that river, and the entire drainage net in a valley area aggregating 17,000 square miles has been rearranged. Recent investigations have shown that the diversion of the Mississippi at Thebes and other diversions of its waters at points now indicated by abandoned gaps in Crowley's Ridge were brought about, not by capture of the river by southward flowing streams, as has been supposed, but by overflow at a time, late in the Pleistocene epoch, when the Mississippi had aggraded its valley with silt derived from the continental ice sheet to a level about 50 feet above the present flood plain. Numerous terraces composed of glacial outwash material afford the principal evidence. The Ohio River also played a part in connection with the diversion of the Mississippi River. It flowed at that time across southern Illinois, through the valley now occupied by Cache River. By paring away the southeastern edge of Crowley's Ridge it beheaded several northwestward draining valleys and thereby created spillways at fairly low levels.

*Archean formations of the Grand Canyon:* IAN CAMPBELL and JOHN H. MAXSON (introduced by John C. Merriam). The oldest rocks exposed in the Inner Gorge of the Grand Canyon comprise a thick and varied metamorphic series (Vishnu schist). These rocks are invaded by granitic intrusives (phantom granite). So complex and so intimate are the relations between the metamorphic series and the igneous rocks that in many instances the resulting formation can only be described as a migmatite. The original sedimentary nature of the schists is shown by the occurrence of quartzite, calcareous members, iron formations and sandstone lentile in slightly altered schists. It is also indicated by retention of such characteristic sedimentary structure, as stratification and cross-bedding. Following the regional metamorphism of the sediments, the phantom granite was emplaced by processes of assimilation and granitization. Different facies of the granite and its associated pegmatites resulted from differing character and intensity of deuteric alteration.

*Some features of flowers and fruit of a new Cordaites:* DAVID WHITE. Fossil plant fragments of Pottsville age discovered in southeastern Illinois by the State Geological Survey disclose leaves, flowers and seeds of a single species of *Cordaites*. Male and female flowers, *Cordaianthus*, are small, bud-shaped and nearly alike. The young seed in the midst of the flower is narrow, soft and is deficient in wing. Stamens, protected like the ovules, by bracts when young, are numerous in the upper part of male flowers, protruding beyond the bracts and arching bouquet-like when mature, with oblong pollen sacs strewn along the upper ends. The base of the stamen seems exactly axillary. The small seeds (*Cardiocarpon*) are longitudinally oval-rhomboidal, with spinose glandular sarcotest, widely dilated as wing and narrow cordate-oval acute "hard" coat. No clearly defined pollen character is noted in the material, consisting of impressions and carbonized residues only. The micropylar canal is distinct, even in immature seeds. In some large seeds, structures, apparently tubular and seemingly continuous with the micropyle, extend, while dilating somewhat, far down into the interior of the endosperm. These structures, which the author is unable to regard as fungal, are interpreted as indicating a stage of development at which the archegonial wall and part of the endospermic center had broken down. No embryo has definitely been recognized in any Paleozoic seed.

*Primitive cephalopods:* AUG. F. FOERSTE (introduced by David White).

*Metaxenia and neophosis, two forms of morphogenetic influence exerted by the generation-complex of the embryo sac apparatus in higher plants:* WALTER T. SWINGLE (introduced by R. A. Harper). [To be printed in SCIENCE.]

*The effect of alternation from spores to vegetative cells on the growth and activity of certain anaerobic bacteria:* E. B. FRED and E. MCCOY. In a study of the factors that govern the growth and activity of bacteria, little consideration has been given to the effect of periodic changes from the spore to vegetative stage. Occasional statements have been made that the spore stage represents a regenerative phase of the cycle and that vegetative cells immediately following germination are of greater vigor and activity. The anaerobic bacteria represented by *Cl. acetobutylicum* and *B. amylobacter* (Bredemann) were chosen for the study of the effect of serial transfer involving periodic change from spores to vegetative cells. At regular intervals of four to five days the cultures were subjected to heat treatment of 1.5 minutes at 90° C. and were then used for subcultures in the usual way. All tests were made in 2 per cent. corn mash, a medium known to be suitable for the growth and sporulation of these organisms. At the present time the experiment has been carried to the one hundred and tenth transfer. Results of the comparison of the first and the one hundredth transfer are now available. The fermentation products of these culture generations have been determined, both as to quantity and ratio of products, but no significant difference has appeared. Vigor of growth has been maintained and, if anything, has become more regular with successive transfers. Comparisons of spore formation of the first and the one-hundredth culture generations seem to indicate an increase in the number of spores produced. This increase may account for the consistent activity which has been obtained. During this long period of time no culture has dropped out of this series because of failure to grow. This is an unusual record for an experiment with an obligate anaerobe.

(*To be continued*)

## BOOKS RECEIVED

ADKINS, HOMER and S. M. MCELVAIN. *An Introduction to the Practice of Organic Chemistry*. Pp. ix + 224. Illustrated. McGraw-Hill. $2.25.

BEEBE, WILLIAM and JOHN TEE-VAN. *Field Book of the Shore Fishes of Bermuda*. Pp. xiv + 337. 300 illustrations. Putnam's. $3.50.

COLBERT, J. C. *Laboratory Technique of Organic Chemistry*. Pp. ix + 341. Illustrated. Century. $2.50.

EHRET, WILLIAM F. *Laboratory Studies in General Chemistry*. Pp. viii + 312. 21 figures. Century. $1.50.

NAYLOR, NELLIE M. and AMY LE VESCONTE. *Introductory Chemistry with Household Applications*. Pp. x + 367. 41 figures. Century. $2.60.

PARSHLEY, H. M. *The Science of Human Reproduction*. Pp. xv + 319. 66 figures. Norton. $3.50.

ISSUE CONTAINING THE PRELIMINARY PROGRAM OF THE CHICAGO MEETING OF THE AMERICAN ASSOCIATION FOR THE ADVANCEMENT OF SCIENCE AND ASSOCIATED SOCIETIES

# SCIENCE

VOL. 77 FRIDAY, MAY 19, 1933 No. 2003

*The American Association for the Advancement of Science:*
*Preliminary Program of the Chicago Meeting:* PROFESSOR HENRY B. WARD ... 461
*Evening Meetings* ... 462
*Entertainment for Ladies* ... 464
*The Century of Progress Exposition* ... 464
*Points of Interest and Excursions* ... 465
*The American Association Press Service* ... 465
*Membership* ... 466
*Business Sessions* ... 466
*Hotel Headquarters and Transportation* ... 466
*Scientific Sessions of Sections and Societies* ... 467
*The Value of Scientific Research to Agriculture:* SECRETARY HENRY A. WALLACE ... 475
*The Significance of Recent Measurements of Cosmic Rays:* PROFESSOR ARTHUR H. COMPTON ... 480
*Obituary:*
*William Henry Holmes:* DR. WALTER HOUGH ... 482
*Scientific Events:*
*The McDonald Observatory; The British Association for the Advancement of Science; The Royal Institution and Sir William Bragg; The American Academy of Arts and Science* ... 483
*Scientific Notes and News* ... 485
*Discussion:*
*The Attraction of a Sphere:* PROFESSOR EDWARD V. HUNTINGTON. *The Movement of Diffusible Substances in Food Products:* JEROME ALEXANDER. *A Louse Feeding on the Blood of its Host:* DR. F. H. WILSON. *Hail Prints and Mud-Cracks of Proterozoic Age:* DR. CARROLL LANE FENTON and MILDRED ADAMS FENTON. *The Need of Opportunity for Exceptional Ability:* DR. J. MCKEEN CATTELL ... 489
*Quotations:*
*The Situation of Jewish Scientific Men and Physicians in Germany* ... 492
*The National Academy of Sciences:*
*Abstracts of Papers Presented at the Washington Meeting. II* ... 494
*Science News* ... 8

SCIENCE: A Weekly Journal devoted to the Advancement of Science, edited by J. MCKEEN CATTELL and published every Friday by

THE SCIENCE PRESS

New York City: Grand Central Terminal

Lancaster, Pa. Garrison, N. Y.

Annual Subscription, $6.00 Single Copies, 15 Cts.

SCIENCE is the official organ of the American Association for the Advancement of Science. Information regarding membership in the Association may be secured from the office of the permanent secretary, in the Smithsonian Institution Building, Washington, D. C.

# THE AMERICAN ASSOCIATION FOR THE ADVANCEMENT OF SCIENCE

## PRELIMINARY ANNOUNCEMENT OF THE SUMMER MEETING TO BE HELD IN CHICAGO FROM JUNE 19 TO 30, IN CONNECTION WITH THE CENTURY OF PROGRESS EXPOSITION

Edited by Professor HENRY B. WARD
PERMANENT SECRETARY

THIS year the summer meeting of the American Association for the Advancement of Science is exceptional in character and importance. It is to be held in Chicago, the great metropolis of the Mid West; it is to cover twice the usual period, the time this year extending from June 19 to 30, inclusive; it welcomes as guests scientists from other lands; it is signalized by programs embracing contributions by leaders in scientific research from the nations of the world.

Recognizing the significance of this occasion, the secretaries of the sections and of the affiliated societies have been for months devoting special attention to organizing programs depicting in each field the progress of science in the past and the outlook for its future service to the nation and the world. No summer meeting previously held in this country has offered to students of science or to the public interested in scientific advancement an opportunity as rich and varied as that embodied in the plans now announced for this meeting.

First of all the location is peculiarly appropriate for such a gathering. A century ago this region was on the edge of the wilderness. In 1833 Chicago was incorporated as a frontier city; this year, as a great metropolis, it celebrates its centenary in a manner calculated to emphasize the tremendous progress which, in common with the nation, it has made in a hundred years. Its marvelous development is based on the advancement of science. The Century of Progress Exposition, conceived, planned and carried to successful realization despite tremendous difficulties in the immediate past, offers to the association concrete demonstrations of the advancement of science in variety and extent heretofore unessayed by any organization or community in the world. The unique character of the exposition will be apparent to all who participate in the meetings.

Working together the Century of Progress and the association issued last year invitations to a selected list of leaders in scientific research throughout the world to visit Chicago and take part in the programs of the meeting. Acceptances were received from about forty and their contributions appear in the general program of the meeting outlined later in this announcement. In consequence of the presence and participation of these foreign guests together with many distinguished men from this continent, the meeting takes the form of an international congress. It affords a rare opportunity for personal contacts and exchange of views on the progress of science here and elsewhere which will be of the highest value to American workers and will stimulate increased activity in these fields.

The list of foreign guests, as already printed in SCIENCE for November 25, 1932 (p. 484), has suffered only slight modification due to various circumstances. The speakers and their topics so far as announced are given later in this article in the record of meetings and general sessions.

The period of two weeks decided upon for the meetings is well filled by the programs of the sections and of the participating societies. While it has not been possible to group together all similar organizations, still the first week in general is being utilized by societies representing pure sciences, whereas those in applied sciences meet in the second week. The number of affiliated societies meeting with the association is unexpectedly large; indeed, the group of engineering societies is so large that this period has rightly been designated as Engineering Week. Relations to the organizations have determined the precise time for certain special groups; thus the meetings of Section N (Medical Sciences) come in the first week, immediately after the convention of the American Medical Association in Milwaukee, and those of Section Q (Education) fall at the end of the second week, thus leading up to the sessions of the National Education Association immediately following.

To a large extent the programs of the sections and the affiliated societies have assumed a special character for this occasion. Many symposia have been organized which merit particular attention, as they include addresses by the foreign guests and by American scientists of distinction. Single addresses and short series of invited papers dealing with particular problems have been preferred to miscellaneous lists of contributed papers. An effort has been made to leave time open, especially in the afternoons, which can be used for group conferences, informal discussions and social affairs.

The evenings have been devoted to a series of general sessions, with programs of wide general interest and speakers in fields commanding present attention. Most of these programs are announced under the auspices of some section and are planned definitely to appeal to the general membership of the association, both by nature of the topics presented and of the speakers. It is the hope of the association that these occasions may also attract such attention from the citizens of Chicago and vicinity as will make known the work of the association and the significance of science as the essential factor in determining progress in the coming century. While the list of events is still subject to slight modification, the series of evening sessions will be substantially as follows.

## EVENING MEETINGS

On Monday evening, June 19, the Century of Progress Exposition will tender a reception to the association and associated societies in honor of the foreign guests. This reception will be held in the Hall of Science on the Exposition Grounds. Admission will be by badge or ticket only. Members should not fail to register sufficiently early to secure the necessary items.

On Tuesday evening, June 20, Section N (Medical Sciences) has organized a general session for the association and its friends. The program will be devoted to the topic of "A Century of Progress in Medicine." The public is invited. The speakers include: Dr. Morris Fishbein, editor of the *Journal* of the American Medical Association, on "Frontiers of Medicine"; Dr. Paul Dudley White, of the Harvard Medical School, on "Heart Disease"; Dr. Max Cutler, of the Michael Reese Hospital, on "The Conquest of Cancer"; Madame Curie, of Paris, will also take part. This meeting will be held in a large auditorium, the location of which will be announced later.

On Wednesday evening, June 21, the general session will be conducted under the auspices of Section B (Physics). The speakers will include Dr. F. W. Aston, of Cambridge, England, on "The Story of Isotopes," and President R. A. Millikan, of the California Institute of Technology, on "New Light on Nuclear Physics."

The same evening Section F has provided another general session, with Dr. Richard Goldschmidt as speaker, on the topic "Some Aspects of Evolution."

Thursday evening, June 22, will be devoted to a

banquet given by the association in the Grand Ball Room of the Hotel Stevens in honor of foreign guests. Members desiring tickets for themselves and friends should make early reservation. Attendance at the banquet is also open to friends of the association, after provision has been made for members desiring to participate. Further details will be announced in the general program.

On Friday evening, June 23, there will be a general session at the Field Museum under the auspices of Section H (Anthropology), in which Professor C. U. A. Kappers, director of the Central Institute for Brain Research, Amsterdam, Holland, will give an address on "The Anthropology of the Near East in Connection with the History of its Population." On this evening the Field Museum will hold an open house for the members of the association and their guests.

Section I (Psychology) sponsors a general session for Saturday evening, June 24, in which Professor Charles E. Spearman will speak on "Recent Advances in Our Knowledge of Human Personality."

On Monday evening, June 26, comes a symposium arranged with the cooperation and support of the Far Reaching Foundation of Denver. The program on the subject "Nationalism" has been worked out by a special committee of Section L (History and Philology). Professor Charles A. Beard, president of the American Historical Association, will present a paper on "Nationalism in American History." Professor Bernadotte Schmitt, of the University of Chicago, will also speak. It is hoped that one or more of the foreign guests will take part.

On Tuesday evening, June 27, Section M (Engineering) and the engineering societies will hold a joint general session in the Grand Ball Room of the Palmer House. Dr. A. P. M. Fleming, of the Metropolitan Vickers Electrical Company, Manchester, England, will address the session on "The Development of Engineering in the Last One Hundred Years."

Wednesday, June 28, is recognized by the Century of Progress Exposition as Engineers' Day. The general banquet of the engineering societies and Section M will be held that evening in the Grand Ball Room of the Hotel Stevens.

Thursday evening, June 29, Section K (Social Sciences) will sponsor a general session. Professor Henry Clay, of Manchester, England, will deliver the address of the occasion.

Friday evening, June 30, the general session is held under the auspices of Section Q (Education). The topic of the evening is "Education for a Democracy." Professor Walter F. Dearborn, of Harvard University, will preside. Miss Jane Addams, of Hull House, Chicago, and President Robert M. Hutchins, of the University of Chicago, will speak.

Certain other special features in the general program merit particular mention. Among these is the conference on "The Diffusion of Scientific Knowledge," organized by Science Service under the leadership of Dr. William H. Howell. The wide-spread and unfortunate failure of the general public to recognize the fundamental importance of research as a *condicio sine qua non* of advancement in the well-being of all nations and the necessity of maintaining and increasing rather than reducing and crippling such activities at the present time make this topic of outstanding importance. The discussion by a group of distinguished foreign scholars from widely different environments is certain to yield results of great value.

The meeting of the American section of the International Union of Pure and Applied Sciences with foreign guests will convene on Saturday morning, June 24, in the International House on the University of Chicago campus, under the leadership of President R. A. Millikan, chairman of the union, and Professor F. K. Richtmyer, of Cornell University, chairman of the section. The program includes papers by Sir Richard Glazebrook, M. Henri Abraham, professor at the Sorbonne, Professor Leigh Page, of Yale University, Dr. George A. Campbell, of the American Telephone and Telegraph Company, Dr. Harvey L. Curtis, of the U. S. Bureau of Standards, and Professor A. E. Kennelly, of Harvard University.

On Tuesday afternoon, June 27, the American Society for Testing Materials has arranged for a joint meeting with Section M (Engineering). On this occasion the Edgar Marburg Lecture will be given by Dr. Herbert John Gough on "The Crystalline Structure in Relation to Failure of Metals, Especially by Fatigue." In 1925 the American Society for Testing Materials instituted the Marburg Lecture for the purpose of securing at annual meetings, by leaders in the respective fields, reports of outstanding developments in the promotion of knowledge of engineering materials. The lecture commemorates the name of the first secretary of the society, through whose development of the technical programs the organization has become widely recognized as a forum for the discussion of properties and tests for engineering materials.

Important symposia and more technical addresses by distinguished foreign guests and others have been developed by many sections and societies and are listed for meetings during the afternoon hours and in connection with society dinners. A record of these items will be found under the programs of the organizations concerned.

On Sunday morning, June 25, members of the association are invited to attend services in the University of Chicago Chapel. The address will be given by Professor Shailer Mathews. It is hoped that special courtesies can be offered to the association on Sunday afternoon also, of which later notice will be given.

### ENTERTAINMENT FOR LADIES

Mrs. Henry Gale, chairman of the Ladies' Committee, has reported the present stage of plans for entertaining the ladies while their husbands are attending the scientific sessions. On Wednesday, there will be an automobile trip up the North Shore, luncheon and visits to two or three private gardens, with tea; on Thursday afternoon, a visit to the University of Chicago campus, with tea at the Ida Noyes Hall; in the late afternoon, probably on Friday, a boat trip on the lake in private boats of Chicago yachtsmen. For at least the first and last of these functions the parties will be limited in number. Plans for registering for them will be announced in the printed programs for the meetings, along with plans for visiting other points of interest in Chicago by individual request, guest memberships at the women's clubs, etc.

## THE CENTURY OF PROGRESS EXPOSITION

(*From the Exposition office through the courtesy of Dr. Philip Fox*)

The Century of Progress Exposition, in addition to having a historical background, will show the latest industrial developments and the basic scientific principles behind them. A replica of Fort Dearborn, Chicago's first building, is seen there, and with a turn of the head the lofty skyscrapers of America's foremost contribution to architecture, which had its inception in Chicago.

The general type of exhibits of the Basic Science Division was outlined by the Science Advisory Committee of the National Research Council. The exhibits are intended to present a unified front of modern science, but for operating purposes they are classified under the following seven heads—Mathematics, Astronomy, Physics, Chemistry, Biology, Geology and Medicine. The exhibits are for the most part presented in the Hall of Science. They are designed to be intelligible and appealing to the uninitiated and at the same time of interest to the specialist.

In the field of biology, every resource at command will be enlisted to present in clear and simple fashion a few of the fascinating problems and principles of that science. Living plants and animals will be used in the demonstration of the principles of genetics, evolution, ecology and animal societies. The rôle of the cell will be emphasized. Cell activities will be demonstrated and illustrated by models of magnified cells. So far as possible the demonstrations will be made by means of moving models, living specimens, moving pictures and transparencies, as well as preserved plants and animals. Among highly interesting presentations will be the embryological exhibits, the models displaying the physical mechanism of speech and thought, the union of plant cells, the production of food in plants, the growth of trees, marine biology, the distribution of plant life over the globe, etc.

Chemistry will be presented as the fundamental science of the transformation of matter. The exhibits will attempt to demonstrate what chemistry is and what it has done to advance civilization. Such phenomena as burning, the rusting of metals, the combustion of fuels, the function of breathing, etc., will be shown as various manifestations of chemical change. The development of the world's raw materials and their production by means of chemical transformation into articles and commodities of vital necessity to mankind will be shown. The principle of catalysis and its application to the production of useful products, the application of the principle of absorption and the study of colloidal matter and the products which have resulted will likewise be portrayed. Important chemical applications of electricity will be demonstrated.

In the geological exhibits the origin and growth of the earth will be traced by means of operating models and other dynamic exhibits. How the processes of deposition and erosion have changed the earth's contours will be shown. The formation of mountain ranges, how volcanoes and geysers occur and the origin and recording of earthquakes will be explained. Petroleum's occurrence in the earth and man's amazing methods of locating it will be shown by a series of exhibits. A geological time clock, which records 2,000,000,000 years of the earth's history within the space of a few minutes, will be another unique feature of this exhibit.

Visitors will be given a broad and comprehensible view of mathematics. This science, for purposes of clarity in the exhibit, has been divided into four major subdivisions: numbers and algebra, geometry, analysis and applied mathematics. Historic apparatus and instruments used by the U. S. Navy in navigation, gunnery and communication will be on display. The contributions of mathematics to the development of other basic sciences will be interestingly set forth.

In the exhibits of physics, visitors will learn of a wide variety of phenomena—how gases can exert high pressure, how gas and steam engines and refrigerating systems operate, how drops of water and other liquids happen to be round, how sounds are produced, transmitted through the air and recorded. Fundamental electrical phenomena will be demonstrated, and the application of electricity and magnetism to industrial uses for man's welfare will be clearly set forth. One of the interesting features of the exhibits of physics will be an optical section which reveals refraction of light by prisms and lenses, colored effects produced in various ways and important spectra.

The astronomical exhibit is housed in the Adler Planetarium and Astronomical Museum, which contains an unexcelled collection of antique astronomical and mathematical instruments for observation and computation. The chief exhibit is the Zeiss Optical Planetarium. No instrument has been devised which has greater versatility in exhibiting the phenomena of any science.

The medical sciences will tell the story of the control of pain, of the doctor's service to the sick, of antisepsis and asepsis in surgery, the discovery of the x-ray, the extension and clarifications of man's vision by means of the microscope, the progress of medicine from the saddle-back doctor of 1833 to the scientific practitioner of to-day. One of the striking features of the medical exhibit will be the transparent man—a heroic model of the human body, showing the skeletal, nervous, vascular, respiratory, digestive and muscular systems.

Outdoor and indoor exhibits will come to tell a complete story of social science, tracing the life of man from earliest times to the present. In the outdoor area groups of Indians will live their native life as closely as possible. This exhibit will culminate in a reproduction of one of the great Maya buildings of Yucatan—the highest development of American aboriginal culture.

The indoor exhibits will be housed in the Hall of Social Science. A central exhibit—the American family—sets the keynote for the stories of education and social work. The dramatic story of anthropology begins a huge relief map showing the nine cultures of North America.

Another display tells how the story of the past is read: once read it becomes history. This in turn leads to the exhibits in psychology and sociology and on to statistics, economics and political science. In the section on education is shown the development of the American School in response to American needs.

The record of agriculture and engineering, too extensive even to be summarized here, is shown in appropriate buildings. To the engineers the exhibits in the Electrical Building and Transportation Building will be of special interest. The type of construction in many of the buildings also presents some novelties. In addition there are separate exhibits by the great industrial concerns.

## POINTS OF INTEREST AND EXCURSIONS

(*By courtesy of the local committee*)

There are numerous points of interest in and about Chicago for its visitors. The city is being built on a definite program, which has as its slogan Daniel H. Burnham's injunction: "Make no little plans." The park and boulevard systems, the forest preserves, the reversal of the Chicago River as an item toward the sanitation of Chicago and the development of the Lakes-to-Gulf Waterway are integral parts of the plan.

One should visit the Art Institute, the Field Museum of Natural History, the Adler Planetarium and Astronomical Museum, the Museum of Science and Industry (which in its present form preserves the beauty of the Fine Arts Building of the Columbian Exposition), the Shedd Aquarium, the Oriental Institute, the Zoological Gardens, the Chicago Historical Society Building, the Museum of the Chicago Academy of Sciences and the educational institutions, principally the University of Chicago and Northwestern University.

If interested in the world's food supply, visit the International Harvester plant, the Stock Yards and the Board of Trade. One may visit also the steel center in South Chicago and Gary, the oil-refining plants in Whiting, the great merchandising plants of Sears-Roebuck and Montgomery Ward, the Merchandise Mart, great stores, of which Marshall Field's is the premier, the banking center of LaSalle Street and the great printing establishment of the Lakeside Press.

The Sand Dunes at the south end of Lake Michigan, Lake Geneva with the botanical gardens and the Yerkes Observatory, or farther, the Dells of Wisconsin, provide attractive excursions; likewise, short lake trips or boat trips across the lake and to Milwaukee.

## THE AMERICAN ASSOCIATION PRESS SERVICE

(*By Austin H. Clark*)

The aim of the Press Service is to assist in presenting to the public through the press a true and accurate story of the development of science in this country. Naturally the development of science, as portrayed in the press from year to year, is to a large extent comparable to a history of the scouts and advance guards of an army rather than to the more methodical progress of the army itself.

When we who are engaged in science delve into history we like to read of the more spectacular events, and we are prone to evaluate history on the basis of a scattered and more or less disconnected series of such events, more or less completely ignoring the more prosaic social trends that gave these events their significance or made them possible.

To one who really knows history the average man's idea of historical events seems just as far afield from a proper conception of the basic fundamentals as science in the press seems to the scientific man. Both science and history, when brought before the public, must be presented in terms that interest the public and that the public understand. The public is not interested in the slow progress of a great army or in the progress of the great mass of scientific workers. But it is interested in results, especially spectacular results.

We who are engaged in scientific work are fortunate in having the results of our labors presented in the press by a corps of able and conscientious writers in whom we are justified in placing complete confidence. If, in order to interest the public, these writers must lay emphasis on points that are quite different from the points that we in talking among ourselves would emphasize, that is their responsibility. So long as what they write is accurate, we have no valid reason for objection. This fact is now very generally realized and appreciated.

At Chicago the functions of the Press Service will be carried on as heretofore. Those who are to present papers are asked to send two copies of their manuscripts, each accompanied by an abstract, to the American Association for the Advancement of Science Press Service, Smithsonian Institution Building, Washington, D. C., as far in advance of the meeting as possible. A single copy of the manuscript will not suffice, and both copies are to be sent to the same address.

The manuscripts sent to the Press Service are not for publication as such. They are solely for the use of the press representatives in the preparation of news items or features. They are regarded as confidential, and except for the properly accredited press representatives no one is allowed access to them.

So far as possible the Press Service endeavors to supply the press with such additional information as will be advantageous in the proper presentation of a news item, and it also aids the press in securing interviews with authors when such interviews are requested.

The press is by far the most important medium for the diffusion of scientific knowledge among the people as a whole. It has become the outstanding factor in the education of those beyond school age and is an increasingly important factor in broadening the knowledge and interests of those still in school.

The press is conscientiously doing its best to make as accurate and as timely as possible the information that it presents. It is becoming increasingly important that we who are occupied with scientific work should do all we can to help it.

## MEMBERSHIP

The unusual privileges accorded members at the Chicago meeting make it desirable for all to register early to receive the full program and the badge which will admit to the various special functions. Registration on this occasion will be handled at the Stevens Hotel and at branch registration offices in Eckhardt Hall, University of Chicago, and in Thorne Hall, McKinloch Campus, Northwestern University.

Since it was felt that many in the Middle West would desire to participate in this meeting and enjoy especially the privileges of contact with the distinguished foreign guests, a special invitation has been extended to those living within 300 miles of Chicago to join the association at this time without payment of the usual initiation fee. Persons desiring to take advantage of this offer should address the Washington office in advance or make application at any registration desk during the meeting.

### Invited Guests

Scientific men or women coming from outside the United States and Canada who are not members of the association may be welcomed as guests for the meeting. Information concerning such persons should be sent to the permanent secretary's office in Washington or later to him at the Stevens Hotel, Chicago. Full data are desired that the cases may be properly presented to the executive committee and official invitations duly authorized and issued.

## BUSINESS SESSIONS

The council is charged with the duty of handling the business of the association and has provided that all matters offered for its consideration be referred first to the executive committee for study and formulation. Any items may be sent to the Washington office up to June 10. After that date they should be sent to the Chicago headquarters, Hotel Stevens, in care of the permanent secretary. The executive committee will meet in the Stevens Hotel on Monday, June 19, at 10 A. M., to review items previously presented and to prepare the agenda for the council. The first council meeting will be held on Monday afternoon at 2 P. M. Subsequent meetings of the council will be held at 9 A. M. on Tuesday and Wednesday, and thereafter if necessary. The executive committee will also meet daily to care for business matters that may demand attention. In view of the difficulties necessarily associated with careful consideration of important questions it is desirable that all proposals be left with the permanent secretary as early as feasible.

## HOTEL HEADQUARTERS AND TRANSPORTATION

Data regarding hotel headquarters were printed in SCIENCE for May 12. Reduced railway rates by the "certificate plan certificate" have been granted by almost all railroads in the United States and Canada. Persons attending the meeting should purchase a first-class one-way ticket to Chicago, securing a "certificate plan certificate" reading "for the American Association for the Advancement of Science and Associated Societies." The certificate must be left at the validation desk in the registration offices to be called for later at the same place. Each person presenting an endorsed and validated certificate may purchase a continuous passage, one way return ticket for *one third* of the regular fare by the same route as that traveled to Chicago. Certificates must be validated before July 4. Tickets to Chicago must be purchased between June 15 and June 28 (both dates inclusive). Return tickets must be purchased by July 4; having purchased the return ticket its holder can remain in Chicago at will, provided he reaches the original starting point within thirty days.

Special fares of varied character have already been announced by certain lines and probably more such will be offered before the date of our meetings. Information about these rates and the precise conditions of issue and use may best be secured from your local agent. Early application is advisable. It is likely that special ten-day rates will be preferable, except for persons desiring to make a longer stay in Chicago.

## SCIENTIFIC SESSIONS OF SECTIONS AND SOCIETIES

Sections are arranged in the order of the alphabetic designations used in the association's records. Affiliated societies are given the letter of the section under which each is listed, together with a distinguishing number. The president and secretary of each society are named, and they represent the organization on the council of the association, unless other representatives have been elected and are present to serve at Chicago. It is hoped that the societies may all be well represented at council meetings in order to facilitate prompt and proper transaction of business.

The programs as outlined are not complete, but they are in the main correct and adequate to give a true conception of the final program.

### *A—Mathematics*

A–1. Section A of the Association. June 21–23.
*Vice-president,* Charles N. Moore; *Secretary,* E. R. Hedrick.

A–2. American Mathematical Society. June 19–23.
*President,* L. P. Eisenhart; *Secretary,* R. G. D. Richardson.

A–3. Mathematical Association of America. June 20–23.
*President,* E. T. Bell; *Secretary,* W. D. Cairns.

The program of the American Mathematical Society will open on Monday, the morning being devoted to registration and the afternoon to a session of contributed papers. On Tuesday morning there will be another session of contributed papers. On Tuesday afternoon the Mathematical Association of America is planning a program at which the following papers will be presented: "The Postulation Method in Mathematics," by Professor E. V. Huntington, of Harvard University; "The Lag of Mathematics behind Literature and Art in the Early Centuries," by Professor H. E. Slaught, of the University of Chicago; "Applications of Mathematics to Real Estate Problems," by Dr. Henry Babcock, of Evanston. On Wednesday morning Section A and the American Mathematical Society will hold a joint symposium, at which Professor Lipot Fejer, of the University of Budapest, will speak on "The Infinite Sequences Arising in the Theories of Harmonic Analysis, of Interpolation and of Mechanical Quadratures," and Professor C. N. Moore, of the University of Cincinnati, will give a paper entitled "On the Use of Cesaro Means in Determining Criteria for Fourier's Constants." One other speaker has been invited to participate in this meeting. Wednesday afternoon will be devoted to a joint session of Section A and the society, at which invited addresses on geometry will be given. Professor Levi-Civita, of the University of Rome, will speak on "Nets on a Surface and Extension of Trigonometry," and Professor W. C. Graustein, of Harvard University, will give a paper entitled "Invariant Methods in Differential Geometry." Two other speakers have been invited to participate. On Thursday morning the American Mathematical Society will hold a meeting devoted to short contributed papers. For Thursday afternoon the Mathematical Association of America is planning a program in which the following men will present papers: Dr. T. C. Fry, of the Bell Telephone Laboratories, on "Fundamental Concepts in the Theory of Probability"; Professor George D. Birkhoff, of Harvard University, on "Mathematics and Art"; Dr. D. H. Lehmer, of the California Institute of Technology, on "A Number Theory Machine." On Friday morning there will be a joint session of Section A and the American Mathematical Society, at which Professor Levi-Civita will give a lecture on "Some Mathematical Aspects of the New Mechanics" and Professor G. D. Birkhoff on "Quantum Mechanics and Asymptotic Series." This meeting will be of special interest to the members of the American Physical Society, although they are not meeting jointly with Section A. For Friday afternoon the American Mathematical Society has arranged for a lecture by Professor L. E. Dickson, of the University of Chicago, on "Recent Progress in Additive Number Theory," which will be followed by short papers on number theory. A dinner for the mathematicians is planned for Friday evening.

*B—Physics*

B–1. Section B of the Association. June 19–24. *Vice-president,* C. J. Davisson; *Secretary,* H. A. Barton.

B–2. American Physical Society. June 19–24. *President,* Paul D. Foote; *Secretary,* W. L. Severinghaus.

B–3. American Meteorological Society. June 19–20. *President,* Herbert H. Kimball; *Secretary,* Charles F. Brooks.

On Monday morning, June 19, Section B and the American Physical Society will have a program of short contributed papers. The American Meteorological Society will hold a meeting devoted to papers on "A Century of Progress in American Meteorology," at which the following papers will be presented: "Pioneers in American Meteorology and the Founding of Weather Services," by Mr. Eric R. Miller, of the U. S. Weather Bureau at Madison; "The Early History of Aerology in the United States," by Mr. S. P. Fergusson, of Harvard University; "History of the Application of Meteorology to Aeronautics with Special Reference to the United States," by Mr. W. R. Gregg, of the U. S. Weather Bureau at Washington; "On the Dynamics of Penetrative Convection," by Dr. J. Bjerknes, of the Geophysical Institute, Bergen, Norway; "Periodicities in Rainfall," by Professor Dinsmore Alter, of the University of Kansas. On Monday afternoon the American Meteorological Society will hold a symposium on "Radiation and General Circulation of the Atmosphere." Dr. H. H. Kimball, of Harvard University, will present a paper on "Solar Radiations as a Meteorological Factor"; Dr. W. J. Humphreys, of the U. S. Weather Bureau at Washington, a paper on "Incoming and Outgoing Radiation as Affected by the Atmosphere"; Dr. J. Bjerknes, on "A Theory of the General Circulation of the Atmosphere." Mr. John Patterson, of the Meteorological Office in Toronto, will also present a paper. On Tuesday morning Section B and the American Physical Society, with Section C as their guests, will hold a symposium on "Application of Quantum Mechanics in Chemistry," with the following speakers: Professor J. C. Slater, of the Massachusetts Institute of Technology, on "Electron Energies in Atoms and Molecules"; Professor Linus Pauling, of the California Institute of Technology, on "Quantum Mechanics of Condensed Ring Systems, Free Radicals and Other Complex Molecules"; Dr. Henry Eyring, of Princeton University, on "Quantum Mechanics and Chemical Reactions"; Professor R. S. Mulliken, of the University of Chicago, on "Band Spectra and Molecular Structure." The American Meteorological Society will hold a symposium on "Dynamics of Extratropical Cyclones." Dr. J. Bjerknes will present a paper on "Vertical Cross Sections through Extratropical Cyclones"; Mr. Andrew Thomson, of the Meteorological Office in Toronto, will present a paper on "The Cyclone of November 18–19, 1931"; Dr. W. J. Humphreys, on "Origins of Extratropical Cyclones"; Mr. K. O. Lange, of the Massachusetts Institute of Technology, on "Atmospheric Soundings for Glider Meets"; Mr. Phil E. Church, of Mooseheart, Illinois, on "Dynamic Climatology from the Massachusetts Institute of Technology Weather Maps"; Professor T. A. Blair, of the U. S. Weather Bureau at Lincoln, Nebraska, on "Interrelations of Seasonal Weather, Pacific Ocean and North America"; an additional paper by Professor C. G. Rossby, of the Massachusetts Institute of Technology. On Tuesday afternoon the American Meteorological Society will hold a meeting devoted to miscellaneous papers. The following men will present papers: Dr. H. H. Kimball, of Harvard University, and Mr. I. F. Hand, of the U. S. Weather Bureau at Washington, on "The Use of Glass Color Screens in the Study of Atmospheric Depletion of Solar Radiation"; Mr. Bernard Haurwitz, of the University of Leipzig, and Mr. Harry Wexler, of the Massachusetts Institute of Technology, "Turbidity of American Air Masses according to Linke's and Ångström's Measures of Turbidity"; Mr. S. P. Fergusson, of Harvard University, on "Anemometer Experiments." Section B and affiliated societies will hear an address by Dr. J. Bjerknes on "Atmospheric Soundings, Methods and Results." On Wednesday morning Section B and the American Physical Society will meet with Section C in a symposium on "Isotopes" (see announcement of Section C). On Wednesday afternoon Section B and the American Physical Society will participate in a joint symposium with Sections C, D and E on "Measurements of Geologic Time" (see announcement of Section E). Following the symposium, Professor Enrico Fermi, of the University of Rome, will give an address on "Theory of Hyperfine Structures." In the evening the American Physical Society will hold a dinner, which will be followed by a general session. On Thursday morning Section B and the American Physical Society with Section D will hold a joint symposium on "Spectroscopy and Astronomy" (see announcement of Section D). On Thursday afternoon Section B and the American Physical Society will meet for a lecture by Professor N. Bohr on "Space and Time in Contemporary Physics." On Friday morning Section B and the American Physical Society will hold a symposium on "Nuclear Disintegration." Professor E. O. Lawrence, of the University of California, will speak on "Recent Work on Nuclear Disintegration at the University of California"; J. D. Cockroft, of the University of Cambridge, England, on the "Disintegration of Light Elements by High Velocity Protons"; Dr. M. A. Tuve, of the Department of Terrestrial Magnetism at Washington, on "Disintegration Experiments on Elements of Medium Atomic Number"; Professor W. D. Harkins, of the University of Chicago, on "Disintegration of Nuclei by Neutrons." The members of Section B will be interested in the program which Section A has arranged for Friday morning. In the afternoon Professor A. Sommerfeld, of the University of Munich, will give an address on "Theory of Metallic Conduction." On Saturday morning Section B is meeting with the American Section of the International Union of Pure and Applied Physics.

*C—Chemistry*

C–1. Section C of the Association. June 19–23. *Vice-president,* Arthur B. Lamb; *Secretary,* J. H. Simons.

C–2. American Chemical Society. June 23.

On Monday morning Section C will hold a joint symposium with Section N on "Colloid Chemistry Related to Biological Problems." Professor Theodor Svedberg, of Upsala University, Sweden, will present a paper on "Sedimentation Constants and Molecular Weights of the Respiratory Proteins." Professor Filippo Bottazzi, of Naples, Italy, will present a paper on "Physico-Chemical Properties of Concentrated Blood Serum." Additional papers will be presented by the following: Professor Edwin J. Cohn, of the Harvard Medical School, on "Electrostatic Forces in Systems Containing Biological Components"; Professor J. W. McBain, of Stanford University, on "Some Experimental Methods Applicable to Biological Problems"; Professor W. J. V. Osterhout, of the Rockefeller Institute for Medical Research, on "Cell Physiology in Relation to Colloidal Structure." On Tuesday morning, Section C will meet in a joint session with Section B and the American Physical Society at a symposium on "Application of Quantum Mechanics in Chemistry" (see announcement of Section B). On Thursday, Section C and the Chicago Chemists Club will have a luncheon at the International House, which will be followed by brief informal and non-technical talks. On Wednesday morning, Section C will hold a joint symposium with Section B and the American Physical Society on "Isotopes"; Dr. F. W. Aston, of Cambridge, England, will present a paper on "Some Measurements of Relative Abundance of Isotopes"; papers will also be presented by Dr. K. T. Bainbridge, Bartol Research Foundation of the Franklin Institute, on the "Masses of Isotopes and the Disintegration of Atoms"; Dr. E. W. Washburn, of the U. S. Bureau of Standards, on "Isotopic Fractionation of Water"; Professor Fred Allison, of the Alabama Polytechnic Institute, on the "Magneto-Optic Method in the Study of Isotopes"; Professor W. D. Harkins, of the University of Chicago, on "Neutrons and Isotopes" and Professor H. C. Urey, of Columbia University, on "Diffusion Method of Separation of Isotopes." On Wednesday afternoon Section C will meet with Sections B, D and E in a symposium on "The Measurement of Geologic Time" (see announcement of Section E). The American Physical Society is holding a dinner on Wednesday evening, which will be of interest to members of Section C. On Thursday morning Section C will hold a session devoted to contributed papers. On Friday morning Section B is holding a symposium on "Nuclear Disintegration," which will interest members of Section C. In the evening Section C and the Chicago Section of the American Chemical Society are holding a dinner at the Midland Club. Professor Theo. Svedberg, of Upsala University, Sweden, will give the principal address on "Sedimentation of Molecules in Centrifugal Fields."

*D—Astronomy*

D–1. Section D of the Association. June 21–24. *Vice-president,* V. M. Slipher; *Secretary,* H. T. Stetson.

D–2. American Astronomical Society. *President,* W. S. Adams; *Secretary,* R. S. Dugan.

On Wednesday afternoon, June 21, Section D and the American Astronomical Society will meet with Sections B, C and E in a symposium on the "Measurement of Geologic Time" (see announcement of Section E). On Thursday morning Section D and the American Astronomical Society will participate in a joint symposium with Section B and the American Physical Society on "Spectroscopy and Astronomy." Professor A. Sommerfeld, of the University of Munich, will speak on the "Present Status of Spectroscopic Theory"; Professor W. S. Adams, of the Mt. Wilson Observatory, on "Spectroscopy as a Tool in Astronomy"; Dr. I. S. Bowen, of the California Institute of Technology, on "Spectra of Highly Rarefied Gases"; Professor Otto Struve, of Yerkes Observatory, on "Matter in Interstellar Space." On Thursday afternoon Section D and the American Astronomical Society will attend the lecture by Professor N. Bohr, of the University of Copenhagen, on "Space and Time in Contemporary Physics." On Friday and Saturday mornings Sections D and the American Astronomical Society will hold sessions at the Adler Planetarium, devoted to miscellaneous papers contributed by members. On Saturday afternoon an excursion will be made to the Yerkes Observatory.

*E—Geology and Geography*

E–1. Section E of the Association. June 20–22.
*Vice-president,* R. T. Chamberlin; *Secretary,* Kirtley F. Mather.

E–2. Geological Society of America. June 20–22.
*President,* Reginald A. Daly; *Secretary,* Charles P. Berkey.

On Tuesday morning Section E and affiliated societies have arranged a session, at which Professor J. J. Sederholm, of Helsingfors, Finland, will speak on "Ultrametamorphism and Anatexis." Dr. R. J. Tillyard, of Australia, will present a paper on "A New Class of Arthropods from the Precambrian of the Adelaide Series, South Australia." Dr. Arthur Bevan, of the University of Virginia, will speak on "Recent Studies of the Paleozoic Formations in Virginia." On Tuesday afternoon Professor J. J. Sederholm will give an address on "Progress and Scope of Precambrian Research." In the evening an informal dinner will be held for geologists and geographers. It is hoped that Sir Douglas Mawson, of England, will be present and that he will speak after the dinner. On Wednesday afternoon Section E will hold a joint symposium with Sections B, C and D on "The Measurement of Geologic Time," at which the following papers will be presented: "General Survey of the Problem," by Dr. Alfred C. Lane, of Tufts College; "Working Formulae for the Age of a Radioactive Mineral," by Professor A. F. Kovarik, of Yale; "The Significance of the Isotopes of Uranium and Lead," by Dr. C. S. Piggot, of the Geophysical Laboratory; "The Actinium Series of Radioactive Elements and the Measurement of Geologic Time," by A. V. Grosse, of the University of Chicago; "The Helium Method, a New Outlook," by W. D. Urry, of the Massachusetts Institute of Technology; "Thorianite from Eastern Pennsylvania," by Dr. R. C. Wells, of the U. S. Geological Survey; "Post-glacial Time Calculations from Recent Geothermal Gradient Measurements in the Calumet Copper Mines," by President W. O. Hotchkiss, of the Michigan College of Mining and Technology, and Professor L. R. Ingersoll, of the University of Wisconsin; "The Radium Content of the Travertine Deposits of Mammoth Hot Springs, Yellowstone Park, as an Index of Their Age," by Dr. Herman Schlundt, of the University of Missouri.

On Thursday morning Section E will hold a joint session with the Geographical Society of Chicago, at which the following men will speak: Professor Charles C. Colby, of the University of Chicago, on "Distribution of World's Major Cities"; Professor Stanley D. Dodge, of the University of Michigan, on "A Plan for the Study of the Regional Geography of the Upper Connecticut Valley"; Professor V. C. Finch, of the University of Wisconsin, on "A Departmental Program for Geographical Research: Plan and Progress"; Professor Wellington D. Jones, of the University of Chicago, on "A Reconnaissance Map of Metropolitan Chicago." On Thursday afternoon there will be another joint session. Professor K. C. McMurry, of the University of Michigan, will speak on "A Geographical Reconnaissance of the Lower Rio Grande Valley of Texas"; Dr. Richard Hartshorne, of the University of Minnesota, on "Geographic and Political Boundaries in an Area of International Tension: Upper Silesia"; Professor Henry M. Leppard, of the University of Chicago, on "Tyneside"; Professor Glenn T. Trewartha, of the University of Wisconsin, on "Results of Field Reconnaissance in Japan"; Professor R. S. Platt, of the University of Chicago, on "An Air Traverse of Central America."

*F—Zoological Sciences*

F–1. Section F of the Association. June 20–23.
*Vice-president,* A. S. Pearse; *Secretary,* George R. La Rue.

F–2. American Society of Zoologists. June 20–23.
*President,* W. C. Curtis; *Secretary,* W. H. Cole.

F–3. Entomological Society of America. June 22–23.
*President,* J. J. Davis; *Secretary,* H. B. Hungerford.

F–4. American Association of Economic Entomologists. June 22–23.
*President,* W. P. Flint; *Secretary,* A. I. Bourne.

On Tuesday morning, June 20, Section F has arranged a symposium on "Physical and Chemical Changes in Nerve during Activity"; in this Section N will join. Professor G. H. Parker, of Harvard University, will preside. Professor A. V. Hill, of London, will give an address on "The Heat Production of Nerve"; Professor W. O. Fenn, of the School of Medicine and Dentistry of Rochester, will speak on "Nerve Respiration"; Professor R. W. Gerard, of the University of Chicago, on "Chemical Activity of Nerve"; Dr. H. S. Gasser, of Cornell University, on "Electrical Phenomena in Nerve." On Tuesday afternoon, Dr. Joseph Barcroft, of Cambridge, England, will address the section on "Foetal Respiration." On Wednesday afternoon Section F will meet with the American Society of Naturalists and Section O in a symposium on "Heredity" (see announcement of American Society of Naturalists). On Thursday morning Section F, the Entomological Society of America and the American Association of Economic Entomologists will meet to hear a lecture by Dr. R. J. Tillyard, of Australia, on "The Evolution of the Insect." The lecture will be followed by a luncheon for members of both societies of entomologists. On Thursday afternoon Section F will meet with the Ecological Society of America in a symposium on "Life in Deep Water" (see announcement of the Ecological

Society of America). On Friday evening the two entomological societies will hold a dinner for members at the Chicago Women's Club. It is hoped that Dr. Royal N. Chapman, of the University of Hawaii, will give an address on some phase of insect life in Honolulu.

*G—Botany*

G–1. Section G of the Association. June 20–22.
*Vice-president*, Karl M. Wiegand; *Secretary*, Sam F. Trelease.

G–2. Botanical Society of America. June 20–22.
*President*, George J. Peirce; *Secretary*, Loren C. Petry.

G–3. American Phytopathological Society. June 20–22.
*President*, F. D. Heald; *Secretary*, F. C. Meier.

G–4. American Society of Plant Physiologists.
*President*, W. E. Tottingham; *Secretary*, W. A. Gardner.

On Tuesday morning, June 20, Sections G and O, the Botanical Society of America, the Ecological Society of America, the American Society of Plant Physiologists and the American Society of Agronomy will hold a joint session. Professor Ludwig Diels, of the University of Berlin, will give an address on "Taxonomy of the Angiosperms"; Sir Daniel Hall, of England, on "Does the Introduction of Wild Plants to Cultivation Induce Variation?" and Professor C. E. Allen, of the University of Wisconsin, on "Polyploidy in the Hepaticae." On Tuesday afternoon the same societies will visit the laboratory and greenhouses of the University of Chicago. For Wednesday is planned an all-day field trip to Warren Forest and Dune Reservation, Michigan. In the morning Sections G and O, the American Society of Agronomy, the American Society of Plant Physiologists and the American Phytopathological Society will hold a meeting devoted to progress in plant pathology during the century. Dr. Jean Dufrénoy, of Brice, France, will present a paper on "Local Immunity in the Plant Cell"; Dr. Neil Stevens, of the U. S. Department of Agriculture, on "The Dark Ages in Plant Pathology, 1832–1872"; Dr. J. C. Arthur, of Purdue University, will speak on "My Memories of Plant Pathologists, 1872–1933." In the afternoon the same societies, under the leadership of Dr. G. B. Ramsey, of the U. S. Department of Agriculture, will take a trip to South Water Markets to study markets pathology problems. For Thursday the Botanical Society of America has planned an all-day field trip to Wychwood, Lake Geneva, Wisconsin, which will be of interest to ecologists. In the morning Sections G and O, the American Phytopathological Society and the American Society of Agronomy will hold a joint session, with Dr. J. C. Arthur presiding. Dr. Otto Appel, of Berlin, will speak. Dr. H. H. Whetzel, of Cornell University, will present a paper on "A Century of Research in Plant Pathology," and Dr. I. E. Melhus, of the Iowa State College, on "A Century of Plant Disease Control." The American Society of Plant Physiologists will hold a symposium on "Radiation and Plant Growth." In the afternoon Sections G and O, the American Society of Agronomy and the American Phytopathological Society will accompany Dr. H. W. Anderson, of the University of Illinois, to the Cook County Experimental Farm to study truck crop diseases.

*F and G—Zoology and Botany*

FG–1 American Society of Naturalists. June 20.
*President*, R. A. Gortner; *Secretary*, E. W. Lindstrom.

FG–2. Ecological Society of America. June 20–23.
*President*, George E. Nichols; *Secretary*, Raymond Kienholz.

FG–3. American Microscopical Society. June 23.
*President*, M. J. Elrod; *Secretary*, James E. Ackert.

FG–4. Phi Sigma Biological Research Society. June 19–21.
*Chancellor*, Paul B. Sears; *Secretary*, A. I. Ortenburger.

On Monday, Tuesday and Wednesday mornings the Phi Sigma Biological Research Society will hold business meetings. Sessions for presentation of contributed papers will be held on Monday and Tuesday afternoons. The annual banquet will be given on Monday evening. On Tuesday morning, June 20, the Ecological Society will meet jointly with Sections G and O, the Botanical Society of America and the American Society of Agronomy (see announcement of Section G). In the afternoon the same societies will make a trip to the greenhouses of the University of Chicago. In the evening there will be an informal dinner for botanists and ecologists at Ida Noyes Hall, at which Professor Ludwig Diels, of Berlin, will speak on "Plant Geography with Reference to the Pacific Flora." The Ecological Society of America and the Botanical Society of America have arranged an all-day field trip for Wednesday to Michigan dunes and Beach Maple Forest, which will be primarily plant ecology, but also animal ecology. On Wednesday afternoon the American Society of Naturalists, with Sections F and O and the American Society of Agronomy participating, has arranged a symposium on "Heredity." Professor F. R. Lillie, of the University of Chicago, will preside. Professor Richard Goldschmidt, director of the Institute of Experimental Biology of Berlin, will talk on "The Influence of the Cytoplasm on Gene-Controlled Heredity." Professor Sewall Wright, of the University of Chicago, will speak on "Physiological and Evolutionary Theories of

Dominance." The Botanical Society of America has arranged an all-day field trip to Wychwood, Lake Geneva, Wisconsin, which will be of interest to ecologists. On Thursday afternoon the Ecological Society, with Section F participating, has arranged a symposium on "Life in Deep Water." Professor August Krogh, of the University of Copenhagen, Denmark, will speak on "Energetics in Great Depths of the Ocean," which will be followed by papers by Professor C. Juday, of the University of Wisconsin, on "The Centrifuge Plankton Content of the Water"; Dr. E. A. Birge, of the University of Wisconsin, on "The Non-Centrifugable Organic Content of the Water"; Professor A. S. Pearse, of Duke University, on "The Ecology of Deep Water Animals"; Dr. P. S. Galtsoff, on "The Biochemistry of the Invertebrata of the Sea." Dr. V. E. Shelford, of the University of Illinois, will lead the discussion. On Friday the Ecological Society of America will take an all-day field trip to Indiana Dunes, primarily for animal ecology.

### *H—Anthropology*

H-1. Section H of the Association. June 22–24. *Vice-president,* T. W. Todd; *Secretary,* W. M. Krogman.

H-2. American Anthropological Association. *President,* F. C. Cole; *Secretary,* J. M. Cooper.

On Thursday morning Section H and the American Anthropological Association will hold a meeting devoted to the subject of ethnology. The following men will speak: Dr. B. Laufer, of the Field Museum of Natural History, on "The Domestication of Animals"; Dr. M. J. Herskovits, of the Northwestern University, on "The American Negro: a Physical, Cultural and Historical Problem"; Dr. A. R. Radcliffe-Brown, of the University of Chicago, on "Studies in Social Organization"; Professor R. Redfield, of the University of Chicago, on "The Maya Indian: a Study in Acculturation." Thursday afternoon will be devoted to visiting anthropological exhibits of A Century of Progress. On Friday morning will be held a symposium on "Archeological Surveys." Dr. A. T. Olmstead, of the University of Chicago, will speak on "Historical and Archeological Method in the Near East." The following papers will be presented: "Archeological Surveys—National Scope," by Dr. Carl Guthe, of the University of Michigan; "Pictorial Survey of the Mississippi Valley," by Mr. Thorne Deuel, of the University of Chicago; "Archeological Survey of Southern Illinois," by Professor Arthur Kelley, of the University of Illinois. At the Friday afternoon session Dr. E. A. Speiser, of the University of Pennsylvania, will speak on "The Ethnic Background of the Early Civilization of the Near East"; Professor Leland W. Parr, of the George Washington University, on "Physiological Approaches to the Study of Anthropology with Special Reference to the Near East"; Mr. Henry Field, of the Field Museum of Natural History, on "Ancient and Modern Inhabitants of Central Mesopotamia"; and Dr. W. M. Krogman, of Western Reserve University, on "Cranial Types of Alishar Huyuk." This meeting will be followed by a special inspection of the new Hall of the Races of Mankind and Hall of the Stone Ages of the Old World at the Field Museum of Natural History. On Friday evening the association will hold a general session on the subject of "Anthropology." The Saturday morning session will be devoted to physical anthropology. Professor C. U. A. Kappers will speak on "Racial Differences in the Human Brain"; Dr. T. Wingate Todd, of Western Reserve University, on "The Brain in Childhood"; Drs. W. H. F. Addison and Henry H. Donaldson, of the Wistar Institute of Biology, Philadelphia, on "The Area of the Sunken Cerebral Cortex as Determined from the Length and Depth of Selected Sulci, in Three Classes of Human Brains: Scholars, Hospital Whites, Hospital Negroes." Professor C. J. Herrick, of the University of Chicago, will lead a general discussion on "The Human Brain."

### *I—Psychology*

I-1. Section I of the Association. June 20–24. *Vice-president,* Walter R. Miles; *Secretary,* John E. Anderson.

For Tuesday morning Section F has arranged a symposium on "Physical and Chemical Changes in Nerve during Activity," which the psychologists will find of interest. On Tuesday afternoon Section I will hold a symposium on "Character," in which will be presented a paper by Professor Emilio Mira, of Barcelona. Professor Mandel Sherman, of the University of Chicago, and several others will also participate. On Wednesday morning there will be a symposium on "New Conceptions of Intelligence." Professor Charles E. Spearman, of London, will speak on "New Conceptions and Test of Intelligence." Following the symposium, Professor Henri Pieron, of the Sorbonne, will give an address on "Sensorial Basis of Knowledge." On Thursday morning a symposium has been arranged on "Reaction Time," in which Professor Henri Pieron will speak. Professor Walter R. Miles, of Yale University, and several others will also participate. At the close of the symposium Professor Emilio Mira will give an address on "New Conceptions of Moral Behavior." For Friday morning a symposium is arranged on Gestalt, which will be discussed by Professor Wolfgang Koehler, of Berlin. Professor Raymond H. Wheeler, of the University of

Kansas, and several others will participate. It is hoped that a symposium on "Clinical Psychology" will be held on Saturday morning. On Saturday evening there will be a general session of the association, with an address by Professor Charles E. Spearman, on "Recent Advances in Our Knowledge of Human Personality."

*K—Social and Economic Sciences*

K-1. Section K of the Association. June 27–30. *Vice-president,* Wesley C. Mitchell; *Secretary,* James Ford.

K-2. American Statistical Association. June 26–29. *President,* Irving Fisher; *Secretary,* W. I. King.

K-3. American Sociological Society. June 26–29. *President,* L. L. Bernard; *Secretary,* L. Wirth.

K-4. Econometric Society. *President,* Irving Fisher; *Secretary,* Charles F. Roos.

On Tuesday evening, June 27, Section K has planned a program devoted to social insurance. Professor Wm. Oualid, of the University of Rome, and Professor G. A. Bagge, of the Social Science Institute of Sweden, will speak. On Wednesday morning, June 28, Section K and the Econometric Society are meeting in joint session with Section O on "Elasticity of Demand for Agricultural Products" (see announcement of Section O). A program of Section K on Wednesday evening will be centered around "Social Trends." The speakers will be Professor W. F. Ogburn and Professor Chas. E. Merriam, of the University of Chicago. On Wednesday or Thursday the Econometric Society will hold a meeting on "Recent Developments in Business Cycle Theory." Section K has arranged the program for the general session of the association on Thursday evening, with Professor Henry Clay as speaker. On Friday afternoon the Econometric Society will meet with the American Society for Testing Materials for a program on "Theoretical Economics in Engineering." Professor Irving Fisher, of Yale University, will preside. Dr. S. Karrer, of the Consolidated Gas, Electric Light and Power Company of Baltimore, will speak on "Economics in the Program of Industrial Research" with discussion by Dr. L. O. Grondahl, of the Union Switch and Signal Company; Dr. C. F. Roos, secretary of the Econometric Society, will speak on "Contributions of the Mathematician to Economics," with discussion by Professor H. Schultz, of the University of Chicago. Professor H. Hotelling, of Columbia University, will speak on "Contributions of the Theoretical Statistician to Economics," with discussion by Dr. R. W. Burgess, of the Western Electric Company. Dean Kimball, of Cornell University, will speak on "The Engineering Economist of the Future." On Friday evening the same societies will meet for a program on "Some Fundamental Problems of Mutual Interest to Scientific Economists and Engineers." Dean A. A. Potter, of Purdue University, president of the American Society of Mechanical Engineers, will preside. Professor Jos. Schumpeter, of Harvard University, will give a discussion "From the View-point of the Scientific Economist"; Dr. F. B. Jewett, vice-president of the American Telephone and Telegraph Company, "From the View-point of the Engineer," and Dr. A. P. Fleming, of the Metropolitan Vickers Electrical Company, of Manchester, England, on "The Internationalization of Scientific Knowledge as a Factor in World Economic Recovery." The American Sociological Society and the Society for Social Research will hold round table discussions on the following subjects: "The Family," L. Guy Brown, of Ohio Wesleyan University, chairman; "Crime; The Community," R. D. McKenzie, chairman; "Prediction and Forecasting," S. A. Stouffer, of the University of Wisconsin, chairman: "Minimum Standards of Training in Research Techniques," W. C. Reckless, of Vanderbilt University, chairman; "Graphic Presentation," Howard W. Green, of the Cleveland Health Council, chairman; "Experimental Social Psychology"; "Collective Behavior in the Depression," Harold D. Lasswell, of the University of Chicago, chairman; "Rural Sociology." Each round table will meet one or two forenoons of the days from June 26 to 29.

*L—Historical and Philological Sciences*

L-1. Section L of the Association. June 26. *Vice-president,* Waldo G. Leland; *Secretary,* Joseph Mayer.

L-2. The History of Science Society. June 26. *President,* J. Playfair McMurrich; *Secretary,* F. E. Brasch.

On Monday evening, June 26, Section L has arranged a symposium on "Nationalism." Professor Charles A. Beard, president of the American Historical Association, will present a paper on "Nationalism in American History." Professor Bernadotte Schmitt, of the University of Chicago, will also speak. It is hoped that one or more of the foreign guests will take part.

*M—Engineering*

*(From N. H. Heck and C. E. Davis)*

The program of Section M is an integral part of a coordinated program of nearly a score of engineering societies meeting in Chicago during the week of June 26. Sessions of the engineering societies will start on Monday morning, June 26, and continue through Friday, Wednesday, however, being set aside for certain joint functions. The outstanding features of the week include a number of addresses by distinguished engineers and scientists. On Tuesday afternoon at half past three Dr. Herbert J. Gough, of England, will present the Edgar Marburg Lecture under the auspices of the American Society for Testing Materials. Dr. Gough's subject has been selected as "Crystalline Structure in Relation to Failure of Metals, Especially by Fatigue." On Tuesday evening, June 27, under the auspices of Section M, Dr. A. P. M. Fleming, of England, will discuss "The Industrial Development of the Century." Outstanding engineers representing the various engineering societies will contribute to the discussion.

The joint functions of Wednesday will include the award of the Guggenheim Medal to Juan de la Cierva, inventor of the autogiro. The ceremony will take place at Soldiers Field, where Mr. Cierva will arrive in an autogiro and be conducted to the platform where the medal will be awarded. The rest of the day will be spent in a visit to the various engineering and scientific features of the exposition. In the evening there will be a joint dinner at the Stevens Hotel with an outstanding national figure as speaker.

On Thursday there will be a joint engineering luncheon under the auspices of the American Society of Military Engineers in honor of General Lytle Brown, chief of the Corps of Engineers. On Thursday evening a boat trip on the lake will give an excellent opportunity to enjoy the spectacular lighting effects of the exposition.

On Friday afternoon and evening there will be sessions under the auspices of the Econometric Society, participated in by the American Society of Mechanical Engineers, the American Institute of Electrical Engineers and the American Society for Testing Materials, which will be devoted to some fundamental problems of mutual interest to scientific economists and engineers. The speakers will be Dr. A. P. M. Fleming, of England, Dr. F. B. Jewett, Dean Dexter S. Kimball and others.

The Society for the Promotion of Engineering Education will celebrate its fortieth anniversary in the same general locale of its origin, in 1893, as the society was founded on the occasion of a previous fair. The program will be devoted largely to a résumé of the progress in engineering education during the life of the society.

Other features of interest include a joint dinner of the boards of direction of the four major engineering societies and a dinner of the National Council of State Boards of Engineering Examiners.

The engineering sessions are planned to cover the entire field of engineering. Approximately four hundred papers will be presented at some two hundred sessions during the week.

### *N—Medical Sciences*

N-1. Section N of the Association. June 19–22. *Vice-president,* C. R. Stockard; *Secretary,* Walter M. Simpson.

On Monday morning, June 19, Section N will meet in a joint session with Section C (see announcement of Section C). On Tuesday morning Section N will hold a joint meeting with Section F (see announcement of Section F). On Tuesday evening at eight o'clock a general session of the association is to be held under the auspices of Section N, commemorating "The Century of Progress in Medicine." On Wednesday morning, June 21, a symposium on "Pathological Physiology" will be held with the following speakers: Dr. Arthur L. Tatum, of the University of Wisconsin, on "Morphine Addiction and Morphine Tolerance"; Dr. C. H. Best, of the University of Toronto, on "Fatty Changes in the Liver of Normal and Diabetic Animals"; Dr. Maurice B. Strauss, of the Thorndike Memorial Laboratory, on "The Etiology of Pernicious Anemia and the Related Macrocytic Anemias"; Dr. William H. Park, of the Department of Health, New York City, on "BCG Vaccination." Madame Curie may also address this meeting. On Thursday morning, June 22, a surgical-endocrinological symposium will be held. Dr. George Crile, of the Cleveland Clinic, will give an address on "A Century of Progress in Surgery—Anesthesia, Antisepsis and Asepsis, Shock, and Careful Handling of Tissues." Dr. Max Ballin, of Detroit, will speak on "Clinical Recognition and Surgical Treatment of Parathyroidism"; Dr. Percival Bailey, of the University of Chicago, will discuss "Surgical Control of Hypophyseal Disorders"; Dr. John de J. Pemberton, of the Mayo Clinic, will speak on "Recent Developments in the Clinical Recognition and Surgical Management of Hyperfunction of the Thyroid Gland." Dr. Evarts Graham, of the Washington University School of Medicine, will speak on "Clinical Recognition and Surgical Treatment of Hypoglycemia Produced by Tumors of the Islets of Langerhans," with discussion by Professor Robert R. Bensley, of the University of Chicago.

### *O—Agriculture*

O-1. Section O of the Association. June 20–28. *Vice-president,* A. R. Mann; *Secretary,* P. E. Brown.

O-2. American Society of Agronomy. June 20–28. *President,* P. E. Brown; *Secretary,* F. B. Smith.

On Tuesday morning Section O and the American Society of Agronomy will hold a joint session with Section G (see announcement of Section G). In the afternoon Section O and the American Society of

Agronomy, with Section G, will visit the greenhouses and laboratory of the University of Chicago. In the evening Section O and the American Society of Agronomy will attend the dinner for botanists and ecologists. On Wednesday and Thursday mornings Section O and the American Society of Agronomy will meet with Section G, the American Phytopathological Society and the American Society of Plant Physiologists for programs on progress in plant pathology during the century (see announcement of Section G). On Wednesday afternoon Section O and the American Society of Agronomy will meet in joint session with Section F and the American Society of Naturalists in a symposium on Heredity (see announcement of American Society of Naturalists). On Wednesday evening Section O will hold a dinner at which Sir Daniel Hall, of England, will speak on "Polyploidy and the Special Question in the Genus Tulipa," and Professor Jean Dufrénoy, of Brice, France, on "Death—The Change of Living Substance within the Cell." On Wednesday morning, June 28, Section O and the American Society of Agronomy will hold a joint session with Section K and the Econometric Society of America on "Elasticity of Demand for Agricultural Products," which will be discussed by Sir Daniel Hall, of England. It is hoped that Professor G. F. Warren, of Cornell University, Mr. Mordecai Ezekiel and Mr. E. J. Working, of the U. S. Department of Agriculture, will also speak.

*Q—Education*

Q-1. Section Q of the Association. June 29–30.
*Vice-president,* Walter F. Dearborn; *Secretary,* William S. Gray.

Q-2. National Society for the Study of Education. June 29–30.
*President,* M. E. Haggerty; *Secretary,* Guy M. Whipple.

Section Q will hold a joint meeting with the National Society for the Study of Education, the Department of Supervisors and Directors of Instruction and the American Educational Research Association. On Thursday afternoon Section Q and affiliated societies will hold a session on "Recent Advances in the Study of Components of Mental Ability." Professor Frank N. Freeman will preside. Dr. Charles Spearman, of the University of London, will report on recent experiments in factor analysis. Dr. Karl Holzinger, of the University of Chicago, will discuss the general theory of factor analysis and Professor Louis L. Thurstone will lead the discussion. A program for Friday morning is being organized around "The Function, Value and Future of Educational Research." Professor Walter S. Monroe, of the University of Illinois, will preside. This will be discussed with reference to research activities (a) in public school systems, by Dr. W. W. Theisen, assistant superintendent of schools, Milwaukee, Wisconsin; (b) in colleges and universities, by Dr. V. A. C. Henmon, of the University of Wisconsin; (c) in departments of education, by Professor Edgar Blake, of Ohio State University. "Dependability and Value of Survey Types of Investigation" will be discussed by Dr. Harl Douglass, of the University of Minnesota. On Friday afternoon there will be a session on "Essentials of an Education," Professor Ernest Horn, presiding. The discussion will be introduced by papers on "Maturation and Its Relation to Instruction." Dr. Charles H. Judd, of the University of Chicago, will speak on "The Application of Maturation to School Organization and Teaching," and Professor C. R. Griffith, of the University of Illinois, will speak on "The Psychology of Maturation." The remainder of the program will consider the essentials of an education in contemporary life at (a) the elementary school level, by Miss Bess Goodykoontz, of the U. S. Office of Education; (b) the secondary school level, by Dr. A. K. Loomis, of the University of Chicago, and (c) the college level, by Vice-president Clarence S. Yoakum, of the University of Michigan. A program is being organized for Friday evening on "Education for a Democracy." Dr. Walter F. Dearborn will preside. Miss Jane Addams, of Hull House, and President Robert M. Hutchins, of the University of Chicago, will speak.

# THE VALUE OF SCIENTIFIC RESEARCH TO AGRICULTURE[1]

By Secretary HENRY A. WALLACE
U. S. DEPARTMENT OF AGRICULTURE

In this series of radio broadcasts it is the custom, as I understand it, for each Cabinet officer to do a little boasting about his own department. I am more than willing to do my share of that on behalf of the Department of Agriculture; but in my remarks to-night I hope not only to discuss the past of this department, but also to consider its future.

Necessarily, that involves the new farm bill. By

[1] Address over a national radio network of the N.B.C. on May 1.

to-night I had hoped to be able to talk in some detail about it, but since the bill has not yet become law, detailed discussion will have to wait. In lieu of that, let me discuss the view that the new bill is the logical next step in the work of the Department of Agriculture in particular, and of all government in general.

In order properly to appraise the work of this far-flung department of the Federal Government, suppose we cut through a tedious underbrush of official and legal language, and set forth, in plain words, what the Department of Agriculture was established to do.

If you have thought about mankind's struggle through the ages to build an orderly society, you will agree that there have been two primary problems: first, to produce enough food and fiber to feed and clothe us all; second, to divide what we produce as equitably as possible.

We have always had to be concerned with production. Whatever else man can do without, he can not live without food. And that was no simple problem back in the days when men lived in tribes in the forests, and when the food supply depended upon a man's skill with crude weapons. When the first faint stirrings of commerce and industry drew men to live in larger groups in cities, the problem of a food supply became even more acute. Those who lived in the ancient cities could not grow their own food and fiber. Those who remained on the farm had the new job of growing enough not only for themselves, but for other families in nearby cities. Thus the dependence of the city dweller upon the farmer is overwhelmingly real. It is the key-log in this structure we call modern civilization.

And there were times when the structure was in danger of collapse, or indeed did collapse, because the key-log weakened and gave way. By reason of abnormal seasons, drought or flood, famines came and wrecked whole segments of human society. It was customary to blame those catastrophes on nature. Man, weak creature, was powerless if nature chose to starve him or drown him or otherwise maltreat him.

Somewhere back in the ages, a few individuals, more daring, more imaginative than the rest, began to wonder whether that was true. They reasoned that though nature could not be ignored, it could be modified. Man began doing that when he learned how to make fire by rubbing sticks together. We have been modifying the behavior of nature ever since, to prevent famine, flood and other disasters, until, as Julian Huxley puts it, man has done more in five thousand years to alter the biological aspect of the planet than nature has done in five million years. By putting nature in harness, so far as possible, we have solved mankind's first great problem—the problem of producing enough food to go round. We have solved it too well, as a matter of fact, but I shall speak of that later.

When it is possible for the farmers of a nation to increase production 50 per cent., while crop acreage is increasing only 25 per cent., we know that science has been at work. That is exactly what has happened in the United States during the past 30 years. In large part it is a result of the scientific work of the United States Department of Agriculture and the cooperating state institutions.

It was for the purpose of putting science to work in agriculture that this Federal Department of Agriculture was established by act of Congress 71 years ago. Washington, Jefferson and Franklin saw the need for it even back in their day. The department was created primarily for scientific research, its main job always has been a research job, and I hope research will always remain a principal duty.

Of course it is not enough to discover facts: a public institution has also the obligation to see that the facts are made available to all who can profit by them.

When a plant breeder in the department develops a variety of wheat that is highly resistant to rust, the job of the department has not ended with that discovery. The new variety has to be tried out in various regions, in the field. Next, the results of those trials have to be made known to wheat growers. That involves publications, both technical and popular, and articles for the press, and radio broadcasting. Then the seed of the new variety has to be made available to farmers. The county extension agent may step into the picture at this point, and suggest that the interested wheat grower sow some of the new seed in a test plot, alongside some of the seed he and his neighbors have been using in the past. And when the old and the new varieties of wheat are up and are harvested, let the neighbors for miles around come in to compare them, and decide whether or not the new variety is better than the old and worth investing in.

That is a thumbnail sketch of the way science is applied to agriculture in this country, and it portrays a system that is the envy of many another nation. Sir Horace Plunkett, Ireland's great authority on agriculture, in 1928 was moved to describe the Department of Agriculture as "the most widely useful department in the world." I am inclined to agree, and I only hope that its future will be as brilliantly successful as its past.

Whether he knows it or not, every farmer in the United States is farming differently to-day—and better—because of the scientific discoveries resulting from state and federal appropriations. The average hour of man labor and the average acre of land is undoubtedly 20 to 30 per cent. more productive to-day because of this scientific work. From the fundamental point of view—that of supplying the food and fiber needed by our modern civilization—the millions of dollars spent by state and federal agencies during the past generation have been abundantly worth while.

I appreciate that it is often difficult for the layman to see any earthly use in many of the things that scientists do and talk about doing. Of what value is it to you and to me, for instance, for a man to spend his time trying to discover the workings of nature? How can a man—we are inclined to say—do anything useful unless he works directly with the things that we all can touch and see, that we know have practical utility?

Well, when confronted by questions like that, I think of men like Faraday and Mendel and some of the scientists in the employ of the Federal Government. About a hundred years ago in England Michael Faraday was what we might call an experimental philosopher. He never concerned himself with the invention of machines. His sole aim was to learn something about the workings of nature. He discovered the principle of electromagnetic induction, and if you remember your high-school science, you will recall that without that discovery, we would to-day have no means of putting electrical energy to work for us. Without Faraday, the amazing inventions of Edison and Marconi would not have been possible, and your radio and your electric lights would not exist.

And Mendel, that cloistered Moravian monk who whiled away the hours studying plants and experimenting with the cross-breeding of varieties of garden peas—of what earthly use was all that? He did it because it interested him. But was it of any use to the rest of us? I can assure you that it was, for the principles he discovered have been employed by the plant breeders of to-day in developing more productive varieties of every plant that feeds and clothes you. Scientists like Mendel and Faraday were working in what we call pure science. They were trying to discover nature's fundamental secrets, but without thought of any practical application of their discoveries. Had some overzealous administrator tried to restrict their curiosity to some specific object, or the immediate solution of some highly practical problem, we would have been deprived, in all probability, of their great discoveries.

It falls upon another group of scientists to apply these basic principles to the pressing problems of the world and turn them to practical account. Thus most of the scientific research in government departments is applied science. The surprising thing, however, is that even in the field of applied science far-reaching discoveries are made, often as a by-product of the immediate task.

One of the most famous examples was the discovery by scientists in the Department of Agriculture some forty years ago, that a microorganism found in the blood of cattle is the cause of splenetic fever, and that the disease is transmitted by the cattle tick.

During the years 1888 to 1893, four men spent most of their time trying to make that discovery. Splenetic fever had become a costly disease of cattle throughout the South. Home-made remedies, treatment by skilled veterinarians, alike proved futile. The disease was costing the live-stock industry, and ultimately the consumer of meat, many millions of dollars.

The four Department of Agricuture scientists, in the employ of the government because they wanted to pursue scientific research without interruption, and at salaries sadly out of line with their worth to the nation—these men kept doggedly on the job despite all sorts of obstacles and disappointments. The joy of achievement was their chief reward. And their achievement proved to be of lasting benefit not only to the live-stock industry, but to all mankind, for their research was the first demonstration that a microbial disease can be transmitted exclusively by an insect host or carrier.

From that came the knowledge, at the hands of other scientists, that yellow fever, malaria, sleeping sickness and other maladies are similarly transmitted. From that flowed the successful control of yellow fever, for instance, which in turn made possible the building of the Panama Canal. So it can truthfully be said that the success of four Department of Agriculture scientists in discovering the cause of a cattle disease was a first step in the construction of the Panama Canal.

These scientists—by name Theobald Smith, Curtice, Kilgore and Salmon—of course had no idea of the far-reaching consequences of their discovery. They were intent on finding the cause of a cattle disease, not in discovering a fundamental principle in medicine. But that happens often in scientific research.

And at other times, a scientist may fail to solve one problem, only to solve another unexpectedly. Not long ago some chemists in the Department of Agriculture were examining molds—fungous growths, that is—to find one that would produce tartaric acid. Patiently they tested one after another, until they had exhausted the possibilities of 149 different molds. Finally the 150th rewarded their long search with success—but not the success they were expecting. Instead of producing tartaric acid, the 150th mold unexpectedly produced gluconic acid. This is now used in making calcium gluconate, the only calcium salt that can be injected between the muscles, without causing abscesses, in treating certain human diseases. This salt used to cost $150 a pound. As a result of this research, it may now be had for 50 cents a pound.

Much of the scientific work of the department, however, calls for more than the ordinary equipment of a scientist. I am thinking of the plant explorers, the men who cut their way through treacherous jungles, or press on across the forbidding deserts of Mongolia in search of plants that we need here at home. Whenever you eat bread made from durum wheat, or enjoy a choice steak or pork chops from cattle or hogs fed on alfalfa and soybeans, or sample a package of dates or a crate of navel oranges from California or the new Satsuma oranges from Florida —whenever you enjoy any of these things, you are reaping the benefit of the work done by a handful of explorers employed by the Department of Agriculture.

If you live in the Gulf Coast region, you probably are familiar with the rise of a new industry down there, the growing of tung oil trees. About 25 years ago tung oil revolutionized the manufacture of varnish, but the oil had to be imported from China. Back in 1905 David Fairchild, plant explorer of the Department of Agriculture, brought the first seeds of the tung trees to the United States from the Yangtze Valley of China. Our plant industry men discovered, after a good deal of experimentation, that the trees do well in the Gulf Coast region, and the new industry is to-day firmly established there.

Not every trip of a plant explorer, of course, is so productive. Every trip has its dangers and its adventures, but frequently the results are slight. Yet the introduction of a navel orange or a useful variety of soybeans or a hardy wheat atones for many unsuccessful trips.

In one way or another, I have said, every farmer in the United States is farming differently to-day because of the scientific discoveries resulting from state and federal appropriations. To be specific and as up-to-date as possible, suppose we run down the list of research achievements reported by one bureau of the Department of Agriculture for the past year. Before me is a summarized report for the Bureau of Plant Industry, and among their accomplishments I find these items:

Established the superiority of five new hybrid lines of corn in Iowa tests; released, for the use of growers, two new lines of hybrid sweet corn that will be resistant to bacterial wilt; released, for the use of growers, a new wilt-resistant variety of tomato, known as the Pritchard; introduced a new blackberry variety, the Brainerd, especially adapted for the West and South, and also introduced three improved varieties of strawberry; developed new root-stocks for Satsuma oranges, and found new disease-resistant stocks for California grape vineyards; introduced a new sugar beet, U. S. No. 1, that is resistant to the costly curly-top disease, and that also greatly outyields older varieties; tested some promising new sugar-cane seedlings, crosses of American and New Guinea varieties; reported distinct progress in breeding alfalfa that will be immune to bacterial wilt; developed a new variety of Egyptian cotton in Arizona.

As another part of its job, this bureau investigates the storing, handling and processing of foods. For the year under report the bureau scientists discovered, among other things, that putting apples in cold storage immediately after picking almost completely prevents soft scald; that adding sulfur dioxide to the sawdust packing of grapes retards the development of mold; and that treating fruits with carbon dioxide before shipment is as effective as pre-cooling in preventing spoilage.

That is a partial report of the research accomplishments of one bureau. It gives point to the statement that research can stabilize crop production and eliminate or reduce those hazards—of disease, of climate, even of soil—which make agricultural production uncertain. For it remains true that though drouth or disease or insect pests may raise the price of a crop by reducing the supply, such higher prices are cold comfort to the particular farmer whose cotton has been destroyed by the boll weevil or whose wheat has been hit by rust. I have, I think, a proper scientific respect for insects and diseases, but I question whether we ought to leave it up to them to determine the size of our crops and the level of our incomes. Nor can I forget that every year, according to Dr. L. O. Howard, the damage wrought by insects nullifies the labor of a million men.

If time and your patience permitted, it would be possible to cite instances to show how research has affected all our major farm crops and classes of live stock, how the patience, the skill and the informed imagination of scientists employed by the Department of Agriculture have altered the agricultural map of this country and modified the farm practises of every farmer in the land. Many farmers are not aware of this, for the results of research reach the individual farm by an intricate, devious path, but they get there just the same.

If you will agree with me on that, I suspect you are at the same moment questioning whether this research has proved to be an unmixed blessing. For science and invention, you will say, have not only made it possible for us to produce enough to go around: they have made it possible for us to pile up towering surpluses, which in turn seem capable of bringing our whole economic system crashing down around our ears.

We can not deny that, when scientists in the Department of Agriculture develop a variety of wheat that produces five bushels more per acre than the variety commonly grown, one result may be, and often is, too much wheat. When our modern knowledge of nutrition enables one bushel of corn to go as far as two bushels did in the pioneer days in feeding live stock, one result may be too much pork and lard.

Of late years the Department of Agriculture and the colleges have been aware of the problem. They have tried to meet it by helping the individual farmer adjust his own production to changing market needs. They have hoped that advice and complete information on supply and demand would suffice.

Where they have been remiss, in my judgment, is in declining to face the fact that the individual farmer can not adjust his production intelligently, unless he knows, with some degree of certainty, that his neighbors will do likewise. And it is to face that fact realistically that the new farm bill has been drafted. The essence of it is collective action, by all the producers, to accommodate their production to the market that actually exists.

Our expenditures for science, our efforts at increasing productive efficiency have in no sense been unwise. Certainly no thoughtful person could approve the abandonment of scientific research, or the relegation of our machines to the ash-heap. To do that would be like abandoning the use of automobiles because we have automobile accidents. As a rule, the fault is not with the automobile, but with the driver.

It is not the fault of science that we have unused piles of wheat on Nebraska farms and tragic bread-lines in New York City at one and the same moment. Rather it is because we have refused to apply science to the development of social machinery, machinery that will regulate our economic system to the end that what we produce can be equitably divided.

I am not one to ask for less efficiency. I want more, and I know that we can get far more. But I want the efficiency to be controlled in such a way that it does more good than harm. I want to see the farmers of the South grow 300 pounds of cotton per acre instead of 150 pounds, and the farmers of the North 50 bushels of corn per acre instead of 35 bushels. I want to see the average milk cow yield 400 pounds of butter fat per year instead of 200. And I see no reason why our hogs eventually should not produce 100 pounds of pork on the average from 6 bushels of corn, instead of from 9 bushels.

These things can all be done. The research now going on will make it possible, and will pave the way for countless new agricultural achievements as well.

Only the other day I learned that research now in progress indicates that crops grown in some regions of the nation have a higher nutritional value than do apparently similar crops grown in other areas. If further study bears this out, the consequences will certainly be far-reaching. We may have a new agricultural map a decade from now.

The research job, far from being done, is only well begun. We shall need new varieties of cereals and grasses to resist diseases better than those we now have. We shall have to keep cutting costs of production by increasing yields per acre. Methods of cultivation, like methods of feeding and managing live stock, must be subject to continuing investigation if we are to keep abreast of the continually changing economic world about us.

When our chemists, not long ago, discovered an economical method by which bagasse, a sugar cane waste, could be made into high-quality cellulose, suitable for rayon, we patted ourselves on the back for an achievement of considerable importance. But over in the Bureau of Chemistry and Soils is a small bottle of a brownish cellulose substance called lignin, which was derived from the corn plant after many years of experimentation. The chemist will tell you that lignin is one of the principal parts of woody plant tissues; that it can therefore be obtained in abundance; and that it may yield a startling new collection of products. Already he has discovered in lignin such compounds as phenol and creosol. Lignin may yet rank, in its rich potentialities, in its influence on disposing of farm wastes, with our major chemical discoveries.

No, the job of scientific research in agriculture is not over, nor will it ever be. But to-day we have a new job, a new field for experimenting—that of social control. Research to increase productive efficiency, to widen markets, must continue. Eliminate the less important research activities, in deference to the need for economy; get rid of the dead wood in our scientific organizations—but keep the men of science at the tasks which will always need doing. And add to the old job the one that has been begun so well, this new job of developing the machinery of social control.

Can we, do you suppose, become as efficient in our social experimenting as we have already proven ourselves in scientific experimenting? If this can be done, we can go ahead into one triumph after another in the scientific world. If it is not done, I fear for the future of our civilization.

The farm bill is an effort in the direction of such social inventiveness. In some ways, it is perhaps as crude as the first automobile. But I believe it is profoundly right in purpose, for it attempts a reconciliation between science and social justice; and I believe it can be made to work, if the rank and file of the people of the United States—the men who grow our food, the men who handle and distribute it, the men and women who consume it—the new machine will work if all these people are genuinely hungry to distribute the fruits of science in a just way.

For that is our great modern problem. Having conquered the fear of famine, with the aid of science, having been brought into an age of abundance, we now have to learn how to live with abundance. Sometimes I think it requires stronger characters, greater hearts and keener minds, to endure abundance than it takes to endure penury. Certainly it requires a new degree of tolerance among competing economic groups and a willingness to subordinate the will of the few to the welfare of the many.

Personally, I think the last twelve years have imprinted this lesson deeply on all of us. I think we are ready, now, to reach out towards a new order. I believe we are ready to attempt to plan our economic life in return for stability and security. If this is true, then we have reached a great moment in the history of mankind. We have determined to become the masters rather than the victims of destiny. We are daring to bring the economic interests of men under conscious human control.

We may make mistakes along the way; we may have difficulty in mastering all the intricacies of an economic system that is full of puzzling contradictions; but if we operate our new social machinery with the spirit of social justice in all our hearts, I believe that it will work.

# THE SIGNIFICANCE OF RECENT MEASUREMENTS OF COSMIC RAYS[1]

By Professor ARTHUR H. COMPTON
UNIVERSITY OF CHICAGO

THREE major methods of observing cosmic rays have been developed. By means of an ionization chamber filled with a gas such as argon under high pressure the cosmic rays can be measured in terms of the conductivity or ionization they produce in the gas. Thus it is found that at high altitudes in a balloon or on a mountain a much greater ionization is observed than at sea-level, while inside a deep tunnel, if the gas is shielded from gamma-rays, ionization is almost completely absent. The cloud expansion chamber, invented by C. T. R. Wilson, makes visible the paths of the ionizing particles associated with the cosmic rays, as they break into ions some of the air molecules through which they pass. Some of these particles seem to be the cosmic rays themselves, whereas others are secondary particles produced by the cosmic rays. Highly sensitive ion chambers, connected through amplifying tubes to electrical recorders, serve to count the cosmic rays as they pass through the chambers. These are known as "counting tubes." By arranging these tubes in pairs, so connected that they will record only when both are excited simultaneously, it is possible to study the direction from which the cosmic rays are coming.

With the help of such devices it has been found that a kind of ray exists which comes from high above the earth and is strongly but not completely absorbed as it passes through the earth's atmosphere. Believing that these rays have originated in the remote parts of space, they have been called cosmic rays. The heat that they bring to the earth is less than that of starlight. But they are the most penetrating rays with which we are acquainted.

Two types of theories have been suggested to account for the origin of these rays. The first type assumes the cosmic rays to be photons, or electromagnetic waves, like light or x-rays or the gamma-rays from radium, but of much shorter wave-length. If the rays are of this type, their observed penetrating power corresponds to the energy of rays that might be emitted by subatomic processes, such as the formation of hydrogen out of helium or the annihilation of hydrogen atoms. Dr. Robert A. Millikan has strongly defended the view that cosmic rays are emitted at the formation of heavy atomic nuclei from groups of lighter nuclei, and has made this a stage in the life cycle of matter in a continuous universe. Sir James Jeans has proposed the annihilation of hydrogen atoms as a source of the most penetrating cosmic rays, and sees this as one way in which the universe is running down.

The second class of theories supposes that cosmic rays are not photons, but electrically charged particles entering the earth's atmosphere from outer space. Dauvillier imagines that these particles are shot out from the sun by intense local electric fields. Swann suggests that they come from the changing magnetic field of sunspots on the hotter stars. But by far the most romantic and by no means the least plausible theory is that of Abbe Georges H. Lemaitre. He attributes them to a primeval explosion of the universe some thousands of millions of years ago, since which time the universe has been expanding, and certain atoms and pieces of atoms that have been flying about in space ever since constitute the cosmic rays which we now observe.

In order that a choice may be made among these theories, it is important that the nature of the cosmic rays be learned. Five methods of approaching this problem may be mentioned:

[1] Based on an address delivered at the dedication of the Eastman Research Laboratories of Physics and Chemistry, at the Massachusetts Institute of Technology, May 1, 1933.

(1) Observations with the cloud expansion chamber described above show that the ionization observed in air is due directly to high-speed particles. When a strong magnet is present these particles curve in both directions, indicating that some are positively and some negatively charged. Some of these particles are certainly secondary rays produced by more energetic primary rays, though certain ones have energies sufficient to carry them through the earth's atmosphere. These experiments thus do not tell us whether the primary cosmic ray is a photon or an electrified particle.

(2) Experiments with the coincidence counters described above, performed by Bothe and Kölhorster in Germany and Rossi in Italy, have shown that these coincidences are due to ionizing particles which are absorbed at substantially the same rate as the cosmic rays themselves. These experiments have been supplemented by recent ones by Johnson and Street which show that the pairs of ionizing particles that are frequently observed are produced by rays which are themselves ionizing particles. Since the only ionizing particles with which we are acquainted are electrically charged, these experiments point strongly toward the cosmic rays as electrically charged particles rather than photons.

(3) Opposed to this conclusion are some early experiments by Millikan and his collaborators which seemed to show no variation of the intensity of the cosmic rays with the position in the earth's magnetic field. Theories, due to Störmer and recently much more completely developed by Lemaitre and Manuel S. Vallarta at the Massachusetts Institute of Technology, have shown that unless they have energies much greater than is supposed, any electrified particles should have their paths bent by the earth's magnetic field, resulting in a diminished intensity near the equator as compared with that near the poles. During the past year a group of our associated expeditions have made measurements at stations widely distributed over the earth. Their combined data show precisely the kind of variation in intensity with latitude predicted by the theory, only the energy of the electrified particles is somewhat greater than had been supposed. More recent experiments by Clay and by Millikan's collaborators have confirmed this result. This indicates definitely that at least a part of the cosmic rays consists of electrified particles.

(4) At those latitudes where the deflection by the earth's magnetic field is sufficient to prevent part of the incoming electrified particles from reaching the earth, there should be a difference between the rays from the east and from the west. If the rays are positively charged, they should come mostly from the west; if negatively, mostly from the east. At these latitudes, numerous experiments have failed to show any appreciable difference. Our geographical distribution curves, however, indicated that as far south as Mexico such differences should appear. Accordingly, Alvarez, from the University of Chicago, and Johnson, from the Bartol Research Foundation, have been working independently in Mexico City during the past month, and have both reported a definite predominance of the cosmic rays from the west. This means that at least a considerable part of the cosmic rays consists of positively charged particles.

(5) The recent high altitude balloon flights have had as their chief objective the study of the ionization due to cosmic rays near the surface of the atmosphere. It can be shown that if the primary rays are photons, the observed ionization should reach a maximum with increasing altitude, and then fall toward zero as the surface of the atmosphere is approached. If, however, the primary cosmic rays are electrified particles, the observed ionization should approach a maximum at the top of the atmosphere. The highest measurements so far performed are those of Regener, whose balloon went to 17 miles above the earth, and his results seem rather definitely to support the electrified particle theory.

Thus every type of direct test that has been devised has indicated the presence of electrified particles in the cosmic rays. We can say definitely that positively charged particles constitute an important part of these rays. The possibility has not been excluded that photons may be present among these rays as they enter the earth's atmosphere; but as yet no direct evidence of such photons has appeared, and it appears probable that, if present, they play a minor rôle.

The experiments thus favor those theories which are based upon the assumption of cosmic rays as electrified particles rather than as photons. Of the electrified particle theories, those which attribute the rays to particles shot from the sun or stars, as Dauvillier and Swann have done, are somewhat difficult to reconcile with the positively charged character of the rays. For while negatively charged thermoelectrons might well be thus produced, the origin of positively charged rays is more difficult to account for. New information on this point may be anticipated if work now in progress shows whether these positively charged cosmic rays are protons or positrons.

In the meantime, all the data so far found fit satisfactorily with Lemaitre's bold "explosion" theory of the rays.

A rapidly growing aspect of the study of cosmic rays is their use as a tool for the investigation of the structure of the atomic nucleus. The most striking result of such experiments is Anderson's recently announced discovery of the positive electron, or "positron." Because of the tremendous energy of the individual cosmic ray, it is capable of producing nuclear disruptions much more violent than those resulting from the most powerful artificial sources. Thus a recent photograph by Blackett shows no less than twenty pieces presumably ejected from the nucleus of a single atom by the action of one cosmic ray. The energy of the particles flying from this burst is not less than several billion electron volts. It will be a long time before the laboratory will produce ten billion volt electrons. Until that time we may expect to find cosmic rays of unique value for studies of nuclear structure.

# OBITUARY

## WILLIAM HENRY HOLMES

WILLIAM HENRY HOLMES, anthropologist, geologist and artist, died April 20 at Royal Oak, Michigan, at the age of eighty-six years. Born near Cadiz, Ohio, on December 1, 1846, his parents Joseph and Mary Heberling Holmes, he received the schooling available in the forties, progressing till he graduated at the Hopedale Normal School. For several years he taught in the district and normal schools, until his preference for art prevailed over other interests.

Dr. Holmes entered into science by a fortuitous avenue which the ancients attributed to destiny or fortune. On a visit to Washington the youth was found in the Smithsonian Institution enjoying himself in drawing birds displayed in a case. One of the ornithologists happened by and saw the drawing, appreciated the evidences of his skill, and got him employment for work at the Institution. From that time on his pencil and brush were requisitioned for illustrations of the various reports. On that horizon Dr. Holmes viewed his future course in the development of his art. With this in view he later studied in Europe at several German schools. In the course of events he was drawn into the work of the U. S. Geological Survey and took the field in 1872 as artist under F. V. Hayden, becoming an assistant geologist in 1874. During this period he produced hundreds of drawings showing the physiographic features, of which those of the Grand Canyon of the Colorado are classics in geology. In charge of the survey of the San Juan region in Colorado, he stepped into a field that was to dominate his scientific life. This region, the homeland of the ancient Pueblo Indians, strewn with ruined pueblos and cliff dwellings, exerted its fascination to Dr. Holmes, and we find him in 1875 writing the first report on these archeological sites, his first contribution to anthropology. Many of these ruins he was the first white man to see, and he entered houses where the dust had not been disturbed for a millennium. Returning in 1889 to Washington he became connected with the Bureau of American Ethnology, pursuing researches on the geological history of man in America, of which subject he was the outstanding student. From 1894 to 1897 he was non-resident and resident professor of anthropic geology in the University of Chicago and curator of anthropology in the Field Museum. During this period he prosecuted an archeological survey of the ruined Maya cities of Yucatan, the report demonstrating his skill as an artist, architect and archeologist. Again returning to Washington, he became head curator of the Department of Anthropology of the U. S. National Museum, and for a few years he devoted his efforts to museum science, building this branch of the museum to an enviable state of excellence.

As a master of museum science Dr. Holmes was without rival. In the harmonious arranging of cases for exhibit he applied the laws of structure implanted in him. To questions near to museums of the time he brought a consummate taste and unerring judgment as to ways and means. The group cases illustrating the races of man were designed by him as pictures telling the story in the most artistic manner. These groups show he had the knack to present science in an instructive and pleasing setting. For these reasons the groups are favorably and widely known as climaxes of achievement in museum installation. In a multitude of objects in the National Museum his taste and near approach to perfection are evident. Mention should be made of the models of ancient temples of Yucatan as examples of this outstanding artistic ability.

In anthropology the branch in which Mr. Holmes was especially proficient was archeology. To this nascent branch he contributed much of the groundwork which has remained unshaken to this day. To his early work in the Southwest he added explorations of ancient works broadly over the whole United States. It remained to him to correlate much of the data secured by personal fieldwork and the work of others. Confining his work to America, he took the leadership in controverting the application of European terminology and sequences to this field, advancing a restricted view as to the antiquity of man in the Western Hemisphere. In the era of sometimes bitter controversy that marked the adolescence of anthropology, Holmes was always to the front with well-reasoned contributions serving to clear up the subjects in question.

The body of anthropological literature contributed by Holmes in extent seems alone a life work. The larger works appeared in the annuals of the bureau. Among these are: Stone Implements of the Potomac-Chesapeake Tidewater Province (15th ann.); Aboriginal Pottery of the Eastern United States (20th ann.); Handbook of American Antiquities. Part 1. Introduction. (Bull. B. A. E. no. 60). During his administration of the Bureau the Handbook of American Indians, Bulletin 30, was brought to completion and published.

Throughout his career he displayed a remarkable ability to grasp a subject at once or to see the implications of a problem as unerringly as his pencil followed the subtle outlines of his model. The driving force that was within Holmes never ceased its urge till near the close of his busy life. Whatever he undertook was carried forward under pressure of his indomitable will. This characteristic is observed in his youth when despite obstacles he trained himself in art.

Many honors came to Holmes during his busy life. He was a member of the National Academy of Sciences, president of the Washington Academy of Science and of the Cosmos Club. He was honorary member of the University of La Plata, Argentina, and prominent in Spanish-American conferences, meetings of the Americanists, and in many other movements. On his 70th birthday he was presented with a magnificent anniversary volume of anthropological essays by his friends and co-laborers.

WALTER HOUGH

# SCIENTIFIC EVENTS

## THE McDONALD OBSERVATORY

DR. OTTO STRUVE, director of the Yerkes Observatory of the University of Chicago, has announced that Mt. Locke, a 6,790 foot peak in the Davis Mountains in southwestern Texas, has been chosen as the site of the new McDonald Observatory.

The McDonald Observatory will be a cooperative enterprise on the part of the University of Texas, which is to build the telescope and observatory buildings from a part of the bequest of the late W. J. McDonald, of Paris, Texas, and the University of Chicago, which is to provide the staff for the observatory. The agreement between the two universities is the first cooperative effort in astronomy made in this country. Although enabling them to build a much larger and effective instrument than would have been possible had two independent observatories been constructed and staffed, the cooperative agreement will mean a saving of over a million dollars to the two universities.

The decision of Dr. Struve to place the McDonald Observatory on Mt. Locke was made following the return this week of an expedition headed by Professor George Van Biesbroeck, of the Yerkes Observatory. This expedition, which spent seventeen nights on Mt. Locke making observations, confirmed the findings of two earlier expeditions made by Assistant Professor Christian T. Elvey last November and by Dr. Struve in December.

A tract of 200 acres, which includes Mt. Locke, has been given the University of Texas for the observatory site. The Mt. Locke site is about fifteen miles from the nearest town, Fort Davis, and Dr. Struve believes that it offers the best conditions for astronomical research to be found in the United States.

Because the solar system is unsymmetrically situated among the stars of the galaxy, and more than nine tenths of the stars and nebulae interesting to astronomers are south of the equator, the farther south an observatory the better the conditions. Were unlimited means available, the McDonald Observatory probably would have been established south of the equator, in New Zealand.

The southern latitude of Mt. Locke, approximately 31 degrees, makes many stars visible which are never above the horizon at Yerkes Observatory at Williams Bay, Wisconsin. Atmospheric conditions are much better in the Davis Mountains also, the nights being uniformly clear and the stars being twice as bright as they are in the latitude of Chicago. The elevation of Mt. Locke exceeds that of the Mt. Wilson and Lick Observatories, and is just a little short of the elevation of Lowell Observatory near Flagstaff, Arizona, but the McDonald Observatory will have a much larger instrument.

Definite specifications for the equipment at the McDonald Observatory have been made and submitted to instrument builders in this country and abroad. Dr. Struve expects that the order for the telescope will be placed in the near future, and completion of the observatory may be possible a year ahead of the contract date of July 1, 1938.

The mounting of the McDonald telescope is to be constructed in such a way that the light of any star may be concentrated in a room of constant temperature, where it may be analyzed with the aid of prisms, photo-electric photometers or other analyzers. There will be a plateholder for the direct photography of comets, stars, planets and nebulae, and several specially designed lenses which will improve the optical definition of the instrument.

Second only in light-gathering power to the 100-

inch mirror at Mt. Wilson, the McDonald telescope will have an eighty-inch mirror made of glass with a low coefficient of expansion and will therefore be suitable to a climate where appreciable changes of temperature during one night are usual.

## THE BRITISH ASSOCIATION FOR THE ADVANCEMENT OF SCIENCE

THE British Association for the Advancement of Science will meet in Leicester from September 6 to 13. The inaugural general meeting will take place at 8:30 P. M. on Wednesday evening, September 6, when Sir Frederick Gowland Hopkins, also president of the Royal Society, will deliver the address of the president on the chemical aspects of life.

The presidents of the sections and the titles of their addresses are as follows:

Section of Mathematical and Physical Sciences, Sir Gilbert T. Walker, "Seasonal Weather and its Prediction"; Section of Chemistry, Professor R. Robinson, "Natural Coloring Matters and their Analogues"; Section of Geology, Professor W. G. Fearnsides, "Structures of Some British Coal-fields"; Section of Zoology, Dr. J. Gray, "The Mechanical View of Life"; Section of Geography, The Right Honorable Lord Meston, subject to be announced; Section of Economic Science and Statistics, Professor J. H. Jones, "The Gold Standard"; Section of Engineering, R. W. Allen, "Some Experiences in Mechanical Engineering"; Section of Anthropology, the Right Honorable Lord Raglan, "What is Tradition?"; Section of Physiology, Professor E. D. Adrian, "The Activity of Nerve Cells"; Section of Psychology, Professor F. Aveling, "The Status of Psychology as an Empirical Science"; Section of Botany, Professor F. E. Lloyd, "The Various Door Mechanisms of *Utricularia* and *Polypompholyx* and their Method of Action"; Section of Educational Sciences, J. L. Holland, "The Development of a National Educational System"; Section of Agriculture, Dr. A. Lauder, "Chemistry and Agriculture."

There will be a large number of symposia and discussions.

Evening discourses to the members will be delivered on Friday, September 8, and Monday, September 11, by Sir Josiah Stamp, general treasurer of the association, on a subject in economic science, to be announced; and by Professor Jocelyn F. Thorpe, on "The Work of the Safety in Mines Research Board." A reception will be held by the Lord Mayor and Lady Mayoress of the City of Leicester (Councillor Arthur Hawkes, J.P., and Mrs. Hawkes), on Thursday evening, September 7; a garden party will be given by the University College on Monday afternoon, September 11; a reception will be given by the Leicester Literary and Philosophical Society in the Museum and Art Gallery on Tuesday evening, September 12. The usual excursions to points of interest, to industrial establishments and to educational institutions have been arranged.

This is the second meeting of the association to be held at Leicester. It met there in 1907, when Sir David Gill, the astronomer, was president, and the occasion was notable as the last on which Lord Kelvin attended and addressed the association of which he had long been an active supporter. The meeting of the association in 1934 will be held in Aberdeen.

## THE ROYAL INSTITUTION AND SIR WILLIAM BRAGG

WE learn from the London *Times* that at the annual meeting of the members of the Royal Institution, which was held on May 1, with the president, Lord Eustace Percy, in the chair, it was announced that the payments in connection with rebuilding had been completed. During the years 1929–32 the managers had been successful in collecting the sum of £96,300 for the rebuilding and research endowment.

The institution's Friday evening discourses and afternoon lectures had crowded the lecture theater on many occasions during the year, and the privilege of free attendance at afternoon lectures by *bona fide* students in London had been much appreciated and used. Professor G. Elliot Smith had succeeded Professor J. B. S. Haldane as Fullerian professor of physiology. On the research side the x-ray investigations under the direction of Sir William Bragg showed steady progress. Lord Eustace Percy was again elected president for the ensuing year, with Sir Robert Robertson treasurer and Major Charles E. S. Phillips secretary.

At the conclusion of the meeting a portrait of Sir William Bragg, the director, by William Nicholson was presented to the institution, where it is to be hung, by the honorary secretary, Major Phillips, on behalf of a group of friends. In a brief speech, as reported in the *Times,* Major Phillips paid a tribute to the artist and expressed the respect and admiration which the members of the Royal Institution felt for the great scientific achievements of their director and their appreciation of the manner in which he upheld its great traditions. All of them regarded him with affection, and it was fitting that his portrait should be hung on their walls with those of the other men who had made the Royal Institution what it was. He read a letter from Sir James Crichton-Browne apologizing for absence and remarking that the portrait showed "the face and figure of a real man, an embodiment of vital and intellectual vigour, a great discoverer, a brilliant expositor and a genial friend."

Lord Eustace Percy, accepting the gift on behalf

of the Royal Institution, said that the portrait was one which the institution might well be proud to possess; it reminded them very warmly and intimately of a man whom they all respected and loved.

Sir William Bragg said that he was proud and grateful that his portrait should be given with such expressions of good will. The institution was an unofficial body, not connected with any government or municipal establishment. It worked on its own and its successes had been due to the devotion of its members, who had always helped it within their powers. In the past 10 years he had always found a prompt response made by any member approached with a request on behalf of the Royal Institution for lectures or other services. He had never had an unfavorable response and hoped he never would. The institution was held in astonishing affection by the country at large. Its members were a friendly body, and in this lay their strength. They were trying to draw together, by personal contact if possible, all those interested in the advance of knowledge. That they had been able in the last three years to pull themselves out of difficulties and rebuild their home was the result of real friendship all around.

## THE AMERICAN ACADEMY OF ARTS AND SCIENCES

At the annual meeting of the American Academy of Arts and Sciences held in Boston on May 10, the following officers were elected:

*President,* George H. Parker; *Vice-president for Class I,* Harry M. Goodwin; *Vice-president for Class II,* Walter B. Cannon; *Vice-president for Class III,* Edwin F. Gay; *Vice-president for Class IV,* Arthur S. Pease; *Corresponding Secretary,* Tenney L. Davis; *Recording Secretary,* Walter E. Clark; *Treasurer,* Ingersoll Bowditch; *Librarian,* Alfred C. Lane; *Editor,* Herbert V. Neal.

Fellows of the academy elected in the natural and exact sciences are:

Class I

Section 1—*Mathematics and Astronomy*

Jesse Douglas, Cambridge.
Marshall Harvey Stone, New Haven, Connecticut.

Section 3—*Chemistry*

Louis Frederick Fieser, Waltham.
George Bogdan Kistiakowsky, Cambridge.
Henry Weeden Underwood, Cambridge.

Section 4—*Technology and Engineering*

Harold Kilbrith Barrows, Winchester.
Arthur Edwin Norton, Cambridge.
Frank Edward Winsor, West Newton.

Class II

Section 1—*Geology and Meteorology*

Charles Franklin Brooks, Milton
Frank Morton Carpenter, Cambridge.

Section 3—*Zoology and Physiology*

Philip Bard, Cambridge
Alden Benjamin Dawson, Cambridge
Frank Rattray Lillie, Chicago, Illinois.
Jeffries Wyman, Jr., Chestnut Hill

Section 4—*Medicine and Surgery*

Reginald Fitz, Brookline
Edgar Erskine Hume, Washington, D. C.
George Burgess Magrath, Boston.
George Cheever Shattuck, Brookline.
Soma Weiss, Cambridge.

Among these elected in Class IV are:

Section 1—*Theology, Philosophy and Psychology*

Gordon Willard Allport, Cambridge.
Howard Crosby Warren, Princeton.
Frederic Lyman Wells, Newton Highlands.

Section 2—*History, Archeology and Anthropology*

Edward Sapir, New Haven

Foreign members were elected as follows:

*Section of Chemistry*

Jaroslav Heyrovsky, Prague.
Fritz Paneth, Königsberg.

*Section of Zoology and Physiology*

Hans Spemann, Freiburg i. B.

*Section of Theology, Philosophy and Psychology*

George Elias Müller, Göttingen.

*Section of History, Archeology and Anthropology*

Sir Arthur Keith, London.

# SCIENTIFIC NOTES AND NEWS

The Rumford Medal of the American Academy of Arts and Sciences has been awarded to Dr. Harlow Shapley, director of the Harvard College Observatory, for "researches on the luminosity of stars and galaxies."

Professor S. A. Mitchell, director of the Leander McCormick Observatory of the University of Virginia, has been elected a foreign associate of the Royal Astronomical Society.

It is proposed to name a Colorado mountain peak after Dr. William Trelease, emeritus professor of botany of the University of Illinois, formerly head of the Henry Shaw School of Botany at Washington University, St. Louis, and director of the Missouri Botanical Garden.

Professor Albert Einstein will deliver the first Gibson Memorial Lecture at the University of Glasgow on June 20. On June 21 the doctorate of laws will be conferred on him.

SIR CHARLES S. SHERRINGTON, Waynflete professor of physiology, University of Oxford, will deliver the Bede Lecture on May 24, on "Mechanism and the Brain."

THE Linacre Lecture was delivered at the University of Cambridge by Professor E. Mellanby on May 6 on "The Nervous System within the Pale of Nutrition."

PROFESSOR H. H. PLASKETT, who was associate and professor of astrophysics at Harvard University from 1928 until 1932, when he was elected to the Savilian professorship of astronomy at the University of Oxford, delivered his inaugural address on April 28 on "The Place of Observation in Astronomy."

THE Italian Eugenics Society recently elected Dr. Jon Alfred Mjøen, Vinderen Laboratorium, a corresponding member. Dr. Mjøen also recently was elected a corresponding member of the Berlin Society for Anthropology and Ethnology.

THE Daniel Guggenheim Medal "for notable achievement in the advancement of aeronautics" for 1933 has been awarded to Commander Jerome Clarke Hunsaker, vice-president of the Goodyear-Zeppelin Corporation of Akron, Ohio. The formal presentation of the medal will probably take place at a meeting of the Society of Automotive Engineers in Chicago in August. Previous Guggenheim medalists have included Orville Wright, Ludwig Prandtl, of Germany, Frederick William Lanchester and Juan de la Cierva of England.

THE Canadian Institute of Mining and Metallurgy has awarded the first platinum medal established for award by any scientific society to John James Denny, of Kingston, in recognition of his contribution to the art of concentrating gold and silver ores. The gift is that of the International Nickel Company of Canada, Limited, in commemoration of the fiftieth anniversary of the discovery of the nickel deposits in the Sudbury district. It was designed by Dr. R. Tait McKenzie, research professor of physical education at the University of Pennsylvania.

THE Colwyn Gold Medal of the British Institution of the Rubber Industry was presented on the occasion of the fourteenth annual dinner, held in London on April 28, to W. H. Paull in recognition of his services to the pneumatic tire industry.

FOUR appointments have been made by Yale University and the Bernice Pauahi Bishop Museum of Hawaii, in their joint program of scientific investigation within the Pacific Ocean area. Dr. Peter H. Buck has been reappointed Bishop Museum professor of anthropology at Yale, and Professor Samuel J. Record, of the Yale School of Forestry, has been selected as the representative of the university to go to Honolulu to consult with the director and trustees of the museum in regard to further collaboration between the two institutions. Arthur C. Smith, associate curator of the New York Botanical Garden, and Laura M. Thompson, of Berkeley, California, have been appointed Bishop Museum research fellows for 1933–34.

DR. C. L. BUTLER, who has been a member of Mellon Institute since 1926, has been appointed senior fellow in pure research in the department of research in pure chemistry.

DR. GEORGE B. RAY, associate professor of physiology in the School of Medicine of Western Reserve University, has been appointed professor of physiology and pharmacology at the Long Island College of Medicine. He succeeds Dr. John C. Cardwell, who retired last June.

CAROL Y. MASON has been appointed assistant professor of geology at Milwaukee-Downer College.

DR. K. G. EMELÉUS, lecturer in physics at the University of Belfast, who is at present in the United States as holder of a Rockefeller fellowship, has been appointed to the chair of experimental physics in succession to Professor W. B. Morton.

THE Committee on Scientific Research of the American Medical Association has made a grant to Dr. Robert Hegner, professor of protozoology in the Johns Hopkins School of Hygiene and Public Health, for the purpose of studying the relation of starch to infections with intestinal protozoa.

PROFESSORS C. J. JOUBERT and M. S. du Toit, of Stellenbosch University in the Union of South Africa, arrived recently at the Citrus Experiment Station of the University of California, at Riverside, and are making an extended study and research in connection with agricultural problems affecting South Africa. Professor Joubert is making a study of the methods of biological control of insect pests, especially in connection with California's control of the mealy bug situation. Professor du Toit is studying methods of reclamation of alkali lands.

DR. KURT LEWIN, acting professor of psychology at Stanford University, sailed recently for Japan. He will travel through Japan and Russia, lecturing at the universities of Tokyo and Moscow. He planned to arrive early in May in Germany, where he will continue his work. Professor Lewin was formerly connected with the Institute of Psychology at the University of Berlin.

Dr. Thomas Barbour, professor of zoology and director of the University Museum at Harvard University, made the principal address at the public opening of Maryland Hall, University of Richmond, on April 28. Maryland Hall completes the group of science buildings at that university.

Professor Charles E. Spearman, of the University of London, lectured before the Society of the Sigma Xi at Northwestern University on May 5, on "Current Psychologies."

At a joint meeting at Washington University of the Academy of Science of St. Louis and the St. Louis Anthropological Society on April 26, Dr. Albert Ernest Jenks, professor of anthropology at the University of Minnesota, delivered an illustrated address on "Minnesota's Glacial-Age Man."

Professor Eliot R. Clark, of the University of Pennsylvania, delivered an address to the faculty and students of the School of Medicine, George Washington University, on April 29, on "The Spontaneous Activity of Capillaries."

Dr. L. A. Wolfanger, of Columbia University, recently gave a series of lectures at Northwestern University on the characteristics, interpretation and economic significance of soils.

Dr. James Ewing, Cornell University Medical College, and director of the Memorial Hospital, New York, will deliver the second Frank Billings Lecture of the Thomas Lewis Gilmer Foundation of the Institute of Medicine of Chicago, on May 26. His subject will be "The Depression: Its Effects on Medicine, Research and Practice."

At the suggestion of Dr. Max Henius, of Chicago, the Danish Government has appointed a committee of the most distinguished scientific men in Denmark to plan and prepare for the Museum of Science and Industry of Chicago a comprehensive series of exhibits to show the evolution of Danish science from the days of Tycho Brahe. The chairman of the committee is Frederik V. Petersen, under-secretary of state, and the vice-chairman is the Danish Ambassador to the United States, Otto Wadsted. Other members include Professor Niels Bohr; Benny Dessau; Dr. Martin Knudsen, professor of physics in the University of Copenhagen; Dr. August Krogh, professor of physiology in the University of Copenhagen; Dr. Svend Lomholt, director of the Finsen Laboratories; Dr. T. Madsen, director of the State Serum Institute; P. M. Michelsen, chairman of the Danish Arts and Crafts Society; Professor A. W. Moerkeberg, director of the Royal Danish Agricultural College; Professor N. E. Noerlund, president of the Royal Danish Science Association; Director Charles H. Olesen, chairman of the Society for the Development of Danish Industries; Professor Valdemar Poulsen, inventor of the radio telephone and other radio devices; Professor S. P. L. Soerensen, director of the Carlsberg Laboratory, and Dr. E. Buch Andersen, professor of physics in Aarhus University.

Formal installation of a new chapter of Sigma Xi was made on April 25, in the University of California at Los Angeles. Fifty charter members, principally faculty and teaching assistants, make up the initial roster of the new chapter. Following the official dinner held in Kerckhoff Hall, the charter members and many prominent guests from outside institutions listened to the formal addresses of the delegates charged with the installation. Professor Chas. J. Chamberlain, of the University of Chicago, and Dr. J. A. Anderson, astronomer and president of the Mt. Wilson-California Institute Chapter, officiated. Officers elected included Dr. Samuel J. Barnett, chairman; Dr. E. K. Soper, secretary, and Dr. Hosmer W. Stone, treasurer. Pending establishment of the long-delayed graduate school in the Los Angeles division of the state university, membership in Sigma Xi will be confined largely to the university staff. Political developments in state legislative circles, however, are said to promise an early recognition of graduate study on the southern campus.

The tenth annual initiation meeting of the University of Virginia Chapter of Sigma Xi was held on May 2. The meeting was addressed by President Joseph S. Ames, of the Johns Hopkins University, who spoke on "Recent Applications of Science in Aviation." The ninth annual award of the President and Visitors' Research Prize of $100 was made to Dr. Carl C. Speidel, of the school of anatomy, Department of Medicine, for a paper entitled, "Studies of Living Nerves; the Movements of Individual Sheath Cells and Nerve Sprouts Correlated with the Process of Myelin-sheath Formation in Amphibian Larvae." The Andrew J. Fleming Prize of $50 for the best paper in biology by a graduate student was awarded to Mr. Chauncey McL. Gilbert.

The fourth annual New York State Public Reforestation Conference was held on May 12 and 13 in Binghamton, N. Y., under the auspices of the New York State College of Forestry at Syracuse and the Binghamton Chamber of Commerce. Among the speakers on the program were Lithgow Osborne, Conservation Commissioner, Albany, New York; Seth Gordon, president, American Game Association, Washington, D. C.; Congressman John D. Clark, co-author of the Clark-McNary act, an important forestry measure; Dean Samuel N. Spring, of the New York State College of Forestry, and William G.

Howard, director of the Department of Lands and Forests in New York.

The Mexican Society of Geography and Statistics recently celebrated its hundredth anniversary with special ceremonies, attended by President Rodriguez, cabinet ministers and members of the diplomatic corps. The celebration, which consisted of two addresses and several orchestra numbers, marked the centenary of the issuance of a decree by President Valentin Gomez Farias in 1833, establishing the "National Institute of Geography," an organization which later became the Mexican Society of Geography and Statistics.

The annual meeting of the British Medical Association will be held for the first time in Dublin next summer under the presidency of Dr. T. G. Moorhead, Regius professor of physic in Trinity College. The annual representative meeting will begin on July 21 and will be continued on the following three week days in the Hall of the Royal Dublin Society, where Professor Moorhead will deliver his presidential address on July 25. The clinical and scientific work is being divided among sixteen sections, which meet on the mornings of Wednesday, Thursday and Friday in Trinity College and University College.

The fourth International Congress of Radiology will be held in Zurich, under the presidency of Professor H. R. Schinz, from July 24 to 31, 1934. Membership of the congress is confined to members of radiological societies and those introduced by such societies. The thirty-two countries which were represented at the third congress in Paris have been invited by the organizing committee to appoint delegates to the international committee and to nominate a speaker to report on the organization of the cancer campaign in his country at the opening session. At the general meetings the following subjects will be treated: x-ray diagnosis of bone tumors, vasography, the development of pulmonary tuberculosis as seen radiologically, radiation treatment of uterus-carcinoma, radiation treatment of malignant tumors of the mouth and pharynx, radiation genetics, mitogenetic radiation (mitogenetische strahlung), structure analysis, identical physical measurement of the dose in x-ray and radium treatment, hard gamma-rays, cosmic radiation, earth-radiation, shortwave therapy (kurzwellentherapie). In addition the sections for x-ray diagnosis, radiotherapy, radiobiology, radiophysics and technic, electrology and heliotherapy will hold discussions and every member of the congress is entitled to present a communication. During the congress an exhibition of apparatus, photographical accessories, chemical products and scientific books will be on view. All radiological societies are requested to send as soon as possible a list of their members to the general secretary, Dr. H. E. Walther, Gloriastrasse 14, Zurich.

The award of five Strathcona Fellowships for the investigation of transportation problems has been announced by Yale University. All five men have had previous railroad experience, two of them being third generation railroad men. The recipients of the fellowships are: Robert A. Emerson, Morden, Manitoba; Stevenson Milne Gossage, Montreal; Thomas M. C. Martin, Warsaw, Wisconsin; Palmer E. Savage, Montreal, and Lyell R. Shellenbarger, Hopkins, Minnesota. The Strathcona fellowships were made possible by the bequest of Lord Strathcona, born Donald Alexander Smith, who came to Canada with the Hudson Bay Company and who is identified with the pioneer days of the railroad on this continent. He served in the Dominion House of Commons, became High Commissioner of Canada in 1896, and was raised to the peerage in 1897. In addition to the fellowships, Lord Strathcona's will provided for two professorships at Yale devoted to the study of transportation, and for the erection of Strathcona Hall with its collocation of offices, classrooms and a special working library for students and instructors making transportation their major interest. The Strathcona professorship of mechanical engineering is held by Professor Samuel W. Dudley, and the Strathcona professorship of engineering mechanics, by Professor Charles J. Tilden.

The first specimens to be received of the new radium and silver ores of Great Bear Lake, Canada, by the Academy of Natural Sciences of Philadelphia, have been placed on exhibition. This discovery of pitchblende, the principal ore of radium, was made on the eastern shores of Great Bear Lake, just below the Arctic Circle, by Gilbert LaBine in 1930. Associated with the pitchblende was much silver. The glaciated surface of one vein of silver was so wide as to rival the famous "silver pavement" of Cobalt, Ontario. So remote is the district that airplanes are the chief method of reaching it and it then is accessible only during a few months of the year. Several tons of pitchblende already have been produced, and are being reduced to radium at a plant just erected at Port Hope on Lake Ontario. A new and efficient process has been developed by the Canadian Bureau of Mines, which greatly cuts down the time needed to recover the radium. Supplementing the exhibit are a large mass of silver from the Eldorado Gold Mines, at LaBine Point, Great Bear Lake; gold from Nova Scotia; labradorite from Labrador; asbestos from Quebec; fluorite from Ontario; and specimens of blue sodalite and nickel ore obtained on a recent expedition to Canada by the Academy of Natural Sciences.

# DISCUSSION

## THE ATTRACTION OF A SPHERE

IT is surprising to find in SCIENCE for April 14, 1933 (page 371), a denial of the well-established theorem that under the Newtonian law of gravitation the attraction between two homogeneous spheres is the same as if the entire mass of each were concentrated at its center. Since the proof of this theorem, while entirely elementary, is often omitted in the text-books, it may be permitted to reproduce it here.

Consider a thin spherical shell of radius $a$ and surface density $\rho$, attracting a particle of mass $m$ at distance $c$ from the center. If the surface is regarded as generated by rotating a circle about the axis of $x$, as shown in the diagram, an element of arc $ds$, rotating through a small angle $d\vartheta$, will generate an element

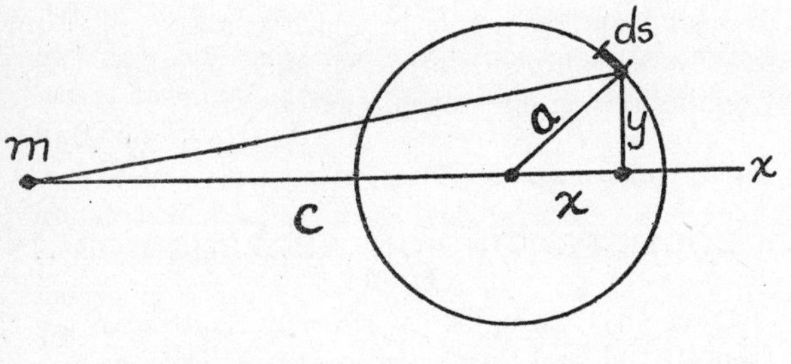


of area $yd\vartheta ds$, which may be regarded as a particle whose mass is $\rho\, yd\vartheta ds$.

According to the Newtonian law, the force exerted by this element on the particle $m$ is $G\,[m\rho\, yd\vartheta ds]\,/\,[(c+x)^2+y^2]$. This force is directed toward the element, and the component along the $x$-axis (which is all that concerns us) is obtained by multiplying by the cosine of the angle, namely, $(c+x)\,/\,[(c+x)^2+y^2]^{\frac{1}{2}}$. Hence, noting that $yds = adx$, and $y^2 = a^2 - x^2$, the element of force along the $x$-axis is

$$(c+x)\ [Gm\rho\, ad\vartheta dx]\ /\ [c^2+2cx+a^2]^{3/2}.$$

Integrating from $\vartheta = 0$ to $\vartheta = 2\pi$, and then from $x = -a$ to $x = a$, we have as the total force acting on the particle $m$ along the $x$-axis,

$$F = \int_{-a}^{a} \frac{(c+x)\ Gm\,\rho\, 2\pi\, adx}{[c^2+2cx+a^2]^{3/2}} \qquad (1)$$

Now suppose that the mass of the attracting spherical surface, namely $4\pi a^2\rho$, were concentrated at a distance $D$ from the particle $m$, where $D$ is as yet undetermined. Then, by the Newtonian law, the force acting on the particle $m$ would be

$$F' = Gm\ (4\pi a^2\rho)/D^2$$

Equating these values of $F$ and $F'$, we have the following equation for determining $D$:

$$\frac{2a^2}{D^2} = \int_{-a}^{a} \frac{(c+x)\ adx}{[c^2+2cx+a^2]^{3/2}} \qquad (2)$$

To evaluate this integral, make the substitution $t = (c^2+2cx+a^2)^{\frac{1}{2}}$, and note that when $x = a$, $t = c+a$, and when $x = -a$, $t = |c-a|$, where the vertical bars indicate the absolute value of $c-a$. Then we find

$$\frac{2a^2}{D^2} = \frac{a}{2c^2}\int_{|c-a|}^{c+a} \left(1+\frac{c^2-a^2}{t^2}\right) dt. \qquad (3)$$

Two cases must now be distinguished, according as the particle $m$ is outside or inside the spherical shell.

Case 1. If $c > a$, $|c-a| = c-a$, and we readily find $2a^2/D^2 = (a/2c^2)\ (4a)$, so that $D = c$.

That is, *the attraction of the spherical shell at an external point is exactly the same as if all its mass were concentrated at its center.*

Case 2. If $c < a$, $|c-a| = a-c$, and we find $2a^2/D = 0$, so that $D$ is infinite. That is, the attraction of the shell at an interior point is zero.

Finally, a solid sphere in which the density at any point is a function only of the distance of that point from the center, may be regarded as made up of a series of concentric homogeneous shells. Since each shell attracts an external particle as if all its mass were concentrated at its center, the same will be true of the sum of the shells. Hence we have the theorem:

*On the basis of the Newtonian law of the inverse square, a homogeneous sphere, or any sphere in which the density is a function only of the distance from the center, attracts an external particle exactly as if all the mass of the sphere were concentrated at its center.*

In view of the recent misunderstanding of this theorem, I trust that this reproduction of the standard proof may not be wholly superfluous.

EDWARD V. HUNTINGTON

HARVARD UNIVERSITY

APRIL 18, 1933

## THE MOVEMENT OF DIFFUSIBLE SUBSTANCES IN FOOD PRODUCTS

WHEN fluids diffuse through substances of capillary structure, they tend to carry solutes with them. Where water is the diffusing fluid, phenomena of hydrolysis, chemical reaction, selective adsorption and differential diffusion may become manifest.[1] Colloids may diffuse, albeit more slowly than crystalloids—a

[1] Jerome Alexander, *Jour. Am. Chem. Soc.*, 39: 84, 1917; SCIENCE, 54: 74, 1921.

fact explicitly stated by Thomas Graham, but often garbled or misstated.

Where evaporation can take place at the exterior surfaces of the mass through which diffusion is occurring, there is a marked tendency for non-volatile solutes to accumulate at such surfaces.[2] Some possible consequences of this movement of diffusible substances in agricultural operations have been pointed out, for plant food is carried with diffusion streams.[3]

Since many of the operations whereby foods are prepared for consumption involve the evaporation of water from exposed surfaces (*e.g.*, the baking of bread, ripening of fruits), it is obvious that various solutes may be separated or segregated to a greater or lesser extent in the process. This led me to include in a paper written several years ago, but still unpublished, a few remarks on "Skins and Crusts," epitomized below.

In discussing with Mr. Robert Whymper a paper he is about to read before a joint meeting of several chemical societies in New York (April 14), it developed that his experimental results dealing with the processing of cacao beans, illustrated this principle of diffusion. We therefore decided to entitle the paper: "The Movement of Diffusible Substances in Food Products. I. Preparation of Cacao," with the expectation that it will be the first of a series of papers dealing with this aspect of food and their preparation.

Apart from the question of economy, skins and crusts are commonly reputed to be "healthy." Children and adults are often urged to eat the skins of baked potatoes, for example. So far as I know, there have been no precise determinations as to what extent salts, vitamins and other diffusible substances accumulate in or near the surface layers of bread, potatoes, and the like; but it seems extremely likely that cooking would result in some marked degree segregation of solutes, which would tend to persist for some time after the cessation of active surface evaporation.

Bechhold showed that plaster of Paris "bricks," soaked in copper sulfate solution and then dried, had practically all the copper salt at or near their exposed surfaces, although when wet they were blue clear through. The slow accumulation of salts at the exposed surfaces of ordinary building bricks is known to every one, for it so often constitutes an eyesore. Mr. Whymper has called my attention to the fact that genuine mummy wheat from Egyptian tombs contains on the average only about 0.7 per cent. of salts, whereas the usual average for wheat today is about 2 per cent. Some old samples from Rothamsted Experimental Station (Harpenden, Herts., England) showed the following:

| | |
|---|---|
| Sample of wheat dating from 1852 | 0.90 % salts |
| " " " " " 1853 | 0.83 % " |
| " " " " " 1854 | 1.14 % " |

Presumably, as moisture is absorbed and given up by the wheat kernel, there is a slow accumulation of salts on the exterior, and much of this extruded salt falls or is rubbed off, thus decreasing the content remaining in the grain itself.[4]

A study must be made of many of the common practises of the kitchen, which are generally based on sound scientific foundations, even though this be unknown to cooks or to scientists. Vegetable soups (*minestra*), and "pot likker (popular in the South), contain valuable solutes, and braised or steamed vegetable would seem to be more desirable than vegetable drained from the water in which it was boiled; for this water, thrown into the sink, contains salts, vitamins and other valuable extractives.

JEROME ALEXANDER

NEW YORK CITY

## A LOUSE FEEDING ON THE BLOOD OF ITS HOST

THAT any Mallophagan can actively remove blood from its host and thus warrant consideration as a possible vector or intermediate host of organisms causing avian disease has been extensively denied.

This writer, while recently studying poultry lice at Cornell University, observed individuals of *Menopon stramineum* Nitzsch. running about on the skin of a white fowl and showing a pigmented substance in the crop, indicative of blood. That this was not obtained from clots from accidental injuries to the host was strongly suggested by the finding of an individual, showing blood in the alimentary tract, with mandibles deeply sunken in the quill of a young feather from which the dermal papilla, bearing blood vessels, had not yet withdrawn. On the removal of the louse blood flowed from the wound. The injury appeared as if two holes, one for each mandible, had been pierced in the quill and then the partition separating them cut out. Examination of the quill showed many scars of the same type of wound as the one from which the louse had been removed. The unfolding barbs showed still older scars, suggesting that this type of feeding was habitual. The louse and feather were removed and preserved.

Similar observations by others working with poultry lice are awaited with interest.

F. H. WILSON

TULANE UNIVERSITY

[2] H. Bechhold, *Kolloid Zeitschrift*, 27: 299, 1920; W. Kraus, *ibid.*, 28: 161, 1921.

[3] Jerome Alexander, SCIENCE, *loc. cit.*, and 56: 196, 1922.

[4] R. Whymper, ''Knowledge,'' 36: 85–138, 1913.

## HAIL PRINTS AND MUD-CRACKS OF PROTEROZOIC AGE

ON page 679 of the second part (1932) of his "Treatise on Sedimentation," Professor W. H. Twenhofel calls attention to the fact that geologists have neglected to record hail prints in rocks more ancient than the Triassic.

Apparent hail prints, with deep pits and elevations opposite the side of impact, occur in the Proterozoic Beltian rocks of Glacier National Park. They are commonest in the basal (Rising Wolf) and uppermost (Rising Bull) members of the Grinnell formation, in the Bighorn Basin of the Two Medicine Valley, and at the western foot of Gunsight Pass. They also occur in Hole-in-the-Wall and Kintla quartzites in the Boulder Pass district, in the northwestern part of the park.

Twenhofel also remarks (page 686) that the commonly assumed three cracks, radiating from a center, seem to be the exception among mud-crack patterns. They are; but such cracks are common in the Rising Bull member in the Two Medicine Valley, and appear in other shallow water formations throughout Glacier National Park, generally being preserved as sand fillings in argillite. We have observed similar cracks in sandy shales of late Medina (Silurian) age in the Niagara Gorge near Lewiston, New York. Specimens are in the collections of the Buffalo Museum of Science.

CARROLL LANE FENTON
MILDRED ADAMS FENTON

WEST LIBERTY, IOWA

## THE NEED OF OPPORTUNITY FOR EXCEPTIONAL ABILITY

PROFESSOR L. W. STERN, of the University of Hamburg, president of the German Psychological Association; Professor Gustav Kafka, of the Dresden Institute of Technology, secretary, and Professor David Katz, of the University of Rostock, member of the council, have been compelled by their colleagues to resign offices which indicate the high standing of Jews in the intellectual life of Germany. Professor Felix Krueger, the successor of Wilhelm Wundt at Leipzig, has been elected president of the association, and the place of meeting has been changed from Dresden to Leipzig.

Shortly after the conclusion of the war I wrote to Professor Krueger proposing that the International Congress of Psychology meet in America to mark the friendly relations of the psychologists of the world,[1] but he opposed the plan. The congress was in fact held at Oxford in 1923, it having been the first international congress after the war (though the physiologists met the same summer); Professor Krueger advised German psychologists not to attend. He did not go to the congress held in Copenhagen last summer and refused to invite the next congress to meet at Leipzig; as Professor Köhler did not want us at Berlin, an invitation from Madrid was accepted.

The announcement to members of the German Psychological Association of the meeting to be held in Leipzig in October, signed by Professor Krueger, is more nearly what might be expected in Soviet Russia or in Italy than in Germany. Its rhetoric is not easy to translate, so I quote:

> Die Erinnerung an Wilhelm Wundt, den Hundertjährigen, paart sich hierbei mit der Zuversicht, das die deutsche Psychologie in lebensvollem Zusammenhange mit ihrer ruhmreichen Vergangenheit stetig und entschieden vorwärts schreiten wird. An alle Mitglieder richtet der Vorstand die Bitte, sich dahin zu vereinigen, das die Leipziger Tagung einen Verlauf nehme, wie ihn die Würde der Wissenschaft und die hohen Aufgaben unserer Gesellschaft erfordern. Aus den Umwälzungen der gegenwärtigen Zeit soll die *Deutsche Gesellschaft für Psychologie,* durch Gemeinschaftskräfte innerlich verbunden, neu gefestigt hervorgehen.
>
> Die bisher vorgesehenen Sammelreferate bleiben in Kraft. Etwaige Änderungen oder Ergänzungen des übrigen Programms sollen vornehmlich die Richtung auf Fragen der *Persönlichkeitsforschung* nehmen. Zugleich soll die *praktische* Bedeutung der Psychologie für Kernfragen des gegenwärtigen deutschen Lebens gebührend zu ihrem Rechte kommen.

It will be noted that stress is laid on work on the problems of individual differences and on the practical applications of psychology in the service of the new political and social developments in Germany. It is a curious circumstance that I made in Leipzig now nearly fifty years ago the first measurements of individual differences and carried out the first quantitative work in applied psychology. Wundt was so much opposed to these experiments that I could not continue them in his laboratory, but was compelled to purchase the needed apparatus and set it up in my own rooms. As late as 1921 when I wrote to

[1] It should be put on record that at a meeting held in Philadelphia in August, 1917, of the Psychology Committee of the National Research Council (which accomplished such useful service for the government during the war) I proposed the following resolution which, as I remember it, was unanimously approved:

*Whereas,* the President of the United States has stated that there is no quarrel and should be no ill-feeling between the people of the United States and the people of Germany;

*Resolved,* that the Psychology Committee of the National Research Council places on record its appreciation of the wisdom of the President's expression of good-will. We recognize our obligations to the German universities and to the great men who have led in the development of psychology. We trust that an early peace may be established and that we may soon again be able to cooperate with German and Austrian psychologists in the advancement and in the useful applications of our science.

Professor Krueger in regard to the Psychological Corporation, which we were establishing to advance the applications of psychology and to place research on an economic basis, he objected emphatically to such uses of psychology.

It should, however, be realized that we are not in a position to cast the first stone at our German colleagues. Communists are as anathema here as there. Jews are not treated on terms of equality, either as teachers or as students, in our eastern universities. The president of the largest of them is said to have given the instruction: "Do not exclude any student because he is a Jew, but do not admit any Jew if it can be helped." Twenty years ago I was compelled to resign from the Century Club because I had objected to the exclusion of Jacques Loeb, one of the world's most distinguished biologists. Professor Edwin R. A. Seligman, the prominent economist, had also been blackballed, and there were in addition to Loeb three other members of the National Academy of Sciences ineligible to membership through race. Yet the Century Club has now brought action in the courts to obtain exemption from taxation on the ground that it is not a social club but an institution devoted to literature, art and science.[2]

We have in America a great race, brought here by force and forming 10 per cent. of the population, to which we do not give political, legal, social or economic equality. We are in no position to play the part of Pharisees, but we can try to better the situation by giving opportunity to those of exceptional ability who are unable to continue their work elsewhere. In 1910 (SCIENCE, November 4) I wrote:

> There were 126 foreign-born men of science on the list of 1903. While the majority came to this country before attaining scientific reputation, a large number were called from Canada, Great Britain, Germany and other countries to fill positions in our universities, of whom seven were among our leading hundred men of science. The members of this group have added greatly to the scientific strength of the country, not only by the research that they have accomplished, but also because they have brought familiarity with the educational methods of other nations, and high ideals of scholarship and of the dignity of the career of the scientific man and university professor. It is surprising and truly most unfortunate that while nine leading foreign men of science have returned to their native countries during the past seven years, only one has come to America—one scientific man among seven million immigrants. There is no way by which the abundant wealth of the country could be used to greater advantage than by bringing to it men of promise and men of distinction.

Psychologically we seem not to have abundant wealth just now; but materially we are far richer than we were in 1910. The market value of stocks and bonds has increased by billions of dollars in the course of the past couple of weeks. Why not take by taxation one of these billions and endow in perpetuity 5,000 of the ablest scientific men of the world with $200,000 each? It would be the most profitable investment ever made.

We have fallen from the high estate when our country offered a refuge to the oppressed of all nations. We have not, however, completely forgotten what we owe to Puritans and Quakers, to refugees from Germany as recently as eighty years ago. Can we not now provide for those of exceptional ability who, owing to race or political views, are unable to do at home work of value to the whole world?

J. McKEEN CATTELL

[2] This note may go too far in the direction of autobiography, but illustrations can best be drawn from personal experiences, which have not been lacking. When I have been asked by publishing houses to write an autobiography, I have replied that it would give them too many libel suits.

# QUOTATIONS

## THE SITUATION OF JEWISH SCIENTIFIC MEN AND PHYSICIANS IN GERMANY

THE political significance of Nazi revolutionary supremacy under Herr Hitler in Germany is outside our field; but the treatment of the Jewish learned and professional classes stands condemned in the eyes of the intellectual world. It is a relapse to the crass repression of the Germany of Heine's day and the *Judenhetze* of Prussia fifty years ago. An outstanding case is the resignation by Professor James Franck, Nobel prizeman with G. Hertz for physics in 1925, of his chair in experimental physics in the University of Göttingen. Professor Franck, it is said, probably would have been spared the forced retirement now operative against Jewish officials, including university professors; but he feels that Germans of Jewish descent are being treated as foreigners and foes of the Fatherland, and asks to be released from his office. Professor Franck served with distinction during the war and received the Iron Cross of the First Class. His action follows fittingly on the retirement of Professor A. Einstein from Germany, and is the logical, indeed the only, reply for a man of his standing to the acts by which Jews are being excluded from the liberal professions and debarred from the universities. This is the achievement of a movement which, ever since the war, has sought to mould the German people to one pan-Teutonic pattern—in accord with neither the facts nor the conclusions of ethnology. In the denial of a part in Germanic culture to any element alleged to be foreign, Jews, liberals and socialists are to be treated alike; but Jews have suffered most.

The Jewish people need no one to hold a brief on their behalf. The contribution of the Jews to the growth of civilization in the Western world speaks for itself. There were Jews in Germany in Roman times, and wherever they were found in medieval Europe, in spite of, or perhaps because of, their disabilities, they were laying the foundations upon which the modern system of finance and commerce was built up. In Italy as bankers, they rivaled the great houses of Lombardy. In the liberal arts, the preservation of much of classical literature and philosophy was due to them. In the later Middle Ages they were largely responsible for the reputation of Spain as a center of intellectual and scientific development. In the middle of the eighteenth century the revival of Jewish learning, which had Mendelssohn for its inspiration and leader, paved the way for the Jewish people to take its place in the intellectual life of the respective countries of their adoption as their disabilities were gradually removed, so that Bunsen could say that in the German universities of his day the greater number of the principal professors were Jews. Everywhere the Jews have won to preeminence in literature, in the arts, especially music, and the drama. Even if it were not admitted that the Jews had contributed to Germanic culture—a contention which could not be accepted without argument—in the world of learning and science it is to men such as Oppert, the classical scholar, Benfey, the Orientalist, and Heinrich Hertz, the physicist, to take three names only, selected almost at random, that she owes her international standing, just as much as to any of her sons of purest German stock.—*Nature.*

News items appearing in the issues of the *Münchener medizinische Wochenschrift* and the *Deutsche medizinische Wochenschrift* for the weeks of April 7 to April 21, inclusive, indicate the following actions in Germany against Jewish and other foreign physicians:

An ordinance of the Prussian Ministry of the Interior of March 29 states that foreigners, even those who received their preliminary education in Germany, can no longer count on receiving licenses to practise in Germany.

Control of the five largest associations in charge of sickness insurance has been placed under the federal ministry of labor.

Dr. Gerhard Wagner, Munich, first chairman of the National Socialist German Physicians' Organization, has been nominated Commissioner of the National Physicians' Organizations, of the Association of German Physicians and of the German Alliance of Physicians' Societies.

The Supreme German Medical Societies (Die deutschen ärztlichen Spitzenverbände) gave out the following ordinance in accordance with their commissar, Dr. Gerhard Wagner (first chairman of the National Socialist Physicians' Union):

> In execution of their resolution to adhere to the spirit and form of the medical societies of the new order, the directors of the Aerztevereinsbund and the Hartmannbund ask their members, with the advancement of German medicine in mind, to take pains immediately to dismiss from committees and boards of directors all Jewish members; all colleagues who can not conscientiously adhere to the new order must be replaced.
>
> Through the directors of the sickness insurance societies it is to be impressed in turn on the directors of the sickness insurance companies and insurance organizations, officials and superintendents to replace immediately Jewish and Marxist confidential consultants.
>
> DR. STAUDER.

> I decree that the foregoing regulation be immediately enforced and notification thereof sent me.
>
> DR. WAGNER.

Dr. Frank, surgeon and member of the board of health, director of the hospital at Fürth, was taken in protective arrest. He was replaced by the internist Professor Weigeldt. Dr. Sponheimer, superintendent surgeon, was granted leave of absence.

The Universities of Leipzig and Bavaria have decreed that no member of the Jewish race will be permitted to matriculate in medicine for the next ten semesters. Enrolment of students for the study of medicine at the University of Munich is to be cut down to 345, at Würzburg to 130, and at Erlangen to 98. Under the terms of these regulations, any one who had one parent or one grandparent of Jewish race is considered Jewish.

The annual session of the German Society for Internal Medicine was scheduled to meet this spring under the presidency of Professor Lichtwitz of Berlin. He resigned from his office and was replaced by Professor A. Schittenhelm, of Kiel. At the forty-fifth Congress of Internal Medicine in Wiesbaden, Dr. Schittenhelm, successor to Dr. Lichtwitz, stated that differentiation must be made between old settled German-Jewish families of high culture and recently arrived eastern Jewish elements, since it is only the latter who bring about a racial taint by intermarriage with Germans. "Men like Ehrlich, Neisser, Minkowski and Wassermann," he said, "should be given great respect by German physicians and people of their talent would in the future undoubtedly be able to succeed in Germany."

In Baden, all Jewish physicians have been dismissed from the public health service and from the sickness insurance organization. In the hospitals they are permitted to treat only Jewish patients and to perform postmortem examinations only on Jewish patients who have died. A similar regulation has been established in Munich.

In Munich, S. Obendorfer and O. Neubauer requested a leave of absence from the Schwabing Hospital. The following Jewish physicians of the main office of public health in Berlin were given leave of absence: Professor Seligmann, Drs. Borinski, Cohn, Wolff, Nussbaum and others. The Jewish physician-in-chief of the cripple welfare station VII in Charlottenburg, Dr. Böhm, was replaced by Dr. Kniekamp of the orthopedic clinic.

The business director of the Berlin ambulatory clinic, Max Edel, and Dr. Friedeberger were placed under protective arrest.

The editor of the *Deutsches Aerzteblatt,* San.-Rat. Vollman, was given a leave of absence by the chairman of the Deutscher Aerztevereinsbund. Dr. K. Walder, of Potsdam, takes his place.

The Committee on Therapeutics of the German National Society of Physicians has made public a list of pharmaceutic preparations manufactured by concerns under Jewish ownership or control with the request that physicians in general do not prescribe such preparations.—*Journal of the American Medical Association.*

# THE NATIONAL ACADEMY OF SCIENCES

## ABSTRACTS OF PAPERS PRESENTED AT THE WASHINGTON MEETING. II.

(*Continued from page 460*)

*The Woods Hole Oceanographic Institution:* HENRY B. BIGELOW. A report is presented to the academy on the history and present activities of the Woods Hole Oceanographic Institution, giving the events leading to the establishment of the institution; reasons for the choice of Woods Hole for the site for its headquarters; descriptions of the laboratory, of the scientific equipment and of the research ship *Atlantis;* the general organization, staff, facilities for visiting investigators, cooperation with other institutions and plans for publication; the reasons for adopting a directed and coordinated program of research; and a summary of investigations now in progress and of the cruises of *Atlantis.*

*The bearing of genetics on the theory of evolution:* THOMAS HUNT MORGAN.

*Phenomena associated with cosmic rays:* W. F. G. SWANN (by invitation). Certain of the investigations in progress at the Bartol Research Foundation in the field of cosmic rays have been summarized by the author and in particular the following were described: (1) Observations of cosmic ray atomic disintegration made simultaneously by ionization methods and by counter methods. (2) Experiments dealing with the detection of individual cosmic rays by direct measurement of the ionization which they produce. These experiments lead to the determination of the ionization per centimeter of path in different gases. (3) Certain possibilities as to the origin of cosmic ray energies, particularly in relation to the origin of electronic cosmic ray energies as a result of electric fields produced by electromagnetic induction in the stars. (4) Observations on electrostatic deflection of secondary cosmic rays.

*Cosmic ray intensities in the stratosphere:* I. S. BOWEN and R. A. MILLIKAN. By sending up recording electroscopes, barographs and thermometers with the aid of sounding balloons in accordance with the technique which we first used in 1922, we have, during the past summer, made three successful flights, one of which reached an altitude at which the pressure had fallen to 16 millimeters of mercury—about 99% of the way to the top of the atmosphere—a second flight reached a height of 21 kilometers and the third the height of 16 kilometers. On two of these flights we obtained reliable records of the cosmic ray intensities as a function of altitude up to 18 kilometers, 92% of the way to the top by weight. At this altitude the cosmic ray intensities are approximately 100 times greater than at sea-level, and the intensity altitude curve is of such a shape as to indicate that the rays entering the atmosphere have not yet got into equilibrium with their secondaries. Three flights thus far made, two by ourselves and one by Regener, are in reasonably good agreement.

*The penetrating power of cosmic rays as a function of altitude:* R. A. MILLIKAN and H. V. NEHER. We have made accurate airplane observations with our new electroscopes, so designed as to give as accurate readings on moving platforms as in a laboratory, reaching altitudes above 29,000 feet. Up to this altitude we have taken readings both without lead shields and with a lead shield, and have thus obtained direct measurement of the penetrating power of the cosmic rays existing in different levels. These rays show a rapid softening with altitude, and essentially the same softening in temperate latitudes as in equatorial latitudes. The observed behavior seems to us to be best interpreted in terms of cosmic ray photon bands of widely differing penetrating power, the less penetrating bands coming into play at the higher altitudes.

*The magneto-optic method of analysis and some recent applications:* FRED ALLISON (introduced by Arthur L.

Day). A very brief outline is given of the magneto-optic method of analysis, the apparatus and its manipulation. The method detects compounds of both inorganic and organic substances. It has proved itself a tool of value in certain problems in qualitative and quantitative analysis, particularly those concerned with compounds existing in very small concentrations, the sensitivity being of the order of several parts in $10^{12}$ and the results being unaffected by the presence of foreign materials. Observations are made on minima of light intensity, the scale readings of which are characteristic of the compounds and are measures of differential time lags in the reaction of the compounds to the applied magnetic fields. The time lags are functions of the combining weights of both the cation and the anion. The method determines the number and the order of abundance of the isotopes of the cation but not of the anion. The scale readings are reproducible by the same and different observers (including the work during the past five years of some fifteen observers on the same and different sets of apparatus) to within about 3 mm, corresponding to 0.01 scale division and to a time lag of $10^{-11}$ sec., while quantitative results can be obtained within an error of 10 per cent. The more recent progress of the work is described, namely, the isotopic constitution of some of the radioactive elements; the isotopes of beryllium and zinc; a slight temperature effect on sensitivity; and investigations on the problem of mutual isotopic influence. Mention is made of a new quantitative technique developed by Professor E. R. Bishop and her students and also of the application of the method to a problem in photosynthesis by Dr. A. L. Sommer.

*The discovery of the free positive electron:* CARL D. ANDERSON (introduced by Robert A. Millikan). During a systematic study by means of a vertical Wilson cloud-chamber of the high energy particles associated with the cosmic radiation, evidence was uncovered which led to the striking conclusion that the free positive electron, heretofore unknown, was present among the cosmic-ray particles. By placing a horizontal lead plate across the center of the cloud-chamber for the purpose of studying the interaction of cosmic-ray particles with matter, photographs were obtained which could be interpreted logically only on the basis of the existence of a particle with positive charge of a magnitude less than twice that of the electron and probably exactly equal to it, and a mass comparable to that of the free negative electron. From the occurrence of the free positive electrons with groups of other tracks it is concluded that they result from disintegration of atomic nuclei. The term positron is suggested to denote the free positive electron when it occurs unassociated with a mass of atomic magnitude. The cloud-chamber, planned in the summer of 1930 by Professor R. A. Millikan and the writer, operates in a uniform magnetic field up to 18,000 gauss. Exposures are automatically taken at the rate of one in 14 seconds. Out of a total of about 25,000 exposures, 1,450 photographs of cosmic-ray tracks have been obtained, which have yielded the following facts. Particles of both positive and negative charge occur in about equal numbers. Their energies range from above a billion volts in a few cases down to energies of a few million volts and less. Groups of associated tracks of both positive and negative particles occur (in our photographs as many as 12 tracks on one photograph) indicating the disintegration of atomic nuclei by the cosmic-radiation; the detailed mechanics of the absorption of the cosmic-radiation is very complex and at present not clearly understood. P. M. S. Blackett and G. Ochialini, using an automatic (tube-counter controlled) cloud-chamber, have obtained additional evidence for the existence of the free positive electron.

*Semi-conductors and their electrical properties:* R. H. FOWLER. By invitation.

*Perfect quality and auditory perspective in the transmission and reproduction of music:* F. B. JEWETT. [Printed in SCIENCE for May 12.]

*Radioactivity and the light nuclei:* R. M. LANGER and R. W. RAITT (introduced by Robert A. Millikan). The fact that the beryllium atom is unstable and disintegrates spontaneously is now established on the basis of the following evidence: (1) Purified Be metal in an ionization chamber produces a current which is about two times as great as that supplied by the thorium family contamination and a hundred times as great as that of the radium family contamination. The Ra and Th measurements were made with the double chamber emanation method capable of detecting an alpha activity one hundred times smaller than that shown by the Be. (2) The range of the particles, assumed to be alpha rays, is about one centimeter, according to Al foil measurements. This range is decidedly shorter than that of any possible contamination. (3) The helium content of beryllium minerals is out of proportion to the uranium and thorium content, but is quite consistent with the rate of decomposition which we have estimated with ionization chamber methods. (4) The excess in mass of $Be_9$ over the mass of two helium atoms and a neutron indicates on very general grounds that it is unstable. If the current theory of alpha-particle disintegration is applied to the case of $Be_9$, one finds a decay rate over $10^{30}$ times larger than that observed. However, this theory is not a general quantum mechanical deduction but depends on a model which pictures the nucleus as a composite of alpha particles. Apparently we must conclude that the Be nucleus is not composed of alpha particles. This is quite in accord with the modern theory of nuclear structure, which has had considerable success with the hypothesis that the structural units of the nucleus are the proton and the neutron.

*An ionization spectrometer for long wave-length x-rays:* F. K. RICHTMYER and S. KAUFMAN. Much of our knowledge of the x-ray spectrum in the region of wave-lengths longer than 1.5 Angstroms comes from photographic measurements. However accurate may be the values of the wave-lengths of spectrum lines determined by photographic means, such measurements are not very trustworthy in determining the shapes and relative intensities of lines and in measurements which involve the determination of x-ray energy. Because of the many problems awaiting study in the long wave-length x-ray region, we have adapted the Siegbahn high-vacuum spectrometer for ionization measurements, using the usual single crystal method. The easily attainable resolving power is such as to give observed widths of the K $\alpha$ lines of Cu(29) only a few per cent. wider than when measured by a two-crystal instrument. There seems to be no difficulty in using this instrument to make ionization-chamber measurements up to 5 or 6 Angstroms, or longer.

*A test of the "momentum transfer" theory of accommodation coefficients of ions at cathodes:* K. T. COMPTON and E. S. LAMAR. In a recent paper, read before the National Academy of Sciences, it was suggested that the accommodation coefficient for positive gas ions on a metal cathode should be less than unity only if the mass of the metal atom exceeds that of the ion. In order to test this hypothesis, experiments already reported for helium ions on molybdenum have been continued for argon ions on molybdenum and on aluminium. The cathode to be studied was the molybdenum or aluminium bob of a glass pendulum, whose deflection gave a measure of the pressure acting, and was immersed in the positive column of a low voltage argon arc. The pressures on the cathode were due to the recoil of those ions which retain some of their kinetic energy after neutralization and to radiometric effects resulting from heating of the cathode by ion bombardment. From an analysis of the data, it was possible to compute an accommodation coefficient for the positive ions. The results indicate an accommodation coefficient of about .79 for argon ions on molybdenum, and an accommodation coefficient of unity on aluminium.

*Evidence that acidosis is not caused by acids:* YANDELL HENDERSON and LEON A. GREENBERG. In recent years acidosis has been one of the most largely discussed topics in relation to illness. This condition, or group of conditions, is important. But the explanation that is now generally accepted is shown by the investigations to be reported in this communication to be erroneous. It is now supposed that the condition called acidosis arises from an excessive formation of acids in the body. This increased formation of acids is supposed to explain the great decrease of sodium bicarbonate and other alkalies in the blood. The acid chiefly concerned is lactic acid. The amount of this organic acid is increased under severe deficiency of oxygen, as in carbon monoxide poisoning, in which an asphyxial "acidosis" develops. It has recently been shown by Lundsgaard in Denmark that animals which are given a small dose of the drug monoiodoacetic acid are rendered incapable of producing lactic acid. Accordingly, in the investigations to be reported to the academy animals were first treated with this drug, and then subjected to such conditions (deficiency of oxygen) as have been found to induce a state of so-called acidosis. The result was that all the features of that state, particularly the diminution of bicarbonates in the blood, were developed, but without the formation of any increased amount of lactic acid. The conclusion that the state called "acidosis" is not due to intoxication by excessive formation of acid in the body is in accord with the fact that the administration of alkalies to patients with acidosis, as in diabetes, has not been found beneficial and has been generally abandoned. The theory that "acidosis" is intoxication by acid is an apparently logical deduction from the conception now prevailing as to the nature of the acid base equilibrium of the blood. It is, however, definitely contradicted by facts, and some other theory will have to be developed.

*Cellular reactions to lipoids from acid-fast organisms:* FLORENCE R. SABIN and KENNETH C. SMITHBURN. The lipoids in acid-fast organisms can be separated into three classes, phosphatides, fatty acids and wax-like materials. The phosphatides are an important factor in the production of the lesions of tuberculosis. They are readily dispersed in water, a property which makes it easy to test their biological reactions. They are phagocytized by monocytes which, in dealing with them, become epithelioid cells. The fatty acids, represented largely in the acetone-soluble material, stimulate all types of connective tissue cells, cause vascular dilatation and hemorrhage and induce adhesions. The wax-like materials have long been considered of great importance because they are responsible for the acid-fastness of the organisms. The wax-like material of the human tubercle bacillus is an alcohol, $C_{94}H_{188}O_4$; the corresponding material from an acid-fast organism isolated from a case of leprosy is a glyceride. These materials can not be wet with water, a property which may account for the fact that the cells deal with them in a manner different from phagocytosis. The purified substances injected in the form of a dry powder cause a multiplication of young connective tissue cells around the particles. These cells are simpler than monocytes and show no signs of being able to phagocytize the wax-like material, but rather they fuse to make foreign body giant cells to surround it. There are then signs of a change in the material which, at first opaque and granular, becomes globular and translucent. If the phosphatide has not been completely removed from the material injected, the monocytes are able to separate it from the wax. These cells then show signs of phagocytosis and become epithelioid cells. Since a single lipoidal substance gives only one type of cellular reaction, the biological tests offer a check on the degree of separation of the lipoids. Although foreign body giant cells occur in tuberculosis, it is probable that they are an accessory phenomenon in the progress of the disease and that the wax-like materials by which they are produced may be classified as biologically inert.

(*To be concluded*)

## BOOKS RECEIVED

JOCHELSON, WALDEMAR. *History, Ethnology and Anthropology of the Aleut.* Pp. v + 91. 27 figures. Carnegie Institution of Washington.

NEAVE, S. A. and others. *History of the Entomological Society of London, 1833–1933.* Pp. xlvi + 224. The Society. 10s. 6d.

# SCIENCE

VOL. 77 FRIDAY, MAY 26, 1933 No. 2004

*Preliminary Report on the Yale North India Expedition:* DR. H. DE TERRA ... 497

*A History of the National Research Council, 1919–1933. III. Division of Engineering and Industrial Research:* PROFESSOR DUGALD C. JACKSON ... 500

*Scientific Events:*
*The Industrial Fellowships of Mellon Institute during 1932–33; The Morris Arboretum of the University of Pennsylvania; The Fourth Annual Conference of Donors at the Johns Hopkins University; Symposium on the Physics of Nuclei and of High Energy Radiations; The Conference on the Diffusion of Scientific Knowledge* ... 503

*Scientific Notes and News* ... 505

*Discussion:*
*Fluorescence of Cells in the Ultra-violet:* DR. A. C. GIESE and PROFESSOR P. A. LEIGHTON. *The Boron Content of Sea Water:* DR. E. G. MOBERG and M. W. HARDING. *Persistent Strands of the Root-rot Fungus in Texas:* HOMER C. MCNAMARA, R. E. WESTER and K. C. GUNN. *The Most Northern Occurrence of Mesquite on the Great Plains:* DR. CHAS. N. GOULD ... 509

*Special Correspondence:*
*The Academy of Natural Sciences of Philadelphia* 512

*Reports:*
*Medals Presented at the Annual Dinner of the National Academy of Sciences* ... 514

*Scientific Apparatus and Laboratory Methods:*
*An Apparatus for Maintaining Artificial Respiration in Laboratory Animals:* DR. W. R. BOND. *A Special Air-chamber for Studying Photosynthesis under Natural Conditions:* PROFESSOR A. J. HEINICKE ... 515

*The National Academy of Sciences:*
*Abstracts of Papers Presented at the Washington Meeting III* ... 517

*Science News* ... 10

SCIENCE: A Weekly Journal devoted to the Advancement of Science, edited by J. MCKEEN CATTELL and published every Friday by

THE SCIENCE PRESS

New York City: Grand Central Terminal
Lancaster, Pa. Garrison, N. Y.
Annual Subscription, $6.00 Single Copies, 15 Cts.

SCIENCE is the official organ of the American Association for the Advancement of Science. Information regarding membership in the Association may be secured from the office of the permanent secretary, in the Smithsonian Institution Building, Washington, D. C.

# PRELIMINARY REPORT ON THE YALE NORTH INDIA EXPEDITION

By Dr. H. DE TERRA
YALE UNIVERSITY

## SCOPE OF THE EXPEDITION PLAN

THE idea that geological and biological sciences may support each other in research on related problems may at first appear strange, especially if they are supposed to cooperate in a task of exploration in a region so little known as the Himalayas. However, for me, who had explored formerly as a geologist in western Central Asia and northern India, it seemed quite obvious that a study of fresh-water life in these highly elevated mountain ranges would help to throw new light on the geographical conditions of the Himalayas during the Pleistocene and postglacial periods. For it was in comparatively young geological times that the Tibetan plateaus and the adjoining highlands were uplifted to form the "Roof of the World," and it was to be expected to find a peculiar faunal character with endemic forms which would reveal faunal relations to Central Asia or to India.

The geological work was to be focused on the study of those diastrophic events which resulted in the earth's highest mountain structure, north of peninsular India. Investigation of such a wide scope which was to be carried out on difficult territory required careful selection of particularly promising mountain sectors. These were to be found in Kashmir proper, where a thick Pleistocene sequence of strata in a structural basin could furnish evidence on Pleistocene orogeny. On the other hand, the eastern Karakoram, north of the Himalayas, seemed to be most profitable for an investigation of the structural outlines of this northern neighbor of the Himalayas. Geomorphological observations were to support the structural studies. A topographical survey was to facilitate this work. Finally, there was a good chance for collecting vertebrate fossils in the richly fossiliferous Siwalik formations south of the Himalayas.

Owing to the great interest which this plan of mine found at Yale, and thanks to the kind support it received by its President, of Professor Ch. W. Warren, dean of Sheffield Scientific School, of Professors R. S. Lull and R. G. Harrison, I could start with the field work on March 1, 1932.

The biological work had been entrusted to Mr. E. G. Hutchinson, assistant professor of biology at Yale; the paleontological collecting to Mr. G. E. Lewis, of the Peabody Museum at New Haven. Temporary additional members of the staff were: Mr. A. M. N. Ghosh, of the Geological Survey of India, and Khan Sahib Afraz Gul Khan, surveying officer of the Survey of India.

### Collecting and Studies in the Salt Range

The first field trip led to the Salt Range in the Punjab, where each of the members pursued their own scientific tasks. Following a personal request from Professor Charles Schuchert, of Yale University, a collection of invertebrate fossils in the well-known and highly fossiliferous Permian and Triassic limestones of the Salt Range was to be made. Owing to the generous help of Dr. L. L. Fermor, director of the Geological Survey of India, Mr. Ghosh from the Survey was made available for this work. He collected first under my supervision and later independently near Warcha, Amb and Chideru. New sections of the Permian formation were also studied at these places, and it is hoped that these new data will throw additional light on the age of the Permian glaciation. In Professor Schuchert's opinion this collection turned out to be very satisfactory, as almost all Waagen's types and additional genera are represented.

Hutchinson studied some salt lakes on the central plateau of the Salt Range northwest of Kushab. The paleontological collecting continued in the area of the upper Soan River until the middle of May.

### Geological and Biological Work in Kashmir

On March 18, my wife, Mr. Hutchinson and I moved from the Punjab to Srinagar, Kashmir. This city through its central location in the Kashmir Valley made a convenient place for expedition headquarters. Here camp and other additional equipment could be purchased for the summer trip to western Tibet and the Karakoram Ranges. Furthermore, all excursions into the Kashmir Valley, be it by houseboat, car or pony caravan, could be arranged from Srinagar. Hutchinson spent from March 24 until May 10 on the large lakes: Dal-, Anchar-, Manasbal- and Wular-lake and on the Jhelum River as well. I could almost devote the same amount of time, though frequently interrupted by preparations for the coming summer trip, to the geological study of the Valley of Kashmir. Middlemiss had already found through former studies that the so-called Karewa formation (Pleistocene) of the Kashmir Valley had been disturbed and folded along the southern flank of the basin. The exact age of these clay, sandstone and gravel series had since Godwin Austin's time always been disputed. Lack of fossil evidence and of a closer field study prevented the stratigraphic classification of these interesting strata which evidently had taken part in Hamalayan diastrophism. During the spring and later again in the fall of 1932, I found several new and highly important fossil localities in the Karewa. In gray fat clays, presumably belonging to an interglacial period (of Illinoian-Wisconsin age), I found three rich plant localities. Prominent amongst the plants are, besides *Alnus, Populus, Quercus,* the genera *Buxus, Trapa* and *Charophytes,* and Cinnamon, indicating a climate similar but somewhat warmer than Kashmir enjoys nowadays. These plant-bearing clays were found overlain by moraine material of the last glacial stage. The upper Karewa beds yielded a great number of fresh-water shells, plants, and the remains of a straight tusked Proboscidian. The latter was found near Sombur, being probably the first Himalayan representative of a mammoth. Only six miles distant from this locality I came across some prehistoric artefacts lying in the upper Karewa beds. On another locality I believe to have found similar, although somewhat doubtful, implements. As not only the lower but also the upper Karewa have been tilted and dragged high upward along the Pir Panjal Range, it seems obvious that a diatrophic phase of late Pleistocene, and even possibly of later date, resulted in renewed uplift of the flanking Himalayan Ranges in the region of the upper Jhelum River. This uplift may be estimated from 6,000 to 8,000 feet.

Hutchinson's work in the lakes in Kashmir resulted in a large collection of fish and various fresh-water forms and in gathering chemical and other biological data. The faunal character appeared to be different from that of the Indian lowlands, with quite a number of endemic forms. As the ancient lake beds of subrecent and Quaternary origin contain a great number of fossil shells, it should be possible to find considerable amount of evidence on the late Pleistocene-alluvial history of the Kashmir Lake basin.

### Expedition Activities in the High Himalayas and Eastern Karakoram

Around the middle of May the expedition members united at Srinagar to prepare for the start to the highlands of western Tibet. A caravan carrying food and biological apparatus was sent ahead to Leh, capital of Ladakh, in the upper Indus Valley. Khan Sahib Afraz Gul Khan, our surveyor, with his two servants, had joined us here and we all left Srinagar on May 16. Within two weeks we crossed the northwest Himalaya on the "High Treaty Road" into Ladakh, and arrived at Leh on June 2. An excursion to the great monastery of Hemis proved to be a unique experience, as we witnessed the lamaistic mystery play. This short trip into a side glen of the Indus Valley brought me also a large collection of old Tertiary plants, of which I had found a few traces during my first journey in 1927. On June 21, we left Leh for the Panggong Lake and crossed the southern Karakoram Ranges, taking the route *via* Digar- and Shakya Pass (18,100 feet) to Tankse and Lukong. The great Panggong lake basin (13,915 feet), extending from Ladakh into the Tibetan province of Rudok, and containing one of the largest, high mountain lakes north of the Himalayas, afforded good possibilities for our geological and biological work. The lake, now salty, must have been a fresh-water lake of considerable depth and extension during the last interglacial period. Shell-bearing lake beds containing fish vertebrae are overlain by morainic boulder. As in the case of the Kashmir Valley, the fossil remains of fresh-water life will help to reconstruct the changes in biological conditions during postglacial times.

From the Panggong an excursion led to the high valley of Koh-lungpa (17,250 feet) and across the main Karakoram Range to Ororotse Tso. This lake (17,383 feet) was found still solidly frozen on July 12, but it proved to be very rich in fresh-water life. The main axis of the Karakoram Range, bending here from a northwest-southeast into a west-easterly trend, was crossed a second time on our way to the upper Chang-Chenmo Valley (17,000 feet). A line of higher snow peaks, all ranging over 21,000 feet in altitude, was found continuing south of this valley toward the Tibetan frontier, where it gradually passes over into a broken line of monadnock-like snow massives surmounting the western Tibetan plateau. This range is regarded by me as the easternmost outpost of the high Karakoram Range. Our route led us from here along the Tibetan frontier *via* Nyagzu back to the Panggong Lake.

The geological structures in this part of the Karakoram are characterized by heaving, folding and steeply inclined thrusts; the latter being between nice granite and metamorphic rocks on one hand, and fossiliferous young Paleozoic to marine Triassic and Cretaceous formations on the other. The pressure of folding must have acted vertically, but from the Mustagh-Karakoram Range on northward it seems to have thrown the folds towards Central Asia. In comparison with my former observations, I am inclined to believe that the southern Karakoram Ranges (Mustagh- and Kailas-) represent "root-zones" of large thrusts, while the adjoining highlands between the northern Karakoram and the K'un-lun Mountains are made of lesser folded portions of the Himalayan region. Evidences of thrusting on a large scale were also found in the northwest Himalayas near Karghil, where thick Triassic limestone series have been moved upon Cretaceous formations. These observations, of which only very little can be related on the occasion, lead me to believe that the geological structure of Himalaya and Karakoram is dominated by thrusting in alpine fashion. Although it still remains to be seen whether this thrusting led to a regular "Deckenstructure," the evidence rather leads to the conclusion that these highest mountain ranges show themselves not only morphologically but also structurally as true alpine ranges, which have been folded up from the bottom of the former Tethys Sea at various times in intervals from the close of the Cretaceous up to the close of the Tertiary period. The geomorphic features of this highest relief are composed of four main elements: (1) Remnants of a preglacial relief consisting of plateau relicts and piedmont levels between 16,000 and 20,000 feet altitude. (2) Glaciated high ranges and massives (20,000 to 22,000 feet), surmounting the former widely extended plateaus. (3) The glacial relief which dominates the landscape. (4) Postglacial features bearing evidence of wide-spread and most intense rejuvenation of rivers through broad uplift at intervals.

It was surprising to find plenty of evidences for a recent rise in the lake level of most high mountain lakes. This became especially apparent along the shores of Panggong and Tso Moriri Lake, where trigonometrical stations, religious buildings, roads and lower beach levels had been inundated by what appears to be a recent increase in precipitation. It is to be hoped that these observations, together with Dr. Haude's meteorological work in Central Asia (Swedish-Chinese Expedition of Sven Hedin), will help toward an ultimate solution of the problem of the "desiccation of Central Asia." From the Panggong we worked our way southward along the Tibetan frontier to the Pongur Tso, to Chushul, the Indus Valley, Moriri Lake in Spiti, and back to Leh.

The total route of 1,300 miles by pony and caravan, with nine important mountain lakes on our way and 4,600 square miles of newly surveyed territory, gave us ample opportunity to follow the original plan of field researches. Much credit for this undisturbed field work has to be given to my companions, my wife and Professor Hutchinson, and to our surveyor, who in spite of his strenuous work was always willing to assist me greatly in expedition matters.

During my geological investigations a great number of invertebrate fossils were collected. Aside from limnological material and a number of smaller mammals a few hundred plants have been gathered by Professor Hutchinson. He also succeeded in getting many data on the ecology of the invertebrate ground fauna at altitudes over 17,000 feet. "It is hoped," he says, "that a study of the zoogeographic realm of the invertebrates living at high altitudes will throw much light on the history of these regions. As far as it is possible to judge at present, the rather large number of species endemic to these elevated regions argues against any wholesale glaciation of the region."

The expedition returned from Ladakh to Srinagar, Kashmir, on October 2.

### Various Activities of the Expedition until January, 1933

During the last five months the various expedition members were busy in Kashmir, the Punjab, Calcutta and the Nilgiri Hills of southern India. Although the latter region was out of the general field of our studies Hutchinson was anxious to get some zoogeographical data on the fauna of the Nilgiris in relation to the "pluvial relict" hypothesis.

Mr. Lewis, who had started back in June to the more promising fields of the Siwalik formations, collected in Bilaspur State in the Simla Hills and adjacent portions of the Punjab. He also worked in the Siwalik Hills proper, from the Sutlej River to the Kaluwala Rao near Dehra Dun (United Provinces). He reports about his results as follows, "An abundance of excellent material was collected in the time available, and in addition to the large vertebrate fauna numerous invertebrates and paleobotanical specimens were secured; all of which will be added to the collections of the Peabody Museum of Natural History of Yale University."

My field work in Kashmir continued until November 23 and was then transferred partly back to the Salt Range and partly to the Siwalik foothills in the Rawalpindi district. The last excursion to the southwestern Salt Range undertaken for the sake of the tilted Pleistocene strata made me come across a prehistoric site. This was discovered first by Mr. Hutchinson, who had done biological work on the salt lake Kalakahar. A second locality was found near-by on an ancient lake terrace with three layers of implementiferous soil containing coup de poing, scrapers and rejects of presumably early paleolithic age. A human skull was found in between the upper two

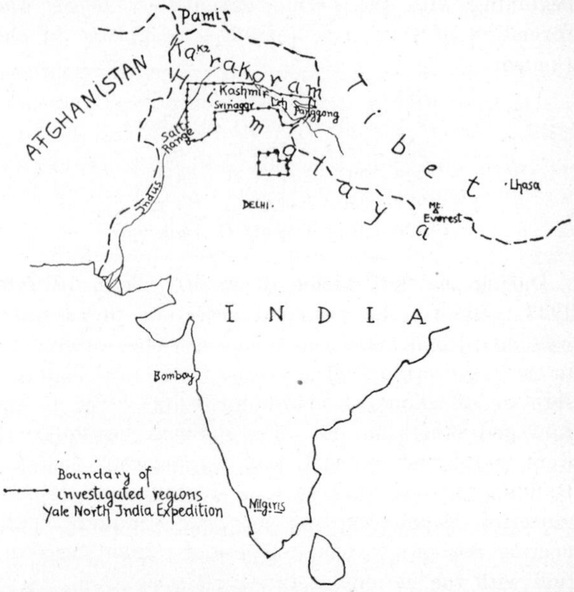


layers. With the kind permission of the director of the Indian Archeological Survey I was able to collect these traces of what appears to be the earliest settlement of prehistoric man in India.

Around the middle of January, 1933, the field work of the expedition was terminated and the members left India shortly after. The scientific collections have safely arrived at New Haven and shall be worked upon by the members of the expedition and with the aid of scientific experts.

As this undertaking was being carried out in countries which offer many natural hindrances to scientific exploration, the success of the expedition was due in great part to the help of the Government of India and various Indian scientific institutions. I greatly appreciate all the support that has been so generously extended toward us by British-Indian government officials.

H. de Terra

Yale University

# A HISTORY OF THE NATIONAL RESEARCH COUNCIL 1919–1933

## III. DIVISION OF ENGINEERING AND INDUSTRIAL RESEARCH[1]

By Professor DUGALD C. JACKSON

CHAIRMAN

The Division of Engineering was established as one of the Council's divisions in 1919 for the purpose of organizing and coordinating engineering research in industry. Its membership consists of representatives

[1] This is the third of a series of ten articles prepared to describe briefly the nature of the activities with which the National Research Council has been engaged during the past fourteen years.

from the national engineering societies and certain members-at-large.

The following persons have served as chairmen, beginning with the period immediately before the formation of the division from a committee of the Council:

1918- —Henry M. Howe
1919–1921—Comfort A. Adams
1921–1923—Alfred D. Flinn
1923–1927—Frank B. Jewett
1927–1930—Elmer A. Sperry
1930–1933—Dugald C. Jackson

During the first period of its life, from 1919 to 1923 inclusive, the principal object of the division was regarded as getting more and better research done in the engineering field, avoiding the rôle of dictatorship or of assuming credit for work which it encouraged others to do. The division headquarters were established in the United Engineering Societies Building in New York City on invitation of the Engineering Foundation and the four Founders Engineering Societies, for the purpose of intimate association with the national engineering societies.

The second period of the division, from 1923 to 1927, was one of transition. Numerous research projects which had their roots in wartime requirements were completed, and their committees were discharged to clear the decks for project activities to meet current needs.

After the Division of Research Extension was merged with the Division of Engineering in 1924, an attempt was made to balance the activities of the division between research projects *per se* and promotional efforts. The organization then was quite unique. It was a pioneering effort, with few precedents. A director and a secretary of the division were selected to guide the work of the division under the supervision of the chairman and executive committee.

In the period 1927–1933, the third of division life, research projects already started have been continued. A variety of new ways has been found for increasing effectiveness in bringing to the attention of the public, and of specialists like industrialists and bankers, the value and benefits of research in the industries. A change in the character of the promotional activities of the division from "why" to "how" do research during this period is also significant.

The major work of the division can be classified best under two main headings: (1) research projects and (2) promotion of research.

The gradual evolution of a research-project policy and the development of procedure in the administration of research projects undertaken for study has been indicated. In the conduct of several of these projects the division has been fortunate in the cooperation of other divisions of the Council. In others its quasi-governmental standing has stood it in good stead in securing the cooperation of governmental departments. It has always had the whole-hearted support and cooperation of the interested engineering societies.

It obviously would be impossible in the space allotted to this report to describe even in brief detail each of the more than fifty research projects which have been completed during the past fourteen years or which are now under way. Two examples (one, the marine piling investigation from the list of completed projects; and the other the Highway Research Board, from current work) are therefore here selected to illustrate project policy, method of conducting project work, and the significance of results obtained.

A section of the San Francisco Bay contained many large and valuable structures, which had been erected on unprotected wooden piles over a period of several decades. In 1914 it was found that a species of shipworm previously unknown in those waters had attacked the dikes at the entrance of Mare Island Navy Yard and other structures in the bay. In 1917 signs of serious damage appeared in the dikes. Within the next four years practically every timber structure in the vicinity was damaged, with losses estimated at $15,000,000.

The National Research Council was requested to organize a study on a nation-wide scale. A national committee was formed to study the preservation of wooden structures from the attack of marine borers, and to conduct an investigation into the value and proper use of various substitutes for timber. Cooperation was secured on a comprehensive scale. Among the governmental agencies assisting were: United States Coast Guard, Navy Department, War Department, Forest Products Laboratory, Bureau of Lighthouses, Bureau of Fisheries, Coast and Geodetic Survey and Chemical Warfare Service. Other cooperating organizations included the American Railway Engineering Association, American Association of Port Authorities, Harvard University, Massachusetts Institute of Technology, University of California, American Museum of Natural History and the Smithsonian Institution. Funds amounting to more than $50,000 were contributed by twenty-eight railroads, steamship lines and industrial companies. In addition to the organizations already mentioned, agencies of state and municipal governments, industries and harbor property owners over the world furnished services and materials. Two other divisions of the Council assisted in this work, namely, those of biology and agriculture, and chemistry and chemical technology.

As a consequence of this coordinated investigation, accurate knowledge is now available of conditions existing in all our ports on the Atlantic, Gulf and Pacific Coasts, including Alaska and our insular possessions. We know the habits of these borers, their life cycle, their breeding seasons, how to prevent their attack, how to preserve structures and also how to counter-attack. The completed report occupies a book of 534 printed pages and was widely distributed and used throughout the world as a reference book.

The Highway Research Board was organized in 1920 to assist in outlining a comprehensive program of highway research and to coordinate activities thereunder, to organize specific projects of highway investigation, and to act in a general advisory capacity.

The value of quasi-governmental standing of the Council is exemplified by the work of this board. The executive order of the President of the United States permits the Department of Agriculture to support and assist this project to a degree which would be impossible were it sponsored under other auspices. In this particular case total cash contributions from various sources have been more than $200,000. The wide-spread affiliations of the board are indicated by the fact that it has direct representation from every state highway department and many of the leading engineering colleges.

Time will not permit the review of other research projects completed or under way, such as those in heat transmission, electric and gas welding, molding sands and fatigue of metals under repeated stress. One special project quite different in character from the foregoing, the World Engineering Congress, is worthy of mention on account of its international character. The congress of 1929 was held in Japan under the auspices of the Kogakkai (Engineering Society of Japan) during the months of October and November. The purpose of these congresses, which are held at intervals of several years, is to advance and diffuse knowledge by presentation of papers and discussions on engineering subjects, to interchange views on various phases of professional engineering work, to promote international cooperation in the application of engineering science, and to cultivate a feeling of fellowship among engineers of the world.

The Division of Engineering and Industrial Research was selected by representatives of the American engineering societies to act as a sponsor body and to initiate activities on behalf of American engineers. Eighty papers by invited American authorities were prepared for the congress under this sponsorship, representing a cross-section of engineering developments in this country. The congress was personally attended by a large delegation from the United States, whose eminence in the profession reflected credit on American engineering and added to international friendships.

The promotional efforts of the division have been adapted in character and purpose to the state of industry. At the outset special attention was given to an exposition of the value of research in the industries. Activities at the present moment include, in addition to the above, special emphasis on "how to do research," on the promotion of research within trade associations for the benefit of their respective fields of industry and trade, and on fuller recognition of the university as a seat for the conduct of research in cooperation with industry.

Two domestic inspection tours of representative research laboratories have been sponsored and arranged for groups of industrial executives and bankers related to various fields of industry and from different geographical areas.

Eighty-five executives, including chairmen of boards, presidents, vice-presidents and general managers of industrial corporations and financial institutions, participated in the first one (1930). The general plan of organization, the type of problems selected for the research laboratory and methods used in their solution were studied. The importance and benefits to the particular industry derived from each laboratory were also discussed. These laboratories were mostly those maintained by large individual companies, but the tour program included the U. S. Bureau of Standards and the laboratory of a trade association.

The second tour of research laboratories was patterned after the first, but emphasized the significant feature that industrial research is not an affair exclusively for large companies. Under the critical financial conditions prevailing in the autumn of 1931, it is significant that nearly sixty representative industrial executives and bankers participated in this tour. While the number was not so large as in the previous tour, the geographical representation from as far west as the Pacific Coast and as far south as New Orleans demonstrated appreciation of the opportunities afforded by these tours.

Encouragement of research by trade associations has included the presentation of suitable addresses before association meetings, arrangement for key executives and research committees to visit successful research laboratories, suggestions as to the formation of research committees, the type of problems to be selected for study, the financing of the research projects, and the selection of laboratory facilities. Such assistance has been rendered to the textile, fisheries, brick and clay, glass-container, motion-picture, porcelain-enamel, steel-construction and aviation industries. A great deal of work remains to be done in this field.

Recognizing the need for promotional efforts designed to demonstrate "how to do research," the division sponsored the preparation of a book entitled, "Profitable Practice in Industrial Research." Fourteen distinguished men in science and in scientific research collaborated in the preparation of this volume, thus making available their experience and achievement in the development of a technique in industrial research.

In order to carry out effectively its promotional efforts, the division has found it necessary to keep at hand various types of information which may be useful to those who are considering the establishment of research laboratories or their proper administration. Examples of these are: bibliographies, surveys, plans for laboratory layouts and the book, "Profitable Practice in Industrial Research."

# SCIENTIFIC EVENTS

## THE INDUSTRIAL FELLOWSHIPS OF MELLON INSTITUTE DURING 1932–33

THE past fiscal year of Mellon Institute, ended February 28, 1933, covered a period of commercial dullness throughout the country. Notwithstanding the severe depression, however, the industrial fellowship activities in the institution were just as extensive and important as in 1931–32.

During 1932–33, 67 fellowships—18 multiple and 49 individual fellowships—were in operation, on which the services of 109 fellows and 28 assistants were required. At the close of the year 55 fellowships—14 multiple and 41 individual fellowships—were active, and 83 fellows and 15 assistants held positions thereon. Twenty-six fellowships have been at work for five years or more, and of this number 14 have concluded 10 years of research and nine fellowships have been operating for 15 years or longer.

In the last fiscal year $616,360 was received by the institute from fellowship donors to defray the cost of scientific investigations carried on for these companies and associations. The money appropriated by donors to the institute during the past twenty-two years amounts to $8,893,378.

Nine new fellowships began operation during 1932–1933, and 12 fellowships concluded their investigational programs in that year. During the calendar year 1932, 2 bulletins, 40 research reports, and 27 other papers were contributed to the literature by members of the institute. Forty U. S. patents and 62 foreign patents were issued to fellows. The total publications for the twenty-two years ended December 31, 1932, have been as follows: 18 books, 107 bulletins, 653 research reports, 961 other articles and 485 U. S. patents.

Many notable advances were made by the fellowships of 1932–33, and releasable facts regarding this investigational progress are presented in the twentieth annual report of the director, Dr. E. R. Weidlein, to the institute's trustees. Especially noteworthy were the research accomplishments of the industrial fellowships on air pollution, coke, commodity standards, food varieties, organic synthesis, packaging, petroleum production, protected metals, shoes and sugar. A large number of new products were developed and many of them were introduced commercially by fellowship donors. The urgent necessity for reviving business has been spurring many manufacturers to try through scientific investigation to evolve novel commodities as well as to improve their plant and merchandising practises. Throughout 1932–33 the very enthusiastic cooperation of donors in need of research results has expedited the work of their fellowships.

In addition to the numerous strictly technologic investigations of its fellowships and the constantly productive activities of its department of research in pure chemistry, the institute is studying the economic and social aspects of industrial research. Staff members of the organization are also aiding unemployed scientific men and engineers in securing professional posts, and are advising and encouraging the many companies that appeal to the institution for technical assistance.

The construction of the institute's new building is being continued despite prevailing business conditions. By the end of 1932 about 80 per cent. of the limestone had been set in place in the exterior, and during the subsequent two months practically all this work was completed. So far 235,000 cu. ft. of limestone and 22,000 cu. ft. of granite have been used, and only a very small amount of stone remains to be placed at the four corners of the edifice. The interior mechanical work is progressing, and it is thought now that the institute can occupy the building in the summer of 1934.—W. A. HAMOR.

## THE MORRIS ARBORETUM OF THE UNIVERSITY OF PENNSYLVANIA

THE Morris Arboretum in Chestnut Hill, which was bequeathed to the University of Pennsylvania by the late Miss Lydia Thompson Morris, will be formally dedicated at exercises to be held there on Friday, June 2.

On Saturday there will be a private viewing of the arboretum by officers and members of various horticultural societies and by others actively interested in the promotion of horticulture, and on Sunday the arboretum will be opened for the first time for inspection by the public.

The program for the dedicatory exercises on June 2 will be opened with a scientific session to be conducted at the arboretum at 11 o'clock, with Dr. Thomas S. Gates, president of the university, presiding.

At this session addresses will be made by President Gates; Dr. Rodney H. True, chairman of the department of botany at the university and director of the arboretum; Dr. A. H. Reginald Buller, professor of botany at the University of Manitoba, and Dr. Robert A. Harper, who is Adrian professor emeritus of botany at Columbia University.

Following the scientific session, officials of other well-known arboretums, distinguished scientists and men prominent in various other fields, who will be among the university's guests, will attend a buffet luncheon at the arboretum.

At a convocation to be held there at 3 o'clock on the afternoon of June 2 an address will be delivered by Dr. A. Lawrence Lowell, president of Harvard University, and three honorary degrees will be conferred. In addition there will be a brief ceremony during which custody of the arboretum will be formally transferred to the university.

Preceding the convocation, over which President Gates will preside, will be a formal academic procession. The Rev. W. Brooke Stabler, chaplain of the university and Boardman lecturer on Christian ethics, will give the invocation, and the ceremony of transferring custody of the arboretum will follow.

In this ceremony Maurice Bower Saul, attorney, will represent the executors and trustees of the Morris estate, while President Gates will accept custody of the arboretum on behalf of the university.

At the conclusion of his address, the degree of doctor of laws will be conferred upon President Lowell, and the degree of doctor of science upon Dr. Buller and Dr. Harper, speakers at the morning scientific session.

For the private viewing on Saturday, June 3, the arboretum will be open from 10 A. M. until 5 P. M. For the public inspection on Sunday it will be open from 1 to 6 P. M.

The Morris Arboretum, which overlooks the picturesque Whitemarsh Valley, consists of two estates of approximately 160 acres upon which Miss Morris, who died on January 24, 1932, and her brother, the late John T. Morris, developed one of the finest collections of botanical specimens in the United States. One of these estates, "Compton," where Miss Morris made her home, lies in Philadelphia County, while "Bloomfield," the adjoining estate, is situated in Montgomery County. Compton includes about eighty-five acres of highly diversified land with hillsides and valleys and several small streams. The original estate on which the residence now stands was first planted by Mr. Morris, but subsequently additional land was purchased and on this land later plantings were made by Mr. Morris and, after his death in 1915, by Miss Morris.

In addition to bequeathing the arboretum to the custody of the university, Miss Morris also left the residue of her property, after certain bequests, to constitute an endowment for the arboretum's maintenance and development.

## THE FOURTH ANNUAL CONFERENCE OF DONORS AT THE JOHNS HOPKINS UNIVERSITY

THE donors of the fellowships established under the National Fellowship Plan of the Department of Chemistry of the Johns Hopkins University held their fourth annual conference at the university on May 5. The program for the day included addresses by Dr. C. E. Kenneth Mees, director of the Eastman Kodak Company, and Dr. Irving Langmuir, Nobel Laureate in Chemistry. Discussion of the fellowship plan, and visits to the research laboratories of the fellowship students also played a part in the program.

Dr. Joseph S. Ames, president of the Johns Hopkins University, opened the meeting in the morning. In the afternoon, discussion of the fellowship plan centered especially about the following points: the value of the selection of candidates by personal interview; the present research work of the fellowship men, and a comparison of the careers of those appointed for the fellowship and those not appointed, based on a statistical report which was drawn from questionnaires returned by the candidates of former years.

President Ames, at this time, announced the developments under the plan for the year 1932–33. He stated that the H. A. B. Dunning Fellowship for Maryland, given by Dr. Dunning, of Baltimore, and the F. G. Donnan Fellowship for England, given by Dr. Walter A. Patrick, have been endowed. Dr. A. R. L. Dohme, of Baltimore, has renewed for a four-year period his lectureship established to bring noted scientists to lecture at the university.

At 2:30, Dr. C. E. K. Mees delivered a short address on "Scientific Research and Industrial Depression" over WBAL broadcasting station. Dr. Mees gave a more extended discussion of this same topic at the university at 4:00. In his address, he sought to defend scientific research against the charge that "the troubles of the modern world are really due to the advance of science."

The evening program of the conference was opened by a dinner at the Baltimore Country Club, given by President Ames in honor of the donors, the chemistry faculty and the speakers of the occasion.

Concluding the program for the day, Dr. Irving Langmuir, who recently received the Nobel award in chemistry, gave an exposition of recent research in the field of "Two Dimensional Gases, Liquids and Solids." His topic was of especial interest to advanced chemists and physicists.—N. E. G.

## SYMPOSIUM ON THE PHYSICS OF NUCLEI AND OF HIGH ENERGY RADIATIONS

THERE was held from May 11 to 26 at the Norman Bridge Laboratory of Physics of the California Institute of Technology at Pasadena, a symposium on "The Physics of Nuclei and of High Energy Radiations," with the following program:

"Some Considerations on Cosmic Rays," Professor P. S. Epstein.
"The Free Positive Electron," Dr. C. D. Anderson.
"The Foundations of Atomic Mechanics," Professor Niels Bohr, of the University of Copenhagen.
"A Review of the Experimental Evidence for Neutrons," Professor C. C. Lauritsen.
"The Foundations of Atomic Mechanics," Professor Niels Bohr.
"Artificial Disintegration of Nuclei," Professor E. O. Lawrence, of the University of California.
"Recent Cosmic Ray Observations," Dr. H. V. Neher.
"The Foundations of Atomic Mechanics," Professor Niels Bohr.
"Spontaneous Nuclear Decomposition," Dr. R. M. Langer.
"The Foundations of Atomic Mechanics," Professor Niels Bohr.
"The Absorption and Scattering of High Energy Radiations," Professor J. R. Oppenheimer.

In addition to his participation in the symposium, Professor Bohr delivered a general lecture on the subject, entitled "'Explanation' in Natural Science." In this lecture he described the gradual change which the idea of mechanical explanation has undergone and the general outlook to which we are led regarding the problems in biology and psychology.

## CONFERENCE ON THE DIFFUSION OF SCIENTIFIC KNOWLEDGE

THE summer meeting of the American Association for the Advancement of Science in Chicago will give opportunity for a unique gathering that deserves the special attention of scientific men. This is a Science Service Conference on the Diffusion of Scientific Knowledge which will be held on Friday, June 23. It will partake of the character of an international conference in which distinguished scientists from other countries will participate. It is hardly necessary to comment on the importance of the widest and most effective possible dissemination of information concerning advances in the scientific field. A few facts regarding the origin and general plan of the symposium will be of interest.

Last January the executive committee of Science Service sought to determine the most appropriate way in which that institution could cooperate with the association and the Century of Progress in the Chicago meeting. Out of that discussion came a plan to hold a conference on the diffusion of scientific knowledge with contributions from representative scientists of the various countries participating in the meetings. The value of such a conference was so clear that the officers in charge of the Chicago program enthusiastically approved the idea. The executive committee of Science Service requested its chairman, Dr. W. H. Howell, to arrange the symposium and to secure speakers from among the foreign guests representing the Scandinavian countries, England, France, Germany and Italy. In this way it is hoped to present a picture of methods employed in various parts of the world to bring scientific research before the public, and to provide an opportunity for scientific men from different countries to express their views in regard to the purposes to be sought and the means to be used in the popularization of science.

The speakers at the conference will include: Professor Joseph Barcroft, professor of physiology, University of Cambridge; Professor Niels Bohr, director of the Institute for Theoretical Physics, Copenhagen University, Copenhagen; Professor Filippo Bottazzi, professor of physiology, University of Naples; Professor Jean Dufrénoy, director of the Station of Agricultural Pathology, Brive (Corrèze), France; Professor Robert A. Millikan, director of the Norman Bridge Laboratory of Physics, California Institute of Technology. Dr. J. McKeen Cattell, president of Science Service, will preside at the conference.

The Science Service conference will be held at a luncheon meeting at the Hotel Stevens, on Friday, June 23, at 12:45 P. M. An invitation is extended to all interested to attend. Tickets will be obtainable at the American Association for the Advancement of Science registration booth, upon arrival in Chicago.—W. H. H.

# SCIENTIFIC NOTES AND NEWS

DR. FRANK SCHLESINGER, director of the Yale University Observatory, has been elected a correspondent of the Paris Academy of Sciences in succession to the late Professor H. H. Turner, of Oxford, England.

DR. HARVEY CUSHING, who was until his retirement last year Moseley professor of surgery at Harvard University, was presented with the Bigelow Medal by the Boston Surgical Society on May 3, for his "contributions to the advancement of surgery." Previous recipients of the medal have been: 1921, Dr. William J. Mayo, Rochester, Minnesota; 1922, Dr. William W. Keen, Philadelphia; 1926, Dr. Rudolph Matas, New Orleans; 1928, Dr. Chevalier Jackson, Philadelphia; 1931, Professor George Grey Turner, Newcastle-upon-Tyne, England, and 1932, Dr. John M. T. Finney, Baltimore.

DR. CARROLL C. PRATT, of the department of psychology of Harvard University, was among those recently elected fellows of the American Academy of Arts and Sciences in Class IV, Section 1, which includes theology, philosophy and psychology.

AT the recent Montreal meeting of the Electrochemical Society the Edward Goodrich Acheson Medal was awarded to Dr. Colin G. Fink, of Columbia University. Lawrence Addicks, chairman of the medal committee, in presenting his report stated that the award was made to Dr. Fink on account of his record of distinction as an original investigator, as an inventor and as a teacher of electrochemistry. The formal presentation of the medal will take place at the fall meeting of the society, Chicago, September 7 to 9, 1934.

*Popular Astronomy* notes that Sir Frank Dyson and Lady Dyson were recently guests of honor at a complimentary luncheon in recognition of the effective service Sir Frank had rendered during a period of twenty-three years as astronomer royal of England and of his attainments and achievements in astronomy. Speeches of congratulation were made by Professor F. J. M. Stratton and Dr. W. A. Parr, presidents, respectively, of the Royal Astronomical Society and the British Astronomical Association.

DR. ARTHUR E. MORGAN, president of Antioch College and president of the Dayton-Morgan Engineering Company, has been appointed by President Roosevelt to be chairman of the Tennessee Valley Power Authority, the supervisory body which is to direct the development of Muscle Shoals.

FRANK W. PECK, director of extension of the department of agriculture of the University of Minnesota since 1921, has been appointed to the staff of the federal farm board under its chairman, Henry Morgenthau, Jr. He has applied to the university regents for a year's leave of absence to take up this work.

WATSON DAVIS, since 1923 managing editor of Science Service, has been elected director. This position has been vacant since the death in 1929 of Dr. Edwin E. Slosson, the first director. The following officers of Science Service were reelected at its recent annual meeting: Dr. J. McKeen Cattell, *president;* Dr. W. H. Howell, *vice-president* and *chairman of the executive committee;* Harry L. Smithton, *treasurer;* Watson Davis, *secretary;* Dr. C. G. Abbot and Marlen Pew, *members of the executive committee.*

DR. DEAN LEWIS, surgeon-in-chief of the Johns Hopkins Hospital, will be installed as president of the American Medical Association in Milwaukee on June 12.

THE new officers for 1933–1934 of the Electrochemical Society elected at the Montreal meeting are: Dr. John Johnston, of the U. S. Steel Corporation, *president;* H. S. Lukens (University of Pennsylvania), E. F. Cone (of *Iron Age*) and S. G. Blaylock (Trail, B. C.) *vice-presidents;* S. D. Kirkpatrick, editor, *Chemical and Metallurgical Engineering,* O. W. Storey, Chas. F. Burgess Laboratories, Inc., and T. F. Baily, Alliance, Ohio, *managers;* Dr. Robert M. Burns, of the Bell Telephone Laboratories, *treasurer,* and Dr. Colin G. Fink, of Columbia University, *secretary.* The Weston Fellowship ($1,000) for 1933–1934 was awarded to Mr. R. D. Blue, a graduate of the University of Indiana. The Electrochemical Society's annual prize to young authors went to Frank W. Godsey, Jr., of New Haven, for his paper on "Electrolytic Condensers."

THADDEUS MERRIMAN, chief engineer of the New York City Board of Water Supply, has been elected president of the Metropolitan Section of the American Society of Civil Engineers. David B. Steinman, consulting engineer, was elected vice-president, and Jacob S. Langthorn was chosen treasurer. Arthur G. Hayden, William W. Brush and E. M. Van Norden were elected directors.

NEWLY elected officers of the University of Cincinnati Chapter of Sigma Xi are: *President,* Dr. Shiro Tashiro, professor of biochemistry in the Medical College; *Vice-president,* Dr. Robert A. Kehoe, director of the Kettering Laboratory; *Secretary-treasurer,* Dr. Saul B. Arenson, associate professor of inorganic chemistry, College of Engineering and Commerce; *New Members of the Nominating Committee,* Dr. Chas. N. Moore, department of mathematics, and Dr. D. A. Wells, department of physics.

MR. CHARLES AUGUSTUS CARLOW was elected president of the Mining Institute of Scotland at the recent annual meeting.

DR. GEORGE F. BUCHAN has been elected chairman of the council of the Royal Sanitary Institute for the session 1933–34, in succession to Dr. Charles Porter, whose term of office has expired.

A GRANT of $500 has been made from the Marsh Fund of the National Academy of Sciences, under which M. K. Elias, of the Kansas Geological Survey, will carry on field studies of fossils of western Kansas, Nebraska and South Dakota. Dr. Elias will begin the field work in Cheyenne, Rawlins, Rooks and Graham Counties.

MISS ANNE HEYMAN was awarded the first prize of $300 for her paper, "The Bacteriology of Goiter," by the American Association for the Study of Goiter at its annual meeting, which was held in Memphis, Tennessee, from May 15 to 17. The prize is awarded annually for the best paper based on original research on any phase of goiter. The present investigation was carried out in the Hygienic Laboratory at the University of Michigan under the supervision of Dr. Malcolm H. Soule.

THE American Medical Association has made a grant to the Research Department of the Barnard Free Skin and Cancer Hospital of St. Louis, to support studies, under the direction of Dr. M. G. Seelig, of the carcinogenic action of scarlet red and dibenzanthracene 1:2:5:6.

THE Daniel-Pidgeon fund for 1933 of the Geological Society of London has been awarded to Mr. J. D. Solomon, for work on the correlation of the Pleistocene deposits of southeastern England with those of the Continent.

THE Carnegie Corporation has recently voted $30,000 to the Research Grant Board of the Union of South Africa to support specific scientific research projects which may be selected by the board. This grant from the corporation's special fund (applicable elsewhere than in the United States) supplements a previous grant of $50,000 voted in 1927. The membership of the board is as follows: Professor Robert B. Young, *chairman;* Sir Spencer Lister; Professor L. Fouche; Dr. J. McCrae, and Dr. P. J. du Toit. Among the projects already carried out are: Lepidoptera of South Africa, by Dr. A. J. T. Janse; Engraved Stones of Bechuanaland and Griqualand West, by Miss M. Wilman; Music and Musical Practises of the Native Peoples of South Africa, by Professor P. R. Kirby.

DR. CURT STERN, of the Kaiser Wilhelm Institut, who has been in this country since 1932, is working temporarily at the laboratory of the Carnegie Institution at Cold Spring Harbor, New York.

DR. PEDRO ARA, formerly director of the Anatomical Institute in Cordoba, Argentina, now of Madrid, Spain, is visiting the United States.

DR. PIERRE LECOMTE DU NOÜY, chief of biophysical chemistry at the Pasteur Institute, Paris, sailed for the United States on May 18. He will be in charge of the Pasteur Institute exhibit at the Chicago exposition.

DR. C. G. ROSSBY, professor of meteorology at the Massachusetts Institute of Technology, will return from Europe early in June, after an absence of eight months, during which he studied the latest advances in modern European meteorological methods.

DR. WALTER STRAUB, professor of pharmacology at the University of Munich, was a recent guest of Dr. Harvey B. Haag, professor of pharmacology at the Medical College of Virginia, Richmond. Dr. Haag worked in Dr. Straub's laboratory several years ago in Munich.

DR. JOHN H. VAN VLECK, professor of theoretical physics at the University of Wisconsin, will give this summer a course of lectures on "The Recent Developments in the Theory of Magnetism" at the University of Michigan.

DR. FREDERICK L. HISAW, professor of zoology at the University of Wisconsin, was the guest speaker at the final meeting of the year of the Iowa Section of the Society for Experimental Biology and Medicine held at the State University of Iowa on May 12. Dr. Hisaw addressed the society on "Hormones Influencing the Primate Endometrium."

MARQUETTE UNIVERSITY has announced the appointment of Dr. Edward J. v. K. Menge, director of the department of zoology, to be international guest lecturer to the national universities of Poland for the summer of 1933. He will deliver a series of six lectures interpreting the science and philosophy of America in its relations to the science and philosophy of Slavic and Latin countries. In 1927 Dr. Menge was international guest lecturer to the national universities and learned societies of Brazil, Uruguay, Argentina and Chile.

BY invitation of the senate and academic council of the University of London, Professor William King Gregory will give a series of lectures on the evolution of man at University College at the end of May. Professor Gregory sailed for England on May nineteenth and will return about the middle of June.

DR. J. BJERKNES, director of the Geophysical Institute, Bergen, Norway, who is the guest of the Century of Progress Exposition and of the American Association for the Advancement of Science for the Chicago meeting, will give a series of lectures on the stratosphere at the Massachusetts Institute of Technology early in June. Dr. Bjerknes is also expected to lecture at the University of Toronto.

PROFESSOR HENRY FAIRFIELD OSBORN sailed on May 19 for a brief visit abroad. Arriving in London on May 25 he expects to read before the Royal

Society of London a paper entitled "Principles of Biomechanical Evolution, Observed in Fossil Mammalia"; on May 29, at a regular weekly session of the Académie des Sciences of the Institut de France, the same communication will be made in French with the title "Aristogenèse, le Nouveau Principe Inductif d'Evolution Biomécanique." These two addresses are the tenth and eleventh in a series on the Origin of Species; the ninth, "Aristogenesis, the Observed Order of Biomechanical Evolution," was presented to the National Academy of Sciences on April 25. Professor Osborn's Aristogenesis conclusions are the results of his scientific observations, chiefly on titanotheres and proboscideans, for the past forty-five years. Returning to England on May 30, Professor Osborn will spend the four days before his departure on June 3 in reexamining the famous Piltdown specimens in the British Museum and comparing with the originals the drawings that were prepared for him by Miss Barbara Hopkins; he hopes also to return with Mr. J. Reid Moir to the Piltdown and Foxhall localities, to make further study of the geology of these regions, in preparation for his forthcoming revision of "Men of the Old Stone Age."

THE one hundred and eighty-sixth regular meeting of the American Physical Society will be held at Chicago from June 19 to 24, as a joint meeting with Section B of the American Association for the Advancement of Science. On Monday morning, June 19, there will be sessions for the reading of contributed ten-minute papers. The remainder of the week will be devoted to symposia, public lectures and other forms of entertainment connected with the Century of Progress Exposition. The titles of the symposia are: "Applications of Quantum Mechanics in Chemistry"; "Isotopes"; "Age of the Earth"; "Applications of Spectroscopy in Astronomy"; "Nuclear Disintegration." Among distinguished foreign guests will be: F. W. Aston, Niels Bohr, J. Bjerknes, J. D. Cockcroft, Madame Curie, E. Fermi and A. Sommerfeld. They will participate in the symposia together with members of the American Physical Society.

THE sixth power show at Chicago previously scheduled for the Coliseum will be transferred to the Exhibition Hall of the Stevens Hotel, the center of "Engineering Week" activities of the Century of Progress. This change in location will permit the engineering profession visiting Chicago to visit the show while attending their meetings, and brings together the "Engineers' Day" banquet and the exhibit in the same building. Approval of participating in "Engineering Week" of the World's Fair has been given already by 19 engineering associations. Others will also participate. The organizations cooperating are as follows: American Association for the Advancement of Science, American Association of Engineers, American Ceramics Society, American Foundrymen's Association, American Institute of Electrical Engineers, American Institute of Mining and Metallurgical Engineers, American Society of Civil Engineers, American Society of Mechanical Engineers, American Society of Municipal Engineers, American Society for Testing Materials, American Society of Agricultural Engineers, National Council of State Boards of Engineering Examiners, Society for the Promotion of Engineering Education, Society of Industrial Engineers, Institute of Radio Engineers, Western Society of Engineers, American Society of Refrigerating Engineers, American Welding Society, National Industrial Advertisers Association, National District Heating Association.

AT the annual meeting of the District of Columbia Chapter, Society of the Sigma Xi, held on May 9, Lyman James Briggs, acting director of the National Bureau of Standards; George Walter McCoy, director of the National Institute of Health, and Matthew William Stirling, chief of the Bureau of American Ethnology, Smithsonian Institution, were presented as members-elect, and an illustrated address was given by Dr. Paul Bartsch, curator of the division of mollusks, Smithsonian Institution, who presented some of the results of his recent exploration of marine life in the deeps near the West Indies. The president-elect for the coming biennium is Dr. Alexander Wetmore, assistant secretary of the Smithsonian Institution.

THREE new buildings have been erected at Bear Mountain for the Trailside Museum of the American Museum of Natural History, which opened for the season on May 1. The buildings were erected by the Commissioners of Palisades Interstate Park under direction of William A. Welch, general manager and chief engineer, and John Tamsen, park superintendent. The wooden craft-house and garage were replaced by buildings of native stone, and a new Geology Trailside Museum, also of native rounded boulders, was built. The new museum will house exhibits of minerals and rocks of the region, relief models, reference collections and a library. New stone steps and bridges have been built along the trail at several points, a new approach has been made to Geology Point overlooking the Hudson River, and more parking space and other improvements have been added.

WORD has been received that the preparation of the English manuscript of the International Rules of Botanical Nomenclature adopted at Cambridge in 1930 has been completed. This draft was sent to Germany and France about February 1 for translation. It is expected that these rules will be published during 1933.

# DISCUSSION

## FLUORESCENCE OF CELLS IN THE ULTRA-VIOLET

THE corpse-like appearance of human skin due to fluorescence in the ultra-violet is familiar to all who recall the mercury lamps formerly used in photography.

Fluorescence of living tissues may have been observed long ago, but it was not understood until after Stokes explained the nature of fluorescence in physical systems in 1852.[1] As early as 1855 Helmholtz[2] had made a careful study of fluorescence of the lens of the eye and considered the wave-lengths 3000–4000A most effective in producing fluorescence. Hertel[3] in 1905 showed that fluorescence of the cornea of the rabbit and of human skin is apparently strongest at 2320A, less distinct from 2320 to 2800A, rather feeble at 3830A, but can be detected even in the visible light at 4480A through a yellow-green filter which absorbs all the reflected 4480A. In 1909 Schanz and Stockhousen[4] reported that fluorescence of the lens of the eye begins in the blue, is more intense in the violet, and becomes most intense in the ultra-violet between 3700 and 4000A, with a maximum at 3850A. Walker[5] summarizes studies on the fluorescence of eye tissues. Stübel[6] in 1911 studied the fluorescence of a great number of other tissues, tissue products, protozoa, bacteria and various organic materials in light screened to give the wave-lengths 3000–4000A. He finds that the color of fluorescent light for different tissues varies from yellow to blue.

It seems of interest to report fluorescence of Paramecium, Oxytricha and a bacterium in the monochromatic light of the wave-lengths of the quartz mercury arc.

Paramecium multimicronucleata and Oxytricha fallax, cultured on a 0.1 per cent. lettuce infusion, were concentrated by centrifuging gently, washed in a balanced salt solution,[7] and again concentrated by centrifuging. They were then pipetted into a quartz-faced cell. Observations were made through a binocular microscope (20x) at right angles to the incident beam of light coming through a quartz monochromator from the arc.[8] The whole set-up was enclosed in a black drape to exclude stray light during observations.

The protozoans fluoresced at all the ultra-violet lines used. At 3660A the fluorescence was of a pale greenish gray shade. At 3350, 3130 and 3020A the color was more of a pale greenish blue. At 2804 and 2654A the protozoans fluoresce with a more whitish light, and as they dart into the beam of light appear like so many fireflies on a dark summer's night. At 2537A the color was again a pale greenish blue. Varying the size of the slit to change the intensity of the lines employed showed that at about equal intensities of incident radiation, fluorescence was of maximal intensity at 2804 and 2654A, of lesser but comparable intensity at 2537, 3020 and 3350A, and apparently minimal at 3130 and 3660A. The intensity of fluorescence was merely judged by the effects upon the eye of the observer.

A pseudomonad bacterium isolated from a lettuce infusion was observed in suspension in the quartz cell placed in the beam of ultra-violet light. A pale blue-green fluorescence occurred throughout the range of ultra-violet wave-lengths, but as the individual bacteria could not be seen in the set-up used, the degree of fluorescence at different wave-lengths could not be compared.

Hertel[3] states that the cornea ceases to fluoresce on death. Renschler[9] says Paramecia killed by the arc light fail to fluoresce. To determine whether death is always followed by cessation of fluorescence, protozoan cells were killed in several ways. Coagulated rapidly by the full light of the arc excluding only the heat, Paramecia showed decreased fluorescence. Killed by low intensities of monochromatic ultra-violet radiation, the Paramecia cytolized rapidly. The medium then became highly fluorescent and it was impossible to determine the nature of fluorescence of partially cytolized Paramecia or of the protoplasmic fragments. Coagulated by adding a few drops of 1.0 N HCl to the cell, the Paramecia showed greatly decreased fluorescence with apparent extinction at 3660A. But when heated until they just coagulated and studied in the ultra-violet light, Paramecia showed slightly increased fluorescence at 2537 and 2654A and little change from 2804 to 3660A. It appears then that fluorescence, of dead protozoan cells at least, depends upon the method employed in killing.

Fluorescence is chiefly of interest as one of the secondary processes following excitation of the electrons in the molecules of protoplasm by absorption of radiation. It will be noted that the abiotic wave-lengths (3000A and shorter) are strongly fluorescent. Part of the energy absorbed is emitted as light of longer wave-lengths probably without producing photochemical effects. Therefore fluorescence should

[1] Stokes, *Phil. Trans.*, p. 558, 1852.
[2] Helmholtz, *Pogg. Ann.*, 94: 205, 1855.
[3] Hertel, *Zeitschr. f. Allgem. Physiol.* 5: 95, 1905.
[4] Schanz and Stockhausen, *Arch. f. Ophthal.*, 73: 561, 1909.
[5] Walker, *Proc. Am. Acad. Sci.*, 51: 760, 1915–1916.
[6] Stübel, *Pflüger's Arch. f. d. Ges. Physiol.*, 142: 1, 1911.
[7] Barker and Taylor, *Physiol. Zool.*, 4: 620, 1931.
[8] Leighton and Blacet, *Jour. Am. Chem. Soc.*, 54: 3165, 1932.
[9] Renschler, SCIENCE, 73: 480, 1931.

be taken into account in any quantitative theory of the effects of ultra-violet light.

A. C. GIESE
P. A. LEIGHTON
STANFORD UNIVERSITY

## THE BORON CONTENT OF SEA WATER

DURING the last few years the concentration of boron in sea water has been the subject of a great deal of interest and not a little speculation on the part of workers concerned with certain phases of oceanographic chemistry. Attention to this element has been directed principally by a number of investigations of the buffer mechanism, *i.e.*, the factors that determine and regulate the hydrogen-ion concentration of sea water. In this mechanism are involved the salts of the various weak acids known to occur in sea water, namely, carbonates, bicarbonates, phosphates, arsenates, silicates and borates. However, according to the information available until very recently, only the salts of carbonic acid, and in a few localities also the silicates, are present in sufficient quantity to require notice in studying the buffer system. Nevertheless, it has been found that the behavior of the buffer mechanism in sea water is not in accord with the theory of carbonate solutions, even when allowance is made for the activity of the ions of the strong electrolytes present. To explain this discrepancy the possibility of the occurrence of buffer salts other than those of carbonic acid in appreciable quantities has been considered but, as previously stated, this possibility has not been supported by the existing analytical data. For the phosphate, arsenate and silicate reliable data have been available for a number of years, but for the borate content only one value has been reported, namely, in 1877 by Dieulafait[1] who estimated that water from the Mediterranean contains approximately 0.0002 g. per liter of boron. This is equivalent to about 0.02 millimoles of boric acid, a quantity of no significance in the buffer mechanism, since it is only 1 per cent. of the molar concentration of the total carbon dioxide.

There was also reason to suspect that the boron content of sea water varied considerably with locality because in 1859 Veatch[2] reported to the California Academy of Sciences that he had detected boron in water from along the coast between San Diego and the Strait of Juan de Fuca, but not in water from beyond fifty or sixty miles off the California coast. He found boron most abundant toward the South and concluded that in certain localities it enters the sea from submarine volcanic sources. The absolute quantities of boron found were not indicated.

[1] L. Dieulafait, *Comptes Rendus*, 85: 605–608, 1877.
[2] J. A. Veatch, *Proc. Calif. Acad. Sci.*, 2: 7, 1859.

The reason that the concentration of boron in sea water has not been adequately investigated long ago is that until recently there has been no satisfactory method for its determination. In 1932 Foote[3] described a titration method suitable for determining small quantities of boron in water but this was soon thereafter modified by Wilcox[4] who used a quinhydrone electrode for detecting the titration endpoint. Foote also determined the boron content of a sample of sea water from Ventura, California, and found it to be 4.27 parts per million.

In this laboratory the electrometric titration method of Wilcox has been used, with minor modifications necessitated by the difference in salt content between sea water and the water for which the method was developed, for analyzing about fifty samples of sea water obtained from various depths from the surface down to 500 meters off La Jolla and to 3,200 meters near the Hawaiian Islands and from the surface in several other localities, including northern California and Tortugas, Florida. In these samples the boron content varied from 4.30 to 4.80 mg. per kilogram, the average being close to 4.50 mg. This variation corresponded very closely with the variation in the salinity of the water, the average ratio between boron and halides being 0.000239, or, stated in other words, boron constitutes about 0.013 per cent. of the total solids in sea water. As boric acid this corresponds to about 0.4 millimoles per liter or, if boric acid is regarded as monobasic, to nearly 20 per cent. of the equivalent concentration of all the weak acid radicals present.

It is therefore probable that boron compounds play an important part in regulating the hydrogen-ion concentration of sea water and that some of the conclusions drawn from previous studies of the buffer system will need to be revised. These matters will be discussed in a subsequent paper.

E. G. MOBERG
M. W. HARDING
SCRIPPS INSTITUTION OF OCEANOGRAPHY
UNIVERSITY OF CALIFORNIA

## PERSISTENT STRANDS OF THE ROOT-ROT FUNGUS IN TEXAS

THE ability of the cotton root-rot fungus, *Phymatotrichum omnivorum* (Shear) Duggar,[1] to remain in the soil in a viable and infectious condition for a period of years, even when the fields are planted to

[3] F. J. Foote, *Ind. and Eng. Chem., Anal. Ed.*, 4: 39–42, 1932.
[4] L. V. Wilcox, *Ind. and Eng. Chem., Anal. Ed.*, 4: 38, 1932.
[1] B. M. Duggar, "The Texas Root-Rot Fungus and Its Conidial Stage," *Ann. Missouri Bot. Gard.*, 3: 11–23, illus., 1916.

nonsusceptible crops or kept in clean fallow, has been a question of much concern to investigators of this disease.

A partial solution of this problem was afforded when King and Loomis[2] announced the discovery of a sclerotial stage of the fungus in 1929. In the same year Dana[3] described the occurrence and infectious nature of smooth or "horse hair" strands following an 18-month clean fallow. Ratliffe[4] also reported upon a prolonged saprophytic stage of the fungus, which had hitherto been regarded by some as an obligate parasite.

During the years of 1931 and 1932 opportunity was afforded on the U. S. Cotton Breeding Field Station at Greenville, Tex., to further study the habits of the fungus in nature. Extensive searches in the soil for the source of carry-over infection was made in a number of infested plots which had been handled under different cropping and tillage conditions, and therefore permitted at least a minimum estimate as to the age and nature of the carry-over infection.

The colloidal nature of the Wilson and Houston clay soils, in which the examinations were made, presented an unusual opportunity for studying both the fungus and plant root development in their natural state of growth. An examination of a very large number of primary centers in continuous cotton plots in 1931 and 1932 revealed the fact that the carry-over infection was not due entirely to sclerotia and that the most of the infection over-wintered in the soil as strands rather than in the sclerotial stage. Examinations in a plot which was in clean fallow for the first year yielded numerous viable strands throughout the summer and fall of 1932. These strands were located, as a rule, along the old dead roots of the plants that they had destroyed the year before, or previously.

On a plot which had been in oats in 1930 and 1931, and kept in clean fallow after the crops were harvested, viable old strands were found throughout the summer of 1932, in and near primary centers of infection. These strands were found *in situ* upon the decayed remains of the old cotton roots which they had destroyed three years or more before. In some cases they were occupying the empty root channels of former plantings. When these strands were removed from the soil and placed in moist chambers, they readily put out new growth. Old strands found interlacing a colony of sclerotia in a plot which had been in clean fallow for 5 years were also viable. The age of the strands associated with colonies of sclerotia can not be determined accurately as they may have been the product of regenerated growth, from the original colony, subsequent to the fallow treatment.

The growth of the hyphae which usually took place from the ends of the old strands was characterized by radiating or parallel growth of elongated cells which freely anastomose during the early growth stages. As this growth developed, the conjugation of cells became less frequent and the more typical type of acicular hyphae with right-angled branches appeared. Histological studies showed that the older strands possessed an outer corticle ring of thick-walled, irregular shaped cells inside of which were large, elongated, thin-walled, septate cells. In younger strands the elongated cells may be smaller and the corticle layer very rudimentary or even absent.

The knowledge that strands of the root-rot fungus, in addition to the sclerotia, remain in a viable and infectious condition in the soil for several years, is worthy of note. In contrast to the more deeply seated infections of the far southwest, the strands at Greenville, Texas, were found most abundant in the surface foot of soil which render them more accessible to tillage operations or to soil disinfectants.

Homer C. McNamara
R. E. Wester
K. C. Gunn
Bureau of Plant Industry
U. S. Department of Agriculture
Greenville, Texas
November 17, 1932

[2] C. J. King and H. F. Loomis, "Further Studies of Cotton Root-Rot in Arizona with a Description of a Sclerotium Stage of the Fungus," *Jour. Agr. Research*, 39: 9, p. 641–676, illus., 1929.

[3] B. F. Dana, "Recent Development in Root-Rot Investigations," *Farm and Ranch*, 48 (46): 22–23, 1929.

[4] G. T. Ratliffe, "A Prolonged Saprophytic Stage of the Cotton Root-Rot Fungus," U. S. Dept. Agr. Circ., 67, 8 pp., illus., 1929.

## THE MOST NORTHERN OCCURRENCE OF MESQUITE ON THE GREAT PLAINS

In 1897, while collecting invertebrate fossils from the Comanche Cretaceous in southern Kiowa County, Kansas, I found a small shrub about five feet in height, which at that time was unknown to me. The next year, 1898, Dr. Lester F. Ward, the noted phytopaleontologist whom I was then assisting in collecting dicotyledonous leaf impressions from the Cheyenne sandstone, identified this shrub as mesquite (*Prosopis*). This was, I believe, the first and, so far as I am now aware, the only recorded occurrence of mesquite growing in Kansas.

The location is in the so-called "Black Hills," about four miles southeast of Belvidere, and ten miles west of Sun City. More specifically, it is in the southeast corner of Township 30 South, Range 16 West, at about 37° 20′ north latitude. Dr. Ward's interpretation of this mesquite growing so far from its natural habitat was that seeds had been carried by cattle from Texas.

The mesquite tree, which reaches its maximum size along Rio Grande River in western Texas and northern Mexico, is quite abundant in southwestern Oklahoma, especially in the counties bordering Red River south of the Wichita Mountains, where it sometimes reaches the size of 10 inches in diameter and 20 feet in height. It occurs sparingly as far east as Coal and Atoka counties, Oklahoma, being found on the prairie between the eastern end of the Arbuckle and the western end of the Ouachita mountains. It also occurs in central Oklahoma as far north as southern McClain County. Both these locations are in the drainage of Washita River.

Queerly enough, mesquite is very rare, if indeed present at all, in the drainage of the two Canadian rivers in the western part of Oklahoma. But it is found in the valley of Cimarron River north of the Canadians in the northwestern part of the state. It is especially abundant in canyons and slopes of the Gypsum Hills and in the flat lands at the foot of these hills south of Cimarron River in Blaine, Major and Woodward counties, where thousands of acres are covered with dense growths of the shrub which here rarely becomes more than eight feet in height. So far as observed, it does not here occur among the sand hills.

Mr. R. C. Tate, a local naturalist of Kenton, Oklahoma, has reported numerous specimens of mesquite shrubs along Cimarron River and its tributaries in northwestern Cimarron County, which is the westernmost of the three counties which make up the Panhandle of Oklahoma, originally known as No Man's Land or the Neutral Strip.[1]

For some years Mr. Tate has been searching for the mesquite in southern Colorado, and under date of November 17, 1932, writes me that he has finally located a specimen about a quarter of a mile north of the Colorado line, in section 15, Township 35 South, Range 49 West. This is in Baca County, 49 miles west of the southeast corner of Colorado and in latitude 37° north.

Tate also reports clumps of mesquite along Carrizo Creek in northeastern New Mexico. The location is section 15, Township 30 North, Range 35 East, about 12 miles west of the Oklahoma line, and about the same distance south of the Colorado line.

It is altogether possible that the plant may occur along the Big Bend of the Cimarron River in Morton, Stevens, Grant or Seward Counties in southwestern Kansas. If in Grant County, the locality may be farther north than the lone shrub which Dr. Ward and I found near Belvidere, southern Kiowa County, 34 years ago.

It would appear that the greater number of observers are inclined to agree with Ward that the seeds of mesquite have been carried northward by cattle. However, it might not be amiss at this time to place on record an observation by the late Colonel Charles Goodnight, famous plainsman and rancher, one of the first men to successfully raise buffalo in captivity. In his opinion the seeds were carried by wild horses or mustangs, rather than by cattle or buffalo. Colonel Goodnight, who was an unusually close observer, is reported to have said that he had frequently noted small mesquite shrubs spring up near piles of horse manure at points far distant from the natural habitat of the plant.

However, the most vexing problem is, why is the mesquite so rare, if not entirely absent, in the valley of both North and South Canadian rivers in western Oklahoma, and so abundant along the tributaries of Cimarron River still farther north? Plant ecologists please answer.

CHAS. N. GOULD
UNIVERSITY OF OKLAHOMA

[1] "Some Observations on the Spread of Mesquite to the North in Cimarron County, Oklahoma," *Proceedings* of the Oklahoma Academy of Science, Vol. VIII, 1928, p. 58.

# SPECIAL CORRESPONDENCE

## THE ACADEMY OF NATURAL SCIENCES OF PHILADELPHIA

IN a review of the 1932 activities of the Academy of Natural Sciences of Philadelphia recently issued, Charles M. B. Cadwalader, managing director, depicts its 121st year as one of marked advances, and calls special attention to new exhibits, a large increase in museum attendance and continued scientific exploration in many parts of our own and other lands.

"We have shared the common decrease in income and contributions," says Mr. Cadwalader, "but have not lessened our efforts to give Philadelphia a free natural history museum of the first order, and to continue the laboratory research that has made the academy world known. During the year we kept the museum open every day, without any change in hours, and we had 113,300 visitors, a 9 per cent. increase over 103,700 in 1931, and nearly three times as many as in 1930. Among these were 2,900 in special classes from Philadelphia schools; 2,200 from private and public schools in New Jersey, Delaware and the metropolitan area, 1,000 Boy Scouts, who entered their names in the register provided for them, and 600 pupils from the School of Industrial Art in the regular Saturday sketching classes.

"Two new animal life-groups, with backgrounds painted by C. Clark Rosenkranz, were opened—one of musk-oxen from East Greenland, the expedition and group a gift from R. R. M. Carpenter, a trustee of the academy; and one of swans from Currituck County, North Carolina, presented by Mrs. Charles W. Henry. We now have eight of these striking exhibits in North American and African Halls, and five additional ones are in course of construction. These include the remarkable giant sable antelope from Angola, West Africa, gift of Prentiss N. Gray, a trustee of the academy; also the rare giant panda from Szechuan Province, China, and the takin, a strange cattle-like mountain antelope from western China, both presented by Brooke Dolan, whose expedition collected the specimens. Two others, now partially completed, await further financing—a waterhole group of fifteen East African animals, which will be the largest in the museum, and a group of American bison, with four unusually fine specimens presented by General Harry C. Trexler, a trustee of the academy.

Additional birds needed for the half-completed display of those found in and near Philadelphia have been secured. This exhibit, which is so popular with school children, teachers and nature lovers, can be finished as soon as funds are provided.

In Mineral Hall was installed the first of a series of instructive exhibits, this one answering the question, "What is Geology?" Other additions include modern cases given by Effingham B. Morris, for effective showing of spectacular minerals; a large "ringing rock" from Bucks County, Pennsylvania; a section of the Kilbourn meteorite, and a clear crystal ball cut from a mass of quartz found in Logan, Philadelphia.

The seventeen expeditions sponsored by the academy included several of outstanding importance. Brooke Dolan, who headed an expedition to western China and Tibet, returned after eighteen months' absence with 200 mammals, 900 birds and numerous mollusks, many of them rare and nearly all new to the academy's collections, the largest and most valuable representation ever received from that part of the world.

M. A. Carriker, Jr., accompanied by H. Radclyffe Roberts, continued his bird survey of Peru, returning from his fourth expedition with 2,000 specimens. Dr. Witmer Stone says: "The importance of this work consists not only in making an inclusive collection of Peruvian birds and discovering new varieties in regions hitherto unexplored by naturalists, but also in securing data on distribution to aid in determining places of origin of the various types. It will shed further light on the development of the Andes Mountains, for our knowledge of the earth's past history is derived quite as much from such sources as from geology."

Other expeditions were as follows: Mr. and Mrs. Rodolphe M. de Schauensee to Siam, and Mr. and Mrs. Sidney J. Legendre to Indo-China, both for birds and mammals; W. Judson Coxey, a fifth expedition to Ecuador for butterflies and moths; Mrs. J. Norman Henry and Miss Josephine deN. Henry to British Columbia for plants, minerals and insects; Miss Mary G. Henry to the famous Meteorite Crater in Arizona; Edgar B. Howard to New Mexico for fossil remains; Wharton Huber to New Mexico for birds and mammals; James Bond, a sixth expedition to the West Indies for birds; Samuel G. Gordon to Canada for minerals; Arthur N. Leeds to Florida for ferns; Bayard Long and Dr. Walter M. Benner to the Carolinas and Georgia for plants, and Dr. and Mrs. Francis Harper to the Okefinokee Swamp in Georgia for plants.

More than 65,000 specimens of mammals, birds, mollusks, insects, moths, butterflies, fishes, reptiles, minerals and plants were added to the laboratory collections, which now total more than 7,000,000 specimens.

Using Cape May, New Jersey, as a base for continued study of bird migration, Dr. Witmer Stone, curator of vertebrate zoology, found an explanation of the curious northward flight of certain birds on their southward autumnal journey. His observations indicate that strong northwest winds at that season cause the birds to fly into the wind to prevent being blown out to sea. When they find feeding grounds, they delay their passage over the wide Delaware Bay until the winds abate.

Henry W. Fowler, curator of fishes and reptiles, completed the sixth and seventh volumes of his monumental work on "The Fishes of the Philippine Seas and Adjacent Waters."

Dr. Henry A. Pilsbry, curator of mollusks, discovered that the Florida pond snails do not serve as temporary hosts to the human blood fluke which causes Schistosomiasis, a serious malady spreading throughout the tropics. Comparing specimens secured by the recent expedition to the Everglades with those from Puerto Rico and the Caribbees, he found that they do not belong to the same genus, as was previously believed.

Mr. Cadwalader calls attention to the inadequacy of funds for maintenance and staff in the academy's library, which now contains 120,000 volumes. He also emphasizes the valuable services rendered during the year by the following voluntary workers: Miss Margaret N. Robins, Miss Mary Allison Reed, Miss Virginia C. Beggs, Mrs. Emmett R. Dunn, Jean Piatt, Miss Betty Shryock, Mark H. C. Spiers, Joseph Wood, Jr., Miss Anne Harbison, Ernest L. Bell, Cyrus H. Chappell, Walter S. Cosgrove, J. W. R. Rehn, Russell M. Wood, Don M. Benedict, William R. Keeney, Mrs. Francis Harper, Edward R. Barnsley, Miss Anne Wistar Comfort, Horace J. Hallowell, Miss Josephine deN. Henry, Miss Mary G. Henry and George Vaux.

A total of 4,500 members and visitors attended the meetings of the seven natural history organizations associated with the academy—the Delaware Valley Ornithological Club, the Philadelphia Mineralogical Society, the Philadelphia Botanical Club, the Leidy Microscopical Club, the American Entomological Society, the Pennsylvania Fish Culturists' Association, and the Pennsylvania State Fish and Game Protective Association.

Fenimore Johnson was elected a member of the board of trustees.

# REPORTS

## MEDALS PRESENTED AT THE ANNUAL DINNER OF THE NATIONAL ACADEMY OF SCIENCES

THERE has been printed in SCIENCE the names of those to whom the medals of the National Academy of Sciences were presented at the Washington meeting. The following statement gives some information concerning the medallists and concerning previous awards of the medals.

*Alexander Agassiz Medal for Oceanography:* Awarded to Albert Defant, of the Institut für Meereskunde, Berlin, Germany, for his studies on atmospheric and oceanic circulation and his notable contributions to theoretical oceanography. This medal is provided through the Murray Fund, a gift from the late Sir John Murray to found the Alexander Agassiz gold medal for the awarding of medals to scientific men in any part of the world, for original contributions to the science of oceanography. Ten previous awards have been made, as follows: Johan Hjort, 1913; Albert I, Prince of Monaco, 1918; C. D. Sigsbee, 1920; Otto Sven Pettersson, 1924; Vilhelm Bjerkness, 1926; Max Weber, 1927; Vagn Walfrid Ekman, 1928; J. Stanley Gardiner, 1929; Johannes Schmidt, 1930; Henry Bryant Bigelow, 1931.

*Public Welfare Medal:* For eminence in the application of science to the public welfare—awarded to William Hallock Park, of New York City, for his work as head of the research laboratories of the New York City Department of Health as a pioneer and leader both in research and in the application of scientific discovery to the prevention of disease. This medal is provided for from the Marcellus Hartley Fund, established in 1913–14 through the gift of Mrs. Helen Hartley Jenkins, in memory of her father, Marcellus Hartley. Ten previous awards have been made, as follows: G. W. Goethals, 1914; W. C. Gorgas, 1914; Cleveland Abbe, 1916; Gifford Pinchot, 1916; S. W. Stratton, 1917; Herbert Hoover, 1920; C. W. Stiles, 1921; Charles V. Chapin, 1928; Stephen Tyng Mather, 1930; Wickliffe Rose, 1931.

*John J. Carty Medal and Award for the Advancement of Science:* Awarded to John Joseph Carty, a member of the academy, since deceased, in whose honor the medal was established for his distinguished accomplishments in the field of electrical engineering, particularly as they have influenced the development of electrical communication, and also his noteworthy influence on the introduction of fundamental science and of the methods of sound scientific research as an integral and powerful tool of industrial development. This is the first award of the Carty Medal, which was established by the American Telephone and Telegraph Company in November, 1930, in recognition of Mr. Carty's noteworthy contributions to science and as a testimonial of the esteem in which he is held by his associates in the Bell System. The terms of the gift provide that the awards shall be made to an individual, for noteworthy and distinguished accomplishment in any field of science coming within the scope of the National Academy of Sciences; either for specific accomplishment in some field of science, or for general service in the advancement of fundamental and applied science.

*Henry Draper Medal:* Awarded to V. M. Slipher, Lowell Observatory, Flagstaff, Arizona (a member of the academy), in recognition of his spectroscopic researches, among the most important of which may be mentioned: (1) The discovery of "stationary" calcium lines in stellar spectra; (2) the development of efficient methods of observations of the spectra of spiral nebulae and the securing of the first observations of their radial velocities; (3) observations of bright lines and bands in the spectra of the night sky. This medal is made possible through the Henry Draper Fund, established by gift of Mrs. Henry Draper in 1883, in memory of her husband, a deceased member of the academy. Twenty-one previous awards of this medal have been made, as follows: S. P. Langley, 1886; E. C. Pickering, 1888; H. A. Rowland, 1890; H. K. Vogel, 1893; J. E. Keeler, 1899; Sir William Huggins, 1901; George E. Hale, 1904; W. W. Campbell, 1906; C. G. Abbot, 1910; H. Deslandres, 1913; Joel Stebbins, 1915; A. A. Michelson, 1916; W. S. Adams, 1918; Charles Fabry, 1919; Alfred Fowler, 1920; Pieter Zeeman, 1921; H. N. Russell, 1922; A. S. Eddington, 1924; Harlow Shapley, 1926; William Hammond Wright, 1928, and Annie Jump Cannon, 1931.

*Mary Clark Thompson Medal:* Awarded to Francis Arthur Bather, of Wimbledon, England, for his distinquished services in the fields of paleontology and geology. His principal scientific contributions are his Crinoidea of Gotland, published in Stockholm in 1893, his work on the Triassic echinoderms of Bakony in 1909, his chapters on echinoderms in Lankester's treatise on zoology, his contribution on the Cystidea from Girvan in 1913, and his studies in the Edrioasteroidea in 1915. These are in addition to many other papers on geological and biological subjects covering the field of fossil invertebrates though relating mainly to crinoids. He also has made important contributions on museum technique. The Mary Clark Thompson Fund, which makes the award of this medal possible, was established by gift of Mrs. Thompson in 1919. Seven previous awards have been made as follows: To Charles Doolittle Walcott, 1921; Emmanuel de Margerie, 1923; John Mason Clark, 1925; James Perrin Smith, 1928; William Berryman Scott, 1930; Edward Oscar Ulrich, 1930, and David White, 1931.

# SCIENTIFIC APPARATUS AND LABORATORY METHODS

## AN APPARATUS FOR MAINTAINING ARTIFICIAL RESPIRATION IN LABORATORY ANIMALS

SOME mechanical device for carrying out artificial respiration in laboratory animals is practically an indispensable piece of equipment in the physiological laboratory. It has not been long since experimenters resorted to hand or foot bellows for the performance of this necessary procedure. These have been gradually replaced by more elaborate mechanical machines, in which the volume and rate of the output may be varied as desired. One of the most popular methods particularly for student experiments, employs an ordinary wind-shield wiper as a means of interrupting a current of air. In some laboratories motor-operated rotary valves are inserted in the air-line leading to the laboratory tables. Still others find it practical to equip each mammalian group with special apparatus for instituting artificial respiration. As desirable as this seems, the facilities of many laboratories do not permit such an expenditure, and therefore, recourse is made to some of the simpler and less expensive methods, except where certain research problems are involved.

For more than eight years the simple device described in this article has been in use in this laboratory, and having given most satisfactory service with practically no attention, it is reported here for whatever value it might be to other laboratories. The Crowell blower, designed for volume output, is probably more desirable than other types of air pumps which are capable of higher pressures. There is little danger of rupturing the lungs from the full pressure exerted by many of these rotary blowers. The tank placed in the line acts as a buffer and serves to regulate the degree of lung inflation, as well as governing the rate of inflation with respect to the total duration of the respiratory phase. As a means of interrupting the current of air an ordinary safety valve, in the line, as shown in the accompanying diagram, is readily adapted. This valve is mechanically operated by a rod connecting to cam C on the speed-reducing gear. The tension of spring H is so adjusted that the

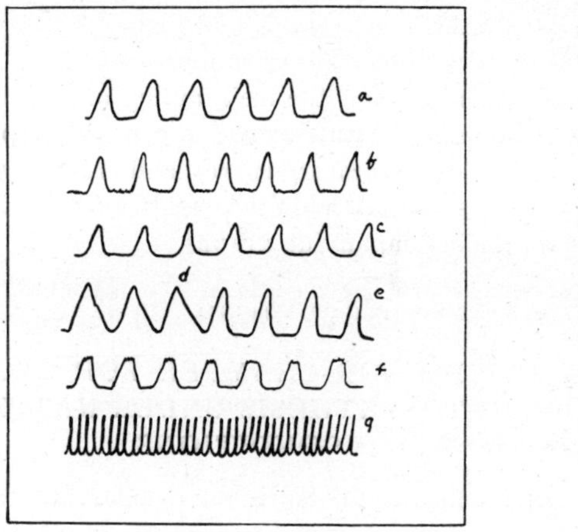


safety valve is held open when the cam is in the "up" position, and the air output of the blower escapes through valve E. The turnbuckle, by adjusting the tension of spring B, regulates the time of closing and opening of the safety valve. By increasing the tension on this spring the safety valve remains closed through a greater arc in the revolution of the speed reducer, and therefore prolongs the inspiratory phase. Valve E regulates the rate of de-

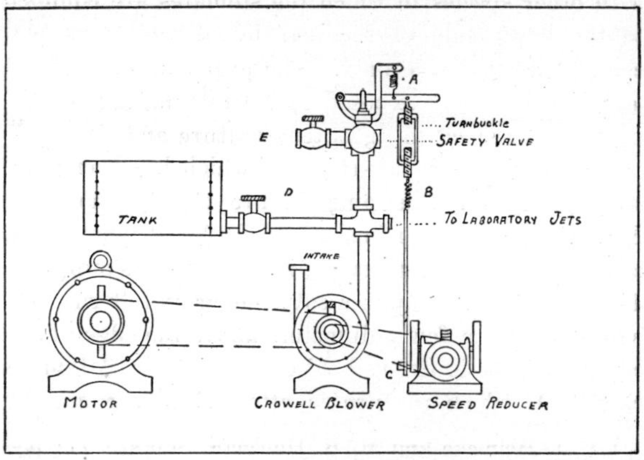


flation or the duration of the expiratory phase. No special valves in the main air line leading to the laboratory tables are necessary, since the resistance of this line is so much greater than through the safety valve, the pressure at the laboratory jets drops practically to zero when the safety valve is opened. By regulating the opening of the air cocks on the laboratory table, the volume of air delivered can be varied according to the requirements of the animal. It may be found necessary, when experiments are conducted simultaneously on a large number of animals, to slightly close valves E and D, and to increase the tension on spring B. The respiratory rate is regulated by means of step pulleys on the motor or pump shaft. Inexpensive reducing gears of 48:1 ratio are available from most dealers in laboratory equipment. A further reduction of 2:1 for motors operating at 1750 R.P.M. is necessary, and gives an approximated respiratory rate of 20 per minute.

That the method for maintaining artificial respiration described in this article is capable of producing a variety of respiratory curves, and is readily adapted to most laboratory requirements, may be readily seen from the accompanying graphs.

W. R. Bond
Medical College of Virginia

## A SPECIAL AIR-CHAMBER FOR STUDYING PHOTOSYNTHESIS UNDER NATURAL CONDITIONS

In studies of photosynthesis under natural conditions with the apparatus recently described by Heinicke and Hoffman,[1] the use of a Cellophane or plastacele envelope as a leaf chamber has distinct advantages over larger containers. However, when the leaf is exposed for a prolonged period to the direct rays of full sunlight, the temperature within the envelope, as in all chambers in which the leaf is wholly enclosed, may rise 6 to 10 degrees C. above that prevailing outside.

This difficulty can be avoided with the apple and with other species in which the stomates are confined to the lower side of the leaf by attaching an air-chamber to that side only. The upper surface of the leaf is thus freely exposed to entirely natural conditions with respect to light, temperature and humidity.

The details of an air-chamber which has been used successfully for this purpose are clearly shown in Fig. 1. The chamber is a modified glass funnel which contains a side arm through which the air is supplied. The leaf (B) rests upon a soft rubber or felt rim (C) which extends a few millimeters above the edge of the cup (D).[2] It is firmly held in place by a flat brass ring (A), which in turn is attached to the cup by

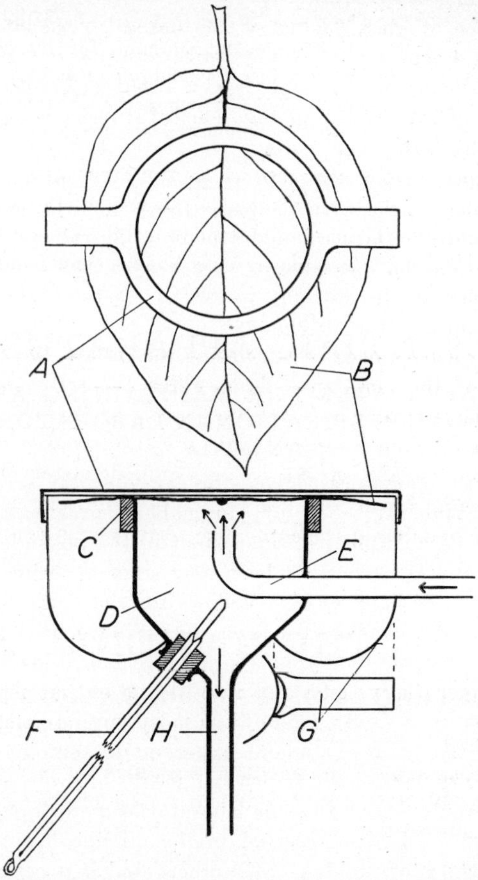


Fig. 1. Diagram of an assimilation chamber used in studies of photosynthesis. The top view is shown above; the cross-section below. The brass ring (A) is used to hold the leaf (B) against rubber cushion (C) of glass cup (D). Air supplied through (E), exhaust through (H). Thermometer, at (F). Top view of spring clamp leading from ring to bottom of cup, at (G).

means of spring clamps (G). The tension of these clamps can easily be adjusted so that the pressure will be sufficient to prevent the free passage of air, but not enough to injure the leaf tissue. The cup is held in position by means of a wire test-tube holder which is attached to the twig or other support. It may be left in place for several days or even for weeks at a time.

The fresh air supply is drawn through a glass tube from the side arm (E) which extends from about 10 cm outside the cup to the middle of the chamber. The end of the tube inside the cup is bent so that the leaf lies parallel to and about 1 cm above the opening. The air thus circulates near the under side of the leaf tissue before it passes through the narrow tube at the bottom of the funnel and thence to the absorption towers.

A similar chamber can easily be made without special technique in glass blowing. This consists of

[1] A. J. Heinicke and M. B. Hoffman, Science 77: 55–58, 1933.

[2] When the rim is coated with a thin layer of soft grafting wax the contact between the leaf and the cup becomes air-tight. The device may thus serve as a porometer for studying the relative size of stomatal aperture at different periods of the day.

a piece of glass tubing of the desired diameter and about 4 cm long. A 3-hole rubber stopper is inserted in one end, and the other end is fitted with a narrow piece of soft rubber tubing, which furnishes a cushion for the leaf. The center hole of the stopper is for the glass tubing through which the fresh air can be supplied. The thermometer is inserted in the second hole and the third will accommodate the exhaust tube. This tube may be bent in such a way that it can be attached to the stem by means of friction tape and thus support the air-chamber.

For convenience in calculating the results, the diameter of the glass tube from which the air-chambers are made should be carefully chosen, so that the area of the opening is exactly 1/10, 1/7, 1/5, or any simple fraction of 100 sq. cm. The inside diameter of the brass ring which holds the leaf in position corresponds to the opening of the cup. The activity of a definitely limited area is thus determined so that it is unnecessary to measure the total leaf surface. Where the same area is used, the air supply can be accurately regulated and held constant in successive determinations. This is important if the carbon dioxide supply is not to become a limiting factor in the results. Where the suction available is not sufficient to supply at least 2 L of air per hour for each sq. cm of leaf surface, an air-chamber with smaller diameter may be used.

The results obtained with these cup chambers have been slightly higher on the average than those obtained with the Cellophane envelopes. This may be due to the fact that no account is taken of the gaseous change that might occur through the upper surface of the leaf, but mainly to the fact that excessively high temperatures are avoided and that the air supply is always adequate for maximum rates.

A. J. Heinicke

Cornell University

# THE NATIONAL ACADEMY OF SCIENCES

## ABSTRACTS OF PAPERS PRESENTED AT THE WASHINGTON MEETING. III.

*(Continued from page 496)*

*Recent studies on chemical mediation of nerve impulses:* W. B. Cannon. Previous studies by Cannon and Bacq proved that a substance, which they called "sympathin," is given off from smooth muscle when it is stimulated by sympathetic nerve impulses. Sympathin is carried in the blood stream and has sympathomimetic effects on denervated structures (salivary glands and cardiac and smooth muscle) elsewhere in the body. Adrenin likewise has sympathomimetic effects; it has been assumed that sympathin is the same as adrenin. The present investigation has shown that sympathin differs from adrenin and that two kinds of sympathin are produced: one from smooth muscle when made to contract, that causes elsewhere only motor or excitatory effects, sympathin E; the other from smooth muscle when made to relax, that causes elsewhere only inhibitory effects, sympathin I. These observations introduce a new phase in our knowledge of chemical mediation of nerve impulses.

*Studies on the function of the adrenal cortical hormone and the cause of death from adrenal insufficiency in dogs:* W. W. Swingle (introduced by E. G. Conklin). The chief function of the adrenal cortical hormone appears to be the regulation and maintenance of a normal circulating volume of fluid within the vascular system. In the absence of the hormone, fluid is continually lost from the circulation, presumably by transudation through the capillary walls, with the result that the adrenalectomized animal is unable to maintain his normal blood volume, and eventually dies from circulatory collapse due to insufficiency of circulating fluid. Accompanying the progressive decrease in blood volume is a progressive fall of blood pressure to the death level. The decline in arterial pressure is apparently a direct result of the decreased volume of circulating fluid. The decrease in blood volume and blood pressure are not terminal phenomena in adrenalectomized animals but first appear within twenty-four to seventy-two hours after discontinuing hormone injections, and before active symptoms of insufficiency appear. Both volume and pressure steadily decline to the death point which may not occur until eight to twelve days later. Hemoconcentration, decreased renal activity, rise in blood non-protein and urea nitrogen, increased blood viscosity and the marked slowing of the circulation which invariably appears, are all directly correlated with and chiefly dependent upon the decline in plasma volume and blood pressure. Adrenalectomized animals, in the absence of the cortical hormone, are apparently unable to draw fluid back into the blood stream through the capillary walls. Following administration of adequate amounts of cortical hormone to prostrate animals, the blood volume, blood pressure and blood constituents return to normal. The animal is able to dilute its blood and build up a normal blood volume and all symptoms of adrenal insufficiency disappear. It is our opinion that all of the manifestations, symptoms and physiological peculiarities, which have been described as occurring in adrenalectomized animals are merely results of a progressively failing circulation due to decreasing volume of circulating fluid in an animal which is unable to compensate (as do normal animals) for its low blood volume and blood pressure by dilution.

*The progressive degeneration of nerve:* G. H. Parker and V. L. Paine. When the lateral-line nerve of the catfish, Ameiurus, is cut near its origin in the fish's head, the nerve degenerates over its whole distal length. If degeneration in the medullary sheath and the neurofibrils is studied, the process is found to take place progressively, beginning near the degenerative cut and spreading away from the region of injury. Degeneration progresses over the nerve at a rate of from three to five centimeters per day and is best seen between six and thirteen days after the degenerative cut has been made. Progressive degeneration of nerve is contrary to the ordinarily accepted view which is based, for the most part, on a study of nerve in warm-blooded animals. Here the rapidity of the process makes it difficult to observe the real operation which is better studied in such a cold-blooded form as the catfish.

*Concerning reticulo-endothelial cells and the utilization of the magnet to procure them:* PEYTON ROUS and J. W. BEARD. Fixed on the walls of the blood vessels of certain mammalian organs are peculiar cells, usually termed reticulo-endothelial, which rapidly remove bacteria from the circulation and destroy them. They also remove damaged blood corpuscles and injected particulate matter, becoming greatly engorged therewith on occasion. It is supposed that these cells constitute a physiological system having various important activities; but of this there is no certainty, because the cells have appeared to be inaccessible to direct study. The authors find that they can be obtained alive from deeply anesthetized animals by injecting particles of highly magnetic ferric oxide into the blood stream; loosening the iron-containing cells afterwards from their principal situation, within the liver, by means of massage and a stream of fluid; and selecting them from the host of other elements in suspension by means of an electromagnet. The reticulo-endothelial cells so procured flourish under suitable conditions outside of the body and behave characteristically, manifesting their recognized activities. Experiments to test their presumptive functions are under way.

*Human insensible perspiration as a laboratory and clinical measurement:* FRANCIS G. BENEDICT. The ordinary person sitting quietly loses in weight about 30 grams per hour, due chiefly to the vaporization of water from the lungs and skin. This insensible loss in weight, the so-called "insensible perspiration," is closely correlated with the total heat production, and hence varies with the size of the individual and with the metabolism. This measurement has important relations to studies in so-called "water balance" and is of significance in cases where the metabolism can not be measured directly. Thus its use for estimating the total heat production of people for twenty-four hours has been of great value.

*Primary and secondary $1n+1$ types, a new unbalance in the jimson weed:* A. F. BLAKESLEE, S. SATINA, A. D. BERGNER and A. G. AVERY. Among the plants of *Datura stramonium* growing in the greenhouse this past winter, there were two small individuals which resembled haploids (1n) in appearance, but which at the same time had peculiarities suggestive of the known effects of extra chromosomes in certain primary and secondary $2n+1$ types. Their preliminary classification as $1n+1$ forms has been confirmed cytologically by finding 13 chromosomes in pollen-mother-cells and root tips instead of the 24 characteristic of normal diploids (2n). Judging from appearance, the first type has the primary $15 \cdot 16$. If this is true, we have identified four types with characters brought about by unbalance of this $15 \cdot 16$ chromosome extra and its formula would be $1n+15 \cdot 16$. The series in order of increasing unbalance would be $4n+15 \cdot 16$, with unbalance of 1 vs. 48; $2n+15 \cdot 16$ with unbalance of 1 vs. 24; $2n+2\,(15 \cdot 16)$, with unbalance of 2 vs. 24 (or 1 vs. 12); and $1n+15 \cdot 16$, with unbalance of 1 vs. 12. The second plant from appearance is probably a $1n+7 \cdot 7$ type. This haploid secondary, if it actually is a secondary, would have twice the numerical unbalance of the diploid secondary $2n+7 \cdot 7$, which was its female parent. It would have an unbalance of two $\cdot 7$ halves vs. 12, which is the most extreme unbalance so far secured in any type of Datura. It is hoped it will be possible to confirm the tentative classification of the extra chromosomes if offspring can be obtained from these extremely weak plants and if a sufficient number of pollen-mother-cells can be secured at the proper stage of division. Lesley and Frost have reported a haploid Matthiola with a small chromosomal fragment extra, but apparently these two $1n+1$ plants in Datura are the first haploids to be reported with a whole chromosome extra.

*Gene constitution and endocrine quality in determining growth reactions:* C. R. STOCKARD. In various crosses between structurally contrasted pure breeds of domestic dogs localized structural peculiarities occur, resulting from the presence of one or more genes which determine a given structural pattern. The growth and pattern in one body region may be quite normal, while a modified pattern is developed in another region in spite of the same chemical or endocrine environment existing in the several regions. A significant example of these facts is shown in the inheritance and development of the short-twisted tail of the English bulldog when crossed with the long-tailed short-legged basset-hound. The bulldog-tail is transmitted as a double recessive in inheritance and its expression is related to two factors probably located in different chromosomes. The homozygous double recessive appears in the second generation in only one in sixteen individuals. Dystrophy in the cartilages of the skull and of the tail vertebrae in the bulldog might be thought of as similar reaction in the two separate regions to a common internal cause. However, some of the second generation hybrid individuals from crosses between the bulldog and basset-hound may show almost normal hound-like heads and yet possess the deformed short-twisted bulldog tail. Such individuals, homozygous for both recessive factors determining "screwtail," develop chondrodystrophy of the tail vertebrae in the same endocrine environment in which the skull and extremities grow and develop quite normally. This would seem to indicate that general endocrine conditions may be ineffective in regulating the type of growth response in opposition to the genetic constitution. For illustration, ordinary individuals may not respond in their growth reactions to pituitary modification in the same manner as might those inheriting acromegaly.

*Retinal rivalry as a neglected factor in stereoscopic vision:* MARGARET F. WASHBURN. This paper argues that a neglected but important factor in stereoscopic vision is, not the combination of two slightly different images on corresponding points of the two retinas, but the alternation of these images in retinal rivalry. That rivalry occurs when the stereoscope is used is well known. This paper demonstrates (a) that it occurs in our ordinary perceptions of solid objects, a fact apparently hitherto unrecorded; and (b) that when similar figures, each containing all the lines of both the right and left views of a solid object, are combined by a stereoscope the figure looks flat, because rivalry is absent, although it contains all the retinal elements for a stereoscopic effect. Since solidity is itself primarily a motor experience, involving the movements of handling and grasping an object, it seems natural that it should be suggested not by a static fusion of retinal images but by an apparent movement. Rivalry occurs both in the stereoscopic slide and in ordinary vision, and as one eye's image becomes dominant over that from the other eye, the apparent movement produced is identical with that which would be produced by part of the object's approaching or receding in the third dimension.

*The "spread" or "scatter" phenomenon in learning:* EDWARD L. THORNDIKE. A satisfying after-effect of a mental connection works back upon it to strengthen it. But this confirming influence of a reward is not entirely concentrated on the one connection to which the reward belongs. The influence strengthens also neighboring connections in the series. Curves are presented showing the extent and amount of this "spread" or "scatter" for several representative sorts of learning. The significance of the discovery of this phenomenon for general theories of modifiability is discussed briefly.

*Basic approaches to a science of music and speech:* CARL E. SEASHORE. Our researches in the psychology of music have revealed the surprisingly close relationship between the science of music and the science of speech, which it is important to recognize in the further organization of research. The paper classifies the types of relationships which have been discovered through experiment, and, on the basis of these, outlines a program for a laboratory of phonetics devoted to the science of these two arts.

*Aristogenesis, the observed order of biomechanical evolution:* HENRY FAIRFIELD OSBORN. This is the author's ninth contribution on the problem of the origin of species and principles of biomechanical evolution observed in paleontology. The term "biomechanical" applies to organic mechanisms. No more apt term than "aristogenesis" can be applied to the observed order of biomechanical adaptation exemplified in the grinding teeth and horns of mammals, as closely observed during the past half century. Aristogenesis is a concrete principle; it has no theoretic significance such as the "entelechy" of Aristotle, the "pangenesis" of Darwin, the "vitalism" of Driesch, the "bathmism" of Cope, the "emergence" of Morgan, the "holism" of Smuts. Like the "biogenesis" of Haeckel signifying recapitulation, aristogenesis signifies adaptive origin. As a process of nature it is not to be challenged as a concept, still less as an explanation, hypothesis or theory. We know how it works, but at present we have no hypothesis as to why it works or as to what its causes are. A definition of aristogenesis is as follows: Aristogenesis is the gradual, secular, continuous, direct, reactive, adaptive origin of new biomechanisms. It is a creative process from the geneplasm, of entirely new germinal characters. It is the orderly creation of some better or more adaptive biomechanism. Certain lines of descent are distinguished by the potentiality of creative origin from the geneplasm of new adaptive biomechanisms. Germinally predetermined origin of new biomechanisms tends toward betterment, and arises independently, in widely separated geographic areas, at same or different aristogenic rates. Aristogenesis is a secular genetic and adaptive reaction rather than an immediate adaptive somatic reaction to new habit or environment as in Lamarck's theory. *Aristogenes* in origin and early development are wholly independent of the natural selection principle of Darwin. Whereas *Aristogenes* are predetermined by germinal potentiality, progressive differences in species arise also through more or less profound changes of form and proportion distinguished as *Allometrons* and expressed in measurements and indices, for example, in the familiar proportional changes of the head expressed in the Greek terms brachycephaly (broad-headed, index 80) and dolichocephaly (long-headed, index 70). Allometrons are relatively rapid in development or temporal, whereas aristogenes are relatively slow or secular. The 19 aristogenes of a lower Miocene mastodont occupy from 10 to 14 million years in rising to the 34 to 37 aristogenes of an upper Miocene mastodont. So far as the modes in which the "origin of species" is defined by biomechanisms we are now on absolutely sure ground. This ground is contra-Lamarckian and contra-Darwinian. It is also contrary to the neo-Darwinian evolutionary hypotheses of the leading biologists and geneticists of our day.

*The general formula of heredity:* HARRY H. LAUGHLIN (introduced by Henry Fairfield Osborn). Most inborn qualities, whether structural or functional, which are constitutionally important in human life, which are essential to well-bred domestic plants and animals, and which are therefore highly hereditary, are not single Mendelian units, nor are many of them based upon so few as two or three genes working additively. For the most part, each such valuable quality is the somatic end-product of many genes, which in development interact in many ways. Many such multi-genic traits are definitely measurable as end-products in the individual, and consequently we can compute the probability that the particular quality developed to a specified degree will appear in a pre-indicated or random-selected offspring. The basis of such prediction is the degree of development of the selected quality in each of the several near blood-kin. The traits or qualities which can be thus predicted may be structural or functional, vital or insignificant, useful or injurious, but they must be measurable as entities in the individual, and they must show a definite tendency to "run in families." For all such traits, the formula of heredity works out mathematically: $K = f(M, R)$. K is the probability that the pre-indicated or random-selected offspring, with a given M or prediction basis, will fall within the selected R or class range of offspring. The mathematical model of this formula is always a "skewed saddle."

*Evidences of man's ancestral history in the later development of the child:* C. B. DAVENPORT. It has long been known that man, in his foetal development, passes through many stages reminiscent of the course of the evolution of the human species. Thus tail, gill-slits, tubular heart, amphibian-like kidney, for example, are ancestral. It is less well appreciated that at birth the child is still far from an adult in proportions of parts, and has still to pass through a series of changes shown by adult primates. At birth of the child the chest is a cylinder of approximately circular cross-section. This is the shape of the chest of the foetus of other primates and many other mammals. It is the generalized, undifferentiated form of the chest. In running quadrupeds, like the gazelle and horse, the depth of the chest becomes greater than the breadth. But in man, the breadth becomes greater than the depth. The circular-cylindrical chest is rather characteristic of adult tree-climbers, and fits them for the undifferentiated movements required in climbing; for specialization in upright walking it is convenient that the arms swing free of the torso, and this result is attained in adult man's broad shoulders; but these broad shoulders are achieved relatively late in development. Again, the upper and lower segments of the leg of the human foetus are, in the early months, very unequal, since the thigh takes the initiative in rapid growth. This appears to be an undifferentiated condition. Later the lower leg grows rapidly so that it approaches equality with the thigh; that is, about 90 per cent. at eleven or twelve years. This is the condition that is rather characteristic of tree-climbers. After this pre-adolescent stage the femur forges ahead, and the leg index falls in the adult condition to about 84 per cent. This long thigh takes the adolescent out of the childish, ape-like class of climbing, jumping, romping animals into that of walkers and runners. The human foot shows remarkable adaptations to supporting the great weight of the body upon the spool-like talus and distributing that weight to the whole foot in the most efficient fashion. But the adaptive changes are completed only as adolescence appears. The infant has a rather low instep, like anthropoid apes. This instep increases to adolescence, and gives a valuable resilience to the step. The human fetal foot is at first long, as compared with the lower leg, just as in the anthropoid ape. This may be regarded as a generalized condition. In later months this foot index diminishes from 95 per cent. to 90 per cent.; in the adult boy to 65 per cent., while it remains at about 90 per cent. in the adult gorilla and chimpanzee. A long heel is a human characteristic. The foetus has a relatively short heel bone, a condition that is retained by adult chimpanzee and orang-utan, but the heel bone increases in childhood up to adolescence. The parallelism of ontogeny and the phylogenetic series is clearly due to the fact that the higher forms pass through the same embryological stages that the lower forms do, but they go beyond the point at which the less evolved species stop their development.

*Racial aspects of the pathology of the ear:* ALEŠ HRDLIČKA. The collections of the division of physical anthropology, U. S. National Museum, include now over 15,000 racial crania, over three fourths of which are American. This American material is largely precolumbian and comprises a number of series ranging from hundreds to several thousands of specimens, including the contents of entire large burial grounds, and these series are not only of great value to anthropology but also to the study of prehistoric American pathology. One of the most interesting categories of pathological conditions shown by the material comprises the defects and diseases of the bony ear structures. The present paper deals with the two most striking conditions of this nature, namely, a complete congenital absence of the external auditory meatus and apparently of the whole tympanic bone; and ear exostoses. In the present communication the speaker reports the results of personal examination for ear exostoses in 7,814 skulls, Egyptian, Eskimo, American Indian, Polynesian, Negro and Melanesian. The abnormalities are shown decisively to be most frequent in certain inland groups of the Indian, and next in the Polynesians. They are never congenital, and rare in childhood, developing essentially during the earlier half of the adult life. They are moderately to considerably more common in the males than in the females, more frequently bilateral than unilateral, and when unilateral they show a tendency to develop more commonly on the left side. They vary much in number, size and shape, and often show more or less symmetry on the two sides. They, the speaker concludes, are not incidental or chance formations, but represent a generalized pathological entity, an oto-exostotic diathesis, which manifests itself in different degrees in different racial and local human groups, according to local checking or favoring conditions.

## BOOKS RECEIVED

DANGEARD, PIERRE. *Traité D'Algologie.* Pp. 441. 380 figures. Lechavalier, Paris.

JEANS, SIR JAMES. *The New Background of Science.* Pp. viii + 301. Macmillan. $2.50.

MORGAN, H. R. *Results of Observations with the Nine-Inch Transit Circle 1913–1926.* U. S. Naval Observatory. Government Printing Office.

NEWMAN, F. H. and V. H. L. SEARLE. *The General Properties of Matter.* Pp. 388. 113 figures. Macmillan. $4.00.

REUTER, E. B. and C. W. HART. *Introduction to Sociology.* Pp. x + 548. McGraw-Hill. $3.50.

# SCIENCE

VOL. 77 FRIDAY, JUNE 2, 1933 No. 2005



*Academic and Industrial Research in the Field of Therapeutics:* SIR HENRY H. DALE 521

*Obituary:*
*Fred E. Brooks:* DR. C. R. CUTRIGHT. *Memorials. Recent Deaths* 527

*Scientific Events:*
*The Scientific Situation in Germany; In Honor of the late Stephen Tyng Mather; Field Conference of the New York State Geological Association; Group Conferences at the Cold Spring Harbor Biological Laboratory; Professor Harrison as Croonian Lecturer* 528

*Scientific Notes and News* 531

*Discussion:*
*Conservation versus Preservation:* DR. V. E. SHELFORD. *Notes on a Sphagnum Bog at Fort Bragg, California:* DR. GEORGE B. RIGG. *Sedimentation and Sedimentology:* DR. HAKON WADELL. *Mechanicism, Vitalism and the Growth of Bacteria:* PROFESSOR JAMES M. SHERMAN and PROFESSOR GEORGE M. CAMERON 535

*Reports:*
*Honors Conferred by the Franklin Institute* 538

*Societies and Meetings:*
*The Ohio Academy of Science:* W. H. ALEXANDER. *The Illinois State Academy of Science:* PROFESSOR HAROLD R. WANLESS. *The Virginia Academy of Science:* DR. E. C. L. MILLER. *The Tennessee Academy of Science:* DR. FRANCIS G. SLACK 539

*Scientific Apparatus and Laboratory Methods:*
*A Telephonic Drop Counter:* DR. CLARENCE F. GRAHAM. *A Disintegrator for Yeast Cells:* DR. WILLIAM F. BRUCE 542

*Special Articles:*
*The Development of Organized Vessels in Cultures of Blood Cells:* DR. RAYMOND C. PARKER. *Laminar Destruction of the Nerve Cells of the Cerebral Cortex:* PROFESSOR J. G. DUSSER DE BARENNE. *Lithium in Sea Water:* BERTRAM D. THOMAS and PROFESSOR THOMAS G. THOMPSON 544

*Science News* 8



SCIENCE: A Weekly Journal devoted to the Advancement of Science, edited by J. MCKEEN CATTELL and published every Friday by

THE SCIENCE PRESS

New York City: Grand Central Terminal

Lancaster, Pa. Garrison, N. Y.

Annual Subscription, $6.00 Single Copies, 15 Cts.

SCIENCE is the official organ of the American Association for the Advancement of Science. Information regarding membership in the Association may be secured from the office of the permanent secretary, in the Smithsonian Institution Building, Washington, D. C.


# ACADEMIC AND INDUSTRIAL RESEARCH IN THE FIELD OF THERAPEUTICS[1]


By Sir HENRY H. DALE

DIRECTOR OF THE NATIONAL INSTITUTE FOR MEDICAL RESEARCH, LONDON, AND SECRETARY OF THE ROYAL SOCIETY OF LONDON


WE have to-day the privilege of assisting at the formal inauguration of these Research Laboratories, which the enterprise of a manufacturing house has brought into being. I know that I can speak for all those who are present, in saying to the directors whose enlightened policy has provided these laboratories, and to the distinguished investigators who will use them, that we wish them all the success which they desire and deserve. And in wishing them success, I have in mind not merely such as will directly increase the efficiency and extend the scope of the industrial enterprise with which these laboratories are associated, though that we may wish them without reserve; but we may also wish them a wider and more enduring success, in adding to the sum of life-saving knowledge, for the benefit of all mankind.

[1] An address delivered at the opening ceremony of the Research Laboratories of Merck and Company, Inc., Rahway, New Jersey, April 25.

The word "research" in relation to industry has been made to do duty over a wide range of meanings. You would probably find some manufacturers who apply the term to the mere experimental control of the details of an unprogressive technical routine, or of the quality of the materials used in it. At the other end of the scale, this great country, in particular, can show conspicuous examples of the far-seeing policy of great industrial enterprises, in providing opportunity for men of world-wide fame in science to follow freely the lead of their own original genius, without any immediate reference to the production of remunerative inventions. Results of the greatest theoretical importance to science have thus been obtained, which any university might be proud to claim as the product of its laboratories of pure research; but in some cases, at least, they have been obtained under conditions which only the technical resources of great industry could provide. I do not think that we can have any doubt that, by such a policy, industry will not only render a proper service to the wider interests of the community from which it draws its support, but will also act in the essential interests of its own success and development. And it will do so, I think, not merely because some of the most important inventions, leading to really new lines of practical development, do in fact arise as incidental results of fundamental researches having no such practical aim, but also because the progress of such free scientific inquiry in any community creates the atmosphere of mental enterprise and the fount of ideas, which enable practical invention to thrive and to come to fruition.

There may be some who will see a danger here, fearing lest the opportunities offered by the research service of industry may come to make too large a draft upon the highest grade of scientific ability, so that the universities may be unable to make good their primary claim upon it, for the training and inspiration of the following generations. The danger is not one which could be treated lightly if there were any good reason to fear its development. For the scientific future of any country, in industry as well as in the academic sphere, must depend on the quality of the recruits which the universities can furnish; and that quality will be determined, not only by the effectiveness and the attractive influence of the formal teaching which they provide, but even more by the opportunity which they afford to their best students, of a living contact with the finest type of ability and achievement in research. If such a danger really existed, we could hardly put the responsibility for it only on industry. The great institutions, supported by private munificence or by public funds, and offering, to men selected for their achievement or promise as investigators, an opportunity to give the whole of their thoughts and energies to research, must share any responsibility of that kind. This country, through the unparalleled and enlightened generosity of its leaders of industry and finance, has led the world in this relatively new development of the endowment of research for its own sake. I myself have the honor now to be associated with an institute thus devoted entirely to medical research, with no formal academic contacts, supported from the public funds by the British Government. Earlier, after a relatively short academic experience, I had charge, for ten of my most active years as a scientific worker, of laboratories also concerned with various aspects of medical research—physiology, pharmacology, immunology, serology—and supported by the head of a great British pharmaceutical firm, Sir Henry Wellcome, who had migrated from your country to mine at an early stage of his career. I allow myself the apparent egotism of these personal details, only to make it clear that I have had the opportunity of viewing, from more than one angle, this problem of the relation between research in the universities, in endowed and public institutes and in laboratories supported by industry. And, so far as this experience has enabled me to form a judgment, I do not believe that there is any real or permanent danger of the universities losing, to whole-time research in endowed institutions or in laboratories associated with industry, the particular kind of scientific leadership and power of inspiration, which, in the interests of all kinds of scientific activity, it is essential that they should retain. So far as I can judge, I believe that, in general, this relatively new growth of whole-time research as a career is already effective, and is likely to become more so, in the reverse direction. In this, as in other spheres of human activity, supply must be largely determined by demand. The universities, in the nature of things, can offer only a limited number of major opportunities in science to their ablest and most enterprising students; and the more numerous the extra-academic opportunities for careers of distinction and of service to the community in research, the more readily will able men be willing to try their ability as investigators, before embarking on careers of professional practise or business; and the wider should be the field thus made available to the universities, in choosing the men they wish to retain and to promote. I do not think, then, that there is any real danger in that direction. Such difficulties as may arise, to hamper the development of the best and most helpful relationship between research in the universities and in the laboratories associated with industry, must come from causes of a different kind. In the field of medical science, which is that of my own direct experience, I am inclined to doubt whether the ideal relationship has yet been everywhere established, between research in the universities and the hospitals, on the one hand, and that associated with the pharmaceutical industry on the other. The finding and acceptance of a proper relationship, however, is vital to the progress of both alike, and to their union in an ordered advance, along the common front of medical science and its applications. It is a matter of special importance to an institution such as this, which starts to-day on its career, with the good wishes and the confident hope of us all. I hope, therefore, that I may be allowed to put briefly before you a few ideas as to the special kind of service which an organization such as this may render to medical science, and as to some of the difficulties which it may have to face.

Let us recognize, in the first place, that investigation in that group of sciences which contribute to medicine entails certain special obligations. The practitioners of medicine are bound, by a tradition of long and honorable history, to place any new knowledge, gained in the practise of their art, freely at the disposal of their professional brethren, without any concealment or any attempt to restrict its use for private advantage. This tradition has no connection with any formal code of professional etiquette governing medical practise. Its basis, I think, is a recognition of an essential condition for the advance of medical science; and in recent years, as such advances have come in increasing measure from the research laboratories, the workers in these, whether medically qualified or not, have in general shown themselves eager to embrace this great medical tradition and to accept this freedom of the great medical brotherhood. Without committing ourselves too hastily in advance to the details of its application over the whole field of enterprise, I think we must accept this tradition as embodying a true ideal, and one which we can not afford to lose or to see obscured. For medical research differs from that in other fields in this respect, that its ultimate aim is the provision of knowledge which will find its application in the relief, the cure or the prevention of human sickness and suffering. Further, while all medical research, however remote from any immediate thought of such application, preserves this ultimate aim, no practical development of the results of medical research can be made, no therapeutic invention can be completed, without a full and frank cooperation with those engaged in clinical practise. Those who are engaged in the task, vitally important to the progress of medical science and practise, of translating the new knowledge of natural laws and principles into terms of practical therapeutics, as the workers in these laboratories will be, require the fullest confidence and cooperation of those, on the one hand, who are freely exploring new avenues of knowledge, without an immediately practical objective, and those, on the other hand, who are directly responsible for the care and the treatment of the sick. And in order that this frank and full cooperation and confidence may be established, between all those engaged in furthering medical discovery and its application at these different stages, they will need to convince one another that they are bound together in a common cause and by loyalty to a common tradition.

I think that we must frankly face the fact that those whose contribution to this common end is made by research in laboratories such as these may find a special difficulty in carrying that conviction. These laboratories have been founded by industry, and their maintenance and progressive opportunity of service to medical science will depend on the extent to which industry receives the proper reward of its enterprise. I have no fear that the directorate responsible for these laboratories will reckon that reward by any narrow calculation, based merely on returns from directly remunerative invention. But you men of science, who have accepted the opportunity which these laboratories offer, will probably find some among your academic or clinical colleagues who will be ready to assume that your researches, henceforward, will be directed merely to the promotion of some trade interest, to securing some advantage to the manufacturing house supporting you over its competitors and not to the advancement of the common cause of medical science. I say that you will probably find some ready to take this attitude, and to regard you as engaged in, at best, an inferior order of medical research; but it may be that I am wrong, and I hope that I am. I was speaking from the analogy, perhaps a misleading one, of my own experience in another country, and now nearly 30 years ago. I suspect, however, that human nature and academic traditions do not exhibit any fundamental differences over those parts of the world where our common language is spoken and that they do not change completely in the course of thirty years. If there is anything in my suspicion, it will be your task, as it was mine, to show these colleagues that they have been wrong in their assumptions; that work in these laboratories supported by industrial enterprise, though differing from theirs, perhaps, in the nature of its immediate objective, can be as genuinely inspired by the ideals of the advancement of medical science, and of service to suffering humanity; and that even in researches undertaken in the interests of some immediately practical development, the alert investigator, given such freedom as you will surely have here, will find the opportunity for making additions to the common fund of scientific knowledge, which may be as fundamentally important as those which come from the academic laboratories. They have had examples before them, indeed, for many years, from other laboratories established and maintained by great pharmaceutical houses in this country; and it must surely be generally recognized that some of the great advances in medical knowledge, which have in recent years come from American universities, have been made possible by the cooperation which only industrially supported research could give. But prejudice dies hard, especially when it has its roots in a tradition which we all acknowledge and respect; and I suspect that you who are to work here will find that there is, for yourselves and your colleagues in other similar institutions, something yet to be won, of the full confidence and cooperation which you need from the academic investigators and which they as certainly need from you. You will win it, when they see that your work differs from theirs, not so much in its quality or its ultimate aim as in the nature of the incentive and in the kind of opportunity offered by the conditions under which it is done.

There is one matter, affecting the question of loyalty to a common medical tradition, which I must mention more explicitly, if only to free myself from the suspicion of shirking a difficulty. I refer to the question of patents for inventions having therapeutic value. I shall make no attempt to conceal my own wish that we could do without them. I am convinced that a general recognition of their use by research workers in the medical field would be unfavorable to open confidence and to the free interchange of experience and materials among such workers, including those whose part in a common investigation is concerned with the human patient. The whole basis of such cooperative work would be endangered by any suspicion that it was being used for the enrichment of some individual or institution, and not for the advancement of medical science for the common benefit.

That being said, I should make it clear that I am not among those who condemn the use of patents in medicine with a kind of dogmatic fervor and without reference to its object and its effect. The object of any patent law is to further the progress of science and its applications, by stimulating invention and by providing the conditions which will make its results available to all who need to use them. I believe that a general use of patents in all parts of the field of therapeutic research and by investigators in all kinds of institutions would definitely hinder, rather than promote, such progress. That belief, however, does not entitle me to suggest that the protection by patent of any kind of therapeutic invention, under any conditions and in any country, must of necessity have that detrimental effect. So far as I can judge the situation, the danger of it seems to me to be greatest in connection with discoveries relating to remedies of the biological type, for which the practical application is apt to present itself as a stage in the general advance of knowledge, to which many, in different institutions and countries, have made essential contributions. I believe that there is a definite danger here from the difficulty of distinguishing between scientific discovery and practical invention, and from the temptation to use the opportunity which a patent affords, not only to endow a particular institution in which a practical development happened to begin, but also to dictate to the whole world an orthodoxy in its application, and thereby to restrict the freedom of further advance. Frankly, I am inclined to regard the medical patent as a peculiarly dangerous weapon when it is wielded by the good intentions of the academic amateur.

On the other hand, I do not see the same danger in the use of patents for inventions related to really new substances of therapeutic value produced by chemical synthesis. I can not ignore the argument that an immediate and complete freedom to all the world for the manufacture and sale of such a substance might have the result of its not being produced at all, because nobody could justify the expenditure necessary to organize its efficient production and to make its value known to those who could use it. I think it could be urged that, under the conditions of modern pharmaceutical industry, in some countries, a patent for a definite invention of this kind may be used in accordance with the very purpose of medical tradition, to make the new knowledge available to all who need to use it. I think that it can also be urged that such a policy may enable an industry to support research leading to further and more important inventions. Without such incentive and guarantee it is hardly likely, I think, that the great pharmaceutical industry of Germany could have embarked on a policy which, after many years, has led to the production of substances representing the first clear advance in the treatment of malaria along new lines since the Jesuit Fathers brought cinchona bark from Peru in the seventeenth century; or that the pharmaceutical industry of this and other countries would have enriched the resources of medicine with all the new general and local anesthetics which now help to reduce the sum of human pain. If the industry of any country tells me that it can only promote research and apply its results, in this synthetic field of therapeutic invention, by the use of patents, I can not presume to contest the statement. But I am certain that patents in the medical field will do no service even to industry, unless they are so used that they serve also the great medical tradition, so that industry wins and retains the confidence of the academic laboratories and the clinics. No invention in the medical field can be completed or brought to use without the cooperation of the physician and his patients. I believe that such cooperation will be readily and properly given so long as it is clear that the aim of industrial research is the real increase of knowledge for the ultimate benefit of mankind and not the promotion of some narrow commercial aim.

The idea of cooperation involves some differentiation of function. It would not be in the general interest of science that the academic institutions and laboratories such as these should be following exactly similar lines of investigation, with the same kind of immediate objective. Broadly, we may distinguish their respective functions, I think, by saying that the primary task of those academic laboratories, which are concerned with the ultimate advancement of therapeutics, is the increase of our fundamental knowledge of the problems involved, without any immediate or insistent thought of its practical application. The function of science in the universities seems to me to be well expressed in the old formula, which, since its foundation in the seventeenth century, has defined the purpose of the Royal Society of London —"the improvement of natural knowledge by means of experiment." That tradition has not needed any artificial importation into the universities of this country. One of the first and greatest of American citizens, Benjamin Franklin, was himself a distinguished fellow of the Royal Society. Your primary task in these laboratories, on the other hand, will be to find applications for the laws governing therapeutic action, as fundamental inquiry reveals them, and to translate them into the practical terms of remedies ready for the treatment of the sick.

Broadly, I think, this differentiation can be made, and I believe it to be important that it should be kept steadily in view. On the other hand, it is natural and proper that, from time to time, these functions should largely overlap. The academic investigator must certainly not be inhibited or called off from his quest, if its natural line of development should lead him to a discovery which is directly applicable to the prevention or treatment of disease. On the contrary, it is right that he should be the more encouraged to pursue his investigation, by the thought of its promise of immediate benefit to mankind. I suppose that we shall agree that the discovery, in the past century, which had the most revolutionary and transforming effect on medical science and practise was that of microorganisms as the cause of infective diseases; and its real starting point was the interest, awakened in the mind of a man of genius, Louis Pasteur, by the relation between the optical rotations of the different tartaric acids and the asymmetry of their crystals. He followed the clue through the differential fermentative action of moulds and of yeasts, to open a new world to investigation, in the bacterial origin of putrefaction and of many diseases. But, out of an unbounded admiration for that great man and for his wonderful gift to mankind, I am sometimes tempted to wonder whether that gift might not have been even greater, and in some of its phases more permanent, if the clamor for practical application had not led him, in later years, so far into the unfamiliar field of therapeutics, and away from his more fundamental inquiries. When Michael Faraday, patiently seeking the improvement of natural knowledge, with an inspired curiosity, discovered the phenomenon of electromagnetic induction, he probably had little thought that it would find any practical application; if he had had any prevision of the kind of civilization which, a hundred years later, would have arisen on his discovery, the thought would probably have appalled him. It will surely happen in the future, as in the past, that free and fundamental researches will often lead to the most important practical discoveries; and we need not grudge his good fortune to the academic investigator whose work has such a result. I do think, however, that there is a definite danger lest he should be diverted by it from his proper task of further free inquiry and should devote his interest to the practical development and application of a discovery already made, which, in many cases, he had better leave to others. The concentration of popular enthusiasm on discoveries which are immediately applicable in therapeutics is natural and intelligible. We need have no fear of its effect, provided that a proper balance of recognition is preserved within the universities themselves, between the achievement of a practical success and the fundamental advancement of knowledge. I have no right, and no desire, to criticize here a particular line of policy, which some of the universities of the North American continent have adopted in recent years, in order to secure to themselves funds for the endowment of further research, from the proceeds of practically useful medical discoveries which have come from their respective laboratories. It is for them to judge their needs and the proper way to meet them. I mention the matter, not from any desire to make or to imply a criticism of action already taken, but because of its direct bearing on a view which I desire to emphasize, namely, that the primary and special function of research in the universities is to build the main fabric of knowledge by free and untrammelled inquiry and to be concerned with the practical uses of it, only as these arise in the course of a natural development. I suggest that we should watch carefully the effect of any line of action which might lead the scientific departments of the universities to give encouragement and promotion to the practical inventor at the expense of withholding it from a potential Michael Faraday or Willard Gibbs. If that should happen, there would be a real danger of the university departments neglecting their own proper part in the cooperative scheme, and encroaching on that more proper to the laboratories supported by industry.

I have suggested, as the primary concern of the laboratories supported by industry, the development to a practical outcome of the fundamental discoveries which the academic and endowed institutions may be expected, in the main, to furnish. But just as the academic worker ought not to be restrained from following freely the line of his inquiry, because it happens to lead to a practical application, the investigator in an industrially supported laboratory ought to have a large freedom, to follow a clue to new knowledge of a fundamental kind, if it presents itself in the course of his practical investigations. Indeed, I think it is probably of great advantage to an industrial laboratory that its staff should have always in hand a substantial body of investigation having no direct relation to any practical development. My own personal experience, if you will pardon a further reference to it, perhaps influences my views unduly. If the head of a great pharmaceutical house, who gave me my first real opportunity as an independent investigator, had been inclined to judge me by my output of therapeutic novelties directly remunerative to his firm, I think he must have concluded that I was a very unprofitable investment. If he did so, he never let me suspect it; on the contrary, I received a steady encouragement to follow, with my colleagues, the natural lead of the problems which our initially practical investigations had presented. And I believe that such a policy is undoubtedly the right one. If necessity is the mother of invention, the spirit of free investigation is most certainly its father. The men who work here will need it, to preserve their active interest in what is happening in the larger world of science, and to maintain their contacts with men of like interests in the academic world.

In a very large proportion of cases, when we come to look at the results, it will be difficult to say whether a particular discovery would come more appropriately from an academic or from an industrial laboratory. Permit me to illustrate the difficulty by an example which has some personal interest for me, as well as for these laboratories. Many years ago my friend, Dr. Reid Hunt, now professor in the Harvard Medical School, thought that he detected the presence, in an animal organ, of some unstable derivative of choline, of greater physiological activity than that substance. An examination of a series of artificial derivatives, with Dr. Taveau, led him to the discovery, in acetylcholine, of a substance having at least one thousand times the activity of the parent base. Some five years later, in the Wellcome Laboratories, I was still following up certain lines of inquiry on the pharmacology of ergot, which had been suggested to me as a subject when I entered that service. A remarkable type of activity showed itself in certain peculiar ergot extracts, and cooperative work with my colleague, Dr. Ewins, led to the isolation of the substance responsible for it, which proved to be acetylcholine. Acetylcholine thus passed from the class of synthetic curiosities into that of natural substances, and a fuller study of its action showed a remarkable relation between its effects on different organs and those produced by parasympathetic nerves. This work, in an industrially supported laboratory, had brought us no nearer to practical therapeutics than Professor Reid Hunt's original discovery had done; but it arose from a chance observation, for which only the industrial connection could have provided the opportunity and of which we were able to take advantage through our association with large-scale work. After another interval, created by the war, the next step was taken in an academic laboratory, when Professor Loewi, in Graz, showed that stimulation of the vagus nerve produces its effect on the frog's heart by releasing something remarkably similar to acetylcholine in its properties; but the quantities were far too small for direct identification. After another interval of years, now in an institute supported by the public funds, another chance observation enabled Dr. Dudley and myself actually to isolate acetylcholine from an animal organ, in quantity sufficient for complete identification. So that now we had evidence that this substance, the most powerful dilator of the arteries of which we have any knowledge, actually occurs as a natural constituent of the body, and almost certainly intervenes in the natural control of its functions. But still its instability, and the consequent evanescent nature of its action, while fitting it supremely for such a natural function, made it of very doubtful value for artificial application in therapeutics. And so the scene shifts again to the industrially supported laboratories, and the systematic search begins for allied esters of choline, with a similar but more persistent action. And already there is news of the discovery of several; of one from the laboratories of the ancestral house of Merck in Germany; of another, apparently of real therapeutic promise, from the research laboratories of this younger house of Merck, for the inauguration of which in their new form we have been invited here to-day. The pharmacological properties of this new substance, however, were first made clear by Simonart, working under academic conditions, in the laboratories of my friend, and for a time my close comrade in research, Professor A. N. Richards, of Philadelphia. I congratulate these laboratories on securing the cooperation and advice of Professor Richards in relation to their activities in fundamental research. The association, as you will see, has a double interest for me; but I take almost as much in tracing the successive stages of this investigation, from the academic to the industrial laboratories and back again, and in finding myself unable to suggest that the nature of the researches at any one stage was specially suited to an academic institution, and at another more appropriate to the function of an industrial laboratory.

I have spoken of the broad differentiation of aim and of function between academic and industrial research, and of the different types of ability and of temperament suited to each. There are men, indeed, of whom we could say with confidence that the associations of academic life are necessary for their happiness and their efficiency in research; and there are others of whom we could say with equal certainty that their best work would be done under such conditions as these laboratories provide. I believe, however, that the men so easily classified are relatively few, and that for a large majority the choice will be determined by the accident of opportunity, rather than by aptitude. For some of this majority, I suspect that the best conditions for the full development and maintenance of their powers of serving science might be provided by a successive or an alternating experience of the conditions of academic and of industrial research. The investigator who has been digging himself to a standstill in an academic groove, might find a new mobility in the less conventional surroundings of an industrial laboratory; while his colleague, whose inventive energies have grown stale from too long contact with a variety of practical problems, might find them refreshed and renewed by migrating for a period to the calmer atmosphere of fundamental research. I believe, then, that a freer interchange of suitable personnel, if it were possible, between the academic laboratories and those supported by industry, might have an invigorating influence on both; but I speak of ideals, without knowledge of practical possibilities. I am sure that even a short experience of the kind of opportunity that these laboratories will afford would make some of your academic colleagues envy the elasticity of organization, the adaptability of equipment and readiness of expansion to a large scale of working which the industrial association can give.

There are several advantages which you will have here over some institutions supported by memorial endowments. I am sure that this country must have had examples of a type of large-hearted testator or pious founder, familiar to us in England. He rightly believes that he can create the most worthy memorial to himself or to those dear to him by the endowment of medical research; but too often he wrongly believes that his generous impulse brings with it a scientific vision and a prophetic wisdom, entitling him to restrict, for all time, the application of his benefaction to research on some particular problem in medicine, which has enlisted his personal sympathies or stimulated his imagination. You who work here will be free to choose your problems, according to the needs of the time and the promise of advance offered by current progress in science; you will be able to give intensive cultivation to the fertile areas, to raise the crops which are likely to give good yield and put in the sickle where the harvest stands ripe for gathering. You will have the great advantage that your buildings can be designed and equipped, with the sole aim of making the most efficient provision for the work which you have in hand or in near prospect. You begin with an equipment perfect for your present needs, and will be able to expand it as your program and your staff expand. I can hardly resist a feeling of envy at the opportunity which Dr. Major, Dr. Molitor, Dr. Engels and their coworkers will have, to concentrate their thoughts on their researches, without distraction by duties of administration or teaching, in laboratories designed so admirably for the needs of research and so readily adaptable to changing requirements.

Whole-time research, however, whether in an endowed or an industrial laboratory, has its own special anxieties and psychological needs. Research workers in an institution such as this can only give of their best, if they can escape from any feeling of isolation from the general scientific community, and can feel an assurance that their work is making an essential contribution to the general advance of medical science and practise. They will need, and I am confident that they will have, all the encouragement and friendly cooperation which their scientific colleagues in the academic laboratories and the clinical centers can give them. We wish them all success, and we congratulate the president, Mr. Merck, and all who have been associated with him, on an enterprise which we now launch, with high hopes, on a career of service to science and to the industry which supports it.

# OBITUARY

## FRED E. BROOKS

FRED E. BROOKS, associate entomologist of the U. S. Bureau of Entomology and nationally known writer on nature subjects, died at French Creek, West Virginia, on March 9. He had been in ill health for several years and the immediate cause of his death was a heart attack. Mr. Brooks' first scientific work was done as associate entomologist of the West Virginia Experiment Station, where he did notable research work with insects affecting grapes. For some time he also worked with small mammals. In 1911 he became associated with the U. S. Bureau of Entomology, where his main work was with wood-boring insects, especially those working on apple. He also conducted research with codling moth, the grape curculio and several nut insects. Most of his research work is published in bulletins of the West Virginia Experiment Station and of the U. S. Department of Agriculture. In addition to entomology he was keenly interested in nature generally and published many papers covering his observations in journals such as *Nature, Country Life in America, The Rural New*

*Yorker* and many others. As an observer he was without a peer and it was in this way that he made his most notable scientific contributions.

C. R. CUTRIGHT

## MEMORIALS

THE memory of John Kern Strecker, curator of the Baylor University Museum, was honored at Waco, Texas, on April 20, in a special service arranged by the Texas Academy of Science and participated in by the entire university. Eulogies were presented by H. B. Parks, of San Antonio, formerly state entomologist and secretary of the academy, and by Dr. Walter J. Williams, professor of mathematics, who was intimately associated with Mr. Strecker. The complete works of Mr. Strecker, assembled by the academy and bound in leather, were presented to the Baylor University Library. Included were ninety-three contributions on mollusks, reptiles, birds and mammals. About twenty papers were incomplete at the time of his death. These will be brought to completion by Dr. Williams and published as soon as possible. Mr. Strecker's death occurred at Waco on January 9.

A JAMES WATT MEMORIAL INSTITUTE was declared open at Birmingham, England, on May 15, by Mr. Alan Chorlton, M.P., president of the Institution of Mechanical Engineers. The premises are a wing of the recently erected York House and include a lecture hall, a library and a committee room. When in 1919 Birmingham celebrated the centenary of James Watt a fund was raised which, after paying the commemoration expenses and the cost of a memorial volume, enabled the trustees to set aside £5,000 for a research scholarship in mechanical engineering in Birmingham University. A sum of £6,000 remained. Sir Gilbert Barling, chairman of the trustees, explained that originally it was hoped to endow a chair of mechanical engineering at the university, which would have required £20,000. Eventually they visualized the erection of a fine building as a memorial home for the various engineering societies in Birmingham. Unfortunately the amount subscribed was very much less than was contemplated. Hence the position had to be reconsidered. Their £6,000 had now grown to £10,000, and as at least £40,000 was needed to erect an appropriate building the trustees decided to proceed in a small way with a view to future development. As a home for engineering societies the purpose of the institute would be educational and scientific. To run it in a fruitful manner they needed about £800 a year, and they were already assured of nearly £700.

*Nature* reports that shortly after the death of Professor John Henry Poynting in 1914 a fund was subscribed by his friends with the object of providing a memorial to him. Part of the money thus raised was used for the publication by the Cambridge University Press of a volume of his "Collected Scientific Papers," of which a copy was presented to every university in the British Empire and to representative universities in foreign countries. Another part of the fund was used for the purchase of a portrait to be presented to the University of Birmingham and hung in the great hall of the university. The remainder, which was invested, together with the accrued interest, has been offered to, and accepted by, the council of the university, for the foundation of a Poynting lecture, to be delivered at intervals of not more than two years by physicists of outstanding distinction.

## RECENT DEATHS

DR. WILLIAM T. COUNCILMAN, Shattuck professor of pathology at the Harvard Medical School until his retirement with the title of professor emeritus in 1922, died on May 27, in his seventy-ninth year.

DR. JOHN CHALMERS DA COSTA, for more than forty years connected with the Jefferson Medical College, Philadelphia, filling the Samuel D. Gross chair of surgery since 1900, died on May 16, at the age of seventy years.

*Nature* reports the death of John Mackereth, a deputy conservator in the Indian Forest Service, on May 5, aged thirty-four years, and of J. T. J. Morrison, emeritus professor of forensic medicine and toxicology in the University of Birmingham, on May 10, aged seventy-six years.

THE recent death of Dr. Halfdan Bryn, Trondheim, is announced at the age of sixty-nine years. A correspondent writes: "With him Norway has lost its greatest anthropologist. Bryn was for some years president of the Norwegian Medical Association and was a member of the Consultative Eugenics Commission of Norway."

# SCIENTIFIC EVENTS

## THE SCIENTIFIC SITUATION IN GERMANY

A WIRELESS to *The New York Times* from Berlin reports that the Kaiser Wilhelm Society for the Advancement of the Sciences, the foremost scientific organization in Germany, which conducts thirty-two research institutes, held its twenty-second annual meeting here on May 23. It was presided over by Professor Max Planck, who said that nowadays no one in Germany could be permitted to stand aside, "rifle at rest." He declared that there was only one watchword—"the consolidation of all available forces for the reconstruction of the fatherland." He read the following message sent by the society to Chancellor Hitler: "The Kaiser Wilhelm Society for the Advancement of the Sciences begs leave to tender reverential greetings to the chancellor and its solemn pledge that German science is also ready to cooperate joyously in the reconstruction of the new national state."

Dr. Wilhelm Frick, Minister of the Interior, told the scientists what the state expected from them if it was to look after them. "It is the nature of scientific thought and research so to engross man as to expose him to the danger not only of becoming severed from the greater whole but actually losing his sense of duty —forgetting that he must serve the community," he declared. "With all respect for the freedom of science, let us postulate that service to science must be service to the nation and that scientific achievements are worthless when they can not be utilized for the culture of the people."

No more scientists of Jewish extraction have been eliminated from the Kaiser Wilhelm Society's institutes, and among the elective members of its governing board three persons of the Jewish faith were reelected.

The investiture of Professor Ernst Krieck with the rectorship of the University of Frankfurt, which was renamed Goethe University last year, took place on May 23. The new rector said that in recent years the universities had lost a central idea, had become sidetracked and "never could have struggled from their paralysis but for the folk renascence. The chief characteristic of this rebirth is the replacement of the humanistic ideal by the national and political. Nowadays the task of the universities is not to cultivate objective science but soldierlike, militant science, and their foremost task is to form the will and character of their students."

A correspondent writes from Holland: "The declaration against Einstein, published by the Prussian Academy of Sciences, was not decided upon at a session of the academy. Tactical motives may have caused the subsequent recognition of the declaration by the academy. The first declaration was signed by the presiding secretary, Heymann, alone. He is, along with the orientalist, Lüders, permanent secretary of the Philosophical-Historical Division. The second declaration was signed by Heymann and Von Ficker. Von Ficker is one of the permanent secretaries of the Mathematical-Physical Division. The other permanent secretary is Max Planck, who was in southern Italy at the time of the declarations."

## IN HONOR OF THE LATE STEPHEN TYNG MATHER

A MONUMENT, erected in honor of Stephen Tyng Mather, first director of the National Park Service, was unveiled by Mrs. Franklin D. Roosevelt, on May 27, at Bear Mountain, New York, at dedication ceremonies on the occasion of the meeting of the National Conference on State Parks, which was held from May 23 to 26. Mr. Mather's widow, a resident of Darien, Connecticut, and his daughter, Mrs. Edward McPherson, of Ithaca, were present at the ceremonies.

Mrs. Roosevelt, before drawing aside the red, white and blue curtain which veiled the plaque, remarked briefly that it was "a joy to have Mr. Mather's work recognized and commemorated." The plaque is a bronze tablet set in the face of a mammoth boulder. Designed by Bryant Baker, it bears Mr. Mather's profile against a background suggestion of mountains and trees, with the dates of his life span, July 4, 1867, to January 22, 1930. Its inscription reads: "He laid the foundation of the National Park Service, defining and establishing the policies under which its areas shall be developed and conserved unimpaired for future generations. There will never come an end to the good that he has done."

The Secretary of the Interior Harold L. Ickes, who flew from Washington for the dedication, said that Mr. Mather's record of achievement was

> as far flung and enduring as the great national parks whose true mission in our national life he first conceived and expressed.
>
> Stephen Mather was a fortunate dreamer of dreams who had the rare chance to follow his dreams and to make them come true. Before he came into our national park system, a park was just a park, an interesting or beautiful expanse of woods and lakes and mountains, without intimate connection with the lives of the people. He conceived the theory that our parks should be made the means of preserving the health and maintaining the morale of the American people.
>
> To do what he did it was necessary not only that he love the mountains and forests and all the beautiful handiwork of nature, it was equally necessary that he should truly love just people. And it is hard to say whether he loved nature more than people or people more than nature. It is probably well within the truth to say that he loved both of them equally and that when he had them in conjunction he loved them both supremely.
>
> It is keeping well within the bounds of truth to say that our great system of national parks and state parks providing, as they do, a means of out-door recreation unequaled in the history of the world, is largely due to the love of humanity and of nature that burned deep within the soul of Stephen T. Mather. He knew all the national parks intimately. He knew every employee in the service. They loved him and knew him as their friend and their affection and loyalty he returned in full measure. To the

extent that so many thousands of acres could feel the personal touch of any man, every section of every national park felt the personal touch of this great conservationist and lover of humanity. And they responded generously to that touch.

## FIELD CONFERENCE OF THE NEW YORK STATE GEOLOGICAL ASSOCIATION

THE New York State Geological Association convened for the ninth annual field conference on May 12, at Newburgh, New York. In the morning thrust contacts of the Precambrian crystallines of the Highlands on the Paleozoic sediments were examined at Snake Hill, near Newburgh, and at Cornwall-on-Hudson, and the Precambrian intrusives were studied at the east end of Bear Mountain Bridge. After stopping for lunch at Mohansic Country Club, the cars were driven along the parkways to northern Manhattan and The Bronx, New York City; exposures of the Fordham gneiss, Inwood marble and Manhattan schist were visited. In the evening, a dinner was held at Columbia University in conjunction with the Geology Journal Club.

On Saturday, May 13, the first stop was at the diabase with included olivine zone along the state road above Edgewater, New Jersey. After crossing the Palisades, the remainder of the morning was spent in the Belmont-Gurnee quarry at Granton, where a contact of Newark sediments and intrusive basalt is well exposed; many specimens of the branchiopod *Estheria ovata* Lea and of ganoid fishes were obtained. After lunch in Jersey City, the party visited the exposures of the Staten Island serpentine and the moraines on Staten Island, New York.

About eighty members, many of them undergraduates in the universities and colleges in the state, attended the excursion. Professor R. J. Colony, of Columbia University, was president.

G. MARSHALL KAY,
*Secretary*

## GROUP CONFERENCES AT THE COLD SPRING HARBOR BIOLOGICAL LABORATORY

As a part of its policy of fostering a closer relationship between biology and the basic sciences, the Biological Laboratory at Cold Spring Harbor is inaugurating a plan, according to which it invites each year a group of mathematicians, physicists, chemists and biologists, actively interested in some one phase of quantitative biology, to carry on their work, and to engage in a group conference at the laboratory during the summer. The aim is that every important aspect of a given subject should be adequately represented from the physical and chemical, as well as from the biological, point of view.

"The Potential Difference at Interfaces and its Bearing upon Biological Phenomena" is the subject this year, and the following men will be in residence.

Harold Abramson, biochemistry, College of Physicians and Surgeons, Columbia University.

David R. Briggs, chemistry, The Otho S. A. Sprague Memorial Institute, University of Chicago.

Barnett Cohen, physiological chemistry, the Johns Hopkins School of Medicine.

Kenneth S. Cole, physiology, College of Physicians and Surgeons, Columbia University.

Stuart Mudd, bacteriology, the School of Medicine, University of Pennsylvania.

Hans Müller, physics, Massachusetts Institute of Technology.

Eric Ponder, biology, Washington Square College, New York University.

In conjunction with this meeting, a series of lectures and symposia will be given by members of the group in residence and by other invited speakers. The latter include:

Robert Chambers, biology, Washington Square College, New York University.

Hugo Fricke, biophysics, the Biological Laboratory.

Herbert S. Gasser, physiology, Cornell University Medical College.

Duncan A. MacInnes, physical chemistry, Rockefeller Institute for Medical Research.

L. Michaelis, physical chemistry, Rockefeller Institute for Medical Research.

W. J. V. Osterhout, botany, Rockefeller Institute for Medical Research.

Donald D. Van Slyke, chemistry, Rockefeller Institute for Medical Research.

The symposia will take place on each Wednesday in July, and on Monday, July 24, and Friday, July 28, beginning at 10 A. M., and continuing, with ample time for discussion, throughout the day. Individual lectures will be given on other days, according to a schedule which may be obtained from the laboratory.

## PROFESSOR HARRISON AS CROONIAN LECTURER

DR. ROSS G. HARRISON, Sterling professor of biology at Yale University, has been invited by the Royal Society to give the Croonian Lecture in London, and will speak on a lectureship which began with Alexander Stuart in 1738, the roster of which includes the distinguished anatomists and physiologists of Great Britain during two centuries, with very few from other countries. A correspondent writes:

Professor Harrison, who last year received the honorary degree of doctor of science from Trinity College, University of Dublin, in recognition of the fact that "in his own science he is one of the most famous discoverers and teachers of the New World," was the first to show that it is possible to remove groups of individual cells from the living body, and grow them in the body juices in such a way that their behavior can be watched under the microscope. This growing of groups of living cells is known as "tissue culture," and has constituted a great step forward in the study of living cells and consequently in the investigation of diseases. He has employed this method to trace the development of embryonic cells into differentiated cells, and his transplantations of pieces taken from an embryo into another place, or even into a different embryo, have elucidated much that was previously obscure.

Managing editor of the *Journal of Experimental Zoology* since its foundation in 1904, Dr. Harrison was the first to observe directly the outgrowth of the nerve fiber, showing that it is a mode of protoplasmic movement. His links with zoologists in this and other countries are many. He is a member of the National Academy of Sciences and the American Philosophical Society, a fellow of the American Academy of Arts and Sciences, and has been honored by scientific societies of Germany, France, Italy, Norway and Austria.

Professor Harrison's most intimate connections, however, are through the students trained in the Osborn Zoological Laboratories at Yale. During his directorship a total of 58 Ph.D. degrees have been conferred upon students from the department of zoology, of whom some forty are now professors in twenty-five institutions. In addition, post-doctoral research students come each year to Yale University to study his technique. In recent years they have included investigators from China, Russia, Belgium, France, Germany, etc.

The lectureship to which Professor Harrison has been invited was founded by William Croone, a successful practising physician and lecturer to the Company of Surgeons in London, who contributed information far in advance of his time on muscular physiology and the embryology of the chick. He was one of the founders of the Royal Society and in the remarkable group of its early members, which included Sir Isaac Newton, Sir Christopher Wren, Halley, the astronomer, and the two great diarists, Evelyn and Samuel Pepys, his contributions to the discussion of the society are noted in the records.

## SCIENTIFIC NOTES AND NEWS

THE University of Wisconsin will confer, at the annual commencement exercises on June 19, the doctorate of laws on Dr. Arnold Sommerfeld, professor of mathematics at the University of Munich, and the doctorate of science on Dr. James Aston, professor of mining and metallurgical engineering at the Carnegie Institute of Technology, Pittsburgh.

THE degree of Sc.D., *honoris causa,* will be conferred by the University of Cambridge on the Marchese G. Marconi and on Sir Frederick Gowland Hopkins, Sir William Dunn professor of biochemistry.

THE University of Liverpool has conferred the degree of doctor of science on Dr. Geoffrey Ingram Taylor, Yarrow research professor of the Royal Society.

FOR the development and promotion of agricultural exploration and the introduction of new and valuable plants into the United States, the committee on the Marcellus Hartley Fund of the National Academy of Sciences has awarded its Public Welfare Medal to Dr. David Fairchild, of the Division of Foreign Plant Introduction, Bureau of Plant Industry of the U. S. Department of Agriculture. The medal is given for "eminence in the application of science to the public welfare."

FOR chemical research work of high significance as pure science and of equally high value in its practical application, two research workers, Dr. F. B. La Forge and Dr. H. L. J. Haller, of the U. S. Department of Agriculture, have been awarded the Hillebrand Prize of the Chemical Society of Washington, for the determination of the chemical structure of rotenone, a new substance used in insect poisons.

DR. DAVID EUGENE SMITH, professor emeritus of mathematics at Teachers College, Columbia University, has been decorated by Persia for his study of the mathematical works and philosophy of Omar Khayyam.

DR. E. D. MERRILL, director of the New York Botanical Garden, was elected a foreign member of the Linnean Society of London at the meeting on May 11.

DR. C. TATE REGAN, director of the British Museum (Natural History), has been elected a foreign member of the Royal Danish Academy.

A WIRELESS dispatch to *The New York Times* states that Professor Albert Einstein, who has received a professorship in the Collège de France, has been proposed for membership in the French Academy of Sciences. After favorable discussion, the proposal was postponed for inquiry as to whether Professor Einstein's election was possible under the academy's rules, which state that before a foreigner can be named as an associate member he must first have served as a corresponding member.

AT a special dinner on May 5 at which the faculty of Harvard University and the governing boards of the university and of the Peter Bent Brigham Hospital were present, a portrait of Dr. Harvey Cushing, who recently retired from the Moseley professorship of surgery at the university and as surgeon-in-chief of the hospital, was presented to the hospital, and a portrait of Dr. Henry A. Christian, Hersey professor of the theory and practise of physic and physician-in-chief to the hospital and from 1908 to 1912 dean of the medical school, was presented to the university.

INFORMAL exercises were held on May 21 in the Chemistry Library at the University of Illinois in connection with the presentation of portraits of three of its distinguished chemists, Professor A. W. Palmer, Professor S. W. Parr and Professor W. A. Noyes, by the Association of Illinois Chemists to the University of Illinois. Professor Palmer was head of the department of chemistry from 1894 to 1904, Professor Parr was professor of applied chemistry from 1890 to 1926, and Professor Noyes was head of the department from 1907 to 1926. Dr. Norman W. Krase, who had charge of the arrangements for the painting of the portraits, presided. Professor Roger Adams, head of the department of chemistry, after speaking briefly of the history of the department and of the accomplishments of Professors Palmer, Parr and Noyes, presented the portraits to the university. President Harry Woodburn Chase accepted the portraits. Professor W. A. Noyes related some of the facts connected with the development of the chemistry department with which he has been so long associated.

PROFESSOR CHARLES F. SCOTT, for twenty-two years chairman of the department of electrical engineering at Yale University, will retire from active teaching in June. His colleagues held a reception on May 19 in his honor, when Professor Russell H. Chittenden, formerly director of the Sheffield Scientific School, presented a collection of letters of congratulation and appreciation.

DR. H. A. BUEHLER was the guest of honor at a testimonial dinner at Rolla, Missouri, on May 10, in celebration of his twenty-fifth anniversary as state geologist of Missouri. He was appointed to this position in May, 1908, and has served continuously since that time. Dr. Buehler's distinguished services to the state and particularly his participation in the development of the mineral industry of Missouri were reviewed by a number of speakers.

DR. FELIX D'HERELLE has resigned from the professorship of bacteriology which he has held at Yale University since 1927. While in residence Dr. d'Herelle confined himself largely to the study of bacteriophagy as a laboratory phenomenon, since suitable clinical material was lacking. It is the hope of elaborating his work in the clinical field, possibly at the new institute for infectious diseases at Tiflis, Russia, which now takes him abroad.

DR. LOREN ROSCOE CHANDLER, of the department of surgery at the Stanford Medical School, has been appointed dean to fill the vacancy caused by the recent death of Dr. Henry G. Mehrtens.

PROMOTIONS at Yale University include Dr. Harry Martin Zimmerman to a professorship of pathology and Dr. Dirk Brouwer to an assistant professorship of astronomy.

THE Senate of Queen's University, Belfast, has appointed Mr. P. T. Crymble to the chair of surgery in succession to Professor Andrew Fullerton.

*Nature* states that Dr. M. Dixon has been appointed to the university lectureship in biochemistry, established in connection with the scheme for the employment of the Rockefeller benefaction to the University of Cambridge, and Dr. E. G. Holmes has been appointed to the university lectureship vacated by Dr. Dixon.

DR. FRITZ KNOLL, of Prague, has been appointed professor of botany at the University of Vienna.

THE following new full-time appointments have been announced in the School of Medicine, George Washington University: Edward Bright Vedder, professor of experimental medicine and executive officer, department of pathology and experimental medicine; Dr. William Henry Waller, instructor in anatomy; Dr. Jesse Harmon, instructor in biochemistry; Dr. Hubert Scott Loring, instructor in biochemistry; Dr. James Leslie Snyder, instructor in pathology, and Dr. John Ralston Pate, teaching fellow in anatomy.

DR. JAMES ANGUS DOULL, head of the department of public health and hygiene of the School of Medicine of Western Reserve University, Cleveland, sailed from Vancouver on May 25, to spend the summer establishing experimental work for the Leonard Wood Memorial Foundation for the Eradication of Leprosy in the Philippine Islands. Dr. Doull will work at Culion and Cebu, where the foundation has leper colonies.

DR. E. D. MERRILL, director of the New York Botanical Garden, will attend the fifth Pacific Science Congress, Victoria and Vancouver, B. C., as an official representative of the U. S. Government, the National Academy of Sciences, the American Philosophical Society and the New York Botanical Garden.

PROFESSOR ARTHUR H. COMPTON gave a public lecture at the University of Iowa on May 12 on "Cosmic Rays on Six Continents." He also gave two technical lectures on May 12 and 13 on "Some Recent Experiments with Cosmic Rays."

DR. OSCAR RIDDLE, of the department of genetics of the Carnegie Institution, on April 28 addressed the Brown University Chapter of Sigma Xi on "Sex and Reproduction," and the Biology Seminar on "Hormones of the Anterior Pituitary."

DR. CHARLES R. STOCKARD, professor of anatomy, Cornell University, gave a lecture at the hospital of Duke University on the "Peculiar Form and Type in Man and Animals" on April 8; on May 3 Dr. Otto H. F. Vollbeahr lectured on old and rare books, and on May 15 Dr. Arthur Steindler, professor of orthopedics in the State University of Iowa, gave a clinic on "The Low Back."

DR. ROBERT P. FISCHELIS, secretary and chief chemist of the Board of Pharmacy of the State of New Jersey, will deliver the commencement address to the graduating class of the Connecticut College of Pharmacy at New Haven, on the evening of June 5. His subject will be "Pharmacy's Contribution to Public Health Service."

THE Bakerian lecture of the Royal Society was delivered on May 25 by Dr. J. Chadwick, who took as his subject "The Neutron."

THE Geological Society of Chicago held its last spring meeting on May 18. The speakers were Dr. Theo. A. Link, Imperial Oil Company, and Professor C. A. Heiland, Colorado School of Mines, whose subjects, respectively, were the exhibits of petroleum geology and of geophysical methods at the Century of Progress Exposition at Chicago.

THE annual initiation dinner and meeting of the New York University Chapter of the Society of the Sigma Xi was held on May 19 at the University Faculty Club. Mr. Barnum Brown, curator of fossil reptiles at the American Museum of Natural History, addressed the society on "Dinosaurs of North America, Particularly Those of the Cretaceous Period." At this meeting twenty-three new members were inducted. Officers were elected for the next academic year as follows: *President,* Professor R. R. Renshaw; *Vice-president,* Professor Charles W. Lytle; *Secretary-Treasurer,* Professor Harry G. Lindwall.

THE luncheon given by Section C and the Chicago Chemists Club at the time of the meeting of the American Association for the Advancement of Science will be at 12:30 on Tuesday, not Thursday as stated in the preliminary announcement.

A SYMPOSIUM on "Nationalism" will be held by Section L of the American Association for the Advancement of Science in the auditorium of the Chicago Historical Society at Chicago on Monday, June 26, at 8:00 P. M. This has been organized by means of assistance generously provided by Dr. Duren J. H. Ward and the Far Reaching Foundation of Denver, Colorado. The presiding officer will be Professor James A. James, of Northwestern University, and the speakers and their subjects will be : Professor Bernadotte E. Schmitt, University of Chicago, "Nationalism in European History Since the Times of Napoleon"; Dr. Charles A. Beard, president of the American Historical Association, "Nationalism in American History"; Dr. Albrecht Mendelssohn Bartholdy, director of the Institute of Foreign Affairs, Hamburg, "Imperialism, Nationalism and International Peace." The discussion will be led by Professors Bernard Faÿ, of the Collège de France, and Charles E. Merriam, of the University of Chicago.

A ONE-DAY conference on problems relating to death from asphyxiation was held at the New York Academy of Medicine on May 24, under the auspices of the Society for the Prevention of Asphyxial Death. Dr. Paluel J. Flagg, president of the society, was chairman of the conference. Dr. Linsly R. Williams, director of the Academy of Medicine, delivered an address of welcome. The speakers included Health Commissioner Shirley W. Wynne, Dr. Harrison P. Martland, medical examiner for Essex County, New Jersey; Albert W. Whitney, associate general manager of the National Bureau of Casualty and Surety Underwriters; Dr. Daniel J. Donovan, chief surgeon of the New York City Police Department, and Dr. Yandell Henderson, professor of applied physiology of the Yale University Medical School.

THE annual excursion of the Physiographers and Geographers Club of New York City took place on May 20 as a bus trip for the purpose of studying the Triassic Basin of New Jersey, under the guidance of Dr. Bertram T. Butler, of the College of the City of New York. All the rock formations of the Triassic were studied in various quarries, the intrusive Palisade and Sourland Mt. ridges were visited as well as the surface lava flows forming the Watchung ridges. The large river systems, including the Delaware, were surveyed. Several volcanic centers, as Cushetunk Mt. and Bellvale, were included. Professor J. E. Woodman, of New York University, is president of the club; the secretary is Dr. Anna Welnitz. An innovation was the taking of moving pictures covering the details of the Triassic structures.

As previously announced, the undergraduate instruction in forestry at Cornell University is to be abandoned, and such work is to be concentrated in Syracuse University. Now it is officially stated that the Syracuse University College of Agriculture is to be discontinued.

THE Board of Estimate of New York City has

voted to set aside a plot of city-owned land in Manhattan Square, near the American Museum of Natural History, as a site for the museum's planetarium, a project to be financed through a Reconstruction Finance Corporation loan. The board stipulated that when the construction cost of the project is repaid through fees collected from the public, the property should revert to the city. The R. F. C. has approved a loan contingent upon the city's providing the site. Trustees of the museum recently organized an American Museum of Natural History Planetarium Authority to direct the project, naming the Mayor and other city officials to serve with officers of the museum.

THE sum of 2,000,000 kronas (about $400,000), has been bequeathed for the purpose of erecting a building for the Technical Museum of Stockholm by the "Knut and Alice Wallenberg Foundation," created by the Swedish banker, Knut A. Wallenberg, and Mrs. Wallenberg. The conditions attached to the donation are that the government should place building space at the disposal of the museum free of cost and that the work in order to reduce unemployment should be begun as soon as possible, in any case before the end of 1934. According to Science Service the Technical Museum of Stockholm is at present temporarily housed in the Royal Swedish Institute for Engineering Research, the head of which is Commercial Counsellor Axel F. Enström, one of its active supporters. The director, T. Althin, has gradually brought together a collection of objects and exhibits illustrating the origin, history and development of the present technical methods and inventions. The majority of these objects owing to lack of space has been stored in different parts of the city, but will now be exhibited in the new museum. It will be constructed in three stories with a floor space of about 8,000 square meters and will, when ready, be the leading institution of its kind in the north. It will also contain spacious lecture rooms and a library.

AN expedition to Guadelupe, an island belonging to Mexico and lying off the coast of Lower California, to hunt specimens of elephant seal, largest of all seals, for a proposed group to be installed at the Field Museum of Natural History, sailed from San Diego, California, on May 28. The expedition is being made aboard the yacht *Velero III,* a 1,000-ton ship about 200 feet long, owned and commanded by Captain G. Allan Hancock, of San Diego, who has placed the vessel at the disposal of the museum for this expedition. Captain Hancock and Dr. Harry M. Wegeforth, president of the Zoological Society of San Diego, have made all arrangements for carrying out the project. Two members of the Field Museum staff, Julius Friesser and Frank C. Wonder, joined the expedition at San Diego. The government of Mexico has issued permits to the expedition to collect the giant seals, which are rare and are under protection to prevent their extermination.

NINETEEN fellowships have been awarded by the New York State College of Forestry for the years 1933–34. Each scholarship carried a grant of $500. Two men have been given a one-semester award in order to complete their work. Six of the scholarships will be for a Ph.D. degree and the balance for master's degrees. These men are considered by the faculty to be especially qualified to take up advanced work. All recipients of the fellowships agree to give instructional assistance or do routine departmental work not to exceed fifteen hours a week. The holder of the fellowship is expected to devote his full time for the period of his appointment as outlined by the committee on scholarships.

*Museum News* states that the Newark, New Jersey, Museum has curtailed its activities as a result of a cut in the city appropriation from $100,000 to $65,000. Eighteen trained staff members and eight other assistants have been dropped from the rolls. Salaries have been cut 25 per cent. The lending work of the educational department, which last year made 32,000 loans of objects to Newark schools, has been discontinued, also the work of the extension department through which loans of small exhibits have been made to stores, churches and other organizations. The museum will be open to the public from 12 to 5 daily, except on Mondays. Daily gallery talks and the hobby work will be continued and the museum's activities centered on making as full use as possible of the museum building and equipment.

THE London *Times* reports that Dr. A. Maher, Keeper of the Irish Antiquities in the National Museum, Dublin, in the course of excavation work at Store Park, Ballyglass, County Mayo, on Saturday unearthed a stone cist, containing the skeleton of a man of powerful build, about 6 feet high. The find turned out to be a cist burial of the early Bronze Age, dating back 3,000 years. In the same cist a small clay-baked urn, which differs from any in the National Museum and is decorated with strange markings, was discovered. From the position of the bones it appears that the man was buried in a crouched position, the typical manner in which the dead were placed in Ireland during the Bronze Age. The skeleton and urn have been acquired for the National Museum, and will be scientifically examined in the near future. This is the second Bronze Age burial to be discovered in this neighborhood in the same week.

# DISCUSSION

## CONSERVATION VERSUS PRESERVATION

THE Yellowstone Park Act of 1872 refers to "preservation from injury or spoilation of all timber, mineral deposits, natural curiosities or wonders within the park, and their retention in their natural condition." It was apparently considered illegal to carry on any "control" measures under the old law. The National Park Service Act, 1916, states that the purpose "is to conserve the scenery and the natural and historic objects and the wild life therein and to provide for the enjoyment of the same in such manner and by such means as will leave them unimpaired for the enjoyment of future generations." The Secretary of the Interior was further authorized to remove timber, control attacks of disease and insects and to provide for the destruction of such plant and animal life as may be detrimental to the use of the parks. This was very unfortunate legislation, as the confidence in beneficial results from such "control" has, since that time, materially weakened.

Many people conceive of the National Park Service as a conservation organization. To conserve, as the term is now most frequently used, means to preserve while in use and it often implics ultimate depletion. In actual practise the operations carried on in the name of conservation are not designed to preserve the natural order but to establish and maintain a different order as regards kind and abundance of plants and animals present. The difference between preservation is well illustrated in a recent publication by Wright, Dixon and Thompson,[1] who advocate the preservation of the birds and mammals in national parks. They point out the importance of dead timber to various birds and mammals, and the need of such timber for numerous invertebrates might well be added. Conservation as usually practised removes dead and mature timber, while preservation lets nature take its course.

In a series of suggestions by the authors mentioned nearly all the ordinary "conservation" views are reversed:

> Every species shall be left to carry on its struggle for existence unaided, as being to its greatest ultimate good, unless there is real cause to believe that it will perish if unassisted.
>
> No native predator shall be destroyed on account of its normal utilization of any other park animal, excepting if that animal is in immediate danger of extermination, and then only if the predator is not itself a vanishing form.

The authors of the report further advocate the encouragement of visitors to see animals; *e.g.*, bears in their natural surroundings rather than about a garbage pile.

The conservation idea may reasonably be extended to cover the preservation processes described in this recent publication. If so, one may conceive of the maintenance of exotic pheasants in South Dakota as very near the zero point of the conservation of nature with most other so-called conservation measures not far above this level. A nature sanctuary in a national park or national forest in which every effort was made to preserve a sample of original nature without disturbance may well stand at the top of the conservation series.

In nature sanctuaries the natural fluctuations of organisms are allowed free play and serve among other things to show what natural fluctuations in abundance are like. There is or has been so much interference with natural processes in the form of "control" of this and that organism that the student of "wild life" management who would seek a basis for more scientific treatment of the animals in his charge, is left without guiding principles or reliable information and will continue thus until the preservation measures advocated by Wright, Dixon and Thompson with additional measures of equal importance are put into effect in as many nature reserves as possible.

V. E. SHELFORD[2]

## NOTES ON A SPHAGNUM BOG AT FORT BRAGG, CALIFORNIA

THE farthest south sphagnum bog which the writer has seen on the Pacific Coast is located about three miles east of Fort Bragg, which is on the coast, about 125 miles north of San Francisco. It is from 200 to 400 feet or more in width and is perhaps three fourths of a mile long. The bog occupies an irregular depression in a flat about 300 feet above sea-level. A creek originates in the bog and flows into the Noya River which flows into the ocean at Fort Bragg. The soil of this flat is almost pure sand known as Mendocino sand.

The bog is in a young stage of development in which the aspect is mainly given by *Ledum columbianum*, forming a dense growth four or five feet tall, and a large sedge (*Carex* sp.) which is a little taller than the Ledum and is equally abundant. Scattered *Myrica californica*, mostly five to ten feet tall, occurs much as in the bogs of the Oregon coast, and a low growth of *Gaultheria shallon* is also found. A robust species of *Sphagnum* forms a dense growth among the *Ledum* and *Carex* and forms many hummocks. The herbs identified are *Drosera rotundifolia, Hypericum anagalloides, Lilium maritimum* and *Gentiana* sp.

[1] "Fauna of the National Parks of the United States," Contribution of Wild Life Survey Fauna Series 1, 1933.

[2] Chairman of the Committee on the Preservation of Natural Conditions, Ecological Society of America.

The forest succession comprises small scattered trees of the three species—*Cupressus pigmya, Pinus muricata* and *Pinus contorta.* The first of these is the dominant one, though the last one shows occasional larger individuals (30 feet or more tall). Young specimens of the dominant tree (3 feet or less in height) are as abundant as the older ones (20 feet or more in height).

The plant community surrounding this bog is a scrubby forest of small trees (mostly 40 feet or less in height) forming a dense growth. It is largely *Cupressus pigmya,* but there is some *Pinus contorta* and an occasional specimen of *Pinus muricata.* The shrubby undergrowth in this forest is largely *Myrica californica, Ledum columbianum* and *Gaultheria shallon.* The first two of these grow much taller in the forest than in the bog. Herbs occurring in both forest and bog are *Lilium maritimum* and *Gentiana* sp. This forest forms a belt about two miles wide on the level stretch of Mendocino sand. Back of this is the redwood forest on good soil.

Borings made in this bog near the origin of the creek show three strata of peat. (a) A surface layer of living sphagnum, under which is dead sphagnum, little disintegrated and much mixed with roots of *Ledum* and *Carex.* This layer of living and dead sphagnum is mostly 12 to 18 inches deep. (b) A layer of sedge peat with many small roots and some wood. The depth of this layer is mostly 1.5 to 2 feet. (c) A mixed layer of mud clay, sand and wood about 4 feet deep. The wood in this layer, like that in (b), is in a fairly good state of preservation. The boundaries between these layers are not very distinct. The borings were made with a Davis peat borer, and the large amount of wood encountered made sampling very difficult.

Evidently this bog has been formed in a relatively flat, shallow ravine by a dense growth of sedges and other swamp vegetation on the accumulated mud, sand, clay and remains of woody plants. The sphagnum is a comparatively recent invader. Drainage in this bog is better than that in most Pacific Coast bogs and this may account in part for its lack of maturity.

Fort Bragg has wet winters and dry summers. The average monthly and annual precipitation in inches (37 years' record) is as follows: January, 7.71; February, 6.89; March, 4.89; April 2.45; May, 1.49; June, 0.42; July, 0.08; August, 0.04; September 0.81; October, 1.80; November, 5.01; December, 6.11; annual, 37.70. The only snow reported during the last 17 years is 1.0 inch in January, 1923. No temperature data are available for Fort Bragg, but the 45 years' record at Eureka to the northward shows an average of 51.40° F. and the 41 years' record of Pt. Reyes of 52.5° F. The monthly data for Eureka are as follows:

| | Jan. | Feb. | Mar. | Apr. | May |
|---|---|---|---|---|---|
| Average ... | 47.1 | 47.6 | 48.4 | 50.0 | 52.2 |
| Highest ... | 77 | 85 | 78 | 79 | 78 |
| Lowest ...... | 20 | 24 | 29 | 31 | 35 |

| June | July | Aug. | Sept. | Oct. | Nov. | Dec. |
|---|---|---|---|---|---|---|
| 54.5 | 55.7 | 56.2 | 55.7 | 53.6 | 51.1 | 47.8 |
| 85 | 76 | 79 | 82 | 84 | 81 | 70 |
| 40 | 43 | 45 | 36 | 35 | 27 | 24 |

The maximum recorded at Pt. Reyes is 98° (September) and the minimum 30° (March). All the above data were furnished by the U. S. Weather Bureau office at San Francisco.

The character of this bog is of interest in the general problem of the occurrence and course of development of sphagnum bogs along the North Pacific Coast of America. It is reported that sphagnum forms considerable growths at various points in the forests of the coast of northern California, but detailed information about bogs formed by it is not available. This bog has much in common with the coastal bogs of Oregon, though it has not reached the somewhat mature stage shown by many of the Oregon bogs. Its forest succession resembles that in bogs of Oregon and Washington in including *Pinus contorta* but differs strikingly from them in the occurrence of *Cupressus pigmya.* The climatic conditions under which it has developed do not differ greatly from those under which the bogs of Western Oregon and Washington have developed.

The writer made his study of this bog on August 26, 1931. His first information in regard to it was received from Mr. W. G. Corbitt, and valued assistance in its study was given by Mr. V. B. Davis. He will welcome further information in regard to the occurrence of sphagnum areas in California.

GEORGE B. RIGG
UNIVERSITY OF WASHINGTON, SEATTLE

## SEDIMENTATION AND SEDIMENTOLOGY

THE terms "sedimentology" and "sedimentation" are subjects of comment by W. H. Twenhofel in the *Bulletin of the National Research Council,* Report of the Committee on Sedimentation, 1930–1932, p. 18. Dr. Twenhofel considers the terms "sedimentation" and "sedimentationist" as more fitting designations than "sedimentology" and "sedimentologist" for "the range of geologic processes concerned in the formation of the sedimentary rocks" and for "a student of sediments," respectively. He rejects "sedimentology" because it contains "roots from two languages."

The choice of terms is perhaps not of great importance for the present. It has seemed advisable, however, to reconsider the question, because, whatever term is now adopted, it will be difficult to change when once entrenched in the literature.

First, a minor correction of Dr. Twenhofel's statement is needed. In my article "Sedimentation and Sedimentology," in SCIENCE of January 1, 1932, "sedimentology" was not proposed as a designation for "the range of geologic processes concerned in the formation of the sedimentary rocks," but as a designation for the subject concerned with these processes.

The term "sedimentology" had previously been so rarely used in geological literature (3 or 4 times), that I believe most geologists were not aware of its existence. After my article appeared in SCIENCE in January, 1932, I learned that the term "sedimentology" was first introduced some ten years ago by Dr. A. C. Trowbridge, who, in "American Men of Science," has listed sedimentology as one of his major subjects.

Etymologically hybrid formations are not uncommon. In my earlier article in SCIENCE, glaciology was mentioned as an analogy to sedimentology. "Sociology," "vulcanology" and "stratigraphy" are hybrid formations which in the past have been used without objection. Since "terminology" itself is a Latin-Greek formation, there seems to be no reason for disqualifying the term "sedimentology," especially since the latter, in the interest of non-ambiguity and logical consistency, is superior to "sedimentation" as a term for the subject. Hybrid formations are also frequently found in the German language, which permits such combinations as *Sedimentgesteine, Sedimentpetrographie,"* etc.

All standard dictionaries state that sedimentation is an act or process of depositing sediments. The use of the term "sedimentation" also for the subject concerned with processes of sedimentation and formation of sediments, ancient or recent, is a violation of the principle of non-ambiguity, and is therefore more objectional than the use of a hybrid formation. There is a distinct difference between the glaciation of North America and the glaciology of North America, or better, the glaciation of Greenland and the glaciology of Greenland. In analogous manner, differentiation should be made, for instance, between the sedimentation of the Mexican Gulf and the sedimentology of the Mexican Gulf.

The choice between "sedimentologist" and "sedimentationist" as designations for a student of sediments is not entirely a matter of taste. The terms "Vulcanist" and "Neptunist" designate two old schools of geologists, *i.e.,* these terms signify advocates or assertors of certain theories rather than students of certain subjects. The sole ending *-ist* does not always signify a student or one versed in a particular subject. There is generally a difference between a socialist and sociologist, a symbolist and symbologist, an idealist and ideologist. Generally, the ending *-logy* signifies a theoretical, scientific, analytical, philosophical study, and the ending *-logist* usually denotes a student or one versed in the subject.

Another objection to "sedimentation" is that it does not readily permit the formation of derivatives corresponding to "sedimentologic" and "sedimentological." These adjectives are useful for such expressions as "sedimentological (or "sedimentologic") research," "sedimentological investigations," "sedimentological theories," etc.

In conclusion, retention of "sedimentation" for the act or process of deposition of sediments, and adoption of "sedimentology" as a term for the subject concerned with these processes will tend toward clearness. A new term entirely of Greek composition is not likely to be accepted.

"Sedimentography" is herewith introduced as an additional term signifying the descriptive branch of sedimentology, *i.e.,* that part which deals with the minute phases, megascopic and microscopic features, textures and classification.

HAKON WADELL

## MECHANICISM, VITALISM AND THE GROWTH OF BACTERIA

MUCH has been written about the chemical nature of growth, and in this connection unicellular and higher cold-blooded organisms have received especial attention. The fact that the rate of growth, metabolism and activity of such organisms increases with a rise of temperature, to the optimum, in a similar manner to the thermal acceleration of a chemical reaction, has justly received emphasis.

It is not the intention of this note to detract from the progress which has been made toward the explanation of life processes on purely physical and chemical bases. Least of all would we wish it to be considered as a partisan contribution to that threadbare discussion of "vitalism" and "mechanism." After all, it is probable that most of the functions of living matter which can not now be accounted for physically or chemically are obscure simply because of the deficiencies in our scientific conceptions.

*Bacterium coli* grows actively at 45° C. and also at 10° C., the rate of reproduction being about thirty times as fast at the higher temperature. It is known that actively growing bacteria continue to grow at the same rate when transferred to sterile medium of the same composition. On purely chemical grounds one would expect that if a transfer were made from an actively growing culture at 10° C. to sterile medium of the same composition at 45° C., growth should immediately be accelerated to the rate characteristic of a culture growing at this temperature. This, however, is not the case. Such a treatment induces a "lag" before growth of the culture can again proceed, and some of the cells die before the adjustment is made. Within one hour, however, reproduction is under way at a rate characteristic of a 45° C. culture.

If an actively growing culture at 45° C. is transferred to sterile medium of the same composition at 10° C., more striking results are obtained. In this case there occurs an extensive mortality among the young bacterial cells—sometimes exceeding 95 per cent. of the total. As is well known, such a drop in temperature has no effect upon "mature" bacterial cells.

A fact brought out by these experiments, which is perhaps new and certainly not generally appreciated, is that abrupt environmental changes within the range of growth of an organism may prove lethal to the young of the species. The "hardening" of young greenhouse plants by subjecting them to low temperatures, so they may later survive freezing, is a practise which rests on conclusive experimental data. But that environmental fluctuations within the natural range of growth may be fatal to the young organism has not been so clear.

A point of more interest is the fact that the young bacteria growing at 10° C. are not so extensively killed when changed to 45° C. as are those growing at the higher temperature when changed to the lower. This indicates a greater hardiness in those grown at the lower temperature. That this is indeed the case has been proved by other methods.

The experiments on which this communication is based constitute a part of a series which was planned in order to test a hypothesis, long held by us, that slow growth should lead to a more perfect adjustment of an organism to its environment and, therefore, to greater viability. While the greater viability of the cells grown at low temperatures, as compared with those grown at higher temperatures, has been established, it is not conclusively proved that the difference is due to the slower growth rate. Proof of this point would convey broad implications.

JAMES M. SHERMAN
GEORGE M. CAMERON
CORNELL UNIVERSITY

# REPORTS

## HONORS CONFERRED BY THE FRANKLIN INSTITUTE

AT the Medal Day exercises of the Franklin Institute of the state of Pennsylvania, held in the hall of the institute in Philadelphia on the afternoon of Wednesday, May 17, fourteen honors which had been awarded during the institute year were presented to their recipients or representatives of them. The medalists were drawn from three foreign countries as well as from the United States. The awards were as follows:

A certificate of honorary membership was presented to Mr. Alfred Rigling, of Philadelphia, Pennsylvania, in recognition of a half century of helpful and intelligent service as librarian and assistant secretary of the Franklin Institute, during which long term of duty well done he has been a pillar of strength to the institute, a source of comfort to the discouraged and of knowledge to the ignorant, a librarian amazingly informed concerning his library and a kindly gentleman skilful and eager in friendly service to his fellow men.

A certificate of merit to Dr. Henry Selby Hele-Shaw, of London, England, in consideration of his development of a superior filtering device involving stream-line principles. The British consul, Mr. Frederick Watson, received the certificate.

A certificate of merit to Mr. Arthur F. Poole, of Ithaca, New York, in consideration of his combination in a battery-operated clock, of known mechanisms, that has produced a clock in which the swing of the pendulum is the driving force of the gears controlling the hands, and also determines the frequency of the impulse, that requires battery renewal at long intervals only and that is an accurate time-keeper.

The fourth presentation of the day was that of an Edward Longstreth Medal—founded in 1890 by Edward Longstreth, of Philadelphia—to Mr. Howard L. Ingersoll, of the New York Central Lines of New York City, in consideration of his development of the locomotive booster to a state in which it gives valuable aid to locomotive performances and railroad service.

A second Longstreth Medal was presented to Dr. Dunlap Jamison McAdam, Jr., of the Bureau of Standards, Washington, D. C., in consideration of the fact that Dr. McAdam has provided information that satisfactorily explains certain structural failures, has developed formulae and diagrams to illustrate the complex relationship of the influences of stress on corrosion, and has done more than any one else to establish the fundamental principles of corrosion fatigue, coupled with the fact that the information provided has already been usefully applied and should have wide future practical application.

Three John Price Wetherill Medals—founded in 1925 by the family of the late John Price Wetherill—were next presented: the first to Messrs. Henry S. Hulbert, Francis C. McMath and Robert R. McMath, of the McMath-Hulbert Observatory of the University of Michigan, Lake Angelus, Michigan, in consideration of their design and construction of novel apparatus for the making of motion pictures of astronomical subjects, which have proven of value in the teaching and popularization of astronomy.

A Wetherill Medal was presented to the Industrial Brownhoist Corporation, of Bay City, Michigan, in consideration of the high degree of ingenuity in design and execution of detail, embodied in a successful machine for cleaning railway ballast resulting in a real contribution to railroading and the solution of a maintenance problem of great moment, especially under traffic conditions of extreme density.

The Wetherill Medal was presented to the Koppers Company of Delaware, of Pittsburgh, Pennsylvania, in consideration of the development of systems for the liquid purification of gases, the success of which is evidenced by the number of such installations in regular use.

A Louis Edward Levy Medal—founded in 1923 by the family of Louis E. Levy, of Philadelphia—was next presented to Mr. Leon S. Moisseiff, of New York City, for his paper entitled "The Design, Materials and Erection of the Kill Van Kull (Bayonne) Arch," published in the May, 1932, issue of the *Journal* of the Franklin Institute.

A George R. Henderson Medal—founded in 1924 by the widow of George R. Henderson, of Philadelphia—was presented to Mr. Otho C. Duryea, of the O. C. Duryea Corporation of New York City, in consideration of the meritorious railway engineering and the novel feature embodied in the invention of the Duryea Railway Car Cushion Underframe.

The Howard N. Potts Medal—established in 1906, by will of Mr. Potts, a Philadelphia lawyer—was awarded to Mr. Igor I. Sikorsky, of the Sikorsky Aviation Corporation of Bridgeport, Connecticut, in consideration of his pioneer work and inventions in the development of multi-motored airplanes of various types, for different uses, including amphibians and the largest combined planes for land and water service, and of his method of direction control of a multi-motored machine by the use of an automatic stabilizer.

One Elliott Cresson Medal—founded in 1848 by Mr. Elliott Cresson, who was very much interested in the work of the Franklin Institute, this award being highly prized and next to the Franklin Medal in importance—was awarded this year to Señor Juan de la Cierva, of London, England, in consideration of the original conceptions and inventive ability which have resulted in the creation and development of the autogiro.

The Franklin Medal was founded in 1914 by Samuel Insull, Esq., of Chicago, Illinois, a long-time member and friend of the Franklin Institute. This medal is to be awarded to those workers in physical science or technology, without regard to country, whose efforts, in the opinion of the institute, have done most to advance a knowledge of physical science or its application.

The Franklin Medals are awarded each year, usually to an outstanding scientist of the United States and to some scientist from some other country. This year the first Franklin Medal was awarded to Dr. Orville Wright, of Dayton, Ohio, in recognition of the valuable investigations carried out by him and his brother, Wilbur, from which they obtained the first reliable scientific data concerning the principles of flight and the design of aeroplanes, upon which they constructed the first heavier than air machine which flew by its own power under human control.

The second Franklin Medal was awarded to Dr. Paul Sabatier, dean of the Faculty of Science of Toulouse University, Toulouse, France, in recognition of his numerous and fruitful contributions to the general field of chemistry and especially to organic chemistry, in which he discovered the catalytic activity of finely divided common metals and devised methods for their use in science and industry. Dr. Sabatier was unable to come to America to receive his medal in person. He was represented by the councillor of the French Embassy in Washington, Monsieur Jules Henry.

On the evening of Medal Day, the Franklin Institute held a dinner at the Bellevue-Stratford Hotel in honor of the medalists of the day. About seventy-five guests were present.

# SOCIETIES AND MEETINGS

## THE OHIO ACADEMY OF SCIENCE

THE forty-third annual meeting of the Ohio Academy of Science was held on April 14 and 15, on the beautiful campus of historic Ohio University, Ohio's oldest university, at Athens, Ohio. To the surprise of many the attendance was probably the largest in the history of the academy, there being some 360 registered members and visitors, besides quite a few who forgot to register.

This meeting concluded the presidency of Dr. R. A. Budington, Oberlin College, Oberlin, Ohio, the two outstanding events of whose very successful administration were the formation of a new section, namely, a section of chemistry, under the inspiration and leadership of Dr. William Lloyd Evans, of Ohio State University, and the sponsoring by the academy of a series of radio talks by members of the academy on various popular scientific topics, made possible through the courtesy of the broadcasting station WEAO at Ohio State University, Columbus.

The general meetings of the academy were favored with four interesting lectures, one on the evening of the 13th by Professor F. J. Roos, of Ohio University, on "Architecture in Ohio"; two on Friday morning, one by Dr. F. C. Waite, of Western Reserve University, on "The Early History of the Microscope" and the other by Dr. S. Charles Kendeigh, of the Baldwin Bird Research Laboratory and Western Reserve University, on "Toleration of Low and High Temperatures by Birds." The fourth was the presidential address given before an overflowing audience on Friday evening at the annual dinner by President Budington on "The Innocence and Guilt of Science." In addition to these general lectures, some 145 papers were read in the eight sectional meetings held on Friday and Saturday, some by distinguished scientists from outside of the state. The attendance at these sectional meetings was very large, in some instances overtaxing the capacity of the meeting place. The demonstrations and exhibits were unusually interesting and elaborate, notably the exhibit of insects of southeastern Ohio.

The organization of a section of chemistry and the presence of a large number of eminent chemists from the leading universities and colleges of the state added much to the success and importance of the meeting. We also note with pleasure the presence of a large number of members of the Central Ohio Physics Club, Professor G. E. Owen, of Antioch College, president.

The following members of the academy were elected to fellowship in the academy, *viz.:* David Dietz, Rush Elliott, Robert A. Kehoe, Roderick Peattie, and William C. Stehr.

At the final business meeting on Saturday morning, 24 new members were received into the academy, and the election of officers for the coming year resulted as follows:

*President,* Dr. E. Lucy Braun; *Vice presidents—zoology,* Neale F. Howard; *botany,* Orville T. Wilson; *geology,* William A. P. Graham; *medical sciences,* Robert A. Kehoe; *psychology,* Richard S. Uhrbrock; *physics and astronomy,* Ray Lee Edwards; *geography,* Roderick Peattie; *chemistry,* William Lloyd Evans; *Secretary,* William H. Alexander; *Treasurer,* A. E. Waller; *Elective Members Executive Committee,* R. A. Budington and James P. Porter; *Trustee Research Fund,* Alpheus W. Smith; *Publications Committee,* F. O. Grover, J. E. Carman and S. W. Williams; *Library Committee,* F. C. Blake; *Committee on State Parks,* Edmund Secrest, H. C. Sampson and Emery R. Hayhurst; *Save Outdoor Ohio Council,* Herbert Osborn and E. N. Transeau.

It is worthy of note that this is the first time in the history of the academy that the academy has honored itself by the election of a woman as its president.

W. H. ALEXANDER,
*Secretary*

## THE ILLINOIS STATE ACADEMY OF SCIENCE

THE twenty-sixth annual meeting was held at the Broadview Hotel and Senior High School, East St. Louis, Illinois, on May 5 and 6. The meeting was attended by nearly 700 persons, including about 150 high-school students, members of high-school science clubs affiliated with the junior section of the academy.

General addresses were given by: Harry F. Ferguson, president of the academy and chief sanitary engineer, State Department of Public Health, on "The Future of the Illinois Academy of Science"; Dr. M. B. Visscher, professor of physiology, University of Illinois College of Medicine, on "Medical Science, its Past, Present, and Future"; Dr. Frank J. Jirka, director of the State Department of Public Health, on "Advances in the Science of Public Health"; Dr. Harry R. Hoffman, director, Behavior Clinic of the Criminal Court of Cook County, on "Psychiatry in the Criminal Courts of Cook County."

There were 105 scientific papers on the program in 10 sectional meetings. The program of the agriculture section, arranged by H. W. Mumford, dean of the College of Agriculture, University of Illinois, was a symposium on the subject, "Problems of the Soybean Industry." The economics section, under the direction of W. H. Voskuil, mineral economist, Illinois State Geological Survey, held a symposium on "Problems of the Illinois Coal Industry."

Six field excursions were held on Saturday, May 6: (1) An anthropological trip to the Cakokia Mounds State Park, under the direction of A. R. Kelly, University of Illinois; (2) a botanical trip to the Missouri Botanical Gardens, directed by H. S. Pepoon, State Natural History Survey; (3) a chemical trip to the Monsanto Chemical Works, directed by Percy J. Hill, East St. Louis; (4) a geographical trip to study the water factors in the geography of the East St. Louis district, directed by Lewis F. Thomas, Washington University, St. Louis; (5) a geological trip, directed by M. M. Leighton, chief, Illinois State Geological Survey, to study the coal measures and glacial geology of the East St. Louis district, the Dupo anticline and oil field, and the limestone mine on the Valmeyer anticline; and (6) a physics trip to the Cahokia Power Plant.

The following resolution was adopted by the academy:

I. *Whereas,* this Academy has at an earlier meeting adopted resolutions concerning the establishing of National Forest units in the State of Illinois, be it resolved that the academy assembled in Annual Meeting on May 5th, 1933, reaffirm its interest in and active support of a policy looking toward the development of forestry conservation within our state. Be it further reaffirmed that this Academy stands ready to offer its support to both State and Federal Agencies in furthering the establishment of adequate programs of forest conservation.

II. As a body of more than one thousand persons interested in science, the Illinois State Academy of Science takes this opportunity to affirm its interest in and concern for the welfare of all scientific work of the various state agencies. Be it therefore

*Resolved,* that this body go on record endorsing the past and projected programs of research and studies carried on by the various educational institutions, scientific surveys and other research organizations under state direction. Be it further *Resolved* that the State Legislature be urged to continue to extend adequate financial support to these organizations. Further be it *Resolved* that the Legislative Committee of this Academy be instructed to work for all matters of legislation favoring these agencies and to oppose all untoward legislation threatening the progress of education and of science in the State.

The following were chosen officers for the year 1933–34:

*President:* B. Smith Hopkins, chemistry, University of Illinois.

*First Vice-president:* Charles H. Behre, geology, Northwestern University.

*Secretary:* Harold R. Wanless, geology, University of Illinois.

*Treasurer:* George D. Fuller, botany, University of Chicago.

*Editor:* Dorothy E. Rose, State Geological Survey, Urbana.

It was decided to hold the twenty-seventh annual meeting of the academy at Decatur early in May, 1934. Dr. J. H. Ransom, of James Millikin University, will serve as chairman of the committee on local arrangements.

HAROLD R. WANLESS,
*Secretary*

## THE VIRGINIA ACADEMY OF SCIENCE

THE Virginia Academy of Science held its eleventh annual meeting at the State Teachers College, Fredericksburg, Virginia, on May 5 and 6, with a registration of 320. In the section of astronomy, mathematics and physics 27 papers were presented; in biology, 37; in chemistry, 17; in geology, 15; in the medical sciences, 15; and in psychology and education, 12, making a total of 121.

The annual prize of fifty dollars was awarded to S. A. Wingard, of the Virginia Polytechnic Institute, for a paper entitled, "The Production of Rust-Resistant Varieties of Beans by Hybridization," and honorable mention was accorded to a paper by A. N. Vyssotsky and Emma T. A. Williams entitled "Color Indices and Integrated Magnitudes of Fifteen Bright Globular Clusters." These awards carry added significance this year because of the unusually high quality of the papers in competition with them.

The research committee reported that during the year the following grants in aid of scientific research had been made: Jesse W. Beams, physics, University of Virginia, $150; J. C. Forbes, biochemistry, Medical College of Virginia, $75; J. M. McGinnis, psychology, Hollins College, $40; C. C. Speidel, anatomy, University of Virginia, $100; N. Beverly Tucker, chemistry, Virginia Military Institute, $50; I. A. Updike, chemistry, Randolph-Macon College, $75.

A noteworthy item in the year's work is the increase in the number of junior (or student) members, the number having increased from 54 to 115. There were also two papers presented by junior members and two exhibits of their work were shown. One was an array of totally cleared anatomical and zoological specimens and the other was an inexpensive, laboratory-built apparatus for the fixation of atmospheric nitrogen.

Dr. William A. Kepner, of the University of Virginia, was elected president for the coming year, Dr. William T. Sanger, of the Medical College of Virginia, president elect, and Professor D. Maurice Allan, of Hampden-Sydney College, member of the council.

Following the meeting rather extensive field trips were made by the committee on the flora of Virginia and by members of the geology section.

E. C. L. MILLER,
*Secretary*

## THE TENNESSEE ACADEMY OF SCIENCE

THE thirty-second meeting of the Tennessee Academy of Science was held at the Reelfoot Lake Biological Station of the academy on April 28 and 29. The feature of the meeting was an address by The Very Reverend I. H. Noe, dean, St. Mary's Episcopal Cathedral, Memphis, in dedication of the John T. McGill Laboratory Building. This building is named in honor of Dr. John T. McGill, professor emeritus of chemistry at Vanderbilt University and secretary-treasurer of the Tennessee Academy of Science. In thus dedicating this building recognition is given to Dr. McGill of his many years of valued work in and for the academy and particularly of his efforts which resulted in the establishment in 1931 by the state of

Tennessee of the Reelfoot Lake Biological Station under the management and control of the Tennessee Academy of Science. The John T. McGill Laboratory is a modernly equipped building containing four laboratories fitted with proper work tables, cabinets, aquaria, etc., several stock and preparation rooms, and a large assembly room. This laboratory, located on the east side of Reelfoot Lake in Obion County, lies in a region which represents well the water and land fauna and flora of the Mississippi bottom. It is a few minutes walk from the comfortable Walnut Log Lodge, where special rates are available for workers at the laboratory. It is the policy of the executive committee of the station to allot free working space in the laboratory for research work of scientific interest. Application should be made to Dr. A. R. Bliss, Jr., University of Tennessee Medical School, Memphis, Tennessee.

In addition to the dedicatory exercises, approximately thirty papers were presented during four sessions of the meeting. These interesting programs were composed of reports on research work on diversified subjects and were presented by representatives of the following institutions: The University of Tennessee, Memphis; Southwestern University; George Peabody College; Vanderbilt University; Tennessee Department of Public Health; U. S. Department of Agriculture; Lambuth College; West Tennessee Teachers College; Freed-Hardeman College; University of Tennessee Junior College, Martin; State Teachers College, Murfreesboro. Numerous groups made field excursions both on the lake and into the surrounding woodlands for the collection of specimens and material from this interesting territory. These trips and the congenial atmosphere of the Walnut Log Lodge contributed not a little to the success of the meeting. The academy is indebted to Dr. A. R. Bliss, Jr., and his committee on arrangements for making possible one of the most pleasant and successful of the academy meetings.

FRANCIS G. SLACK,
*President*

# SCIENTIFIC APPARATUS AND LABORATORY METHODS

## A TELEPHONIC DROP COUNTER

THE drop counter here described operates on the mechanical contact principle, but uses a telephone transmitter as the contact mechanism in place of the conventional metal vane making contact in a pool of mercury. The small current variations of the transmitter are amplified by a powerful vacuum tube relay, which gives a large current output sufficient to operate any type of recording apparatus.

Fig. 1 represents a Western Electric telephone transmitter with the rubber mouthpiece removed. A triangular vane of thin mica or celluloid, about 5×7 cm, is fastened at its center to a light celluloid spindle some 7 cm long, and the lower end of the spindle is cemented to the diaphragm of the transmitter with celluloid-acetone cement. The vane is mounted parallel to the diaphragm and about 5 cm above the top of the transmitter to allow a layer of sound-deadening cotton to be spread over the transmitter. The transmitter is laid in a boxful of cotton to prevent outside vibrations from actuating the mechanism, and the pipette is adjusted so that the drops fall on the vane.

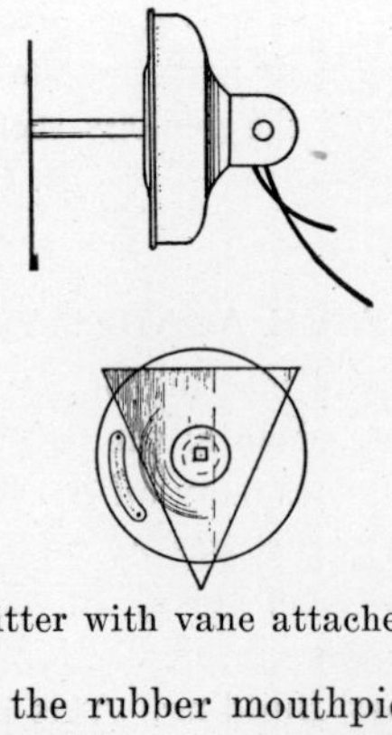

FIG. 1. Transmitter with vane attached to diaphragm.

Fig. 2 shows the electrical system used to amplify the current variations of the transmitter. A is the transmitter, B a $1\frac{1}{2}$ volt dry cell, C a microphone transformer with a 60 to 1 ratio between secondary and primary, D the bias battery of 9 volts made of two $4\frac{1}{2}$ volt C-batteries in series, E is the amplifying tube, F the filament supply transformer, G the output connections and H the 110 volt supply leads.

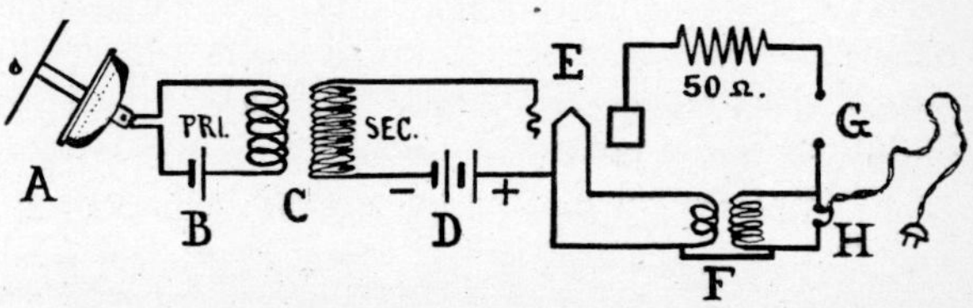


FIG. 2. The amplifying system of the apparatus.

The amplifying tube is a General Electric Thyratron FG-17, a mercury ionization vacuum tube of peculiar properties which operates on raw 110 volt alternating current and requires no B-battery. In this device the plate current does not follow the grid voltage up and down as in the ordinary amplifying tube, but no plate current at all flows until the grid voltage reaches a certain value, when the mercury vapor suddenly ionizes and an output of about 50 watts results. The tube consequently is an excellent off-and-on relay, and is well adapted to many recording and controlling processes in the laboratory. The output is half-rectified alternating current, which operates most direct current magnets satisfactorily. The tube fits an ordinary 4-prong radio tube socket, but the plate connection is made to the metal knob on top of the tube instead of the plate contact on the base. Filament current at 2.5 volts and 5 amperes is supplied by a small transformer to be had at any radio supply store, and no rheostat is necessary. The output circuit of the tube should contain a 50 ohm resistance to limit the current flow to 0.5 ampere in case of a short circuit, since the filament can be ruined by excessive current passed through the tube.

In operation the current to the Thyratron is turned on, and the tube allowed to heat for 3 or 4 minutes until the contained mercury is vaporized. The microphone battery is then connected and the apparatus is ready to work. As the current through the transmitter and primary of the transformer may amount to 25 milliamperes, the microphone battery should be disconnected when not in use, and for long runs one 2-volt cell of a storage battery may be used for economy's sake. There are no adjustments to be made when the apparatus is in operation. The response of the Thyratron to each drop can be made longer or shorter by a decrease or increase in the negative bias impressed on the Thyratron grid by the bias battery D, so that the length of time the current continues for each impulse can be set for the inertia of the moving parts in any recording apparatus. The value of 9 volts for the bias battery is an average which will give a quick magnet response to drops falling as rapidly as they can without coalescing into a stream.

The apparatus is not at all critical in its adjustment; in fact, the transmitter has a great excess of sensitivity, and with its normal battery voltage of 4.5 volts and a small negative bias in the grid circuit will operate the Thyratron when a sheet of paper is rustled before the uncovered mouthpiece. The wires from the transmitter to the amplifying set and the wires of the output circuit can be made of any convenient length, since moderate resistance or capacity affects these circuits but little. It is convenient to mount the pipette at the edge of a table and let the drop fall about 30 inches to the transmitter resting on the floor.

The use of the apparatus is not confined to drop counting, but it can be adjusted to make a record of the fall of any body large enough to shake the diaphragm. When adapted to sound recording by an increase in the sensitivity of the transmitter, it can be used to pick up the ticks of a pendulum and send out time signals, to respond to a single note when the transmitter is placed in a tuned resonator, to record sounds in general, or to operate mechanical devices at a definite level of sound-intensity. Laboratory workers may find the apparatus useful in ways not contemplated in the present application.

CLARENCE F. GRAHAM

ALBANY, N. Y.

## A DISINTEGRATOR FOR YEAST CELLS

A SIMPLE device to break up yeast cells is desirable in order to obtain certain growth-promoting factors which are not available without rupture of the cell wall. Such an apparatus can be made from glass rod and tubing with a few rubber connections and a suitable motor. The accompanying diagram shows the structure of the apparatus.

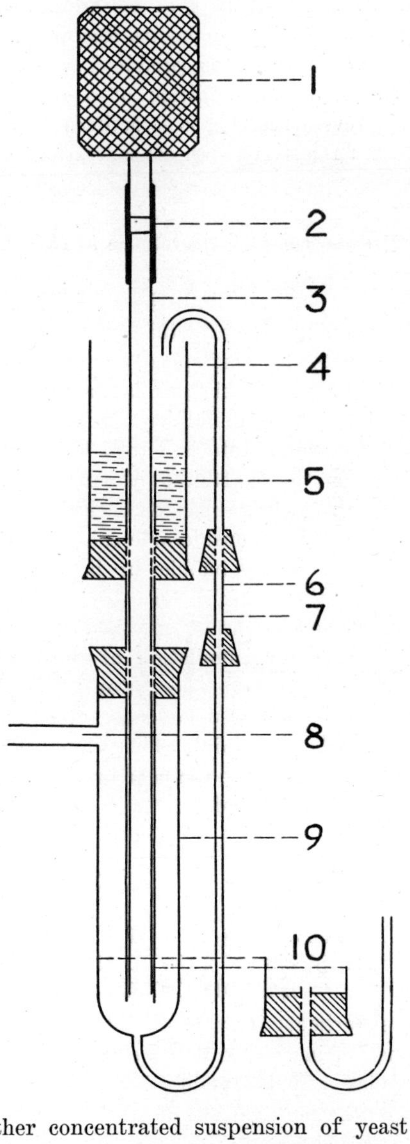


A rather concentrated suspension of yeast placed in the reservoir (4) flows by gravity through a long bearing (5) in which a vibrating shaft (3) is revolving. As the material drops from the bearing into the receiver (9), it is transported by a current of inert gas through a return tube (7) to the reservoir (4) from which it may again flow between the shaft and bearing. This continuous circulation and regrinding is maintained until an examination of the material in the reservoir by the hanging drop or Gram stain methods shows that sufficient disintegration has occurred.

A number of details are essential to the success of the operation. A smooth bearing and shaft running without vibration at high speed have very little effect on the yeast cells. The surfaces of the bearing and shaft must be roughened by rubbing them with moist carborundum powder (100 mesh) before assembling the apparatus. About 0.1 g of the abrasive is added to 20 cc of suspension to insure keeping these surfaces rough. Vibration is produced by a vibrating joint. The occasional addition of a drop of octyl alcohol to prevent foaming is sometimes very effective in securing a relatively high concentration of the desired factors. Pyrex glass is used throughout to avoid the marked change in acidity which is caused by soft glass and to increase the life of the apparatus. It is desirable, although not essential, to permit the bearing to project part way into the liquid in the reservoir. An opening blown in this tube just above the stopper prevents any dead space. A current of nitrogen, air or other suitable gas is passed through a bubble counter and humidifier containing distilled water. A convenient rate is 3 to 5 bubbles per second; but when the shaft and bearing have become worn, a more rapid rate may be desirable to prevent the formation of any considerable column of liquid in the return tube. If gas bubbles up between the shaft and bearing, either the clearance between the two is too great or the current of gas has not been rapid enough to prevent accumulation of fluid in the receiver and return tube. The motor is run at 3,000 to 4,000 r.p.m.; the speed depends somewhat on the action of the vibrating joint, which should not become violent enough to damage the bearing.

The average length of run has been five hours. Examination showed that 50 to 75 per cent. of the cells had disappeared within 90 minutes and 90 per cent. in 300 minutes. The disintegration is most efficient with the more concentrated suspensions, since the rate at which the cells are ruptured depends apparently on the probability of a cell being pinched between the rotating, vibrating rod and the rough bearing surface. After centrifugation and filtration through a Berkefeld filter, the turbid sterile filtrate is used without undue delay. The apparatus may be used for disintegration of other biological materials and for securing intimate contact and mixing in chemical reactions involving combination of a gas with a suspended solid where continuous exposure of new surface is desired.

EXPLANATION OF THE DIAGRAM

The dimensions given are those of an apparatus which gave consistently satisfactory results, but there is no apparent reason why many of them could not be altered: (1) Motor—a "Sew motor" with its rheostat was used; (2) vibrating joint: a 2 inch length of glass tubing connected securely to the shaft of the motor with rubber tubing and to (3) with a two inch length of heavy rubber tubing; (3) disintegrator shaft, a straight rod or capillary tube 27 cm by 7.8 mm; (4) reservoir, a 12 cm by 3 cm glass tube attached to the bearing by a number 6 rubber stopper; (5) bearing, a straight tube 22 cm by 10 mm outside diameter, wall thickness, 1 mm; (6) return tube in three sections, 3 mm outside diameter; (7) gas outlet, identical with (6); (8) gas inlet; (9) receiver, constructed from a $6 \times \frac{3}{4}$ inch side arm test-tube either by sealing a 17 cm section of the return tube to the base as illustrated, or (10) by cutting off the base of the tube smoothly, flanging the edge, and using a number 4 stopper to connect the return tube.

WILLIAM F. BRUCE
THE ROCKEFELLER INSTITUTE FOR MEDICAL RESEARCH
DEPARTMENT OF ANIMAL AND PLANT PATHOLOGY
PRINCETON, N. J.

# SPECIAL ARTICLES

## THE DEVELOPMENT OF ORGANIZED VESSELS IN CULTURES OF BLOOD CELLS

IN an experiment in which blood cells were placed for incubation in culture flasks containing a mixture of blood plasma and Tyrode solution, the usual technique for the cultivation of the leucocytes[1] was slightly modified in that coagulation was allowed to take place spontaneously and without the customary addition of embryonic tissue juice. Later, the cultures were found to contain numerous, highly organized, tubular processes that projected out from the original explant. A year ago, Hueper and Russell[2] reported

[1] A. Carrel and A. H. Ebeling, "Pure Cultures of Large Mononuclear Leucocytes," *Jour. Exp. Med.*, 36: 365, 1922.

[2] W. C. Hueper and M. A. Russell, "'Capillary-like Formations' in Tissue Cultures of Leucocytes," *Arch. f. exp. Zellforschung*, 12: 407, 1932.

the appearance of similar structures in a certain percentage of "leucocyte" cultures,[3] some of which had been prepared in the same manner as those referred to above. The phenomenon was but casually studied by them, however, and no attempt was made to determine the conditions under which it occurred. It seemed necessary, therefore, to study the matter anew and to ascertain the exact conditions under which the structures arise. It is the purpose of this communication to present the information thus far obtained.

The cells were taken from blood drawn from the carotid of adult chickens according to the procedures regularly employed in the preparation of plasma. After centrifugation, and the subsequent removal of the cell-free plasma yield, the thin superficial layer of plasma containing the buffy coat of leucocytes was coagulated by the addition of a drop or two of embryonic tissue juice. A few minutes later, this layer could then be removed as a disk and cut into small fragments for the preparation of the cultures. Each fragment consisted of a layer of white cells together with such red cells as remained adherent to them. In some cases, the red cells were separated, as completely as possible, from the fragments and discarded. In other cases, a considerable quantity of them was allowed to remain.

The fragments were placed in flasks to which plasma and Tyrode solution had previously been added. In a few instances, the plasma was replaced by serum, thereby eliminating all possibility of coagulation. In certain experiments in which plasma and Tyrode solution were used, a trace of embryonic tissue juice was added in order to induce rapid coagulation. In others, substances were introduced that would stimulate the cells to great activity without the immediate coagulation of the medium, as, *e.g.,* tryptic digest of fibrin. Some of the cultures comprising these various experiments were allowed to remain for a time at room temperature prior to incubation at 37° C. Others were placed in the incubator the moment they were prepared.

These experiments have disclosed the fact that the formation of the capillary-like structures is, in the beginning, a purely physical phenomenon dependent upon the response of the cells to gravity, the consistency of the medium, and the surface peculiarities of the individual cells. As soon as fragments containing both red cells and leucocytes have been placed in a plasma mixture that does not coagulate immediately, certain cells, in passing from a higher to a lower level, initiate a general outflow from the central mass into the surrounding medium. Red cells have smooth surfaces and easily shift their position. Leucocytes, on the other hand, being capable of independent locomotion, adhere to one another and to solid structures. They may, however, be swept along in a current of red cells.

The configuration assumed by the outflowing blood cells depends upon the consistency of the medium and the elevation of the fragment above the general level of that medium. If the medium is composed of serum, the cells flow out from all sides as when a vessel bursts that contains a viscous fluid. In the presence of plasma, however, the outflowing cells may take every conceivable form ranging from broad, fan-like disseminations, through short, stalky, bud-like projections to long, slender ones. It will not be possible at this time to describe more than one type of formation, namely, that which results in the subsequent development of a long, slender tube.

At one or more points on the margin, a few cells become dislodged and break away from the fragment. Their places are taken by those behind. If the proximal impact is great, these cells are also pushed out into the medium. A general streaming begins. Each cell that is forced out follows in the wake of those that have gone before. They may proceed in single file, or abreast of one another, but always over exactly the same route. This route assumes the nature of a tunnel-like passage through the plasma. As long as the cells in the lead are being pushed forward by those from behind, they will continue to advance through the medium until it coagulates. The moment coagulation occurs, however, the cells in the lead, being unable to make further progress, come to a stop. If coagulation occurs before the proximal outflow has ceased, the passage will remain open and unobstructed, despite the fact that the cells in transit may be widely separated If the pathway is only partially filled with cells, they may be made, at any time, to flow in either direction by manipulating the flask. After this happens, the force of the outflowing cells may still be so great that a large spherical expansion is formed at its distal end. Enlargements may also appear elsewhere along the tube. Very often it may be completely ruptured, and occasionally, short branches are found.

All this may occur within half an hour after the cultures have been prepared. As soon as the surrounding medium has become firmly coagulated, however, now further change occurs either in the length of the tube or in its diameter. The structures do not, as Hueper and Russell[2] have reported, continue to grow upon further incubation.

Up to this point, the development of the tubules depends solely upon the rapidity with which the plasma coagulates. A culture held at room tempera-

[3] Although not implied by the title of their report, these cultures contained every cell type present in the circulating blood.

ture develops tubules in greater number and of greater length than a sister culture incubated immediately. Their development is not suppressed by substances that enhance cell activity unless they induce, at the same time, the immediate coagulation of the medium. Embryonic tissue juice prevents their formation by producing immediate coagulation.

So far, the tubules have no definite walls. These begin to be formed very shortly after coagulation has taken place in the medium. The walls do not arise as a direct transformation of the fibrin clot. Instead, they are formed by the activity of living cells, or cell products, the so-called thrombocytes, that have been deposited along the course of the tubule. Where there are gaps between the cells confined in the tubule, these minute bodies may be seen to spin out fine hair-like filaments at the interphase between the lumen of the tubule and the surrounding coagulum. It is believed that the fibrin of the plasma clot serves as a supporting structure upon which the thrombocytes lay down their fiber-like strands. Out in the surrounding medium, these small corpuscles produce similar strands, but here at random. The majority of them tend to agglutinate. Very often, the agglutinated masses become joined together by numerous threads.

After a few days, the red cells within the capillary-like formations become progressively phagocytized by the macrophages. Eventually, these in turn escape into the surrounding medium, sometimes through definite breaks in the walls, but more often by way of their proximal ends. When the tube has become empty, as may occur after 4 or 5 days, any number of macrophages may remain spread out over its outer surface. In this position, they bear striking resemblance to the much discussed cells of Rouget. At times, they are so numerous that their undulating membranes seem to fuse with one another, giving the impression of an unbroken syncytium. If the cultures were fixed and stained at this moment, their nuclei might easily be mistaken for nuclei present in the wall. This apparently accounts for the statement of Hueper and Russell[2] that the wall itself becomes nucleated. This has not been confirmed. When, as may eventually happen, these Rouget-like cells wander away, they leave a fibrous wall that is quite devoid of any cellular structure whatsoever.

Occasionally, the wall is incompletely formed, the fibrillar strands being laid down over a single portion of the original pathway. At other times, a single cord of fibrous material may extend along one side of it, or even this may be absent. Invariably, however, its lumen remains open and filled with the clear fluid that has diffused in from the medium.

To summarize: Isolated blood cells, in a plasma substratum, are capable of constructing highly organized channels that are analogous to the blood capillaries of the organism.

Raymond C. Parker

The Rockefeller Institute for Medical Research
New York City

## LAMINAR DESTRUCTION OF THE NERVE CELLS OF THE CEREBRAL CORTEX

One of the structural characteristics of the cerebral cortex is that it is composed of a number of layers of nerve cells. Generally a fundamental subdivision in six layers is accepted nowadays.

Very little is known as yet about the functions of these various layers. It is known that in the giganto-pyramidal area of the cortex (field 4 of Brodmann) the giant pyramidal cells of the fifth layer give rise to most of the nerve fibers descending into the spinal cord as the fibers of the pyramidal tracts. It is assumed on the basis of histological evidence that the three or four outer layers are predominantly receptive in function and that the two inmost layers more particularly subserve efferent functions. Perhaps a few additional, although indeed less probable assumptions could be made, but that would be all. Our factual knowledge of the functions of these various layers is as yet very restricted. This is largely due to the stupendously complex structure of this tissue, but also to the fact that until now no method has been available which permitted an experimental attack upon the various layers of the cortex, and by that a direct approach to their respective functions.

In this preliminary paper I want to describe briefly a simple method which makes possible destruction, at will, of consecutive layers of the nerve cells of the cerebral cortex, *i.e.,* of either its first two superficial layers, or of the first four, or of all the six layers. This is possible by applying heat locally to the exposed cortex for a very short period. It was found that heating to 90°–100° C. for five seconds results in death of all the nerve cells in the heated area throughout the whole thickness of the cortex, and that, by heating it to about 70° C. for from one to two seconds, it is possible to kill the nerve cells of only the two superficial layers.

The apparatus used in these experiments is very simple. The copper tip of an ordinary electric soldering-iron is sawed off so that a rectangular surface of appropriate size ($5 \times 7$ millimeters) is obtained. This surface can be heated to any temperature suitable for our purposes, by taking off the proper voltage from a potentiometer-rheostat (of f.i. 600 ohms, 1 Amp.) plugged into a power outlet. For special purposes copper tips of various size and shape are used, which can be screwed into the stem of the soldering-iron. A series of settings of the rheostat was established for a few suitable temperatures (60, 70, 80, 90, 100° C.) for each type of copper tip used. The temperatures of the tips were determined in the usual way with thermocouples and a ballistic galvanometer. These experiments were performed on monkeys (*Macacus rhesus*) under sterile conditions; the animals were killed after one or two weeks and the changes in the cerebral cortex studied by the Nissl method.[1]

The lesions are found to be strictly localized to the heated area. It shows as an encapsulated area, sharply marked off from the surrounding normal cortex by a wall of proliferated connective tissue and blood-vessels. The nerve cells within this area have all disappeared; those immediately outside this wall of connective tissue show a normal Nissl picture. Of great interest is the fact that the neuroglia inside the damaged area is not killed, but is found to have reacted to the heating by proliferation. Even a temperature of 130° C. applied for ten seconds does not kill the cortical neuroglia.

This method of laminar thermo-coagulation of the cerebral cortex, as it might be called, results, therefore, within a wide range of temperatures, in a sharply localized, selective destruction of the nervous elements. By selecting a suitable temperature and a suitable period of application of the heat it is possible to destroy, at one's discretion, the nervous elements, the nerve cells and their processes, in consecutive layers of the cortex.

Details can not be given in this preliminary paper; suffice it to point out that this method permits a new attack upon many important problems in the fields of physiology, anatomy and experimental pathology of the cerebral cortex.

J. G. DUSSER DE BARENNE

YALE UNIVERSITY

## LITHIUM IN SEA WATER

COMPARATIVELY little is known concerning the distribution of the rarer alkali metals in nature in spite of the intrinsic interest of the subject. Beyond the fact that the order of occurrence is probably Na, K, Li, Rb, Cs, Va, no quantitative data are available to enable us to assign numerical ratios to this series. Even in the case of sea water, which has been extensively studied by so many investigators since the beginnings of chemistry, quantitative determinations of the alkalies, lithium, rubidium and caesium are practically non-existent, and virginium has only recently been discovered. Analyses by Schmidt,[1] frequently quoted in works on oceanography and geochemistry, give values as high as 0.04 per cent. of rubidium in sea salt, but examination of Schmidt's original paper shows that his results are based upon indirect analysis with a very high probable error. Grandeau,[2] who found rubidium in beet root, failed to detect the element in sea water and also mentions Bunsen's failure to find it.

So far as the authors know there is no published account of even the detection of caesium in sea water. In some works on oceanography its identification is attributed to Sonstadt, but in every such case the writer has overlooked Sonstadt's[3] admission that the spectrum lines he thought were due to caesium were actually given by strontium.

As far as is known, the authors report in this paper the first quantitative determination of lithium in sea water. In this procedure a liter sample is used. The calcium and magnesium are removed by precipitation with sodium carbonate. This precipitate is dissolved and reprecipitated in order to avoid the possibility of loss of some of the lithium with the carbonates.

The filtrates from the two precipitations are combined and evaporated, the magnesium carbonate which continues to precipitate as the solution evaporates being removed by filtration from time to time. When the volume is about 100 ml the solution is filtered and acidified with hydrochloric acid. The evaporation is then continued in the acid solution.

When sodium chloride begins to separate the solution is cooled, and an equal volume of ethyl alcohol is added, which precipitates much of the sodium chloride. This is filtered off, washed with a little 50 per cent. alcohol and evaporation of the filtrate continued. The sodium chloride is reserved for subsequent treatment.

When sodium chloride again begins to crystallize from the solution, the above procedure is repeated, and this is continued until the volume is about 10 ml. The precipitation may also be accomplished with hydrogen chloride gas.

At this point all the sodium chloride which has been removed is dissolved in water and reprecipitated by the same process of alternate evaporation and addition of alcohol until the volume of solution remaining is about 5 ml. This is added to the 10 ml of filtrate from the first procedure. Reprecipitation of the sodium chloride is necessary to avoid loss of some of the lithium with the sodium chloride.

An equal volume of alcohol is added to the combined filtrates and the solution is saturated with dry hydrogen chloride. The greater part of the remaining sodium chloride and sulfate and some potassium is removed by this operation, and the solution is evaporated to dryness.

It is now necessary to remove the remainder of the magnesium. The residue from evaporation is dissolved in 20 ml of 50 per cent alcohol, 2 ml of normal sodium carbonate solution is added, and the solution is boiled. The precipitate is filtered off, dissolved and reprecipitated to avoid any possible loss of lithium. The combined filtrates from the two pre-

[1] I am greatly indebted to Dr. Harry M. Zimmerman, of the department of pathology, for the preparation and help in interpretation of this histological material.

[1] Schmidt, *Bull. Acad. St. Petersburg*, 24: 231, 1878.

[2] Grandeau, *Comp. Rend.*, 53: 1100, 1861.

[3] Sonstadt, *Chem. News*, 22: 25, 1870; *ibid.*, 22: 44, 1870.

cipitations are acidified with hydrochloric acid and evaporated to dryness. The residue is dissolved in a minimum amount of water, alcohol is added until the volume is 10 ml and the solution saturated with dry hydrogen chloride, filtered and the sodium chloride washed with absolute alcohol. The filtrate and washings are evaporated to dryness.

The residue, weighing a few milligrams, consists largely of potassium chloride and sulfate, some sodium and magnesium chlorides, and contains the lithium.

Complete separation of the lithium and its direct determination is impracticable, but it may be estimated by use of the spectroscope with comparative ease. The authors use an atomizer (zerstäuber) especially designed to spray a solution into the air inlet of a blast lamp so that the spectrum may be observed continuously.

The solution rises by capillary action in the tube A (Fig. 1) which is open at the point B and sealed off

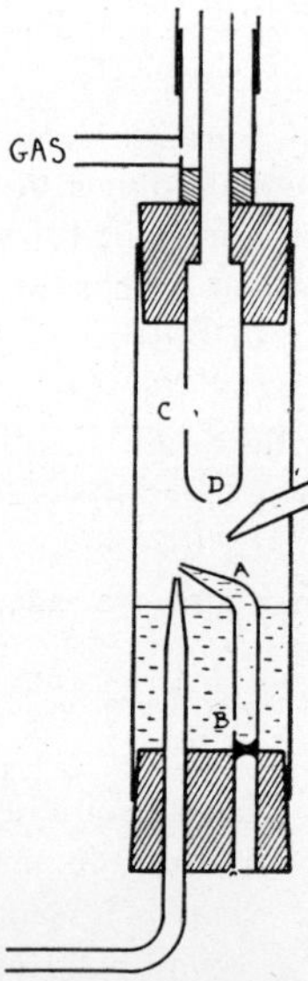


FIG. 1. Apparatus used in the quantitative spectrum analysis for lithium.

just below this point. The air blast produces a fine spray, and a small quantity of this is carried up through C into the burner. The opening at D permits any excess to drain back without interfering with the passage of the spray into the tube. The tube sealed into the side allows solutions to be added during the course of the analysis. The lower part of the apparatus is made of glass, but the burner proper is of brass.

The residue containing the lithium is moistened with a drop of hydrochloric acid, dissolved in two milliliters of water and washed into the reservoir of the atomizer with an additional two milliliters of water. Then, while the spectrum is being observed, a 3 N solution of potassium chloride is added until the red potassium line at 7666 Å is of sensibly the same intensity as the red lithium line 6708 Å. This requires some skill and judgment, since the lines are of somewhat different color. With practise, however, results with known quantities of lithium can be duplicated with an accuracy comparable with other methods of quantitative spectrum analysis.

This method is also useful for estimating small quantities of strontium in the presence of much calcium, using the blue lines of the two elements.

The solution is removed quantitatively from the atomizer (the quantity which was used in the burner is negligible), evaporated, and the residue weighed as potassium chloride.

This entire procedure is duplicated with a synthetic sea water containing a known quantity of lithium and a ratio established between the lithium and potassium, which will give equal intensity to the two lines. This ratio will depend upon the apparatus and to some extent upon the experimenter. The authors found a value of 2:10,000. Since the quantity of potassium chloride actually weighed is relatively large, the results are unaffected by the small amounts of sodium and magnesium which may be present.

In this way the lithium in sea water of ordinary concentration (chlorinity = 19 $^0/_{00}$) has been determined to be 0.1 mg per liter.

The importance of lithium in the economy of the sea is not known. No quantitative estimations of the element in the various organisms have been made, although it has been reported qualitatively by many. Possible variations in the quantity of lithium present in sea water, due to marked growth of plankton, are also unknown. The accuracy of the method does not permit, nor does its tediousness encourage, the determination of such fluctuations.

BERTRAM D. THOMAS
THOMAS G. THOMPSON
OCEANOGRAPHIC AND CHEMICAL LABORATORIES
UNIVERSITY OF WASHINGTON

## BOOKS RECEIVED

BRINKLEY, STUART R. *Principles of General Chemistry.* Pp. x + 585. 160 figures. Macmillan. $5.50.

PATTERSON, THOMAS L. *Comparative Physiology of the Gastric Hunger Mechanism.* Pp. 56–272. 94 figures. New York Academy of Sciences.

POWDERMAKER, HORTENSE. *Life in Lesu.* Pp. 352. Illustrated. Norton. $4.00.

RABER, ORAN. *Principles of Plant Physiology.* Pp. xv + 432. 29 figures. Macmillan. $3.00.

SMITH, GEORGE McP. *Quantitative Chemical Analysis.* Pp. xii + 199. Macmillan. $2.25.

WILLARD, HOBART H. and N. HOWELL FURMAN. *Elementary Qualitative Analysis.* Pp. viii + 406. 35 figures. Van Nostrand. $3.25.

# SCIENCE

VOL. 77 FRIDAY, JUNE 9, 1933 No. 2006

*The National Academy of Sciences:* DR. W. W. CAMPBELL 549
*A History of the National Research Council, 1919–1933. IV. Division of Chemistry and Chemical Technology:* PROFESSOR CHARLES A. KRAUS 552
*Scientific Events:*
*Chicago Program on Radiation and Plant Life; Mathematics at the Chicago Meeting; Chemistry at the Chicago Meeting; The Medical Sciences at the Chicago Meeting; The American Society and Journal for Pharmacology and Experimental Therapeutics; Obituary* 554
*Scientific Notes and News* 557
*Discussion:*
*Meaningless versus Significant Terms in Geological Classification:* DR. FRANK LEVERETT. *Three Prehistoric Parasites:* DR. GALE E. WILSON. *The Distribution of Serapias Helleborine in Central New York:* DR. VERNON A. YOUNG. *I-inositol in Citrus Fruits:* E. K. NELSON and GEORGE L. KEENAN 560
*Special Correspondence:*
*The Leonard Wood Memorial for the Eradication of Leprosy:* F. P. G. 562
*Societies and Meetings:*
*The Iowa Academy of Science:* DR. JOSEPH C. GILMAN. *The Kansas Academy of Science:* DR. GEORGE E. JOHNSON. *The Texas Academy of Science:* H. B. PARKS 563
*Scientific Apparatus and Laboratory Methods:*
*A Simple Aquarium Aerator:* DR. ERNEST C. DRIVER. *A New Stop-cock Clamp:* DR. ALDEN F. ROE 565
*Special Articles:*
*The Action of the Parenteral Administration of Sugars on the Hydrogen-ion Concentration of Normal and Malignant Tissues in Living Animals:* PROFESSOR CARL VOEGTLIN, DR. H. KAHLER and DR. R. H. FITCH. *Solar Variations and Atmospheric Pressure:* H. H. CLAYTON 567
*Science News* 8

SCIENCE: A Weekly Journal devoted to the Advancement of Science, edited by J. MCKEEN CATTELL and published every Friday by

THE SCIENCE PRESS

New York City: Grand Central Terminal

Lancaster, Pa. Garrison, N. Y.

Annual Subscription, $6.00 Single Copies, 15 Cts.

SCIENCE is the official organ of the American Association for the Advancement of Science. Information regarding membership in the Association may be secured from the office of the permanent secretary, in the Smithsonian Institution Building, Washington, D. C.

# THE NATIONAL ACADEMY OF SCIENCES[1]

By Dr. W. W. CAMPBELL

UNIVERSITY OF CALIFORNIA

ONE year ago, our committee on program and arrangements for the annual meeting of 1932 asked me, as the then new president, to deliver an address, of a specified length, at the annual dinner, and I did so. To the best of my knowledge, that was an innovation—a supplement to the prevailing type of dinner program. This year the committee repeated the invitation, perhaps largely because last year I respected the wisely specified time limit, with three minutes to spare. But I have a purpose in these preliminary remarks. As two points fix the direction of a straight line, so two presidential addresses in successive years may go far in establishing a custom. Fortunately, the membership of the academy is highly individualistic, and is always ready and quick to express its views. I need say no more.

It was gratifying, last week, to observe that the deep depression in the curve representing the recent course of financial and economic events in our country is apparently not matched by a similar depression in the curve depicting the output of new knowledge, achieved through research, in the domain of the physical and biologic sciences. The number of papers offered for the program of this week's meeting was uniquely large, and to accommodate them it was found necessary to hold duplicate sessions, one in this auditorium and the other in the lecture room, on all our four half days, as you will have observed. The high quality of the papers anticipated from the authors' names has been amply confirmed in their reading. These facts in relation to the academy's program are, I believe, in accord with the advance in knowledge made in our nation, as a whole, through research, as indicated by papers and volumes, rich in contents, published in the last year or two. I take special delight in adding that we have been extremely fortunate in the qualities of the papers presented in response to personal invitations issued to several guests by the academy's committee on program: Professor Vegard, professor of physics in the University of

[1] Address of the president at the annual dinner of the National Academy of Sciences, Washington, D. C., April 25, 1933.

Oslo, Professor Swann, director of the Bartol Foundation for Research in Physics, Philadelphia, Dr. Allison, head professor of physics in the Alabama Polytechnic Institute, Dr. R. H. Fowler, professor of mathematical physics in Cambridge University, and Dr. F. E. Matthes, of the U. S. Geological Survey; and I tender them this more comprehensive expression of the academy's gratitude than was possible in the several sessions. We are likewise deeply indebted to our former president, Professor Thomas Hunt Morgan, of the California Institute of Technology, for his admirable lecture of last evening.

I have been speaking of research activities and research results of the present and of the recent past; but what of the future, even of the immediate future? They threaten to be very different. A condition of intense anxiety on this subject exists in nearly all our universities, in the research institutions, in the learned societies in general, in the research organizations supported by the government of the nation, and with countless thousands of public-spirited and wide-awake citizens who have a fair comprehension of what scientific discovery, through experimentation and research, has done for humanity. In many universities, especially state universities, where research, sympathetically nurtured and supported through the years, has brought forth new knowledge of tremendous importance to the welfare of the nation, the degree of existing anxiety as to what may happen can be said to have approached, here and there, the stage of fear. The legislatures of the majority of our states are now in session, and they have the duty of appropriating funds for the support of their respective educational institutions through the next two years. The attitude of many, perhaps nearly all, of the legislatures toward research at public expense may fairly be described as unsympathetic and, in some cases, I am informed, as severely hostile. I need not say to this audience that a university, shorn of its research activities and deprived of the scholarly atmosphere that research develops, will eventually differ but little in character from what we may call a higher high school. The name "university" will remain, but the qualities special to a real university will dwindle and disappear. The Book of Great Wisdom, tried and proved through the centuries, says that "Where there is no vision, the people perish." Equal confidence may be placed in the thesis, "Where there is no research, the universities perish." The governments, the universities and the peoples in Europe and in many other parts of the world understand this principle perfectly. The universities in those countries, with few exceptions, are national, or state, or municipal universities, financially supported in major degree by their governments.

No American citizen in possession of his senses questions for a moment the absolute need for reduced appropriations. Wisdom in the immediate present, and our welfare, both our public and our private welfare, in the future, demand the prompt balancing of budgets—national, state, county, municipal budgets, and personal budgets as well; and all good citizens are ready to lend their approval to proposals for reductions made circumspectly and in accord with the inherent needs and the inherent merits of the services that would be thereby affected.

There is a large amount of valuable research now conducted, under the government, in the city of Washington, or with Washington as its administrative center. It is, for the most part, work that the states and the universities—both the state universities and the private universities—in their happiest days, and the research institutions existing and actively operating in this country, could not undertake, for reasons partly financial and for other extremely important and vital reasons that are not financial. For example, how could the state of Nevada or Colorado or Tennessee or Vermont undertake to contribute, individually, to the plans now being carried out by the U. S. Coast and Geodetic Survey? The investigational work conducted by our government is more or less in parallel with, but not unnecessarily duplicating, research activities supported on a large scale by the government of Great Britain, including Canada and the other dominions, the government of France, the government of Germany, the government of Italy and the governments of many of the other and smaller nations. The financial support of our national government for the researches in Washington and elsewhere in the United States has been obtained, for the most part, upon the basis of need and merit, and not at all by political log-rolling, not to any extent whatsoever by the threats of an "organized minority," tacit or vocal, to the effect that the congressman or the senator who does not vote the financial support asked for will be defeated at the next election. The researches referred to are conducted, it is absolutely unnecessary for me to say, by able, conscientious men who spent many years and much money in their later 'teens and their early twenties preparing in colleges and universities and graduate schools, many of them in England, France or Germany, to do this work—in fact, devoting several decades of each of their precious lives to fitting themselves for carrying on their present investigations. Many of the research organizations, under the government, to which they are attached, have had long and glorious histories; their high standards are being maintained; and their accomplishments continue to be valuable in commendable and worthy degree. At this point I must say that I am in possession of no knowledge that would justify me in thinking, for one moment, that any executive officer of the government is proposing or intending to cut appropriations for the support of existing research activities in unjust or catastrophic degree. It is difficult for me to anticipate or fear that arbitrary cuts will be made, in the course of the conscientious governmental administration of our country, even though the power so to proceed unquestionably exists.

The Act of Incorporation of the National Academy of Sciences, adopted by the Congress and approved by President Lincoln in the year 1863, makes the academy an official agency of the government, as expressed in the following language, quoted from the act: ". . . the Academy shall, whenever called upon by any department of the Government, investigate, examine, experiment, and report upon any subject in science . . . , but the Academy shall receive no compensation whatever for any services to the Government of the United States." When an American citizen, necessarily a successful scientist, accepts election to membership in the academy, he tacitly agrees to heed every such summons, and to serve his government to the best of his ability, in the manner described, and without expectation or hope of receiving compensation. The academy has responded many times, and promptly, to the government's call, and it welcomes such duty.

If this address should happen to be published—this may or may not be the case—there would be opportunity to *read* the passage just quoted from the Act of Incorporation, and to comprehend better its significance. The reader could not fail to observe the limitations imposed upon the academy's freedom of action. The connection between the government of the nation, on the one hand, and the National Academy of Sciences, on the other, is not in the nature of a broad avenue with lines of trees and a strip of lawn in its center and a roadway on either side. It is rather a street, and it is not for me to say how wide is that street. The specification reads that "the Academy shall, whenever *called upon* by any department of the Government," and this corresponds to the definition of a one-way street.

In this connection a few very special things should be said, and even emphasized. Here I am speaking as a member of the academy, and not in commitment of the academy to any views or policies—I have not that authority or power—but in the light of my membership and experiences and observations in relation to the academy extending back through thirty-one years.

(1) The academy is composed of 265 members, whose chief interests throughout their lives have resided in the natural sciences and the biologic sciences. They have all had wonderful opportunities—in many cases opportunities of their own making—to advance human knowledge in their several fields, through research and discovery, and they have been successful in their quest for the truth; otherwise, they would not be members of the academy. They are men (and two women) of strong character who have found happiness and satisfaction in their work. They have extended knowledge and, in many cases, have applied new knowledge to the daily affairs of the world, all with incalculable advantage to the human race. On such questions as government appropriations they have no "axes to grind." Their judgment would be devoid of self-seeking and, after due consideration of the facts, wholly in accord with the public welfare.

(2) The academy's interest in scientific research, of high merit, whether conducted in universities, research institutions or under government auspices, is very deep; but the academy would not and could not give its support to pseudo-research—that is, research in name that is not research in fact.

(3) The academy could not by any possibility lend its moral support to poor or faulty or uninspiring systems of research administration, or to systems or plans financially extravagant.

(4) I can not doubt that the academy would hold to the view that existing organizations, or their substitute organizations in other departments, charged with responsibility for the conducting of research, should be prepared to accept such reasonable subtractions from their financial resources as are based upon the thorough consideration of all elements involved.

I am not called upon to set forth here, of all places in the United States, and especially before this audience, the importance of research, the incomparable values of its accomplishments, the need for its continuance in strength diminished in no greater degree than is unavoidable. In my opinion, the products of research and invention in the domain of the physical and biologic sciences have been more potent in advancing the state of civilization on the earth from its low level of the fifteenth century to its high level in the twentieth century than have all other forces combined. I do not expect universal acceptance of this thesis, but I am prepared to defend it. There is no question that many other forces, both idealistic and practical, have been exceedingly influential and powerful in behalf of the nations and their peoples, but in the main those forces would not have existed, or certainly could not have operated, if the physical and biologic sciences had not provided the mental and moral attitudes, the opportunities, the open sesame that permitted them to go out into the great world and exert their effective and beneficent influences.

Neither is there need for saying to this audience that the desirable cultivation of the fields of knowledge represented in the research activities of universities and governments has been but little more than begun. Our great commercial organizations recognize this fact in the existence of their research departments. They know that the discovery of fundamental knowledge and the application of the finest methods of scientific research are the essential and powerful aids to industrial progress. These commercial organizations control and apportion the appropriations in support of their several departments of activity and endeavor with rare acumen and judgment, and we shall not learn that any of those organizations, successful in large degree, will reduce their financial support of research for the year beginning on July 1, 1933, in percentages exceeding those relating to their administrative divisions. Their boards of trustees are too wise for that. I do not know of any good reason why research activities conducted in universities and under governments should not be supported in accordance with the same policy. We know that such research activities have earned and paid priceless dividends through the years, the decades and the centuries of the past, and I do not have the slightest lack of confidence in the correctness of the thesis that further research activities, continued through the years, the decades and the centuries ahead, will be equally fruitful in results that the human race should have and will use to its tremendous advantage.

# A HISTORY OF THE NATIONAL RESEARCH COUNCIL 1919--1933

## IV. DIVISION OF CHEMISTRY AND CHEMICAL TECHNOLOGY[1]

By Professor CHARLES A. KRAUS

CHAIRMAN

THE Division of Chemistry and Chemical Technology is a representative organization of American chemists. Its membership in the main consists of representatives from the different societies of American chemists and members-at-large nominated by the division itself. In addition, it acts through numerous committees, the membership of which is unrestricted. The division is, therefore, under the control of American chemists acting through representatives chosen by their own organizations.

Its chairmanship has been held by the following persons since the organization of the division in 1918:

1918 —John Johnston
1919–1920—W. D. Bancroft
1920–1922—F. C. Cottrell
1922–1923—E. W. Washburn
1923–1924—J. Enrique Zanetti
1924–1925—James F. Norris
1925–1927—William J. Hale
1927–1928—Frank C. Whitmore
1928–1929—George A. Hulett
1929–1930—James E. Mills
1930–1931—Harry A. Curtis
1931–1932—Henry K. Benson
1932–1933—Charles A. Kraus

The division acts as agent in cooperation with other similar national agencies on all problems of international concern. It recommends the appointment of delegates to the International Union of Chemistry, votes on matters requiring decision *ad interim*, receives and distributes reports of committees of the union, and assists in organizing American committees supplementary to committees of the union. In a field such as chemistry there are many questions that can be settled only by international agreement. The division, owing to its wide affiliations, is in a position to give expression to the opinions of American chemists.

Following the war, there was great need for reliable values of physical and chemical constants. Indeed, a thoroughly satisfactory tabulation of such constants had not theretofore been made. At the request of the International Research Council, the Division of Chemistry and Chemical Technology, acting conjointly with the Division of Physical Sciences, undertook the stupendous task of publishing "International Critical Tables of Physical and Chemical Constants." The publication of these tables entailed the critical examination of the vast amount of data collected in the literature up to that time. The division organized an editorial staff, including ten foreign representatives; and arranged for the detailed analysis of all available data by collaborating experts in the various fields. The first volume of the Tables appeared in 1926 and the seventh volume in 1930. These seven volumes totaled 3,404 pages.

[1] This is the fourth of a series of ten articles prepared to describe briefly the nature of the activities with which the National Research Council has been engaged during the past fourteen years.

One of the defects of practically all existing tables of constants has been the lack of satisfactory indexes. The division accordingly undertook to provide an index to the Critical Tables. This index, comprising some 330 pages, will appear from the press in April of the present year.

The "Survey of American Chemistry" was brought out in 1926, in order to provide a general view of the state of research progress in America. This survey developed into an annual publication, the seventh volume of which is now in press. Chapters dealing with various fields of chemistry are contributed by authors who themselves are active in those fields. Originally all fields were reviewed each year, but with the last volume of the Survey it was decided to review some fields only every second or third year. To any one who is interested in following the development of research in chemistry generally throughout the country, the Survey has proved very helpful.

The division has been of assistance in providing avenues for publication of important results in many different ways. Various chairmen of the division have contributed monographs on timely subjects, journal publications have been assisted, and reports of numerous committees have been made available. The division was helpful in establishing *The Chemical Review,* a bi-monthly journal, and there might also be named the Chemical Monograph Series, which now comprises some 50 volumes.

The division, through various committees, has administered research funds provided for special investigations. Among these may be mentioned the investigation carried out at the Bureau of Standards on the preservation and permanence of records. As the result of this investigation it has been found that the life of all record papers is greatly influenced by conditions such as light, humidity and atmospheric impurities. Corrective measures have been suggested and libraries are already making use of the results of this investigation. This work has also done much to stimulate further investigation of problems relating to the permanence of record papers. Important investigations were also carried out under the auspices of the Committee on Chemical Research on Medicinal Substances, with funds provided for the purpose from various sources. The division also cooperated with the Central Petroleum Committee in organizing petroleum research under a grant of $500,000, which was administered by the Petroleum Institute.

Much of the work of the division is carried out through its committees, the membership of which includes not only members of the division but also chemists throughout the country.

The Committee on the Chemistry of Colloids was organized in 1919 and has ever since been active in promoting colloid research. This committee was instrumental in arranging for the publication of several books and of numerous monographs, the earliest of which were published in mimeographed form by the National Research Council. In 1923 the committee was instrumental in organizing the First Colloid Symposium. This symposium has since been continued each year in cooperation with the Colloid Division of the American Chemical Society. The papers read at these symposia have been published in monograph form.

The Committee on Contact Catalysis was organized in 1920. Its first report was published in the *Journal of Industrial and Engineering Chemistry* in 1921, and subsequent reports have been published each year in the *Journal of Physical Chemistry.*

The Committee on Photochemistry was organized in 1927, and has published reports in the *Journal of Physical Chemistry.* The Committee on the Construction and Equipment of Chemical Laboratories was organized in 1924. Its final report was published in book form by the Chemical Foundation in 1930. This committee has been reorganized and is continuing its work in collecting data relating to laboratory construction and equipment. The Committee on Explosives Investigation was very active and rendered much valuable service for some years following the war. Among its other activities, it carried on a study of the utilization of surplus military explosives, and prepared a descriptive list of hazardous chemicals and explosives. The Committee on Research Chemicals was active for a number of years following the war, collecting data on research chemicals available in this country. Lists of research chemicals were published in the Reprint and Circular Series of the National Research Council.

Other committees, such as the Committee on Pharmaceutical Research, on Methods of Organic Analysis, on Medicinal Substances and on Petroleum Chemistry, have been active in stimulating research. The Committee on Chemical Research on Medicinal Substances was formed in 1923. It continued until its functions were taken over by the Annual Survey of American Chemistry, after its members had published 144 papers and three United States patents. Research results valued at many millions of dollars have been credited to the activities of this committee. The Central Petroleum Committee was constituted in 1926 with the cooperation of the Divisions of Physical Sciences and Geology and Geography, to plan a research program on the chemistry, physics and geology of petroleum, in conjunction with the American Petroleum Institute. This program has contained 41 separate projects, some of which have been completed, while others are still active.

Each year as funds permitted the division has undertaken conferences for the initiation and coordination of chemical research. Such conferences have been held on the subjects of permanence of printed records, on the coordination of chemical literature, on biological nomenclature, and on farm waste and chemistry of soils. The results of these meetings have been intangible in part, but the mere bringing together of eminent men interested in a certain phase of chemistry is important.

The division has from time to time collected pertinent data relating to chemistry. Since 1922, the division has each year made a census of graduate students in chemistry throughout the country, and this census has been published in the journals. The division also conducted a study of conditions of chemical research in the Southern States. The report of this study was published by the Chemical Foundation. Other activities include cooperation between academic and industrial research, and a list of research problems in various fields of chemistry.

One of the important activities of the division has been the administration of the grants in aid of research. During the past four years 42 grants have been made to 37 individuals. Many papers have been published as a result of these grants and many capable research workers have been encouraged in their work. Particularly during the last few years, the grants-in-aid have proved invaluable to research workers who have found themselves handicapped through lack of funds.

Another important activity of the Research Council and of the Division has been in connection with the National Research Fellowships. Since their foundation, 257 fellowships in chemistry have been awarded to 150 individuals. While it is true that some will profit more than others from the opportunities afforded by these research fellowships, there can be no question that the National Research Fellowships have produced tangible results.

Through meetings of the division and of committees, and through other contacts afforded by the division, those interested in various fields of chemistry are brought together and contacts are established. It is from these contacts that we may expect some of the major benefits in the course of time.

# SCIENTIFIC EVENTS

## CHICAGO PROGRAM ON RADIATION AND PLANT LIFE

THE American Society of Plant Physiologists has joined with Sections G and O and their affiliated organizations in the programs of June 20 and 21. On the morning of June 22, however, a special symposium has been arranged for plant physiologists who are attending the meetings. The meeting will be held in the Civic Opera Building, Chicago, in the rooms of the Lighting Institute at 10:00 A. M. The meeting will be open to all visiting botanists and to professional growers of plants. The titles of the papers are as follows:

"Influence of Radiation on $CO_2$ Absorption by Plants": W. H. Hoover, Smithsonian Institution.

"The Interrelated Effects of Light and Temperature on Plant Growth": A. D. Davis, University of California.

"Growth as a Criterion for Physiologic Response to Radiations": E. S. Reynolds, Missouri Botanic Garden.

"Photoperiodism and its Practical Application to Greenhouse Crops": Alex Laurie, Ohio State University.

"Responses of Certain Plants to Artificial Radiation Factors Applied as Supplements to Daylight": R. B. Withrow, Purdue University.

"The Response of Greenhouse Plants to Electric Light Supplementing Daylight": Laurenz Greene, Purdue University.

"Experimental Work at Pennsylvania State College on Radiation as Applied to Plants": H. W. Popp, Pennsylvania State College.

"Chemical Responses of Certain Plants to Solar Ultra-violet Radiation": W. E. Tottingham, University of Wisconsin.

"Some Growth Responses of Plants to X-ray Treatments": C. A. Shull, University of Chicago.

The program will be continued in the afternoon, if necessary, followed by a round table discussion.

CHARLES A. SHULL

## MATHEMATICS AT THE CHICAGO MEETING

THE preliminary program of the Chicago meeting of the American Association for the Advancement of Science and Associated Societies, printed in the issue of SCIENCE for May 19, contains information concerning the programs of the different sections, but it may be well to repeat here a summary of the plans of the mathematicians given in the announcement of the American Mathematical Association.

It reports that the American Association and associated societies will present unusually attractive programs in connection with the Century of Progress, the week of June 19 being devoted chiefly to pure science and the next week to applied science. There will be numerous addresses by prominent foreign scientific men who have been specially invited for these meetings. These programs and the many interests offered at the Century of Progress exposition add unusually attractive features to our usual pleasant summer meetings.

The society will hold a session on Tuesday afternoon in Mandel Hall at which Professor Tullio Levi-Civita, of the University of Rome, will speak on "Some Mathematical Aspects of the New Mechanics," and Professor G. D. Birkhoff, of Harvard University, will speak on "Quantum Mechanics and Asymptotic Series." At a symposium at ten o'clock Wednesday morning in Mandel Hall, Professor Lipót Fejér, of the University of Budapest, will speak on "The Infinite Sequences Arising in the Theories of Harmonic Analysis, of Interpolation, and of Mechanical Quadratures," this to be followed by addresses by Professor C. N. Moore, of the University of Cincinnati, "On the Use of Cesàro Means in Determining Criteria for Fourier's Constants," and Professor Dunham Jackson, of the University of Minnesota, on "Certain Problems of Closest Approximation." A second symposium will be held at two o'clock on Wednesday in the Italian Building on the Fair Grounds; addresses will be given by Professor Levi-Civita on "Nets on a Surface and Extension of Trigonometry," by Professor W. C. Graustein, of Harvard University, on "Invariant Methods in Differential Geometry," and by Professor Enrico Bompiani, of the University of Rome, on "Deformations of Higher Species of Surfaces and Manifolds." At two o'clock on Friday, in Eckhart Hall, an address will be given by Professor L. E. Dickson, of the University of Chicago, on "Recent Progress in Additive Number Theory," following which there will be a session of short papers on number theory. Sessions for the reading of short papers will be held on Monday afternoon and Thursday and Friday mornings.

Among the addresses of the week by physicists will be the following: At 4:30 Tuesday, at the Fair Grounds, Dr. Bjerknes, Geophysical Institute, Bergen, Norway, on "Atmospheric Soundings, Methods and Results"; at 4:30 Wednesday, in the Italian Building, Enrico Fermi, University of Rome, on "Theory of Hyperfine Structures"; at 8:00 P. M. Wednesday, place to be announced, Dr. F. W. Aston, University of Cambridge, on "The Story of Isotopes" and Dr. R. A. Millikan, California Institute of Technology, on "New Light on Nuclear Physics"; at 4:30 Thursday, in the Italian Building, Professor Niels Bohr, of the University of Copenhagen, on "Space and Time in Contemporary Physics." Other addresses by the visiting scientists will be announced in the current issues of SCIENCE.

The joint dinner of the mathematicians and their guests will be held on Friday evening at 6:30 at Judson Court. On Monday evening the American Association and its associated societies will hold a general reception on the grounds of the Century of Progress. The American Association will hold a dinner on Thursday evening at which the visiting scientists will be guests.

## CHEMISTRY AT THE CHICAGO MEETING

ACCORDING to an announcement sent out by the American Chemical Society, joint sessions with the sections of the medical sciences, physics and geology and geography of the association have been arranged by the Section of Chemistry, of which Professor Arthur B. Lamb, of Harvard University, president of the American Chemical Society, is chairman.

Professor Francis W. Aston, of the University of Cambridge, England, Nobel prize winner in chemistry for 1922, and Professor The. Svedberg, of the University of Upsala, Sweden, Nobel prize winner in chemistry for 1926, will head a contingent of foreign chemists who will take part.

Professor Aston and Professor Robert A. Millikan, of the California Institute of Technology, Nobel prize winner in physics for 1923, will deliver addresses at a public meeting Wednesday night, June 21. Professor Aston will speak on "The Story of Isotopes," a subject which has thrown new light on the structure of atoms, building blocks of the universe, and Professor Millikan will discuss nuclear physics.

American chemists from universities and government and industrial bureaus of research will detail advances in the application of mathematics to chemistry's problems and gains in chemistry's war on disease.

Two recipients of the Langmuir Medal of the American Chemical Society, annually awarded to the young chemist who shows most promise of achievement, will present papers. They are Professor Linus Pauling, of the California Institute of Technology, first medal winner, and Dr. Oscar K. Rice, of Harvard University, second medal winner. Dr. Henry Eyring, of Princeton University, who was awarded the prize of the American Association for the Advancement of Science for 1932, will also participate.

A symposium devoted to the earth's age will bring together the sections of chemistry, physics and geology and geography on Wednesday afternoon, June 21, at two o'clock in Rosenwald Hall. The secretary of the section is Professor J. H. Simons, of Northwestern University.

Because of the importance of chemistry to medicine, the Section of Chemistry will meet jointly with the Medical Section on Monday morning, June 19, at 9:30 o'clock in Thorne Hall for a symposium on the relation of colloid chemistry to biological problems.

Professor Svedberg, who won the Nobel prize for his work in colloid chemistry, will describe a new investigation into the sedimentation constants and molecular weights of the respiratory proteins. Professor Filippo Bottazzi, Istituto di Fisiologia, Naples, and Professor W. J. V. Osterhout, Rockefeller Institute for Medical Research, will address the session.

The subject of a third symposium, to be held at the International House on Wednesday morning, June 21, with the Chemistry and Physics Sections jointly participating, will be "Isotopes." Professor Aston, who received the Nobel prize for his work in isotopes, will give measurements of the relative abundance of isotopes.

Quantum mechanics in chemistry will be discussed at a symposium of the Chemistry and Physics Sections and the American Physical Society, Tuesday morning, June 20, at 9:30 o'clock in the International House. The speakers will include Professor J. C. Slater, of the Massachusetts Institute of Technology; Professor Pauling; Dr. Eyring, of Princeton University, and Professor R. S. Mulliken, of the University of Chicago.

Many chemists are expected to attend the joint session of the Section of Physics and the American Physical Society on Friday morning at 9:30 o'clock in the International House, which will be devoted to the breaking down of matter. The speakers include: Dr. J. D. Cockroft, of the University of Cambridge; Dr. M. A. Tuve, of the Carnegie Institution; Professor W. D. Harkins, of the University of Chicago, and Professor E. O. Lawrence, of the University of California.

The dinner of the Chicago Section of the American Chemical Society, in conjunction with the Section of Chemistry of the association, will be held on Friday night, June 23, at the Midland Club. Professor Svedberg will deliver the principal address, "The Sedimentation of Molecules in Centrifugal Fields," at a supplementary meeting in the Field Museum. A luncheon of the Chicago Chemists Club and the Section of Chemistry of the association will be held on Tuesday, June 20, at 12:30 o'clock in the International House. Brief informal and non-technical talks will be made.

## THE MEDICAL SCIENCES AT THE CHICAGO MEETING

THE *Journal* of the American Medical Association reports that at the summer session of the American Association for the Advancement of Science in Chicago, June 19–23, Section N (the medical sciences) will sponsor four symposiums and a public meeting. Headquarters will be at the Knickerbocker Hotel. Monday morning, June 19, the section will join with Section C (chemistry) at Thorne Hall, Northwestern University, for a symposium on colloid chemistry as related to biologic problems, with the following speakers:

Dr. Edwin J. Cohn, Harvard Medical School, Boston, "Electrostatic Forces in Systems Containing Biological Components"; Professor Theodor Svedberg, Upsala University, Sweden, "Sedimentation Constants and Molecular Weights of the Respiratory Proteins"; Professor Filippo Bottazzi, Naples, Italy, "Physicochemical Properties of Concentrated Blood Serum."

Tuesday morning, June 20, Section N will combine with Section F (zoology) in a symposium with the following speakers:

Professor Archibald V. Hill, London, England, "Physical and Chemical Changes in Nerve During Activity"; Dr. Wallace O. Fenn, University of Rochester, "Nerve Respiration"; Dr. Ralph W. Gerard, Chicago, "Chemical Activity of Nerve"; Dr. Herbert S. Gasser, New York, "Electric Phenomena in Nerve."

Wednesday morning a symposium on pathologic physiology will be held at Northwestern University, in which the following will participate:

Dr. William H. Park, New York, "B C G Vaccination"; Dr. Charles H. Best, Toronto, "Fatty Changes in the Liver of Normal and Diabetic Animals"; Dr. Arthur L. Tatum, Madison, Wisconsin, "Morphine Addiction and Morphine Tolerance"; Dr. Maurice B. Strauss, Boston, "Etiology of Pernicious Anemia and the Related Macrocytic Anemias."

Thursday morning, June 22, a surgical-endocrinologic symposium will be presented at Northwestern University by the following:

Dr. George W. Crile, Cleveland, "A Century of Progress in Surgery: Anesthesia, Antisepsis and Asepsis, Shock and Careful Handling of Tissues"; Dr. Max Ballin, Detroit, "Clinical Recognition and Surgical Treatment of Parathyroidism"; Dr. Percival Bailey, Chicago, "Surgical Control of Hypophyseal Disorders"; Dr. John deJ. Pemberton, Rochester, Minnesota, "Recent Developments in the Clinical Recognition and Surgical Management of Hyperfunction of the Thyroid Gland"; Dr. Evarts A. Graham, St. Louis, "Clinical Recognition and Surgical Management of Hypoglycemia Produced by Tumors of the Islets of Langerhans."

It is expected that Madame Marie Curie, Paris, codiscoverer of radium, will address some of these meetings.

A public meeting celebrating a century of progress in medicine will be held Tuesday evening, June 20, in Thorne Hall. The program arranged is as follows:

Dr. Morris Fishbein, Chicago, editor, the *Journal* of the American Medical Association, "Frontiers of Medicine"; Dr. Paul Dudley White, Boston, "Heart Disease"; Dr. Max Cutler, Chicago, "The Conquest of Cancer."

## THE AMERICAN SOCIETY AND JOURNAL FOR PHARMACOLOGY AND EXPERIMENTAL THERAPEUTICS

THE annual meeting of the society was held at the University of Cincinnati from April 10 to 12. The following officers were elected for next year:

*President,* Wm. de B. MacNider
*Vice-president,* A. L. Tatum
*Secretary,* V. E. Henderson
*Treasurer,* O. H. Plant
*Council,* C. M. Gruber
G. B. Roth
*Membership Committee,* J. Auer

The most important business before the society was the offer of Dr. J. J. Abel, who founded the *Journal of Pharmacology and Experimental Therapeutics* and who, with Dr. Carl Voegtlin and Dr. Reid Hunt, formed the original corporation, to turn over the journal to the society as its official organ. This offer was unanimously accepted by the society, and the following resolution was adopted by the society as the means of expressing its appreciation to Professor Abel:

*Be it Resolved,* that the Secretary of the Society for Pharmacology and Experimental Therapeutics be instructed to write to Professor Abel and to the members of the Corporation of the *Journal of Pharmacology and Experimental Therapeutics,*

(a) That the Society wishes to express to them its deep gratitude and thanks for their most gracious and very generous offer to transfer the Journal free of all encumbrances to the Society.

(b) That the Society records its grateful appreciation of Dr. Abel's long and faithful service in furthering the advancement of Pharmacology in this country by promoting and editing the Journal.

(c) That the Society wishes to assure Dr. Abel that every effort will be made to maintain and extend if possible, the high standards of excellence as set by the Journal during the twenty-four years it has been under his control.

(d) That the Society is deeply touched by the devotion shown by Dr. Abel to its interest in returning from Baltimore to this meeting in order to aid in completing the arrangements for the transfer of the Journal to the Society.

The necessary steps were taken by the society for giving effect to this transfer.

V. E. HENDERSON,
*Secretary*

## OBITUARY

DR. EDGAR HENRY SUMMERFIELD BAILEY, professor emeritus of chemistry at the University of Kansas, where he was a member of the faculty for fifty years, died on June 1 at the age of eighty-four years.

PROFESSOR WILLIAM P. RYAN, head of the department of chemical engineering at the Massachusetts Institute of Technology and director of its school of chemical engineering practise, died on May 31 at the age of thirty-eight years.

FREDERIC POOLE GORHAM, professor of bacteriology at Brown University, died suddenly on June 4. He was sixty-two years old.

# SCIENTIFIC NOTES AND NEWS

WE are informed by cable that there was organized in London on June 1 the Academic Assistance Council with Lord Rutherford as chairman. Its object is to provide positions or other aid for university professors and scientific men who because of "religion, political opinion or race are unable to carry on their work in their own country."

DR. ISAIAH BOWMAN, director of the American Geographical Society, has been elected chairman of the National Research Council, to fill the position occupied until his recent resignation by Dr. Vernon Kellogg. Dr. Bowman will remain director of the American Geographical Society and will devote half his time to the work of the National Research Council. There has been created in the National Research Council the office of honorary vice-chairman to which Dr. William H. Welch, of the Johns Hopkins University, has been elected. The honorary chairman is Dr. George Ellery Hale, honorary director of the Mount Wilson Observatory.

DR. HAROLD WILLIS DODDS, professor of politics at Princeton University and chairman of the administrative committee of the Princeton School of Public and International Affairs, has been elected fifteenth president of the university to succeed the late Dr. John Grier Hibben. Dr. Luther P. Eisenhart, professor of mathematics and dean of the faculty, has been elected dean of the Graduate School to succeed Dr. Augustus Trowbridge, who resigned last year, and Dr. Robert Kilburn Root, Woodrow Wilson professor of literature and chairman of the department of English, succeeds Dr. Eisenhart as dean of the faculty. Since the resignation of Dr. Hibben in June, 1932, Edward D. Duffield, president of the Prudential Insurance Company and trustee of the university, has been acting president.

DR. GEORGE DAVID BIRKHOFF, professor of mathematics at Harvard University, has been elected Perkins professor of mathematics to succeed Professor William F. Osgood, who on September 1 retires with the title of professor emeritus.

PROFESSOR WILLIAM H. TALIAFERRO, associate dean

of the Division of the Biological Sciences at the University of Chicago, has been appointed chairman of the department of hygiene and bacteriology to succeed Dr. Edwin O. Jordan, who retires on October 1 after being associated with the university for forty-one years.

DR. SIMON FLEXNER, director of the Rockefeller Institute for Medical Research, was the speaker on June 1 at a luncheon at the Bankers Club, given in his honor by the Bond Club of New York.

THE Dutch Red Cross Society, under the presidency of Prince Hendrik, awarded its gold medal on April 19 to Dr. Karl Landsteiner, member of the Rockefeller Institute for Medical Research, for his discovery of the blood groups in relation to blood transfusion.

THOSE on whom honorary degrees are to be conferred by the University of Cincinnati on June 10 include Professor Herman Schneider, dean of the College of Engineering and formerly president of the university; Dean Roscoe Pound, of the Harvard Law School, and John Adam Fleming, director of the Department of Terrestrial Magnetism, Carnegie Institution of Washington.

DR. WILLIAM DE BERNIERE MACNIDER, Kenan research professor of pharmacology at the University of North Carolina Medical School, on May 30 was awarded the honorary degree of doctor of science during the commencement exercises closing the ninety-fifth session of the Medical College of Virginia, Richmond.

DR. HUGH H. YOUNG, clinical professor and visiting urologist at the Johns Hopkins Hospital, will sail on June 20 to receive the honorary degree of doctor of philosophy from Queen's University, Belfast, Ireland.

SIR WALTER MORLEY FLETCHER, secretary of the British Medical Research Council, and Dr. Samuel Smiles, Daniell professor of chemistry at King's College, University of London, will receive the degree of D.Sc. from the University of Belfast.

PROFESSOR HENRY B. WARD, who is retiring as professor of zoology and head of the department of zoology at the University of Illinois, was given a "surprise party" at his home on the evening of May 27. Seventy of his colleagues and friends were there and presented him with a canoe and boat house, and a volume of letters from one hundred and twenty-five friends and associates. Professor Ward has become permanent secretary of the American Association for the Advancement of Science under conditions which permit him to continue research work.

BOSTON surgeons and members of the Italian Medical Society on June 3 paid tribute to Dr. Alberto Alessandri, professor of surgery at the University of Rome, at a dinner given in his honor at the University Club. Dr. Alessandri is in Boston as part of his tour of the country, during which he is studying American hospitals and surgical methods.

DR. ERNEST E. IRONS, dean of the Rush Medical College, has been appointed chairman of the department of medicine at the University of Chicago, succeeding Dr. George F. Dick. Dr. Dick continues as professor in the department of medicine at the college and as professor and chairman of the department of medicine in the Division of Biological Sciences of the University of Chicago.

OWEN STANLEY GIBBS, professor of physiology and pharmacology, University of Georgia School of Medicine, has been appointed professor of physiology at Georgetown University School of Medicine, Washington, D. C.

DR. ISIDOR MORRIS HEILBRON, at present Heath Harrison professor of organic chemistry in the University of Liverpool, has accepted an invitation to a chair of organic chemistry in the University of Manchester.

MR. ROBERT RAE, of Queen's University, Belfast, has been appointed to the professorship of agriculture at the University of Reading, in succession to Professor S. Pennington.

THE chair of physiology at Edinburgh University, which becomes vacant on September 30 of this year by the retirement of Sir Edward Sharpey-Schafer, has been filled by the appointment of Dr. Ivan de Burgh Daly, professor of physiology in the University of Birmingham.

AT the University of Dublin Sir Charles Arthur Kinahan Ball has become the Regius professor of surgery in succession to the late Sir William Taylor, and John Purser has been appointed to the chair of civil engineering, which had become vacant by the death of Professor David Clark. Mr. Purser is assistant professor of civil engineering at the City and Guilds (Engineering) College and reader in civil engineering in the University of London.

DR. WALTER J. WILLIAMS, of Baylor University, Waco, Texas, was recently appointed curator of the university museum. The death of John K. Strecker, who had held this position since 1903, occurred on January 9. Dr. Williams had been closely associated with him since 1924.

DR. DANIEL F. JONES, who is a member of the board of overseers of Harvard College, has been elected president of the American Surgical Association.

PROFESSOR GEORGE H. PARKER, director of the zoological laboratories of Harvard University, was chosen on May 29 *president* of the Harvard Chapter of Sigma Xi for the coming year; Dr. James B. Conant, the newly elected president of the university, was elected *vice-president;* Professor Kirtley F. Mather, *secretary;* Dr. L. Don Leet, *assistant secretary,* and Professor William L. Crum, *treasurer.*

DR. ALEXANDER WETMORE, assistant secretary of the Smithsonian Institution, has been elected president of the District of Columbia Chapter of Sigma Xi.

THE following have been elected as officers of the Chicago Chemists Club for the year 1933–34: *President,* Gustav Egloff; *First vice-president,* E. C. Leamon; *Second vice-president,* C. O. Miller; *Secretary,* C. D. Lowry, Jr.; *Treasurer,* E. A. Dieterle, and *Trustee,* Bruce K. Brown.

AT the annual general meeting of the Royal Geographical Society, London, to be held on June 19, the council will propose the election of Major-General Sir Percy Cox as president of the society in succession to Admiral Sir William Goodenough, whose term of office expires in November. Sir William will then become a vice-president. Sir Percy Cox has been a fellow of the society since 1895, was a vice-president in 1926 and is at present a member of the council.

PROFESSOR C. U. ARIENS KAPPERS, director of the Central Institute for Brain Research at Amsterdam, arrived in New York on May 29. He is a guest of the Century of Progress Exposition and the American Association for the Advancement of Science. After the meeting he is expected to give lectures in New York and Toronto. Dr. Ludwig Diels, director of the Botanical Garden and Museum at Berlin, also a guest of the exposition and the association, arrived on April 16. The *Bulletin* of the New York Botanical Garden states that he planned to spend a month in botanical exploration in the southeastern states, to visit Washington and Boston and to spend some time in New York before going to Chicago about the middle of June.

DR. ERNEST O. LAWRENCE, professor of physics at the University of California, will be visiting lecturer in physics at the summer session at Cornell University. Dr. Lawrence will give a course of lectures on "The Theory of Electric Discharges" and will conduct a discussion course dealing chiefly with "Nuclear Phenomena."

DR. ALFRED LANDÉ, professor of physics at the Ohio State University, delivered on May 26 the annual Sigma Xi address on "Determinacy in Physics and Biology" before the University of Cincinnati Chapter.

DR. D. B. DILL, of the Fatigue Laboratory, Harvard University, recently addressed the Massachusetts State College Sigma Xi Club on "Capacity for Work." On May 2 Dr. C. C. Little, of the Roscoe B. Jackson Memorial Laboratory, Bar Harbor, Maine, addressed the club on "Recent Researches on Cancer."

THE officers of the "Notgemeinschaft der deutschen Wissenschaft" have presented their resignations. They include Dr. Friedrich Schmidt-Ott, formerly "Kultus" minister, president since its foundation; Dr. Walter von Dyck, professor of mathematics at the Munich Institute of Technology; Professor Fritz Haber, who recently resigned as director of the Kaiser Wilhelm Institute for Physical Chemistry, and Dr. Heinrich Konen, professor of physics at the University at Bonn, vice-presidents.

THE Pacific Science Congress opened at Victoria, British Columbia, on June 1, with 160 men of science from thirty nations bordering on the Pacific in attendance. Lieutenant-Governor J. W. Fordham Johnson welcomed the convention to British Columbia, and Dr. H. M. Tory, of Ottawa, president of the congress, responded. Among the speakers at the opening session were Professor Paul Chavier, of the Paris Academy of Sciences; Professor G. I. Taylor, of the Royal Society of London; Dr. S. Hatai, of the Imperial Japanese University, Tokyo; Professor G. Van Eferdingen, spokesman for the Netherlands Government, and Dr. H. E. Gregory, director of the Bernice P. Bishop Museum at Honolulu. On Monday, June 5, the entire group adjourned to Vancouver, B. C., where the meeting will continue until Wednesday, June 14. After the close of the congress, the members will take a four-day tour through the famous Canadian Rockies, to Calgary and return.

IT has been found advisable to cancel the 1933 meeting of the National Conference on Weights and Measures which normally would be held early in June. After considering the entire situation the executive committee of the conference has decided by a unanimous vote that it would be unwise to attempt to hold a meeting this year. When the 1932 meeting was abandoned it was hoped that one could be held as usual in 1933, but continuance of abnormal economic conditions has made it certain that but few people would have been able to attend.

THE one hundred and first annual session of the British Medical Association will be held in Dublin, July 21–29. The annual representative meeting will begin Friday, July 21, and continue the next three week days. The annual general meeting will be held Tuesday afternoon, July 25, and the scientific sessions will occupy the next three days. Saturday,

July 29, will be devoted to excursions to places of interest. Dr. Thomas G. Moorhead, regius professor of physic, Trinity College, Dublin, is the incoming president of the association.

THE date of the meeting of the Phi Sigma Society is June 26, 27 and 28, not June 19, 20 and 21, as announced in the preliminary program of the Chicago meeting of the American Association.

THE fiftieth anniversary of the founding of the Wisconsin Agricultural Experiment Station was observed at the Farm Field Day in Madison on June 3. The Babcock film, a talking picture taken by the U. S. Department of Agriculture while the late Dr. S. M. Babcock was still living, was shown for the first time to a Wisconsin audience. It shows Dr. Babcock in his laboratory explaining the test and the machine which he developed which is used generally wherever dairying is carried on. Dr. Eugene Davenport, formerly dean of the College of Agriculture of the University of Illinois, was the principal speaker. The departments of the College of Agriculture, carrying on research, arranged an exhibit to show recent developments and findings as they apply to practical every-day farm and home problems.

# DISCUSSION

## MEANINGLESS VERSUS SIGNIFICANT TERMS IN GEOLOGICAL CLASSIFICATION

IN the February 10, 1933, issue of SCIENCE there appears a brief article by Dr. M. M. Leighton on "The Naming of the Subdivisions of the Wisconsin Glacial Age," in which he proposes the substitution of certain meaningless terms—Tazewell, Cary and Mankato—for the significant terms, Early Wisconsin, Middle Wisconsin and Late Wisconsin, which have been in general use for considerable time, and are readily understood by any one reading geological literature, denoting as they do successive parts of the Wisconsin glacial stage. The incentive for suggesting the new names seems to have its basis in a newly acquired view of Dr. Leighton that the deposition of the Iowan drift came only a short time before that of the Early Wisconsin drift, and so it may properly be included in the Wisconsin stage.

Whether the Iowan should be so included, if the entire field is taken into account, is far from being clearly established. This has been made forcibly apparent in a recent report by Dr. W. C. Alden on eastern Montana and adjacent areas (Professional Paper 174, U. S. Geological Survey, issued in 1932). There are deposits in Montana and the Dakotas which Dr. Alden is inclined to refer to the Iowan, but he considers them too old to be included in the Wisconsin stage. These are discussed by him under the heading "Illinoian or Iowan." But he thinks they do not appear to be as old as the Illinoian of Illinois.

Inasmuch as the entire series of drifts classed as Illinoian, Iowan and Wisconsin fall in the last quarter of the Pleistocene Period the distinctions in age aspects are less striking than between these drifts and those of middle and early Pleistocene age, known as Kansan and Nebraskan. This being the case, it seems advisable to let the terms that are in general use stand, especially where they have significance, and are self-explanatory, and not replace them by a set of meaningless terms.

FRANK LEVERETT

ANN ARBOR, MICHIGAN

## THREE PREHISTORIC PARASITES

IN 1916–17 an expedition of the Peabody Museum of American Archaeology and Ethnology of Harvard University excavated Basket-Maker Indian remains from desert caves in the northeastern portion of Arizona. Several human bodies were recovered and these have been described in the museum report[1] and elsewhere.[2]

Besides the human remains, two dogs were also found in undisturbed burial cists dug into the hard pan of the so-called "White Dog" cave. With the larger dog were found the bodies of many thousand flies. These flies were identified at the Museum of Comparative Zoology at Harvard as being *Caliphora coloradensis.*

Just recently a thorough microscopic examination has been made of uncontaminated skin and hair taken from the larger dog, and in a surprisingly well-preserved state have been found the eggs and young adults of a louse (*Trichodectus*), eggs and adults of a flea (*Sarcopsylla penetrans*), and numerous colonies of a fungus (*Trichosporum giganteum*) growing upon the hair shafts.

The only claim to fame of these insignificant parasites is their age, which has been conservatively estimated to be between six and ten thousand years.

GALE E. WILSON

SEATTLE, WASHINGTON

## THE DISTRIBUTION OF SERAPIAS HELLEBORINE IN CENTRAL NEW YORK

*Serapias Helleborine* L.—classified in the past as *Epipactis Crantz; E. latifolia* All.; *E. viridiflora*

[1] S. J. Guernsey and A. V. Kidder, "Basket-Maker Caves of Northeastern Arizona," Peabody Museum papers, Vol. viii, No. 2, 1921.

[2] G. E. Wilson, "A Study in American Paleohistology," *American Naturalist*, Vol. lxi, 1927.

Reichenb.—is believed to have been introduced from Europe. Its range was first reported in the immediate vicinity of Syracuse, New York, and later Buffalo, New York, and Toronto, Ontario. A more recent study shows it occupies a wider but limited range and is rare in each locality where found.[1]

Since *Serapias Helleborine* was first observed in the vicinity of Syracuse, the only region of the eastern United States where the hart tongue fern, *Scolopendrium vulgare,* grows, botanists suspected that its distribution would be limited to the same general areas. The orchid, however, has been a persistent invader of new areas in central New York, rapidly increasing as it adapts itself to the environment. Especially is this true in the Cayuga Lake Basin, where *Serapias Helleborine* was rare 15 years ago but to-day is a rather common plant, growing from roadsides to deep woods.[2] During the past year, 1932, this orchid has invaded in large numbers highly diversified areas both in natural and cultivated habitats in central New York. One of the areas invaded was a highly domesticated habitat in a residential district of Syracuse. This habitat, a heavy, sodded, well-kept residence lawn, supported seven vigorous plants approximately 2½ feet tall. These plants were growing in four unusual positions in the lawn, which saved them from the cutting blades of the lawn mower until their growth revealed a pleasing form to the eye of the caretaker, who permitted them to grow unmolested. Three of the above plants were growing in a very heavy lawn sod slightly higher in elevation than the surrounding ground. One grew in the shade of a hedge, where its roots mingled among those of the hedge plants, and three in close contact with a cement walk. These plants all produced many blossoms and a heavy seed setting followed. According to the statement of the property owner, this is the first season this plant has appeared in the lawn or in the immediate neighborhood. This observation covered a period of 25 years. Another interesting appearance of *Serapias Helleborine* this year for the first time was in a residential area on the shores of Cazenovia Lake, 16 miles east of Syracuse. Here the orchid grew abundantly in the back yard of a summer home. Furthermore, it has been found growing abundantly the past season in the bottomlands of various lakes in the vicinity of Syracuse, where in the past it occurred only sparingly.

The finding of this once rare orchid growing so luxuriantly in domesticated, as well as in natural habitats, is indeed interesting. If the present year's distribution is a reliable criterion for the future, flower lovers of central New York may realize a lifetime desire and see orchid plants as abundant in their back yards as some of the more common plant species of the region. This assumption may be purely speculative, however, since so many factors not fully understood may play an important rôle in the growth and distribution of an orchid species in a specific region during any particular year. Nevertheless, the occurrence of *Serapias Helleborine* in domesticated habitats definitely indicates that it may ultimately adapt itself to such environments. With this in mind, the writer as well as others interested in the distribution habits of this plant gathered its seed during the present year, to be scattered and planted in such cultivated habitats as lawns, flower plots and shrub areas. In addition, the seeds have been sent to individuals in various regions of the United States in the hope that more information relative to its environmental demands and adaptations can be gathered.

*Serapias Helleborine* is not as spectacular in its beauty as several other species of the Orchidaceae; nevertheless, the tall leafy stem with its dense-flowered raceme is very attractive. Therefore, should this orchid prove itself to be adaptive to widely divergent habitats, nature will have again added an attraction to the home lot.

VERNON A. YOUNG
NEW YORK STATE COLLEGE OF FORESTRY

[1] Gray's Manual, 6th and 7th editions; also Britton and Brown, 1st and 2nd editions of "Illustrated Flora of the Northern United States and Canada."

[2] A report from Dr. A. J. Eames, of Cornell University, Ithaca, N. Y., in personal correspondence.

## I-INOSITOL IN CITRUS FRUITS

IN the isolation of ascorbic (hexuronic) acid from citrus fruits there is always obtained a residue insoluble in methyl alcohol which can be recrystalized from water.

This substance melts at 225–226°. A mixture with i-inositol gives no depression in melting-point, and the optical-crystallographic properties are identical with those of i-inositol. The optical-crystallographic properties of anhydrous i-inositol, recrystallized from water at the temperature of the boiling-water bath, were found to be as follows: substance occurs as irregular colorless fragments when crushed for study by optical-immersion method. The indices of refraction are: $\alpha = 1.525$, $\beta = 1.555$, $\gamma = 1.570$, all $\pm$ 0.003. The double refraction is strong, $\gamma - \alpha = 0.045$. Biaxial interference figures common; optic sign −; 2 E not large.

The yields of i-inositol from ten liters of juice were as follows: Lemon = 1.24 g., orange = 0.47 g., grapefruit = 0.28 g.

E. K. NELSON
BUREAU OF CHEMISTRY AND SOILS
GEORGE L. KEENAN
FOOD AND DRUG ADMINISTRATION

# SPECIAL CORRESPONDENCE

## THE LEONARD WOOD MEMORIAL FOR THE ERADICATION OF LEPROSY

THE Leonard Wood Memorial for the Eradication of Leprosy does more than memorialize in its name a great soldier, physician and humanist. It exemplifies and continues one phase of the work in which Leonard Wood himself was greatly interested in the Philippines, in common with other measures designed to safeguard the health of the native population. Lepers had been segregated and cared for through the humanitarian efforts of Franciscan monks for over three hundred years in Manila, but little progress had been made either in their care or in the understanding of the age-old disease from which they suffered not only in this locality but in the world in general. The Philippine Health Service in 1906 began to exercise greater and more intelligent care in the segregation and treatment of lepers, particularly through the establishment at Culion of a modern colony for them.

In 1922 Dr. H. W. Wade, who had long been active in the study of leprosy in connection with the Philippine Health Service, was sent as pathologist to Culion. No less important in the forward movement which has already begun to bear the fruit of progress in the study of this ancient disease was the fact that Dr. Wade's wife, Dorothy Paul Wade, was with him in this station on the fringe of the world. It became evident to both these inspired and devoted helpers of humanity that their countrymen should be informed of the little that was actually being done for these unfortunate victims of one of the oldest maladies in the world and how their fate might be bettered and their numbers decreased. With the active support and authorization of General Wood, Mrs. Wade came to the United States in 1925. Through the influence of General Wood's personal friends and admirers, and by her vivid and tireless presentation of this great humanitarian project throughout the length and breadth of the country, two million dollars was pledged from over fifty thousand subscribers. Additional sums are needed and continue to be offered even in these difficult times.

The men who volunteered their services as an Executive Committee of the Leonard Wood Memorial as it was then formed, the personnel of which has changed but little since that time, did much to inspire confidence in the public that the money subscribed would be wisely used. Their names include: Hon. Robert L. Bacon, Mr. Perry Burgess, Mr. Eversley Child, Hon. Dwight F. Davis, Mr. Robert W. DeForest, Dr. John H. Finley, General James G. Harbord, Hon. Charles Evans Hughes, General Samuel McRoberts, Mr. Arthur Page, Mr. Kermit Roosevelt, Hon. Henry L. Stimson, Mrs. Dorothy Paul Wade, and Mr. Owen D. Young.

It was decided from the very beginning that the money so generously given should not be spent simply in the care of lepers, which is the business of local public health agencies, but more particularly in searching for the causes of the disease, the means of its prevention and finally its more certain cure. In spite of the fact that leprosy has been differentially recognized since biblical times, far too little is known of any of its fundamental aspects. The horror which the unhappy plight of the victim naturally arouses has been confused with the possible danger of contagion. Although the disease is directly or indirectly dependent on contact, the precise mode of its transfer is by no means known.

It seemed, first of all, that additional material facilities in the way of buildings were necessary in order that a more careful study of the disease could be made in the Philippines where it is so prevalent and whence this great investigative project took its origin. For this purpose something like $400,000 was expended in the construction of an entirely new leprosarium in Cebu, pronounced by many leprologists the finest in the world, and at Culion in extensive construction in preparation for the memorial's research program. These buildings, which comprise new laboratories, research wards, housing facilities for the nurses and scientific personnel and a cabin cruiser to facilitate transportation, have been completed and handed over to the Philippine Government.

It soon became evident that a medical board was essential in any development of this sort. For that purpose recognized medical authorities, not only in this specific disease, but in general problems of health and disease prevention, have volunteered their services and include at the present time the following individuals: Dr. William H. Welch, *chairman,* Surgeon General H. S. Cumming, Dr. Victor G. Heiser, Professor W. G. MacCallum, Dr. Earl B. McKinley, Dr. Theobald Smith, and Dr. H. W. Wade. This board continues to advise on the general problems of expenditure of the funds which, in addition to the buildings already mentioned, have taken the form of the development of working possibilities in research in the Philippines and certain attempts at an arrival of an international understanding as to what the problem of leprosy means throughout the world.

Thus the memorial has rendered possible the calling of the first international conference on leprosy which took place in Manila in 1931, and an international *Journal of Leprosy* is about to be published by the International Leprosy Association with the financial aid of the Leonard Wood Memorial. Dr. Wade has been made medical director of the research aspects of the study in Culion and sent on a world tour of leprosaria in 1931–32. A recognized Philippine authority in the disease, Dr. José Rodriquez, was sent for special study in epidemiology to the Johns Hopkins University and has now returned to the Philippines.

The ultimate objective of the fund must be a direct attack through intensive investigation of the disease itself and perhaps in several centers where it exists. It was obvious from the first that highly trained experts must be chosen for this work and the choice of these experts and of the problems that they might propose to investigate in connection with leprosy were so important that it was judged necessary in 1932 to ask the cooperation of an advisory committee on research, consisting of the following members: Dr. Frederick P. Gay, *chairman,* Dr. J. A. Doull, Dr. Ernest W. Goodpasture, Dr. Esmond R. Long, Dr. Earl B. McKinley, Dr. Thomas M. Rivers, Dr. Malcolm H. Soule, and Dr. Hans Zinsser.

Before proceeding to the recommendation of problems and personnel, this advisory committee on research felt it essential to be placed in touch with the situation throughout the world, since most of them were chosen not in virtue of a direct and recent participation in the leprosy problem itself but rather through their broader contacts with research in the innumerable problems of epidemiology, pathology, bacteriology and immunology. For this purpose it is planned to send members of this group, as their time permits, either to the more thoroughly established stations in the Philippines or elsewhere for the first-hand investigation of specific problems, the detailed carrying out of which they may wish to recommend to the memorial for determined and prolonged study. During the current year Dr. Doull, Dr. Soule and Dr. Gay are to visit the two stations in the Philippines for the purpose of this survey and for actual work for a limited time in the problems of leprosy as they perceive them. Additional tours of inspection are not as yet provided for, but it may safely be foretold that the personal knowledge acquired and the international interest inspired by the contact which this group of scientists sets up will do much to pave the way for the eventual solution of this great problem.

F. P. G.

# SOCIETIES AND MEETINGS

## THE IOWA ACADEMY OF SCIENCE

THE forty-seventh annual meeting of the Iowa Academy of Science was held with Coe College at Cedar Rapids on April 21 and 22, with 268 members and visitors in registered attendance.

The presidential address, "Some Biological Contributions to Recreation," was presented by Professor H. E. Jaques, of Iowa Wesleyan College. Other papers of general interest were: "The Occurrence of Mottled Teeth in Iowa," by Carl T. Ostrem, D. A. Greenwood, H. A. Wilhelm and V. E. Nelson, of Iowa State College; "Suggestion as to Structure in Ionic Solutions," by G. W. Stewart, of the State University of Iowa, and "Note on the Purchase Price of a Bond," by John F. Reilly, of the State University of Iowa. The annual academy lecture was presented by Professor H. J. Gilkey, of Iowa State College, on "Building the Hoover Dam."

The following officers and section chairmen were elected for the forthcoming year: *President,* E. J. Cable, Iowa State Teachers College; *Vice-president,* Edward Bartow, State University of Iowa; *Secretary-Treasurer* and *American Association for the Advancement of Science Representative,* J. C. Gilman, Iowa State College; *Editor,* Mrs. F. W. Nichols, Ames; *bacteriology* and *botany,* W. F. Loehwing, State University of Iowa; *chemistry, general* and *physical,* R. W. Getchell, Iowa State Teachers College; *chemistry, organic* and *biological,* V. E. Nelson, Iowa State College; *geology,* D. B. Gould, Cornell College; *mathematics,* J. F. Reilly, State University of Iowa; *physics,* E. P. T. Tyndall, State University of Iowa; *psychology,* Thomas McConnell, Cornell College; *zoology,* J. H. Bodine, State University of Iowa.

The academy convened in eight sections for the presentation of 152 papers of special interest. The retiring section chairmen made the following reports of their respective meetings:

*Bacteriology and Botany:* C. H. Werkman, *chairman.* The bacteriology and botany section presented a program of thirty-one papers and conducted a symposium on teaching under the chairmanship of Dean C. E. Friley, of Iowa State College. All meetings were well attended and the quality of the papers was high.

*Chemistry:* Leo P. Sherman, *chairman.* Papers were presented before the organic and biological section by Henry Gilman and students, V. E. Nelson, and H. L. Keil, G. H. Coleman and others, J. B. Culbertson, L. Chas. Raiford, L. C. Bauguess and C. P. Berg, N. A. Clark, H. S. Olcott, H. Gregg Smith[1] and W. H. Seegers, on such widely diverse topics as: "The Progressive and Step-wise Decarboxylation of Furantetracarboxylic Acid" (Gilman); "The Effect of Substituents in the Formation of Thio-carbanilides by Various Methods" (Raiford); "The Rôle of Liver in Growth, Reproduction and Lactation" (Smith and Seegers); and "The Determination of Manganese in Biological Material" (Clark). The meeting was well attended and close attention was given to all the thirteen interesting papers. A joint dinner for all the chemists was ably presided over by Dr. Ben Peterson, of Coe College, who called upon Drs. Culbertson, of Cornell College, and F. E. Brown, of Iowa State College, for short addresses.

*Geology:* John E. Smith, *chairman.* The meeting of the geology section was instructive and well attended. Among the papers on stratigraphic geology were: "Section at Ft. Dodge Limestone Company's Mine"; "Stratigraphy of the Hopkinton Formation in Jones, Jackson and Clinton Counties"; "Iowa Stratigraphy on Methodical Scheme"; "The Kansas City Formation in the Pammel Park Area"; "Some Buried Pictured Rocks"; "The Structure of the Des Moines Series at Redfield, Iowa." On glacial geology were presented papers on "Contrasted Till Relief" and "Pleistocene Geology of Central Iowa." Papers related to geology were: "Possible Migration in the Very Dawning Period of Pueblo Culture" and "The Carbon Dioxide Cycle in Nature." An excellent paper on "The Status of the Devonian Beds at Middle Amana" was also presented.

*Mathematics:* L. M. Coffin, *chairman.* In addition to a number of papers on the history and teaching of mathematics, papers were presented on number theory, potential theory, geometry, differential equations, statistics, probability theory, mathematics of finance and mechanics. The joint dinner was addressed by Professors Smith, Rietz, Rusk and McGaw.

*Physics:* H. J. Plagge, *chairman.* The physics section of the Iowa Academy of Science met at Coe College, Cedar Rapids, Iowa, on April 21 and 22. All sessions were unusually well attended, and twenty-five papers, covering recent developments and investigations, were presented. At the annual dinner, held at the Roosevelt Hotel, Friday evening, Dr. G. W. Stewart spoke on the subject "Physics 'round the World," basing his lecture on his recent tour around the globe.

*Psychology:* Leigh C. Douglass, *chairman.* A total of twenty-eight papers, covering a wide range of subjects, was presented in the psychology section. These papers, when classified, are as follows: abnormal, 3; art, 2; child, 3; education, 8; emotions, 2; music and speech, 5; physiological, 5. One of these papers, by Professor C. A. Ruckmick, of the State University of Iowa, on "What We Don't Know about Emotions," in which he summarized the research work that has been done in this field and charted the fields to be explored, was presented at the dinner meeting.

*Zoology:* Elery R. Becker, *chairman.* There were fifteen papers presented in the zoology section. Of these, three were concerned with the physiology of sex, two were purely physiological, four were anatomical in nature, two dealt with the parasitic protozoa, one presented the life history of the firebrat, two may be classified as ecologic, and one was of a systematic nature. One noticeable feature of the program was that most of the papers were given by the younger workers.

JOSEPH C. GILMAN,
*Secretary*

## THE KANSAS ACADEMY OF SCIENCE

THE sixty-fifth annual meeting of the Kansas Academy of Science was held at the Kansas State College, Manhattan, from April 13 to 15. The program consisted of approximately 160 papers given in general sessions on Friday and Saturday forenoons, April 14 and 15, and in the sectional meetings. Sectional programs in biology, chemistry, physics, psychology and junior academy were held on Friday afternoon. The entomology sectional program was held on Saturday afternoon under the auspices of the Kansas Entomological Society. A total attendance of 293 was recorded at the programs.

Dr. Philip Fox, director of the Adler Planetarium, Chicago, delivered the main address on April 14, at 8:15 P. M., under the auspices of the Science Club and Sigma Xi at Kansas State College. His subject was "The Architecture of the Heavens." At the annual banquet earlier in the evening the retiring president of the academy, Dr. Robert Taft, of the University of Kansas, delivered the presidential address on "Old Photographs, a Brief Review of the History of American Photography in the Period 1840–1880." Dr. Paul B. Lawson, of the University of Kansas, opened the annual meeting by a lecture on spiders in the evening of April 13.

The officers elected for 1933–34 were: *President,* J. W. Hershey, McPherson College, McPherson; *First Vice-president,* W. H. Matthews, Kansas State Teachers College, Pittsburg; *Second Vice-president,* E. A. Marten, University of Wichita, Wichita; *Secretary,* G. E. Johnson, Kansas State College, Manhattan; *Treasurer,* H. A. Zinszer, Fort Hays Kansas State College, Hays. The chairmen of sections are: *Biology,* H. E. Crowe, Friends University, Wichita,

[1] Deceased.

and (vice-chairman) Elsa Horn, Kansas State College, Manhattan; *chemistry,* W. W. Floyd, Ottawa University, Ottawa; *physics,* G. W. Maxwell, Kansas State College, Manhattan; *psychology,* J. B. Stroud, Kansas State Teachers College, Emporia; *entomology,* P. A. Readio, University of Kansas, Lawrence; *Junior Academy,* Hazel E. Branch, University of Wichita, Wichita. Additional *members of the executive council* are: Robert Taft, University of Kansas, Lawrence; F. U. G. Agrelius, Kansas State Teachers College, Emporia; L. Oncley, Southwestern College, Winfield. Dr. F. C. Gates, of the Kansas State College, Manhattan, was reappointed editor.

State aid to the extent of $300 a year was reported by the chairman of the state aid committee, Dr. W. J. Baumgartner, of the University of Kansas at Lawrence. The 1934 meeting will be held in Wichita.

GEORGE E. JOHNSON,
*Secretary*

### THE TEXAS ACADEMY OF SCIENCE

THE summer meeting of the Texas Academy of Science was held at College Station, where it was the guest of the Agricultural and Mechanical College. At the banquet on May 19, a class of thirty-three new members, all from the faculty of the college, was introduced to the membership. Following the banquet Dr. Mark Francis, widely known for his work on Texas tick fever and for his interest in the paleontology of the Gulf Coast, delivered an illustrated lecture relative to his findings in Texas. At the conclusion Dr. E. N. Jones, president of the academy, presented Dr. Francis with a certificate of life fellowship. Saturday was given over to three field trips. The botanical section under Dr. R. G. Reeves, of A. and M. College, visited locations where the local flora was best represented. The geological section, headed by Dr. H. B. Stenzel, of A. and M. College, and Professor and Mrs. F. B. Plummer, of the University of Texas, visited some newly discovered fossil deposits near the college. The third section represented a combination of interests and made a tour through the eastern part of the state, visiting various points of biological and historical interest. At the meeting of the executive committee arrangements were made for the annual meeting to be held at Dallas on October 20 and 21, and the invitation of Dr. Edwin F. Carpenter, secretary-treasurer of the Southwestern Division of the American Association for the Advancement of Science, for a joint meeting in May, 1934, was referred to the regular session of the executive committee for consideration.

H. B. PARKS,
*Secretary-Treasurer*

## SCIENTIFIC APPARATUS AND LABORATORY METHODS

### A SIMPLE AQUARIUM AERATOR

IN the course of the school year it is frequently desirable to maintain aquaria, both of fresh and salt water, for intervals of a week or two. In order to accomplish this some system of aeration is usually necessary, but in many cases one feels that the purchase of an electric pump is hardly justified. Several fairly simple and efficient aerating devices have been described (Schaeffer,[1] Walker,[2] etc.), but they require that running water be available and limit the location of aquaria to within a few feet of a sink. The writer has been using, quite successfully, a very simple aerator, which can be constructed in a few minutes from materials available in most laboratories, requires no electricity or running water to maintain it, needs only a few minutes' attention a day, can not misbehave in such a way as to injure the contents of the aquarium or flood it with tap water, and allows the aquarium to be placed almost anywhere in the room.

Two lengths of glass tubing, one of one eighth inch diameter, the other a size larger; a Y tube preferably the size of the smaller glass tube; some rubber tubing for connections; and a screw tubing clamp are needed. The larger tube is bent in the form of a "constant level" siphon, as shown in the diagram, the inlet end

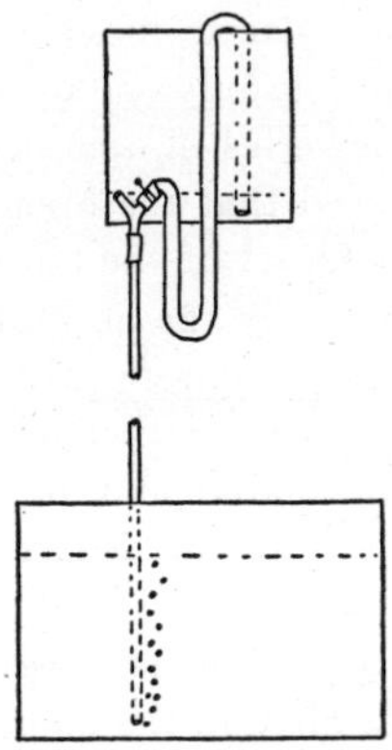

being bent slightly to one side so that water can enter freely, even when this end rests on the bottom of a container. The Y, preferably a glass one, especially if sea water is to be used, is connected to the outlet end of the siphon by just enough rubber tubing so that the screw clamp can be fitted on between the end of the siphon and the Y. The open end of the Y should stand a little above the intake end of the

[1] A. A. Schaeffer, SCIENCE, 31: 955, 1910.
[2] J. H. Walker, SCIENCE, 73: 709, 1931.

siphon, and as near the level of the top of the outlet bend as possible. The siphon will then need no starting after it has once been put in operation. The second glass tube—the smaller one—is then closely connected to the stem of the Y. This tube should be at least eighteen inches long, for best results. Its length determines the depth to which air can be carried below the surface of the water in the aquarium below, and this drop tube should reach almost to the bottom of the aquarium, so that the bubbled air may come in close contact with as much of the water as possible. A vessel of some kind—a battery jar serves well—is now stood on some convenient support above the aquarium and is filled with water from the aquarium. The apparatus can be started easily by slipping a piece of rubber tubing about two feet long over the open end of the Y and sucking on it. As soon as the water starts to flow through the siphon, this tubing is removed and the screw clamp tightened until water no longer drips from the open end of the Y, but instead a series of air bubbles is sucked in. Once started, the only attention required is an occasional replenishing of the water supply from the aquarium below. Care must be taken, of course, that no debris which might clog the Y is transferred. With this piece of apparatus an aquarium can be kept near a window where the aeration will be supplemented by the photosynthetic activity of the plants, and by manipulation of the window a reasonably low temperature can be maintained. Under such conditions, if the aquarium is not overstocked, filling the reservoir two or three times a day will suffice to keep the water sufficiently aerated.

If desired, several aquaria can be placed in tiers, and an aerator be placed in each, leading to the aquarium below, so that only one upper reservoir need be filled to keep the series in operation. In that case care must be observed that the open end of the Y is at the normal water level of the aquarium. Any surplus water brought in by the aerator above will then serve to operate the aerator for the aquarium below.

This device has proved particularly useful when the tap water was chlorinated and it was necessary to bring pond water into the classroom. Also with marine material, when the amount of sea water available was limited, it has still been found possible to keep the animals alive in the laboratory for several weeks.

ERNEST C. DRIVER

SMITH COLLEGE

## A NEW STOP-COCK CLAMP

SOMETIMES it is necessary that glass valves be made relatively more leak-proof than the binder in the valve lubricant can assure. This is especially true if valves in a system are subject to pressure over considerable periods of time. To overcome such difficulties in leakage, a spring clamp was devised and is herewith described.

A stiff collar is cut from sheet copper (.5–.7 mm thick) in a form similar to the drawing. It is then cut half across and opened to admit the neck of the glass plug. The ends of the collar are then turned down but so that they still clear the seat portion of the valve.

If the closed spring coil, which is used, can not be purchased, it may be made by winding No. 2 music wire[1] on a stiff iron wire or small rod held in the chuck of a breast drill—the latter clamped in a vise. After a 2–3 cm length of coil has been wound, it should be set by heat (in a flame) before removal from the small rod on which it is wound.

The spring tension on the collar varies, depending on the size of the cock and its use. However, as a

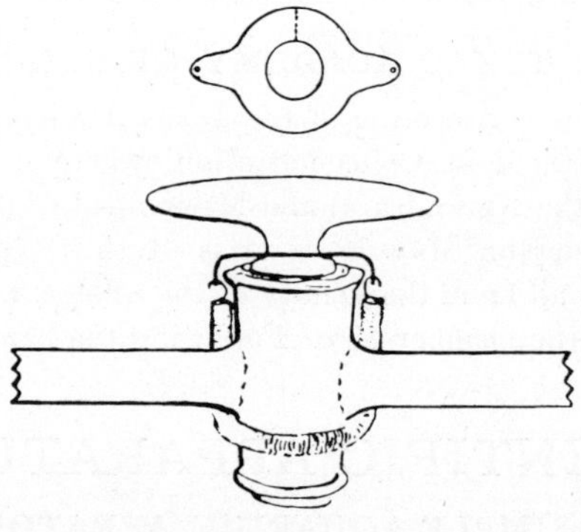

criterion for the usual size cock, an adjustment to give a pull of 100–200 g is found to be satisfactory. A moderate tension on the plug will not force the lubricant out appreciably and cause freezing of the valve if a good lubricant, as "Lubriseal," is used. The clamp may be plated if subject to corrosive vapors.

One notes that the collar of the clamp rests upon the shoulder of the glass plug but still permits its perfect freedom of movement; and that the plug may be removed and cleaned readily by extending the spring over the end of the plug seat.

This clamp has found satisfactory application on stop-cocks of manometers, vacuum pump distributors, gas analyzing burettes and other apparatus. Two stop-cocks at the base of one of the gas-analyzing machines—a multiple bulb side-arm type burette—supporting a meter column of mercury, were found to remain functional and leak-proof for weeks without cleaning.

ALDEN F. ROE

THE GEORGE WASHINGTON UNIVERSITY
SCHOOL OF MEDICINE

[1] Obtained from large hardware stores.

# SPECIAL ARTICLES

## THE ACTION OF THE PARENTERAL ADMINISTRATION OF SUGARS ON THE HYDROGEN-ION CONCENTRATION OF NORMAL AND MALIGNANT TISSUES IN LIVING ANIMALS[1]

THE principal factors—biochemical and physiological—which control the acid-base equilibrium of the blood of animals are well known. Very little is known, however, concerning the regulation of the acid-base balance in the tissues. Even in the case of the voluntary muscle, which has been subjected to intensive investigation during the last twenty years, it has so far been impossible to gain an adequate picture of the factors which may control the hydrogen-ion concentration of muscle tissue in living animals. Data obtained on isolated tissue have only limited value, inasmuch as the conditions prevailing in the body can not be duplicated accurately. Attempts to apply the customary colorimetric and electrometric methods to extracts or macerations of tissues have yielded figures differing by as much as one pH unit for one and the same tissue. This is due to serious technical errors, such as acid production during the preparation of the material, loss of $CO_2$, interference of oxidation-reduction systems in electrometric estimations by means of metal electrodes, etc. More satisfactory results were obtained by Rous, who applied pH indicators to exposed tissues of living animals and, by noting the color change, obtained an approximate estimate of the hydrogen-ion concentration.

About a year ago we described a technique for the continuous measurement of the pH of the tissues in living animals, which makes use of a specially constructed capillary glass electrode in conjunction with a quadrant electrometer and potentiometer.[2] Further improvements in this method have been made since. A great advantage of the glass electrode over other electrodes is that it permits pH measurements in the presence of the oxidation-reduction systems which occur in all tissues. However, there is one objection to the method in that the electrode makes contact not with a single morphological tissue unit, but with the different cells comprising the tissue as well as tissue lymph. Direct contact with blood can be avoided by careful insertion of the electrode into the tissue.

Recognizing this limitation we believe from our extensive experience that the method is of real value in the study of various problems. We have applied it to the study of the nature of cancerous growth. The work is based on the fact that certain tissues are known to ferment glucose with the formation of lactic acid. As a normal tissue we chose the voluntary muscle of rats, because of the ease with which it produces acid upon slight injury, a fact which from a technical standpoint furnished a severe test of the reliability of the method. On the other hand it was shown by Warburg and coworkers by experiments *in vitro* that lactic acid production is especially pronounced in malignant tissues, even in the presence of oxygen. Furthermore, Cori and Warburg have found that venous blood coming from a malignant tumor has a lower glucose and a higher lactic acid content than normal venous blood. The same investigators have also shown that the lactic acid formation in tumor tissue *in vitro* and *in vivo* can be increased by increasing the glucose supply.

We were therefore interested to ascertain whether it is possible to force the lactic acid production in voluntary muscle or malignant tissue by means of injection of glucose to such a degree as to cause an increase in the hydrogen-ion concentration. Having found that this was easily possible with malignant tumors, we decided to study also the action of other natural sugars obtained in pure form through the kindness of Dr. C. S. Hudson and his collaborators. The sugars were injected mostly intraperitoneally but sometimes subcutaneously as a 20 per cent. solution in doses of 600 mg per 100 g body weight. The animals—rats and mice—were deprived of food for 24 hours before the beginning of the experiments. They received pentobarbital in doses to produce a light anesthesia. The following tissues were studied: voluntary muscle of rats, Jensen rat sarcoma, Flexner-Jobling rat carcinoma, Walker rat sarcoma 325 and the spontaneous mammary mouse carcinoma of the New York State Institute for Malignant Disease.

In order to ascertain whether the observed increase in hydrogen-ion concentration is accompanied by increased lactic acid retention, Dr. J. M. Johnson, after the last pH measurement, analyzed the tissues for lactic acid by the method of Friedemann, Cotonio and Shaffer. The results indicate that there was always more acid present when the tissue had shown an acid drift as measured electrometrically. This means that there is an increased acid production throughout the tissue and not just locally at the electrode. In view of the relatively high dissociation constant of lactic acid it is not surprising that the tissue buffers are unable to prevent an increase in the acidity of the tissue. Whether or not other organic acids besides lactic are concerned in the production of the observed acid drift can not be decided on the basis of the present evidence.

[1] Read before the National Academy of Sciences, April 24, 1933.

[2] Carl Voegtlin and Herbert Kahler: SCIENCE, 75: 362, 1932.

We conclude, first, that the new method yields reliable data; second, that the buffer action of the tissues studied, particularly the malignant tumors, can be overcome by injection of relatively large doses of certain natural sugars and that the acid-base equilibrium is therefore a function of carbohydrate metabolism.

As to the possible significance of these results, it may be pointed out that the pH controls many important biochemical reactions, such as the action of proteolytic, glycolytic and other enzymes; oxidation-reduction; the state of tissue colloids, etc. The work of Jacobs and others, furthermore, suggests that lactic acid, being an organic acid, may have a peculiar action owing to its ease of penetration into cells. We have found that there is an acidity gradient: tumor-surrounding tissue-normal tissue. We therefore may well ask the question whether the excessive local production and accumulation of lactic acid represents an important factor in the destructive action of malignant tumors upon the surrounding normal tissue and upon the tumor cells themselves. Work along this line is under way.

CARL VOEGTLIN
H. KAHLER
R. H. FITCH
U. S. PUBLIC HEALTH SERVICE

## SOLAR VARIATIONS AND ATMOSPHERIC PRESSURE[1]

THE Smithsonian Institution has been measuring for 20 years, or more, the amount of solar radiation reaching the earth and computing from the observed data the value outside the atmosphere. These values prove to be variable, and it was deemed worth while to compare these variations with variations of atmospheric pressure on the earth in order to ascertain what relationships, if any, might be disclosed. For this purpose the formulas of correlation were used such as is now the custom to use in the comparison of variables.

The Smithsonian Astrophysical Observatory recently published a table giving the monthly means of the preferred solar values from three widely separated observatories for the interval 1921–1930. The monthly means for the 120 months included were compared with the monthly means of pressure for the same interval at 162 stations scattered over the earth's surface. These data were obtained from the various weather services of the world for publication in "World Weather Records" and were supplemented by means derived from daily charts of pressure for the North Pacific and North Atlantic Oceans.

[1] Read before the National Academy of Sciences, Washington, D. C., April, 1933.

The computed correlations disclosed the following relationships:

(1) With an increase of solar radiation the pressure increases in regions of the earth where the pressure is normally high and decreases in regions where it is normally low. In other words, the normal pressure gradients are increased and the normal circulation speeded up. It has been shown by previous investigations that with high solar radiation the low pressure band at the equator widens and the high pressure belts and centers in middle latitudes move nearer the pole, this displacement being proportional to the intensity of the solar radiation increase.

(2) The centers of greatest minus correlation are in regions of high vapor content and plus correlations in regions of low vapor content, indicating that the absorption of solar heat by water vapor plays an important part in determining the effect of increased solar radiation on the atmosphere.

(3) The centers of greatest minus and plus correlations change positions with the seasons, following the change in position of the areas of high and low water vapor; thus further proving the intimate relation between these conditions.

(4) In the regions of greatest minus correlation of pressure with increased solar radiation, the temperature and rainfall show plus correlations at least for solar radiation changes of short period.

(5) The computed amount of change of pressure and of temperature agree with expectancy.

(6) In considering the effect of solar radiation changes on the atmosphere there are evidently three factors to be considered, namely, intensity of the solar change, the seasonal changes in the atmosphere and progressive movements similar to atmospheric waves. It is possible also that temporary shifts in ocean currents and changes in water temperatures influence the results.

H. H. CLAYTON

## BOOKS RECEIVED

ADAMS, LEVERETT A. *An Introduction to the Vertebrates.* Pp. v + 414. 290 figures. Wiley. $3.50.

BARNES, ERNEST W. *Scientific Theory and Religion.* Pp. xxiv + 685. Macmillan. $4.00.

DILLAVOU, E. R. *Business and Law.* Pp. xv + 494. McGraw-Hill. $1.40.

FOLEY, ARTHUR L. *College Physics.* Pp. viii + 759. 453 figures. Blakiston. $3.75.

ROMER, ALFRED S. *Vertebrate Paleontology.* Pp. vii + 491. University of Chicago Press. $5.00.

SCHAUINSLAND, HUGO H. *The Great Enigma.* Pp. 93. Dutton. $1.25.

WASHBURNE, CARLETON and HELUIZ WASHBURNE. *The Story of Earth and Sky.* Pp. x + 368. Illustrated. Century. $3.50.

WHEELER, WILLIAM M. and THOMAS BARBOUR. *The Lamarck Manuscripts at Harvard.* Pp. xxi + 202. Harvard University Press. $2.50.

# SCIENCE

VOL. 77 FRIDAY, JUNE 16, 1933 No. 2007

*The Rôle of Analysis in Scientific Investigation:* PROFESSOR DOUGLAS JOHNSON ... 569

*Scientific Events:*
*Unification of Radio Research Facilities in Great Britain; The Annual Meeting of the Royal Institution; National Research Fellowships in the Biological Sciences; Summer Conference in Spectroscopy; Psychology at Chicago* ... 576

*Scientific Notes and News* ... 579

*Discussion:*
*The Problem of Twisted Trees:* DR. MAURICE COPISAROW. *Chlorpicrin Injurious to Greenhouse Plants:* DR. G. H. GODFREY. *The Anniversary of the Normal Curve:* CHARLES J. MARSH. *Questions:* DR. FREDERICK S. HAMMETT ... 581

*Reports:*
*Public Service as an Element in the Life of the American Scientist:* PROFESSOR YANDELL HENDERSON ... 584

*Scientific Apparatus and Laboratory Methods:*
*A Low-cost Laboratory Unit for Lighting and Appliances:* DR. SAMUEL E. POND and OTTO MEIER, JR. *A Simple Sub-surface Thermometer:* PROFESSOR G. F. SLEGGS. *A Specimen Mount for Insects and Other Objects of Natural History:* PROFESSOR HERBERT OSBORN ... 585

*Special Articles:*
*The Absolute Motion of the Solar System and the Orbital Motion of the Earth Determined by the Ether-drift Experiment:* PROFESSOR DAYTON C. MILLER. *The Phosphorescence of Solid Nitrogen and its Relation to Crystal Structure:* L. VEGARD. *Coupled Reactions in Biological Systems:* HERMANN F. SCHOTT and HENRY BORSOOK. *Some Aspects of Intermediary Protein Metabolism:* DR. ERWIN BRAND and DR. MEYER M. HARRIS ... 587

*Science News* ... 6

SCIENCE: A Weekly Journal devoted to the Advancement of Science, edited by J. MCKEEN CATTELL and published every Friday by

THE SCIENCE PRESS

New York City: Grand Central Terminal

Lancaster, Pa. Garrison, N. Y.

Annual Subscription, $6.00 Single Copies, 15 Cts.

SCIENCE is the official organ of the American Association for the Advancement of Science. Information regarding membership in the Association may be secured from the office of the permanent secretary, in the Smithsonian Institution Building, Washington, D. C.

# THE RÔLE OF ANALYSIS IN SCIENTIFIC INVESTIGATION[1]

By Professor DOUGLAS JOHNSON

COLUMBIA UNIVERSITY

CUSTOM decrees that the chairman of your section should, at the interval of a year following his presidency, deliver before you an appropriate address. It has seemed to me that I could best command your interest in some field of discussion where every one of us, geographer and geologist alike, has had experience. So I have selected the broad field connoted by the highly inclusive term, "scientific investigation"; and I would direct your attention, not to any particular results of such investigation, but to a concrete problem of method which I suppose must concern every scientific worker. This problem can briefly be stated as follows: What is the precise rôle of analysis in a properly conceived and successfully executed scientific investigation?

It goes without saying that I am not competent to speak of methods of research in chemistry and physics, where experiment plays a far larger rôle than in geology and geography. So also the biologist, the astronomer and investigators in other fields must speak for themselves. For this reason the title of my address may seem unduly ambitious. Yet I prefer the broader, more inclusive term "scientific investigation" to the more restricted if more accurate "geologic and geographic investigation," because it seems to me probable that some of the principles here discussed may find application beyond the limits of my particular field.

It is a pleasure to express here my indebtedness to several of my Columbia colleagues, Robert S. Woodworth, professor of psychology; Adam Leroy Jones, associate professor of philosophy; Sam F. Trelease,

[1] Abbreviated form of address as retiring vice-president and chairman of Section E—American Association for the Advancement of Science, delivered at Atlantic City, on December 27, 1932. The address will be published in amplified form, with fuller illustration from shore line studies, in the *Bulletin of the Geological Society of America.*

professor of botany; and George B. Pegram, professor of physics; also to Professor William Morris Davis. All these were good enough to read the address in manuscript form and give me the benefit of helpful criticisms.

The dictionaries tell us that analysis is the process of separating a thing or a concept into its constituent parts, in order to arrive at the essential or ultimate elements, causes or principles; that it is the tracing of things back to their sources; and that it is designed to clarify and test knowledge. The chemist analyzes a complex substance to determine its precise composition. For the purposes of our discussion I would define scientific analysis as "the process of separating observations, arguments and conclusions into their constituent parts, tracing each part back to its source and testing its validity, for the purpose of clarifying and perfecting knowledge."

I am persuaded we can pursue our discussion most easily if I illustrate my observations, so far as feasible, by reference to some concrete example. For sake of simplicity I shall select a common phenomenon found on the rocky shores of many lands, and in tracing the part played by analysis at each stage of a comprehensive scientific investigation, shall illustrate my points freely by referring to the study of this phenomenon, the origin of which is still a subject of dispute. Those who follow this discussion should not attach undue importance to the particular example selected for illustrative purposes, nor to the statements made concerning it. I have purposely selected a debatable matter, the study of which is not yet completed. Our concern here is not with the origin of the phenomenon, but with the method of investigating its origin.

Along the rocky shores bordering the sea are found nearly horizontal platforms or benches from a few feet to a few hundred feet in width, cut in solid rock. At their seaward margins these benches terminate in relatively abrupt slopes which descend toward or even into the water. From their inner or landward margins rise steep slopes or rocky cliffs. In elevation the benches range from 1 or 2 feet above ordinary high tide indefinitely upward, often several hundred feet above the same datum plane.

The combination of bench and cliff bordering the sea might arouse no significant reaction in the mind of the ordinary observer. But such a combination instantly excites the brain of the geomorphologist to activity. Memory recalls text book diagrams, explanatory titles under photographs of similar features, discussions of the origin of such features in geological and geographical treatises, perhaps earlier field examination of such forms. Rapidly the mind compares the forms, the situations, the mutual relations of the assembled features in the various cases called before it by observation and memory, and before the observer is conscious of the process he has leaped to an inductive inference: that both bench and cliff were cut into the margins of the land by wave erosion. In this case the inductive inference involves an explanation. But it is only a partial explanation. If the bench is wave-carved, why is it exposed to view above the level of the sea? The mind rushes on: Perhaps the land has been raised since the bench was carved. Perhaps the sea level has dropped.

The observer must now be on his guard against a dangerous tendency of the human intellect—the tendency to accept as valid a plausible explanation, and then to look for facts in support of that explanation. He must deliberately repress the tendency toward premature conclusions, and begin the task of gathering all the facts upon which alone can a satisfactory explanation be based. As already stated, we are not primarily concerned with the course of his particular investigation of these interesting forms, nor with the conclusions he may reach respecting their origin. But we shall draw freely upon this imaginary hypothetical study, to illustrate the uses of analysis in scientific research.

## I. Analysis in the Stage of Observation

The initial stage in scientific investigation is normally that of observation. The first employment of this mental process may be made incidentally, perhaps almost passively. But once the investigator realizes that the observed facts present a problem, for the solution of which additional facts are desirable, he becomes an active inquirer, seeking to discover all facts bearing on the problem. He observes as widely and as accurately as possible, the observed facts being automatically recorded in his memory; but also, since the memory is notoriously fallible, deliberately recorded in his note book if he be a prudent investigator.

Since we are here concerned merely with the recording of external facts observed by the eye, it might appear that analysis has no rôle to play in this initial stage of an investigation. But let us dissect the matter and scrutinize its parts, first turning our attention to the material facts which are the object of observation. Can the analytical powers of the mind be brought to bear upon the facts themselves in such manner as to aid the investigator?

Let our hypothetical student of coastal benches answer. Having observed one such bench, and had his curiosity aroused to investigate, he begins his search for other examples. Very soon he is confronted by the necessity of discriminating coastal benches of the type described above from other forms similar in some respects yet different in others. He needs a name by which to designate the type forming the particular object of inquiry, and tentatively calls them elevated marine benches or simply "marine benches," because of their resemblance to submarine benches formed by wave abrasion and because of their apparent marine origin.

The question then arises: What constitutes a marine bench in the sense in which he is using the term? Is it any nearly level surface in the vicinity of the shore, terminated seaward by an abrupt descent, and landward by cliffs which rise steeply to higher levels? This combination of slopes appears repeatedly in nature, as the product of a variety of causes. The non-critical investigator, who welcomes every shelf and scarp facing the sea as one more link in the chain of facts he seeks to explain, is almost sure to accumulate, without knowing it, an assortment of unrelated observations, many of them irrelevant to his problem. His investigation is seriously compromised from its very beginning. How can he explain the origin and history of elevated marine benches if he unwittingly bases his reasoning on a confused mixture of wave-carved surfaces, benches due to differential weathering, rock terraces cut by a river before drowning brought in the sea, notches cut by a glacial stream flowing between waning continental ice and the sloping hillside, and terraces due to landslides, faulting or monoclinal warping. As all these features are found in the immediate vicinity of the shore in different places, and as all of them have repeatedly been ascribed to wave erosion, it is clear that the field data must in the first instance be subjected to rigid scrutiny.

The facts can not be lumped. They must be separated into their constituent parts, and each part tested as to its relevancy to the problem under investigation.

Thus far we have discussed the necessity of analyzing the things observed. But the investigator must probe more deeply than that. He must analyze the observational process itself. Does he really see what he thinks he sees? Not unless he is constantly on guard against the well known dangers to which observation is subject. Chief among these, perhaps, is the tendency to include inference with fact, to confuse theory with observation. The observer thinks he sees a bench cut in granite, when in fact all he really observes is a few scattered outcrops of granite protruding through the soil; from these he infers, and perhaps erroneously, that the vastly larger invisible mass is likewise granite. Another investigator may report that he saw a wave-carved bench which did not bevel the rock layers. All he really saw was a shelf or bench parallel to the rock layers. He inferred it was wave-carved, when in fact it may have been produced by differential weathering of weaker beds overlying a more resistant layer.

Another danger to which observation is subject is that of ocular deception. This danger looms large when one is looking for certain specific forms in the landscape. The power of suggestion is greater than many realize, and one looking for marine benches is in danger of finding them in faint undulations or irregularities of the terrain which under other circumstances would not impress him as significant. If he is looking for benches which he expects to be horizontal, the inclined position of something he mistakes for such a bench may quite escape his eye, even when the inclination is so marked as to be quite obvious to another who is without preconceptions as to what should be observed.

Incompleteness of observation is another common danger. The eye tends to pick from the landscape that which seems to it for the moment significant, and fails to note much that later stages of the study may show to be vitally important. Even where the initial observation is fairly complete, the benefits which should be derived from it may be lost through failure to record permanently in memory and in note book all the facts observed.

No one is wholly free from the dangers of defective observation. But one who acquires the habit of analyzing his observational powers and processes is less exposed to these dangers than are those who give no conscious attention to this initial step of a scientific investigation. In research, as in other things, to be forewarned is to be forearmed; and the investigator who is conscious of the dangers inevitably associated with the observational process will be on his guard against those dangers.

## II. Analysis in the Stage of Classification

Is there any need for employing analysis in the second stage of an investigation, the stage of classification? Let us note first that the analysis involved in stage one led to a sort of rudimentary classification, the separation of observed facts into those which were relevant and those of doubtful relevancy. We at once suspect that analysis must likewise be involved in any further effective classification of the facts of observation surviving the analysis of stage one.

The investigator is not content merely to exclude from consideration every doubtful bit of data. For example, our hypothetical student does not rest when he has excluded from his study every topographic form which does not certainly belong in the group of elevated marine benches. He raises the question as to whether all these benches need necessarily have had the same history. For he takes cognizance of the fact that if the benches were carved at different times, and some of them were affected by events, such as continental uplift, which did not affect the others, a serious difficulty may be introduced into the attempt to explain their history. The investigation, to be successful, must deal with a group of facts which are comparable. A simple hypothesis competent to explain benches five feet above high tide may conceivably be quite incompetent to explain benches fifteen feet above high tide.

### III. Analysis in the Stage of Generalization

Classification paves the way to the third stage of investigation, in which generalization occurs. Thus in our hypothetical study of marine benches, it is only when classification has been effected that the investigator can make significant generalizations; such, for example, as that in one group the benches have a narrow range in altitude, are always close to the sea, present no evidence of weathering of the rock surfaces, and are free from debris; that in a second group the benches have higher altitudes but equally narrow range in altitude, present evidence of moderate weathering and have small quantities of debris near their inner margins; while in a third group the benches are still higher, vary extensively in altitude and have surfaces which are deeply weathered and prevailingly covered with debris.

We have now to inquire whether the analytical faculties of the investigator can serve any useful purpose in the stage of generalization. Let us first note that the empirical generalizations stated above, free from any explanatory element, had their roots in the careful analysis that made effective classification possible. But it is when inducing generalizations which involve more or less of explanation that the analytical process can render greatest service. Such generalizations, like those free from explanation, must be rooted in the facts and represent a normal outgrowth of them. They must be legitimate inferences induced from the facts themselves. As we shall see in a later section, the investigator may formulate conceptions involving explanation which are not an immediate normal outgrowth of the facts, but the products of invention. As these two types of explanation, the induced and the invented, have somewhat different standing before the court of the intellect, it is important that they be not confused. It is in making this discrimination that the investigator must again employ his analytical powers. The nature of the facts, the nature of their distribution, their relationships, and other pertinent elements must critically be examined, to the end that only legitimate inferences may be induced from them.

For example, the first two groups of classified facts described above, in both of which uniformity of altitude above sea level is a characteristic of the benches, may properly give rise to the generalization that after the benches were carved the sea level dropped. Uniformity of bench altitude suggests this as a legitimate inference involving explanation. But no such generalization may be based on the third group of facts, in which great variation in elevation is an outstanding characteristic of the benches. Such heterogeneity in elevation does not suggest either uniform drop of sea level or systematic differential uplift of the land. Perhaps the facts can be explained on the basis of one or the other of these explanations, or on both combined; but if so the explanations must be deliberately invented and applied to the facts. They are not normal outgrowths of the facts.

### IV. Analysis in the Stage of Invention

In the fourth stage of our hypothetical investigation the inquirer takes the classified facts and the generalizations concerning their nature, and uses them as a basis for invention of as many explanations of the facts as may be possible. It is here that "the scientific use of the imagination," as Tyndall has happily phrased it, comes most prominently into play. The invention may be deliberate, the result of conscious effort. Often it springs unexpectedly into consciousness, the result of a mind well equipped with pertinent knowledge repeatedly "mulling over" the facts in variable combinations. If others have anticipated our inquirer in the inventive process, as is usually true in greater or less measure, he welcomes every idea of alien origin which offers a possible explanation of the facts, and accords it just as hospitable treatment as those born of his own intellect. If the generalizations of stage three involved explanation of the facts, the investigator seeks additional and independent explanations. Where generalization involved but partial explanation, or merely paved the way for an explanation, the investigator employs his inventive powers to complete the unfinished task; and then moves forward to the invention of alternative explanations.

The process of invention is not fully understood. It resembles induction to the extent that the mind starts with concrete facts, and from them passes to conceptions of broad application which take the form of tentative explanations of the facts. But the mind has far greater liberty in the stage of invention than in the preceding stage of generalization. The relation to facts is here less close. A proper generalization, being an outgrowth of the facts, must have its roots well grounded in them. An invention may spring from "thin air," the rarefied atmosphere of more abstract reasoning. The stimulus to invention comes from the facts, and the thing invented must not palpably be contradicted by the facts; but it need not be a normal outgrowth of the facts. Thus, the conception of a uniform drop of sea level was, as we have seen, wholly improper as a generalization based on the third group of facts, relating to marine benches of widely varying altitude, since nothing in this group of facts could rightly give birth to such a conception. But the same conception may properly be invented, "out of thin air," and offered as a possible explanation of the facts in that group, since none of them necessarily contradicts the explanation.

We have noted the greater liberty enjoyed by the mind in the stage of invention. But it is not wholly free. Since the explanations induced in stage three and those invented in stage four are to serve as working hypotheses in the deductive operations of stage five, they must conform to certain fundamental requirements governing the formulation of hypotheses. In the first place, it is essential that the tentative explanations should be so precisely molded that specific deductions may be derived from them. If an explanation is so vague in its inherent nature, or so unskilfully molded in its formulation, that specific deductions subject to empirical verification or refutation can not be based upon it, then it can never serve as a working hypothesis. A hypothesis with which one can not work is not a working hypothesis.

Again, the explanation as formulated must be possible, for explanations clearly contradicted by well-established natural laws waste time and energy without advancing the investigator toward the true goal of his researches. On the other hand, it is manifestly dangerous to exclude explanations which merely appear incredible or absurd because they run counter to established opinions. Many a door to truth has thus prematurely been closed and long remained closed. The hypothesis of continental glaciation seemed incredible in 1840, as did the hypothesis of evolution in 1860.

How then shall the inventive mind properly mold its hypotheses and distinguish between explanations which appear plausible but are really unsound and those which immediately provoke distrust yet merit hospitable consideration? It seems to me that here the analytical process offers us an instrument of incalculable value. Let us dissect each tentative explanation into its component elements, trace each element back to the assumptions and inferences which lie hidden behind it and test the reasonableness of the whole by testing the validity of each part.

## V. Analysis in the Stage of Verification and Elimination

On entering the fifth stage of the investigation our hypothetical inquirer possesses, let us suppose, some half dozen tentative explanations which have survived the analytical processes applied in the preceding stage. He now treats each of these in turn as a working hypothesis, and reversing the mental processes employed in the third stage, endeavors by deductive reasoning to determine as precisely as possible just what features should characterize the shore platforms in case the particular hypothesis for the moment under scrutiny be the true explanation of these forms. His object is to verify, so far as possible, the competence of some hypotheses and to eliminate others which critical tests show to be manifestly incompetent.

He secures the required tests by an appeal to facts. After deducing the reasonable consequences of a working hypothesis, he confronts these by such facts as are already in his possession, drawing upon memory, upon his field notes and upon the published observations of others. If the consequences logically deduced from the hypothesis are in accord with the facts, he accepts this as verification of the competence of the hypothesis to explain the facts already in hand. Where deduced consequences find no counterpart in observed facts, he feels justified in eliminating the hypothesis from further consideration.

To what extent, if any, can analysis serve the investigator in this stage of verification and elimination? Since effective use of the deductive process depends upon one's ability to make logically correct deductions, it is expedient that the investigator should subject his own mental processes to careful scrutiny. There are fallacies in reasoning which must be avoided. These are treated in works on logic and need not be discussed here. But some study of logic will direct conscious attention to one's mental habits, and help to secure the precision and completeness requisite for careful deduction.

The investigator must realize that if his deductions are false, it matters little whether observed facts correspond to them or not. The conclusions are in any case invalidated, and he may either reject a perfectly valid hypothesis or embrace one which is invalid, on the basis of false reasoning. Saftey lies only in analysis. Deductions, like inductions, must be separated into their component parts, and each part scrutinized and its validity tested. Let us illustrate what this involves by turning once again to the problem of the shore platforms.

Let us suppose that our investigator has accepted as one working hypothesis the tentative explanation of storm-wave erosion under present conditions of land and sea level. From this hypothesis he deduces certain expectable consequences, among which let us consider only one. If the platforms are the product of storm waves operating at the present time, he reasons, then there should be found upon their surfaces rock debris constituting the cutting tools with which waves accomplish their erosive work. Turning to his record of field observations, he finds that many of the platforms are remarkably free from debris. Indeed, their outer edges commonly drop abruptly into moderately deep water, so that it is difficult to see how much debris could be cast upon the platforms or maintained there. The facts in hand conspicuously fail to match the expectations deduced from the hypothesis, so our investigator rejects the hypothesis of storm-wave erosion as incompetent. In doing so, he rejects a perfectly valid hypothesis solely because he failed to examine his deductions critically before using them as tests of the competence of the hypothesis.

Let us suppose, however, that our investigator was so fully convinced of the value of analysis as an instrument of research that he would neither accept nor reject a hypothesis until he had subjected each deduction derived from it, and each test of its correspondence with the facts, to such rigid scrutiny as he was able to make. Under these circumstances he would first have examined the deduction relating to the expected presence of wave-cutting tools on the platforms. He would have asked: Upon what does the deduction rest? Evidently upon the assumption that waves of water unarmed with debris can not effectively erode the coast. And on what, in turn, does this assumption rest? Current geologic opinion may run this way, and geologic text books may assert that waves without cutting tools are feeble. But current opinion and the text books have often proved fallible guides. So our investigator would have gone back to the sources on which both opinion and textbook should be based; the actual recorded evidence as to the nature and causes of damage accomplished by waves. Here he would have found much information concerning havoc wrought by waves under conditions which seem clearly to preclude the effective intervention of debris. The terrific impact of the water itself, the force of the currents it generates, the direct pressures exerted upon air and water imprisoned in crevices in the rock, the sudden expansion of air in crevices and pore spaces when the rapid retreat of a wave creates a partial vacuum outside, all these are described as effective causes of damage by waves, on the basis of concrete and seemingly reliable evidence. Our investigator must then have concluded that while shore debris is presumably a highly important factor in wave erosion, there is no reason to exclude the possibility that waves relatively free from debris, and striking with a force varying from hundreds to thousands of pounds per square foot, may accomplish much erosive work. He would therefore have rejected, not the hypothesis of storm-wave erosion, but his tentative deduction respecting the necessity of finding debris on the platforms; and would have looked for other deductions from the same hypothesis which he could use as a more reliable basis for testing its validity.

### VI. Analysis in the Stage of Confirmation and Revision

From the fifth stage of the investigation the inquirer should emerge with a much depleted stock of working hypotheses. In some cases only one will remain as apparently competent to explain all the recorded facts. In other cases two or more may survive thus far. If but one, the cautious investigator will seek confirmation of its validity before utilizing it in his ultimate interpretation of the facts. If more than one, he pushes his studies further to discover which one represents the true explanation of the facts or whether they are jointly responsible for a complex result.

Whether one or several hypotheses survive the tests applied in the preceding stage, the survival is almost always in an "unfinished" state. The tests remain incomplete, and therefore inconclusive, because not all the desired facts are available, and perhaps not all the desirable deductions have been made. The investigator, let us imagine, has deduced five reasonable expectations from a certain hypothesis, of which three only are matched by facts in his possession. On the other hand, he has five categories of facts, of which three only correspond to expectations thus far deduced. He has two deductions having no counterpart in observed facts, and two groups of facts which are disturbing because not related to anything thus far deduced from the hypothesis. Just what these discrepancies mean, he does not know. They may mean that observation was incomplete and that new facts remain to be discovered. They may mean that deduction was incomplete or imperfect. In either of these two cases the hypothesis may be valid as it stands. But there are other possibilities. The discrepancies may mean that the hypothesis is invalid and must ultimately be rejected; or they may mean that it only requires a certain amount of revision to bring it into harmony with all the facts.

It is the task of the investigator in the stage of confirmation and revision to find out just what the discrepancies do mean. He searches for the missing facts which, if found, will constitute logical proof of the validity of the generalization involved in the hypothesis. Here the extraordinary value of the deductive processes of stage five becomes apparent. The observation of stage one was a wandering, unguided observation. But the renewed observation of stage six is skilfully directed observation. He now knows what to look for, and hence how and where to look. If, like the geologist or geographer, he is dealing with facts to be found in the field, directed observation will materially shorten his field work and greatly increase its fruitfulness. He goes directly to the places where the new facts should be found. If, like the physicist, chemist or modern student of biology, he must discover new facts through experimentation, skilfully directed experiment will replace the vague gropings of a less advanced stage of research. The deductive process has added new interest to the quest for truth, and has enormously increased the probabilities of finding it.

Directed observation has another great value. It is apt to lead to the discovery of facts wholly unanticipated by the deductions which direct the search. As Davis has well said, the investigator's outsight on the facts is sharpened by his insight into the nature of his problem. Things which formerly made no impression on eye or mind now instantly arrest his attention, some because they are expected, but others for the very reason that they are quite unexpected. The discovery of facts that are wholly unanticipated, but which none the less find full explanation in a hypothesis under investigation, has exceptionally high value as confirmation of the hypothesis.

Where none of the deductions of stage five fully account for certain of the facts already in hand; or where newly discovered facts fail to find any counterpart in previous deductions; or, again, where some of the facts which should occur, according to a hypothesis otherwise well substantiated, can not be found, revision of the hypothesis is strongly indicated. Lack of completeness in deduction is especially apt to cause difficulty, and proper revision to include some new consequences not previously foreseen may bring complete harmony out of partial discord.

The process of securing the requisite confirmation, revision or rejection of hypotheses makes new and heavy demands upon the critical faculties. Especially is this true of the process of revision and rejection, which carries the investigator back over previous stages of the investigation in a search for some weak link in his chain of reasoning, some factor overlooked, or some item improperly included. If, as we have seen, analysis had a rôle to play in each of these preceding stages, how much more important is it that the analytical faculties should be on the alert in a review of one's reasoning in search for error. If previous work has been carefully performed, the error is not apt to be obvious. More likely it is obscurely involved in some apparently sound procedure, in which case it will continue to escape detection unless each bit of evidence, each argument and each conclusion are separated into their component parts and subjected to critical scrutiny. It is such analysis as this which must, in the circumstances detailed above, determine whether certain apparently incongruous facts should be rejected as irrelevant to the problem or included as fully pertinent; and in the latter case, whether a given hypothesis must be rejected or merely revised, before deduction and observation are brought into harmony.

## VII. Analysis in the Stage of Interpretation

Let us suppose that the investigator has reached the seventh and final stage of his labors, in which he proceeds to formulate for publication his interpretation of the origin of shore platforms. Can he at last dispense with analysis, the instrument which has served him so well at every previous step in his labors?

Not wholly, I think. In any event there must remain with him a caution inspired by his full understanding of the nature of the proofs with which he is dealing, an understanding which comes only from critical analysis of both evidence and arguments. Rarely can geologist or geographer offer mathematical demonstration of the truth of his conclusions. He can, as a rule, go no further than to show that a given proposition has a high degree of probability. Certain facts carefully observed and properly classified prompt the invention of various hypotheses. The deduced consequences of one of these hypotheses alone is matched by all the facts, including some which are newly discovered and highly peculiar. The investigator therefore has much confidence that an interpretation based on this hypothesis will be valid. But he realizes there is still opportunity for error. He may not have thought of all possible hypotheses. He may not have deduced all the reasonable consequences of those hypotheses considered. He may not have discovered all pertinent facts. Some future contribution to knowledge may throw unexpected light on his problem and radically affect his conclusions. He therefore wisely regards his present interpretation as highly probable theory, rather than as demonstrated fact.

In previous stages an error led only one investigator astray, and that one could retrace his steps and repair damage by embarking on some new line of reasoning. But in this final stage an error committed to the printed page may lead many astray and may show wholly unexpected vitality and power for evil. The printed statements must go far enough; but they must not go farther than the evidence and fully tested reasoning warrant. A given interpretation must not be applied to all shore platforms before it has been completely demonstrated that there are no such platforms for which it is not the most satisfactory explanation. It must not even be asserted as the sole cause of any platforms, unless and until it has been clearly proven that no contributing cause has played a part in their formation.

In these and other ways the investigator must be on his guard against overstatement, understatement, erroneous statement of his results. Analysis is the weapon with which he defends himself against too broad generalization and other errors which are wont to intrude themselves into the final stage of an investigation. Each sentence he scrutinizes, each conclusion he dissects, checking here and verifying there, to the end that the formulation of his interpretation shall contain no less, and particularly no more, than critically observed facts and carefully tested reasoning may justify. An interpretation thus cautiously reached and conservatively formulated will surely command the serious consideration of scientific men.

CONCLUSION

Have we, in the method of multiple working hypotheses, applied with the aid of rigorous analysis something which will guide us unfailingly to the discovery of truth? We are compelled to answer this question in the negative. No device, however perfect, can wholly deprive the human intellect of its capacity for making mistakes. De Leon searched in vain for the fountain of youth. Can we hope for a magical fountain of truth?

The most for which we may reasonably hope is by correct methods of research to reduce the chances of error to a minimum and to raise to its maximum the probability of discovering the real causes and relations of things. This we have done, so far as lies within our power, when we are accurate in observing facts, careful in classifying them, cautious in generalizing from them, fertile in inventing hypotheses, ingenious and impartial in testing their validity, skilful in securing their confirmation or revision and judicial in formulating ultimate interpretations.

Multiple working hypotheses as a method, employed in connection with critical analysis as an instrument of precision, offer us, in my opinion, the best guarantee of success in scientific research.

# SCIENTIFIC EVENTS

## UNIFICATION OF RADIO RESEARCH FACILITIES IN GREAT BRITAIN

THE facilities for radio research carried out by the British Department of Scientific and Industrial Research on the advice of their Radio Research Board have been improved by the unification of the Wireless Division of the National Physical Laboratory and the department's Radio Research Station at Slough into a new radio department of the National Physical Laboratory. Mr. R. A. Watson Watt, hitherto the superintendent of the Radio Research Station, is the superintendent of the new department.

Under the new arrangements the Radio Research Board continues to be appointed as at present by the lord president of the council, and its constitution and functions remain unchanged except that the opportunity has been taken to remove the anomaly by which the general work on the maintenance of radio standards at the National Physical Laboratory was a responsibility of the board. In the future the executive committee of the National Physical Laboratory will assume direct responsibility for these standards in the same way as it assumes responsibility for other national standards.

On the formation of the Radio Research Board in 1920, the National Physical Laboratory was entrusted with all work which required a laboratory equipped with instruments of the highest precision. Such work included the development of radio frequency standards, the study of problems of selectivity, aerial arrays and the generation of extremely short waves, as well as methods for the measurement of fundamental quantities necessary in accurate circuit design. Owing, however, to its situation and the proximity of other electrical work, the National Physical Laboratory was considered unsuitable for the conduct of radio research work requiring measurements in the field or on isolated sites. For work of this character facilities were provided by the department at the Radio Research Station erected on land adjoining the Admiralty Compass Observatory at Ditton Park, near Slough. Practically the whole work carried out on behalf of the Radio Research Board was thus divided between the Radio Research Station, Slough, and the National Physical Laboratory.

Although the Radio Research Station and the National Physical Laboratory have closely cooperated in the past, the unification which has taken place gives the Radio Research Board much greater freedom in planning its program as a single unit. The amalgamation of the staff of the two sections under a single direction is in the interests of efficiency and economy, and enables the increasing number of inquiries from industry to be made to one single establishment.

## THE ANNUAL MEETING OF THE ROYAL INSTITUTION

THE annual meeting of the members of the Royal Institution was held on May 1, the president, Lord Eustace Percy, being in the chair. According to the report in *Nature* the annual report of visitors for the year ended December 31, 1932, testified to a year of considerable activity. The membership had been well maintained. The privilege of free attendance at the afternoon lectures by *bona-fide* students in London had been much appreciated and used. The report on the progress of the researches in the Davy Faraday Laboratory gave a good indication of the considerable extent of the research organization which is at work under the direction of Sir William Bragg. Some sixteen or eighteen workers are engaged, the majority on problems related to the x-ray determination of structure. Mention was made of Dr. J. M. Robertson's determination of the structure of anthracene, of Dr. A. Müller's work on the long-chain compounds, and of the growth in accuracy and capacity of the large experimental x-ray plant in the hands of Dr. Müller and Mr. R. S. Clay. The capacity of the apparatus is calculated to be about 50 kw.; as yet it has worked well up to 10 kw. The treasurer's report and accounts showed a very satisfactory position, in spite of the heavy demand on the financial resources of the institution caused by the recent reconstruction. After a total expenditure in connection with the rebuilding of more than £100,000, a diminution in the invested funds of the Royal Institution of about £2,000 is shown. This gratifying result is a consequence of many generous donations to the Building and Research Endowment Fund raised by the institution in the past three years. The donations and other receipts to this fund have been sufficient to defray almost the entire cost of the rebuilding, and to go a considerable way towards completion of the program of permanent endowment of research which the managers of the institution have as one of their principal objects. The following officers for 1933–34 were elected: *President,* the Right Hon. Lord Eustace Percy; *Treasurer,* Sir Robert Robertson; *Secretary,* Major Charles E. S. Phillips.

## NATIONAL RESEARCH FELLOWSHIPS IN THE BIOLOGICAL SCIENCES

THE annual meeting of the Board of National Research Fellowships in the Biological Sciences, for the award of 1933–34 appointments, was held in Washington on April 28 and 29, 1933. The board made twenty-six reappointments and forty-one new appointments, as follows:

REAPPOINTMENTS

*For Domestic Study*

Bond, R. M.—Zoology
Boughton, D. C.—Agriculture
Burkholder, P. R.—Botany
Casida, L. E.—Agriculture
Fry, Glenn A.—Psychology
Glass, H. B.—Zoology
Hopkins, E. W.—Agriculture
Jackson, T. A.—Psychology
Kelly, Isabel T.—Anthropology
Kerr, Thomas—Botany
Miller, E. S.—Botany
Morsh, J. E.—Psychology
Mowrer, O. H.—Psychology
Phelps, Austin—Zoology
Riley, H. P.—Botany
Shaw, Luther—Agriculture
Smelser, G. K.—Zoology
Smith, Wm. K.—Agriculture
Taylor, G. W.—Zoology
Tharp, Wm. H.—Botany
Wald, George—Zoology
Walls, Gordon L.—Zoology
Wolfe, J. B.—Psychology
Zirkle, R. E.—Botany

*For Study Abroad*

Hill, R. T.—Zoology
Sparrow, F. K.—Botany

NEW APPOINTMENTS

*For Domestic Study*

Abbe, Ernst C.—Botany
Barker, Horace A.—Zoology
Clark, Harold E.—Agriculture
Day, Harry G.—Zoology
Dyk, Walter—Anthropology
Edelman, Edward E.—Psychology
Gardner, Wm. U.—Agriculture
Goddard, David R.—Botany
Hamlett, Geo. W. D.—Zoology
Harrison, Carter M.—Agriculture
Hooker, Charles W.—Zoology
Hulse, Frederick S.—Anthropology
Hunt, Joseph McV.—Psychology
Jeffers, Katharine R.—Zoology
Krechevsky, Isadore—Psychology
Leeper, Robert W.—Psychology
Livingston, Luzern G.—Botany
Mackinney, Gordon—Botany
Misbach, L. E.—Psychology
Moyer, Laurence S.—Botany
Needham, J. G.—Psychology
Pady, Stuart M.—Botany
Park, Thomas—Zoology
Peckham, Robert H.—Psychology
Rosenfels, Richard S.—Botany
Rudnick, Dorothea—Zoology
Seltzer, Carl C.—Anthropology
Spence, Kenneth W.—Psychology
Steinbach, H. Burr—Zoology
Sumwalt, Margaret—Zoology
Williams, H. H.—Agriculture

*For Study Abroad*

Barron, Donald H.—Zoology
Baxter, Dow V.—Forestry
Birkeland, J. M.—Botany
Ehrlich, John—Forestry
Graham, Roy—Botany
Lindsley, D. B.—Psychology
Neatby, Kenneth W.—Agriculture
Snyder, Wm. C.—Agriculture
Wells, John W.—Zoology
Wilcox, A. N.—Agriculture

## SUMMER CONFERENCE IN SPECTROSCOPY

ONE of the features of the summer research gathering of spectroscopists to be held at the Massachusetts Institute of Technology this year is to be a Spectroscopic Conference scheduled for the week of July 17–22. Each of the five days of the conference will be devoted to some particular branch of spectroscopy, the mornings being devoted to the presentation of papers and the holding of discussion groups, while the afternoons are to be left free for informal discussions, laboratory inspections, and sight-seeing and recreation.

While the program is not yet complete, the following papers have already been scheduled:

Monday, July 17: *Quantitative Spectroscopic Analysis of Materials*

C. C. Nitchie, Bausch and Lomb Optical Company, "Some Practical Applications of the Spectrograph."

W. F. Meggers, Bureau of Standards, "The Physical Basis for Quantitative Spectrochemical Analysis."

F. Twyman, Adam Hilger, Ltd., "The Rôle of the Instrument Maker in Spectrum Analysis."

C. E. K. Mees, Eastman Kodak Company, "Photographic Plates for Spectroscopy."

Keivin Burns, Allegheny Observatory, leader of Discussion on Spectrochemical Analysis.

Tuesday, July 18: *Biological and Photochemical Applications of Spectroscopy*

W. A. Noyes, Jr., Brown University, "The Correlation of Research in Spectroscopy with that of Photochemistry."

P. A. Leighton, Stanford University, "Photochemistry and the Schumann Region."

F. Twyman, Adam Hilger, Ltd., "Basic Principles in the Design of Spectrophotometers."

G. B. Kistiakowsky, Harvard University, "Molecular Dissociation Energies from Spectroscopic Data."

Wednesday, July 19: *Physical and Astrophysical Aspects of Spectroscopy*

D. H. Menzel, Harvard University, "The Spectroscope in Astrophysics."

G. H. Dieke, The Johns Hopkins University, "Astigmatism of the Concave Grating."

F. H. Crawford, Harvard University, "The Present Status of Research on the Zeeman Effect in Molecular Spectra."

Thursday, July 20: *Analysis of Complex Spectra*

A. G. Shenstone, Princeton University, "Incompletely Analyzed Spectra."

W. F. Meggers, Bureau of Standards, "The Structure of Rare Earth Spectra."

G. H. Dieke, The Johns Hopkins University, "The Present Status of Wave-length Standards."

Keivin Burns, Allegheny Observatory, "Wave-length Standards."

Friday, July 21: *Spectroscopy and Atomic Structure*

(To be arranged), "Status of Theoretical Calculations of Atomic Energy States."

G. R. Harrison, Massachusetts Institute of Technology, "Status of Calculations of Spectral Line Intensities."

D. R. Hartree, University of Manchester, "Numerical Calculation of Atomic Properties."

J. C. Slater, Massachusetts Institute of Technology, "Analytical Calculations of Atomic Properties."

A number of other papers which have been tentatively scheduled are not listed because of uncertainties which had not been cleared up at the time of going to press. It is planned to follow each set of papers by extended discussion of the present status and future possibilities of each branch of spectroscopy considered.

## PSYCHOLOGY AT CHICAGO

Members of Section I of the American Association for the Advancement of Science will meet in Chicago from June 20 to 23, in connection with the Century of Progress. Four psychologists from abroad will be present. Each of these will lead a symposium and in addition special lectures are scheduled. American psychologists will also participate in the symposia, the topics and leaders of which are as follows:

June 20, "Gestalt": Wolfgang Köhler, Berlin.

June 21, "Intelligence": Charles E. Spearman, London.

June 22, "Sensory Psychology": Henri Piéron, Paris.

June 23, "Character and Personality": Emilio Mira, Barcelona.

In addition to regular sessions the special symposia and lectures given in other sections of the association are of interest to psychologists. For example, the following may be mentioned:

June 20, forenoon, Dr. A. V. Hill, London, Symposium on Nerve Activity.

June 21, afternoon, Dr. R. Goldschmidt, Institute of Experimental Biology, Berlin, Symposium.

June 23, evening, Dr. C. U. A. Kappers, Brain Institute, Amsterdam, General Address.

The preliminary program follows:

Tuesday, June 20, 2:00 P. M. Symposium on Gestalt Psychology: Wolfgang Köhler, Berlin; R. H. Wheeler, University of Kansas; Heinrich Klüver, Institute for Juvenile Research.

Wednesday, June 21, 9:30 A. M. Symposium on Intelligence: Charles E. Spearman, University of London; Florence L. Goodenough, University of Minnesota. 11:30 A. M. Address: Henri Piéron, Paris.

Thursday, June 22, 9:30 A. M. Symposium on Sensory Psychology: Henri Piéron, Paris; Walter R. Miles, Yale University; Alvhh R. Lauer, Iowa State College. 11:30 A. M. Address: Emilio Mira, Barcelona.

Friday, June 23, 9:30 A. M. Symposium on Character and Personality: Emilio Mira, Barcelona; Mandel Sherman, University of Chicago; John E. Anderson, University of Minnesota.

Saturday, June 24, 8:00 P. M. General Address before the Association: Charles E. Spearman, University of London.

Dr. Walter R. Miles, of Yale University, is chairman of the section and Dr. John E. Anderson, of the University of Minnesota, is secretary. The meetings will be held in Thorne Hall and Lincoln Hall, McKinlock Campus, Northwestern University.

# SCIENTIFIC NOTES AND NEWS

As has been fully reported in this journal, the American Association for the Advancement of Science and associated societies meet in Chicago from June 19 to 31. The Century of Progress Exposition has given the fundamental sciences the central place of honor, with the applied sciences radiating from it. The American Association and the societies devoted to the fundamental sciences will meet during the first week. These meetings will be followed by Engineering Week and the next week will be occupied by the National Education Association and its associated organizations. The full preliminary program of the meeting of the American Association and associated societies will be found in the issue of SCIENCE for May 19. The foreign scientific men who will take part in the meeting of the American Association as guests of the association and the Century of Progress Exposition are as follows: Dr. Otto Appel, of Berlin, agriculture; Dr. F. W. Aston, of Cambridge, chemistry; Dr. G. A. Bagge, of Stockholm, economics; Dr. Joseph Barcroft, of Cambridge, physiology; Dr. A. Mendelssohn Bartholdy, of Hamburg, political science; Dr. Jakob Bjerknes, of Bergen, meteorology; Dr. Niels Bohr, of Copenhagen, physics; Dr. Filippo Bottazzi, of Naples, physiology; Dr. Ludwig Diels, of Berlin, botany; Dr. Jean Dufrénoy, of France, agriculture; Dr. Leopold Fejér, of Budapest, mathematics; Dr. Enrico Fermi, of Rome, physics; Dr. A. P. M. Fleming, of Manchester, engineering; Dr. R. Goldschmidt, of Berlin, zoology; Dr. Herbert J. Gough, of London, engineering; Sir Daniel Hall, of London, agriculture; Dr. A. V. Hill, of London, physiology; Dr. C. U. A. Kappers, of Amsterdam, anthropology; Dr. Wolfgang Köhler, of Berlin, psychology; Dr. August Krogh, of Copenhagen, physiology; Dr. Tullio Levi-Civita, of Rome, mathematics; Dr. Emilio Mira, of Barcelona, psychology; Dr. William Oualid, of Paris, political economy; Dr. Henri Piéron, of Paris, psychology; Dr. J. J. Sederholm, of Helsingfors, geology; Dr. Charles E. Spearman, of London, psychology; Dr. The. Svedberg, of Upsala, chemistry, and Dr. R. J. Tillyard, of Australia, entomology and paleontology.

THE Royal Society, London, has elected as foreign members Professor Harvey Cushing, of the Harvard Medical School and the Peter Bent Brigham Hospital; Professor Peter Debye, director of the Institute of Physics at the University of Leipzig; Professor Friedrich August Ferdinand Christian Went, director of the Institute of Botany and of the Botanical Garden at the University of Utrecht, and Professor Vilhelm F. K. Bjerknes, professor of mechanics and mathematical physics at the University of Oslo.

DR. WILLEM DE SITTER, director of the Leiden Observatory, has been elected a correspondent of the French Academy of Sciences in the section for astronomy.

THE doctorate of science was conferred on Dr. William Morton Wheeler, professor of entomology at Harvard University, at the recent commencement exercises of Columbia University.

NEW YORK UNIVERSITY conferred at its commencement on June 1 an honorary doctorate on Dr. Florence Rena Sabin, member of the Rockefeller Institute for Medical Research.

THE University of Oxford will confer on June 21 the honorary degree of doctor of science on Dr. John Scott Haldane, fellow of New College and honorary professor and director of the mining research laboratory at the University of Birmingham.

THE original building of the New York State College of Forestry, which was opened in 1917, has been named in honor of Dr. William L. Bray, professor of botany and dean of the Graduate School of Syracuse University, who was the first head in 1911 of the College of Forestry. This designation was recommended by the faculty and authorized by the Board of Trustees of the College of Forestry on June 1. Since the early days of the college when he gave the first courses in forestry at Syracuse, Dean Bray has conducted courses in botany at the summer camp of the college on Cranberry Lake.

DR. OSWALD T. AVERY, of the Rockefeller Institute for Medical Research, has been elected president of the American Association of Pathologists and Bacteriologists.

LORD MELCHETT has been elected president of the British Science Guild, in succession to Sir Samuel Hoare, whose three-year term of office ends on June 19.

ACCORDING to *Nature,* Professor A. N. St. G. H. Burkitt, Challis professor of anatomy in the University of Sydney, has been elected president of the Linnean Society of New South Wales.

DR. EDGAR ALLEN, professor of anatomy and dean of the University of Missouri School of Medicine, will succeed Dr. Harry Burr Ferris as professor of anatomy and head of the department of anatomy at the Yale University School of Medicine.

DR. AUGUSTUS G. POHLMAN has resigned as research professor of anatomy and dean of the University of South Dakota School of Medicine to accept an appointment as professor and head of the department of anatomy at Creighton University School of Medicine, Omaha, Nebraska.

PROFESSOR G. HADFIELD, professor of pathology in the University of London, has accepted an invitation to fill the chair of pathology at the University of Bristol to succeed Professor Walker Hall.

DR. A. K. KURTZ, formerly of the U. S. Civil Service Commission, has joined the staff of the Industrial Relations Division of the Procter and Gamble Company as statistician.

AMONG those who will work during the coming year in the School of Mathematics of the Institute for Advanced Study at Princeton are: Drs. A. A. Albert, University of Chicago; K. Gödel, University of Vienna; Jessen, University of Copenhagen; L. S. Pontrjagin, University of Moscow; Meyer Salkover, University of Cincinnati; T. Y. Thomas, Princeton University; E. R. van Kampen, Johns Hopkins University; R. L. Wilder, University of Michigan, and W. E. Bleick, Johns Hopkins University.

DR. RALPH W. CHANEY, head of the department of paleontology at the University of California, has left for northeastern Asia, where he will spend several months. He will return for the fall semester opening in August.

DR. J. BJERKNES, of the Geophysical Institute, Bergen, Norway, who is visiting the United States as the guest of the Century of Progress and the American Association for the Advancement of Science, addressed students of meteorology at the Massachusetts Institute of Technology and eastern Massachusetts members of the American Meteorological Society, June 9, on "The General Circulation of the Atmosphere." Several meteorologists took part in the discussion which followed.

SIR ALMROTH WRIGHT delivered the John Mallet Purser Lecture on "Immunization—the Old Doctrine and the New" at Trinity College, Dublin, on May 17.

THE first of a series of lectures, instituted by the British Science Guild for the purpose of directing attention to the importance of research—both purely scientific and technical—and the utilization of its results in the service of mankind, was given by Sir Harold Carpenter on May 16. The subject of the lecture was "Metals in the Service of Human Life and Industry."

DR. CHARLES F. BROOKS and Mr. S. P. Fergusson, of the Blue Hill Observatory, Harvard University, addressed the New Hampshire Academy of Science, at its annual meeting, June 3, on "Scientific Value of the Work of the Mt. Washington Observatory." Members of the academy drove up the mountain and inspected the observatory, which was established last fall following a grant from the academy. Mr. Fergusson will spend two months this summer on the summit, flying kites and captive balloons carrying recording instruments to show the effect of the mountain on the local wind velocity, temperature and humidity.

RECEIPT of a fund of $300 to pay for the first season of a new series of lectures at Northwestern University to be known as the U. S. Grant memorial lectures in honor of the late Professor U. S. Grant, who was head of the department of geology and geography, was recently announced by Dr. W. H. Haas, professor of geology and geography. The first lectures, probably next November, will be given by Dr. W. H. Collins, director of the Canadian Geological Survey. Dr. Collins has carried on work closely related to that of Professor Grant. The donor of the gift prefers to remain anonymous. It is a tribute from one scientific man to the memory of another. A gift of $150, also anonymous, for a scholarship to be known as the Grant graduate scholarship in geology and geography has also been announced.

THE annual initiation and banquet of the Michigan State College Chapter of the Society of the Sigma Xi was held at Michigan State College on June 1. Twenty-four new members were initiated. The public address was given by Dr. I. F. Huddleson on "Undulant Fever." The officers for the next academic year are: *President,* Dean R. C. Huston; *Vice-president,* Dean Marie Dye; *Secretary,* Professor V. G. Grove; *Treasurer,* Professor R. E. Marshall, who continues his office for another year.

THE Sigma Xi Club of Peking held its annual meeting and dinner on May 5. The speaker on the occasion was Dr. H. B. van Dyke, professor of pharmacology at the Peiping Union Medical College, who spoke on "Correlation among Glands of Internal Secretion." The officers elected for the coming year are: *President,* Dr. H. B. van Dyke; *Vice-president,* Dr. Toh Liu, dean of the College of Science, Normal University; *Secretary-treasurer,* Dr. Adam P. T. Sah, professor of physics, Tsing Hua University. The membership of the Sigma Xi Club in Peking has grown to over fifty. There is said to be evidence that the old capital, now called Peiping, is becoming increasingly important as a research center. Four universities, the Peiping Union Medical College (Rockefeller Foundation), the National Geological Survey and two research institutes are pursuing intensive scientific research programs. The local Sigma Xi membership, which is about one fourth American and three fourths Chinese, is distributed among these eight institutions.

DR. C. E. MCCLUNG, professor of zoology at the

University of Pennsylvania, and managing editor of the *Journal of Morphology,* who, as previously announced, is spending next year in Japan, requests that during his absence manuscripts for the *Journal,* until further notice, be sent directly to the Wistar Institute, Philadelphia.

THE South Carolina Legislature, in an act approved on May 13 and effective on that date, provided that "the property and duties of the State Food Research Laboratory at Charleston shall be associated with the State Medical College." The trustees of the Medical College have announced that, due to heavily reduced appropriations, it will be impossible to continue the laboratory, which has been engaged for some years on investigations in foods and nutrition. Present members of the laboratory staff are Drs. Roe E. Remington and Harold Levine, and Messrs. Harry von Kolnitz and F. Bartow Culp.

THE 150-foot ship that will carry Lincoln Ellsworth to the Antarctic is being prepared for its departure from Norway about the first of August for New Zealand. The ship is to leave New Zealand for the Bay of Wales about November 1, and will arrive at its base about December 15. The expedition is planning a 3,000 mile round trip non-stop flight over the Antarctic Continent.

THE California Institute of Technology has recently named a room in honor of Dr. Leon L. Watters, of New York. The room is in the Norman Bridge Laboratory of Physics and bears the following inscription: "The Watters Generator: The equipment in this room is the gift of Dr. Leon L. Watters, of New York, to the atomic structure research of the California Institute of Technology. It is designed to facilitate the generation of a steady potential of 300 KV, an energy available for x-rays ten times greater than any other equipment up to the present date." The apparatus will be employed to further the work begun by Dr. DuMond regarding which both Professor Einstein and Professor Millikan predict results of great importance.

THE Santa Barbara Museum of Natural History is building a children's loggia in memory of the former director, Ralph Hoffman. It is an addition to the east and south sides of the seismographic building, open in summer and glass-enclosed in winter, equipped with shelves and lockers and with water for modelling work. The design is by Carleton Winslow.

THE *Journal* of the American Medical Association states that negotiations for the organization of a school for public health nurses in Prague to be opened in 1934 have been completed. Construction is to start immediately. The preliminary education required for admission is to be graduation from a secondary school. Training in bedside nursing will be included in the two years course as well as a knowledge of social legislation applicable to field work. Half the cost of the construction of the school was promised to the Czechoslovakian government by the Rockefeller Foundation. The school will be erected on the grounds of the state institute of public hygiene in Prague. Bedside nursing will be practised in the near-by state hospital. Another feature of the school is that it will be for pupils both of the Czech and of the German language. The practical training in the field will be done for the Czech candidates in one of the demonstration districts of Prague, the one for German candidates in a demonstration district in northern Bohemia. The school will accommodate 100 pupils in its dormitory. It is hoped that it will create a type of field worker having the advantages of a trained nurse and at the same time knowledge necessary to understand social problems.

THE Institute of Medicine of Chicago offers a prize of $500 for the most meritorious investigation in medicine or in the specialties of medicine. The investigation may be also in the fundamental sciences, provided the work has a definite bearing on some medical problem. Competition is open to graduates of Chicago medical schools who have received the degree of M.D. during the year 1931 or thereafter. Manuscripts must be submitted to the secretary of the Institute of Medicine of Chicago, 122 South Michigan Boulevard, Chicago, not later than December 31, 1933. In the case of a paper submitted by more than one author, it is stipulated that all the authors must qualify, and that the prize paper be published under the same authorship as that under which it was submitted. The winner of the prize will be expected to present the results of his investigation before the institute at some meeting in 1934, the time to be designated later. If no paper presented is deemed worthy of the prize, the award may be withheld at the discretion of the Board of Governors.

# DISCUSSION

## THE PROBLEM OF TWISTED TREES

SURVEYING the various contributions to this subject, which have recently appeared in SCIENCE, the *Journal of Heredity, Journal of the New York Botanical Garden* and *Nature,* we find fair accord on the following essential points: (1) The wide distribution of the regular tree twisting or spiral grain formation; (2) the aptitude of particular plant species to this structural form, and (3) the prevalence of tree twisting in certain localities. No agreement, however, is found as to the causes underlying this phenomenon.

Now, if we view the problem before us, in conjunction with such biological occurrences, as the curling and twisting of wool fibers, silk worm and spider's web, as well as the spiral growth of the bacterial colony filaments—we realize not only its general character but also that its solution is to be sought in the fundamentals underlying the evolution of organized matter.

Again, considering the fact that (1) the tracing of an organism's form and functions to some more primitive type of organic life is basic to our conception of evolution, (2) many fundamentals of organic life are but a reproduction of some characteristic property of the inorganic constituents (mineral medusa, mushroom and arboreal forms[1]) and (3) spiral formations are general throughout the inorganic world,[2] we may take it that the problem before us ultimately finds its foundation in the general principles of periodicity.[2]

Reviewing these principles, we find (I) periodic structures are the material record of an undulatory movement in a mobile magma. This movement characterizes generally the relationship of matter and energy and is expressible in terms of wave-mechanics. (II) as a record of change or transition periodic precipitations are determined by the relation existing between the frequency amplitude of undulation and the boundaries of the system and (III) periodic precipitations are in general not confined to physical or chemical phenomena only and are not restricted to any specific state or phase of matter or to any definite number of components.

In considering the problem of periodic precipitation, we must bear in mind, however, the fact that whilst the fundamental principles of periodicity and its material records are not limited to any state or phase, the actual type and complexity of each periodic precipitation is determined by all the properties of the particular phase of matter involved in the phenomenon. This is specially the case with the colloidal state capable of functioning as either a system-boundary, medium or component or even all these rolled together, thus evolving the mineralogical and biological periodic structures in all their ramifications.

Turning our attention to organized matter we find that minerals constitute an intrinsic component in every organic cell extending from the iron and sulfur bacteria up to the highest floral and faunal complexities.[3]

The alkaline earth group, together with some silicates, represents the material which imparts protection, rigidity and form to living matter. This function is the direct outcome of the physical and chemical properties of these substances, and therefore we may expect to find in the mineral world some primitive skeleton outline of the organic structural forms. Actually the salts of calcium, barium and strontium as well as silicates produce arboreal growth, such as creeper, bush and tree like forms.[1]

This stabilizing tendency—both in their inorganic condition and in organized matter—is undoubtedly due to the transitory colloidal state of these substances and the particular character of osmosis resulting from it. A more detailed study has shown that this characteristic is even more specific and the growth is typical to each individual radical or group.

So we find the calcium salts yield tree-like formations with a corrugated surface, barium salts give straight growth with a spiral surface, strontium salts form beautiful spirals, of a smooth tape-like growth, whilst silicates produce bamboo-like formations.

Again, our experience with the introduction of such groupings as sulfates, carbonates, phosphates and oxalates shows that the increase in constitutional complexity of the radical combinations, especially organo-metallic associations, is followed by a remarkable impetus in arboreal growth and general functional augmentation. Also, synthetic arboreal growth in the ferrocyanide, arsenate and arsenite groups finds probably a basic expression in the presence of hydrogen cyanide and arsenic in the organism, the assimilation of arsenates and arsenites by plants and the great therapeutic influence of arsenic on animals.

The gradual substitution of these substances by one another in the organism without impairing general metabolism seems to be well established. The silicious matter of the lower organism gave way to calcium carbonate, which in its turn was substituted by calcium phosphate in the higher forms. Our study of bacterial culture media, general nutrition and such plants as loco-weed, tobacco leaves, etc., shows that this substitution is applicable to barium and possibly strontium.

In the light of these facts it would seem that tree twisting is primarily due to local soil peculiarities which eventually modified the structural constituents of the plants. In the course of evolution the contact and inductive influences transformed the mineral efflorescence and arboreal growth into new structures more complex both in form and substance.

[1] Hatschek, *Proc. Roy. Soc.*, 95A: 303, 1919; Copisarow, *Jour. Chem. Soc.*, 233: 1927; *Koll. Zeits.*, 47: 60, 1929.

[2] Copisarow, *Koll. Zeits.*, 54: 257, 1931; *Jour. Phys. Chem.*, 36: 752, 1932.

[3] Copisarow, *Chemical News*, 134: 305, 323, 338, 1927.

The coming into being of organo-metallic and organic associations brought with it differences not only in composition but also in constitution resulting ultimately in the separation of optically active isomers by a process of gradual elimination.[4] The arboreal growth, retaining certain basic features of form inherent in their structural mineral radicles or groups, lost its arbitrary direction and became definitely orientated in accordance with the predominating stereo-isomeric form of its constituents.

The alteration in the direction of twist with age, recorded by several observers, is not really surprising. The great enzymatic transformation during embryonic development, ripening of fruit, as well as the intimate connection existing between enzymes and the cell nucleus—naturally involve a radical change in all plant constituents, which may of course be followed by a corresponding reversal of the helix.

Thus we find that the cause of the general twisting of trees is two-fold—internal and external. The internal factor is found in the specific character of the plant constituents (fusion products of heredity and environment) which determine the type of capillary spiral movement of its fluid nutrients and fibrillar depositions operating on the general principles of periodicity. In the case of young non-rigid plants these internal influences are enhanced or retarded (as the case may be) by light tropism and prevailing air currents. The systematic effect of these contributing external causes is however reduced to a minimum in old rigid formations.

Here, temperature, pressure, winds, sunlight as well as various parasitic and toxic influences may affect stature and produce structural abnormalities but do not participate in the evolution of the regular twisting in trees.

MAURICE COPISAROW

RESEARCH LABORATORY,
145 ALEXANDRA RD.,
MANCHESTER, ENGLAND

## CHLORPICRIN INJURIOUS TO GREENHOUSE PLANTS

IN view of the promising indications for chlorpicrin as a soil fumigant for nematode control, reported elsewhere,[1] recent evidence of the capacity of small concentrations of this gas in the air to injure greenhouse plants may be of special interest to investigators.

In an experimental fumigation of a plant bed just outside one of the Plant Pathology greenhouses at the University of California, Berkeley, California, some of the gas escaping from the soil found its way into the house and caused severe injury to tobacco, strawberry, coleus and other plants. The actual concentration of the gas as it became diffused into the greenhouse atmosphere was very low, probably not greater than 20 parts per million. It was detectable by a smarting of the eyes but not by odor. Details of the arrangement of the fumigated plot with relation to the greenhouse, together with illustrations and descriptions of the signs of injury produced upon the plants, will be presented in another paper, probably in *Phytopathology*. This preliminary statement is made as a warning to other investigators who may be contemplating making applications of chlorpicrin to greenhouse soils to control nematodes. If applications are made in benches or beds inside the house with growing plants elsewhere in the house, such plants may become severely injured from the escaping gas, even though they may be some distance away from the site of fumigation.

G. H. GODFREY

UNIVERSITY OF CALIFORNIA

[4] Mills, Brit. Assoc. Adv. Science, York meeting, 1932.

[1] M. O. Johnson and G. H. Godfrey, "Chloropicrin for Nematode Control." *Indust. and Eng. Chem.*, 24: 311–313. 1932. Other papers on this subject have been submitted for publication.

## THE ANNIVERSARY OF THE NORMAL CURVE

THE two hundredth anniversary of the discovery of the normal probability curve falls this year. It is interesting to note that the discovery of the curve was made by a man whose name is seldom, if ever, attached to it. It is also significant that the discoverer thought that his contribution was to pure or abstract mathematics and that the most practical use that could ever be made of his discovery was in connection with games of chance.

The man was DeMoivre. He published his findings on November 12, 1733. Since that time such wide use has been made of the curve that the above date becomes a landmark of considerable importance, especially in the social sciences.

In a recent book on the history of statistics[1] the following treatment of the event is found:

> The intensive study which DeMoivre gave to this work, together with his applications of the binomial theorem, led him a few years later—probably about 1721—to discover a formula for the ratio between the middle term and the sum of all the terms of $(1-1)^n$, and thus become the discoverer of the normal curve. Many of the recent treatises on probability and sampling approach the matter by a method quite similar to DeMoivre's use of the binomial expansion.
>
> This formula, first published November 12, 1733, is the *fons et origo* of the normal curve. In 1730 DeMoivre had brought out his *Miscellanea Analytica* and

[1] Helen M. Walker, "Studies in the History of Statistical Method," pp. 13–14. Williams and Wilkins: Baltimore, 1929.

three years later he presented privately to a few friends a brief paper of seven pages with the title *Approximatio ad Summam Terminarum Binomii $a - b^n$ in Seriem Expansi.* The discovery of this exceedingly rare document is due to Pearson. . . .

In this obscure treatise on abstract mathematics, written in Latin nearly two centuries ago, and supposed by its author to have no practical implications outside the realm of games of chance, in this brief supplement now so rare that only two copies have been reported extant, we have the first formulation of the momentous concept of a law of errors.

CHARLES J. MARSH

STANFORD UNIVERSITY

## QUESTIONS

IF tomatoes grown in greenhouses have vitamins, does it mean that ordinary window-glass transmits ultra-violet radiations: or does it mean that plants can build up vitamins without the help of ultra-violet?

If sunlight is essential for chlorophyll formation by plants, how did it happen that sprouted seeds with primary and secondary roots, a stem and fully chlorophyllated cotyledons and primary leaves were found *inside* an opened Spanish succulent yellow gourd which had been in the shade in the house for eight months?

FREDERICK S. HAMMETT

PROVINCETOWN, MASS.

# REPORTS

## PUBLIC SERVICE AS AN ELEMENT IN THE LIFE OF THE AMERICAN SCIENTIST[1]

IT has been said truly, that our universities magnify the advantage of the individual at the expense of humanity. Few that leave academic halls with degrees in their pockets carry with them any considerable sense of public duty or think of anything beyond their own personal advancement. Recognition of the duty of parentage, for instance, is an essential element in any lasting civilization; but any sense of such a duty is almost entirely lacking among our collegiate young men and women. What professor in his lectures, what college president in his baccalaureate ever mentions that subject? Yet to teach and to practise public service, and service to humanity are especially the duties of scientific men.

Ours is the most humane and altruistic of professions. Yet we commonly fail, I believe, rather grievously in respect to public service. I shall deal with this subject quite concretely, as it is illustrated in a great social, political, moral and toxicological question now before the American people. I refer to the public duty resting upon American physiologists, biochemists, pharmacologists and pathologists in relation to the alcohol question.

Through an odd chain of events I became during the past year virtually, although of course unofficially, consulting toxicologist to the Congress of the United States. It is mainly on my advice that legal beer is to be 4 per cent. by volume and 3.2 by weight. The volume of such a beverage that must be taken to induce even the lowest slightly intoxicating concentration of alcohol in the blood (one milligram of alcohol per cubic centimeter of blood) is at the limit of the capacity of the human stomach.

The studies which this service involved led me to read practically all the testimony on this subject that has ever been given before Congressional Committees by scientific witnesses. And the more I read the more I was exasperated by the attitude that we scientists generally take when called on by legislators for advice; and the more tolerant and even sympathetic I become toward those much maligned bodies of men, the members of Congress and of the legislatures.

Legislators are necessarily called upon to decide a vast number of questions in all fields of human activity. On many of these questions even the most broadly educated man, unless he has specialized on that one subject, can have only superficial information. Legislators are not specialists. But they can and do call upon scientific men who have specialized on each particular question.

In this case the question is the toxicological properties of alcoholic beverages. What do they get in reply? One scientist says, "Alcohol is a food." Another says, "Alcohol is a powerful narcotic drug." Others add other facts. All these statements are true scientifically. But what is the poor legislator, anxious to do his duty and to legislate wisely, to make out of such raw facts? Scarcely any scientific witness seems to realize that what is actually needed is that he himself shall emphasize the practical significance of the scientific facts, and shall show the legislators to what conclusion and to what policy these facts point in relation to the public welfare.

I know that many scientific men will disagree with me on this. One of our most eminent colleagues, when I presented this view to him, offered the objection that what I proposed "involves more than the scientist's function; it requires him to speak as a citizen." To this I would reply that one does not escape the responsibilities of a citizen merely because he is a scientific expert.

As to the alcohol problem it is surely clear that the American people have made a woeful failure to control its evils both before and under prohibition;

[1] Part of an address at the dinner of the Federation of American Societies for Experimental Biology, at Cincinnati, April 11, 1933.

and that without scientific guidance a third experiment may not turn out any better. Is it not clear that this failure in the past, and possibly in the future, is due to the popular ignorance as to the underlying scientific facts? Is it not also true that it is only such scientific men as we who are gathered at this meeting that can supply and interpret the facts?

You may not believe it, but it is true, that a large, conscientious, determined and utterly ignorant element among our fellow citizens honestly believes that "beer is more intoxicating than distilled spirits." Not one legislator in a hundred realizes, until it is explained to him, that to allow spirits to be dispensed under the same conditions as the merely fermented beverages is equivalent to allowing tobacco shops to sell morphine and cocaine under the same conditions as tobacco.

Our British colleagues have served their nation much better. They have the great tradition and institution of royal commissions and similar advisory bodies that in England are so effective in the fundamental direction of national policy. On the alcohol question the facts and their meaning have certainly never been put more clearly than they were by a committee that reported a few years ago to the British Liquor Control Board. On that committee were such men as Cushny, Dale, Newman, Mott, McDougal and Sherrington. What they reported was virtually nothing more nor less than that the mass law of chemistry applies to alcoholic beverages. Those beverages that are concentrated are powerful and harmful in their effects. Those that are dilute are relatively innocuous. So clear was their report both in its presentation of facts and in the inference derived from those facts, that the Judiciary Committee of the Senate embodied the whole British statement in its own report.[2]

I have not the time in a mere after-dinner speech to develop this topic in detail. I have done so, however, in an article soon to appear in a general journal.[3] But is it not clear, when we face the facts known perfectly well to all of us here at this meeting, that the line of public policy and legislation that should be followed, that must be followed, if the evils of alcohol are to be minimized, is that of substituting the more dilute for the stronger alcoholic beverages?

I ask your cooperation in teaching the American people, and particularly the legislators, the mass law in its application to alcoholic beverages.

YANDELL HENDERSON

YALE UNIVERSITY

# SCIENTIFIC APPARATUS AND LABORATORY METHODS

## A LOW-COST LABORATORY UNIT FOR LIGHTING AND APPLIANCES

A LABORATORY table lighting unit has been designed for individual or class use to provide a satisfactory artificial light source for both high power microscopy and table or stage dissection, providing also outlets for electrical appliances. It is believed that the improvements incorporated will be of extended use where economy (*i.e.*, construction, installation charges and operation) must also be taken into consideration. The major points concerning the fixture are the utilization of the recently developed inside frosted blue daylight lamps in the larger sizes, suitable for use in naked fixtures without color filters or globes, and the convenience-outlets so often beyond reach but here made a part of the lighting fixture.

(1) Provision is made for interchangeable use of lamps from 150 to 300 watts, maintaining the center of illumination within the fixture by socket extensions for the 150 watt and 200 watt sizes, and employing the medium-screw "skirted" base for the largest size. Inside frosted Mazda blue daylight lamps are recommended for the reasons indicated in paragraph 3.

(2) Beam intensity values at the table top and 30 inches from the base of the unit, with the lower edge of the reflector hood 17 inches above the table top, for three sizes of inside frosted blue daylight lamps with same position of light-center, are as follows:[1]

| Lamp size in watts | Socket extension | Intensity in ft. candles at 30° from plane of table[2] | Intensity in f-c in plane of table |
|---|---|---|---|
| 150 | 3 | 23 | 9 |
| 200 | 2 | 30 | 13 |
| 300 | 0 | 41 | 16 |

(3) The quality of the light from the inside frosted blue daylight lamp matches average daylight suitably well for general use, and for those who are accustomed to studying by the latter medium this quality is an appreciable gain over the inside frosted white or the clear daylight incandescent lamps.

Normal lamp life is anticipated in the ordinary operation of the inside frosted blue daylight lamp in the fixture. It is pointed out, however, that the color

[2] Senate Report No. 1105, 72nd Congress.

[3] *Harper's Magazine* for June, 1933.

[1] Measured with Weston Model No. 603 Photronic Illumination meter, equipped with a green-yellow filter so that the color sensitivity of the instrument matched that of the human eye.

[2] Ca. angle of microscope mirror.

quality, intensity of the light and the life of the lamp are dependently related. For a closer approach to average daylight the lamps may be operated at from 100 to 105 per cent. of their rated voltage. When the average line-voltage during normal operation is 115 volts (*i.e.*, at full-load conditions of the circuit being used) lamps having a rated voltage of 110 volts may be used. This results in 60 per cent. of lamp life, 107 per cent. watts consumed, 116 per cent. light intensity and a color quality richer in the blue. The cost of operation (lamps plus energy) under these conditions is not an increase per unit of light, and permits the use of smaller bulbs for the same intensity and of a whiter light.

(4) The fixture-unit (see Fig. 1) has been sturdily

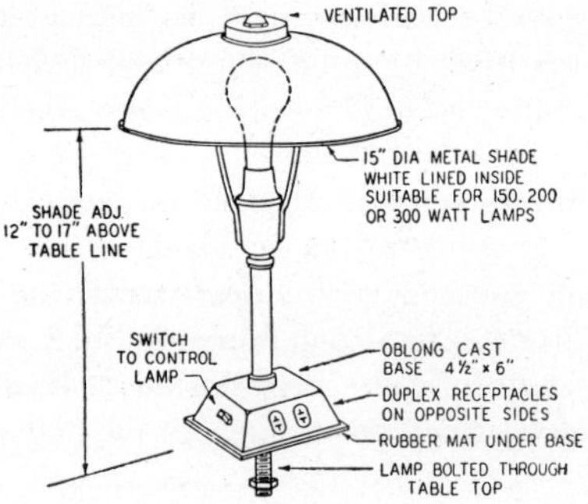


FIG. 1

built. It is flexible in construction, with parts readily accessible. The height of the unit may be adapted so that the lower edge of the reflector hood is fixed at some arbitrary distance above the table top; *e.g.*, 12 inches for tables using one or two microscopes and up to 17 inches for tables using 6 microscopes. The reflector hood is ventilated to provide better lamp life. Its stem is intended to be rigidly connected to the table top to facilitate concealed table wiring; but this may be modified at a slight additional cost to permit surface wiring or use as a portable unit. A rubber guard is placed between the base of the unit and the table top to protect the wiring from liquids accidentally spilled around the base.

(5) The duplex receptacle outlets have been located in the lamp base convenient for simultaneous use of four electrical appliances, such as stage warmers, micro incineration outfits, etc. A separate toggle switch controlling the lamp only is also located in the base of the unit.

(6) Finish of the unit is made durable by a dull black bakelite coated surface; but may be altered to match other requirements. The interior (*i.e.*, reflecting) surface of the hood is a matte white having a coefficient of reflection of 94 per cent. in comparison with a standard magnesia test surface.

The reflector hood is proportioned and located to minimize direct glare from the unit itself and also from units on neighboring tables. The lamp proper is placed in the "base-down" position and only a portion of the neck of the lamp is visible. When the inside frosted blue daylight lamp is used, this visible neck portion of the lamp is free from objectionable glare.

(7) Low cost is obtained because of the simplified design, use of standard fittings and standard lamps. This low initial cost is accompanied by decreased wiring costs when making the installation because both the lighting and receptacle outlet loads are furnished from the same branch circuit, thus making it unnecessary to provide one complete branch circuit for the lighting and another complete branch circuit for the receptacle outlets. This unit may be installed in an existing laboratory without prohibitive rewiring costs.

Laboratory replacements are in progress using this new fixture at the Marine Biological Laboratory, Woods Hole, Massachusetts, with the cooperation of the Biddle-Gaumer Company, Philadelphia, and the laboratory facilities of the Moore School of Electrical Engineering, University of Pennsylvania.

SAMUEL E. POND
OTTO MEIER, JR.
UNIVERSITY OF PENNSYLVANIA

## A SIMPLE SUBSURFACE THERMOMETER

IN order that fishermen may take advantage of the findings of recent research into the relationship of fish to water temperature it is necessary that a subsurface thermometer be used in the course of fishing operations. The difficulty so far has been to devise an instrument of low cost. The apparatus described here entails only the purchase of an ordinary minimum thermometer. Since reversals of temperature gradient are comparatively rare, especially in water of less than 50 fathoms, the minimum thermometer can be used for practical purposes to give the temperature at the greatest depth to which it may be lowered.

The precaution necessary in its use is that it must be maintained in the horizontal position throughout the operation of lowering and hauling; otherwise the double-headed pin may slide. As a rule the pin is not very sensitive and will usually stand a tilt of as much as 30° without sliding. The accompanying illustration shows the means of maintaining the thermometer in the horizontal position.

It is suspended between the opposing pulls of a submerged float and a weight. The lifting power of the float is considerably less than the sinking power of the weight. The figure shows the apparatus resting on the sea-bottom, the usual position at which a temperature will need to be taken. The hauling

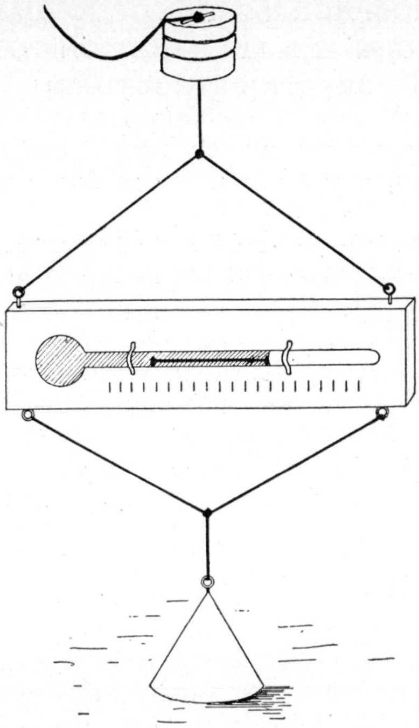

line is slack. Before lowering, the thermometer must be tilted so that the pin touches the meniscus. As the column contracts it is drawn back and left behind on subsequent expansion of the column as the thermometer reenters a zone of higher temperature. In the figure the size of the thermometer is exaggerated. In practice the distance from the thermometer to the sinker should be about a yard. On lowering, the bottom will be felt as in an ordinary sounding; and the observer has merely to wait a few minutes and haul up, the pull of the float maintaining the horizontal position throughout.

G. F. SLEGGS

MEMORIAL UNIVERSITY COLLEGE,
NEWFOUNDLAND

### A SPECIMEN MOUNT FOR INSECTS AND OTHER OBJECTS OF NATURAL HISTORY, ETC.

THE following description of a method of making permanent mounts of natural history specimens is based on work done at the Bermuda Biological Station in January to March in 1933, the plan being adopted during January with trials of different manipulations and with tests of the availability of each.

A dry cell is made by punching the center of a cardboard, bristol-board or similar material of different thicknesses or, where necessary, by building up to desired thickness by assembling several together, and then gluing a proper sized sheet of Cellophane to one side with duco or Cellophane adhesive, making a cell of sufficient depth to accommodate the object to be preserved. The cell and the object are dried by warmth and then the cell closed by applying adhesive to the upper side of the card and drawing the Cellophane down over the cell and pressing it to make a smooth adhesion and, if desired, turning a lap over on the under side and closing the ends by laps of the Cellophane. This makes a mount that is completely enclosed by moisture-proof Cellophane protected from mold, moisture, insect pests or other sources of deterioration and is especially applicable for insect or other collections in tropical or humid climates. Specimens so mounted are available for immediate and convenient examination or study with lens or microscope, either compound or binocular, and can be studied from either side or even at a considerable angle, since the thin layer of Cellophane does not interfere with extremely close study. Records or labels placed on the cards before sealing are also permanently protected by the transparent covering. Specimens mounted in this manner during January and exposed for a number of weeks to the attacks of ants, cockroaches and other pests and also to molds have shown no traces of injury, and it is believed that they will maintain their condition for an indefinite period. Delicate insects like mosquitoes and parasitic hymenoptera as well as insects of larger size are kept in perfect condition.

These mounts have been observed by a number of workers at the Bermuda Biological Station and have also been shown to a number of other specialists and all have agreed that the method seems to have a wide application and to be worthy of special notice.

HERBERT OSBORN

OHIO STATE UNIVERSITY

# SPECIAL ARTICLES

## THE ABSOLUTE MOTION OF THE SOLAR SYSTEM AND THE ORBITAL MOTION OF THE EARTH DETERMINED BY THE ETHER-DRIFT EXPERIMENT[1]

THE ether-drift experiment, first suggested by Maxwell in 1876 and made possible by Michelson's invention of the interferometer in 1881, though capable of being applied to the detection of the general absolute motion in space of the earth, was actually arranged for detetcing only the known orbital component of the earth's motion. For the first time, in 1925 and 1926, at Mount Wilson, the writer made observations of such extent and completeness that they were sufficient

[1] Read before the National Academy of Sciences, Washington, D. C., April, 1933.

for the determination of the absolute motion of the earth. These observations involved the making of about 200,000 single readings of the position of the interference fringes, and lead to more than 25,000 single values of both the right ascension and declination of the apex of the motion.

The ether-drift effect in the interferometer, as is well known, is a second order effect, and the observations correctly define the line in which the absolute motion takes place, but they do not determine whether the motion in this line is positive or negative.

At the Kansas City meeting in December, 1925, before the completion of the Mount Wilson observations, a report was made showing that the experiment gives evidence of a cosmic motion of the solar system, but which failed to identify the effects of the orbital motion, though it seemed that the observations should have been quite sufficient for this purpose.[2]

In the autumn of 1932, a reanalysis of the problem was made, based upon the alternative possibility that the motion of the solar system is in the cosmic line previously determined, but is in the opposite direction, being directed southward. This gives wholly consistent results, leading for the first time to a definite quantitative determination of the absolute motion of the solar system, and to a positive detection of the effect of the motion of the earth in its orbit.

The apex of the cosmic motion of the solar system is located in the right ascension of 4 h., 56 m., and in declination 70° 30′ south, diametrically opposite the apex previously announced. The velocity of the cosmic motion is determined by comparison with the known velocity, 30 kilometers per second, of the earth's orbital motion, and has the value of 208 kilometers per second. For some unexplained reason the observed displacement of the interference fringes in the interferometer corresponds to about one twentieth of the full velocity. This might be accounted for by an incomplete Lorentz contraction, or by Stokes's theory of a dragged ether.

The location of this apex is in the southern constellation Dorado, the Sword-Fish, and is about 20° south of the star, Canopus, the second brightest star in the heavens. It is in the midst of the famous Great Magellanic Cloud of stars. The apex is only about 6° from the pole of the ecliptic; thus the indicated motion of the solar system is almost perpendicular to the plane of the ecliptic. This suggests that the solar system might be thought of as a dynamic disk which is being pulled through a resisting medium, and which therefore sets itself perpendicular to the line of motion.

DAYTON C. MILLER

CASE SCHOOL OF APPLIED SCIENCE

[2] SCIENCE, 63: 433–443, 1926.

## THE PHOSPHORESCENCE OF SOLID NITROGEN AND ITS RELATION TO CRYSTAL STRUCTURE[1]

IN 1924 it was shown that solidified nitrogen, when exposed to electric rays, emitted an intense luminescence, consisting of bands, a number of which remained in the afterglow. Thus we have the case of a chemical element having the properties of a phosphorescent body.

When the temperature is raised above 35.5° K, solid nitrogen passes over from the phosphorescent α-form to another modification β, which has lost its phosphorescent power.

This phenomenon gives an important point of attack for the elucidation of the phosphorescent process. For this purpose the luminescent phenomena were analyzed and interpreted, and secondly the crystal structures of the two modifications of solid nitrogen were analyzed by means of Röntgen rays.

The analysis of the luminescent band-spectra led to the view that the bands appearing in the afterglow are due to "forbidden" electronic transitions from metastable molecular states. Thus the ε-system emitted from solid nitrogen corresponds to an electronic transition from the metastable A-state to the normal state of the nitrogen molecules.

The Röntgen-ray analysis gave for α-nitrogen a cubical structure, where the atoms of the molecular elements are arranged according to the space group $T^4$ and where the molecular axes have fixed positions in the space lattice. This structure lets us understand that the metastable states (which in the gaseous form are soon destroyed) in the α-form may be left undisturbed for a time sufficiently long for the forbidden transition to take place.

The analysis of the β-form was even more difficult, but finally it was found by us and independently by Ruheman that β-nitrogen has a hexagonal structure and that the elementary cell has dimensions nearly corresponding to a hexagonal closest packing of spheres.

For our problem it was of importance to go a step further and try to find out the positions of the individual atoms; but it appeared that the Röntgen reflections could only be accounted for by assuming the centers of the two atoms of a molecular element fall in the center of the molecules. This means that the individual atoms have no fixed positions and that the molecules rotate in the lattice. The rotating molecules require more space, which is seen from the fact that

[1] Read before the National Academy of Sciences, Washington, D. C., April, 1933.

the molecular volume by the transformation increases from 45.37 $Å^3$ to 47.12 $Å^3$. The rotating molecules also explain the rapid fall of the Röntgen-ray reflections with increasing deflection-angle. That molecular rotation can occur in the solid state is evident from the two modifications of hydrogen, and the problem has been theoretically treated by Paceling. In this connection, it is of interest to mention that the oxygen modification, stable above −229.5, was recently found by us to have a cubical lattice with rotating molecules. On the basis of our interpretation of the luminescence, we immediately see the reason why the β-modification has lost its phosphorescent power.

The rotational motions of the molecular elements of the lattice will disturb the metastable states just as in the gaseous system before the forbidden transitions can take place.

Reasons are given for the view that the excitation consists in a kind of dissociation process and that recombination takes place through certain metastable states. The phosphorescence, at any rate in our case, should be closely related to chemiluminescence, the main difference being that in the case of phosphorescence the reacting chemical substances are first to be formed through the excitation process.

L. VEGARD

## COUPLED REACTIONS IN BIOLOGICAL SYSTEMS

THE following is a summary of some preliminary investigations of two coupled reactions in biological systems: (1) The reduction of pyruvate to lactate by means of the energy of the anaerobic oxidation of formate to bicarbonate, and (2) the reduction of fumarate to succinate through the anaerobic oxidation of lactate to pyruvate. Toluene treated *B. coli* served as enzyme system for both reactions.

It was found in both instances that an intermediate substance was necessary which could be reduced at the locus where the one metabolite was oxidized, and reoxidized where the other was reduced. The intermediate substances were methylene violet for the lactate-pyruvate-formate-bicarbonate system, and methylene blue for the succinate-fumarate-lactate-pyruvate system. Without these mediators no reaction occurred.

These findings support the hypothesis of active centers proposed by Quastel.[1] They indicate that "half reactions" can not occur, and therefore the necessity for mediators, or carriers of energy from the point where energy is liberated to the point where it is used, when the energy-liberating and energy-absorbing mechanisms are separate; *i.e.*, that in the toluene treated *B. coli* there is no mechanism corresponding to metallic conduction. They show also that toluene treated *B. coli* contain no mediators capable of serving in the two systems studied.

Further, these experiments suggest that when oxygen is used *in vivo* the centers at which oxygen is bound must be intimately associated with the dehydrogenase mechanisms, or that one or more mediators similar in their function to reversible dyes intervene between the oxygen binding and the dehydrogenase mechanisms. These alternatives are not mutually exclusive. They may co-exist and even supplement each other, as possibly, for example, in the case of the non-iron-containing respiratory ferment system described by Warburg and Christian.[2]

HERMANN F. SCHOTT
HENRY BORSOOK
CALIFORNIA INSTITUTE OF TECHNOLOGY

[1] J. H. Quastel, *Biochem. Jour.*, 20: 166, 1926.

[2] O. Warburg and W. Christian, *Biochem. Zeits.*, 258: 496, 1933.

## SOME ASPECTS OF INTERMEDIARY PROTEIN METABOLISM

THE exogenous origin of creatine was first demonstrated by Levene and Kristeller in 1909 in their protein feeding experiments with cases of muscular dystrophy. In 1929, we reported[1] that glycine fed to patients with muscular dystrophy produced a marked rise in creatine excretion (confirmed by Thomas *et al.*,[2] and others), whereas glutamic acid and cystine had no effect. Studies with a number of other amino acids and various other substances were also reported. The effect of the removal of glycine and of glutamic acid from the metabolic mixture through the feeding of benzoic acid and phenylacetic acid, respectively, was investigated. It was found that the former produced a marked drop in creatine, while the latter was without effect. We are inclined to infer from our experiments that the feeding of brombenzene, which removes cysteine from the metabolic mixture, would be without effect on creatine excretion. Owing to the possible toxicity of the substance we intend to carry out suitable animal experiments instead. The chart shows only the essential results of a few representative experiments.[3]

*Hippuric acid, phenylacetyl glutamine and bromphenyl mercapturic acid formation:* The finding that the feeding of benzoic acid and phenyl acetic acid in proper amounts may have no effect upon the total nitrogen catabolism, although there are appreciable amounts of glycine and glutamic acid, respectively, lost to the body as a result of "Abfang" processes,

[1] *Am. Jour. Physiol.* 90, 296.

[2] *Z. physiol. Chem.* 214, 121.

[3] The significance of our detailed nitrogen and sulfur studies can not be discussed here, due to lack of space.

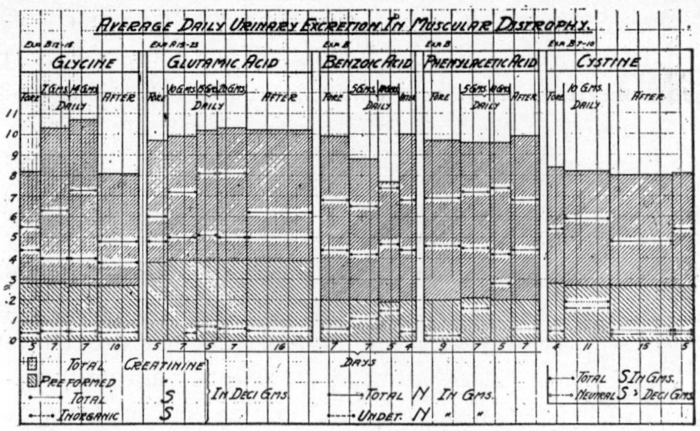


we believe, would indicate that these amino acids are originally present in the metabolic mixture in appreciable amounts and not especially synthesized for detoxification. This view is substantiated by our findings that creatine is markedly reduced by the benzoic acid and uninfluenced by the phenyl acetic acid and also by our observations regarding the respective influence of glycine, glutamic acid and cystine upon the excretion of creatine.

*The rôle of glutathione in intermediary protein metabolism:* It is a surprising fact that the only three amino acids—glycine, glutamic acid and cysteine—which seem to be available for processes of detoxification in the human are the same as those which form glutathione.[4] If glutathione supplies the amino acids for these processes of detoxification, then the unaltered level of protein catabolism accompanying such processes would seem to indicate that an appreciable part of normal protein catabolism goes *via* glutathione. It is possible that this view may be further supported by the finding that methionine replaces cystine in cystine deficient diets (Jackson and Block) and by the observation regarding the influence of methionine on the detoxification of brombenzene in such diets (White and Lewis).

One may conceive that the substances, which are being detoxified, first combine with the glutathione, thereby rendering it more unstable, as a result of which the detoxified compound splits off in combination with part of the original glutathione molecule. This change in stability would be in keeping with our findings regarding factors which influence the lability of the glutathione and cystine molecules.[5]

*E.g.,* phenylacetic acid would combine with the α-amino group of the glutamic acid radical of glutathione, following which the side chain splits off completely at the α-carbon of the cysteine liberating phenylacetylglutamine.

Shiple and Sherwin have called attention to the obviously close relationship between phenylacetylglutamine excreted by man and phenylacetylornithine excreted by birds. Ornithine in this latter compound may be conceived as derived from glutathione by a process in which the distant carbonyl group of the glutamic acid radical is reduced to form a nor-valine radical, which if split off together with the α-amino group of the cysteine would yield ornithine. Such mechanisms may have some bearing on uric acid and pyrrole formation. The possibility of glutathione being a source of ornithine is of interest in connection with the work of Krebs on urea formation and the reported activation of arginase by glutathione. The glutamic acid linkage in glutathione, which linkage is not easily split by enzymes, has long been considered as unusual. The reactivity of the distant carbonyl group of the glutamic acid radical in glutathione hardly has been investigated.

Bromphenyl mercapturic acid referred to above contains an acetyl group, which may be a remnant of the glutamic acid radical of glutathione, rather than the result of acetylation.

*Creatine formation:* Our experiments indicate that the guanidine group of creatine is synthetic in origin and that glycine is involved in creatine formation. Since glutathione is now known to contain glycine, its possible relation to creatine formation is obvious.

*Creatinine formation:* Creatinester hydrochloride and related compounds spontaneously form their respective anhydrides upon neutralization, the free esters apparently being quite unstable (unpublished experiments by Failey and Brand). This behavior of creatinester might suggest that in the animal organism creatinine is formed from a creatine compound in which the carboxyl group of creatine is not free but linked up as an ester, thioxy ester or amide.

Our finding in cystinuria[6] regarding an unusual creatinine metabolism accompanying this disturbance in sulfur metabolism is of interest in this connection. Studies regarding the therapeutic and metabolic effects of glutathione and of mixtures of its constituent amino acids in myopathies are being planned.

We shall consider more fully some of the conceptions of protein metabolism outlined above and their implications in a more detailed publication of our experiments.

This work was aided in part by a grant from the Chemical Foundation.

ERWIN BRAND
MEYER M. HARRIS

NEW YORK STATE PSYCHIATRIC INSTITUTE AND HOSPITAL

[4] This view has been expressed previously by others (Waelsch, H., *Arch. Exp. Path.* 156, 356; Power, F. W., Washington Meeting, Am. Chem. Soc. (1933)).

[5] *Jour. Biol. Chem.*, 70, 381.

[6] *Jour. Biol. Chem.*, 86, 315.

# SCIENCE

VOL. 77 — FRIDAY, JUNE 23, 1933 — No. 2008

*Electricity Released from Matter:* DR. KARL K. DARROW ... 591
*The Electron Theory of Metallic Conduction:* PROFESSOR J. C. SLATER ... 595
*Obituary:*
*Frederic Poole Gorham:* PROFESSOR H. E. WALTER. *Harry Hayward Charlton:* PROFESSORS EDGAR ALLEN, DEA B. CALVIN and M. D. OVERHOLSER ... 597
*Scientific Events:*
*International Museums Conference at Madrid; The Wawona Road Tunnel in the Yosemite National Park; Reduction in Federal Aid for the Land Grant Colleges; Curtailment of Scientific Work under the Government* ... 599
*Scientific Notes and News* ... 601
*Discussion:*
*An Electric Analogue of Vowel Production:* DR. HUGH SKILLING. *Nomenclature of the Vegetable Weevil:* PROFESSOR E. O. ESSIG. *Nomenclatorial Notes on Gastrotricha:* DR. CHARLES H. BLAKE. *Malvaceous Plants as a Cause of "Pink White" in Stored Eggs:* F. W. LORENZ, DR. H. J. ALMQUIST and PROFESSOR G. W. HENDRY. *Incomplete Nuclear Divisions in the Tapetum of the Eusporangiate Ferns:* DR. W. N. STEIL ... 604
*The Fourteenth Annual Meeting of the American Geophysical Union:* DR. JOHN A. FLEMING ... 607
*Scientific Apparatus and Laboratory Methods:*
*Mouth Pipette and Containers for Smaller Organisms:* EARL H. MYERS. *Microscope Lamp for Biological Laboratories:* DR. RICHARD M. HOLMAN 609
*Special Articles:*
*Infection in Mice Following Instillation of Vesicular Stomatitis Virus:* DR. PETER K. OLITSKY, DR. HERALD R. COX and DR. JEROME T. SYVERTON. *Active Immunization to Anthrax by Means of Heterophile Antigen:* GEORGE E. ROCKWELL ... 611
*Science News* ... 6

SCIENCE: A Weekly Journal devoted to the Advancement of Science, edited by J. MCKEEN CATTELL and published every Friday by

THE SCIENCE PRESS

New York City: Grand Central Terminal
Lancaster, Pa. — Garrison, N. Y.
Annual Subscription, $6.00 — Single Copies, 15 Cts.

SCIENCE is the official organ of the American Association for the Advancement of Science. Information regarding membership in the Association may be secured from the office of the permanent secretary, in the Smithsonian Institution Building, Washington, D. C.

# ELECTRICITY RELEASED FROM MATTER[1]

By Dr. KARL K. DARROW
BELL TELEPHONE LABORATORIES, NEW YORK, N. Y.

IN this situation I am reminded of something written a few years ago by Dr. Keen, the noted surgeon of Philadelphia. Dr. Keen was born in 1837 and he remembers men who were in their eighties when he was a child. Those men were born about 1760, and they in turn remembered men who were born around 1700 and whose lives therefore overlapped the life of Isaac Newton. So short is the history of physical science that three human lives suffice to span the entire time from our days back to the founder of modern physics! This is an extraordinary fact to think of, and no less extraordinary is the fact that *two* human lives suffice to cover almost the whole of the history of electrical science. One of these is the lifetime of our distinguished guest.

[1] Address delivered at the Massachusetts Institute of Technology, March 29, 1933, in connection with the celebration of Professor Elihu Thomson's eightieth birthday.

Try to think back, not 80 but 160 years, to the year 1773. Then, there was hardly anything deserving the name of electrical science—little more than an orderless assortment of quaint scraps of information about static charges, sparks and permanent magnets. Only one great electrician whose name we all remember lived wholly before that time; he was, of course, Gilbert. One other did most of his electrical work before that year, though he lived long past it; that, of course, was Benjamin Franklin. Now try to recall all the names of early electricians you possibly can. Unless you have lately been reading the history of electricity, I would wager that every one of them will belong to the 80 years following 1853. You will doubtless begin by running over the names of the electrical units. Well, Volta, Coulomb, Ampere, Gauss, Weber, Faraday and Henry all flourished in that period; and so did Galvani, Oersted, Cavendish and Davy.

These were the men who organized the science of electricity. They discovered the laws of attraction and repulsion of charged pithballs; the laws of attraction and repulsion of current-carrying wires; the laws of electrolysis. Above all, they achieved the synthesis of electricity and magnetism. Their work was so thorough and their results so extensive that one is amazed to-day to realize that they never had a chance of studying electricity outside of dense matter. Electricity to them was a mysterious and reticent entity which normally lurked in the depths of liquids and solids. It never seemed to want to come out into the open, and if it was forced into the open by the processes of thunderstorms or static machines, it hastened straight back into shelter with the utmost speed and violence.

Imagine a physicist who wants to study the nature and properties of water, but never has any at his disposal, except in damp sponges, moistened blotting-paper and crystals containing water of crystallization. Suppose him forbidden to squeeze the water out of the sponges, or steam it out of the blotting-paper, or distil it out of the crystals. This unfortunate person would be in somewhat the same position as the electrician of a century ago, except with regard to the spark. To find an image for the spark, we must concede him one more privilege: we must allow him to pump water out of a hidden reservoir through a pipe into a tank. He would like to be able to draw it off from the tank through a spigot in a small slow stream which he can easily observe and use. But, owing to some strange handicap, he can not do this; he can only pump water steadily into the tank until finally it gives way and bursts wide open and all the accumulated liquid rushes out in one terrific torrent, flooding all the neighborhood and threatening to drown the observer.

As usual, the simile is imperfect and has to be amended. We must suppose that the wall of the tank heals itself as soon as all the water has rushed out, and remains impervious until the internal pressure has mounted up again to a great height. Evidently what our physicist needs (since he can not have a spigot) is a tank which will crack open when there is only a little water in it, so that the outflow will be slow, and preferably just as slow as the influx of new water from the hidden reservoir which the pump is sending up. Now in my parable the tank is one of two metal electrodes which are connected to opposite poles of a battery. If the electrodes are separated by air of normal atmospheric density, the charge on the negative electrode can not burst out until it is built up to a hugely excessive amount. Then the wall of the metal is breached and the charge pours out with great violence until it is nearly all gone, after which the wall is closed and no more charge escapes until a new great excess is crowded into the electrode.

What can be done to persuade the charge to come out earlier? to come out gently and gradually and slowly, so that the flow can be steady, and easy to observe and to control? The answers to this question form all together one of the greatest achievements of the 80 years just past. I will recall them briefly to you.

The first answer was: form an arc in the open air between carbon or metal pole-pieces. This was given by Davy about 1815. It is not a convenient solution for one who wants to study electricity released from matter, because the electrical particles get badly tangled up with the molecules of the air almost as soon as they escape from the negative electrode.

The next answer was: put the electrodes into a tube and pump out the air until what is left has only about a thousandth of the normal atmospheric density. This is an admirable solution. Faraday made a good beginning, but for some reason or other relinquished this field of research. It was not properly developed until the eighteen-sixties and the eighteen-seventies. We ought first to remember the name of the man who made the tubes, for in 1860 the injunction "seal the electrodes into a tube" was not so easy to obey as now. This man was an itinerant glass-blower who earned his living by wandering from college to college in Germany and blowing such glass-ware as the professors of chemistry and physics might happen to want; his name was Geissler. In Bonn he found a professor who wanted low-pressure discharge-tubes for spectroscopic purposes, as the science of spectroscopy was then just coming into being. Reserving the spectra for himself, this professor turned over the task of studying the electrical properties of the discharge to one of his pupils. This pupil, whose name was Hittorf, obtained the chair of chemistry and physics in a small and half-starved college, where he stayed for fifty years. In 1869 he published the first of his great papers; I will quote its opening sentence: "The darkest part of the science of electricity to-day is incontrovertibly the process by which current is conducted through gases." Nowadays we should say just the opposite, and for that we should thank Hittorf; and also Crookes, and others after them, but Hittorf first of all.

When the density of the gas in the tube is about a thousandth of atmospheric density, there is a very striking and lovely pattern of colored lights and shades, luminous clouds and intervening gulfs of darkness; but these are signs that the electrical particles are getting tangled up with molecules of the gas, as in the arc. When the density is ten or a hundred times lower, they disappear and opposite the cathode one may see a green fluorescence spread over the glass wall of the tube. This is due to electrical rays proceeding from the cathode. They travel in straight lines perpendicularly outward from the cathode surface, for if a metal emblem is put in front of the cathode one sees its shadow black and sharply bounded upon the green expanse. If the cathode is bowl-shaped they are focused at the center of curvature of the bowl, and here they will melt even a metal like platinum, which proves that they carry energy with them. If a negatively charged object is brought up close to the tube (with certain precautions) the green flare moves off, showing that the rays are pushed away by the negative charge. If a magnet is brought up, the rays are shifted as a wire would be if it were carrying negative charge straight outward from the cathode.

These cathode rays are therefore a stream of negative charges, pouring out of the cathode and acquiring such energy and such momentum that they hammer themselves against the opposite wall of the tube. So rarefied is the gas that many of them go clear to the opposite wall unimpeded and unintercepted. It is because of the haste of their flight and the tenuity of the gas that they are able to move in straight lines across the hollow of the tube, and reveal themselves by making the glass of the wall fluoresce, and respond to magnets and to distant charges in ways which make their nature manifest. It is because of the haste of their flight and the tenuity of the gas that they remain what they are when they quit the metal: free negative electricity, released from dense matter, disconnected from atoms, unburdened and discarnate.

Rarefied as the gas may be in these experiments, it is actually responsible for the escape of electricity from the cathode. To use my former metaphor, it is the gas which breaks down the wall confining the electrical corpuscles inside the metal. It is preferable, however, to change the metaphor and to say that the gas helps the electricity over the wall. It does this best when its density is neither too high nor too low; at atmospheric density we get only the violent sparks, at very low density, nothing at all. Why this should be so, and how the gas achieves the feat of helping the electricity out of the metal, are very intricate questions to which the answers are only just beginning to be clear. Fortunately it happens that there are two ways of persuading electricity to come out of a metal, which involve no gas at all and are easy to understand. Both of these were discovered in the eighties. You know the agents involved; they are heat and light.

As for the efficacy of heat: various early savants observed phenomena which we with our riper knowledge can explain by it, but there is strong reason for giving the honor of discovery to a man who, as chairmen say, "needs no introduction"—Edison. He in 1884 was working with his carbon-filament lamps, these pre-war "incandescent lights" which nowadays, I suppose, must look as quaintly old-fashioned to people in their twenties as a kerosene lamp to people in their forties. The filament of carbon, enclosed in a pear-shaped bulb evacuated to the degree then called "high vacuum," rose in a single fragile arch from its leads in the socket, and the current was meant to flow the entire length of the arch. Edison, however, noticed that a good share of the current was evading its duty, leaking out of the negative end of the arch and sneaking across the hollow of the tube to the positive end. This he proved by making lamps with an extra lead, connected inwardly to a metal plate projecting into the hollow space between the bases of the arch, outwardly through an ammeter to the positive filament lead; there was a flow of current through the ammeter.

This was one of the great observations of history. On its result repose essential portions of the art and science of telephony over long distances, whether by wire or wireless; broadcasting; many devices for remote control; a thousand ingenious feats of engineering, ten thousand delicate aids to detection of light and sound and electricity, to measurement and research. In the electric lamp a mere annoyance, this "thermionic effect" is the vital principle of those other dimmer lamps not meant for lighting, the tubes of the radio sets now almost as familiar as electric light itself.

At this point of the narration almost any layman would assume that Edison himself went onward and discovered all these things. Not so! this was one of the occasions when the race was not to the swift, nor the battle to the strong. The keen inventor thought so little of this thing which had lain across his path that he showed it to a traveling British electrical engineer named Preece, and not only showed it to him but made up some extra tubes for him to take home and study at his leisure. Preece and Fleming studied the effect with care; but, so foreign to the human mind was then the idea of free electricity, they could not shake off the idea that the carbon filament must be projecting its own substance forth into space, with negative charges clinging to the atoms. Crookes entertained the same idea about the cathode rays in his low-pressure discharge-tubes. There are animals which are obliged to live successive stages of their growth in different media, first water and then air. Somewhat the same destiny was imposed on the thermionic effect as a division of human knowledge; born in the workshop of an inventor, started in life by electrical engineers, it attained to maturity in the academic world.

J. J. Thomson fostered the study of the effect at the English Cambridge, but turned it over in the main to his pupil, Richardson, as in an earlier generation Plücker had entrusted the low-pressure discharge to Hittorf. Richardson discovered the major laws of the effect and showed that they permit a beautifully lucid theory. We are to think of the metal as populated by a swarm of corpuscles of negative charge—henceforth I will no longer avoid the word "electrons"—which rush about in thermal agitation and beat in an incessant patter against the wall of the metal. This "wall" is a metaphor for the force of attraction whereby the positive charges moored to the atoms of metal pull back on the electrons which are trying to escape, and which is in fact confined to a thin region along the surface of the metal. Some of the electrons are moving rapidly enough to overcome this pull, and they climb over the wall; but at room temperature their number is imperceptibly small. As the metal is warmed up, its heat is shared by the electrons, and the fraction which is able to escape increases steadily. Eventually the outflow becomes a perceptible current which rises rapidly with further rise of temperature. Its law of increase is like that of the vapor pressure of a liquid or a solid, and thus we are justified in saying that electrons evaporate out of a metal.

To expel electrons from a metal by heating the entire bulk is an effective way, but in a sense it is crude; we lavish quantities of energy on the atoms of the metal in order that the particles of electricity also may receive some. It would be neater to impart the energy directly to the electrons without wasting any of it upon the atoms. A distant approximation to this ideal is attained by sending a beam of light against the metal. It consists of corpuscles of energy, the so-called "photons"; and every now and then one of these will dive through the surface and yield up its total energy to an electron. This is the so-called "photoelectric effect."

The energy of the photons is greater, the smaller the wave-length of the light, and is calculable from the wave-length. With light of the visible spectrum, what the electron receives is not sufficient to help it over the wall unless the metal is one of those which have walls abnormally low—the alkali metals and their alloys, and a few others. With light of the remote ultra-violet, the photons have energy enough to enable electrons to climb out of any metal whatever. The necessary energy, or (to preserve the metaphor) the height of the wall, can be determined by observing the wave-length of the light which is just able to release electrons from the metal; for the energy of the photons of this light is the same as the quantity in question and it is calculable from the wave-length. The height of the wall can also be estimated from the rate at which the thermionic current increases with rise of temperature. The estimates by the two methods agree very well and this contributes very much to our confidence in the theoretical picture. The establishment of this picture by the study of the photoelectric effect is largely due to a happy alliance of the insight of Einstein with the experimental skill of Richardson, K. T. Compton and Millikan.

Now a few words about the qualities of negative charge when it has been released from matter and is available to our experimental arts. You are of course aware that it consists of corpuscles, the electrons of which I have already spoken, of which the charge and mass are definite and known. The exact evaluation of this charge and this mass, $e$ and $m$ as they are familiarly called, has been a great experimental problem of the early twentieth century. To be precise, its period overlaps slightly with the nineteenth century (J. J. Thomson having made the earliest fairly good estimates, towards 1895), and also with the future, since measurements are still being made; but probably the first quarter of the twentieth century will always be remembered as the time of the achievement. Both $e$ and $m$ are very small by ordinary standards; upwards of $10^{19}$ electrons are required to make up the charge which passes per second through the filament of an incandescent lamp, and upwards of $10^{27}$ to make up the mass of a gram. The eighteenth-century savants who spoke of electricity as a "subtle fluid" were well inspired, in so far as they meant negative electricity; its particles are the most nimble, agile, penetrating and insinuating of all that are known, except perhaps the corpuscles of light, which belong to another category of existence altogether.

Electrons in their passage through vacuum are of course invisible; they are perceived only when their flight has come to an end, as, for instance, by striking upon a fluorescent screen or a photographic plate or entering a metallic collector. Unimpeded flight is like a dreamless sleep, perceived only because it was unperceived while it lasted, known only when it is over. Nevertheless we can trace the paths of electron-streams through vacua with confidence, by noting where they end. It is interesting also to know that the paths of electron-streams may be made visible by using a suitable small density of gas. Occasional corpuscles elicit flashes of light from atoms which they strike, and these mark out the path which the main body of unimpeded corpuscles is following, as the path of an army through a hostile country by night could be marked by the flashes of shots fired by natives on whom occasional troopers happened to stumble.

The most pleasing feature of these corpuscles is that, in large-scale electric and magnetic fields such as we can make in the laboratory, they behave just in the way they should in order to account for the fundamental laws of electricity in dense matter discovered in the eighty years preceding 1853. Electrons repel one another like negatively charged pithballs; electrons dashing past a magnet are displaced like a current-carrying wire. (Indeed it is only because of this that we are able to define and measure the charge and mass of an electron). Perhaps this sounds self-evident, hardly worth the verifying, let alone the saying. However, there is no law of nature to the effect that things which seem self-evident are necessarily found to be true. I will tell you of a case where something not self-evident occurred.

Suppose we send a beam of electrons against a crystal. The crystal is an assemblage of atoms regularly arranged. Each atom is a collection of electric particles roaming in vacant space. The sizes of these particles are so small compared with the spaces between them that each atom may be regarded for the present purpose as a narrow empty region where there is an electric field (and also a magnetic field) varying rapidly from point to point. The crystal is an assemblage of these narrow concentrated fields, tens of millions of them to the linear inch. We might say that it is a region of space occupied by a rhythmic pattern of field strengths. This is traversed by the electron-stream, which behaves in a most remarkable way, as Davisson and Germer found. It behaves as though it were attended by a train of waves, and the crystalline pattern seized upon these waves and guided them according to the well-known laws of wave motion, while the corpuscles trailed along after them.

This is a notion difficult to admit, for we are not accustomed to water-waves or sound-waves dragging massive bodies with them, although there is a striking analogy to be found in the phenomena of light. One immediately inquires whether the concept of the waves would serve in the cases of electron-streams traversing large-scale electric and magnetic fields, such as we know so well in the laboratory. So it does; the deflections of electron-streams in such fields as these can be explained by supposing that the fields act directly upon wave-trains, which accompany the corpuscles and steer them. In these cases by themselves the idea of waves would be superfluous, since we can explain the phenomena as well without them. But when electrons pass through crystals the waves are necessary to account for the phenomena, and this obliges us to imagine them always. It is by no means easy to adapt one's thought to the conception of corpuscles guided by waves, nor to the further and highly abstracted refinements which this notion has undergone in the last few years. But I came here with the intention of speaking to you not of the perplexities of theory, but of the clarities of experiment; and I must not continue to impair your memories of these.

# THE ELECTRON THEORY OF METALLIC CONDUCTION[1]

By Professor J. C. SLATER

MASSACHUSETTS INSTITUTE OF TECHNOLOGY

ELECTROMAGNETIC theory may be broadly divided into two parts: the theory of electric and magnetic fields and the theory of the electrical structure of matter, of conductors, insulators, magnetic bodies, charges, currents. Both branches have undergone profound changes since the time of Maxwell. The electromagnetic field has been of interest particularly in cases of very rapid oscillations, the waves of light and x-rays. There, from the photoelectric effect and other similar phenomena, has arisen the idea that in some respects light seems to behave in a corpuscular way, its energy being concentrated in particles of energy or photons. The electromagnetic waves of Maxwell and Hertz have but a statistical connection with the motion of these photons. The discreteness of the photons is shown beautifully by such a device as a Geiger counter, which can be made to register each photon as it comes along. In weak radiation of high frequency, as x-rays or gamma rays, no one after seeing the experiment can doubt the corpuscular nature inherent somewhere in the phenomenon. But the photons get smaller and smaller as the frequency decreases, the energy of a photon being proportional to the frequency, according to Planck's famous equation

$$\text{energy} = h\nu.$$

Thus by the time we reach the frequencies with which practical electricians deal, frequencies which even in these days of short wave radio are only about $10^{11}$ cycles per second, the photons are so excessively small that any electromagnetic field of reasonable strength contains enormously many photons, so many that their individual effect is entirely lost. We deal with them only statistically, and we may without error replace the discrete photons by the continuous field of Maxwell. For this reason, unless he is dealing with photoelectric cells or some such device, the electrical engineer need hardly come in contact with the theory of photons.

The developments of the other side of electrical theory, the electrical structure of matter, on the other hand, are, and even more promise to be, of great

[1] Address delivered at the Massachusetts Institute of of Technology, March 29, 1933, in connection with the celebration of Professor Elihu Thomson's eightieth birthday.

practical importance. But three examples need be mentioned to make this clear: the development of magnetic theory and magnetic materials, with application to submarine cable construction, the development of the theory of dielectrics, with application to insulating materials, and the development of the theory of electrical conduction and of electrical emission from conductors, with application to vacuum tubes. It can not be claimed that these developments have all been direct results of the theories, but at least they have all had theoretical guidance, and as theory becomes more powerful, as it is doing all the time, it may be expected to serve more and more usefully in suggesting practical advances.

The whole theory of the electrical nature of matter, of course, goes back to the discovery that matter is made of electrons and nuclei. It was really an enormous gain, in clearness of thinking as well as in more practical ways, when it became possible to think of particles of electric charge, instead of states of strain in the ether and such ideas. And physicists lost no time in developing electron theories of matter. Lorentz, doing most of his work shortly before and after 1900, was a leader in this, as were Drude and others. The essence of Lorentz's theory was extremely simple. An electric current consists of the flow of electrons. Since conductors carry current, then, they must contain electrons, free to move from point to point. Experiments on electrons in a vacuum show that they obey the ordinary laws of mechanics, their acceleration being proportional to the force acting on them. Then if there is a difference of potential between two points in a metal, and consequently a force acting on the electrons, they would accelerate, speeding up without limit, if there were not some other force to balance the field. Lorentz made the natural assumption that this other force was of the nature of a viscous resistance, resulting from collisions between the electrons and the atoms. If molecules of a gas, representing the electrons, were moving through a region filled with fixed atoms, the collisions would exert a resistance proportional to the velocity of drift of the electrons, whose magnitude is easily calculated. The motion of the electrons is then very much like the falling of raindrops under gravity. Starting from rest, they are at first rapidly accelerated, but soon they come to a constant speed of fall, in which the gravitational force just balances the viscous force of resistance of the air. This latter force is proportional to the velocity, for small speeds. Hence the external force is proportional to the speed of drift. Similarly in the metal there is proportionality between the electric field and the drift velocity or electric current, and this is the origin of Ohm's law. Lorentz was able by arguments similar to those used in kinetic theory in discussing viscosity, to find the conductivity in terms of the mean free time of electrons between collisions and other simple properties of the system. Thus, let the mean free time be $T$. Since the acceleration measures the increase of velocity per unit time, the velocity of each electron will increase by an amount $aT$ in the direction of acceleration during its free time. The mean additional velocity imparted by the field will be half this, or $aT/2$. But by Newton's law the force, which is $eE$, if $e$ is the charge on the electron, $E$ the applied electric field, will equal the mass times the acceleration. Hence $a = eE/m$, the mean velocity of drift is $\frac{eT}{2m}E$, and the electric current density, which is the number of electrons per unit volume times the charge of an electron times the mean velocity, is $\frac{Ne^2}{m}\frac{T}{2}E$. The factor multiplying $E$ is just the conductivity. Lorentz's actual derivation differs from this simple one only in taking account of the variation in free time from one electron to another, the fact that they move in all different directions with different speeds, and such refinements.

In explaining conductivity, Lorentz's theory was perfectly successful, though without independent methods of finding the quantities $N$ and $T$ it could not lead to any new predictions. But there was one rather fatal difficulty with it. Lorentz assumed the electrons to be just like the molecules of a perfect gas, and in particular to have the same temperature, energy and specific heat as a perfect gas. Yet experimentally the specific heat of metals was found to be such that the electrons could have practically no specific heat. That is to say, the experiments indicate that the energy of the electrons does not vary appreciably with temperature, since the specific heat is the increase of energy per degree rise of temperature. This was entirely at variance with Lorentz's theory. It was also in apparent disagreement with the next important experimental and theoretical advance in the theory of metals after Lorentz, namely, the discovery of thermionic emission and its explanation by Richardson.

It was discovered by Edison that metals heated to red heat or beyond emitted electrons, the number increasing very rapidly with the temperature. Richardson provided an explanation of this. He supposed that electrons, like molecules evaporating from a liquid, were pulled back into the metal by a surface force if they tried to escape. As a result, only the fastest electrons could escape, those whose energy was greater than a certain minimum, the energy lost in passing through the surface, or heat of evaporation, since even after escaping the electron must have some energy left. Now the number of electrons with energy greater than a given value $\varphi$ increases very rapidly as the temperature increases, according to a formula containing the factor $e^{-\phi/kT}$, where $k$ is Boltzmann's constant, $T$ the temperature, and this factor is the leading term in the experimental equation giving the thermionic current as function of temperature. This equation is deduced on the basis of electrons sharing in the temperature energy, as the molecules of a gas or liquid would, from which we get our analogy of evaporation. And thus its success in predicting the results of experiment seemed to provide a verification of just that feature of Lorentz's theory which was shown by the experiment of the specific heat to be untenable. For some time the theory of metals was in a very difficult and contradictory state, on account of these facts.

The difficulty was solved by means of the wave mechanics, through the work of many physicists, including Pauli and Sommerfeld. The deduction from the specific heat is shown to be essentially correct: the energy of the free electrons is practically independent of temperature, the electrons possessing even at the absolute zero of temperature a rather large amount of kinetic energy, of the order of magnitude of fifteen volts. The principle leading to this result is the same principle, developed by Pauli, which leads to the structure of the atoms, and the periodic table of the elements. An atom contains electrons in a number of shells, some of low energy near the nucleus, some of the higher energy farther out toward the periphery of the atom. We should naturally suppose that at the absolute zero of temperature all electrons would fall into the shell of lowest energy, to liberate all the energy available. They do not do this, however, and this is explained by Pauli's exclusion principle, which limits the number of allowable electrons in each shell, excluding further electrons from entering the shell. The result is that even at the absolute zero the electrons of the atom contain much kinetic energy. The exclusion principle similarly prevents the electrons of the metal from losing all their energy at the absolute zero. Further, a result of the distribution of velocities is that the electron speeds are practically independent of temperature, as the electrons in an atom are practically independent of temperature. Thus the low specific heat of electrons is explained.

The low specific heat, and at the same time the possibility of thermionic emission, are most easily shown to be compatible by using Fermi's distribution of velocities, which is found to be correct rather than Boltzmann's, which is at the basis of the ordinary statistics. The ordinary formula, on which, for instance, Richardson's equation is based, states that the chance of finding an electron with energy $E$ is proportional to $\sqrt{E}\, e^{-E/kT}$. But Fermi's formula is $\frac{\sqrt{E}}{e^{(E-E_0)/kT}+1}$, reducing to the other if the term $+1$ in the denominator is neglected. For any low temperature, the exponential is practically zero if $E$ is less than $E_0$, infinite if $E$ is greater than $E_0$, so that the formula gives $\sqrt{E}$ for $E$ less than $E_0$, zero for $E$ greater than $E_0$. This is a distribution independent of temperature, explaining the lack of specific heat. The few fastest electrons, however, which could escape, are those for which $E-E_0$ is so great that the exponential is large compared with 1, the formula reducing to Boltzmann's for these fast electrons, so that Richardson's derivation of the thermionic equation can be used practically without change. Some changes are encountered, however, when we try to apply the theory to such things as emission from coated filaments.

The theory as we have sketched it removes the great difficulty with the previous treatment. But in its present development it goes far beyond this. For the first time, it is now proving possible to connect the theory of metallic conduction with the atomic structure of the metal. We are beginning to get some idea of how the electrons actually move between the atoms, what sort of collisions they make, how their behavior is connected with the particular sort of metal we are considering. This theory is far from usable at the present time, but it is rapidly developing, along with similar theories of magnetism and of other electrical properties. It can not be doubted that in a very few years the theory of metallic conduction will be so well worked out that we can describe the mechanism with a great deal of certainty and apply the results in practical ways. The theory is bound to become of more and more use in electrical engineering, and electrical engineers, taking their guidance as in the past from the fundamental discoveries and advances of physics, will not be slow to take advantage of it.

# OBITUARY

## FREDERIC POOLE GORHAM

FREDERIC POOLE GORHAM, pioneer in bacteriology, nationally-known authority in sanitation and public health, faithful civic servant for many years and great teacher, died suddenly of a heart attack on June 4 in his sixty-third year.

For forty years Professor Gorham served his Alma Mater as teacher, administrator and director of research. He has left his enduring mark on literally thousands of Brown men, particularly on many generations of freshmen, who, entering the class in "Biology 1, 2," oftentimes with hesitancy or indifference, soon came under the spell of his sane enthusiasm.

Of the fifty-six students who have attained the Ph.D. degree at Brown University during the past thirty-two years, twenty-six did their thesis work under his immediate direction. No other member of the Brown faculty has equalled this record. A similar percentage of those who have been granted the master's degree owe their inspiration to his scholarly and sympathetic guidance. These advanced students of biological science have gone out to occupy positions of service and responsibility and they form a living monument of ever-increasing importance to Professor Gorham's memory.

The various extra-academic services to city and state which he has rendered in his long career have been signalized by continuous effectiveness to the very end. For thirty-four years he was bacteriologist for the Providence Department of Health; since 1914 he has been deputy milk inspector for the city; for twenty years he has been an active member of the Rhode Island Shellfish Commission; he was president of the R. I. Tuberculosis Association and secretary of the board of directors of the R. I. State Sanatorium at Wallum Lake; from 1925 to 1931 he served on the Metropolitan Park Commission, and since 1913 he has organized and directed the control of the mosquito nuisance in Providence, expending in this work over a quarter of a million of dollars to the satisfaction of every one concerned.

In all these different exacting activities, which have absorbed vacation-time as well as lengthened every day of the university year, in the face of frequent discouraging lack of appreciation and in spite of the inevitable interference of petty politics, Professor Gorham has steadily and serenely gone ahead with singleness of purpose and unquestioned integrity in the execution of his unselfish philosophy of life.

To quote Dr. H. L. Barnes, superintendent of the state sanatorium, "The time and abilities which he devoted to the State Sanatorium from a busy life, and without compensation, set the highest standard of disinterested public service." And Dr. C. V. Chapin, with whom he worked for years in the health department of Providence, said of him, "He was a man of wonderful judgment and thoroughly grounded in public health work. The beginning of practical bacteriology was Professor Gorham's examination of throats in 1895 for diphtheria control. His knowledge and advice were invaluable in the development of bacteriology. I couldn't say too much for Professor Gorham's work."

He was a fellow of the American Public Health Association and of the American Association for the Advancement of Science. He was chairman of the laboratory section of the American Association of Pathologists and Bacteriologists; past president (1907) of the Society of American Bacteriologists; president of the R. I. Tuberculosis League; member of American Naturalists; Washington Academy of Sciences; Boston Bacteriological Club; Providence Engineering Society, and honorary member of the Rhode Island Medical Society and the Providence Medical Association. Since 1926 he has been the head of the biological department in Brown University.

Among his colleagues and the many students everywhere who have known him intimately it is not so much what he has accomplished during his long useful career, important as that has been, which will be retained in precious memory, as the character of the man himself, a buoyant soul, a true gentleman, a faithful friend.

H. E. Walter

## HARRY HAYWARD CHARLTON

Dr. Charlton, since 1920 a member of the staff of the department of anatomy of the University of Missouri, died suddenly on the evening of May 31, from complications following an operation. His death came on the eve of his appointment as chairman of the department of anatomy.

Dr. Charlton was born at Allston, Massachusetts, on May 18, 1887. His childhood was spent in Nova Scotia. He then returned to the United States, and his high-school work was done in Lowell, Mass. He received his A.B. degree from Lebanon Valley College, Pennsylvania, in 1914 and the degree of master of arts at Yale in 1916.

During the war Dr. Charlton was retained at Yale as technical assistant in pathology, associated with the Gas Defense Service in the Yale Army School. He served as head of the department of anatomy of Fordham Medical School in 1918–19. He returned to Yale and completed his work for the degree of doctor of philosophy in 1920. He was appointed assistant professor of anatomy at the University of Missouri in 1920, associate professor in 1922 and professor in 1931. He served as secretary of the Missouri Anatomical Board from 1922 to the time of his death.

Dr. Charlton's principal interest in research was concerned with the comparative anatomy of the brain, to which study he made several worth-while contributions. He spent several summers in study at the Biological Laboratory, at Woods Hole, Mass., and spent a year on sabbatical leave at Professor Ariens-Kappers' Neurological Laboratory in Amsterdam.

Dr. Charlton will be remembered by his students as a sincere, conscientious teacher, exacting but always fair in his evaluation of students' work.

He is survived by his widow, Mary Polson Charlton, and a daughter, Barbara.

EDGAR ALLEN
DEA B. CALVIN
M. D. OVERHOLSER
UNIVERSITY OF MISSOURI

# SCIENTIFIC EVENTS

## INTERNATIONAL MUSEUMS CONFERENCE AT MADRID

ACCORDING to *Museum News*, the international museums conference at Madrid has been moved from the fall of 1933, as previously announced, to April 4, 1934. It will continue for about ten days and will consider problems of museums and collections of art, archeology, history and popular art.

The subjects to be discussed have been announced by the International Museums Office as follows:

Museum Architecture: (1) General principles of construction, plans and materials, special requirements imposed by purposes of the particular museum, site, environment, arrangements for expansion. (2) Construction of a museum in a historic architectural ensemble. (3) Adaptation of old buildings for museum use.

Arrangement: (1) Exhibition halls. (2) Conference rooms and auditoriums, children's rooms, information and sales rooms. (3) Courts and gardens. (4) Libraries and document rooms, offices. (5) Laboratories, shops for making casts, for photography and restoration. (6) Storage and handling. (7) Caretakers' rooms.

Special Questions: (1) Natural and artificial lighting. (2) Cleaning, heating, ventilation, air conditioning. (3) Protection against fire, theft, earthquake, etc. (4) Custodian service. (5) Floor covering. (6) Coat rooms, buffets, seats, rails and other comforts for visitors.

Presentation of Collections: (1) General considerations in regard to effective exhibition, dimensions and orientation of halls, covering and color of walls, etc. (2) Permanent and temporary exhibitions, exhibits within and without the museum. (3) Presentation of collections—as a whole, selected objects, paintings, combination of paintings, sculpture, furniture, etc., chronological presentation, period rooms and reconstitution of architectural and other ensembles, new acquisitions. (4) Problems caused by enlargement of collections by purchase, gift and bequest, and periodical disposal of unnecessary material. (5) Organization of stored, reserve and study collections. (6) Plans and signs for guidance of visitors. (7) Numbering and labeling. (8) Exhibit material—moldings, cases, hanging methods, protection against vibration, frames, pedestals, movable partitions, rails, etc. (9) Classification and conservation material for drawings, prints, coins, medals, textiles, etc. (10) Publications.

Loans and Exchanges between Museums: Possibilities of collaboration between museums of the same country and between museums of different countries.

An Exhibition of Museum Documents: Plans, photographs, sketches, publications, posters, publicity material.

## THE WAWONA ROAD TUNNEL IN THE YOSEMITE NATIONAL PARK

THE recently completed 4,230-foot Wawona Road Tunnel in Yosemite National Park, California, was formally dedicated on June 10. Secretary of the Interior Harold L. Ickes was unable to be present at the ceremonies, but by means of electrical transcription those gathered in Yosemite National Park heard his message of greeting as delivered in Washington.

The new Wawona Road, which extends from near the foot of Bridal Veil Falls to the Mariposa Grove of Big Trees, is approximately 28 miles in length, is on a six per cent. grade, has wide, easy curves, and can be traveled any day in the year. It was built jointly by the National Park Service of the Department of the Interior and the Bureau of Public Roads of the Department of Agriculture.

The driving of the Wawona Tunnel was begun in January, 1931, and was completed in one year. Blasted through cliffs of solid granite, it is 28 feet wide and 20 feet high. The tunnel has three ventilating shafts drilled horizontally to the cliff face. The largest shaft is at the center of the tunnel and contains three large electrically-driven fans which operate automatically, according to the percentage of carbon monoxide gas in the air. These fans are capable of handling 300,000 cubic feet of air per minute. Lights of 4,000 lumens set in deep-bowl reflectors in the roof of the tunnel to within 180 feet of each end give a warm mellow light free from glare. For 180 feet at each end, bulbs of 6,000 lumens give a brighter light to permit vision adjustment.

Parking space for a hundred cars is available near the east portal of the tunnel.

One of the main features of the dedicatory ceremonies was a historical pageant of progress, portraying the evolution of transportation in the Yosemite since its discovery in 1851. The pageant included aboriginal Indians on foot, prospectors with burros, the first tourist horseback parties, lumbering wagons and horse stages, motor stages and 1933 automobiles.

## REDUCTION IN FEDERAL AID FOR THE LAND GRANT COLLEGES

ACCORDING to a report by Science Service, federal grants for science and education made to the states are reduced by $3,917,000 through the reorganization order sent to the Congress by President Roosevelt. The payments for agricultural experiment stations, the cooperative agricultural extension work and the endowment and maintenance of colleges for the benefit of agricultural and mechanic arts, all educational and research funds granted to the states and territories by the federal government are reduced or "abolished" by 25 per cent. These payments, as authorized for the fiscal year 1934 to begin on July 1, amount to $13,119,096 from the Department of Agriculture and $2,550,000 from the Department of the Interior, a grand total of $15,669,096. Under the curtailment ordered to be effective 60 days from the date of the order, June 10, the funds available will be $11,750,000 in round figures.

Under the federal grants for experiment stations much of the scientific research for agriculture accomplished in the various states in the past three decades has been carried on. The appropriations lost to experiment stations under the order amount to $1,095,222. The extension work done cooperatively with the states, supported in part by the federal funds now reduced by 25 per cent., carried the results of the scientific research to the farmers. County agricultural agents are the embodiment of this educational service. The loss is $1,018,000.

The state universities that have carried higher education to thousands in the opening years of this century are supported in part by the Morrill and Smith-Lever Acts, the funds of which are now cut by a quarter of the appropriated amount. Loss to this educational work is $1,804,024.

Federal aid to land-grant colleges has flowed partly through the Department of Agriculture and partly through the Department of the Interior, the latter having been made the agency of a flat sum of $50,000 for the support of instruction in agriculture and the mechanic arts in each state. It seems probable that the curtailment of these funds, which are of long-standing authorization under the Morrill, Hatch, Smith-Lever and other acts, was made by executive order rather than under other provisions of the economy act passed early in the Roosevelt legislative program because by making it a matter of reorganization the 25 per cent. cuts can be made effective for subsequent years rather than just for this year.

## CURTAILMENT OF SCIENTIFIC WORK UNDER THE GOVERNMENT

A FURTHER wire report by Science Service states that under the economy act, Budget Director Lewis Douglas, acting for President Roosevelt, is directing still further cuts in the funds for science and education. This results in certain scientific bureaus having for 1934 less than half of what they had two years ago. Inevitably this will mean separations for many highly trained scientific workers engaged in work of great public benefit and extreme salary reductions for many of those who retain jobs. The exact cuts that will go into effect on July 1 are difficult to ascertain, as in some instances even bureau chiefs do not know what funds they will have for the fiscal year that begins in a couple of weeks.

It is known that Secretary of Agriculture Wallace and Assistant Secretary Tugwell are making a strenuous fight to continue the present scientific research for agriculture that they consider to be as necessary for agriculture's return to health as the economic measures being put into effect.

In the Department of Commerce, the U. S. Coast and Geodetic Survey is likely to have its funds cut but little under the figures of the 1934 appropriation bill and it may be selected to administer some of the public works appropriations available under the act just passed. The Bureau of Fisheries will have some cuts, but these are not believed to be serious.

But the Bureau of Standards seems to have been selected for heavy cuts, to such an extent that that bureau may have only about 40 per cent. of the money that it had in 1932. About $3,000,000 spent in 1932 is reduced to $1,336,000 for the 1934 fiscal year, the budget bureau demanding about a third reduction in the slightly more than $2,000,000 available in 1934 appropriation bill.

The Bureau of Mines, also in the Department of Commerce, is to be trimmed to about $1,100,000, whereas the appropriation bill for 1934 carried $1,514,300, and these appropriations for 1934 now reduced were considerably less than the 1932 funds spent for the benefit and safety of the important and valuable mining industry and its resources.

The Geological Survey in the Department of the Interior is also likely to suffer heavily. In 1932 it spent $3,141,000; the 1934 appropriation act provided $1,992,000 and eliminated funds for some of the geological research work of greatest fundamental importance. It is understood that the economy cuts will leave only $1,476,000 available. Some of the important work in topographic mapping, water resources and mineral resources may be salvaged by utilization of public works funds, but it is feared that many of the staff will have to be dismissed and 25 to 30 per cent. of the personnel will be lost through dismissal, retirement or that they will be forced to take unusual amounts of leave without pay.

A weakening of our national defenses against disease is imminent through cuts in the U. S. Public Health Service. A fund of $333,650 for prevention of epidemics is scheduled for reduction to $157,000 and similar cuts in other research funds are contemplated.

# SCIENTIFIC NOTES AND NEWS

DR. ALBERT EINSTEIN, who has been visiting the University of Oxford as a research student of Christ Church College, delivered the Herbert Spencer Lecture on June 10 on "The Method of Theoretical Physics." Dr. Einstein will lecture in Belgium during the summer vacation.

THE committee of the Paris Academy of Sciences has voted to present the name of Dr. Pieter Zeeman, professor of physics at the University of Amsterdam, for election to the academy.

THE Academy of Sciences at Heidelberg has elected to membership Dr. Ludwig Aschoff in pathology and Dr. Ernst Zermello and Dr. Gustav Doetsch in mathematics, all of the University of Freiburg.

THE degree of doctor of science was conferred at the commencement of Brown University on June 16 upon Dr. Niels Bohr, professor of physics in the University of Copenhagen, and upon Dr. Lipót Fejér, professor of mathematics at the University of Budapest. The address, made by Dr. Bohr, was entitled "Explanation in Natural Science." He also gave a lecture on "Measurements in Atomic Physics" at the convocation of the Graduate School.

THE Massachusetts State College has conferred the doctorate of science on Dr. Joseph B. Lindsey, who was a member of the staff of the Massachusetts Agricultural Experiment Station for forty-two years and vice-director for twenty-three years, and on Dr. Homer J. Wheeler, Upper Montclair, New Jersey, who was formerly director of the Rhode Island Experiment Station.

WASHINGTON COLLEGE, of Chestertown, Maryland, has conferred the degree of doctor of laws on Dr. Howard A. Kelly, emeritus professor of gynecology at the Johns Hopkins University.

THE degree of doctor of science was conferred at the commencement of Ursinus College on Dr. Guilliam H. Clamer, of Philadelphia, known for his contributions to non-ferrous metallurgy and for his development of electric furnaces.

THE University of Sheffield has conferred the doctorate of science on Professor E. J. Garwood, of the University of London, past-president of the Geological Society of London, and on Professor J. B. Leathes, dean of the Faculty of Medicine of the university.

AT the annual banquet of the Minnesota Chapter of Sigma Xi, held on June 7, the chapter presented to Dr. William J. Mayo, of the Mayo Foundation, Rochester, and to Dean Guy Stanton Ford, dean of the Graduate School of the University of Minnesota, illuminated testimonials in recognition of their service in furthering science and scientific research in Minnesota. The awards were presented by Dr. Louis B. Wilson, national president of Sigma Xi.

THE Distinguished Flying Cross, posthumously awarded to Glenn Hammond Curtiss "for outstanding service rendered to aviation" has been presented to Mrs. Lua Andrews Curtiss, his mother. The presentation was made by Major General Benjamin D. Foulois, chief of the U. S. Army Air Service, at the aviation base at Chapman's Field, Miami.

DR. ALFRED PHILIPPSON, professor of geography at Bonn, and Dr. Erich von Drygalski, professor of geography at Munich, have been awarded Richthofen gold medals. Dr. Ernst Tiessen, professor of geography at Berlin, has received the silver medal.

THE nomination of Dr. Lyman J. Briggs as director of the Bureau of Standards has been confirmed by the Senate.

DR. DUDLEY S. CONLEY, professor of surgery in the School of Medicine of the University of Missouri, will succeed Dean Edgar Allen, who recently resigned to become professor of anatomy and head of the department of anatomy at Yale University.

DR. CHARLES ZELENY, professor of zoology, University of Illinois, has been appointed head of the department to succeed Dr. Henry B. Ward, who has become permanent secretary of the American Association for the Advancement of Science under conditions which permit him to continue research work.

CHARLES JUDSON HERRICK, professor of neurology in the department of anatomy at the University of Chicago since 1907, has been appointed chairman of the department. He succeeds Dr. Robert R. Bensley, who retires with the title of professor emeritus. Dr. Bensley, who went to the university in 1901 as assistant professor of anatomy, has been professor since 1907 and chairman of the department since 1913. He will offer graduate work in the department next year.

CHARLES E. JACKSON has been appointed by President Roosevelt Deputy Commissioner of Fisheries. Since November, 1922, Mr. Jackson has been with Senator E. D. Smith, serving in the capacity of secretary. He succeeds Dr. Lewis Radcliffe, who resigned on April 30, after twenty-six years service with the bureau.

PROFESSOR JUNIUS HENDERSON, of the University of Colorado, curator of the museum since 1903, has retired at the age of sixty-eight years. He was given a farewell banquet by the informal senate of the university, when speeches were made by the vice-president, the dean of the graduate school and heads of various departments. Dr. Henderson plans to spend a year in California. He is succeeded by Hugo G. Rodeck, who will hold the academic rank of assistant professor.

AT the University of Bristol Dr. J. F. Baker, technical officer to the British Steel Structures Committee, has accepted an invitation to fill the chair of civil engineering in succession to Professor A. J. S. Pippard, who resigns at the end of the current session, and Professor A. E. Trueman, professor of geology at University College, Swansea, has been appointed Chaning Wills professor of geology in succession to Professor S. H. Reynolds, who retires at the end of the year.

DR. ALEXIS CARREL, of the Rockefeller Institute for Medical Research, sailed for France on June 10.

DR. JOHN C. MERRIAM, president of the Carnegie Institution of Washington, gave the commencement address on June 12 at the Carnegie Institute of Technology, Pittsburgh.

THE first public meeting of the new chapter of Sigma Xi in the University of California at Los Angeles was addressed on May 24 by Professor Niels Bohr on "Space-Time Relations in Atomic Physics."

DR. HERBERT DINGLE, professor of astrophysics in the Imperial College of Science and Technology, London, and research fellow in the California Institute of Technology, 1932–33, on June 7 lectured on "The Nature of Scientific Thought" at the University of California at Los Angeles, under the auspices of the department of astronomy.

SIR HENRY HADOW gave the Romanes lecture for 1933 at the University of Oxford, on May 31. The title of the lecture was "The Place of Music among the Arts."

PROFESSOR OTTO HAHN, the George T. Baker non-resident lecturer in chemistry at Cornell University during the spring semester, delivered three lectures at the University of Minnesota on June 5, 6 and 7—before the Minnesota Section of the American Chemical Society on "Gaseous Radioelements and their Application in Chemical Research," before the Colloquium of the School of Chemistry on "Co-precipitation and Adsorption Processes" and before the annual meeting of Sigma Xi on "From the Ponderable to the Imponderable." Professor Jan Heyrovsky, of the Charles University of Prague, gave three lectures before the colloquium on the "Theory and Practise of the Polarigraphic Method" on June 8, 9 and 10.

THE *Journal* of the American Medical Association reports that the Gorgas Medical Society of New Orleans has awarded honorary fellowships as follows: to Dr. Arthur Vidrine for his work in surgery; to Dr. Joseph Rigney D'Aunoy for his work on electrocardiography and to Dr. Richard Ashman for achievement in research. The awards are made to those "who have distinguished themselves in medical science and research." Dr. Vidrine is dean of the medical center of the University of Louisiana, Dr. D'Aunoy is professor of pathology and bacteriology and executive secretary of the center and Dr. Ashman is professor of physiology. These fellowships are the first to be awarded by this society, which was organized last year by Dr. Clyde Brooks, professor of pharmacology and experimental therapeutics.

THE twenty-first Wilbur Wright memorial lecture was read by Colonel F. P. Lahm, Air Corps, U. S. Army, on May 30, before the Royal Aeronautical Society at its meeting held in the Royal Institution. Before the lecture the following medals were presented by the president, C. R. Fairey: the gold medal of the society, to Sir Richard Glazebrook, on his retirement from the chairmanship of the Aeronautical Research Committee, which he has held since the foundation of the committee in 1909; the Simms Gold Medal, for the best paper read before the society on any science allied to aeronautics, to Mr. P. Salmon, for his paper on catapults; the Wakefield Gold Medal, for inventions or apparatus tending towards safety in flying, to Mr. L. G. Frise, for his invention of the Frise aileron; the Taylor Gold Medal, for the most valuable paper of the year, to Dr. G. V. Lachmann, for his paper on "Control beyond the Stall"; the Silver Medal, for advance in aeronautical design, to each of the following: Señor J. de la Cierva, for his work in the design and development of the autogiro; Mr. A. H. R. Fedden, for his work on the air-cooled engine, resulting in the attainment of a record height of over 40,000 feet in September, 1932; Mr. D. L. Hollis-Williams, who was responsible for the design of the Fairey long-range monoplane which holds the world's long-distance record of 5,309 miles. The newly-founded British Silver Medal for Aeronautics, to Flight Lieutenant C. F. Uwins, for reaching the world record height in September last, and to Squadron Leader O. R. Gayford and Flight Lieutenant G. E. Nicholetts, who flew non-stop from Cranwell to Walvis Bay in the long-distance monoplane.

ACCORDING to the *Journal* of the American Medical Association, at the general meeting of the Imperial Academy of Japan, the special committee announced the awards of the imperial prizes and others for 1932. The imperial prizes were given to Dr. J. Tsuji, of the Physical and Chemical Research Institute, for his researches on the elasticity of light, and to Professor B. Suzuki, D.Sc., of the Kyoto Imperial University, for his work on fatty acids. The academy prize was awarded to Professor M. Ishimoto, of the Tokyo Imperial University science department, for his seismological observations. The emperor's wedding commemoration prizes, contributed by the Osaka *Mainichi,* were given to Professor S. Kusano, of the Tokyo Imperial University, for his work on fungi; to Professor C. Oguchi, of the Nagoya Medical College, for his research on Oguchi's disease, to Professor Y. Furutake, of the Osaka Imperial University, for his discovery of kynurenin, a crystal chemical compound, and to Professor H. Nomura, of the Sendai University, for his study on the pungency of ginger.

ACCORDING to the *Astronomische Nachrichten,* the division of the Astrophysical Observatory in Potsdam that has been called the Einstein Institute will by decree of the ministry be hereafter known as the Institute for Solar Physics.

ANNOUNCEMENT has just been made at Harvard University that the Institute of Geographical Exploration has been given a valuable library collection which includes several rare accounts of early voyages of exploration and discovery in America. The collection is stated to be the most important single addition which has yet been made to the library on geographical exploration. Numbering nearly 1,000 separate items, the collection has been presented to the university by Mrs. Joseph Tuckerman Tower, of Millbrook, New York. It includes principally books, maps and documents which were collected by her son, Joseph Tuckerman Tower, Jr., of the Harvard College Class of 1921, who died in Mexico in 1931. Before his death Mr. Tower had planned the gift of his collection to the institute at Harvard. In addition to many rare and valuable old books on early voyages, the library includes sections dealing with Arctic exploration, exploration in Alaska, Iceland and in the Hudson Bay region.

THE Board of Governors of the Institute of Medicine of Chicago recently authorized an appropriation of $1,455 to compile a combined card catalogue of the literature in the medical libraries of Chicago (John Crerar, Rush Medical College and the medical colleges of the universities of Chicago, Illinois, Loyola and Northwestern). The plan was organized and the work is being carried out under the supervision of Otto F. Kampmeier, professor of anatomy at the University of Illinois, and chairman of the committee on coordination of medical libraries in Chicago. The union index will be completed in six to eight months, and will be placed in the John Crerar Library because of its central location in the city.

AN additional one hundred and ninety acres of marsh and prairie land have been added to the University of Wisconsin arboretum. Funds made available by the Tripp estate have made acquisition of this land possible. The new tract adjoins the present arboretum land on the south and west, and increases the total area of the arboretum to slightly more than 400 acres. Addition of the new area to the present arboretum gives the university and the State of Wisconsin an excellent opportunity for experimentation in reforestation and propagation of wild life. Acquisition of several tracts deemed essential to the project permitted the Board of Regents to establish the Wisconsin arboretum last August, after nearly six years of constant work on the part of regents, university officials and public-spirited Wisconsin citizens. No state appropriated funds whatever have been used on the project. Acquisition of the original tract of 235 acres was also made possible through use of the residue of the estate of the late J. Stephens Tripp, who left his entire estate to the university. Other groups of citizens donated land also. The committee in charge of the arboretum consists of Professors E. M. Gilbert, George Wagner, James G. Dickson, Chancey Juday, N. C. Fassett, Leon J. Cole and J. W. Jackson, Associate Franz A. Aust, Instructor F. B. Trenk, Superintendent A. F. Gallistel, Secretary M. E. McCaffrey. In addition to this active committee the president has appointed an advisory committee consisting of Dr. E. A. Birge, Dr. H. L. Russell, C. P. Winslow, Aldo Leopold, Paul D. Holleter and Professor Raphael Zon.

THE thirty-seventh annual report has been issued of the New York Zoological Society, which maintains the Zoological Park in the Bronx, the Aquarium and the tropical research station. The report of finances states that the City of New York appropriated $418,891 toward the maintenance of the Zoological Garden and the Aquarium during 1932. During the year the society expended $227,730. The endowment and other funds are $4,123,637, of which $4,035,386 is represented by securities carried at cost or gift value. The market value on December 31 was $3,157,173. "For the continuation of its work," according to the report, "the society requires the immediate addition of $2,000,000 to its general endowment, and desires the constant attention of its members and friends to the needs of its library, extension of its scientific research work, heads and horns collection, publications and gallery of animal paintings."

As the result of a proposal made by Dr. Schaffernak, of Austria, at the World Power Conference at Berlin in 1930, that "an organization be established for the purpose of interchanging, in the field of hydraulic engineering, the results of laboratory research and of observations of natural conditions corresponding thereto," the American committee of the World Power Conference asked the Bureau of Standards last January to serve as the exchange agency for the

United States. The object of the proposed organization is to afford promptly to all the hydraulic laboratories throughout the world information as to the nature of the research which each is undertaking, thus permitting a closer coordination of the work. The first step in organizing this service nationally in the United States was to compile and distribute to the hydraulic laboratories in this country a report covering the activities of these laboratories. As a result of the prompt cooperation of the individual laboratories, it was possible for the bureau to issue on April 1 its first report of this kind, a mimeographed bulletin entitled, "Current Hydraulic Laboratory Research in the United States." The second report will be issued on July 1, and succeeding numbers will appear quarterly. In addition to the above service, the bureau will compile and issue annually a description of the hydraulic laboratories in the United States, their equipment and facilities for research in so far as the heads of the laboratories will furnish the necessary information. It is planned to issue the first report of this kind on June 1.

# DISCUSSION

## AN ELECTRIC ANALOGUE OF VOWEL PRODUCTION

It is of interest to examine the results of the remarkable if somewhat bizarre experiment of Travis and Buchanan,[1] which relates to the production of sound frequencies in the voice, in the light of our knowledge of analogous electric circuit behavior. The mathematics of the electric circuit is remarkably well developed, and since in many cases a strict analogy may be demonstrated between sound vibrations and electric vibrations, it is hoped that in the present study a consideration of this mathematics will prove significant.

First, the possible appearance in the output of vibration frequencies that are entirely absent in the motive force should be considered, that is, the appearance of frequencies in the voice that would not appear in the vibration of vocal cords in the open. Or, in terms of this particular experiment, the change of wave-form when a pure sine wave is passed into the resonating cavities.

There is no doubt that such a change is possible. It is the result of non-linear response of some of the elements involved in the propagation of sound, and appears when a strictly sinusoidal stress does not result in a strictly sinusoidal strain in either the vibrating medium or the containing walls. The irregularity of the vocal passage and the non-homogeneity of the walls make a somewhat non-linear response certain, but the amount of the change of wave-shape is unknown. The amount of the change at any one point may be small, but if any of the chief frequencies thereby introduced should find a resonating cavity of the same natural frequency, the amplitude of such frequency will be greatly increased. It should also be noted that the vibration of the vocal cords is not entirely independent of the resonant system in which they operate, although for practical purposes it is very nearly so. It is to be expected that the distortion of loud sounds is greater than that of soft ones.

[1] SCIENCE, 77: 121, January 27, 1933.

Second, the magnification, in the output, of small irregularities in the input must be considered. An abrupt change in the input motion, a discontinuity, will produce resonance in all cavities, but in amounts varying with the natural frequency, location and size of the cavity. An irregular, or non-sinusoidal input will have a similar effect. So will a wave whose steady-state condition is sinusoidal, when it is starting or stopping. All three of these means of producing resonance will doubtless occur in the normal voice. Only the second will be appreciable in the experiment, as described, with the oscillator; but it is evident that the input can not be mathematically exact even under the most favorable experimental conditions, and there is no mention of a determination of the exact wave-form in detail.

Finally, the relative amounts of frequencies introduced by the two means should be considered. The first, the distortion due to non-linear response of the vocal passages, can produce energy of one frequency only at the expense of decreasing energy of another frequency. The more audible a frequency is, the more it is being damped by losing energy as output. From these considerations, and from the nature of the system, it is improbable that resonance in the sinusoidal steady-state condition could introduce frequencies with amplitudes of more than a few per cent. of the fundamental.

The second type of distortion, due to transient conditions or to non-sinusoidal input, will give resonant vibrations that depend for their energy on a component vibration of their own frequency in the input. Hence, as they also are damped by the output, their amplitude with an approximate sine-wave input may be of the same order of magnitude as the steady state distortion.

So both "steady-state" and "transient" production of resonant frequencies appear to be possible. In either case a small amplitude may be magnified to many times its original amount by resonance, and from the published data it seems impossible to tell which type of distortion produces the resonance detected by Travis and Buchanan.

HUGH SKILLING
STANFORD UNIVERSITY

## NOMENCLATURE OF THE VEGETABLE WEEVIL

THIS interesting weevil is one of the many insects which has recently emerged from natural obscurity and has appeared as an economic pest on three continents during the past twenty-five years, it having originated on a fourth. Its native habitat is the southern half of South America, from which area it has been carried by commerce to Australia, North America and Africa.

The first specimens were collected more than one hundred years ago on Magellan Strait and were described as *Listroderes costirostris* by the Swedish entomologist Schoenherr[1] in 1826. An aberrant form was later named *L. obliquus* by Gyllenhal[2] in 1834. There appears to be some confusion regarding the authority of *L. costirostris,* for in this latter publication, "Schoen. Gen. et Spec. Curcul.," vol. 2, p. 277, 1834, by L. Gyllenhal, and also in vol. IV, p. 189, 1842, by C. H. Boheman, the species is credited to Gyllenhal rather than to Schoenherr. L. L. Buchanan, U. S. Bureau of Entomology, very kindly looked up the original descriptions by Schoenherr and furnished the following information:

In 1826, Schoenherr ('Curculionidium disposito methodica . . . ,' page 158) erects *Listroderes* as follows:—'Genus 82. *Listroderes* nob.—*Merionus* Dej. *Character generis*:—' (12 lines of descriptive matter). Then, '*Descriptio*:' (Remainder of page 158 and more than half of page 159 taken up with a detailed description). Then, '*Typus*: *Listrod. costirostris* Gyllenh. n. sp. Schoenherr's purpose here evidently was simply to describe a new genus, but the description, being based on one species, really amounts to a combined generic description of *Listroderes* and a specific description of *costirostris.* Under these conditions, it seems to me proper to consider *costirostris* as having been described by Schoenherr in this paper.

In 1881 Berg[3] gave some additional information regarding the weevil and listed it from the region of the Rio Colorado in central Argentina, but wrongly listed *Listroderes robustus* Waterhouse as a synonym of *L. costirostris.* Hustache[4] credited the species to Gyllenhal, and to its distribution adds Buenos Aires with the statement that the range extends northwards to meridional Brazil. His figure of *L. vicinus* Hust., pl. II, is very much like *L. costirostris.*

In 1908 this same weevil was discovered in South Australia, where it was described as a new species, *Desiantha nociva,* by Lea[5] in 1909. Along the eastern and southern coasts of that continent it soon became known as a pest of considerable economic importance to vegetable crops and to fruits and was generally called the buff-colored tomato weevil.[6] It was not until years later that the weevil was known to be of South American origin.

On the North American continent the weevil was first recognized as a newly introduced pest of truck crops at McHenry, Mississippi, on March 28, 1922, and was determined as the Australian tomato weevil and first listed as *Listroderes* (*Desiantha*) *nociva* (Lea).[7] Later it was designated scientifically simply as *Desiantha nociva* Lea.[8] Further studies and comparisons with known species convinced Chittenden that the weevil was *Listroderes obliquus,* which he credited to Fabricius.[9] It was also known as *Listronotus obliquus,* and is not to be confused with the American species by that name.[10] In 1926 the same species was discovered attacking vegetables at San Jose, California, and within a few years was known to occur in much of the San Francisco Bay region.

The very same weevil was recorded in South Africa in 1924, having been previously introduced into Port Elizabeth,[11] where it was found to be injuring turnips.

This rapid and wide distribution has no doubt been due to the transportation of infested vegetables from South American seaports used in ships' stores, and it is not unlikely that all these different foci of infestation have a more or less common origin.

Although the insect has generally been scientifically known as *Listroderes obliquus* (Gyll.),[12] Schenkling

1 C. J. Schoenherr, "Disp. Meth. Curculionidum," p. 158. 1826.

2 L. Gyllenhal, "Schoen. Gen. et Spec. Curcul.," vol. 2, pt. 1, p. 277. 1834.

3 C. Berg, "Entomologisches aus dem Indianergebeit der Pampa." *Stett. Ent. Zeit.*, 42: 62, fig. 10. 1881.

4 A. Hustache, "Curculionides de la Republique Argentine." *Ann. Museo Nacionale de Hist. Nat.*, Buenos Aires, 34: 199. 1926.

5 A. M. Lea, *Trans. and Proc. Royal Soc. So. Austr.*, 33: 174–175. 1909.

6 C. French, Jr., Handbook Destr. Ins. Victoria, pt. V, pp. 41–43, Oct., 1909; W. W. Froggatt, "The Buff-colored Tomato Weevil (*Desiantha nociva*)," *Agr. Gaz. N. S. W.*, Sydney, xxvi: 1065–1066. 1915.

7 R. W. Harned, "A New Potato Weevil in Mississippi." *Quart. Bul. State Pl. Bd. Miss.*, 2: 1–2, pp. 6–8, 11–12. 1922.

8 E. K. Bynum, "Controlling the Australian Tomato Weevil, *Desiantha nociva.*" *Ibid.*, 3: 1, pp. 22–24 (1923); F. H. Chittenden, "The Australian Tomato Weevil, Introduced in the South," U. S. Dept. Agr., Dept. Circ. 282, 8 pp., 6 fig. July 31, 1932.

9 F. H. Chittenden, "An Introduced Weevil Related to the Vegetable Weevil." *Proc. Biol. Soc. Wash.*, 39: 71–74, pl. 1. 1926.

10 An entirely different weevil, *Listronotus obliquus,* was described from Texas in 1876 by J. L. LeConte. *Proc. Am. Philos. Soc.*, 15: 128, 129. 1876.

11 *Jour. Dept. Agr., Union South Africa,* 8: 3, pp. 264–265. 1924.

12 E. O. Essig, "The Vegetable Weevil." "A History of Entomology," pp. 203–206, figs. 78–81 (Bibliography). New York: Macmillan. 1931. O. H. Lovell, "The Vegetable Weevil, *Listroderes obliquus.*" *Calif. Agr. Expt. Sta., Bull.* 546, 19 pp., 5 figs., December, 1932.

and Marshall,[13] in 1931, corrected the systematic nomenclature and have listed the species as *Listroderes costirostris* Schoenherr. As to the advisability of adopting this specific name in America, Buchanan has also kindly given his views as follows:

> The citing of *obliquus* in the Schenkling catalogue as an aberration ('ab.') indicates that the compilers regard it as some sort of a subordinate form, but not an absolute synonym, of *costirostris;* and, until the two are found to be synonymous through an examination of the type specimens or through other means, it would seem preferable to continue the use of the name *obliquus* Gyll. in North American literature, either as *obliquus* alone or as *costirostris* ab. *obliquus.*

The common name, vegetable weevil, was approved by the American Association of Economic Entomologists in 1931.[14]

E. O. Essig

University of California

## NOMENCLATORIAL NOTES ON GASTROTRICHA

(1) The genus *Dactylopodola* Strand:

*Dactylopodella* Remane, 1926, *Zeits. Morph. ökol.*, 5: 664 non G. O. Sars, 1905, Crust. Norway, 5: 131 (Copepoda).

*Dactylopodola* Strand, March, 1929, Acta Univ. Latv., 20: 5.

*Dactylopodalia* Remane, 30 May, 1929, Kükenthal and Krumbach, Handb. Zool., 2 (4): 130.

Professor Embrik Strand kindly informed me personally of the month of publication of his paper. As a consequence of the above synonymy it is necessary to form the new family name Dactylopodolidae in place of Dactylopodellidae Remane 1927 and Dactylopodaliidae Remane 1929, and also the new combinations *Dactylopodola baltica* (Remane) and *Dactylopodola typhle* (Remane).

(2) *Lepidodermella* nom. nov.:

*Lepidoderma* Zelinka, 1889, *Zeits. wiss. Zool.*, 49: 300 non Reuss, 1856, Denks. Akad. Wiss. Wien, 10: 83 (Eurypterida).

As I can not find that this homonym has ever been corrected, I propose here as a substitute the name *Lepidodermella.* We have, hence, the new combinations *Lepidodermella squammata* (Dujardin), *Lepidodermella concinna* (Stokes), *Lepidodermella ocellata* (Metschnikov) and *Lepidodermella zelinkai* (Konsuloff).

Charles H. Blake

Massachusetts Institute of Technology

[13] S. Schenkling and G. A. K. Marshall, "Curculionidae: Cylindrorrhininae." Coleopterorum Catalogus (Berlin, Junk, 1931), pars. 114, p. 7, Feb. 12, 1931. (Bibliography.)

[14] *Jour. Econ. Ent.*, 24: 1291, 1303. 1931.

## MALVACEOUS PLANTS AS A CAUSE OF "PINK WHITE" IN STORED EGGS

A type of deterioration in stored eggs in which the egg white becomes pink, and the yolk becomes large, salmon colored and watery in consistency, but turns rubbery when cooked, has caused severe losses in the United States in past years. Eggs from hens fed raw cottonseed products have been known to suffer the same or a similar type of deterioration, but most examples of "pink white" eggs on the market have come from flocks to which cottonseed products were not available.

It was discovered in this laboratory that the extracted yolk fat of "pink white" eggs, and also of fresh eggs from hens fed cottonseed oil gave the Halphen test for cottonseed. It was also discovered that seeds of certain members of the family Malvaceae (other than cotton) notably *Malva parviflora, Lavatera assurgentiflora* and *Althaea sp.* gave positive Halphen tests. Consequently, groups of hens were fed rations containing seeds of *Malva parviflora* and of *Lavatera assurgentiflora.* Eggs from these birds gave a positive Halphen test and also turned pink after a period of storage, while eggs from the same birds, before the seeds were added to the rations, gave a negative test and did not turn pink after the same period of storage.

It is concluded that these and possibly other members of the family Malvaceae when eaten by laying hens may become responsible for "pink white" deterioration in stored eggs. *Malva parviflora* is a common weed in poultry districts and is more available to poultry than other members of the family, so that this species is probably the important cause of "pink white" deterioration.

F. W. Lorenz
H. J. Almquist
G. W. Hendry

University of California

## INCOMPLETE NUCLEAR DIVISIONS AND NOT AMITOSIS IN THE TAPETUM OF THE EUSPORANGIATE FERNS

In 1913 the writer began an investigation of the nature of the nuclear divisions in the tapetum of *Botrychium virginianum* (L.) Swarz. He was soon led to the conclusion that the nuclei undergo incomplete divisions similar to those described by him in *Nephrodium hirtipes* Hk.[1]

As a result of this investigation, extending over a period of two decades, the writer has been convinced that the amitotic divisions described by some workers as occurring in the tapetum of the *eusporangiate* filicales do not take place.

[1] W. N. Steil, "Apogamy in *Nephrodium hirtipes* Hk." *Ann. Bot.*, 33: 109–133, 1919.

The incomplete nuclear divisions, which begin in the young tapetum, result in the formation of nuclei of irregular form, commonly, dumb-bell and kidney-shaped, which have suggested to some workers that the nuclei divide amitotically. The nuclei, as a result of successive incomplete divisions, are polyploid and of unusually large size.

The organization of chromosomes, the presence of spindle fibers and various stages in the reorganization of the resting daughter nuclei are some of the evidences that incomplete divisions, and not amitotic divisions, occur in the tapetum.

The incomplete nuclear divisions herein described have been studied in two *eusporangiate* ferns, namely *Botrychium virginianum* (L.) Swarz and *Ophioglossum vulgatum* L.

A detailed discussion of these nuclear divisions in the tapetum of the ferns studied will be presented in the near future.

W. N. STEIL

MARQUETTE UNIVERSITY

# THE FOURTEENTH ANNUAL MEETING OF THE AMERICAN GEOPHYSICAL UNION

THE fourteenth annual meeting of the American Geophysical Union and the sessions of its sections were held at Washington, D. C., on April 27, 28 and 29.

Progress-reports on geodetic work in the United States and Mexico were presented before the Section of Geodesy, as also papers on gravity-work, on application of radio to astronomical longitude-determinations of the Geodetic Survey of Canada, on the moon's influence on latitude and on the expansion and developments in the time-service at the U. S. Naval Observatory.

The Section of Seismology of the union held a joint meeting with the Eastern Section of the Seismological Society of America. An interesting series of progress-reports, papers and informal communications, totaling 39, was presented at the three sessions of this joint meeting, including, among others, progress-reports on developments of seismological instruments and on the work of various seismograph-stations in the United States and Mexico; papers relating to recent earthquakes, to discussion of methods in seismological determinations, and to precise geodetic measurements and their relation to seismological investigations; and an informal discussion of earthquake-code.

At its meeting the Section of Meteorology had the privilege of hearing a paper by Dr. L. Vegard, of Norway, on the auroral spectrum, in addition to papers by members of the union and other guests on meteorological problems in relation to radiation, on trade-winds of the eastern Caribbean, on reduction of meteorological data from Cruise VII of the *Carnegie,* on interesting facts concerning warm and cold waves, on the value of cloud-observations, on the Giao theory explaining the formation of precipitation in relation to fundamental concepts of the polar-front theory, on turbulence-factors of Linke and Ångstrom and their practical applicability, and on the time, type and areal distribution of tornadoes in the United States.

The reports and papers presented before the Section of Terrestrial Magnetism and Electricity included progress-reports on the year's investigations and projects in the United States, Canada and Mexico and on the International Polar Year of 1932–33, while the papers related to cosmic rays, to earth-resistivity measurements, to ozone and the sunspot-cycle, to cosmic radio correlations and to effect of magnetic activity upon secular change.

As in past years, the meeting of the Section of Oceanography consisted mainly of the progress-reports of eight governmental bureaus and private research organizations engaged in oceanographic work in the United States and Canada. Besides these reports, there were papers on the submarine valleys of the Bahamas, on submarine mock valleys, on investigations of submarine valleys, on monthly sequence of sea-surface temperature on the New York-San Juan steamship route, on air- and water-temperatures in the West Indian region, on development of our conception of the Gulf Stream system and on data from borehole on New Providence Island, Bahamas.

In the Section of Volcanology the papers dealt with volcanic explosions and overthrusts, with the Tertiary Volcano at Cripple Creek, Colorado, and the volcano of Santa Maria in Guatemala, with some features of volcanic sequence in the Cascade Region in Oregon, and with volcanic history of the Magdalena District, New Mexico.

The Section of Hydrology devoted three sessions to hearing reports of its nine permanent research committees and 25 papers covering numerous investigations and developments in scientific hydrology throughout the United States. These brought out clearly the effective cooperation existing between the various hydraulic stations and laboratories of the federal government, of the state governments, of universities and of consulting engineering organizations.

At the business session of the general assembly the general secretary reported a total membership of 355, as of April 28, 1933. Among other things, the general secretary also reported briefly on relations of the union with the international body and on the progress of the International Polar Year of 1932–33. His report showed that interest in geophysics during the past year has continued its rapid growth—a growth to which the union has made substantial contribution.

The following nine resolutions were unanimously adopted:

(I) *Resolution on the death of Robert Lee Faris,* proposed by the Sections of Geodesy and Terrestrial Magnetism and Electricity:

WHEREAS, By the death of Robert Lee Faris on October 5, 1932, the American Geophysical Union has lost one of its original members and a former Chairman of the Section of Geodesy, and

WHEREAS, Captain Faris was interested in many departments of geophysics and helped to advance scientific knowledge not only by his personal efforts in field and office, but also by the influence he was able to exert through the numerous and important administrative positions held by him, and not least by means of his personal character, which won for him the respect and friendship of those with whom he came in contact, therefore be it

*Resolved,* That the American Geophysical Union, in general meeting assembled, hereby expresses and places on record its sense of loss through his death; and be it further

*Resolved,* That copies of this resolution be sent to Mrs. Faris, to the Director of the U. S. Coast and Geodetic Survey, and to Chairman of the Mississippi River Commission.

(II) *Resolution on the death of John Ripley Freeman,* proposed by the Sections of Seismology and Hydrology:

WHEREAS, In the death of John R. Freeman the American Geophysical Union has lost a pioneer in the fields of hydrology, geology, and seismology as related to engineering problems, and

WHEREAS, He has rendered notable services to his profession by his generosity in providing traveling scholarships in hydraulics and in financing the translation and publication of foreign books and papers on hydraulics, and by his untiring efforts toward the establishment of a National Hydraulic Laboratory, and

WHEREAS, He through publication and otherwise has greatly stimulated interest in seismology, especially in applications toward saving life and property; therefore be it

*Resolved,* That the American Geophysical Union expresses its sense of great loss in the death of John R. Freeman, not only because of his high engineering and scientific attainments, but also because of his outstanding personal qualities and his earnest and continuous efforts to advance the profession to which his whole life has brought honor; and be it further

*Resolved,* That a copy of this resolution be sent to Dr. Freeman's family.

(III) *Resolution on the death of Harlan Wilbur Fisk,* proposed by the Section of Terrestrial Magnetism and Electricity:

WHEREAS, In the death of Harlan Wilbur Fisk the American Geophysical Union has lost a member long identified with the affairs of the Union and active especially, as both member and officer, in the Section of Terrestrial Magnetism and Electricity, and

WHEREAS, He rendered important service to the advancement of geophysics, particularly through his extensive participation in the magnetic survey of the Earth and through the interpretation of the results thus obtained; therefore be it

*Resolved,* That the American Geophysical Union records this expression of its sense of profound sorrow on the death of Harlan Wilbur Fisk; and be it further

*Resolved,* That a copy of this resolution be sent to Professor Fisk's family, to the President of the Carnegie Institution of Washington, and to the Acting Director of the Department of Terrestrial Magnetism.

(IV) *Resolution on the death of Louis Winslow Austin,* proposed by the Section of Terrestrial Magnetism and Electricity:

WHEREAS, The death of Louis Winslow Austin has removed from the American Geophysical Union a member always actively interested in the affairs of the Union and one who made notable contribution to geophysics through radio-transmission research and its interpretation in relation to terrestrial magnetism and other geophysical phenomena; therefore be it

*Resolved,* That the American Geophysical Union records this expression of its sense of great loss in the death of Louis Winslow Austin; and be it further

*Resolved,* That a copy of this resolution be sent to Dr. Austin's family, to the Secretary of the Department of Commerce of the United States, and to the Director of the United States Bureau of Standards.

(V) *Resolution on International Polar Year,* proposed by the Section of Terrestrial Magnetism and Electricity:

WHEREAS, The American Geophysical Union regards with satisfaction and approval the progress made in carrying out the International Polar Year program and appreciates the great value of the results that have been and will be obtained during the Polar Year; therefore be it

*Resolved,* That the American Geophysical Union expresses the hope that the International Polar Year Commission will be able to find means for complete analysis, discussion, and distribution of the geophysical data resulting from this magnificent international effort, and that the United States, through its government or otherwise, will be able to assume its proper share in this work; and be it further

*Resolved,* That copies of this resolution be sent to the President of the International Polar Year Commission and to the President of the National Academy of Sciences with the request that the latter make such disposition of this resolution as he may find most effective.

(VI) *Resolution on cosmic rays,* proposed by the Section of Terrestrial Magnetism and Electricity:

WHEREAS, The importance of studies of cosmic rays is steadily increasing and the need for their continuous registration has been demonstrated; therefore be it

*Resolved,* That the American Geophysical Union recommends that support wherever possible be given to the plan of the Carnegie Institution of Washington and cooperating agencies to establish at certain fixed observatories apparatus and equipment for recording cosmic rays photographically and continuously; and be it further

*Resolved,* That a copy of this resolution be sent to the President of the Carnegie Institution of Washington with the request that he furnish copies to the cooperating agencies.

(VII) *Resolutions proposing an International Commission on the Hydrology of Snow and Ice,* proposed by the Section of Hydrology:

WHEREAS, The hydrology of snow and ice and the methods of making snow-surveys constitute an important field in the science of hydrology, with a considerable number of research workers in the subject wisely distributed in different parts of the world, and

WHEREAS, There is at present no international commission that covers this field; therefore be it

*Resolved,* That the American Geophysical Union hereby expresses the hope that the International Association of Scientific Hydrology will take appropriate steps at the forthcoming meeting in Lisbon to create a Commission on the Hydrology of Snow and Ice; and be it further

*Resolved,* That a copy of this resolution be sent to the Secretary of the International Association together with copies of the annual reports for 1932 and 1933 of the Committee on Snow of the Section of Hydrology of the American Geophysical Union.

(VIII) *Resolution on appropriations for scientific investigations by the Federal Government,* proposed by the Section of Seismology:

WHEREAS, There are certain types of investigation which can be carried on effectively only by the Federal Government, and

WHEREAS, Large economies accrue to the Government itself from those investigations, and

WHEREAS, Private engineers, geophysicists, and others are almost absolutely dependent on the results of those investigations for the continuance of their own work; therefore be it

*Resolved,* That the American Geophysical Union expresses its hope that the scientific work of the Federal Government will not be too much curtailed under the stress of economic conditions; and be it further

*Resolved,* That a copy of this resolution be sent to the President of the National Academy of Sciences for such use as the Academy may think proper in its capacity as official advisor to the Federal Government.

(IX) *Resolution on Naval Observatory time-signals,* proposed by the Section of Seismology:

WHEREAS, Accurate time-signals sent out from a strong radio broadcasting station many times daily are necessary for seismological and other geophysical observations, and

WHEREAS, The United States Naval Observatory is now broadcasting such signals seven times daily; therefore be it

*Resolved,* That the American Geophysical Union expresses its appreciation and gratitude for this service; and be it further

*Resolved,* That this resolution be printed in the transactions and that a copy be sent to the Superintendent of the United States Naval Observatory.

The scientific session of the general assembly was devoted to a symposium on relations of hydrology to other branches of geophysics, and included the following papers: (a) "The Relation of Hydrology to the Botanical Sciences," by R. E. Horton; (b) "Relation of Meteorology to Hydrology," by N. C. Grover; (c) "Distribution of Precipitation in the Cumberland and Tennessee Basins," by M. W. Hayes; (d) "Glaciers and Geophysics," by Harry Fielding Reid; (e) "Some Relations between Ground-water Hydrology and Oceanography," by D. G. Thompson; (f) "Oceanography and Hydrology," by G. F. McEwen; (g) "Relation of Seismology to Hydrology," by N. H. Heck; (h) "Geophysical Interpretation of Ground-water Levels," by O. E. Meinzer; (i) "Associated Problems in Hydrology and Terrestrial Electricity," by O. H. Gish.

The marked success of the fourteenth annual meeting of the union and of its sections hinged largely upon the excellent program developed by the committee on meetings, consisting of Messrs. H. A. Marmer (*chairman*), R. M. Field, R. E. Gibson, F. W. Sohon, S.J., and H. F. Johnston.

The manuscript for the planographed volume of the complete *Transactions* of this meeting is already in preparation, and it is hoped that the volume may be issued during July.

JNO. A. FLEMING,
*General Secretary*

# SCIENTIFIC APPARATUS AND LABORATORY METHODS

## A MOUTH PIPETTE AND CONTAINERS FOR SMALLER ORGANISMS

A BIOLOGIST frequently encounters choice specimens for microscopic study in such materials as plankton, bottom deposits or mixed cultures of protozoa. But because of the time required to separate the desired forms from the mass of debris by the ordinary means at hand the specimens are usually sacrificed. For the same reason mixed cultures of protozoa are often tolerated. In my investigation of the soft parts of the foraminifera, many thousands of individuals ranging in size from 40 to 500 μ were isolated. In the preparation of stained materials, it was necessary to change reagents without contamination. It was also necessary to avoid loss, or injury to the fragile protoplasmic parts after decalcification. The pipette illustrated (A) has given several years of satisfaction

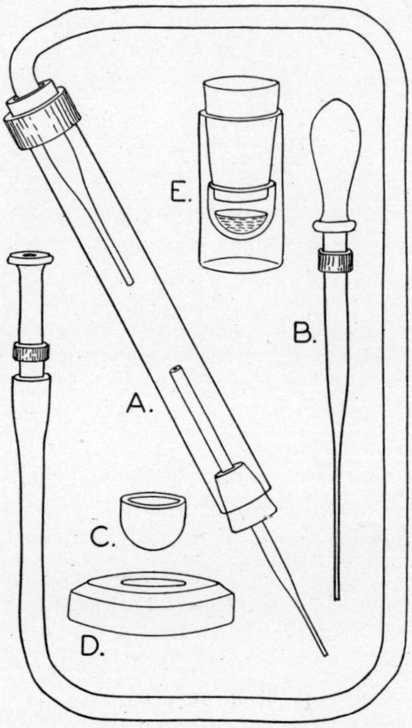


FIG. 1

and is to be recommended for the manipulation of living or fixed organisms of the magnitude mentioned.

The barrel is as convenient in size and weight as that of a fountain pen. Small organisms are drawn into the pipette by capillary attraction controlled by releasing the pressure of the tongue which is held against the end of the mouthpiece. The pipettes require a minimum of material, time and skill to prepare, and can be easily replaced in the barrel. Sterile pipettes of graduated sizes may be conveniently stored in test-tubes. Coating the pipette with paraffin prevents rhizopods and other adhesive organisms from sticking to the walls of the pipette.[1] While changing reagents the barrel constitutes a trap with a capacity of about 8 ml and may be held in any position without contaminating the mouthpiece, or filling the pipette with the contained fluid. By holding the barrel in a vertical position, pipette uppermost, the pipette stopper may be removed and the contents emptied.

At least three holders were necessary in my work. These were marked with bands cut from rubber tubing as follows: white for living material, red for general reagents and black for anhydrous solutions. It is very convenient to mark hand pipettes (B) in the same manner. A rack of suitable height and capacity for the pipette holders, attached to a ring stand or built above the microscope table, is very convenient.

Small or rare organisms were handled to advantage in containers made from the bottoms of bacteriological test-tubes (C) cut with a hot wire and ground flat on top with a carborundum stone. Supports (D) for these containers were made of plaster of Paris similar to the illustration. For storage these containers may be stoppered and placed in shell vials (E) as illustrated. Large or more abundant organisms may be collected in embryological watch glasses.

The following materials are necessary in the construction of the described pipette and holder: $5\frac{1}{2}$ inches of 14 mm glass tubing; 10 inches 7 mm glass tubing; 18 inches $\frac{1}{4}$ inch rubber tubing; several 00 rubber stoppers; 4 mm thin-walled soft glass tubing is essential for the pipettes.

EARL H. MYERS

SCRIPPS INSTITUTION OF OCEANOGRAPHY
LA JOLLA, CALIFORNIA

## MICROSCOPE LAMP FOR BIOLOGICAL LABORATORIES

THE lighting units used on the students' tables in the elementary botanical laboratories of the Life Sciences Building at the University of California have occasioned so much comment from visiting botanists and zoologists and have brought so many requests for specifications that publication of a brief description of these lamps seems advisable. Besides having proven so completely satisfactory as sources of artificial illumination for microscopic and other laboratory

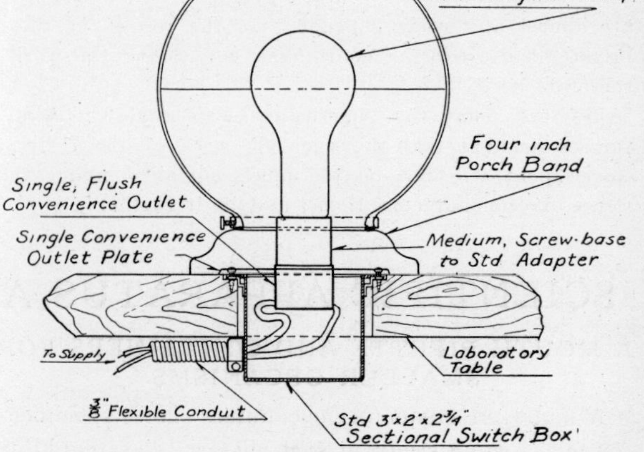


FIG. 1

[1] Suggested by Dr. Kofoid.

work, the cost of these lights is only a fraction of that of the table lamps supplied for similar purposes by the optical and laboratory supply companies.

Along the middle line of each of the laboratory tables, which are 9 feet, 10 inches by 42 inches, and 30 inches high, and which are designed to accommodate three students on each side, three such lamps are fixed. For the installation of each lamp the following parts, which can be secured from any jobber of electrical supplies, are needed:

1 Single flush convenience outlet.
1 Single convenience outlet plate.
1 Medium, screw base to standard adapter.
1 Sectional switch box.
1 Four inch porch band.
1 C. R. I. (crystal rough inside) glass ball, 8 x 4 inches.
1 100-watt ''daylite'' lamp.
2 1-inch round head brass screws.

Connection of the lamps to a wall outlet is through a wire attached to the under surface of the table top; current is supplied to the convenience outlets, which are sunk in holes in the table top.

The total cost of these items per lamp at the time of our installation was slightly less than $2.75. We have found the illumination sufficient for the use of the binocular dissection microscope and for standard compound microscopes for all magnifications up to that supplied by the 2 mm oil immersion objective and ocular 10. If the diffuse illumination coming directly to the user's eyes from the upper part of the lamp proves unpleasant, which in practise it seldom does, the upper part of the ball may be painted on the inside surface with white, opaque paint. If for any reason it is desired to remove the lights so that the table, entirely free from obstructions, may be used for other purposes, it is only necessary to remove the two wood screws from the "porch ring" and slip the adapter with the daylight bulb out of the receptacle.

RICHARD M. HOLMAN
UNIVERSITY OF CALIFORNIA

# SPECIAL ARTICLES

## INFECTION IN MICE FOLLOWING INSTILLATION OF VESICULAR STOMATITIS VIRUS

WE have previously stated[1,2] that intracerebral inoculation of anesthetized white mice with the virus of vesicular stomatitis of horses uniformly induces characteristic lesions in the organs of the central nervous system. Recently Webster and Fite[3] have succeeded in transmitting a fatal infection to mice by means of intranasal instillation of louping-ill virus.

Regular transmission to mice of a lethal infection has also followed nasal instillation of the Indiana and New Jersey[4] strains of vesicular stomatitis virus. The cerebral tissue, aseptically removed from mice succumbing to the experimental infection induced by intracerebral injection of the virus, was ground in a sterile mortar with hormone broth of pH 7.5 to a 1:10 suspension and filtered through a Seitz disk, and instilled intranasally in doses of 0.04 cc by means of a tuberculin syringe fitted with a blunt needle. The nasal tissues were not injured.

Within four to six days, the animals developed hyperesthesia, tremors, incoordination, spastic paralysis most marked in the posterior extremities and prostration, followed by death on the fifth to eighth day. The series of nasal infections was carried through twelve passages—in each transfer the brain of nasally infected mice having been used as the inoculum.

The pathological changes are similar to those occurring in guinea-pigs and mice[1,4] inoculated intracerebrally with neurotropic vesicular stomatitis virus. The nerve cells of the hippocampus in the brain and the anterior gray matter of the cord contain typical intranuclear inclusion bodies, such as are found in the epithelial cells of the guinea-pig pad inoculated with the virus of vesicular stomatitis or of foot-and-mouth disease and in the nerve cells of the guinea-pig inoculated intracerebrally with the virus of vesicular stomatitis.

In addition to the effective brain tissue in dilutions as high as $10^7$, the virus in the 26th generation of tissue cultures[2] in dilutions of $10^6$ and in the filtrates of affected guinea-pig pads was found to be active when instilled nasally in mice. The question arises whether in the field vesicular stomatitis may be conveyed by nasal inhalation of the incitant.

It appears, therefore, that the virus of vesicular stomatitis is strikingly active in a minute quantity (1 to 10 million dilution) in the nasal passages of mice and that the uninjured nasal mucosa is as sensitive to infection as is the injured brain or pads of animals.[5]

These experiments suggest that the closely related

[1] H. R. Cox and P. K. Olitsky, *Proc. Soc. Exp. Biol. and Med.*, 30: 654, 1933.
[2] H. R. Cox, J. T. Syverton and P. K. Olitsky, *Proc. Soc. Exp. Biol. and Med.*, 30: 896, 1933.
[3] L. T. Webster and G. W. Fite, *Proc. Soc. Exp. Biol. and Med.*, 30: 656, 1933.
[4] H. R. Cox and P. K. Olitsky, *Proc. Soc. Exp. Biol. and Med.*, 30: 653, 1933.
[5] All operations were done under ether anesthesia.

virus of foot-and-mouth disease may also be infective in high dilution through intranasal inhalation.

Peter K. Olitsky
Herald R. Cox
Jerome T. Syverton
Laboratories of the Rockefeller Institute for Medical Research
New York

## ACTIVE IMMUNIZATION TO ANTHRAX BY MEANS OF HETEROPHILE ANTIGEN

Since the work of Forssman[1] showing the existence and action of heterophile antigens and antibodies, subsequent investigations have shown these to be widely distributed in animals and bacteria. Recently, Combiesco, Satamtesco, Nestoresco and Adam have demonstrated this antigen in anthrax bacilli.[2]

The work of Bailey and Shorb,[3] and that of Powell, Jamieson, Bailey and Hyde,[4] indicates that the heterophile antibodies play an important rôle in the protection, treatment and recovery in pneumococcus infections.

Thus the following experiment was done to determine whether or not heterophile antibodies play any rôle in anthrax infections.

Two rabbits were inoculated with boiled sheep corpuscles. After a period of two weeks had elapsed from the last injection, a small amount of blood was removed from the ear vein and a titration made to determine their heterophile antibody content. Then these two rabbits, along with two controls, were given subcutaneous inoculations of a virulent anthrax bacilli. The results are shown in Table 1.

TABLE 1

| Previous treatment of rabbits | Heterophile Titer* | Amount of turbid suspension of virulent Anthrax bacilli inoculated | Results |
|---|---|---|---|
| None | none | 0.2 cc subcutaneous | Died in 3 days |
| None | none | 0.2 cc subcutaneous | Died in 4 days |
| 5 intraperitoneal injections of 5 cc of 20 per cent. solution of boiled sheep corpuscles. | 800 units per cc | 0.2 cc subcutaneous | No ill effect. Observed for a month |
| 5 intraperitoneal injections of 5 cc of 20 per cent. solution of boiled sheep corpuscles. | 3200 units per cc | 0.4 cc subcutaneous | No ill effect. Observed for a month |

* Heterophile unit is defined as sufficient antibodies to hemolyze in the presence of complement 0.1 cc of washed erythrocytes diluted 1 plus 3 in terms of whole blood concentration.

From the above experiment it is evident that immunity developed by stimulation with the heterophile antigen in sheep's corpuscles protects rabbits from anthrax infection.

Since heterophile antibodies can be produced by oral administration of the antigen,[5] this method of anthrax immunization might be adaptable to the protection of individuals whose occupation exposes them to anthrax infection. Such individuals as wool sorters and tannery workers might be protected from anthrax infection by oral administration of the heterophile antigen in sheep corpuscles.

The use of heterophile antiserum in the treatment of anthrax infection is being studied, and will be reported later.

George E. Rockwell
Department of Bacteriology and Hygiene
University of Cincinnati

1 J. Forssman, *Biochem. Zeitschr.*, 37: 78, 1911.

2 D. Combiesco, S. Stamatesco, N. Nestoresco, and C. Adam, *Compt. rend. Soc. de Biol.*, 104: 712–717, 1930.

3 G. H. Bailey and M. S. Shorb, *Amer. Jour. Hyg.*, 13: 831–856, 1931; *ibid.*, 17: 329–411, 1933.

4 H. M. Powell, W. A. Jamieson, H. Bailey and R. R. Hyde, *Amer. Jour. Hyg.*, 17: 102–121, 1933.

5 H. M. Powell, *Amer. Jour. Hyg.*, 5: 228–229, 1925; *Proc. Ind. Acad. Sci.*, 34: 261–263, 1926.

## BOOKS RECEIVED

Carnegie Institution of Washington. *Catalogue of Publications.* Pp. xlii + 129. Carnegie Institution of Washington.

Daly, Reginald A. *Igneous Rocks and the Depths of the Earth.* Pp. xvi + 598. 190 figures. McGraw-Hill. $5.00.

Fowler, Henry W. *The Fishes of the Families Banjosidae, Lethrinidae, Sparidae, Girellidae, Kyphosidae,* etc. Collected by the U. S. Bureau of Fisheries Steamer "Albatross." Pp. vi + 465. 32 figures. Smithsonian Institution. Government Printing Office.

Kellogg, W. N. and L. A. Kellogg. *The Ape and the Child.* Pp. xiv + 341. Illustrated. Whittlesey House, McGraw-Hill. $3.00.

Lindsay, Robert B. *Physical Mechanics.* Pp. x + 436. Illustrated. Van Nostrand. $4.00.

Löhnis, F. *Handbuch der landwirtschaftlichen Bakteriologie.* Band I, Teil 1. Futtermittelbakteriologie. Pp. 105. 10, 50 RM. Band II, Teil 1. G. Ruschmann. Düngerbakteriologie. Pp. 158. Gebrüder Borntraeger, Berlin. 15,—RM.

Norris, James F. *Experimental Organic Chemistry.* Third edition. Pp. xiii + 233. McGraw-Hill. $1.50.

Noyes, Katharine Macy. *Jesse Macy.* Pp. xix + 192. Illustrated. Charles C. Thomas. $2.00.

Reck, Hans. *Oldoway.* Pp. 308. Illustrated. F. A. Brockaus, Leipzig. M. 10.50.

Rose, M. *Faune de France.* Pp. 374. 456 figures. Lechevalier, Paris.

Schuchert, Charles and Carl O. Dunbar. *A Text-Book of Geology.* Part II: Historical Geology. Third edition, revised. Pp. vii + 551. 332 figures. Wiley. $4.00.

Tôhoku Imperial University. *Science Reports.* Pp. 199. Illustrated. Maruzen, Tokyo.

# SCIENCE

VOL. 77 — FRIDAY, JUNE 30, 1933 — No. 2009

*William Thomas Councilman:* DR. HARVEY CUSHING 613

*A History of the National Research Council, 1919–1933: V. Division of Geology and Geography:* PROFESSOR W. H. TWENHOFEL 618

*Scientific Events:*
*Establishment of the Office of National Parks, Buildings and Reservations; The British Academic Assistance Council; Honorary Degrees Conferred at Yale University; The Chicago Meeting* 620

*Scientific Notes and News* 622

*Discussion:*
*A Grand Master Key to Biological Literature:* DR. DONALD REDDICK. *Swarming and Mating of Ants:* DR. C. C. GUTHRIE. *Goiter Prevention with Food Plants Grown on Iodized Soil:* DR. KARL G. ZWICK. *A Bacterial Gall Disease of the Douglas Fir:* DR. H. N. HANSEN and PROFESSOR RALPH E. SMITH 625

*Quotations:*
*Academic Assistance* 629

*Reports:*
*Field Conference of Pennsylvania Geologists:* DR. BRADFORD WILLARD 629

*Scientific Apparatus and Laboratory Methods:*
*A Simple String Electroscope:* PROFESSOR BENJAMIN ALLEN WOOTEN and WILBUR T. HARRIS 630

*Special Articles:*
*Effect of Inhibiting Factor from Normal Tissues on Spontaneous Tumors of Mice:* DR. JAMES B. MURPHY and ERNEST STURM. *Fundamental Limits to the Sizes of Clastic Grains:* DR. CHESTER K. WENTWORTH 631

*Science News* 6

SCIENCE: A Weekly Journal devoted to the Advancement of Science, edited by J. MCKEEN CATTELL and published every Friday by

THE SCIENCE PRESS

New York City: Grand Central Terminal

Lancaster, Pa. — Garrison, N. Y.

Annual Subscription, $6.00 — Single Copies, 15 Cts.

SCIENCE is the official organ of the American Association for the Advancement of Science. Information regarding membership in the Association may be secured from the office of the permanent secretary, in the Smithsonian Institution Building, Washington, D. C.

## WILLIAM THOMAS COUNCILMAN

### JANUARY 1, 1854–MAY 26, 1933

By Dr. HARVEY CUSHING

THROUGHOUT his long life Councilman was a man of ardent and generous enthusiasms. It was this quality, combined with his utter informality, which made him such an inspiring teacher for the young and such a delightful companion both for young and old. There was a picturesque ruggedness in his personal appearance, an unexpectedness in his turn of thought, a shrewdness and independence in his observations concerning people, things and events that set him apart from the common mould. He had escaped from early educational and environmental inhibitions by which many persons come to be afflicted and subdued. Combined with an utter unconsciousness of self, there was about him a certain sturdiness of mind, frankness of opinion and honesty of purpose which were no less disconcerting to the self-complacent than refreshing to those who appreciated his outspoken sincerity.

He was born on a busy farm which straddled the Reistertown turnpike not far from Baltimore, and he always regarded it as fortunate that his early years were passed in such an environment. There he learned to plow, to swing a cradle, to bind sheaves of grain and do other things that were unforgettable, like the gathering of Spring simples.

The very earliest thing I can remember [he wrote in one of later-year addresses] is being taken by my grandfather when he set out in the first warm days of early spring with a grubbing hoe (we called it mattock) on his shoulder to seek the plants, the barks and roots from which the spring medicine for the household was prepared. If I could but remember all that went into that mysterious decoction and the exact method of preparation, and with judicious advertisement put the product upon the market, I would shortly be possessed of wealth which might be made to serve the useful purpose of increasing the salaries of all pathologists. . . . But, alas! I remember only that the basic ingredients were dogwood bark and sassafras root, and to these were added *qu. s.* bloodroot, poke and yellow dock. That the medicine benefited my grandfather I have every reason to believe, for he was a hale, strong old man, firm in body and mind until the infection came against which even spring medicine was of no avail. That the medicine did me good I well know, for I can see before me even now the green on the south hillside of the old pasture, the sunlight in the strip of wood where the dogwood grew, the bright blossoms and the delicate pale green of the leaf of the sanguinaria, and the even lighter green of the tender buds of the sassafras in the hedgrow, and it is good to have such pictures deeply engraved in the memory.

Sent off to school at St. John's College, Annapolis, he left there at the age of sixteen and for the next six years 'led an independent existence, raised side whiskers, considered himself a very ripe individual and did pretty much as he chose.' That he was always something of a rebel and disinclined to do anything which did not interest him, he in after years frequently confessed. But at the age of twenty-two, the determination struck him to follow in the footsteps of his father, a country doctor "who had never lost the childish desire to find things out by observation and the test of experiment."

He entered the Medical School of the University of Maryland which was no better nor worse than most schools of the period, the two-year course consisting largely of a series of lectures. The dissecting room, however, provided the contact with Nature for which he yearned, and the form and structure of the body soon fired his curiosity. Fully to satisfy this, the farm provided an excellent opportunity and, beginning with the mole, he proceeded to make a comparative study of the skulls of all available animals until the collection finally threatened to crowd him out of his bedroom. So engrossed did he become in this occupation he largely neglected his second-year course of lectures; and it was not wholly a misfortune that one day during his absence a little nephew 'with a good business head' sold the whole collection for a few cents to an itinerant bone merchant. This grievous episode, by driving him back to his lectures, made it possible for him to attain, in March of 1878, the degree 'qualifying him to exercise the art of medicine which he had so laboriously learned for the advantage of the public.'

Then something notable happened and what this was can be best told fragmentarily in his own words, though properly to do so the scene must be shifted and the calendar advanced to 1921, a full forty-three years.

As the Christmas recess drew near, it was noised about in the Harvard Medical School that on December 19th Professor Councilman was for the last time to conclude his course of lectures on pathology for the second-year class. Entering the large amphitheater to find it packed to the doors by members of all classes, his face became suffused at the burst of applause and then, abandoning his intended discourse, with his engaging hesitancy of speech slightly more pronounced than usual, he said in effect:

"It is plain to see that you regard this as an occasion marking an epoch in my life, and there is a tendency to regard an epoch as an excuse for remarks. The three great epochs of life are birth, marriage and death, and they are often accompanied by certain remarks. At the wedding breakfast many have suffered from these remarks and some of us have made them. The present is a sort of intermediate epoch and though my talk is usually desultory I may take advantage of the occasion to be even more vague and desultory than usual."

By good fortune someone wrote down his impromptu ruminations and though they can not be quoted in full, interesting as that would be, some excerpts will serve to show what it was that happened after his graduation in March of 1878.

> . . . I heard that there was at the Johns Hopkins University a new sort of institution called a laboratory. I vaguely knew of the Johns Hopkins University but not a great deal about it. It had opened in 1876 and Huxley came on to give the opening address; my father drove in from the country and heard this address and he came back and told us what an impression it had made on him. . . . There seems something remarkable about the opening of this University. . . . The men, Martin, Rowland, Brooks, and Remsen, were young men, and as young men they felt no hampering traditions. Traditions may be very important, but they can be extremely hampering as well, and whether or not tradition is of really much value I have never been certain. Of course when they are very fine, they do good, but it is very difficult of course ever to repeat the conditions under which good traditions are formed, so they may be and are often injurious and I think the greatest progress is made outside of traditions. So the Johns Hopkins University started without traditions, and started with young men, full of vigor and enthusiasm, as its leaders. The University at its beginning made provision for twenty fellowships, each fellow being paid five hundred dollars; and *the idea of going to a university and being paid for it* made an impression!

He then went on to tell of Martin's permitting him to join his small class in the biological laboratory for the next three months and how thrilled he was with the informal spirit of the place and with the method of teaching through observation and experiment. That summer he became assistant to the quarantine officer, bought a cheap microscope with his first small earnings, and began with its aid to study such histological preparations as he could find time to make in the intervals of his routine work. And when that autumn Martin offered him the assistantship in physiology for the following year his cup was overflowing.

For the first paper he ever wrote (an experimental study of inflammation of the cornea) he was given a prize of one hundred dollars and with this encouragement he might well enough have been tempted to take up biology as a career. But something else proved a greater lure: for during the summer months of the three years since his graduation he had been at work, partly at the Marine Hospital and partly at the Bayview Asylum (the city almshouse and hospital) meanwhile becoming ardently interested in histological pathology. Properly to pursue this subject further, he decided that he must go abroad, which his frugal savings permitted him inexpensively to do.

He could scarcely have gone at a more fortunate time, for almost daily new discoveries were being made and new methods developed. In 1880 German medicine was approaching its heyday, under the stimulus of the new cellular pathology and the cultivation of pathogenic bacteria, both greatly aided by the increasing use of analine dyes in the study of tissues and micro-organisms. His longest sojourn was passed in Vienna under men who had been brought up in the tradition of Rokitansky. For a considerable time he was with Recklinghausen in the new school at Strassburg. He was working under Cohnheim and Weigert in their active laboratory at Leipzig when in April 1882 the exciting news was brought of Koch's discovery of the tubercle bacillus. And a year later he is found with Hanns Chiari, a man of his own age, whom he had first known in Vienna but who now held the chair of pathology in Prague. From this place under the date of July 16, 1883 a certain "correspondent," W.T.C., sent off to the *Medical News* an entertaining letter largely given over to a vivid description of the ordinary mid-day meal served in that part of the world.

So in his final lecture—to which, from this digression we may again turn—he went on to say:

> I came back from Europe very full of all the things which I had learned and with a more or less definite idea of . . . practising medicine. But I put off later and later the putting up of a sign showing that I was willing to serve, and finally never put it out, because it seemed to me there were so many other interesting things to do. And as long as one saw the possibility of doing these interesting things without actual starvation, there was no question of the choice, and there should never be a question of the choice. I reasoned that if worse came to worst I had a few acres of good land on which I could raise all the food I required and something over, . . . but I never had to resort to agriculture for a living. I speak of this because at that time there seemed to be no possibility of earning a living by teaching pathology, and Welch in New York and I were probably the first two men in the country who tried it. I rather think Dr. Welch took the greater risk because he had not my agricultural resources, though a training and mental capacity far greater than mine.

For the next few years after his return from abroad in 1883 he engaged in various tasks, doing the autopsies at Bayview, teaching in the two local medical schools, helping John S. Billings prepare his National Medical Dictionary, writing articles for encyclopoedias, and for a year serving as Coroner's physician to the City. This position paid him three hundred dollars, but it 'tied him down too much to places and dates' and 'being of a rather roving disposition' he 'did not care to be at a certain place at a certain time,' so he surrendered the job to another physician who had a greater political pull.

Meanwhile, in 1886 he had joined Welch and the early group of workers in the newly erected pathological laboratory which was to form part of a great hospital still in slow process of erection. And with the opening of the Johns Hopkins Hospital three years later there came another period as remarkable, he believed, as the first period, that of the opening of the University. To prepare himself for this event, in which he was slated to take part, he had gone abroad in 1888 for another year of study; and then for the two years prior to the establishment of the Medical School, in close intimacy—

> There lived together in the hospital a group of men, all young, all very good fellows, all working very hard, and all having a very good time. It is an important thing that people should be happy in their work, and if work does not bring happiness there is something wrong; and both at the University and at the Hospital there was that wonderful happiness in work.

All others who shared in that cloistered, carefree, hard-working and stimulating life in the Johns Hopkins Hospital during those two early years have expressed themselves in similar vein and there may never be anything quite like it again. Of this 'mutual admiration society,' as it was dubbed by visitors who had enjoyed its warm hospitality, the acting resident pathologist with the title of Associate Professor was one of the conspicuously unique figures. And it is natural that he should have been among the first of many to be called away by other institutions which were eager to capture something of the local spirit, hoping that it might prove transplantable.

Accustomed as a second-year student to the formal lectures then in vogue at the Harvard Medical School, the writer well remembers what an impression was made by the addition in 1892 to a somewhat austere faculty of this breezy informal pipe-smoking man, unmistakably sloping toward the sunny side, who was said to have been the first 'outsider' ever appointed to a professorial chair in the School. Accustomed to work elbow to elbow with others, those of us who cared to do so and knew enough to take advantage of the opportunity were welcome to a chair and a desk and a problem in his laboratory.

Indelible pictures of him must remain etched on the memory of all who had even casual contact with him in those early days in Boston when mayhap target practice was being held in the laboratory on a Sunday morning. He was a deadly shot for a thumbtack in a plank at twenty paces; and could swear at a golf ball as could few others. He was one of those rare people able without giving offence to punctuate quiet speech with oaths (even when talking to himself); and he depended upon and made considerable fuss over his occasional tipple preferably of Maryland rye. The growing up, later on, of his devoted children hampered him considerably in the first of these diversions—at least when at home; and what he thought of the Volstead Act and its necessary subterfuge does not bear repeating.

As can be seen from some of the quotations that have been given, he did not always necessarily expect to be taken seriously, particularly when in one of his pessimistic moods usually precipitated by examples of human selfishness he had happened to observe. But even these occasional outbursts had their amusing aspects, which would make him laugh (and swear) both at himself and the world. Someone has said that his attitude toward life and its varied experiences was more like that of Mark Twain than of anyone else he had ever known. And not to misjudge the lessening optimism and buoyancy of his later days, it may without impropriety be said that for sixteen years before his sudden end he had been victimized by increasingly severe attacks of angina pectoris.

But let us return again to the valedictory remarks of the retiring Professor of Pathological Anatomy on that December day of 1921, and we find him saying in conclusion:

> It seems to me that the most important thing for the teacher is to awaken interest and enthusiasm in his students and to provide them with opportunities of following the interest which is aroused, for in this way we progress. Knowledge can not be given, it must grow and be slowly formed through one's own efforts. It is of no importance whatever to be talked to. I have always rather enjoyed lecturing, I like to talk, and I have gotten I am sure more out of the lectures than any of my listeners, because a lecture is often an important discipline to the teacher. It enables him to classify things in his mind; through the lecture he often acquires new ideas. I know that sometimes as I have been lecturing I have seen an unscalable wall rising before the trend of my argument, and I have realized that if I said the next two or three sentences I would run against that wall, and one acquires a nimbleness of wit in finding a way around to the other side. I have enjoyed all that, and I think lecturing is an intellectual stimulus and comparatively harmless to the audience . . . it does not really very much matter what the lecturer says.

During those thirty years of consecutive teaching in a school which profited greatly by his ferment, he engaged in many time-consuming researches; and much as he loved to play, when once on a scientific quest he pursued it relentlessly and lived with his problem. While his independent papers deal with a large number of significant and timely subjects, he was more interested in fostering the work of his associates and pupils than in communicating the results of studies carried out by himself alone. Hence, the names of one or more collaborators appear on most of his major publications. Thus his early work on malaria (1885) was shared with A. C. Abbott; his monograph on amoebic dysentery (1891) with H. A. Lafleur; that on epidemic cerebrospinal meningitis (1898) with F. B. Mallory and J. H. Wright; the studies of 220 fatal cases of diphtheria (1901) with F. B. Mallory and R. M. Pearce; a syllabus of pathology for students (1904) with F. B. Mallory; and the several important studies on variola and vaccinia (1891–92) were subsequently brought together (1904) in a monograph under the names of his several coworkers, G. B. Magrath, W. R. Brinckerhoff, E. E. Tyzzer, E. E. Southard, R. L. Thompson, I. R. Bancroft, and G. M. Calkins.

Obviously what fostered the making of the larger number of these conjoint investigations was the opportunity, which contemporary epidemics afforded, of intensively studying the several diseases with which these papers deal; but at the same time sight was not lost of the opportunity for public service to the community in which the epidemics were causing alarm.

On the opening in 1913 of the Brigham Hospital to which he was appointed pathologist, the scope of his work was greatly enlarged though at the same time his responsibilities were doubled. The larger part of his time came to be passed in the hospital and the departmental protocols of the day are models in their thoroughness of detail. The lengthened number of hours he was obliged to spend in the microscopical study of dead tissues may possibly have served to accentuate—if anything could—his love of the outdoors and his interest in growing things.

Disturbed by the architecturally unadorned exterior of the new hospital, he personally selected, planted and during his odd hours cultivated the well chosen varieties of rambler roses that still surround it; and when so engaged, nothing gave him greater delight than for passers-by to mistake him for the official gardener. He had a gift for making things grow and was forever planting and tending shrubs and flowers somewhere. One of his chief joys was the Arnold Arboretum and his knowledge of every shrub and tree in that marvellous place was scarcely exceeded by that of his greatly admired friend, Charles S. Sargent, the Director. The horticultural interests now shown by certain members of the hospital staff of those days can probably be traced to the Sunday morning rambles in the Arboretum or elsewhere through the country in company with Councilman and Pasco, his devoted bulldog, who scarcely ever left his side.

By nature a close observer, this quality was further developed by the exercise of his profession and it was inevitable that he should look about him with greater keenness and more curiosity than most persons. Though a wide and discriminating reader, what he saw with his own eyes he questioned and interpreted in his own terms. He was, in its broad sense, a naturalist, and all things interested him. Two unusual opportunities came to him to gratify his fondness for travel and desire at first hand to study the unfamiliar flora of other regions. In 1916, he accompanied the Rice Expedition to the Amazon; and two years after his retirement at Harvard, having been invited temporarily to join the staff of the Pekin Union Medical College, he took advantage of this to go around the world. He had a gift of description and was a most facile writer of highly entertaining letters which, usually undated, he would dash off on the sheets of ruled yellow paper which he kept ready at hand.

It might be supposed, by the unthinking, that those whose chosen occupation is the study of disease and death would in time become callous and indifferent to life. On the contrary, it is more apt to lead to an abhorrence of suffering of any kind and to a peculiar tenderness toward living things. In his difficult and often baffling search for the cause of disease by the examination of the dead body, by the microscopic study of the tissues and by the experimental reproduction of its processes in lower animals, the pathologist is laying the foundation on which its recognition, alleviation or possible cure by physician or surgeon during life is alone possible. It is a task requiring optimism, patience, intelligence and self-sacrifice of unusual degree. And to show what outlet a pathologist may have, this inadequate tribute to one of them may well close with an allusion to something else.

On relinquishing his chair and with it his hospital position, Councilman merely shifted his attention from the diseases of man to those of plants, and his last printed paper, issued from the Arnold Arboretum, was the result of a microscopic study of the relation of the fungi of its essential humus to the root-system of *Epigaea repens.* As befitted its place of publication in the *Proceedings of the National Academy of Sciences,* it was a detailed presentation of a novel and little studied subject couched in scientific terms. But it was characteristic of him that he could not leave the trailing arbutus without unburdening himself in regard to its "fatal gift of conspicuous beauty" even though his feelings must be relegated to the footnote in which he says:

> The Epigaea repens is one of the most beautiful and interesting of plants. Its blossoms which are among the earliest of the spring flowers are white or pink with a waxy texture and a delicious spicy odor and are borne at the extremities of the stems. The pale green hairy leaves and the pale pink or green stems streaming from the centre close upon the surface of the soil add to the attractiveness. The environment of dead brown leaves, mosses and low plants give a perfect setting. It is unfortunate that these wonderful qualities should be those which are ensuring the destruction of the plant. Large quantities are gathered in the spring and hawked around the city streets, the unfortunate city dwellers seeking to satisfy atavistic and misunderstood yearnings for woods and green dales by purchasing the bunches. . . . The automobile by rendering remote places easily accessible has contributed greatly to its destruction, but the most powerful agency is the commercial exploitation which is ruthless and the traffic of great extent. Where the plants are abundant a family even selling them at wholesale can often earn $25.00 a day . . . but the plant is of slow growth and the relation of leaf and root is so finely adjusted that recovery after considerable loss does not take place and the stimulation to effect new growth cannot act on the plant and the fungus at the same time. By great care and skill plants can be transferred to other suitable localities and may even be propagated by seed but there is little prospect of its ever becoming a garden habitant. . . . I have known it to disappear completely from localities where formerly common and probably no plants can now be found within a dozen miles of any of the large cities. This desire to save the plant is not a mere matter of sentiment. No plant is more suitable for . . . the awakening in children through its study the all important wonder and curiosity. . . .. Apparently like all wild beautiful things which man covets it must go but the loss of such things is a serious loss for man.

Thus Councilman went through life observing, studying, recording and speculating on things small and on things large, but always with consuming interest in the quest that engaged him and living up to his maxim that the chief happiness lies in work. When uprooted from his warm and fertile Maryland soil and transplanted to the rugged shores of Puritan New England, there must have clung to him some of the 'essential native humus' which guaranteed more than a precarious foothold. Though 'deeply engraved on his memory' was the bursting springtime of his boyhood home, he came to appreciate no less the beauties of a slower year's awakening. So it is suitable to leave him—engrossed in the study of the tiny Mayflower and vigorously championing its right to survive.

# A HISTORY OF THE NATIONAL RESEARCH COUNCIL 1919--1933

## V. DIVISION OF GEOLOGY AND GEOGRAPHY[1]

By Professor W. H. TWENHOFEL

CHAIRMAN

THE Division of Geology and Geography was organized in 1918 for the purpose of assisting in the prosecution of the war and was reorganized in 1919 to serve the interests of the sciences in time of peace. The membership of the division at first was placed at twenty-six and later twenty-seven, of which nine members were to be elected at large, one as the representative of the Division of Federal Relations of the National Research Council, and the others chosen by the national societies of geology and geography. Experience soon demonstrated that a large membership was too expensive for the work of the division and also too large for efficient work, and in 1928 steps were taken to reduce the membership gradually to nineteen, which was completely effected by 1932. Since this reduction it has seemed that still greater efficiency and less expense would be attained by further reduction, and this view coincided with the recommendations of the Committee on Policies of the National Research Council, which urged that the executive members of the divisions be reduced to a number not greater than twelve. This reduction in membership is now in process and it is planned, beginning July 1, 1933, to have three members-at-large and nine members chosen by the national societies. It is felt that this reduction will permit centering more responsibility upon the members of the division and thus, in turn, lead to greater interest on the part of the membership.

The division does its work very largely through committees, but there is also much work done through personal contacts of the officers and members of the division with other geologists and geographers. The committees are concerned with a wide range of objectives. The number has varied through the years and at the present time there are twenty-four, the membership of a committee ranging from four to twenty. The motive prompting the appointment of a committee is one of hope of development of a neglected or backward branch of geology or geography through having a group of students interest itself with the branch of geology or geography concerned. In this way advance to a notable degree has been made in several fields of geology and geography, among which are: batholithic problems, studies of the clay minerals, isostasy, measurement of geologic time, micropaleontology, oceanography, paleobotany, petroleum geology, processes of ore deposition, sedimentation, shore-line investigations and tectonic geology. Two recently appointed committees are those on stratigraphy and the accessory minerals of crystalline rocks, and it is confidently expected that substantial advances will be made in those fields. At the present time over 200 geologists and geographers are centering attention on the work of the twenty-four committees, and great credit is due to the chairmen and members who give time and energy to the work of the division.

The roster of chairmen since the organization of the division is as follows:

1918 —John C. Merriam
1919–1922—E. B. Mathews
1922–1923—Nevin M. Fenneman
1923–1924—Andrew C. Lawson
1924–1927—David White
1927–1928—Waldemar Lindren
1928–1931—Arthur Keith
1931–1933—W. H. Twenhofel

The extent of the advance in the work of a committee rests on several factors, among which are, first and most important, the initiative, leadership and industry of the chairman, and, second, the nature of the problem. A committee is discontinued when its work has been concluded through solution of the problems upon which its attention was centered or through development of interest on the part of another organization prepared to assume responsibility for continuation of the work. The division does not attempt duplication of work, and when it is found that a competent organization is prepared to assume responsibility for further development of a project the division willingly retires from the field.

[1] This is the fifth of a series of ten articles prepared to describe briefly the nature of the activities with which the National Research Council has been engaged during the past fourteen years.

Some years ago the division found that not a great deal was being done in oceanography and a committee was appointed in 1922 to develop this field. This committee studied the problems for a decade and through excellent annual reports of progress stimulated interest in oceanographic problems. Ultimately the work carried on by the committee was undertaken by other organizations that had entered this field both in the United States and abroad, and in June, 1932, the committee brought its activities to an end. A committee on state geological surveys was appointed in 1928 and was discontinued in June, 1932, on the completion of a résumé of the activities since 1910 of the state and federal surveys. A committee to assist in the study of pioneer belts was appointed in 1925 and discontinued in 1928, at which time support for the project was assumed by other organizations and the work has continued under their auspices.

The work of the division may be classified as that of research, education and organization, and its various committees direct attention to one or more of these activities. Some committees, as those on measurement of geological time, clay minerals, tectonics and micropaleontology, are concerned almost entirely with research. Others, as the committees on sedimentation and paleobotany, are concerned with research pertaining to sediments or paleobotany and to education in these fields. The work of the committee on the state geological surveys may be considered essentially educational, and the work of the committees on bibliography of economic geology, conservation of the scientific results of drilling, field data of earthquakes, and the International Geographical Union as that of organization.

The research work of the division has resulted in the publication of several bibliographies, of numerous reports which appear in whole or in part in the annual reports of the division, of bulletins published by the National Research Council, of articles published in geological or geographical journals, and of books published by commercial concerns. Research work carried out on grants made by or through the division is usually published in various scientific journals, and in some instances in the publications of a geological survey.

In addition to the work of committees, the division has assisted in the preparation of bibliographies, in the compilation of maps, in surveys of the fields of work of geology and geography, in cooperative work with other research organizations, and it has served as a liaison body between the scientists of the United States and some of the international geographical and geological congresses.

The division has no direct funds of its own other than an annual allotment from the Research Council to take care of its administrative expenses. Some of the committees, as those on measurement of geologic time, studies in petroleum geology, and sedimentation, through their own efforts have acquired funds for aiding research in the fields concerned. These funds have been derived from various sources and from them, from time to time, small grants have been made to individual workers to assist in the solution of particular problems.

The division participates in the allocation of the funds administered by the Committee on Grants-in-Aid of the National Research Council, the committee being composed of the chairman of the Council and the chairmen of the seven technologic divisions. To date sixty grants for geologic and geographic projects, totalling $36,913.50, have been made to fifty-one individuals by this committee. Through these grants three seismographs have been erected in three different places in the United States, aid has been given to paleontologic and stratigraphic studies over many parts of the country, ranging from the Atlantic to the Pacific and from Canada to the Gulf, and aid for studies in these fields has been extended to include territory in several foreign countries. Mineralogy and petrography have received aid for both field and laboratory studies, and work in geography has been made possible in the United States, Greenland, Mexico, Brazil, Japan, and elsewhere. Applications for grants have been numerous and many have been denied because of insufficient funds, or because the projects presented were of such a nature that they did not come within the bounds of the policies under which the grants-in-aid are administered. It is felt that the two fields of learning represented by the Division of Geology and Geography have been greatly benefited through support derived from these funds, and the records of results are extremely creditable.

For the past three years the division has had the administration of from four to six pre-doctorate fellowships, known as the Storrow fellowships, a fund of $5,000 having been given annually to the division for this purpose. These are granted to students of geology and geography, and the allotment per student per annum has been from $800 to $1,000. For the fellowships given for the year 1932–1933 there were sixty-five applicants, or thirteen applicants for each one chosen, thus clearly showing the needs for fellowship support for geology and geography. The fellows study in any institution approved by the fellowship committee of the division. The division is greatly in need of post-doctorate fellowships in order that students of marked ability in research need not be compelled to accept minor commercial or educational positions to have an income necessary for subsistence.

With several well-supported post-doctorate fellowships the most gifted of the younger geologists or geographers of the country could be retained for one or more years in study and research before settling down to some permanent position. It is believed that in this way very great advance could be made.

During the period 1926–1931 the division, together with the Divisions of Physics and Chemistry, cooperated through the Central Petroleum Committee of the Research Council with the American Petroleum Institute in organizing the work and selecting the personnel for the projects financed by the institute under its five-year program of fundamental research in petroleum. Descriptions of these projects and lists of papers which resulted from these studies have been published in the bulletins of the institute.

One of the bibliographic projects now in progress under the auspices of the division is that of the "Annotated Bibliography of Economic Geology." Sufficient funds were raised by the committee to cover the editorial expenses for a period of about seven years, after which it is hoped that the bibliography will have sufficiently demonstrated its usefulness to enlist further financial support.

As noted in a previous paragraph, records of the work of the division are given in numerous publications. In the annual report of the division for 1931–1932, a history is given which includes an annotated list of some 64 projects undertaken by the division since its permanent organization in 1919. In this history are given details and results of the work of the division not possible of presentation in this short paper. These are tangible results that are possible of measurement. In addition there are the intangible results which are difficult of discovery and equally difficult of evaluation. The several division chairmen, the many different members of the division and the personnel of the committees have stimulated research as they have been brought in contact with their colleagues through membership in the National Research Council or its committees, and they themselves in turn have been stimulated by such contacts. To those familiar with the results of the work accomplished, the record seems an enviable one.

The future of the division is of course unknown, but everything seems favorable for continued development along the paths it has already opened. In the early days there was no doubt much uncertainty as to what the division might do, but, measured by its past record, it has more than justified its founding, and, basing itself on its accomplishments, it may look confidently to the future. As in the past there will be required devoted and loyal workers. The division in part can provide for these in the election of members-at-large and the selection of its committee chairmen, but for the greater part of the membership it must rely upon the societies by which these members are chosen.

# SCIENTIFIC EVENTS

## ESTABLISHMENT OF THE OFFICE OF NATIONAL PARKS, BUILDINGS AND RESERVATIONS

THE reorganization order of President Roosevelt, establishing the Office of National Parks, Buildings and Reservations, will take effect sixty days from June 10, the date of issue. It is as follows:

All functions of administration of public buildings, reservations, national parks, national monuments and national cemeteries are consolidated in an office of national parks, buildings and reservations in the Department of the Interior, at the head of which shall be a director of national parks, buildings and reservations; except that where deemed desirable there may be excluded from this provision any public building or reservation which is chiefly employed as a facility in the work of a particular agency. This transfer and consolidation of functions shall include, among others, those of the National Park Service of the Department of the Interior, and the national cemeteries and parks of the War Department which are located within the continental limits of the United States. National cemeteries located in foreign countries shall be transferred to the Department of State, and those located in insular possessions under the jurisdiction of the War Department shall be administered by the Bureau of Insular Affairs of the War Department.

The functions of the following agencies are transferred to the office of national parks, buildings and reservations of the Department of the Interior and the agencies are abolished:

The Arlington Memorial Bridge Commission, the Public Buildings Commission, the Public Buildings and Public Parks of the National Capital, the National Memorial Commission and the Rock Creek and Potomac Parkway Commission.

Expenditures by the Federal Government for the purposes of the Commission of Fine Arts, the George Rogers Clark Sesquicentennial Commission and the Rushmore Commission shall be administered by the Department of the Interior.

## THE BRITISH ACADEMIC ASSISTANCE COUNCIL

THE formation of the Academic Assistance Council, with Lord Rutherford as president, has been reported in SCIENCE. The official announcement of its objects, issued from the rooms of the Royal Society at Burlington House, London, is as follows:

Many eminent scholars and men of science and university teachers of all grades and in all faculties are being obliged to relinquish their posts in the universities of Germany.

The universities of our own and other countries will, we hope, take whatever action they can to offer employment to these men and women, as teachers and investigators. But the financial resources of universities are limited and are subject to claims for their normal development which can not be ignored. If the information before us is correct, effective help from outside for more than a small fraction of the teachers now likely to be condemned to want and idleness will depend on the existence of large funds specifically devoted to this purpose. It seems clear also that some organization will be needed to act as a center of information and put the teachers concerned into touch with the institutions that can best help them.

We have formed ourselves accordingly into a provisional council for these two purposes. We shall seek to raise a fund, to be used primarily, though not exclusively, in providing maintenance for displaced teachers and investigators, and finding them the chance of work in universities and scientific institutions.

We shall place ourselves in communication both with universities in this country and with organizations which are being formed for similar purposes in other countries, and we shall seek to provide a clearing house and center of information for those who can take any kind of action directed to the same end. We welcome offers of cooperation from all quarters. We appeal for generous help from all who are concerned for academic freedom and the security of learning. We ask for means to prevent the waste of exceptional abilities exceptionally trained.

The issue raised at the moment is not a Jewish one alone; many who have suffered or are threatened have no Jewish connection. The issue, though raised acutely at the moment in Germany, is not confined to that country. We should like to regard any funds entrusted to us as available for university teachers and investigators of whatever country who, on grounds of religion, political opinion or race, are unable to carry on their work in their own country.

The Royal Society have placed office accommodation at the disposal of the council. Sir William Beveridge and Professor C. S. Gibson, F.R.S., are acting as Honorary Secretaries of the Council, and communications should be sent to them at the Royal Society, Burlington House, W.1. An executive committee is being formed and the names of trustees for the fund will shortly be announced. In the meantime checks can be sent to either of the honorary secretaries.

Our action implies no unfriendly feelings to the people of any country; it implies no judgment on forms of government or on any political issue between countries. Our only aims are the relief of suffering and the defense of learning and science.

Lascelles Abercrombie, S. Alexander, W. H. Beveridge, W. H. Bragg, Buckmaster, Cecil, Crawford & Balcarres, Winifred C. Cullis, H. A. L. Fisher, Margery Fry, C. S. Gibson, M. Greenwood, J. S. Haldane, A. V. Hill, George F. Hill, W. S. Holdsworth, F. Gowland Hopkins, A. E. Housman, J. C. Irvine, F. G. Kenyon, J. M. Keynes, A. D. Lindsay, Lytton, J. W. Mackail, Allen Mawer, Gilbert Murray, Eustace Percy, W. J. Pope, Robert S. Rait, Rayleigh, Charles Grant Robertson, Robert Robinson, Rutherford, Michael E. Sadler, Arthur Schuster, C. S. Sherrington, George Adam Smith, G. Elliot Smith, J. C. Stamp, J. J. Thomson, G. M. Trevelyan.

## HONORARY DEGREES CONFERRED AT YALE UNIVERSITY

Degrees conferred in the sciences by Yale University on June 21 included the doctorate of science on Dr. Ernest William Brown, Josiah Willard Gibbs professor of mathematics emeritus at the university, and on Dr. Alfred Newton Richards, professor of pharmacology at the University of Pennsylvania. The doctorate of laws was conferred on Dr. Hugh S. Cumming, Surgeon-General of the United States. The degree of master of science was conferred on Dr. William Bosworth Castle, assistant professor of medicine, Thorndike Memorial Foundation, and Boston City Hospital; on Lincoln Ellsworth, New York City, explorer, and on Dr. Alfred Lee Loomis, physicist, director of the Loomis Laboratories.

Candidates for the honorary degrees were cited by Professor William Lyon Phelps, while the degrees were conferred by Dr. Angell.

The citations made in conferring the degrees on Professor Brown, Professor Richards and Surgeon-General Cumming were as follows:

ALFRED NEWTON RICHARDS, SC.D.

*Professor Phelps:* Professor of pharmacology, University of Pennsylvania. Dr. Richards took his B.A. and M.A. at Yale, and began his career in the Sheffield Scientific School Laboratory of Professor Chittenden. Then he taught at Columbia, later at Northwestern, and in 1910 was made professor at Pennsylvania. During the World War he was attached to the staff of the British Medical Research Committee. In connection with the wide-spread studies of shock he made outstanding observations regarding the occurrence of histamine in minute quantities in the organism and its relation to the behavior of the blood vessels. More recently he has highly developed a unique field of research in regard to kidney function. He has trained many competent investigators, the publications coming from his laboratory being highly important. For many years he has been a guiding influence in the development of academic medicine in Philadelphia. Here is a man whose researches have added to organized knowledge and to the welfare of mankind.

*Dr. Angell:* Distinguished investigator in a most difficult and important field, inventor therein of delicate and invaluable techniques, a recognized leader in your special department of research, your *alma mater,* proud of your accomplishments, confers upon you the degree of Doctor of Science and admits you to all its rights and privileges.

ERNEST WILLIAM BROWN, SC.D.

*Professor Phelps:* Professor Brown was born at Hull, England, and received in 1887 his B.A. degree at Christ's College, Cambridge, where two centuries earlier an English poet paid a compliment to Galileo. Professor Brown has won many prizes and is a member of learned societies in America and abroad. In 1891 he became professor of mathematics at Haverford, where he remained until 1907, when he was called to Yale. He became professor emeritus in 1932. His publications on lunar theory and celestial mechanics have given him an international reputation and have added to the glory of Yale. His Tables on the Motion of the Moon is a monumental work and has brought him a blizzard of degrees, medals, prizes and honors. He is an excellent chess player and an amateur humorist of high reputation. In his youth he expected to be a concert pianist, but later took up the music of the spheres. His versatility is additionally shown in that, although he is a specialist on the moon, in the year 1925 in the city of New Haven he arranged a personally conducted total eclipse of the sun.

*Dr. Angell:* In grateful and affectionate acknowledgment of the luster shed upon her by your brilliant scientific achievement during a long and distinguished service on her faculty, Yale University gladly confers upon you the degree of Doctor of Science, admitting you to all its rights and privileges.

HUGH SMITH CUMMING, LL.D.

*Professor Phelps:* Born in Virginia, taking his degree of Doctor of Medicine at the University of Virginia, Dr. Cumming was appointed Assistant Surgeon in the United States Public Health Service in 1894, and became Surgeon-General in 1920. In earlier years he made creditable contributions in the field of public health research, particularly in regard to the sanitary conditions of the shellfish industry, but his finest achievements have been during the last thirteen years, in the administration of Public Health Service. When he took control it was a rather undistinguished organization; he gradually transformed it into an institution of which our country is proud, an institution equalled perhaps in no other country except England. Benchwarmers have been progressively lifted and their places taken by able investigators, with the result that during the last five or six years substantial and far-reaching contributions have been made in the study of such nutritional diseases as beriberi, in the investigation of tularemia, Rocky Mountain spotted fever and endemic typhus; in studies on silicosis, and other aspects of industrial hygiene; also in the field of pure science, where researches in the chemical composition of sugars have attracted attention. All these technical remarks simply mean that Dr. Cumming is a first-rate citizen.

*Dr. Angell:* Eminent representative of a noble profession, essential architect and builder of the Public Health Service of the United States, everywhere recognized as one of the most beneficent of all agencies dedicated to the public weal, in grateful recognition of the intelligence, devotion and skill which you have brought to your duties, Yale University confers upon you the degree of Doctor of Laws, admitting you to all its rights and privileges.

## THE CHICAGO MEETING

THE notable meeting of the American Association for the Advancement of Science and the associated societies, which opened in Chicago on June 19 and continues to June 30, will be fully reported in SCIENCE. The meeting was held on the invitation of the Century of Progress Exposition, which, together with the American Association, invited as guests a number of the most distinguished foreign men of science. Those who accepted the invitation and took part in the general sessions and conferences are the following:

OTTO APPEL, Agriculture, Berlin
F. W. ASTON, Chemistry, Cambridge
JOSEPH BARCROFT, Physiology, Cambridge
A. MENDELSSOHN BARTHOLDY, Political Science, Hamburg
JAKOB BJERKNES, Meteorology, Bergen
NIELS BOHR, Physics, Copenhagen
FILIPPO BOTTAZZI, Physiology, Naples
LUDWIG DIELS, Botany, Berlin
JEAN DUFRÉNOY, Agriculture, France
LEOPOLD FEJÉR, Mathematics, Budapest
ENRICO FERMI, Physics, Rome
A. P. M. FLEMING, Engineering, Manchester
R. GOLDSCHMIDT, Zoology, Berlin
HERBERT J. GOUGH, Engineering, London
SIR DANIEL HALL, Agriculture, London
A. V. HILL, Physiology, London
C. U. A. KAPPERS, Anthropology and Physiology, Amsterdam
WOLFGANG KOEHLER, Psychology, Berlin
AUGUST KROGH, Zoology, Copenhagen
TULLIO LEVI-CIVITA, Mathematics, Rome
EMILIO MIRA, Psychology, Barcelona
WILLIAM OUALID, Political Economy, Paris
HENRI PIERON, Psychology, Paris
J. J. SEDERHOLM, Geology, Helsingfors
CHARLES E. SPEARMAN, Psychology, London
T. SVEDBERG, Chemistry, Upsala
R. J. TILLYARD, Entomology and Paleontology, Australia

# SCIENTIFIC NOTES AND NEWS

DR. HARVEY CUSHING, who recently retired as Moseley professor of surgery at Harvard University and surgeon-in-chief at the Peter Bent Brigham Hospital, has been appointed first Sterling professor of neurology at Yale University. The chair has been founded through a gift of $300,000 from the estate of John W. Sterling.

DR. JAMES FRANCK, professor of physics at the

University of Göttingen, who refused the offer of the Nazi government to let him retain his position there, has been appointed for the coming academic year Speyer guest professor at the Johns Hopkins University.

AT the commencement exercises at Harvard University the degree of doctor of science was conferred on Professor Harlow Shapley, director of the Harvard College Observatory, and on Dr. George David Birkhoff, professor of mathematics. In conferring these degrees, President Lowell made the following citations: "Harlow Shapley—An astronomer of renown, whose spirit, searching for the center of the universe and the nature of the ultra-galactic nebulae, chafes at observing only from this paltry planet." "George David Birkhoff—First in our land among masters of mathematics, that great tool of science; greater still in the realm of pure imagination."

AT the commencement exercises at the University of Pennsylvania the degree of doctor of science was conferred on Professor Charles W. Burr, of the Graduate School of Medicine.

THE doctorate of science has been conferred by Brown University on Professor Harlow Shapley, director of the Harvard College Observatory, and on the late Frederic P. Gorham, at the time of his death chairman of the department of biology at the university.

DR. HERBERT S. JENNINGS, director of the zoological laboratory of the Johns Hopkins University, received the degree of doctor of science at the commencement exercises of Oberlin College.

THE honorary degree of doctor of science was conferred by the Ohio State University at its commencement, on June 12, on Dr. Edward Francis, of the National Institute of Health, Washington, D. C.

SIR WILFRED THOMASON GRENFELL delivered the commencement address at the ninety-sixth commencement of the University of Louisville on the evening of June 6. The honorary degree of doctor of science was conferred upon him by the university.

DR. C. U. ARIENS KAPPERS, director of the Zentral Institut für Hirnforschung at Amsterdam, received the honorary degree of doctor of laws from the Chicago Medical School, at its eighteenth annual commencement, in recognition of his work in neuropsychiatry.

DR. A. A. BENEDETTI-PICHLER, of the department of chemistry, Washington Square College, New York University, has received the Pregl Prize, awarded annually by the Vienna Academy of Sciences for distinguished work in microchemistry.

DR. ROBERT P. BIGELOW, professor of zoology at the Massachusetts Institute of Technology, who has been connected with the institute since 1893, retires at the end of the academic year with the title professor emeritus. He will be an honorary lecturer at the institute next year.

DR. CHARLES H. RICHARDSON, for more than twenty-five years professor of mineralogy and head of the department at Syracuse University, has retired with the title of professor emeritus of mineralogy. He will continue as director of the natural science museum and will give part of the time to lecturing at the university. On June 19 he received the honorary degree of doctor of science from Norwich University, Northfield, Vermont.

SIR ARTHUR KEITH, who has been for twenty-five years conservator of the museum and Hunterian lecturer of the Royal College of Surgeons, will shortly retire, but will continue his connection with the college. He will have charge of the two laboratories of the college, recently built at Down, in Kent, where Charles Darwin lived. They are endowed by Sir Buckston Browne and are for experimental work in surgery. Sir Arthur will supervise the work of young surgeons who will live and work in Down.

DR. E. MELLANBY, professor of pharmacology at the University of Sheffield, has resigned.

DR. G. A. CLARK, lecturer in physiology at the University of Sheffield, has been promoted to a professorship in succession to Professor J. B. Leathes.

AT a meeting of the court of the University of St. Andrews on June 2, John Anderson was appointed professor of surgery in succession to the late Professor L. Turton Price.

AT the annual meeting of the New Orleans Academy of Sciences, the following officers were elected: Robert Glenk, curator, Louisiana State Museum, *president;* H. H. Beard, Ph.D., biological chemist, Louisiana State University Medical Center, *first vice-president;* E. C. Faust, M.D., parasitologist, Tulane University, *second vice-president;* E. L. Demmon, chief, U. S. Forest Experiment Station, *secretary,* and Dr. D. S. Elliott, dean of the department of physics, Tulane University, *treasurer.*

OFFICERS of the Minnesota chapter of Sigma Xi for the coming year are as follows: *President,* Dr. Samuel C. Lind; *Vice-president,* Dr. Frederic K. Butters; *Secretary,* Dr. Frederick B. Hutt; *Treasurer,* Dr. George A. Thiel; *Board of Electors,* Dr. John E. Anderson, Dr. C. H. Bailey, Dr. Charles A. Mann and Dr. Owen Wangensteen.

AT Syracuse University on May 29, Sigma Pi

Sigma, honorary physics fraternity, installed its twenty-sixth chapter when twenty students, alumni and faculty members were initiated into the society as the Alpha-Beta Chapter. The installing officers were: Dr. Marsh W. White, Pennsylvania State College, *executive secretary,* and G. D. Collins, Cornell University, *national vice-president.* The formal installation was followed by a dinner at the University Inn, in honor of the installing officers, visiting members of Sigma Pi Sigma and administrative officers of the university. After brief speeches by Dr. Royal A. Porter, head of the physics department at Syracuse, and others, Dr. White delivered an address on "New Frontiers in Contemporary Physics."

THE Textile Foundation has authorized a survey into the personnel and facilities for textile education. A committee consisting of Dr. Karl T. Compton, president of Massachusetts Institute of Technology, E. C. Brooks, president of North Carolina State College, and R. E. Doherty, dean of the School of Engineering, Yale University, has been appointed to inquire into the possibility of such a survey, and upon their recommendation the work will begin.

THE appointment of an advisory committee on sanitation to serve the Baltimore Health Department, especially on matters of environmental hygiene, has been announced. Dr. William H. Howell, director emeritus of the Johns Hopkins School of Hygiene and Public Health, is chairman of the committee. Wilmer H. Schulze, who since 1929 has been chief of the division of chemical technology, was made director of the new bureau of environmental hygiene in the health department.

DR. GLENNON GILBOY, associate professor of soil mechanics in the department of civil engineering at the Massachusetts Institute of Technology, has sailed for Copenhagen, where he will attend the sessions of the World Power Conference as a delegate of the United States. The conference opened in Copenhagen on June 26, continues in Stockholm from June 28 to July 6 and will end in Oslo on July 8.

COLONEL CHARLES F. CRAIG, of the Department of Tropical Medicine, Tulane University, spoke on "The Factors Influencing the Transmission of the Malarial Fevers" at the recent meeting of the New Orleans Academy of Science.

AFTER completing a series of lectures at the University of London in May, Professor William K. Gregory gave a lecture on June 6 at the University of Oxford on "The Evolution of Jaws and Teeth in Primates." Dr. Gregory has now returned to the United States.

THE annual Boyle lecture of the Junior Scientific Club at the University of Oxford was delivered on June 2 by Lord Rutherford, who took as his subject "The Artificial Transmutation of the Elements."

THE fifth congress of the International Society of Urology will be held at the Royal Society of Medicine, London, from July 10 to 15, under the presidency of Sir John Thomson-Walker.

THE fifteenth annual meeting of the American Society of Mammalogists was held at the Biological Institute of Harvard University, from May 9 to May 13. Sixty-six members were present from ten states and one Canadian province. Forty-one papers were presented. Several resolutions were passed, among them one urging that the black bear be taken off of the bounty list in New Hampshire, and another stressing the importance of preserving the elk herd in the Olympic Mountains. The officers elected for the coming year were: *President,* Vernon Bailey; *Vice-presidents,* T. S. Palmer, H. E. Anthony; *Recording Secretary,* Robert K. Enders; *Corresponding Secretary,* Robert T. Hatt; *Treasurer,* Mrs. Viola S. Snyder; *Directors,* class of 1933–1935, Joseph Grinnell, A. Brazier Howell, Remington Kellogg, W. E. Saunders, Harold Coolidge, Jr. Edward A. Preble continues as chairman of the editorial board in charge of *The Journal of Mammalogy.* The next annual meeting will be held at the American Museum of Natural History in New York City.

THE United States Civil Service Commission has announced open competitive examinations for the positions of senior highway construction supervisor, salary $4,600 to $5,400; senior highway design engineer, salary $4,600 to $5,400, both with the Bureau of Public Roads, Department of Agriculture, Washington, D. C.; junior park naturalist, Department of the Interior, salary $2,000 a year. The salaries carry a provision for a 15 per cent. reduction as a measure of economy and a $3\frac{1}{2}$ per cent. deduction for retirement.

MORE than $2,000,000 has been bequeathed to the University of Chicago by the late W. G. Zoller to establish and maintain a free dental dispensary, according to the Chicago *Tribune.* The income will be used by the university "for the purpose of equipping and maintaining dispensaries and laboratories and to supply competent and skilful dental service, including diagnostic aids to the needy and poor, free of charge, in such manner that the greatest number of people may secure skilful treatment to enable them to be relieved, and to prevent the numerous ills which result from neglect of the teeth."

WE learn from the *Journal* of the American Medical Association that ceremonies were held on April 21 dedicating the George Eastman Dental Clinic at Rome, a gift to the Italian government from the late

Mr. Eastman, of Rochester, New York. Harvey J. Burkhart, D.D.S., director of the Rochester Dental Dispensary, founded by Mr. Eastman, formally presented the building to the government and Dr. Amedeo Perna, director of the new institution, accepted it. A bust of Mr. Eastman, presented to the clinic by Italian citizens of Rochester, was unveiled by Mrs. Burkhart, following an address by Dr. Joseph Carlucci, Rochester. The Honorable John W. Garrett, ambassador from the United States to Italy, read a cable of congratulation from President Roosevelt. Premier Mussolini inspected the building during the day. The Rome clinic is the second of five dental clinics in European cities for which Mr. Eastman set aside gifts of $1,000,000 each. The first was opened in London two years ago. The corner-stone for the third, in Stockholm, was laid on April 29, at ceremonies in which the crown prince and princess of Sweden and Dr. and Mrs. Burkhart participated. It is expected that this clinic will be finished by September, 1934, and that the corner-stones for similar buildings in Paris and Brussels will be laid this autumn.

THE *Journal* of the American Medical Association reports that the All-India Institute of Hygiene and Public Health, Calcutta, a gift of the Rockefeller Foundation to the government of India, was opened recently; addresses were made by Sir John Anderson, governor of Bengal, and Lieut. Col. Alexander D. Stewart, director of the institute. The school will be operated in cooperation with the Calcutta School of Tropical Medicine, where basic subjects will continue to be taught, while the institute deals purely with public health subjects related to Indian requirements. It will later be affiliated with the University of Calcutta, through which a doctorate in public health will be offered. The building, which harmonizes with the school of tropical medicine, has four stories, with facilities for teaching, laboratory work and lectures. A number of rooms will be artificially cooled.

THE Franklin Institute of Philadelphia, on May 17, 1933, conferred a John Price Wetherill Medal on The Koppers Co., Pittsburgh, "in consideration of the development of systems for the liquid purification of gases, the success of which is evidenced by the number of such installations in regular use." The Koppers Research Department, working at the Mellon Institute and at the company's plants, developed a purification process using a liquid absorber. In this process the hydrogen sulfide is first absorbed, and then removed from the absorbing solution by activation with air. This air, containing the hydrogen sulfide, is either discharged into the atmosphere or utilized through combustion in boilers, gas producers, or coke ovens. Later modifications were made in the process whereby sulfur could be recovered from the hydrogen sulfide.

ACCORDING to press reports Colonel Charles A. Lindbergh, technical adviser to the Pan-American Airways System, may take charge of survey flying in Greenland and Iceland this summer. Juan T. Trippe, president of the system, states that an expedition would carry on further studies of the northern transatlantic flying route. If it is possible for him to be away, Colonel Lindbergh may later join the expedition by plane. A chartered vessel, the *S. S. Jelling,* of 3,500 tons, will carry a technical staff headed by Major Robert A. Logan, of the airline, to Labrador and Greenland. It will have on board equipment for meteorological study, including an airplane. The vessel will also serve as a base for the expedition. The expedition aims to supplement the data on the route already assembled. The work is being carried on in association with European international airlines, including Imperial Airways and the French Aéropostale. It is planned that an airplane, flying from New York, shall join the expedition later in the summer to carry out special surveys and photographic work.

# DISCUSSION

## A GRAND MASTER KEY TO BIOLOGICAL LITERATURE

BIOLOGY long since has grown to unwieldy proportions and has split into several groups of more workable size and presumably of greater community of interest. These groups in turn have undergone or are undergoing a disintegration. At Atlantic City, for example, was held the first annual meeting of the Genetics Society of America with a program of 45 papers. A new Mycological Society of America emerged at the same time. Under the four headings of Agriculture, Botany, Medical Sciences and Zoology, 19 organizations held meetings at Atlantic City and in most of them simultaneous sessions were held to dispose of the mass of papers offered. Furthermore, the Atlantic City meeting was not one of the "big" meetings, and many societies met elsewhere. Truly biology has spawned a diversified progeny and the end is not yet.

Some of the new organizations indicate clearly the need for realignments—the old cleavage lines are now unnatural. This was recognized 18 years ago by the Ecologists and more than a year ago by the Geneticists. In other cases the need is extant, witness simultaneous sessions dealing with virus diseases in the Medical Sciences and in the Phytopathological Society, not to mention papers in three different societies dealing with problems of immunity.

The literature of biology is a relatively permanent thing. It will be extant long after the scientist and his presentation at the "annual meeting" are gone and all but forgotten. This literature unfortunately appears in a much greater variety of places than the fairly large number of societies would indicate, even after multiplying that number by the number of nations in which scholarly work is being done. In fact, over 5,000 serial publications are examined for biological publications by the corps of workers of *Biological Abstracts*. Little wonder that a worker in some narrow field of biology hesitates to comment on biology in general or on work in some other cubicle of the science. For some of these cubicles workable keys to the literature exist, but for some others there is no key or the keys have become rusty or are either temporarily misplaced or perhaps lost. Biologists have not been unmindful of the confusion that exists and for several years past have been trying to do something to improve the situation. The monthly accretions of *Biological Abstracts* only serve to intensify and emphasize the necessity for a grand master key. Most fortunately it now appears that the key is going to be available to any one who wishes it. Dr. McClung's modest announcement in SCIENCE of May 27, 1932, indicated that support had been found for the publication of indexes, and the appearance of the index for volume 2 of *Biological Abstracts* in December with the promise of an index for volume 3 within a few months is tangible evidence that this most important need of biology is going to be met.

Ordinarily an index volume can be inserted at its proper place in a file to be examined when needed. A volume which is to form a part of the grand master key to recent biological literature is worth examining most critically. Is it really going to work? The undersigned, of course, can apply the test only in a limited way, but it is easy to see that the index to the biological literature of the year 1928 makes a volume of nearly 500 pages, pages the same size as the one on which these words are printed, six point type, the first quarter with four columns to the page and the remaining three quarters with three columns to the page. Truly, there are a large number of references here, an almost unbelievably large number, but in the very first line the consultant is reminded that "this volume covers only a part of the literature published in the period during which the volume was issued. Succeeding volumes . . . must be consulted. . . ." As one reads on for four pages it becomes evident that the compilers of the volume are biologists, that they speak in terms readily understood by their coworkers, that the problems of making a useful index have been studied most carefully. Upon glancing through the four pages of "introductory guide to the indexes" it becomes apparent that they are pages to be read again. One needs to understand exactly what is said here in order to appreciate how ambitious is the pretension of these index makers. It sounds almost too good to be true. Even the mechanics of construction and composition of such a table will arouse the curiosity of the editorially minded.

But the proof of the genuineness of this master key lies in the actual tests. Does it actually turn the lock of this cubicle and that? The writer has made some tests in a field with which he is familiar. Of course, an author index is largely a matter of alphabet, but in this index each joint or junior author rates a full entry with his name in boldface type. The most notable thing about the subject index is the fact that the words in common usage by workers appear there in proper alphabetic sequence. There is no necessity to speculate about the system of logic employed by the compilers. Generous use is made of "see also" and "see under." The Systematist doubtless will be pleased with the separate systematic index, but this index is also made useful to those who are only mildly concerned with systematics. Each generic name in the subject index is set in italics and is followed by a reference to the systematic index. By turning to the systematic index one is able to orient himself quickly, and he can find there the names of organisms in closely related genera. Furthermore, there is a geographical index and a geological index to paleontological material. By a judicious and intelligent use of the whole index it is possible to cull out from the index alone the papers that might have interest. The abstracts may be consulted then to find out more about the original papers.

It is to be noted that the subject index is based upon an analysis of the abstract and not merely the title. The master key goes no farther than the abstract, but there is increasing evidence that the title "grand master key" is about to be justified. The number of abstracts prepared by the authors themselves appears to be increasing from volume to volume and what is even more important the quality of the abstract is positively improving. Collaborators are learning by experience how to prepare the most useful kind of abstract. In one test case pursued by the writer it was found that an author abstract was actually more useful than the original paper. The original is a long, intricate account of experiments and deductions. The abstract is a short concise statement of results prepared by an author in whose accuracy and integrity a personal acquaintance, at least, places absolute confidence. This suggests, incidentally, that if a limitation of space had been imposed by the editor of the research journal a more readable original might have resulted. Biologists generally are most assuredly under great obligation to the editors who are constructing this grand master key to our literature, and especially are they indebted to the Rockefeller Foundation, which through its support is making this fine work possible. It is indeed encouraging that a great foundation recognizes the fundamental importance of such instruments in the progress of science, especially with the increasing complexity of the literature, and is facilitating their development through a broad program of support. Few opportunities present themselves where limited funds accomplish so much for the general welfare of the science.

DONALD REDDICK
CORNELL UNIVERSITY

## SWARMING AND MATING OF ANTS

VARIOUS kinds of ants are present on lawns in Columbia, Missouri, including large black and brown forms measuring about 1 cm in length and the smaller ones 2 to 5 mm. For 30 years it has been observed that they swarm between August 15 and 20 each year, the average date being near the 20th. This usually takes place about 4 o'clock in the afternoon and it has frequently happened that the swarming has occurred following rain the previous night or forenoon. All varieties swarm at this time, and the start, heralded by the expulsion of the queens to the surface of the ground, is remarkably simultaneous between the different colonies. Once started, within the space of a few minutes, the surface of the ground for a foot or more surrounding the comparatively inconspicuous nest, as judged by the entrance or chimney, is occupied by scores or hundreds of queens, each queen being in charge of several workers who groom her for her flight. Intermingled with the queens and workers are many male ants nervously darting about. Soon after the first queens are expelled from the chimney by workers pushing and pulling—the grooming process is completed and she takes wing. Likewise the male ants take wing. At varying distances the queens alight, as do also the males, but no individual queen is followed by males. After alighting the queen mounts some object as a blade of grass where she is found by a male and the mating process is accomplished in a minute or two and the male departs. After a short interval of quiescence the female becomes nervously active and in a minute or two while clinging to a blade of grass or similar object—by means of her legs she detaches her wings. Immediately she descends to the ground and rapidly searches for a place to begin burrowing. In the average case this is accomplished in a very short time and she starts a tunnel for a new colony. In size the male is much smaller, while the queens are many times larger than the ordinary worker.

Last August while observing a small colony of small brown ants possessing not more than a dozen queens, which had just been removed to the surface and were being groomed for flight, a large black worker ant joined the group—whether by accident or design not being apparent—and instantly a remarkable change in the colony's activities occurred. The queens instantly were seized by several workers and rushed underground, while a mob of other workers attacked the intruder, literally overwhelming it, almost concealing its body. Within less than a minute it was stretched flat with the earth—each appendage, as the limbs, being grasped near the end by an ant which in turn was grasped posteriorly by another ant which in turn was similarly grasped by another ant, so that each limb was stretched by three or more ants which formed radiating lines from the victim's body. Within another minute apparently the victim was dead or rendered harmless, for all but two or three workers abandoned the carcass and retired to the colony, which at this time showed little evidences of activity, the only inhabitants on the surface being the two or three workers engaged in dragging the carcass to the entrance of the colony. The episode was a miniature, but thrilling enactment, with exaggerated ferocity, of Gulliver's experience in Lilliput.

C. C. GUTHRIE
UNIVERSITY OF PITTSBURGH

## GOITER PREVENTION WITH FOOD PLANTS GROWN ON IODIZED SOIL

BEAUMONT and Karns[1] have recently published analyses indicating that the iodine content of turnips can be increased by the application of potassium iodide to the soil. "The iodide-treated plants contained 441 and 950 parts per billion of iodine in the roots and tops, respectively, against 165 and 441 parts in chloride-treated plots."

In connection with this "large relative increase in iodine content" the authors raise the question as to "whether these quantities of iodine in food have therapeutic value."

The answer to this question is of considerable practical interest, in view of the well-recognized pathologic changes in the thyroid gland dependent upon a deficiency of iodine in the soil of certain rather extensive regions of the United States sometimes called the "goiter zones."

A significant contribution concerning the prophylactic value of iodide fertilization of the soil is the extensive study carried on by H. Hunziker,[2] in Swit-

[1] A. B. Beaumont and Geo. M. Karns, SCIENCE, 76: 567, 1932.
[2] H. Hunziker, *Schweiz. Woch'schr.*, 45: 2, 1920.

zerland, a country where thyroid pathology constitutes a national problem.

In a preliminary field experiment Hunziker determined (1916) that application of a small amount of iodide of potassium to the soil did not affect the yield of grass unfavorably.

During the following 3 years (1917 to 1919 inclusive) iodide of potassium was added to the fertilizer used for the garden from which Dr. Hunziker's family was supplied with such vegetables as spinach, rhubarb, cabbage, lettuce, beans, etc. (In 1918 the amount of KI applied to the soil was 17 grams to 1,200 square-meters; in 1919 about 20 grams to the same area.) The iodized vegetables were served to his 5 children (2 boys, 3 girls) ranging in age, at the beginning of the experiment, from 3 to 8 years.

As a control 5 children (2 boys, 3 girls, from 7 to 12 years old) from another family were supplied with vegetables raised on soil which was not iodized.

Hunziker's graphs of the measurements of the circumference of the neck in the thyroid region show plainly the influence of the iodized vegetables on the growth of the thyroid gland. (For the exact mode of the measurements and for the construction of the graph I refer the reader to Hunziker's publication.[2])

The effect of the iodine deficiency of the food was so decided that in July, 1919, after the experiment had lasted 2½ years, the oldest girl of the non-iodized food-group asked that she be treated for a rapidly enlarging struma.

Hunziker's results are corroborated by the findings of von Fellenberg,[3] in Switzerland, and of McClendon and Hathaway,[4] in the United States. According to these authors the development of goiter may be prevented in goitrous zones by administering food-plants raised in goiter-free regions.

Hunziker did not determine the amount of iodine in his vegetables which prevented goiter formation in his children, but McClendon and Hathaway state that 1 part of sodium iodide in 100,000,000 parts of water suffices for this purpose.

It is of historic interest in this connection that in 1850 a commission appointed by the Academy of Science in Paris refused to concur in A. Chatin's[5] conclusion that deficiency of 1/400 milligram of iodine *pro die* might result in goiter development.

I would like to add that Dr. Hunziker carries on his investigations of the goiter problem, while engaged in an active and arduous medical practise in a small country town. Fifteen publications dealing with various aspects of the problem attest his zeal.

Being on the subject of iodized alimentation (under which heading I include the ingestion of the condiment, iodized salt) I take occasion to mention an observation gathered in the field of my specialistic medical endeavor, that is to say, dermatology. I refer to the phenomenon that, due to an existing idiosyncrasy or a developing sensitization (allergy?), the administration of even such minute quantities of iodine as are needed for goiter prophylaxis may be followed, in certain individuals, by a follicular eruption of pustular character. Etiologically, these cutaneous lesions must be differentiated from the juvenile form of acne, which they resemble. Iodide acne seems to occur more frequently since our drinking water is chlorinated, a circumstance which is not surprising, as all the halogens act as follicular irritants ("poisons des follicules," according to Thibierge).

KARL G. ZWICK

CINCINNATI, OHIO

3 von Fellenberg, *Biochem. Ztschr.*, 142: 246, 1923.

4 McClendon and Hathaway, *Jour. Am. Med. Assn.*, 82: 1668, 1924.

5 A. Chatin, *Compt. rend. Academ. d. Sciences*, 30: 82, 1850.

## A BACTERIAL GALL DISEASE OF THE DOUGLAS FIR

A GALL disease of the twigs and stems of the Douglas Fir (*Pseudotsuga taxifolia* Doug.) has been observed quite commonly in parts of Napa, Lake, Santa Cruz, Amador and Siskiyou Counties in California, in marginal localities for the growth of this tree. Infection apparently takes place only on younger trees (about 3 to 15 years old), more abundantly in stands of thrifty, crowded and shaded reproduction. Galls once started on the main stem may continue to live and increase in size for many years. Young trees are sometimes killed by the disease or may have dead tops (spike top) due to girdling by a gall.

The galls are globular in shape, varying in size from a pin head to several inches in diameter, with a rough, spongy, fissured surface breaking out in typical, more or less cross-shaped patterns. The gall is composed of hypertrophied tissues, involving both stele and cortex, and is very similar in structure to the olive tree galls produced by the bacterial pathogene *Bacterium savastanoi* E. F. S.

The causal organism occurs in and among the hypertrophied gall cells and is very easily isolated in pure cultures. It is a non-motile rod averaging $1.9–3.9 \times 0.5–1.5\ \mu$, frequently occurring in pairs. The colony is white with a metallic sheen, rather smooth surface and undulate margin.

Inoculation of the twigs of Douglas Fir trees with this organism gave rise to typical galls from which the organism was again isolated.

H. N. HANSEN
RALPH E. SMITH

UNIVERSITY OF CALIFORNIA, BERKELEY

# QUOTATIONS

## ACADEMIC ASSISTANCE

UNDER the name of the Academic Assistance Council a number of men and women of high distinction have banded themselves together in the interest of those university teachers on the Continent of Europe who have lately been deprived, on political grounds, of their posts and their livelihood. The appeal addresses itself to an ancient and justly cherished English tradition of tolerance. We are accustomed in this country to trust the free working of the intellect. We may claim that our trust is based, not on any underestimate of the disruptive power of thought, but upon a faith in the essential soundness of our own institutions, sufficient to be willing to submit them to the severest of tests without fear that anything will be dissolved away but that which is superfluous, unworthy or outworn. That confidence comes only to a society that has driven its roots very deep into history; and the builders of self-consciously new polities do not possess it. Hence it comes that every revolution makes martyrs in the homes of thought. This is no question of the rightness or wrongness of a political creed. Bolshevist, Fascist, Nazi—all alike have sent professors into exile. The claim of all these exiles upon the hospitality of Englishmen is in every case the same—not the claim of the anti-Bolshevist or the anti-Nazi, but simply that of the seeker after truth.

The immediate need that the Academic Assistance Council seeks to meet is of course that of the refugees from the present régime in Germany. The council has collected a long list of names. Many, but by no means all, are the names of Jewish scholars. That is clearly of importance to Herr Hitler; it is of none whatever to Englishmen. Here we are not concerned with whether a professor is Jew or Gentile, but whether he is to be bond or free—subservient to opinions imposed from above, or claiming the right of learning to follow whithersoever the argument may lead. In vindicating that essential liberty of the mind it is to be hoped that Great Britain will always be ready, not only with applause, but with the material help that is its corollary. British universities will no doubt be swift to offer harborage to our guests in such forms as will enable them to carry on their learned vocations. But universities are for the most part but inadequately endowed even for their own necessities. Reverence for "humaner letters" is not confined to the ranks of professional scholarship, and all who feel that sentiment should respond to the appeal now made. This is not unproductive "charity." It has been the experience of history that the persecution of learning has been the occasion of its special flourishing in the lands that have given it sanctuary. The Byzantine scholars dispersed by the Turks in 1453 sowed the seeds of the Renaissance in Western Europe, and thus repaid a hundredfold the patrons who befriended them. In some such manner we may expect value to be returned for the money which it is now proposed to collect.—*The London Times.*

# REPORTS

## FIELD CONFERENCE OF PENNSYLVANIA GEOLOGISTS

THE third annual meeting of the Field Conference of Pennsylvania Geologists was held at Harrisburg, Pennsylvania, over the week-end of May 27, 28 and 29. The total attendance of about sixty members and guests included, besides Pennsylvanians, representatives of the profession from Maryland, New Jersey, New York, Virginia and West Virginia. The Pennsylvania Topographic and Geologic Survey was host to the conference. The entire staff, consisting of George H. Ashley, *chairman,* Stanley H. Cathcart, Charles K. Graeber, William O. Hickok, IV, Forrest T. Moyer, Marchant N. Shaffner, Ralph W. Stone and Bradford Willard, *secretary,* served as the local committee and planned and carried out the two and one-half day program, a brief summary of which follows.

Those who arrived by Saturday noon, May 27, were given a choice of three trips. The first, under Mr. Graeber, went to the Cornwall iron mines and spent the afternoon there collecting minerals and studying the geology of this historic mining center. Dr. Hickok led a second trip, whose members, after a shorter visit to Cornwall, saw some of the Triassic igneous and sedimentary rocks near-by and certain metamorphic phases caused by Triassic igneous intrusions of the Triassic sediments and Lower Paleozoics. This trip concluded with a visit to the once famous but now abandoned brownstone quarries at Hummelstown. The third Saturday afternoon trip was in charge of Dr. Ashley. This party climbed Third Mountain about ten miles north of Harrisburg to see the overturned syncline of Pottsville conglomerate there exposed as the western tip of the Southern Anthracite Coal Field. This party also observed important physiographic features of the Susquehanna Valley region with particular reference to peneplanation.

On Sunday, May 28, the whole conference united for a sixty-five mile tour of the Susquehanna and Juniata valleys. Dr. Willard was in charge of this excursion. The entire Paleozoic column from the Middle Ordovician through complete Silurian and Devonian exposures up to and including the Upper Mississippian was seen, Appalachian structures were observed, stratigraphic problems discussed and fossiliferous localities visited. Dr. Ashley drew the attention of the party to points of physiographic interest and to the river terraces and gravels of Pleistocene or Recent ages. This trip covered in a more extended form the Middle and Upper Paleozoic section to be visited by the International Geological Congress next July on Trip 1–B.

A choice of two trips was offered on Monday, May 29. Mr. Stone and Dr. Hickok led a party through portions of Cumberland and Adams counties where the chief interests were in economic geology including tile and ornamental stone works. Much also was seen of the Precambrian complex of South Mountain, and visits were made to certain ancient iron mines long since in disuse. Simultaneously with the foregoing, Dr. Willard conducted a second trip on Monday. Observations on this tour dealt entirely with stratigraphic problems. Those selecting this excursion visited several Silurian sections in Perry County, paying particular attention to the Ordovician-Silurian relations observable at points along Blue Mountain. The presence of Dr. Frank M. Swartz, of Pennsylvania State College, added greatly to the interest of the trip because of his thorough knowledge of the problems of the Silurian and the Helderberg, which he discussed at a number of localities.

The annual dinner was held at the Hotel Harrisburger on Saturday evening. After the meal, followed a discussion of the local geology by members of the Survey staff. On Sunday evening informal gatherings took place at the residences of Dr. Ashley and Mr. Stone. During a brief business session after the dinner an invitation was extended to the conference from its members residing in or near Pittsburgh to visit that area a year hence. The invitation was accepted by unanimous vote. The date for this meeting is tentatively set for the last week-end in May, 1934.

BRADFORD WILLARD
*Secretary-Treasurer*

# SCIENTIFIC APPARATUS AND LABORATORY METHODS

## A SIMPLE STRING ELECTROSCOPE

THE instrument described below was developed while the authors were making a study of certain transient electrical phenomena. While there are instruments in use that are similar in general to this one, its simplicity and ease of manipulation, together with its general adaptability, seem to make a short account of it worth while.

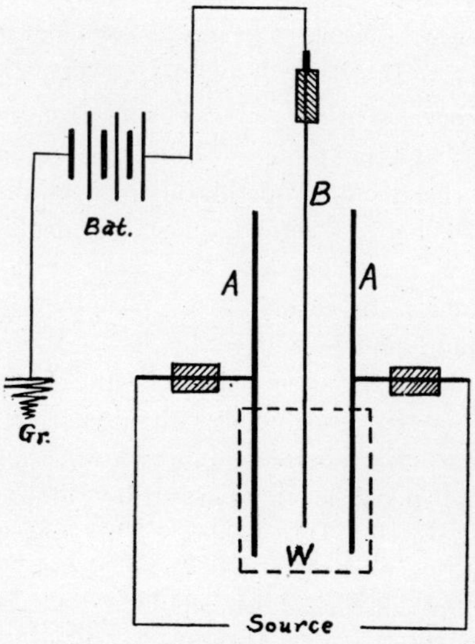


FIG. 1

A A in Fig. 1 are parallel brass plates about 8 cm long and 4 cm wide. They are mounted in the case of the instrument by the projecting rods as shown, so that the distance between them may be adjusted. These rods are supported by insulators of cast sulfur,[1] so that each plate is insulated from the case.

B is a silvered glass fiber[2] approximately 12 cm long hung midway between the plates from another sulfur insulator. It will be noted that the bottom end of the fiber is free.

W is a window in the case of the instrument through which the fiber may be viewed or its image projected.

In visual work the fiber may be observed through a low-powered microscope with a scale in the eyepiece. If the window is illuminated by a small arc, a sharp shadow of the fiber on a bright field may be projected

[1] Cast sulfur has proven to be excellent for this work. It is inexpensive and easily shaped and its insulating value is high. It deteriorates with age, and insulators made from it should be recast at intervals of 6 months or a year.

[2] The use of glass fibers has been surprisingly satisfactory. They are easily and quickly made and they last in service indefinitely.

by means of a cylindrical lens, on a slit in front of a drum carrying a sensitized film. As the drum rotates the film behind the slit is blackened, except where it is protected by the shadow of the fiber. Thus a record of the motion of the fiber may be made in the usual way.

This instrument may be used as a voltmeter and as an oscillograph.

(1) When used as a voltmeter for constant differences of potential the fiber may be connected to a dry cell battery of perhaps 200 volts, and the plates to the source to be measured.

When so connected (Fig. 1) the sensitivity may be varied by changing the distance between the plates and by changing the potential on the fiber. Fig. 2

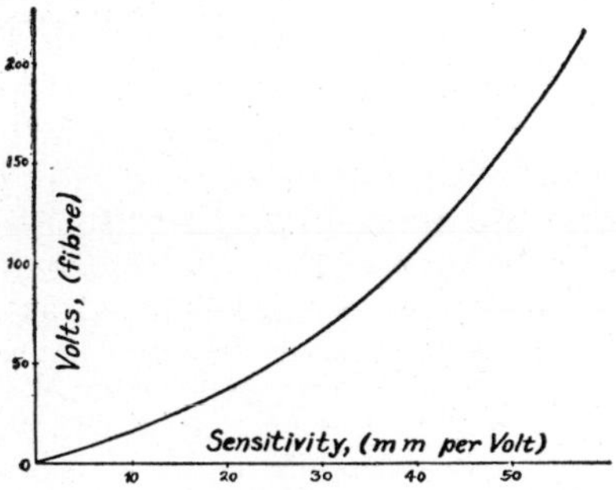


FIG. 2

is a typical curve showing the relation between sensitivity in mm of deflection per volt and fiber potential in volts. The sensitivity through a wide range is very evenly proportional to the potential gradient of the field between the plates. With properly chosen fibers the sensitivity may range from 200 or more mm per volt on the plates to 10 volts per mm, and it may be accurately controlled.

If, instead of connecting the fiber to a battery of dry cells, the fiber is connected through a resistance to one of the plates, the instrument will give steady deflections for alternating differences of potential. When used on differences of potential of this sort, it is very sensitive and readings may be repeated with accuracy.

The fiber should be drawn from ordinary sodium glass tubing and silvered. Its diameter should be something like .2 mm and for voltmeter work should be uniform throughout the whole length. The fact that it is a hollow cylinder insures high elasticity and small inertia, and these properties give high damping in ordinary air and a short period to the moving member. Fibers of this sort usually come to rest at the position of maximum steady deflection in less than .1 second.

(2) When used as an oscillograph a differently shaped fiber is required.

If the instrument as described above is used on alternating differences of potential with the uniform fiber charged from the battery as in Fig. 1, it is easily possible to set up nodes and loops like those in a vibrating rod in the fiber. While not useful in this condition for the study of wave forms, it is very good for the study of vibrations of rods and the like. It lends itself nicely to projection before a class, and when used with a stroboscope it shows the vibrations of the fiber clearly and distinctly in detail.

If the fiber is drawn so as to taper from a reasonable thickness (perhaps .5 mm) at the upper end to hair-like thinness at the free lower end, the stiffer upper part will not vibrate, but the lower fourth or thereabouts will, because of its extreme lightness, follow the variations of the field with no period of its own.

In this condition the fiber will follow audio frequency waves with fidelity when the plates are connected across a source. In connection with a microphone and a one-stage amplifier, voice currents, etc., may be recorded with great nicety. Records have been made of complex waves from various sources, such as organ pipes, orchestral music through the radio, the human voice, etc.

Since the moving part of this instrument is very small and light its motion in the field between the parallel plates disturbs the uniformity of the field very little. Therefore the source of the potential under measurement has to supply a very small charging current to the plates, and consequently very little energy. The exceedingly small amount of energy required to operate the instrument makes it useful in work where the source under investigation is very weak.

Because of the fact that its current requirement is so small, the authors have spoken of the instrument somewhat loosely as an "electrostatic oscillograph."

BENJAMIN ALLEN WOOTEN
WILBUR T. HARRIS
UNIVERSITY OF ALABAMA

# SPECIAL ARTICLES

## EFFECT OF INHIBITING FACTOR FROM NORMAL TISSUES ON SPONTANEOUS TUMORS OF MICE

IN a previous communication evidence was presented which indicated that a factor or substance could be extracted from mouse placenta and embryo skin which had a definite inhibiting action on the growth of transplanted mouse carcinoma. It has also been shown that an inhibiting factor isolated from a fowl sarcoma which was capable of neutralizing the causative agent of this tumor also inhibited the growth of transplantable mouse sarcoma. It was suggested that these factors were related to the substances which control the growth tendency of normal cells. The present report is an account of the effect of the normal tissue factor on the spontaneous mouse tumors.

*Material:* The animals used in the tests all came from inbred families of mice with high mammary cancer rates. The source of the inhibitors tested was late term mouse placenta and the skin of embryos of the same period. The tissues were finely minced, spread in a thin layer and dried *in vacuo* at sub-zero temperature. After desiccation was complete the material was powdered, thoroughly extracted with water (0.1 gm to 1 cc) and the larger particles removed by centrifugation.

*Group I:* This series was made up of 59 mice having a total of 85 primary mammary tumors, which were classed as medium to large size. The tumors were removed by operation and the operated field washed with embryo skin or placenta extract. In 57 of the animals, two grafts were taken from the removed tumor, one immersed in the test fluid and the other in Ringer's solution, and then both were inoculated into the mouse from which the tumor had been removed. Only those animals living over five weeks after the operation are included in the following table. For controls tumor mice from the same families were operated on and grafts returned without treatment to the field of operation or to the tumor grafted to another site.

TABLE I

FATE OF AUTOGRAFTS

| | Grew Per cent. | Doubtful or no growth Per cent. |
|---|---|---|
| 20 tumors removed: | | |
| Autografts treated with embryo skin extract | 50.0 | 50.0 |
| Autografts not treated | 75.0 | 25.0 |
| 37 tumors removed: | | |
| Autografts treated with placenta extract | 21.6 | 78.4 |
| Autografts not treated | 78.4 | 21.6 |
| 64 tumors removed: | | |
| Autografts, no treatment to graft or wound | 96.9 | 3.1 |

LOCAL RECURRENCE FOLLOWING OPERATION

| | | Per cent. |
|---|---|---|
| 27 treated with skin extract | 3 recurrences | 11.1 |
| 58 treated with placenta extract | 3 recurrences | 5.2 |
| 89 with no treatment | 44 recurrences | 49.4 |

Judged by the marked reduction in local recurrences and the large number of treated autografts which failed to grow the results seem definite. The average length of life is sometimes over 80 days with 18.6 per cent. still living. There is a suggestion in the above table of some generalized action of the inhibitors in that the untreated autografts grew less well in animals which had received a certain amount of the inhibitor in the operated wound and with the treated graft (75 and 78.4 per cent.) than the autografts in animals receiving no treatment (96.9 per cent.). It is of interest to note that in a control series 32 per cent. of the 50 mice developed new primary tumors, while in the treated group only 4, or 6.8 per cent., had new tumors.

*Group II:* The more crucial test of the inhibiting action would be its effect on the spontaneous tumor undisturbed by operative procedure. To eliminate any possible local interference with blood supply to the tumors the injections of the test fluids were made intraperitoneally at weekly intervals. The group includes 91 mice with 127 well-established primary tumors, all from inbred stocks with high mammary cancer rates. Of these 40 were treated with embryo skin extract and 51 with placenta extract. The average size of these tumors was somewhat smaller than those used in the operated series. The results are given in Table II.

TABLE II

| | | | Per cent. |
|---|---|---|---|
| Number of tumors in mice treated with embryo skin extract | 60 | | |
| Continued growth | 20 | | 33.3 |
| Stationary or slight retrogression | 17 | 28.3 Per cent. | 66.7 |
| Marked retrogression | 7 | 11.7 " " | |
| Complete absorption | 16 | 26.7 " " | |
| Number of tumors in mice treated with placenta extract | 67 | | |
| Continued growth | 21 | | 31.3 |
| Stationary or slight retrogression | 16 | 23.9 Per cent. | 68.7 |
| Marked retrogression | 17 | 25.4 " " | |
| Complete absorption | 13 | 19.4 " " | |

The figures given above, where only 33.3 per cent. of the tumors in one series and 31.3 per cent. in the other continued to grow after treatment was started, may be compared with our experience with hundreds of untreated tumor animals from the same stocks followed in this laboratory. Steady, progressive growth is the rule, with temporary cessation of growth or retrogression a rare occurrence, and the absorption of an established tumor of such unusual occurrence as to require no consideration in the analysis of the above figures. The average time the treated animals have been under observation has been about 60 days, with a number still living.

There seems to be little doubt that the extracts of the two tissues which have previously been shown to reduce the takes of transplanted cancer have an influence on natural or spontaneous cancer. This inhibiting action is evident not only on the local post-operative recurrence, and the growth of autografts where there was direct contact between the extracts and the cancer cells, but is observable likewise on untreated or unoperated tumors at a distance when the inhibiting materials were injected into the peritoneal cavity.

We do not consider that the results stated necessarily establish the hypothesis on which the experiment was based, for the complexity of the materials makes it quite possible that this explanation is not the correct one. The general relations between the factors which influence the origin and growth of spontaneous tumors, the balancing mechanism of normal tissues, and the inhibitor which has been isolated from the chicken sarcomas can not be seriously discussed until further knowledge is available.

A more detailed report, including data on histological types of the tumors, metastasis occurrence, etc., will be published later. At present the results recorded here are considered of only theoretical importance.

JAMES B. MURPHY
ERNEST STURM

ROCKEFELLER INSTITUTE FOR MEDICAL RESEARCH, NEW YORK

## FUNDAMENTAL LIMITS TO THE SIZES OF CLASTIC GRAINS

TEN years ago the writer presented a scale of size limits for the terms boulder, cobble, pebble, granule and sand, silt and clay grains.[1] The scale was based on average prevailing opinion and stated in units to conform to certain sieve openings in the mechanical analysis scale first used extensively by Udden.[2] With growing precision in terminology and increasing use of quantitative methods of analysis of detrital materials, the usage suggested by the writer has been generally accepted, with only occasional modification of certain terms.

Names for the unconsolidated and consolidated aggregate were also proposed and differ from the fragment names chiefly in the bracketing of the aggregates of boulders, cobbles, pebbles and granules under the single name "gravel." In this usage there is tacit implication that the materials gravel, sand, silt and clay are of equal rank in classification. Aside from purely arbitrary division into classes of equal width on an arithmetic or geometric scale, equality of rank would result only from the use of limits having coordinate natural or genetic significance.

Recently, the writer was led to further consideration of these terms and the conclusion was reached that the seeming narrow unity of the materials sand, silt and clay and the wide size range in the gravel class probably represent an unconscious recognition by man, layman as well as geologist, of certain genetic units based on the several fundamental modes of transport by running water and on several modes of derivation from parent rocks. This interpretation is shown in the following table:

TABLE I

| Mode of transport | Usual source | Name of aggregate |
|---|---|---|
| Traction | All available hard rocks | Gravel |
| Inertia suspension | Mono-mineral grains of phanerites (chiefly) | Sand |
| Viscous suspension | Mono-mineral grains of any rocks (chiefly) | Silt |
| Colloidal suspension | Molecularly decomposable materials | Clay |

In Table I there are listed four distinct modes of handling which occur in running water. Both traction and inertia suspension take place approximately in accordance with the so-called Sixth Power Law, which postulates a complete transfer of kinetic energy from water to particle and which makes no allowance for the subsidiary effect of viscous drag. Viscous suspension, on the other hand, accounts for the transport of finer particles in which the surface effect is greater relative to the mass. The size-velocity relationship in this range is defined by the well-known Stokes Law.[3] Still smaller particles are kept in suspension chiefly by the kinetic effects found in dispersed systems, *i.e.*, colloid systems.

It should, of course, be recognized that none of the lines of demarcation between these modes of transport are sharp and that water-transported detrital materials occur in a continuous series from large boulders to clay particles. However, it appears that each of the processes of transportation has an optimum range in nature and that only partial overlapping occurs. Where more than one of the

[1] C. K. Wentworth, "A Scale of Grade and Class Terms for Clastic Sediments," *Jour. of Geology*, 30: 377–392. 1922.

[2] J. A. Udden, "Mechanical Composition of Clastic Sediments," *Geol. Soc. Amer. Bull.*, 25: 655–744. 1914.

[3] G. G. Stokes, "On the Effect of the Internal Friction of Fluids on the Motion of Pendulums," *Trans. Cambridge Philos. Soc.*, Vol. 9, part 2, pp. 8–106, espec. sec. 4, pp. 48–57, 1851.

processes is carried on concurrently by the same stream, the processes are either found quite distinct in different parts of the stream, or the conditions of flood and tumultuous flow are obviously ill-adapted to effective segregation of the grains by sizes.

If the thesis here implied be correct, the several processes are sufficiently distinct, in spite of overlapping due to variation in velocity, so that detrital materials found in natural deposits occur more abundantly well within the individual coarseness ranges represented by gravel, sand, silt and clay, than in the ranges transitional between those classes. The assumed arrangement of these modes is shown in the figure.

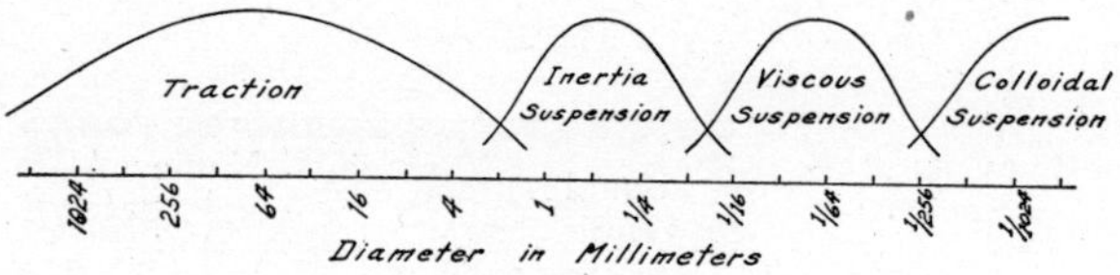


FIG. 1

Column two of Table I suggests a possible further natural contrast of sizes. It is thought that phanerites with grain sizes from ½ mm to 2 or 3 mm are enormously more abundant than similar rocks of coarser grain and that these furnish quartz grains preponderantly in the sand sizes. Among acid rocks, those of finer grain than ½ mm are subordinate to the coarser ones.[4] Aphanitic basic rocks are exposed over far larger outcrop area than coarser basic rocks. Few basic rocks yield mono-mineral grains of sufficient durability to exert any important effect in fixing sand sizes. By far the most important control exerted by the grain size of igneous rocks is due to the predominant sizes of quartz grains in granites.

In the calcareous detrital sediments of certain beaches, the sizes of shells or of other parts of particular species of animals locally give rise to somewhat homogeneous, well-sorted sediments. In particular, one may note the opercula of turbo snails, segments of sea-urchin spines and the tests of foraminifera.[5] These are, of course, much too localized to have been significant in fixing the established concept of sediment grades.

Some may point out that the foregoing discussion is based on the assumption that detrital sedimentary materials have been chiefly sorted by water. The reply is that materials chiefly assembled by other agencies are mostly not readily classifiable in the common terms. For example, glacial till requires a name of its own, the material of kames and eskers deposited by water under somewhat unusual conditions is commonly a somewhat indeterminate mixture of sand and gravel.

Loess, derived perhaps largely from glacial silt and deposited by the wind, does not correspond exactly either with sand or silt or clay. Most soils are also cases in point. Materials accumulated through imperfect action of water are commonly difficult to classify, such as many of the deposits of arid regions and terrace materials deposited by streams excessively flooded by glacial or other waters.

We are forced to recognize that the gravel-sand-silt-clay scale is an aqueous scale and there appears to be a true genetic, even if complex, basis for the grades represented by our common size terms. Wind action may result in superior sorting of sands originally accumulated by aqueous agencies. Whether a well-sorted, well-rounded, mature sand has ever been produced exclusively by the action of wind on the debris from a granite or other suitable rock may well be doubted. If such derivation has taken place, it must be very exceptional and very local.

CHESTER K. WENTWORTH
WASHINGTON UNIVERSITY, ST. LOUIS

[4] R. A. Daly, ''Igneous Rocks and Their Origin,'' pp. 42–52, 1914.

[5] C. K. Wentworth and H. S. Ladd, ''Pacific Island Sediments,'' Univ. of Iowa Studies in Natural History, Vol. XIII, No. 2, pp. 19–23, 1931.

## BOOKS RECEIVED

Institute of the Aeronautical Sciences, Inc. *Proceedings of the Founder's Meeting, 1933. Pp. 85.* The Institute.

LUCK, JAMES MURRAY, Editor. *Annual Review of Biochemistry.* Vol. II. Pp. vii + 563. Stanford University Press. $5.00.

MACPHERSON, HECTOR. *Makers of Astronomy.* Pp. 244. Illustrated. Oxford University Press. $2.50.

*National Plan for American Forestry.* Report of the Forest Service of the Agricultural Department on the Forest Problem of the United States. Vol. I. Pp. x + 1050. Vol. II. Pp. 1051–1677. U. S. Government Printing Office. $1.75 for two volumes.

ROBBINS, WILFRED W. and FRANCIS RAMALEY. *Plants Useful to Man.* Pp. vii + 428. 241 figures. Blakiston. $3.00.

SMITH, GILBERT M. *The Fresh-Water Algae of the United States.* Pp. xi + 716. 449 figures. McGraw-Hill. $6.00.

STEJNEGER, LEONHARD and THOMAS BARBOUR. *A Check List of North American Amphibians and Reptiles.* Third Edition. Pp. xiv + 185. Harvard University Press.

STUHR, ERNST T. *Manual of Pacific Coast Drug Plants.* Pp. 192. Science Press Printing Company. $2.65.

*Svenska Linné-Sällskapets Årsskrift.* Årgang XVI, 1933. Pp. 152. Illustrated. Almqvist & Wiksells, Uppsala.

SYDENSTRICKER, EDGAR. *Health and Environment.* Recent Social Trends Monographs. Pp. xii + 217. 50 figures. McGraw-Hill. $2.50.

VALLANCE, ALEX and MARSHALL E. FARRIS. *Principles of Mechanism.* Pp. vii + 335. 302 figures. Macmillan. $3.50.

WEEKS, MARY E. *The Discovery of the Elements.* Pp. iii + 363. Illustrations Collected by F. B. Dains. Journal of Chemical Education, Easton, Pennsylvania.

WOOTTON, H. A. and C. W. R. HOOKER. *A Text-Book of Chemistry.* Pp. xi + 488. Cambridge University Press, Macmillan. $1.75.

# SCIENCE NEWS

*Science Service, Washington, D. C.*

## COSMIC RAYS

Two of America's leading physicists discussed facts and theories about cosmic rays before the American Association for the Advancement of Science at Atlantic City on December 30.

About most of the experimental facts, they agreed. About the deductions from thousands of experiments performed by scores of investigators ranging the world, they largely disagreed.

Dr. Robert A. Millikan, of the California Institute of Technology, upheld strongly as a fact his conclusion that the cosmic rays that enter the earth's atmosphere are photons, like x-rays and gamma radiation of the same family as light and heat.

Dr. Arthur H. Compton, of the University of Chicago, found "no way of reconciling the data with the hypothesis that any considerable portion of the cosmic rays consists of photons." He concludes that cosmic rays come from outer space as high-speed electrified particles, either negatively charged electrons or positively charged protons.

As to what causes the discharging of the sensitive electrical instruments used in detecting the effects of cosmic radiation, Drs. Compton and Millikan agree. Very energetic electrified particles produce the effect, but whereas Dr. Compton considers them the original rays, Dr. Millikan advanced evidence that they are secondary radiation produced in the earth's air by photons smashing into the hearts of air atoms.

To account for the very penetrating radiations that Dr. Millikan and others have observed in the depths of lakes, Dr. Compton countered with the suggestion that electron cosmic rays produce photons in the earth's atmosphere just as electrons striking an x-ray tube target produce x-rays.

His argument fell in line with experimental evidence for a new process of ionization presented to the same session by Dr. Gordon Locher, a national research fellow at the Bartol Research Foundation, near Philadelphia. According to Dr. Locher x-rays are produced in the gas of a detecting chamber by the passage through of swiftly moving particles like electrons.

Reporting the results of airplane flights this past summer in the United States, Canada and Peru, at altitudes up to twenty-one thousand feet, Dr. Millikan explained that a new type, very sensitive, recording electroscope showed differences in cosmic ray readings at high altitudes that may possibly be explained by a new cause, a modification of the earth's electrical field connected with some secondary influence of sunlight. Changes in the earth's negative electric field such as occur between day and night would change the resistance to the inflow of the secondary negative particles generated by the cosmic rays. But the rays that get down to sea-level are so hard that the earth's electrical field does not affect them. This fits in with a lack of latitude variation in cosmic-ray readings made at sea-level by Dr. Millikan and others recently and in past years.

Dr. Compton and his associates in a world-wide survey during the past eighteen months found large variations with latitude in cosmic ray intensities at sea-level and on the tops of high mountains. This he attributes to the effect of the magnetic field of the earth, since the earth's magnetism would theoretically keep electrified-particle cosmic rays from reaching the equatorial regions where the Compton experiments show cosmic rays to be less.

As to the energies of cosmic rays, there is difference of opinion. Dr. Millikan cited the experiments of his colleague, Dr. Carl D. Anderson, to show that observed cosmic ray energies lie largely below five hundred million volts and that less than a tenth reach the billion volt range.

Dr. Compton advanced an energy of seven billion volts for the electron cosmic rays that are so feeble as not to reach the equator, and he set thirty billion as the figure for a more penetrating component of high-speed electrified particles. Dr. Compton holds that the high energy portion is not affected by the earth's magnetic field.

As to the way in which cosmic-ray effects vary with increase in height over the earth's surface, there is little difference in the experimental results, but both Dr. Millikan and Dr. Compton see the experiments bolstering up their theories.

The question of the origin of the cosmic rays, a moot question upon which there is little experimental evidence except the fact that they come from outer space, was left for future meetings.—Watson Davis.

## MEASUREMENT OF UNITS OF HEREDITY

The unit of heredity known as the gene, that controls physical characteristics and passes them on from generation to generation in man and other living things, has been measured. Its largest size is one quintillionth of a cubic centimeter. This is just about the volume that fifteen protein molecules, one of the largest of the organic chemical aggregations, could crowd into.

This determination of the size limits of the bearers of heredity, announced at Atlantic City to the American Association for the Advancement of Science by Drs. John W. Gowen and E. H. Gay, of the Rockefeller Institute for Medical Research, is considered an important fundamental step in the development of biology.

Genes are the units within the chromosomes which determine the development of physical characteristics when, through the union of male and female germ cells, a new individual is created. Chromosomes can be seen readily with the microscope, but the single gene is probably too small to be seen by the eye even when aided by the most powerful optical means. The gene is as important to biology as molecules, atoms or electrons are to the physical sciences.

"We postulate the existence of the gene because of the properties it gives to aggregates of other matter," Drs. Gowen and Gay explained. "Size is a fundamental structural characteristic. The measurement of size, even though it may be crude, has, if we may judge by our sister sciences, always led to further progress."

The Rockefeller investigators based their discovery of the gene's size upon the discovery made several years ago that x-rays will smash into genes and change the bodily characteristics that they transmit. They used the drosophila fruit flies that have been experimented upon to contribute so much to the new knowledge of heredity obtained since the turn of the century. Pure x-rays specially produced were used to bring about the changes in genes that are known as mutations. Thousands of flies were used in the experiments. The magnitude of the average gene was found by dividing the amount of chromatin, or material in the chromosome, by the number of genes estimated by the mutations observed.

The total number of genes in any one cell was shown to be not less than fourteen thousand three hundred eighty. This corresponded to a largest gene size expressed numerically in cubic centimeters as one tenth visualize this extremely small volume, one quintillionth multiplied by itself eighteen times. In attempting to of a cubic centimeter, it may be helpful to remember that a centimeter is a little more than a third of an inch.

These gene size determinations check approximately with those reported several months ago by Professor Oswald Blackwood, of the University of Pittsburgh.—WATSON DAVIS.

## KING TUT'S PURPLE GOLD

BEAUTIFUL purple surface films on golden sequins found in the tomb of Tut-Ankh-Amen have been proved to be due to the presence of iron in the gold, by Professor R. W. Wood, of the Johns Hopkins University. Professor Wood reported on his examination of these ancient ornaments before the American Association for the Advancement of Science.

The sequins have been the subject of much discussion ever since they were first discovered. Some investigators have claimed that the Egyptians knew an art for coloring gold surface purple, while others have believed that the purple sheen was a kind of patina due to the great age of the ornaments. Professor Wood, using the methods of a physicist, has shown the color to be due merely to the presence of iron in gold which has been first hammered and then heated. He even made duplicates of the sequins by hammering out a gold-iron alloy into thin flakes and heating the latter over a flame. One of his modern purple-gold sequins has been sent to the Cairo Museum, to be displayed along with the originals.

A modern beauty aid helped in the solution of the riddle of the purple film. Professor Wood found he could remove the film by coating the gold ornaments with celluloid varnish such as is used in fingernail polish, and then peeling off the varnish, leaving the underlying gold of a bright yellow color. There was no sign of the film on the peeled-off varnish layer, but the film could be made to reappear by redepositing gold on the side to which the film was attached by vaporizing gold in a vacuum. Then the purple could again be seen by reflected light. The problem in physical optics presented by this phenomenon is still under examination.

Subjected to spectroscopic examination, the stripped-off film proved to be principally iron, probably an iron oxide. Professor Wood then suspended one of the sequins from which the purple film had been removed between the poles of a strong electromagnet. It was attracted toward one of the poles, demonstrating the presence of iron in the gold.

Etching the surface of the gold with acid showed a very marked crystalline structure, such as is found only when rolled or hammered sheet gold is subsequently heated to nearly a red heat. Microscopic examination showed on the surface numerous small globules of gold standing out in high relief, conclusive evidence that the sequins had been heated to a high temperature after having been hammered into shape. It was after having learned these facts that Professor Wood took gold and iron and duplicated the product of the "lost art" of the ancient Egyptian court jewelers.

The microscopic globules Professor Wood believes to be due to melting of the gold out of a gold-orpiment mixture experimentally tried by the Egyptian artist. Orpiment is a bright yellow arsenic-sulphur compound known to the Egyptians and used by them in tomb wall decorations. Lumps of it were found in Tut-Ankh-Amen's tomb, some of which Professor Wood received from the Cairo authorities.

Melting gold with this orpiment, and rolling the resulting bead out into a plate, Professor Wood heated it over a flame and obtained gold globules exactly like those on the sequins. He also hammered out small nuggets of California gold, which had been in his family since '49, and on heating the resulting plates he again obtained the globules. No purple film appeared, however, for the California gold is free from iron.

## MOTION PICTURES OF THE GROWTH OF NERVE FIBERS

MOTION pictures demonstrating how nerve fibers grow through living tissue, and how they repair themselves when injured, were shown before the meeting of the American Association for the Advancement of Science by Professor Carl C. Speidel, of the University of Virginia. Professor Speidel was the winner of the Association's $1,000 prize at the midwinter meeting at New Orleans last year, and the report he rendered constituted a summary of his work up to that time and of advances made since then.

As pictured and explained by Professor Speidel, nerve growth is pioneered by what are known as "growth cones" on the ends of the nerve fibers. These are thickenings of the tips, which probe their way through the tissues, constantly sending out and retracting tiny processes from their surfaces, like finger-tips feeling their way. As the nerve progresses, special cells develop along its course. They hug its sides closely, though they take no part in its actual growth process, nor in its function as a nerve. These are known as the "sheath cells." Finally, as the nerve becomes more mature, it develops around itself a layer of fatty material called the "myelin sheath."

All these developments were shown in the motion pictures. In life, the growth process is rather slow, but by taking only one picture in two seconds and then projecting them at normal movie speed of sixteen to the second, the apparent rate of growth was speeded up 32 times. Another portion of the film was taken at the rate of one frame in eight seconds, giving them a speeding-up effect on the screen of 128 times the natural rate.

Growth after injury, as well as normal growth, was studied. It has long been a disputed point whether a severed nerve grew together again or started afresh from the cut end nearest the central nervous system. Evidence apparently supporting both views has been produced in the past. Professor Speidel's studies showed that where the two cut ends apparently grew together again, there was an anastomosis, or anatomical detour, connecting them by another path. A cut end really quite separated from the central nervous system degenerates and disappears and a new nerve fiber grows out to replace it.

Professor Speidel's first studies were conducted by watching the growth of nerve fibers in the transparent tissues of a frog tadpole's tail. During the past year he has also been studying nerve fiber growth in salamanders, which are rather remote zoological cousins of the frogs. He finds that the growth processes in this order of animals are essentially the same as those he observed in the tadpole tails.

## GROWTH OF PLANTS STIMULATED BY X-RAYS

X-RAYS can cause plants to grow faster, blossom earlier, form more chlorophyll, and in general speed up their life processes. But if they get too much of a dose of the rays, they become cripples. This in brief summary is what Professor Charles A. Shull, of the University of Chicago, has found in experiments which he reported at Atlantic City before the meeting of the American Society of Plant Physiologists.

Professor Shull exposed corn, wheat, oats and sunflowers to x-rays for periods of from one to five minutes, inclusive, under screens to take out the harmful parts of the x-ray spectrum, and also for ten minutes without the benefit of screening. He compared the growth of these plants with "control" plants that were not x-rayed at all.

All the rayed plants except the ten-minute lot apparently were stimulated by the treatment. In some cases they became juicier, or more succulent, as well as larger. In corn a considerable increase of the green food-making substance, chlorophyll, was noted, running from 20 to 60 per cent. above the controls. X-rayed seeds carried on their respiratory processes with greater energy, the data indicating from 30 to 50 per cent. increase.

The three-minute treatment seemed to be most beneficial especially in the case of the sunflowers. Pots of the young plants ranged side by side mark off a curve with the graduated heights of their tops: good at one minute, best at three, not so good at five, and disastrous for the ten-minute treatment without a screen. The plants were in bud at about the same time, but the three-minute group blossomed first.

The condition of the ten-minute group indicated emphatically the effects of too much of a good thing. It was badly burned, and pocked all over the leaves, as though with a mosaic disease. The leaves were irregularly lopsided, an effect not observed at all in the plants given shorter rayings under screens.

## ITEMS

THE earth and the moon were born out of the parent spiral nebula that fathered not only the sun but all the other stars of the Milky Way, is the suggestion of Dr. Harlow Shapley, of Harvard College Observatory, made at the meeting of the American Association for the Advancement of Science. This theory makes the moon, planets and sun all the same age, the progeny of a "secondary swirl or eddy of the parental spiral nebula out of which the local galaxy or Milky Way may be supposed to have generated." The conventional theory is that the earth and planets were born when a passing star pulled matter out of the sun, and some have theorized that the moon was cleaved off the earth at an even later time.

THE planetary nebulae, globes of glowing gas that can be seen in various parts of the sky, are not the light airy things they seem. According to Dr. Adrian van Maanen, of the Mount Wilson Observatory, who reported to the American Astronomical Society, the nuclei of these structures are something like 250 times as massive as the sun, and about a fifth its diameter. This has been found from studies of the motions of these bodies, from which their distances have been determined.

ULTRA-VIOLET rays change the viscosity, or "thickness," of protoplasm by causing it to let go of calcium which it contains. This conclusion is indicated by experiments reported before the American Society of Zoologists by Professor L. V. Heilbrunn and Kathryn Daugherty, of the University of Pennsylvania. They exposed one species of amoeba to the action of ultraviolet radiation. Afterwards they whirled the animals in a centrifuge, which enabled them to measure the changes in their protoplasmic viscosity. They found that the interior protoplasm had been made more viscous, while the originally fairly stiff outer protoplasm had become more fluid. They knew from previous experiments that ultra-violet raying causes a loss of calcium from protoplasm. The changes in the amoebae they ascribed to a release of calcium from the originally stiff, calcium-rich outer layer, which calcium then diffused into the inner mass of protoplasm, originally fluid, causing it to become more viscous.

# SCIENCE NEWS

*Science Service, Washington, D. C.*

## THE AGRICULTURAL APPROPRIATION BILL AND REPRESENTATIVE LAGUARDIA

REPRESENTATIVE Fiorello LaGuardia, Republican lame-duck from New York, has just emerged as one of the most fiery and eloquent defenders of scientific research, in the lower House.

During the debate on the Agricultural Appropriation bill, Representatives Allgood of Alabama, Summers of Washington, Snell of New York, Tabor of Ohio, McGugin of Kansas and others sought to pare or eliminate altogether item after item which would have dealt the scientific work of the department several severe blows.

Due to the masterly defense of Representative LaGuardia and others who joined him in his work, the majority of these amendments to the bill were defeated on the floor.

"Science knows no politics," declaimed the brilliant Italian-American from New York City. "Are we, in the frenzy of economy, brought about by those who control the wealth of this country, seeking to put a barrier on science and research? . . . Science will go on when existing political parties will long have been forgotten."

At another point in the discussions when it seemed that the appropriation for dry land agricultural stations was in danger, Representative LaGuardia defended the past accomplishments of this branch of the Bureau of Plant Industry, and said: "The most humble research scientist in the Department of Agriculture is at this time contributing more to his country than the most useful Member of Congress. The most humble engineer in the General Electric Laboratory or the Radio Corporation of America laboratory is more useful to humanity than the most brilliant orator of this House. The trouble is that the legislative branch of the government has not kept abreast with science. Government has lagged, science has advanced. We have permitted an unbalanced system of distribution to continue while science has increased production. We are living in the paradoxical state where there is great overproduction, on the one hand, and want and misery, on the other. This is not the fault of science. This is the fault of government."

Among the amendments offered by congressmen who saw in the scientific items a place to save money, were:

An attempt to reduce the item for cereal crops and diseases from $488,200 to $465,915; cotton production and diseases from $200,000 to $100,000; foreign plant introduction from $163,574 to $50,000; elimination of the entire amount of $209,955 for forest pathology; genetics and biophysics from $33,617 to $20,000; entire amount for rubber, fiber and other tropical plants, $69,474, because, said Representative Allgood, "This is a subsidy to Ford and other rubber manufacturers"; entire amount of $130,000 for western irrigation agriculture; general administrative expenses in Forestry Service, from $327,819 to $250,000. All these were voted down by the House.

An amendment offered by Representative Summers, of Washington, reducing the $215,000 in the bill for forage crops and diseases to $201,014 was accepted by the House, Summers explaining that the reduction would be applied to work on the corn borer, which he termed the "bogy-man of agriculture."

Other amendments offered and rejected were one to cut Bureau of Chemistry and Soils' Washington appropriation from $1,095,695 to $750,000 (by Allgood, Democrat, of Alabama); another to cut federal highway aid to states from $35,000,000 to $10,000,000.

An amendment accepted by the House was offered by Representative Summers, of Washington, eliminating an item of $25,000 for the development of mechanical equipment for corn borer control by the Bureau of Agricultural Engineering.

Barring slight alterations, however, the bill passed the House, substantially as reported out from the House Appropriations Committee.

## SUPPORT OF COLLEGES URGED AT NATIONAL CONFERENCE

BECAUSE of the value of the scientific research being conducted in institutions of higher learning and because of the training they afford for modern complex life, the support of colleges and universities was strongly urged by a special committee of the Citizens Conference on the Crisis in Education, meeting in Washington.

From these institutions has come a large proportion of the trained personnel of the established professions and the leadership of our complex industrial and social life, the report pointed out.

Furthermore the results of the scientific research carried on by such institutions have been of well-nigh incalculable worth to the economic life of the nation. When viewed from these two standpoints alone the general scheme of higher education of the country must be regarded as a principal, productive asset, the conservation and further development of which are matters of permanent concern for the states and for the nation.

No reduction of the extent to which the youth of the nation is given education at public expense was recommended by this committee.

The effective, economical and non-political operation and adaptation of the plan of popular education, at all levels, from the elementary schools through the universities, are fundamental obligations of the American state.

During a period of economic stress such as that now existing, there is imposed upon all of those in positions of responsibility, whether in government, industry or cultural activity, a clear responsibility of affirming the inherent basis of our American plan and of promoting confidence among the people in their educational institutions.

With the rapid changes occurring throughout the world and especially in our own country, we face problems vastly more numerous and more difficult and more immediate than those we have faced in the past. There will consequently rest upon the publicly supported higher institutions a greatly increased responsibility for research and guidance. Adult education in particular should open opportunities for preparation for a new civic era. It is imperative that nothing should be done now to impair the service of our higher institutions in this field of all important democratic education.

## THE VIENNA MEDICAL FACULTY ON YEAST TESTIMONIALS

MEMBERS of the Vienna medical faculty who have given medical testimonials in favor of yeast have been "officially sharply reproved by the dean," that official, Professor Dr. Ernst Pick, has just informed the American Medical Association. All members of the faculty were forbidden to give any testimonials intended for advertising purposes in the future.

The statement to the American Medical Association was signed by both Professor Dr. Pick, dean of the medical faculty and director of the pharmacological department, and by Professor Dr. Roland Grassberger, formerly dean of the medical faculty and director of the hygienic department.

An investigation by the faculty showed that not a single member of the Board of Professors (heads of departments) of the medical faculty is involved in the yeast testimonials, and that the only ones concerned were seven privat-docents not included on the board, not one of whom has the official position of teacher or is in charge of a department.

Privat-docents, according to the statutes of the universities of Austria, explains the American Medical Association, are not appointed by the state but merely permitted by the state to teach.

The Vienna medical faculty statement contended that the testimonials favoring yeast were "spread and misused for advertising in American illustrated and other magazines in quack-fashion."

The medical faculty is concerned lest through the impropriety of these advertisements the reputation and esteem of the Vienna Medical School be seriously affected among the medical profession and people in America, and requested the American Medical Association to spread the explanation of the situation among its members and also publicly.

## DEFICIENT DIET AND MENTAL EFFICIENCY

THE fear that a diet deficient in essentials might have an immediate effect on ability to do mental work may be groundless, if results of an experiment with rats apply to human beings.

The ability of white rats, 90 to 100 days old, to do the mental task of threading a maze, when they were suffering the effects of faulty diet, was tested by Dr. Martin F. Fritz, of the Iowa State College.

The 148 animals were divided into three groups, only one of which had a normal diet of bread and milk. One group received a diet containing too much iron salt and iodine and too little chlorine. The diet of the third group was also deficient in vitamin B.

The animals having the faulty diets took somewhat longer to find their way through the maze, but there was very little difference between the groups in number of errors. Even those animals who died during the experiment showed no significant differences from others in the same group.

Dr. Fritz makes three suggestions as possible explanation of this preservation of mental ability in the face of physiological breakdown. Storage, he said, may be an important factor. Since the rats were 90 days old, they had had opportunity to store vitamin B in the liver.

There is also the possibility that in mature rats the nervous system is afforded a certain amount of protection so that a breakdown in other parts of the physiological organism resulting in death will occur before there are marked effects upon the nervous system, he said, and cited an experiment which showed that the muscles of a starved cat had lost 30 per cent. while heart, brain and cord lost only 3 per cent.

Finally, it may be that even though the nervous system is subject to degeneration, only a part of the fibers are necessary to carry on the task.

## THE WORLD'S LARGEST SHIP

WHEN the *Normandie* puts to sea, the French merchant marine will more than recapture its position lost by the tragic burning of the *Atlantique,* the world's twelfth largest steamship.

The *Normandie* is the largest vessel in the world, clearly exceeding the *Leviathan* and the *Majestic* in both tonnage and length. She was launched during the past fall at St. Nazaire to be put in transatlantic service in 1934.

France now has only one vessel larger than the *Atlantique,* that is, the *Ile de France* of 43,153 registered tons, the tenth largest steamship, according to Lloyds. It is exceeded in both tonnage and length by the *Leviathan,* U. S.; *Majestic* and *Berengaria,* British; *Bremen* and *Europa,* German; *Olympia* and *Aquitania,* British, and *Rex* and *Conte di Savoia,* Italian.

The *Normandie* has an overall length of 1,027 feet, 963 feet between perpendiculars, and will be rated at approximately 75,000 gross tons. The *Leviathan's* registered tonnage is approximately 60,000, more than the *Majestic's* 56,000, but her length between perpendiculars is only 907 feet 6 inches compared with 915 feet 5 inches for the *Majestic.*

The *Normandie's* breadth of 119 feet 6 inches accounts chiefly for her greater tonnage. The vessel is a little more than 19 feet wider than either the *Leviathan* or the *Majestic.*

In addition to excessive size, the *Normandie* will contain the largest electric motors ever built. Rated at 40,000 horsepower each, the new motors will give the vessel a total horsepower of 160,000; but even then she will not be the most powerful ship. The U. S. S. airplane carriers *Saratoga* and *Lexington* bear this title with 180,000 horsepower plants in each. Each contains eight motors rated at 22,500 horsepower, connected in pairs to four propelling shafts.

The *Normandie's* claim to fame would probably not be so clear-cut had work on the new British Cunard liner, *R–534,* continued. But, because of economic conditions, construction was suspended almost a year ago on this vessel which, it was announced, would be rated at 73,000 tons and would have a length of 1,018 feet.

The *Normandie's* hull is divided into 12 water-tight compartments. There are eleven decks, five of which are continuous from stem to stern. Accommodation will be provided for 930 first-class, 680 tourist and 560 third-class passengers, which, with 1,320 officers and men, will allow the ship to carry 3,490 persons.

The turbo-electric machinery has been designed for a service speed of 30 knots to enable the vessel to cross the Atlantic from Havre to New York by way of Plymouth, under all conditions, in less than five days.

## ITEMS

COSMIC rays raining on the meeting of the American Physical Society at Atlantic City were seen as flashes of light on a novel electric sign arrangement devised by Dr. Thomas H. Johnson, of the Franklin Institute. To sensitive cells which were discharged electrically whenever they are hit by an incoming electric ray, Dr. Johnson connected neon flash lamps in such a manner that they were lighted whenever a cosmic ray hit. The "hodoscope," as he called the new detector after the Greek for "way" and "aim," had a panel of 58 lamps and the direction from which the rays came was shown by the streaks of light upon it.

FOR the first time, evidence on the possible shape of the active particles in the filtrable viruses that cause such diseases as smallpox, yellow fever, hog cholera and plant mosaics was placed before a scientific body, when Drs. William N. Takahashi and T. E. Rawlins, of the University of California, presented their report to botanists attending the meeting of the American Association for the Advancement of Science. If the invisible, filter-passing particles in these viruses have the shape of tiny rods they should present a bright appearance if light waves arranged all in one direction fall on them at the proper angle. Accordingly, a beam of polarized light, in which all wave-fronts are parallel, was directed on a solution of a virus flowing from a small tube. The solution did present a bright appearance, confirming the hypothesis.

COMPLETE success in protecting dogs and other animals against distemper is claimed in the final report of "The Field" Distemper Council, of which the Duke of Portland is president, as the result of ten years' research and subsequent enterprise of commercial laboratories. A virus, a vaccine and an anti-serum have been produced, and a healthy dog can be given lasting protection against distemper infection by the inoculation of vaccine followed a fortnight later by one of virus. If the anti-serum, used alone, is given sufficiently early in the disease, it will lessen the severity of an attack of distemper. A survey of the results with the vaccine-virus method showed that, where exposure to infection was certain, the incidence of distemper among 650 foxhounds belonging to 23 hunting packs was only 1.4 per cent., and the deathrate 0.3 per cent. Without inoculation the incidence among young foxhounds is nearly 100 per cent., and the deathrate frequently 50, and sometimes more than 75 per cent.

AN epidemic of plague may break ont in London sooner or later if present conditions continue. This suggestion was made by one of England's eminent professors of medicine, Dr. W. Langdon Brown, Regius professor of physic at Cambridge University. The plague-carrying flea lives on rats, but black or dark rats are a worse plague menace than brown ones. In Britain black rats are gradually increasing. If they are allowed to continue to multiply a plague epidemic in London is likely to follow. In big cities such epidemics tend to break out as soon as carriers of the germ become sufficiently numerous. London's freedom from plague epidemics since the "Great Plague" of 1664–5 has been due to the dominance of the brown rat, which came to England on ships, bred very rapidly and almost exterminated its natural enemy, the black rat. During recent years, however, there have been so many campaigns against rats in general that millions of the brown rats have been destroyed. The race of black rats has thus been able to make headway.

WHATEVER may be the cause of common colds, bad weather brings on epidemics of them, scientific studies have shown. "Keeping dry is an elementary precaution in avoiding colds," the Metropolitan Life Insurance Company advises. Officers of the company offer the following explanation of how chilling of the body from clothing that has become wet during stormy weather may induce a cold: "A child who goes out in a storm without proper protection collects a certain amount of water in his shoes and clothing. If he has just had a good meal and is well nourished, during the time he is physically active, he generates enough heat from his food or stored-up energy to compensate for the extra demand which the evaporation of this water makes. At the end of his journey to school, his shoes and stockings may carry a large quantity of water. From a condition of marked physical activity, he becomes relatively quiet. His heat output decreases just at the time that evaporation of the water in his shoes and stockings—the drying process—calls for extraordinary quantities of heat. This unusual demand comes at a time of decreased production and evidently places a strain on the body's heat-regulating mechanism so great, at times, as to break down the ordinary defense, and a cold frequently follows."

# SCIENCE NEWS

*Science Service, Washington, D. C.*

## THE STRUCTURE OF EARTH'S INTERIOR

How earthquakes and other natural events help geologists and geophysicists to form ideas of the inaccessible interior of the earth was related by Professor R. A. Daly, of Harvard University, in his presidential address before the meeting of the Geological Society of America in Cambridge, Massachusetts.

Ordinary rocks, like granite, sandstone and limestone, forming the forty-mile-deep crust of the earth, are aggregates of larger or smaller crystals. Below the crust and all the way to the center of the globe the temperature is too high to permit crystals to form. Down to the depth of about 1,800 miles the material is vitreous, or glass-like. On account of the dead-weight pressure, increasing from 15 tons to 7,000 tons on the square inch, this glassy ''rock'' is on the average more rigid than steel. Hence it can transmit earthquake waves of the ''shear'' or ''shake'' kind.

This thick shell of rigid glass overlies a core, which, in spite of a minimum pressure of 7,000 tons on the square inch and maximum pressure of 22,000 tons on the square inch, seems to a number of expert seismologists to act like a true liquid; if so, the core can not transmit the shear waves. It is generally regarded as essentially a huge ball of metallic iron, chemically like the meteoritic iron of our museums of natural history. If the core is liquid, it must be at a temperature much higher than that of the electric arc.

The thin, crystallized crust itself is layered, lighter rock resting on heavier rock. Similarly the thick, vitreous shell is layered, with a downward step-wise increase of density. At the depth of 1,800 miles the material is more than twice as dense as granite, but at that deep level the density rises abruptly so as to be nearly four times that of granite or ten times that of water.

The great heat of the interior was explained as largely primitive, inherited from the earth's beginning. A fraction of the heat is of radioactive origin and has been generated by the violent explosions of atoms in the rocks, particularly within the thin crust itself.

Because more than 97 per cent. of the earth is too hot to crystallize, its body is extremely weak. True strength is almost, if not entirely, confined to the crust, which, being so thin, must bend if over wide areas it becomes newly loaded with glacial ice, ocean water or deposits of sand and mud. It must bend in the opposite direction if widely extended loads of such material be removed.

Professor Daly's theory of the earth thus accounts for some of the major reshapings of the planet during its long history. The theory seems best to account for the continued existence of dry land; for the origin of chains of high mountains; for the rise of molten rock, or lava, into the crust or all the way to the earth's surface, as volcanoes, and for the great chemical variety of of the world's lavas.

Yet Professor Daly was careful to point out that, in spite of support from modern conclusions about the earth's origin, from earthquake studies, from the record of temperatures found in deep mines and bore-holes, from the nature of volcanic action, and from the myriad facts now known about ''igneous'' rocks, the general theory he described is best regarded as a working hypothesis, a useful guide to research during the decades to come.

## ABBE LEMAITRE ON COSMIC RAYS

Professor Albert Einstein has given his scientific blessing to the ingenious theory proposed by Abbé Georges Lemaitre that cosmic rays are birth cries of the universe and the radiations from the super-radioactive primeval matter that existed when the universe was young.

Abbé Lemaitre, the young Belgian priest-cosmologist, first proposed this idea of cosmic ray origin in 1931. He has now expounded it to investigators at Pasadena with Professor Einstein in his audience.

The father of relativity commented upon the Lemaitre ''birth cries of the universe'' theory by saying that ''if matter is short-lived Lemaitre's theory is inevitable'' and that besides no other theory agrees so well with all observations.

Abbé Lemaitre stated that cosmic radiation contains a thousandth of the total existing energy. He views the commonest elements as analogous to alpha rays that are emitted by radium.

The difference of interpretation of the nature of cosmic rays existing between Dr. Robert A. Millikan and Dr. A. H. Compton was touched upon by Abbé Lemaitre. He explained that beta particles or electrons must show latitude effect which moreover seems to exist. This upholds the Compton idea. But Abbé Lemaitre added that experiment shows that a preponderance of cosmic rays consists of photons or radiations like light rays. This upholds the Millikan idea.

The original energies of the ''universe's birth cries'' radiation have been greatly degraded by the red-shift effect, Abbé Lemaitre explained. This is the effect that when observed in the spectra of the far-distant nebulae indicates that the universe is expanding at a tremendous rate. Abbé Lemaitre was the first to enunciate the expanding universe theory later sponsored by De Sitter, Einstein and other ''universe makers.''

## METHYLENE BLUE AS AN ANTIDOTE

Several thousand persons are killed each year by carbon monoxide gas and by cyanides. If half this number could be saved by the newly-discovered antidote, methylene blue, Dr. Matilda M. Brooks and Dr. J. C. Geiger, of San Francisco, would have made an epochal contribution to medicine and the welfare of mankind.

For Dr. Brooks, working in the department of zoology,

University of California, hit upon the idea of using the common bacteriological stain as an antidote for these two poisons, and Dr. Geiger, director of public health, promptly put the idea into use and two lives have already been saved.

Dr. Brooks was carrying on research in biology, working in pure science when she made the methylene blue discovery. She knew that earlier investigators, chief among them Professor Otto Warburg, of the Kaiser Wilhelm Institute for Biology, Berlin, found in connection with work on yeast cells and other organisms, that methylene blue counteracts the effect of cyanide and of carbon monoxide on living tissues. Dr. Brooks took the next step and tried the effect of methylene blue on animals that had been poisoned with carbon monoxide or with cyanide. She found it a successful antidote with small mammals, such as mice and guinea-pigs, and in a report of her work to the Society for Experimental Biology and Medicine in April, 1932, she suggested the use of methylene blue in human cases of cyanide or carbon monoxide poisoning.

When Dr. Geiger called on Drs. P. J. Hanzlik and C. D. Leake, professors of pharmacology at Stanford University and the University of California, respectively, for modern methods of treating poison cases, they suggested to him, among other methods, the methylene blue method for cyanide and carbon monoxide.

As a result of its successful use, methylene blue may become part of professional first aid kits, such as those carried by fire and police rescue squads. The method used at the Park Emergency Hospital at San Francisco consists of injecting into the patient's vein a one per cent. sterile aqueous solution of methylene blue, which is listed in the U. S. Pharmacopoeia as methylthionine chloride. In the first cyanide poisoning case reported, 50 cubic centimeters, or nearly two ounces, were used. The patient stated that he had taken 15 grains of potassium cyanide in about 4 ounces of water.

## A NEW VARIETY OF BARLEY

A NEW type of barley that is more disease-resistant, that will yield more, and that incidentally will make a finer and more potent brew for beer, has been perfected at the University of Wisconsin by Professor Benjamin Donald Leith, and was one of the five crops that was awarded a place in the "Hall of Fame" of the International Livestock Exposition at Chicago, Illinois.

In 1918 Wisconsin annually raised 38 million bushels of barley, most of which went into the huge beer vats of the state. It was famous as a good "beer barley," but it had one serious drawback. On its stalk were hundreds of little inpointing barbs. These stalks would get into the harvesters' clothes and would creep up and up, despite frenzied efforts to get rid of them. Things got so bad that the farmers' helpers refused to harvest barley crops, and there was a general appeal to the university for help.

Professor Leith was set at work to discover a new barbless type of barley, and it was only a month or so ago that he announced the completion of his work. The new barley has been given the official name of Wisconsin Barbless Barley, Pedigree 38. It is almost entirely resistant to striped disease, the scourge of barley. An increase of from ten to twenty bushels to the acre has been made in its yield.

Gustave W. Pabst, a well-known Milwaukee brewer, has tested over 5,000 bushels of it at his own expense and has found that for brewing purposes it is a vast improvement even over the old barley.

Seed for the Pedigree 38 barley has been distributed over the entire United States by the university agricultural department and preparations are all made for a colossal comeback of the barley crop—provided Congress legalizes beer.

## FACIAL EXPRESSIONS OF THE BLIND

THE pantomime of smiling for politeness' sake, and of putting on an expression of fear or concern when a friend tells of a slight mishap, is a language of which the blind know scarcely "a single word."

This is the report of M. Georges Dumas, who has studied the quiet, often apathetic faces of the blind in French institutions, to find out whether they mimic expressions at all, as seeing persons do. His studies, reported in the *Journal of the American Braille Press,* shed light on the origin of the social art of looking pleasant.

The blind laugh or look sad when genuinely stirred. But those interviewed by M. Dumas did not know how their faces changed in emotion, nor how to produce these expressions at will.

One blind man, accustomed to self-analysis, said: "I know perfectly well what you ask me, but I do not know how joy, sorrow or anger are expressed on my face."

The same man said that he did not feel that his happy, laughing face was different from his face when sad.

M. Dumas attributes the absence of mimicry in blind people to their inability to observe other people and to imitate their expressions. Before his study of the blind, he said he had thought it likely that human beings learn mimicry by a different method from imitating others. He had speculated "that we imitate voluntarily in our own spontaneous expression after becoming conscious of it through our own muscular and cutaneous sensibility."

M. Dumas concludes: "It would obviously be a great service to the blind to teach them mimicry which would make them seem more like ourselves. It would draw us nearer them and at the same time help to adapt them to community life from which their blindness isolates them."

## ITEMS

REPORTS received at the U. S. Public Health Service indicate that influenza is decreasing throughout the country, both in the number of cases and in the number of deaths. For the week ending January 7, the latest for which figures are available, there were 72,241 cases reported throughout the country. This is almost twenty thousand less than the previous week's total. Deaths for 85 cities of the country have also decreased from 14.7 per thousand to 13.6. While the epidemic is not yet over, no more great rise in the number of cases is expected. Health authorities have pointed out, however, that little waves of increased influenza prevalence always follow a large outbreak, and such small waves may continue for the rest of the winter.

BORON is the latest chemical atom to be smashed at the Cavendish Laboratory, Cambridge, by Drs. J. D. Cockcroft and E. T. S. Walton, who last year succeeded in smashing lithium in a similar manner with a release of atomic energy. Bombarding boron atoms with speedy hydrogen atomic hearts, they obtained electrically charged helium atomic hearts or alpha particles. Twenty-five times the number of helium atoms were obtained from the boron bombardment than had previously been obtained with lithium. But as yet the atom smashing is not a useful process in a practical way since roughly only one alpha particle is emitted for every two million proton hydrogen hearts flung at the boron by an electrical potential of 500,000 volts. The Cambridge physicists wrote to *Nature:* "The ionization produced by the particles suggests that they are alpha-particles and the energy of the main group would support the assumption that a proton enters the boron nucleus (of atomic mass eleven) and the resulting nucleus breaks into three alpha-particles."

THE first steps toward making a female sex hormone in the chemical laboratory seem to have been taken by two British investigators, Dr. J. W. Cook, of the Cancer Hospital, and Dr. E. C. Dodds, of the Middlesex Hospital, London. They have produced a chemical compound which, when injected into castrated rats, has an appreciable oestrogenic action similar to that of the sex hormone, oestrin. In their report to *Nature,* Drs. Cook and Dodds give the following formula for their compound: one keto, one, two, three, four tetrahydro phenanthrene. Phenanthrene is a coal-tar product used in the artificial production of dyes and drugs. The rest of the new compound's name tells the chemist the way in which additional hydrogen and oxygen are combined with the phenanthrene. At least four female sex hormones have been reported in recent years from research centers in the United States, Canada, England and Germany. They have been obtained from human placental material and from the kidney secretions of expectant mothers.

MADE visible by invisible light, dials on an aviator's instrument board will glow in darkness so that the pilot may see distant beacons without being blinded by close-up lights. This lightless, yet efficiently usable airplane "dashboard," has been described before the Illuminating Engineering Society by S. G. Hibben, of the Westinghouse Lamp Company, as a new application of ultraviolet light. The dial figures are to be covered with a special paint which fluoresces under ultra-violet light.

THE time designations of A. M. and P. M. will be obsolete and the hours run from 0 to 24 in British post offices if a proposal before the House of Lords finds approval. The movement for continuous numeration of the hours has the support of Sir F. W. Dyson, who recently retired as astronomer royal, who says that there is no valid objection against the 24-hour system which is less confusing and has been in use on the European continent for a long time. Astronomers already use the 24-hour notation, with 0 at midnight and 13 o'clock corresponding to old-fashioned 1 P. M.

THE germs that cause colds in the head are harmless at certain times even if they reach a human being in food, water or air. This is the theory advanced by Dr. E. C. Rosenow, of the Mayo Clinic, and reported to the Society of American Bacteriologists. Colds and other respiratory diseases occur when germs belonging to the ever-present streptococcus family acquire peculiar virulence and other properties. Contact with persons suffering from colds is not of prime importance in the spread of this or other respiratory ails. In these studies Dr. Rosenow used his newly-developed method of identifying peculiar properties of disease organisms by their electric charges. In this way he found streptococci of the same charges and disease-producing potency for animals in the throats of persons suffering from the usual colds and allied ailments of early autumn, from the raw milk and water supplied, and from flies.

EYES act as glands, in certain animals at least, secreting a substance that causes the contraction of color-bodies in their skins and thus controls their chameleon-like color changes. Experiments pointing to this hormone-production by eyes were reported by Professor Lloyd M. Bertholf, of the University of Western Maryland and the University of Munich, in a paper before the American Society of Zoologists. The animals furnishing the color-changing extract were crustacea. The hormone was found in the stalks on which their protruding eyes are mounted. The eye-stalk extract, when injected into the body, produced color changes not only in crustacea, but in frog tadpoles and several species of fishes—animals far removed in the zoological realm from the invertebrate crustacea.

GRASSHOPPERS will not cause major crop damage in the West during the coming summer, unless unexpected weather conditions favoring them should occur. This is predicted as a result of the annual grasshopper survey of the bureau of entomology of the U. S. Department of Agriculture, which has just been completed. The field research men of the bureau examine the soil in trouble-promising areas, counting grasshopper eggs and judging as well as they can the climatic conditions that favor or hinder their development when warm weather returns. In only one state, North Dakota, is the egg-count higher than it was in the fall of 1931, though there are local "bad spots" in a number of other states. In these places the farmers may again have to spread poison bran bait for the young 'hoppers, unless a cool, moist spring favors the development of parasites and fungus diseases and thus keeps the numbers of the insects down by natural means.

# SCIENCE NEWS

*Science Service, Washington, D. C.*

## ARTIFICIAL PRODUCTION OF NEUTRONS

Artificial production of neutrons in larger quantities than the world has hitherto known has been achieved by Drs. Charles C. Lauritsen, Richard Crane and Andrew Soltan at the California Institute of Technology.

This is considered the greatest step in atomic physics since British experimenters, Drs. J. D. Cockcroft and E. T. S. Walton, of Cambridge, disintegrated lithium last year and released atomic energy. It shows that possibilities lying within the nucleus of the atom are practically unlimited, in the opinion of those who have analyzed the work.

In the experiments just performed the metal beryllium was disintegrated with artificial alpha rays or hearts of helium atoms. These were given a push of half million volts. Slow neutrons, which probably have under a million volts of energy but which nevertheless penetrate two inches of lead, were produced.

The neutrons were measured with a small electroscope about the size of a fountain pen which was devised by Dr. Lauritsen. Paraffin was used as a detector, the neutrons, or electrically neutral particles, plunging into this substance and giving rise to radiation that affected the roentgenometer or small electroscope.

This experiment was the first time that neutrons had been produced without use of radioactivity. This means that the quantities and intensities of neutrons to be produced in the future will undoubtedly be much greater as the bombarding radiation can be supplied by extremely high voltage apparatus that is now being built in not one, but several, laboratories. The alpha particles used were accelerated by one of the institute's giant high voltage tubes.

The ranges of neutrons and protons so produced will soon be measured accurately and this will mark the beginning of the spectroscopy of the nucleus of the atom. Far-reaching developments are expected from this new field comparable with the advances brought about by the exploration of the outside portion of the atom in the past decade.

## PROFESSOR EINSTEIN AND ABBE LEMAITRE

*(Copyright, 1933, by Science Service)*

"Can you explain, Professor Lemaitre, in simple terms without too many mathematical symbols, the important features of your theory?" That is exactly the question asked by Professor Einstein at a symposium on relativity at the California Institute of Technology. It was a gathering of scientific men interested in relativity, and a small crowded room contained an imposing set of personalities: Professor Einstein, Abbé Georges Lemaitre, Professor P. S. Epstein, Dr. H. Bateman, Dr. E. T. Bell, Dr. R. C. Tolman and Dr. T. von Kármán.

First Professor Epstein presented an interpretation of the so-called cosmical constant. This was promptly attacked by the others but successfully defended by Professor Epstein. Finally he himself dealt a death blow to his suggestion.

Then the Abbé Lemaitre took the floor, and Professor Einstein asked his question. It was not entirely facetious, for Professor Einstein thinks about the fundamental ideas before he worries about questions of technique which he can later develop with ease.

The essence of the discussion was the use of the cosmical constant. Professor Einstein had introduced it into relativity, but when Dr. Edwin Hubble, of Mount Wilson Observatory, found that light coming from distant nebulae was considerably reddened, he no longer found it necessary. His present position is that if one can get along without this constant it might be better to do so. However, Abbé Lemaitre contended that while he could not prove the constant was an absolute necessity for a consistent theory, it was certainly legitimate and would moreover lead to useful results. Thus with its help he could explain the formation of the nebulae. This was exactly what Professor Epstein had just concluded was impossible on any classical non-relativistic basis. He had tried to do this twenty years before, but the present discussion brought out the deficiencies of the method.

Professor Einstein pointed out that it might nevertheless be possible to explain the formation of nebulae with a relativity theory, but without a cosmical constant. He also mentioned that this constant played a part like matter of negative density. It moreover expressed the instability of a uniform or even distribution, so that if a hole was formed it would push matter away from itself and thus enlarge; it is like a negative gravitational force or a repulsion.

Abbé Lemaitre countered that he felt it would be impossible to construct such a theory, but he said he could not rigorously substantiate his feeling. However, he added a very important argument in his own favor. He showed that without the cosmical constant, designated by the small Greek letter lambda, it would be extremely difficult to explain the rapid development of the universe. This on classical grounds would require a thousand million million years ($10^{15}$) while only about ten billion ($10^{10}$) are available. On the other hand, it might be mentioned that lambda is responsible for the recent short estimates of the age of the universe.

Next Professor Tolman warned against possible neglect of complications which occurred in nature. It is very hard to tell which are unimportant and which are significant.

The discussion took place in three languages. Professor Einstein usually began to speak in adequate English. He would generally feel hampered and soon go on in German. Abbé Lemaitre showed slight difficulty with that and then Professor Einstein burst out in French, which came much more easily than his English.—R. M. Langer.

## CLOUDS IN THE STRATOSPHERE

THE existence of clouds at heights from 15 to 19 miles above the earth, a region of the atmosphere where clouds have never before been believed to exist, has been established recently by observations made in Norway by Professor C. Störmer with the photographic equipment he has successfully used in measuring the height of aurora.

These high clouds have been called "Mother of Pearl Clouds" on account of the pureness of the spectral colors with which they glow and the concentric arrangement of their coloration in band after band similar to the color scheme inside a clam shell. Shades of pink, lilac, purple and blue occur, but generally reddish hues predominate. These colors shine about as bright as in an average rainbow and may be seen only near sunset, increasing rapidly in brightness immediately after the sun sets.

Mother of Pearl clouds have been reported most frequently after the passage of a center of low pressure, but have not been observed generally, on account of the thick low cloud obscuring their view. On the lee-side of mountains, however, the föhn winds dissolve these rain and storm clouds, permitting a view of the extremely high cloud. Mother of Pearl clouds have been found to remain stationary for hours and on other occasions to move with velocities up to 100 miles per hour. On January 13, 1929, they were observed to fall steadily a distance of one mile in an hour and a quarter.

The origin and constitution of these clouds has not so far been explained. The highest cirrus clouds formed from floating ice crystals are only eight miles high in these latitudes and until these Mother of Pearl clouds were discovered, the stratosphere was considered cloud-free except for the noctilucent clouds about fifty miles high and supposed to be associated with volcanic ejecta.

Observers in states and provinces just east of the Rockies would appear to be favorably situated to observe these extraordinary brilliant clouds especially during chinooks. The observer should note the time, arrangement and brilliance of colors as well as the direction and velocity of the cloud.—ANDREW THOMSON.

## FOUCAULT EXPERIMENT

DELEGATES to the annual meeting of the Royal Astronomical Society of Canada, held in Toronto, saw a new version of a celebrated experiment which demonstrates the rotation of the earth, using only an iron ball and a long wire as the apparatus. It was shown by the President, Dr. R. K. Young, who is associate professor of astrophysics in the University of Toronto.

Known as Foucault's pendulum, from the name of the French physicist who devised it, the experiment created a sensation when it was first shown in the Pantheon in Paris in 1851. Foucault suspended a heavy cannon ball at the end of a 200-foot wire, fastened in the ceiling. Attached below the bob was a pointer, sweeping out a track in a layer of sand. The scientist gave the ball a push, starting it swinging. It drew a line in the sand each time the motion reversed. As the hours passed, the line slowly rotated, an effect attributed to the earth's rotation. The pendulum continues to swing in the same plane in space in which it is started, while the earth turns beneath it.

The demonstration here removed anomalies from the original experiment. It has been found that the pointer on the iron ball usually traces a narrow ellipse in the sand, instead of reversing in a straight track, a behavior not previously explained. Dr. Young suggested a reason for the looping. He hung the suspension wire through a small, rigid ring, which took out the side-play through friction. He said: "The tendency for the ball to travel in an ellipse may be due to the flattening of the earth at the poles.

"When the pendulum is not moving, it hangs perpendicular to the earth's surface. If the earth were a perfect sphere, the pendulum line would pass through its center. But the world is not exactly round. A perpendicular to its surface at intermediate latitudes does not go through the middle.

"This fact introduces an additional small force, which encourages the Foucault pendulum to move in an ellipse."

At Toronto the pendulum path turns through a complete circle in about 35 hours. A pendulum hung over the equator does not deviate from its original path. At the North or South Pole the track would turn once every 24 hours. The rotation of the tracks of other pendulums, many of which are in constant operation in the museums of the world, can be calculated from the latitude in which the ball is swinging.

## AN EXPLANATION OF STUFFY ROOMS

SIR LEONARD HILL, the well-known English physiologist and writer on public health subjects, finds that certain heat rays (infra-red rays) given off by dark or dull-red sources of heat cause the nostrils to contract and thus interfere with breathing. He believes that this is the chief reason for the stuffiness that we experience in an overheated room.

In a lecture given in London at the recent Public Health Congress he showed that this effect is not due to a direct action of the heat upon the nostrils, but that it is a reflex effect from the sensory nerves of the skin. He described the particular heat rays that give this effect as "nose-shutters."

Their action is especially marked in persons whose breathing is already partially obstructed, those with a deflected septum of the nose, for example, or a person suffering from catarrh, asthma or hay fever.

The effect can be neutralized by fanning the skin of the face with an electric fan, or by the action of certain other rays, which he speaks of as nose-openers, that are given off especially by luminous sources of heat. They may also be absorbed by water vapor and he suggests that this is the explanation of the efficacy of a bowl of water placed in front of a heater in relieving the stuffiness of a room.

He finds also that these nose-shutting rays cause a diminution in the secretion of the mucous membrane of the nose, and since these secretions may be supposed to protect us from infecting organisms in the air, it is possible that the nose-shutters increase the risks of respiratory infections.

From experiments made at Bedford College, London, he found that 60 per cent. of the persons examined experience difficulty in breathing when exposed to heaters that give off these nose-shutting rays and that in over 25 per cent. of the cases the obstruction to breathing was so marked that it could be demonstrated in records of the respiration made upon a suitable apparatus.

## CHOLESTEROL AS SOIL FOR THE GROWTH OF CANCER

CHOLESTEROL, an important chemical compound found in animal tissue, "prepares the soil" for the growth of cancer. This new theory of a cause of cancer is suggested in a report by Dr. A. H. Roffo, of Buenos Aires, in the current issue of the *American Journal of Cancer.*

Cholesterol is found in all animal fats and oils and in many organs of the body. It is related chemically to ergosterol, from which vitamin D is formed by the action of sunlight.

In the case of skin cancers, Dr. Roffo believes that cholesterol is accumulated in the skin by the effects of exposure to light and in turn acts as a condition for the production of cancer. It prepares the soil, as he expresses it, probably because under the influence of light it itself becomes photoactive, emitting emanations which affect the surrounding tissue.

As evidence for these views he presents such facts as these: Cancerous tissues show an increased cholesterol content compared with normal tissues, especially as regards the skin; tumor cells show a tendency to absorb and fixate cholesterol from the blood, or, in the case of cell cultures, from the surrounding medium.

In the skin a fixation of cholesterol in the tissues is favored by exposure to light. His analyses show that in the face and other parts of the skin exposed to light more cholesterol is present than in those parts protected from the light by clothing. He finds in this relationship an explanation of the fact that skin cancers are frequent on the face and rare where the skin is covered by clothing.

So far as skin cancers are concerned he sums up his views in the statement that "cholesterol prepares the soil for subsequent malignant growth by acting as an accumulator of light."

## ITEMS

THE anti-neuritic vitamin B has been produced by the action of ultra-violet rays on adenine sulphate, B. C. Guha and P. N. Chakravorty, of the Bengal Chemical and Pharmaceutical Works, Calcutta, have reported by cable to *Nature.* Thus it appears that two vitamins are produced by activation of a chemical with ultra-violet light. Scientists found several years ago that rickets-preventing vitamin D is formed by the action of ultra-violet light on ergosterol. Vitamin B is found naturally in the bran layers of cereals, in vegetables, milk, eggs, liver and pancreas. Professor Adolf Windaus, of the University of Göttingen, isolated the vitamin in pure form a year ago and gave it the chemical formula, $C_{12}H_{17}N_3OS$. The Indian report indicates that the vitamin is the type of compound known as a purin.

FURTHER exploration of the cave at Choukoutien, China, where the Peking skull was found, has disclosed a small wrist bone not appreciably different from that of modern man and also a piece of collar-bone about the average of the length of the collar-bone of an adult male in North China to-day. Describing these discoveries, Professor Elliot Smith said that the feet of Peking Man showed that he must have walked like an ape, with in-turned toes, but there is no evidence that he shared the apes' ability to grip with his feet. The shape of his hands leaves no room for doubt that this member of the human family had already gained the skill and intelligence which stamp him as genuinely human.

THE mystery that for forty years has surrounded the highly fatal Peruvian disease known as Oroya fever is finally being penetrated, it appears from a report in the current issue of the *Journal* of the American Medical Association. Dr. Ramón E. Ribeyro, professor at the National University of San Marcos of Lima, Peru, has finally shown that the outlook in this disease is good unless it is complicated by infection with an organism known as paratyphoid B bacillus. It is this complication which is responsible for the deaths that occur in cases of Oroya fever.

THE positions of all the large thunderstorms which occur over Europe and the North Atlantic can now be determined by radio apparatus in the British Isles, independently of weather reports. This is announced by R. A. Watson Watt, superintendent of the Radio Research Station of the British Department of Scientific and Industrial Research. Atmospherics produced by the thunderstorms are so exactly analyzed by cathode ray oscillographs that with two radio stations working in cooperation it is possible to calculate trigonometrically the positions of the storms to within about a hundred miles. The two stations used are the Radio Research Station, near London, and the Leuchars Aerodrome Station, in Fifeshire, Scotland. These stations are about four hundred miles apart, and they enable thunderstorms to be located within a radius of 3,000 miles.

EFFORTS to raise antelope in captivity have at last succeeded in Alberta, with the growth of a herd of 42 to nearly 500 animals. The raising of this most timid of wild animals without its being conscious of captivity was accomplished by Canadian Government big game specialists, when they decided to save the antelope from the extinction which threatened it not long ago with the advance of settlements. A small herd of 42 animals was found grazing near Medicine Hat. The area on which it was living was fenced in, unknown to the antelopes, and now the shy animals will come to be fed. The preserve is one of two established in southern Alberta to save this once numerous animal.

# SCIENCE NEWS

*Science Service, Washington, D. C.*

## SOME PAPERS PRESENTED AT THE ATLANTIC CITY MEETING

THE distance between the United States and England appears to vary each day as the moon moves across the sky. If the hypothesis advanced to the American Astronomical Society by Dr. Harlan T. Stetson, director of the Perkins Observatory at Delaware, Ohio, and Alfred L. Loomis, of the Loomis Laboratory, Tuxedo, New York, is correct, the change in distance is about 63 feet. They make this suggestion to account for surprising variations in British and American time which have been uncovered by Mr. Loomis' researches. With what is probably the most complete installation of the latest type of precision clocks in the world, and automatic radio sets, to record time signals from a number of national observatories, he has found that the times do not agree. The time is determined at both places by observing the instant that a star crosses the meridian. Therefore, if the two observatories are shifting slightly in longitude, the star will cross slightly early when it is west of the average, and late when it is to the east. In the absence of any other satisfactory explanation, Dr. Stetson and Mr. Loomis have adopted the idea that such a shift does take place. The Loomis-Stetson hypothesis to explain this variation in step with the moon's position is that there is a natural stretching or shifting in the earth's crust, within its elastic limits, which would yield and recover periodically under the stress of the moon's gravitational pull. Another result of the studies is the indication that the radio wave takes twice as long to cross the Atlantic as would a beam of light traveling the same distance.

A NEW theory of the origin of cosmic rays was suggested to the American Physical Society by Dr. Ross Gunn, of the U. S. Naval Research Laboratory. Out in the stars that are still young there are born in great "star-spots," like sun-spots on our sun, negatively charged ions or electrons which are given great energies. These pass through the outer layers of the star and each picks up a positive ion, and the two together form an energetic neutral pair of some 10 to 100 thousand million electron volts. When such particles hit the earth they become separated in the upper atmosphere by electromagnetic forces or collisions and become the cosmic rays. Such neutral pair particles which are fathers to cosmic rays are uniformly distributed in space, Dr. Gunn believes, thus accounting for the cosmic radiation coming from all directions. The sun-spots give rise to weaker neutral radiation which gives rise to the aurora and magnetic storms but are not powerful enough to generate cosmic rays.

A NEW process of x-ray generation, caused by the passage of a swiftly moving electrified particle through gas, was reported to the American Physical Society by Dr. Gordon L. Locher, National Research Fellow at the Bartol Research Foundation of the Franklin Institute. Dr. Locher discovered the new process of ionization while investigating the nature of the cosmic rays. Part of the charge in an ionization chamber such as used for measuring the cosmic radiation is caused by characteristic x-radiation generated by the passage of the cosmic radiation particle through it.

THE new type electrostatic high-voltage generator, invented by Dr. R. J. Van de Graaff, and constructed by the Massachusetts Institute of Technology at Round Hill, Massachusetts, with a Research Corporation grant, will develop a steady direct current potential of 10,000,000 volts with a continuous power output of about 20,000 watts. One of the first tasks of the generator will be atom-smashing. To provide a portable high-voltage machine, Dr. Van de Graaff and E. H. Bramhall have designed a rugged machine mounted on rubber-tired casters that will develop 1,500,000 volts. Both generators work on the principle of the old-fashioned static electricity generator and belts carry the electric charges to large discharging spheres.

DISCOVERY of 236 stars in the northern Milky Way with layers of glowing hydrogen surrounding them was announced to the American Astronomical Society by Dr. Paul W. Merrill and Cora G. Burwell, of the Mount Wilson Observatory. These are known as type Be stars, and are of interest to astronomers because of some of their peculiar properties. Astronomers at Mount Wilson have been making a search for them, using the spectroscope to study the lines in the stars' spectra. As a result, the total of known Be stars has been raised to 408.

ULTRA-VIOLET radiation is much more damaging to bacteria than it is to the filtrable virus class of disease causes. This is indicated by researches reported to the Botanical Society of America by Professor B. M. Duggar and Alexander Hollaender, of the University of Wisconsin. Cultures were exposed of the virus of tobacco mosaic and of three kinds of bacteria to the action of ultra-violet rays of a certain narrow range of wave-lengths. It was found that the virus resisted radiation up to 150 times the amount that sufficed to kill one of the bacterial species. The spores or resting-stages of the bacteria were more resistant to ultra-violet than were their vegetative cells.

FOR the first time, evidence was brought forward on the possible shape of the active particles in the filtrable viruses that cause such diseases as smallpox, yellow fever, hog cholera and plant mosaics by Drs. William N. Takahashi and T. E. Rawlins, of the University of California. If the invisible, filter-passing particles in these viruses have the shape of tiny rods they should present a bright appearance if light waves arranged all in one direction fall on them at the proper angle. Accordingly, they directed a beam of polarized light, in which all wave-fronts are parallel, upon a solution of a virus flowing from a small tube. The solution did present a bright appearance, confirming the hypothesis.

A CHANCE mosquito bite of a chicken or a monkey may be an unsuspected source of malarial infection. Studies showing that chickens may be infected by certain strains of malaria were reported by Professor Reginald D. Manwell, of Syracuse University. It has not been known generally that such large birds as chickens could get malaria. This is because the disease runs a short, mild course in the barnyard bird and so is not recognized. Professor Manwell's discovery that chickens could be infected resulted from efforts to find a more suitable bird than the canary for his studies of the disease. Since chickens can be infected artificially, Professor Manwell questioned whether they and other animals hitherto supposed to be not susceptible to malaria may not also be infected in nature. It that case they would serve as unrecognized reservoir hosts, their blood containing enough malarial parasites to infect other mosquitoes but not enough for detection by ordinary microscopical methods. It is quite conceivable that monkeys or other mammals might in this way contribute to the perpetuation and spread of human malaria.

DR. MICHAEL LEVINE, of Montefiore Hospital, New York City, reported to the American Phytopathological Society that, after many vain attempts, he had finally succeeded in inducing a cactus to develop crown gall, a form of plant tumor caused by a microorganism. His efforts to produce the disease in smaller cacti, like the familiar prickly-pear, were not successful, but when he inoculated young specimens of the Sahuaro, or giant tree cactus of the Southwest, he obtained the characteristic abnormal growths. However, the resistance apparently natural to cacti appeared partially even here, for the internal structure of the plant tumors on the Sahuaro was not that of fully developed crown galls, but remained in a more or less juvenile or embryonic condition.

MOTION PICTURES demonstrating how nerve fibers grow through living tissue, and how they repair themselves when injured, were shown by Professor Carl C. Speidel, of the University of Virginia. Professor Speidel, who was the winner of the $1,000 prize of the association at the midwinter meeting at New Orleans last year, gave a summary of his work up to that time and of advances made since then. As explained by Professor Speidel, nerve growth is pioneered by what are known as "growth cones" on the ends of the nerve fibers. These are thickenings of the tips, which probe their way through the tissues, constantly sending out and retracting tiny processes from their surfaces. As the nerve progresses, special cells develop along its course. They hug its sides closely, though they take no part in its actual growth process, nor in its function as a nerve. These are known as the "sheath cells." Finally, as the nerve becomes more mature, it develops around itself a layer of fatty material called the "myelin sheath."

THE exact way in which a single tuberculosis germ multiplies into three or more new germs has been observed by Professor Morton C. Kahn, of Cornell Medical College, New York. Bacteria or germs have a life cycle something like the egg, the pupa and the butterfly. Professor Kahn was the first to work out that cycle for the tubercle bacillus. He considers that the question of how disease-producing bacteria reproduce, or multiply into more bacteria, is one of the most important problems confronting present-day bacteriologists. The rod-shaped tuberculosis germ cleaved into three or more oval bodies which became further reduced in size to extremely fine granules. From these tiny granules very small and delicate rod-shaped types developed. These rods finally elongated and thickened until they became the same size and shape as the tubercle bacillus from which they started. These new, rod-shaped tuberculosis germs were able to produce typical tuberculosis in guinea-pigs. Contrary to the claims of some investigators, Professor Kahn did not find that the tubercle bacillus, even in the form of the almost sub-visible granules, could pass through fine-pored filters. He did find that some of the fine young granules and rods formed from the original tubercle bacillus lost the family characteristic of retaining certain aniline stains even after exposure to acid.

DR. ROSEBURY and his associates at the College of Physicians and Surgeons, Columbia University, have found that they could produce or prevent dental fissure caries in rats at will by changing the size of the particles of uncooked rice in the rat diet. No tooth decay occurred when cooked rice replaced uncooked rice in the diet. The type of tooth decay thus produced is so much like the dental caries of the fissures or crevices of human teeth that it is assumed that the same causes produce the condition in man and in rats. The tooth decay may be produced in healthy, well-grown rats that are on an adequate diet with plenty of vitamins, minerals and other food essentials, and that have teeth free from structural defects. Rats on adequate diets, however, have less tooth decay than rats on deficient diets. Dr. Rosebury pointed out that there are several kinds of tooth decay to be found in rats. Not all of them are comparable to human caries. Failure to distinguish between the different types of rat caries has caused much confusion in experimental studies of tooth decay in the rat.

A CHANCE that diabetics may be freed from the hypodermic injection method of taking insulin and may be able to take it by mouth instead is indicated by the chemical study of the hormone reported by Dr. Hans Jenson, of the Johns Hopkins Medical School. The activity of insulin may be due to a peptide composed of cystine and glutamic acid. It that case it might be possible to give it by mouth. Insulin itself, whether extracted from the pancreas or whether prepared in chemically pure form, is destroyed by the enzymes of the stomach and intestines. That is why it must be given by injection under the skin to be effective. If a peptide or similar protein compound of low molecular weight could be found having the insulin effect, probably enough of it could be absorbed from the stomach to make it possible to give it by mouth.

DR. W. R. COE, of Yale University, outlined the sex life of the oyster. He said in part: "It was formerly believed that the commercial oyster of our Atlantic coast

was of separate sexes and that the sexuality of any individual remained unchanged during its entire lifetime. Recent studies, however, have shown that this is not entirely correct, for it has been proved that an individual that has functioned as one sex during one spawning season may assume the opposite sex the next year. But only a small proportion of the adult oyster population shows this change in any one year, the majority of individuals retaining the same type of sexuality for two years or more. And it is not improbable that some—perhaps many—individuals retain the same sex throughout life or, at least, after passing through an initial male phase during their first or second year.''

MANY seeds of trees, shrubs and other plants of commercial or ornamental value are wrapped up in coats so highly resistant that it takes months or years for them to germinate. Professor J. Nelson Spaeth, of Cornell University, reported to the Botanical Society that seeds of linden or bass wood did not germinate in two years if left untreated. Chilling them at various temperatures, even as low as that of liquid air, failed to have much effect on their torpidity. But when seeds were treated with concentrated sulfuric acid for from twelve to twenty minutes, they showed 49 to 63 per cent. germination in four months. Florence Flemion, of the Boyce Thompson Institute for Plant Research, experimented with the stubborn seeds of Rhodotypos, an ornamental shrub of the rose family. These appear to need a period of ''after-ripening'' in order to germinate and grow properly. By peeling off the seed coats, she induced a few of them to grow without this after-ripening period, but they developed very slowly, and the young plants have the appearance of being dwarfs.

THE forest of Alaska is marching northward. Its front is made of young trees, none of them over a hundred years old, though a few miles to the rear there are plenty of specimens that can boast three centuries. This and other evidence of advancing tree line in the North was presented before the Ecological Society of America by Professor Robert F. Griggs, of the George Washington University. His observations in Alaska are supported by similar studies made by other botanists in the Scandinavian countries. Professor Griggs's most striking observations were made at Kodiak, which is now just beyond the timbered area, though old records indicate that areas now heavily forested were treeless a few generations ago. ''The trees at the edge of the forest are small and squat, suggesting an adverse climate,'' he said, ''but when examined they were found to be growing as rapidly as the same species a thousand miles within its borders to the southeastward. They are likewise reproducing freely.''

THE machine age may starve to death in the near future, victim of to-day's profligate use of metals, coal and oil. In his presidential address before the American Society of Naturalists, Professor Ross Aiken Gortner, of the University of Minnesota, observed that precious, irreplaceable stores of natural resources absolutely essential to modern industrial civilization are disappearing into the maws of industry and dissipated wastefully over the earth. ''In the last hundred years this lusty infant, applied science, has increased its food consumption perhaps a thousand fold,'' he said, ''and unfortunately for mankind already the shelves in some of nature's cupboard show signs of exhaustion of specific food supplies.'' Professor Gortner warns that the coal and oil supplying this energy will be exhausted within the next thousand years. More menacing is the approaching exhaustion of copper, antimony, tin, lead, zinc, chromium, manganese, nickel and iron stored in parts of the earth accessible to man. In the past hundred years the tools of science have wrested from the earth from a tenth to half of the available natural resources. Man has enjoyed them for a moment, then destroyed them or cast them aside in a form useless to coming generations. Water power, alcohol from vegetation and solar energy are totally inadequate to replace oil and coal.

## INDEX TO ADVERTISEMENTS

Ainsworth & Sons, Inc., William 17
Akatos, Inc. 5
Allegany School of Natural History 25
American Chemical Products Co. 16
American Instrument Co., Inc. 19
American Professions Supply Co. 21
American Telephone and Telegraph Co. 6
Angel & Co., Inc., H. Reeve 12
Biddle Co., James G. 19
Biological Laboratory, Cold Spring Harbor 25
Boston Univ. School of Medicine 25
Bramhall, Deane Co. 19
Breeding and Laboratory Institute 18
Brooklyn Botanic Garden 34
Cargille, R. P. 22
Carnegie Institution of Washington 34
Carver, Fred S. 7
Central Scientific Co. 15
Chicago Apparatus Co. 9
Columbia Univ. Press 32
Denver Fire Clay Co. 13
Donaldson, Henry H. 35
Douredoure, Ernest V. B. 4
Eastman Kodak Co. 35
Emerson, J. H. 20
Fiala Outfits 20
Fish-Schurman Corp. 22
Freas Thermo-Electric Co. 17
Gaertner Scientific Corp. 16
General Biol. Supply House 15
General Electric X-Ray Corp. 13
Gradwohl School of Laboratory Technique 25
Hellige, Inc. 20
Hoke, Inc. 18
Holt & Co., Henry 29
LaMotte Chemical Products Co. 19
Lea & Febiger 31
Lee Sales Co., S. C. 21
Leeds & Northrup Co. 3
Login & Son, Inc., B. 35
Loring, J. Alden 21
McGraw-Hill Book Co., Inc. 27
Macmillan Co. 38, 39, 40, 41, 42, 43
Martini, Walter F. 20
Mead Johnson & Co. 22
Meylan, A. R. and J. E. 18
Minnesota Press, Univ. of 32
New York Biol. Supply Co. 8
Oxford Univ. Press 33
Rochester Univ., School of Medicine and Dentistry 25
Rockefeller Institute for Medical Research 34
Sargent & Co., E. H. 20
Saunders Co., W. B. 1, 2
Science Press, The 14, 21
Science Press Printing Co., The 23
Spindler & Sauppe, Inc. 18
Standard Scientific Supply Corp. 14
Stechert & Co., G. E. 36, 37
Stylograph Corp. 35
Thomas Co., Arthur H. 24
Triarch Botanical Products 11
University Presses 32
Ward's Natural Science Establishment, Inc. 10
Wiley & Sons, Inc., John 44, 45, 46, 47
Wilmot Castle Co. 12
Wistar Institute of Anatomy and Biology 35
Zeiss, Inc., Carl 48

# SCIENCE NEWS

*Science Service, Washington, D. C.*

## THE NEW QUANTUM MECHANICS

By Dr. R. M. Langer
California Institute of Technology, Science Service Correspondent



Professor Albert Einstein's first paper on the new quantum mechanics is soon to appear under the title: "Semivectors and Spinors." He has allowed his colleagues in theoretical physics at the California Institute of Technology to have an advance view of some of the ideas contained in this forthcoming paper which will be published in the *Proceedings* of the Prussian Academy at Berlin with Dr. Walter Mayer as the collaborating author.

Professor Einstein is careful to explain that most of the results had already been discovered by other workers. But he wrote the forthcoming paper at the request of his friend, Professor Paul Ehrenfest, of Leiden, to clarify this little known subject.

His discussion with the theoretical physicists was, of course, technical. To make it easier for his American listeners Einstein spoke in English. This is the first extended discussion that he has delivered in English. Usually he speaks in German in order to express himself more precisely and clearly. His English is, however, quite good.

Semivectors are related to vectors in somewhat the way that imaginary numbers are related to real numbers. The spinors are restricted semivectors. The vector concept is fundamental in relativity because it enables one to avoid irrelevancies. Thus it helps to discover new laws.

The semivector may suggest new physical laws also, for it has the same simplifying properties as the vector. As in the case of the vector, the semivector can furnish tensors. The famous equations of Lorentz can be written for semivectors, but no important change is involved. The Dirac equation for an electron can be derived in an elegant manner, but Professor Einstein pointed out that it was not the simplest case of its type.

He said that it would be interesting to study the simplest case. Then he went on to say that semivectors could be used to advantage in generalized relativity, but that unlike vectors they led to complicated equations.

When Professor Richard C. Tolman, of the California Institute of Technology, asked for a physical description of a semivector, Professor Einstein confessed that he had been unable to think of any geometrical or physical picture, but added that with mathematical analysis the subject could be handled with great ease.

## THE UNCERTAINTY THEORY AND THE ELECTRIC FIELD OF A PARTICLE

Abbé Georges Lemaitre, the Belgian priest-professor of the University of Louvain, who has been visiting here, has extended the uncertainty theory of physics to the electrical field of a particle.

Professor W. Heisenberg, the German physicist, by developing his uncertainty principle, which held that it was impossible to know accurately the place and speed of an object at the same instant, introduced a concept of wide philosophical consequences.

Now in a letter to the *Physical Review,* Abbé Lemaitre develops formulae which allow him to conclude that for instantaneous determinations the electromagnetic field of an electron, proton or atomic nucleus is practically undetermined. To know the instantaneous field of such a fundamental particle of matter to within one part in a hundred, Professor Lemaitre computes that its charge must be at least 60,000,000 (sixty million or 6 times $10^7$) times the fundamental charge on the electron which physicists designate as small letter e. This is a relatively large quantity although it is small when translated into volts.

The atom as originally visualized by Professor Neils Bohr, the Danish physicist, was considered by Professor Lemaitre in the light of these new computations of the uncertainty principle.

"Bohr was right," Professor Lemaitre said, "when he considered the field of the atomic nucleus as determining the orbit of the electron, since this field is static and remains significant when averages are taken over long periods of time. He was also right in neglecting the radiation of the moving electron, because we see now from the uncertainty principle that the only determined field is the average field during a time in which the electron has made more than 10,000,000,000 (ten billion or $10^{10}$) revolutions."

## FEDERAL "ECONOMY" AND MINE RESCUE WORK

The nation's "mine rescue squads" and the preventive and research work that protects 1,700,000 men and $14,000,000,000 of capital in the country's mining industry are threatened with the Congressional economy ax.

If recommended federal appropriation cuts urged by the House Committee are made, the U. S. Bureau of Mines of the Department of Commerce will have $127,000 less in funds to support the mine rescue cars, train miners in rescue and safety, operate an experimental mine and perform research on equipment and method to aid the states in preventing mine disasters.

At the present time $741,000 is provided for this work. This is only one two-hundredth of one per cent. of the nation's investment in the mining industry—an infinitesimal price to pay for protection. The budget pared the recommended funds for 1933–34 to $664,000 and now the House bill proposes only $614,000.

The eventual abolition of this fundamental research and service to the mining industry is threatened by the House Committee report just made. The committee reported its opinion that the investigations had been unavailing in many instances because the states have not made public nor acted upon the findings of the bureau. Unless the states secure improved conditions in the mines, the committee does not favor continuance of the federal work. Evidently viewing the task of making mines safe as a static one, the committee then said, in effect, that if the mines are made safer, the rescue and safety work can be abolished.

During the past fiscal year, the Bureau of Mines aided mines and states in connection with 33 explosions in which 87 persons were killed and 59 injured; with 21 fires which took one human life, and with 40 miscellaneous accidents which claimed a toll of 58 persons killed and 156 injured.

The mine rescue cars of the Bureau of Mines have acted as the "Rescue Squads" of the mining industry. Ten such cars have been maintained, equipped and ready to speed at an instant's notice to the rescue of trapped victims of a mine disaster. They have been kept at strategic points throughout the mining territory of the country. When not needed for emergency work they were kept in constant use, traveling continuously from mine to mine giving instruction and exhibitions of first-aid and mine rescue methods. In the event of a mine disaster, the nearest car drops its training at once and proceeds to the scene of the accident, where the crew gives its valuable trained assistance in rescue and recovery operations.

Reduction of funds last year made necessary the withdrawal from service of four of these ten rescue cars. This year's slash in funds will require the withdrawal of more cars and, what is more vital in the long run, about half the curtailment will be from research.

## RECLAIMING RIVER-BOTTOM LANDS

PRESIDENT-ELECT ROOSEVELT'S project for reclaiming river-bottom lands for agriculture, while marginal upland farms are returned to forest, is in a sense a return to the world's earliest recorded planned farming systems, those of Egypt and Babylonia. For in both these ancient lands the river bottoms were farmed and the uplands let alone.

In Egypt this was necessarily the case, for the uplands were deserts. But even if there had been hill lands available, they probably would have been neglected in favor of the richer lands nearer the river.

River bottom lands the world over are usually more fertile than the adjacent uplands. This is as true in the Tennessee Valley as it is in the lands of the Nile and the Euphrates and Tigris, and for the same reasons. The recurrent floods of rivers carry down the best surface soil from the uplands nearer the head of the river, as well as decayed plant and animal remains from the forests, and spread it over the inundated lowlands. In time, thick deposits of easily worked, exceedingly rich alluvial soil are formed.

It was on this alluvial land, collected as a geological tribute from vast uninhabited territories in Africa and Asian highlands, that the world's first farming civilizations rose. And it is to such a neglected wealth of river-bottom land, which now contains much of the fertility that a century of rains have washed down from the hillside farms and denuded forest areas, that President-elect Roosevelt hopes to see poor hill farmers and possibly landless men from cities transplanted.

In Egypt the annual inundations of the Nile were an almost unmixed blessing; the only great misfortune that could visit the land was that the flood might not rise high enough. In Babylonia floods were sometimes disastrous, but the twin rivers of that land were usually controlled by mighty engineering works and a network of distributing canals for irrigation. In the Tennessee Valley, and in the other lowlands to which Roosevelt's ultimate vision extends, floods will be no blessing and must be kept under control by diking, by impounding flood waters in power reservoirs, and by holding head-water streams to a more even flow by means of new forests on the hills.

## THE ALUMINUM AGE

THE exhaustion of iron and steel of the present age of metals forebodes no evil for civilizations-to-come, in the picture of the future given the American Institute of Electrical Engineers at a recent meeting by Professor Colin G. Fink, of Columbia University, inventor and authority on electrochemistry.

For the next age will be that of aluminum, Professor Fink predicted. And aluminum is the most abundant common metal in the earth's crust, being even more common than much-used iron, which it is expected to supplant for many purposes.

"The keynote of the coming new era will be the large number of new products and devices," according to Professor Fink. "Among the metals the one metal to enter the widest variety of new fields will be aluminum —aluminum for railway equipment, aluminum for roofs and buildings, for food containers, for transmission, for airplanes, for tank cars, pipe lines, fencing, etc. Finally we should mention the new aluminum plate, superior to tin plate in many respects, developed at the electrochemical laboratories at Columbia.

"Whereas the supply of raw material for many of our metals is comparatively limited in years, the supply of bauxite or aluminum ore is almost limitless. Thus, for example, whereas copper at the 1929 rate of consumption will last but forty or fifty years, the aluminum ore reserves will satisfy our demands for many hundred years."

In the relative abundance of the common metals in the earth's crust, taking the parts by weight, aluminum leads with 80,000, iron is second with 50,000, while copper is seventh with only twenty. For every pound of copper in the earth's crust there are 4,000 pounds of aluminum.

## VITAMIN $B_2$ AND PERNICIOUS ANEMIA

ONE cause of pernicious anemia may be lack of vitamin $B_2$ in the diet, Dr. William B. Castle, of the Thorndike Memorial Laboratory, Boston City Hospital, and the Harvard Medical School, reported to the American College of Physicians meeting in Montreal. His studies also suggest a new idea of the relation between certain vitamins and the conditions caused by their lack.

Dr. Castle received the John Phillips Memorial Prize of the college. Associated with him in the anemia research were Drs. Wilmot C. Townsend, Clark W. Heath and Maurice B. Strauss, of the Thorndike Memorial Laboratory, and Dr. C. P. Rhoads, of the Rockefeller Hospital.

Liver may be a means of curing pernicious anemia, but lack of liver in the diet is not the cause of the disease. Pernicious anemia develops in those people whose stomachs can not make their own supply of liver extract from a normal diet. When vitamin $B_2$ is fed to a normal human being, his stomach makes it into something that acts like liver extract because of a reaction with what Dr. Castle calls the intrinsic factor in the stomach juice. It is chiefly lack of this intrinsic factor which causes the usual cases of pernicious anemia and also some of those occurring in mothers before the birth of a child. After the child is born, however, the intrinsic factor reappears to a certain extent, as it did in one exceptional case of pernicious anemia following liver treatment.

Vitamin $B_2$ is found in meat, milk, eggs, the outer layer of rice, and yeast. It is lack of this factor in the diet which produces the type of pernicious anemia found in the tropical disease, sprue, and in celiac disease, an intestinal ailment of children. The vitamin factor in the cause of pernicious anemia Dr. Castle calls the extrinsic factor.

A third important factor in the development of this disease is what Dr. Castle calls "defects of absorption." Even if the vitamin is eaten in abundance and the intrinsic factor is present in the stomach juices, the body may fail to absorb the product formed by the interaction of these two factors. This is seen in certain cases of pernicious anemia or sprue in which enormous doses of liver extract have little effect when given by mouth, whereas the usual dose given by hypodermic produces a typical response.

Dr. Castle's researches have thus shown that there are three ways in which the formerly fatal disease, pernicious anemia, may be caused. It is a deficiency disease in a novel sense, since the deficiency is not so much a lack of vitamins in the diet as the failure of a reaction with a vitamin in the digestive tract or elsewhere in the body.

## ITEMS

A NEW compact electrical impulse generator hurling 3,000,000 volts is reported to *Nature,* from the Metropolitan Vickers Laboratory, Manchester. The new high voltage machine is only five feet in diameter and ten feet high. It contains parallel charged, oil impregnated condensers with all spark gaps segregated in an air column with the air under high pressure. It thus combines the advantages of both air and oil gaps. The engineers who constructed the new generator were: T. E. Allibone, F. S. Edwards and D. B. MacKenzie.

THAT all neutrons do not have the same mass or weight is predicted by Dr. A. v. Grosse, of the Kent Chemical Laboratory, University of Chicago, in a communication to *The Physical Review.* Electrons, or beta rays, given off from a disintegrating atomic heart, do not always have the same energies. This has worried physicists so much that some have suggested that the principle of conservation of energy be abandoned in considering the emission or capture of electrons in the atomic nucleus. Dr. Grosse suggests instead that the masses of all neutrons are not identical, but vary according to the energies of the beta rays that are actually observed. The neutron was the atomic building block, similar to the proton or hydrogen atom heart except for its electrical neutrality, which was discovered by Dr. J. Chadwick, at Cambridge, England, last year.

LITHIUM atoms have been disintegrated by bombardment with streams of protons or positive electrical particles at relatively low voltage, by three German physicists at the Institute for Experimental Physics at Kiel, Drs. H. Rausch von Traubenberg, A. Eckardt and R. Gebauer. They sought the threshold, or point of lowest electrical energy, at which the atom-breaking phenomenon would take place. When first performed last year by Drs. J. D. Cockcroft and E. T. S. Walton at Cambridge University, the energy used amounted to 600,000 volts. With a specially constructed apparatus the workers at Kiel obtained definitely detectable atomic breakdowns with an input of only 29,000 volts, less than a twentieth of the energy used in the English experiments. The work is summarized in a report to *Die Naturwissenschaften.*

ENOUGH iodine to supply the entire present American market could be produced at the end of a year's expansion program of a new chemical plant recently established at Los Angeles to extract this widely used element from California oil-well brines. Its present production is several hundred pounds of iodine a day, but it can be expanded to produce 350 tons a year, the present American consumption, if this should prove necessary. The plant has already wrecked the monopoly price formerly maintained by the Chilean nitrate corporation, which obtained iodine as a by-product of its fertilizer production. Some months ago the Chilean corporation cut its former price of $4 a pound to $3; within the past few weeks a further cut was made to the present prevailing price of $1.95 a pound. The new American firm has met all its rival's price cuts, and it is reported they are able to face any price competition which Chilean iodine may offer.

VIGILANT sentinels of science on all the borders of the United States stopped over twelve thousand invasions of American territory by insect pests and fungus diseases of plants in a single year. A detailed report of the period covered—July 1, 1931, to June 30, 1932—has been published by the U. S. Department of Agriculture. At least eight distinct species of fruit flies were stopped, as stowaways on a long list of fruits and vegetables from an even longer list of foreign ports. Most prominent among them was the Mediterranean fruit fly, whose outbreak a few years ago in Florida caused a serious situation and was suppressed only with much labor and expense. This world-distributed pest was detected on fruits from Algeria, France, the Azores, Bermuda, Hawaii, Italy, Spain and Venezuela.

# SCIENCE NEWS

*Science Service, Washington, D. C.*

## IRREGULAR DISTRIBUTION OF DISTANT GALAXIES IN EVOLUTIONARY GROUPS

THE distant galaxies, those clouds of stars far beyond our own galactic system, which includes the sun and all the stars that we ordinarily observe in the sky, seem to be irregularly distributed in space. This is the opinion expressed by Dr. Harlow Shapley, director of the Harvard College Observatory, in an Observatory Bulletin that has just appeared. Furthermore, he suggests, these irregularities are the result of some evolutionary process in the higher system of which the galaxies themselves are the units.

These galaxies appear on the photographs taken through great telescopes as faint nebulae, and they show in greatest numbers in regions far from the Milky Way, for there the stars in our own galaxy, and the associated dark matter, obscure them. But even in the regions where they are most numerous, there is considerable irregularity in their distribution. The question was whether or not this is real, or whether they too are partly hidden by dark material in space. The nebulae studied by Dr. Shapley are those nearer than 25 megaparsecs. A megaparsec is the biggest unit of distance employed by astronomers. It is the distance that a beam of light will travel in 3,260,000 years.

Dr. Shapley's research was to determine whether there was any correlation between the distribution of these galaxies, and that of the faint stars. These stars are presumably the most distant in our own Milky Way system, and so, if the sparseness of the galaxies was the result of dark matter in our own system, the stars should be affected similarly. However, he finds that there is no correlation whatever. The stars are also distributed very irregularly, but in some regions where they are thick, the galaxies are very scarce, and *vice versa*. There are other cases where the two happen to be most numerous in the same regions.

"From these simple tests," states Dr. Shapley, "it appears that the distribution of external galaxies is wholly independent of the distribution of faint stars, and we deduce therefrom that if obscuring matter is involved it is external to our own galactic system. A much more reasonable assumption, of course, is that the irregularities in apparent distribution are real and indicate groupings of external galaxies. The irregularities are obviously too pronounced to be attributed to chance; they are rather a demonstration of evolutionary tendencies in the metagalactic system."

This idea would fit in with earlier researches by Dr. Shapley which indicated that distant space is reasonably transparent, in that it is not filled with a sort of mist. This was shown by a study of the relation of the size of the galaxies to their surface brightness. If space is transparent, the distant ones would be faint merely because they seem smaller than those which are nearer. If space were filled with some sort of obscuring fog, however, the brightness of a certain area of the distant galaxies would be less than that of a corresponding area in a nearer one. However, he found that the average surface brightness was fairly constant regardless of distance. If there were actual dark clouds that obscured all the light if they obscured any, the surface brightness would not be affected. But in the absence of any evidence that there are such clouds beyond our galaxy, it is more reasonable to assume, as Dr. Shapley suggests, that the irregularities are real.

## EOANTHROPUS AND NEANDERTHAL MAN

DR. HANS WEINERT, anthropologist at the Kaiser Wilhelm Institute, Berlin, has examined the original specimens of Eoanthropus, the Dawn Man of Piltdown, England, and is convinced that Eoanthropus is more human than Neanderthal Man and that he is probably not as old as he has been considered by earlier investigators.

Dr. Weinert's argument turns to a considerable extent on the Dawn Man's teeth and lower jaw, which were found separately from the fragments of the upper skull. These have hitherto been considered to be definitely apelike, contrasting strongly with the massive, but just as definitely human cranium. So great has this contrast appeared to earlier workers that some of them would not believe that jaw and cranium belonged to the same being, but held that the skull was a man's, the jaw an ape's. But the German investigator finds that the teeth are human after all, and is of the opinion that the jaw and skull do belong together.

The Eoanthropus fossils consist of two fragmentary crania, half of a lower jaw containing two molars, a loose eye tooth and a loose molar. The pieces of one skull, the jawbone and the loose eye tooth were found in a gravel pit at Piltdown, Sussex, between 1909 and 1913; the pieces of the second skull and the loose molar in the same neighborhood, at a distance of about two miles, in 1915. In the gravel stratum were many bones of extinct animals, including mastodon, hippopotamus and rhinoceros. These animals were identified as being of early Ice Age date, so that the human fossils were assumed to be of equal antiquity, although it was recognized that the gravel deposit, bones and all, might be secondary, that is, washed in from elsewhere.

Now, Dr. Weinert states, the English investigators agree with him in regarding the animal remains as older than the human fossils, so that the great antiquity heretofore assigned to Eoanthropus is at least open to question.

As for the likelihood that the skull and the teeth belong to two different creatures, he points out that the coincidence would have to be twice repeated, since the loose molar was found near the second group of skull fragments, just as the jawbone-piece and the loose eye tooth were found near the first. He feels that the probability of the pieces really belonging to each other is greater than the chances of a double coincidence of the remains of the same kind of man and the same kind of ape being found in the same place. As for the apelikeness of the jaw teeth, he says, "the lower jaw is not so pronouncedly anthropoid as has been assumed; the teeth are human; what appears apelike about them can be found in other human teeth as well."

Stating that he intends soon to publish his detailed findings in a leading German anthropological journal, he adds, "If my work finds acceptance, then Eoanthropus is no 'Anthropus' and no ape, but a 'Homo' (man), indeed more 'Homo'—and therefore more truly human—than the Neanderthaler."

Dr. Weinert's preliminary conclusions are contained in a communication to *Forschungen und Fortschritte.*

## CLIMATIC FACTORS IN THE DEVELOPMENT OF CIVILIZATION IN RUSSIA

RUSSIA'S sprint to overtake and pass the western cultures, under the spur of Soviet leadership, is foredoomed to failure, in the opinion of Dr. Ellsworth Huntington, research associate in geography at Yale University. In an address before the Franklin Institute, he based his prediction on the depressing effects of Russia's dry, cold, monotonous winters, as contrasted with the more varied and stimulating climates of western Europe and the northeastern United States. January and February, called "Russia's best generals" in the days of the Napoleonic invasion, are according to this view also Russia's worst enemies.

Dr. Huntington has for many years maintained a thesis of the dominant importance of climatic factors in the development of civilizations, often in the face of strong disagreement on the part of other scientists.

"According to my theory Russia would be expected to be more inert and less progressive than countries like Germany, France and England, which surround the North Sea," said Dr. Huntington. "This does not preclude the rise of men of extraordinary genius and energy, but it does mean that we should expect such men to be poorly supported in their efforts at progress. The vital point is whether a new social system, led by great organizers but imposed on people under an environment with cold winters of depressing dryness, low temperatures and lack of variability, can cause Russia to rise above the level that would be expected on the basis of its climate.

"Thus far nothing of the kind has happened. In spite of the five-year plan industry in Russia has not quite reached the level that it would normally have reached if there had been no war and revolution.

"This may seem like an extraordinary statement. Nevertheless, the curves of production of coal, iron, petroleum, cotton goods, sugar and other commodities all show that if the rate of progress that prevailed from 1880 to 1913 had continued, Russia would to-day be better off industrially than is actually the case.

"In the same way, although a vast number of Russians have learned to read, the real question is what proportion are really doing any intelligent reading, and how this compares with the proportion in Germany, for example, or with the proportion that would be thus reading if the pre-war rate of progress had continued."

Dr. Huntington's remarks on Russia were made in illustration of his general theme, that climate operates through three main factors in influencing the development of human cultures. First in importance is the mean temperature. Human beings do their best physical and mental work at temperatures around 63 degrees Fahrenheit, and too wide a departure in either direction is depressing. Furthermore, the plants and animals man has domesticated find their optimum temperatures near man's own.

Contrary to common assumption, Dr. Huntington continued, high humidity of the air is beneficial, not harmful, at the moderate temperatures best for human life; it is bad only at excessive temperatures. Finally, a variable climate is more favorable for the development of initiative and energy than is an equable one. Thus the moderately stormy American climate is better than the monotonous cold of the Russian winter, or the monotonous warmth of the tropics.

## REFORESTING OF SLOPES TO CONSERVE WATER SUPPLY

PRESIDENT-ELECT ROOSEVELT'S project for reforesting the uplands of the Tennessee Valley will arouse interest among foresters for more than its possibilities toward a restoration of the nation's timber supply. Long before any wood can be harvested from the new forests, they will have begun to pay for themselves in the improvement of the region's water supply and in the checking of the land's deterioration through erosion.

The significance of reforestation in the conservation and regulation of water was exhaustively discussed at a recent meeting of the Society of American Foresters, by Director C. L. Forsling, of the Intermountain Forest and Range Experiment Station at Ogden, Utah. Although Mr. Forsling's immediate work is in the West, the general principles he discussed are regarded as valid for any region. His discussion will be reported in detail in the forthcoming issue of *The Journal of Forestry.*

Denudation of upland forest areas brings in its train a whole chain of evils, as outlined by Mr. Forsling. The ground loses the sponginess given to it by the dead leaves and forest litter, and hence will not hold the water and let it trickle down into the soil to the underground run-off channels. Instead, the run-off goes along the surface, washing away the valuable top soil, choking streams with floods and then as suddenly leaving them almost empty, clogging irrigation and water-power conduits, fouling domestic water supplies, killing fish and leaving loads of unwanted silt on bottom lands after inundations.

The destruction of tree cover, especially of conifers, also permits a more rapid melting of snow in spring, wasting water that would be valuable later and causing early floods. In the special case of the Tennessee River, which flows northward into the Ohio River near its mouth, these spring floods can be especially damaging, because the snow melts off its upper watershed in the

South while it is still winter in the lower Ohio Valley, thereby increasing the suffering of the people driven out of their homes into the cold of late February or early March.

All the evils of denudation have been operative in the Tennessee Valley and in other river valleys in the East and Southeast for over a century, so that much of the farm land has already lost its value as such and must soon be abandoned. Mr. Forsling called attention to the Little Pigeon Creek Valley in Indiana, where Abraham Lincoln's father cleared virgin timber to make a farm in 1816. The farms of this region, he said, are already being abandoned, their fertility exhausted or their top soil eroded away.

The project of President-elect Roosevelt promises to be an experiment in the rehabilitation of both forest and farm lands on a scale hitherto undreamed of, and for this reason foresters and water conservation engineers will watch its progress with intense interest.

## THE BALD EAGLE

THE bald eagle, hailed in a thousand patriotic orations as America's bird of freedom, is very much in need of protection if it is not to be exterminated from the land. Only five states of the forty-eight grant it legal immunity by special act, and there is no federal legislation whatever for its protection, notwithstanding the fact that it is the official emblem of the United States of America.

So declares the National Association of Audubon Societies, which defends the bird against charges commonly made to its disparagement. The bald eagle's occasional choice of dead fish, which sometimes replaces fresh fish in its diet, has been used as a slur on its character, but this trait, the association points out, is actually in the eagle's favor, making it useful as a cleaner-up of beaches and stream-banks. Scientific records show that the bald eagle does little harm as a predator. It belongs to a class of large and picturesque birds that have been for many years the object of an ignorant prejudice although few do more harm than good, while the great majority are either harmless or positively beneficial in their food habits.

The bald eagle, especially, has been too long misunderstood and misrepresented. Most people fail to realize the character of the actual eagle, but carry in their minds an impression of a false and imaginary bird, a fabulous creature that is an angel to politicians, a devil to game wardens and a mythical feathered ogre out of "Grimm's Fairy Tales" to the rest of us.

Franklin's tirade against the bald eagle doubtless was based on pique, since Congress refused to adopt his own candidate, the wild turkey, as the emblematic national bird. Audubon, in quoting Franklin, was evidently striving to paint a colorful, well-rounded portrait, for his account likewise contains a classic appreciation of the noble bird's many admirable points.

## ITEMS

BY allowing the heart of a helium atom to "tune in" on the heart of an aluminum atom, creating in it a sympathetic vibration, physicists of the Carnegie Institution's department of terrestrial magnetism at Washington have smashed the aluminum heart or nucleus. This achievement by Dr. L. R. Hafstad was announced by Dr. M. A. Tuve in a lecture before the Franklin Institute. The first experiments on the resonance smashing or disintegration of atoms were performed by Dr. M. Pose in Germany, and Drs. Hafstad and Tuve have now confirmed this work and carried it further. It is found that when the attacking alpha particle or wave, which is the helium heart, has the proper energy it penetrates the other atom's nucleus. In this case, the alpha particles of mass four from radium joined with aluminum of mass 27 and formed silicon of mass 30 and released hydrogen of mass one in the form of a proton or wave-particle of positive electricity. Using high voltage apparatus generating 600,000 volts, Drs. Tuve, Hafstad and O. Dahl repeated the experiments of Cockcroft and Walton at Cambridge, England. Hydrogen hearts, or protons, were flung at lithium and boron and helium obtained from the disintegration.

SOME seventy years ago Alexander Lagerman, one of Sweden's greatest inventors, was penniless and lacked the means for completing his foremost invention, the automatic match-making machine, which is one of the principal causes of Sweden's supremacy in the match industry. Shortly afterwards the Swedish Academy of Science recognized his merits and gave him a sum of 3,000 kronor to enable him to finish his invention. Lagerman, who died twenty-eight years ago, in his will donated a fund for the benefit of inventors in need of economic support. A few days ago eleven young Swedish inventors among some sixty applicants received varying sums from the Lagerman Fund to enable them to complete their promising inventions. These include an accumulating fuel pump for Diesel engines, a new protective device for railway crossings, household and agricultural appliances, etc.

CATERPILLARS can hear. They hear sounds audible to human ears, according to a report read before the American Society of Zoologists by Dr. D. E. Minnich, of the University of Minnesota, who outlined experiments demonstrating his point. He held tuning-forks of several pitches within the range of the middle piano keyboard over a sound box in which were caterpillars of fourteen different species. When he struck the forks the caterpillars served notice that they heard, either by stopping their movements or by vigorously contracting their longitudinal muscles.

"GEOGRAPHY 36." This is the prosaic title of a new course in aerial photography offered during the second half of the present school year at Harvard University. The instruction will be under the direction of four Army officers, Captain A. W. Stevens, Captain D. M. Reeves, Captain B. C. Hill and Lieutenant J. F. Phillips, on leave from Wright Field, Dayton, for the purpose. The latest photographic equipment, including a five-lens camera, will be used and plans are being considered for actual aerial work by students toward the end of the course. The course is open to qualified undergraduate students as well as graduates.

# SCIENCE NEWS

*Science Service, Washington, D. C.*

## FREE POSITIVE ELECTRONS

"POSITRON" is the name with which the newly discovered positive electron will be christened by its discoverer, Dr. Carl D. Anderson, of the California Institute of Technology, Pasadena, as soon as the existence of the free positive electron becomes fully established. Dr. Anderson announced in SCIENCE last September the existence of the positive electron from cosmic ray studies, and experiments in Cavendish Laboratory, Cambridge, have just confirmed his work.

When the London correspondent of Science Service cabled the news of the confirmation by the British physicists, the news was specially relayed by telegraph to Dr. Anderson with the suggestion: "Why not christen your new particle 'positron'?"

"With regard to your suggestion," Dr. Anderson wired in reply, "we have already discussed here negatron and positron.

"Historically and derivatively the word, electron, denotes the unit charge, positive or negative, without any reference to the associated mass. The discovery that there exists a positive charge which, like the free negative electron, is unassociated with any mass of atomic magnitude, requires the introduction of a new term to distinguish it from the proton which is used to denote the positive electron associated with the mass of the atom of hydrogen. We have been discussing in the laboratory for some months past the desirability of calling the free positive electron, positron, and then using the similar contraction, negatron, for the free negative electron. This makes a logical and systematic notation which should be introduced if and as soon as the existence of the free positive electron becomes established.

"If the observations obtained here, part of which are already published, are actually due to positrons then we have new experimental evidence that in passing through matter positrons lose energy more rapidly than do negatrons."

The demonstration of the existence of a positive electron, as a fundamental particle of matter, positively charged but with the mass of the familiar negative electron, throws atomic structure theory into at least a momentary state of confusion. And since the positive electron was found in cosmic rays it may prove to be helpful in explaining the nature of this radiation.

Physicists are presented with the fourth of the fundamental particles of matter or bricks out of which atoms might be built. Two years ago there were only two, the positive particle, or proton, and the negative particle, or electron. In 1931, Dr. J. Chadwick in the Cavendish Laboratory of the University of Cambridge forged the last link in the chain of experimental evidence for the reality of the neutron, the close combination of electron and proton that carries no electrical charge. Now out of the same famous laboratory, presided over by Lord Rutherford of Nelson, has come the demonstration of the reality of the positive electron, confirming the suggestion issued last September by Dr. Carl D. Anderson as the result of cosmic ray track photography in Dr. R. A. Millikan's laboratory at the California Institute of Technology.

WATSON DAVIS

## REPORTING EARTHQUAKES

CHINA'S Christmas earthquake disaster, whose 70,000 deaths in Kansu Province are just being reported by cable, after the news had slowly filtered out of the interior, sent its own reports by much faster methods, and they were read and correctly interpreted by scientists on the day of the catastrophe itself.

Within a few hours after the earthquake occurred, eight seismological stations in widely separated parts of the world wired and radioed the facts of their instrumental records to Science Service. Investigators at the U. S. Coast and Geodetic Survey interpreted the data, and stated that they indicated a "very severe earthquake that was probably extremely destructive to life and property" in the interior of China. The latitude and longitude as thus calculated correspond exactly with the locations now being reported by cable.

This is the second time that a disastrous earthquake in that same region has sent its own report, via the sensitive instrument in seismological observatories, weeks ahead of the delayed cable news. On May 22, 1927, an even greater catastrophe, in which a hundred thousand Chinese perished, occurred in Kansu, and within eighteen hours its location had been determined and the statement made that loss of life and property would probably be very heavy. At the end of July, a missionary priest finally found his way through a ruined and bandit-infested region to a telegraph wire and sent the first verbal confirmation of the scientists' prediction.

Similar "beats" have been scored by scientists and seismographs over reporters and telegraphs in several other notable earthquakes during recent years. Data for these reports are gathered by Science Service and interpreted by the U. S. Coast and Geodetic Survey and the Jesuit Seismological Association, acting in cooperation with many seismological observatories in universities and other institutions in the United States and foreign countries.

In the case of the Chinese quake, the first wave was recorded on the nearest reporting seismograph, that of the Philippine Government Observatory at Manila, 6.5 minutes after the quake started in China. The second wave arrived 10.9 minutes after the shock. The difference in time between these two records indicated to scientists of the U. S. Coast and Geodetic Survey that the quake was about 2,220 miles from Manila. Similar time gaps were interpreted to signify distances of 4,200 miles from Strasbourg, in Alsace; 4,470 miles from West Bromwich, near London; 7,020 miles from the headquarters of the Jesuit Seismological Association in St. Louis, Mo., and 8,250 miles from the U. S. Coast and Geodetic

Survey observatory in San Juan, Puerto Rico. Similar reports were received from Tucson, Arizona, and the University of Vermont, Burlington, Vt. All the data were relayed through Science Service, which acted as a clearing station.

## THE PREVENTION OF RANCIDITY BY MALEIC ACID

MALEIC acid, a cheaply and easily produced synthetic compound, has been found to be a good thing to add to edible fats and oils to keep them from getting rancid. Dr. G. R. Greenbank, of the U. S. Department of Agriculture, who made the discovery, has applied for a public service patent on its use for this and similar purposes, which it is expected will be granted soon. Under such a patent, the product can be used freely by anybody, and no one can establish a monopoly.

Dr. Greenbank was led to his discovery by a project in chemical research, with the object of finding why some oils and fats kept naturally better than others. He did not succeed in learning this, but did learn that the natural "better keepers" had extremely minute quantities of unidentified organic acids in them.

Then he tried adding acids of known composition to oils and fats, and soon found that maleic acid, added in a proportion of one part to ten thousand of the oils to be preserved, would enable it to stand without turning rancid for about three times as long as untreated samples of the same oils. The better the quality of the oil the longer it would be preserved by the maleic acid; the best oils had their natural life extended five times instead of the average three.

Dr. Greenbank has tried this method on many fats and oils used as food and in the industries, including butterfat, butter, lard and the oils of cottonseed, peanuts, corn and sesame. He has also tried it on such food products as milk powder and pie-crust, and he believes it will be useful in the cereal industries.

The chemistry of maleic acid's efficiency in preventing rancidity is not yet known. Dr. Greenbank thinks it possible, however, that it operates by stopping the formation of peroxides, which are intermediate steps in the respirational-digestive processes of the bacteria and other fermentive organisms that oxidize fats and oils, thereby splitting off the acids that give them the rancid odors.

Maleic acid is chemically related to malic acid, one of the mild acids found in apples and other fruits. It can be made from malic acid, though in commercial practise it is obtained synthetically in other ways. At present it is made by the chemical firms manufacturing photographic reagents, who make it so cheaply that they can sell it for a few cents an ounce.

## ITEMS

A COMET that may become visible to the unaided eye was discovered early Thursday, February 16, in the northern evening sky by Leslie C. Peltier, an amateur astronomer of Delphos, Ohio, the Harvard College Observatory has been informed. It is at present eighth magnitude and sufficiently bright to be visible through small telescopes or high-powered field glasses. It lies between the constellations of Cepheus and Cassiopeia in the region of the Milky Way and it is moving southeastward. Further observations may be expected to show whether the comet is a newcomer to the heavens or an old comet returning to the vicinity of the sun. Mr. Peltier is a veteran comet discoverer. He reports the astronomical position of his latest discovery as right ascension 22 hours 48 minutes and north declination 62 degrees.

FOSSIL bones of a forty-foot plesiosaur, the largest and most complete specimen ever found in Australia, have been brought back to the Harvard Museum of Comparative Zoology by William E. Schevill, who has recently returned from an eighteen-months' expedition to that country. The bones are now being examined and prepared for permanent mounting.

CANCER will soon be treated at Mercy Hospital, Chicago, with a giant x-ray tube, with a voltage of 800,000 and a radiation output equivalent to radium worth $75,000,000. The new tube is about to be shipped from the General Electric laboratories, Schenectady, New York. The new 800,000-volt tube has several times the energy rating of the cancer-treating tube installed about two years ago in Memorial Hospital, New York. The tube itself is 14 feet long and it is being installed in such a manner as to assure the comfort and safety of patients and the hospital staff.

FISH livers have a new use—as treatment for pernicious anemia. This is announced by Professor L. S. P. Davidson, of the University of Aberdeen, in a report to the *British Medical Journal.* Professor Davidson found that an extract from livers of cod, haddock and whiting is effective in treating pernicious anemia. Beef liver is now widely used for this purpose.

"LACE CRABS," strange, delicately-constructed fossil creatures that lived in the primal seas half a billion years ago, may have been merely the "soft-shell" stages of trilobites, extinct relatives of lobsters and crayfish that dominated the waters of that long-gone epoch. This new solution for an old riddle of geology has been suggested by Dr. Rudolf Ruedemann, of the New York State Museum. Working with a specially constructed microscope, Dr. Ruedemann has found evidence that the "lace crabs" had shed an outer shell, as lobsters and crabs shed their shells to-day. In this "soft-shell" stage they looked like creatures of an entirely different order, with wide-apart eyes on their unprotected heads, and the delicate lacy limbs that have given this fossil group its name. The principal deposits of "lace crabs" have been found in fine-grained shales, hardened out of the mud into which the unprotected moulting trilobites settled for shelter while their new shells were forming, and where many of them were trapped and killed by pockets of water over-charged with carbonic acid. The "lace crabs" were first described by the late Dr. Charles D. Walcott, secretary of the Smithsonian Institution. Dr. Ruedemann's suggestion that they were "soft-shell" trilobites is set forth in a recent Smithsonian publication.

# SCIENCE NEWS

*Science Service, Washington, D. C.*

## INAUGURATION DAY

WHATEVER the uncertainties of Washington weather may bring Mr. Roosevelt's inauguration as president, he can look forward with reasonable assurance to January 20, 1937, for a day of settled weather. On that day, when, according to the Twentieth Amendment, future presidential inaugurations will take place, he can probably begin his second term (if the fortunes of politics so ordain) under kindlier skies than Washington usually provides around the stormy beginning of March.

An examination of Weather Bureau records for the past ten inauguration years, from Cleveland's second, in 1893, to Hoover's in 1929, shows that only one of the January twentieths in that time had any measurable snow or rain. That was the first of the series, January 20, 1893, which was a chilly, rainy day with a little snow. Contrasting with this, the March fourths during the same series provided rain or snow seven times out of ten chances. Cleveland's second inaugural took place in a snowstorm, and Taft rode to the White House through a veritable blizzard that dumped nearly ten inches of snow on the streets of the capital. The most recent inauguration day, Mr. Hoover's in 1929, brought a cold, disagreeable rain that began just before the oath of office was administered and lasted all the rest of the day.

January 20 inaugurations not only promise fairer, more settled weather, if past performance can be construed as promise, but they will probably not bring severe cold. The Weather Bureau's records for January 20 in all inauguration years from 1892 to 1929 show mean temperatures above the freezing mark on all but three of the days. Those were January 20, 1893, with 20 degrees; January 20, 1897, with 30 degrees, and January 20, 1901, with 25 degrees. The highest mean temperature of the series was January 20, 1913 (Wilson's first inaugural), with 49 degrees. Since the principal ceremonies of the inauguration usually take place during the warmest part of the day, the mean temperature can be expected to be bettered considerably in most years.

Weather probabilities for March 4, the last inauguration day under the old dispensation, are totally unpredictable as yet, according to Weather Bureau officials. During the past few weeks changes have been taking place so rapidly that not even the most tentative guess can be made of possible tendencies. It is possible to say only that the first week of March is an unsettled period, when anything may happen.

## SECRETARY OF AGRICULTURE WALLACE

HENRY A. WALLACE, who is to be Secretary of Agriculture in Mr. Roosevelt's cabinet, brings to his office the combination of practical farming and equally practical science that has become a tradition of the Department of Agriculture. Born to the editorship of the great farm paper, *Wallace's Farmer*, which his grandfather had founded and his father continued, Henry Wallace was given the best training that the Iowa State College at Ames afforded. He came out with his baccalaureate in science in 1910, both a "dirt farmer" and a "dirt scientist."

Among other things, he calls himself an agronomist, which means a scientist of field crops. His outstanding agronomical work, however, has been in plant breeding, specifically in corn breeding. Before his time, Dr. George H. Shull, now at Princeton University, had applied the principles of Mendel to the production of "pure lines" in corn, isolating desirable characters in specially developed strains of plants, even though in doing so he made them unpromising runts in all other respects. Then he recombined his "pure lines" at will to build up a mosaic of characters of exactly the kind he wanted.

Dr. Shull had become interested in other plants and let his corn work drop. Henry Wallace took it up and carried it out on a much larger scale, producing numerous new strains of corn on his farms around Des Moines. The best of these high-yielding offspring of crossed "pure lines" have revolutionized corn production in the Midwest. Paul DeKruif, in his book, "Hunger Fighters," has brilliantly summarized the work of Shull and Wallace.

But corn breeding, and botany applied to the problems of the cornfield, are by no means all of Henry Wallace's scientific accomplishments. He has given much thought to the economic problems of the farmer as well, building up a considerable reputation as an agricultural economist. And since both plant breeding and economics require the expert handling of numerical data, he has become a statistician, as much at home behind a calculating machine as he is behind his editor's desk or among his experimental corn-rows.

The titles of his three published books reflect his threefold scientific interest: "Agricultural Prices," published in 1920; "Corn and Corn Growing," in 1923, and "Correlation and Machine Calculation," in 1924.

## THE NEUTRON

THE neutron is not a mere close combination of electron and proton acting like a fundamental particle of a nature, but it actually is an elementary particle itself.

This is the conclusion of Dr. Franz N. D. Kurie, twenty-six-year-old research fellow in the Sloane Physics Laboratory, Yale, after experiments on atomic collisions in which neutrons take part.

When Dr. J. Chadwick, of Cambridge, England, last year discovered the neutron, it was held that it is an electrically neutral combination of the more familiar electron and proton.

By measuring the angles at which protons are ejected from nitrogen atoms, Dr. Kurie found that the neutron does not conform to the configuration described by physicists. Two views of neutrons have been held: that it is either like a dumbbell, with a positive and negative charge separated by a small distance with their effects cancelled; or is like an onion, with a sphere of one kind of electricity surrounded by a layer of the other kind so that again the charge is cancelled.

The direction in which either of these models of the neutron would eject protons has been calculated, and it has been found that the dumbbell type should eject them all perpendicularly to its own path, while the onion type would eject some straight ahead, with about ten times as many being thrown off perpendicularly.

Dr. Kurie's experiments with neutrons did not confirm either of these theories and he believes that the neutron is not built according to either of the accepted models. He concludes that the neutron is an elementary particle possessing an individuality and discrete qualities as do the electron and proton.

Dr. Kurie performed his experiments with a Wilson cloud chamber, a device which makes visible the track of a swift-moving proton somewhat as an aviator can see the wake of a boat which is itself too small to be seen.

Of the three thousand neutrons which pour throughout the chamber each second, but which can not be seen since they do not disturb the molecules of the gas within, one neutron occasionally hits a proton, the nucleus of a nitrogen atom. This proton, carrying an electrical charge, disturbs the molecules in the chamber and leaves a track which Dr. Kurie photographed with a special camera which he perfected while obtaining his doctorate at Yale University under the direction of Professor Alois F. Kovarik. The angle at which the proton has been ejected can thus be measured since the direction in which the neutrons are moving is known.

## RAT-CATCHING CATS

Selective breeding of rat-catching cats is the best way to keep down rats in the opinion of Dr. Adrian Loir, medical officer of the port of Le Havre, France.

Dr. Loir's interest in the subjects of rats and cats arises from the fact that rats may spread bubonic plague. France, like other countries, keeps hourly guard on her ports lest plague-stricken rats, with infected fleas ready to pass on this scourge to human beings, gain entrance.

Dr. Loir recently reported the success of his cat breeding to the French Academy of Medicine, the most important forum of medical science in France. He discoursed before this gathering of learned men on such an apparently frivolous topic as his cat, Poupette, and another rejoicing in the name of Lico.

Lico is a champion and is first holder for 1930 of the cup of the Rat-catching Cat Club of Normandy. The Rat-catching Cat Club was founded by Dr. Loir, with its chief object the breeding of cats with a constant and intense craving for catching rats. Not all cats chase rats. Some establish a tacit neutrality pact with rats, with whom they may be seen in some streets at night, the one ignoring the other studiously. Such is not the case with Dr. Loir's cats, however.

In one dock area in Le Havre, in 1930, where as many as 145 rats were caught in only 8 days, there are now no more rats. Five rat-catching cats, one of whom is Lico's son, patrol this area which the rats of Le Havre have learned to dread more than the plague itself.

One day Herriot, formerly Prime Minister, paid a visit to Le Havre, where he was so impressed by Dr. Loir's initiative that he begged a cat of him for the benefit of the town of which he was mayor, Lyon. It seemed that the abattoirs of Lyon were overrun by rats. It was the story of Dick Whittington all over again.

As Dr. Loir told the story, the Mayor of Le Havre was not deaf to this appeal. Le Havre was to come to the rescue of Lyon. A special credit was opened to allow the director of the abattoirs to réceive Le Havre's envoy with the necessary distinction. Her name was Poupette, and the litter of kittens to which she gave birth shortly after her arrival was a practical gesture indicative of her appreciation of the hospitality she had enjoyed. On November 24, 1932, the director of the abattoirs wrote: "I wish to tell you that the abattoir of Lyon is completely rid of rodents of every size."

## BACTERIA-FERMENTED BEER

Beer made by the fermentive action of a special bacterial culture instead of the customary yeast, and drunk, bacteria and all, is an excellent remedy for disorders of the digestive organs as well as a palatable drink. So states Professor Paul Lindner, of the Berlin Agricultural College, who made the discovery in the course of an endeavor to determine the identity of "soma," the sacred drink of the ancient Persians and Indians. Professor Lindner's preliminary report is given in the German scientific weekly, *Forschungen und Fortschritte*.

"Soma" had long been supposed to be merely ordinary beer, with the addition of some kind of plant, not now identifiable with any certainty. But the health-giving properties of the brew are so lauded in the ancient literature that Professor Lindner suspected that the well-being induced by it was more than the ordinary pleasant delusion of a successful Bierabend.

He had for many years been familiar with the Mexican drink "aguamiel," made from the juice of the century plant, and sometimes called "milk of the green cow" because it was drunk by the Mexicans while it was still white with its active fermentation. He had discovered that the fermentive organism in this drink is not a wild yeast but a bacterium, which he called *Termobacterium mobile,* or for convenience simply Tm. The same organism has been found in other fermented drinks produced in the tropics, and where it is present it predominates to the exclusion of yeast.

Professor Lindner suspected that it was the bacteria rather than the beverages they produced that brought about the excellent digestive and assimilative health of the drinkers. To test this theory, he centrifuged out about a tablespoonful of the organisms from some fermented liquid and swallowed them "straight." They did have a most beneficial effect.

He then undertook scientifically controlled brewing, using Tm bacteria instead of yeast. He found that the products of such fermentation were pure ethyl alcohol with a very little lactic acid, but no fusel oil, supposed to be the prime cause of the "Katzenjammer" following indiscreet indulgence in yeast-fermented beverages. For one thing, the bacteria apparently can not ferment malt sugar, but only glucose, and hence produce a beer of quite low alcoholic content, but high food value.

He induced a commercial brewery in Sweden and one in Vienna to produce bacteria-fermented beer on a moderately large scale, and with the cooperation of Dr. Leo Kaps, of the Wilhelmina Hospital in Vienna, tried it on a large number of patients. When given with the bacterial cloudiness still in it, the beer induced excellent conditions in the digestive tract. The same beer filtered, however, was merely an agreeable drink and had no therapeutic value.

## ENERGY FROM COAL, OIL AND GAS

Oil and gas will have increasing use as energy sources in the United States and by 1950 they will account for nearly half of the expanded fuel requirements of the nation.

A forecast of the relationship between coal and petroleum in the future and a survey of future energy requirements was presented to the American Institute of Mining and Metallurgical Engineers meeting in New York by Professor W. Spencer Hutchinson, of the Massachusetts Institute of Technology, and August J. Breitenstein, Ashland, Pennsylvania, engineer.

In 1950 it is estimated that 499,500,000 tons of coal will be used, compared with 517,018,000 tons in 1930. The situation is reversed for petroleum, with 1,419,000,000 barrel consumption predicted for 1950 and 868,484,000 barrels consumed in 1930.

Total energy *per capita* demanded in the United States shows a consistent growth, the engineers were told, and it increased at a faster rate than the population. Chief sources of energy to-day are the mineral fuels, coal and petroleum, which between them account for more than 90 per cent. of the demand, with water-power supplying only 10 per cent.

A marked change has occurred in the relative proportion of energy obtained from coal and oil. Only 30 years ago 91 per cent. of the country's horsepower came from coal, and only 4 per cent. from oil and natural gas, but in 1930, horsepower from coal had dropped to 60 per cent. while the proportion furnished by oil and gas had risen to 31 per cent. By 1950 it is estimated that coal would furnish only 46 per cent. of the country's power, while 45 per cent. would come from oil and gas, and 8 per cent. from waterpower.

Consumption of coal in this country reached its zenith in 1917, with 6.08 tons *per capita*. From this year the decline was rapid. It was only 4.2 tons in 1930.

Other findings of the study by Professor Hutchinson and Mr. Breitenstein are:

Whereas, in 1930, the effective energy supply in the United States, expressed in trillions of British Thermal Units, was 9,031, it will have risen to 14,500 by 1950.

In 1930, the energy supply *per capita*, expressed in millions of British Thermal Units, was 73, while in 1950, it is expected to be 94.

Whereas, bituminous and anthracite coal accounted for 60.3 per cent. of the total energy derived in 1930, it will account for only 46.6 per cent. in 1950.

Petroleum and its natural products, including also natural gas and natural gas gasoline, will show a marked rise. Accounting for only 31.6 per cent. of the total energy derived in 1930, they will account for 45.3 per cent. in 1950.

Waterpower will account for exactly the same percentage of the total energy derived in 1950 as in 1930, namely, 8.1, although the energy applied by hydropower will be greater than in 1930.

## ITEMS

The earthquake that caused excitement and alarm in Peru on February 23 had its epicenter near the western boundary of Bolivia, according to a report of investigators for the U. S. Coast and Geodetic Survey made after examining seismological data telegraphically collected by *Science Service* from a number of American and Canadian observatories. The approximate location was given as 19 degrees south latitude, 68 degrees west longitude. Since the reports indicated a violent earthquake, destruction of property and loss of life may have occurred in case the epicenter happened to coincide with a populated region. Direct reports may not come out immediately, due to the lack of telegraph lines and other means of communication in the interior.

Peltier's comet, discovered by an Ohio amateur astronomer, will not become visible to the unaided eye. A parabolic orbit solution made at the University of California by Anderson and Wyse under the direction of Professor A. O. Leuschner shows that the comet approached closest to the earth on February 25 and that it was then only slightly brighter than when discovered. Its brightness will now decrease. The comet's orbit resembles that of certain other comets, but not closely enough to identify it as an old comet paying a return visit. The comet is ninth magnitude in brightness and it has a slight condensation but no stellar nucleus.

A new national monument has been set apart on the Grand Canyon of Arizona, about fifty miles down-river from the point in Grand Canyon National Park now most visited by tourists. The new area, which will be known as Grand Canyon National Monument, comprises a total of 392 square miles, and has one magnificent vantage-point from which one can look down on the Colorado, winding its way at the bottom like a silvery ribbon. From most points on the rim in the present Grand Canyon National Park the river is quite invisible. Another feature of the new National Monument is a volcanic cone, thrown up in some long-past time and now wholly extinct. It bears the imposing name of "Vulcan's Throne." National Monuments, as distinguished from National Parks, are areas which are either less accessible to the public or for one reason or another are not suitable for immediate development and administration on the regular National Park scale.

# SCIENCE NEWS

*Science Service, Washington, D. C.*

## MEASUREMENT OF THE SPECTRUM PHOTOGRAPHS OF STARS

THE radiometer has now been used to study the spectrum photographs of stars, which show their composition. This application has been made by Dr. Sinclair Smith and Olin C. Wilson, Jr., of the Mount Wilson Observatory.

The common form of radiometer, which was the invention of the great English physicist, Sir William Crookes, consists of four small vanes balanced on a pivot in a partially evacuated bulb. One side of each vane is polished, the other blackened, and the black side of one faces the polished side of the next. When heat radiation, either from the sun or an artificial source, falls on the vanes, they start moving in the direction of the polished sides. The reason for this is that the black side absorbs more of the radiation than the other, and is heated more. The molecules of the small amount of gas remaining in the bulb are constantly in motion. When they hit the warmer side, they bounce off with a greater kick than those hitting the polished side, and so they push the vanes around.

In the arrangement developed by the Mount Wilson scientists, two tiny vanes are used, suspended from a fiber of quartz. Thus they can not turn completely around, as they twist the fiber. To the upper part of the fiber is attached a small mirror. A beam of light falls on this mirror and is reflected to a moving photographic film. As a greater or less amount of radiation falls on the vanes, the fiber twists more or less, and the reflected spot of light moves back and forth, leaving a trace on the film.

The spectrum photographs to be studied are negatives, and show a series of parallel clear lines, of which the relative brightness and widths are significant, as well as their positions. To study them, a strong light is focused to a narrow line on the plate, which is then steadily moved by an electric motor. The light that passes through, and the heat that accompanies it, varies with the intensity of that part of the spectrum plate. This heat falls on the radiometer, and thus the moving spot of light reflected from the mirror traces on the film a record of the intensities of the spectral lines.

Such a device is called a registering spectrophotometer, and previous ones have used either thermocouples or photoelectric cells to detect the light changes. The former converts the heat into electric energy, while the latter makes a similar conversion of light. Dr. Smith states that the new device avoids the electrical difficulties accompanying each of these, and that it is more sensitive than the thermocouple. He also says that it is much simpler, and that many institutions might build one, though unable to afford the other and more expensive instruments.

## COLLOID GOLD

GOLD dispersions in water, known to the ancients as ''aurum potabile,'' have been purified here by a special method of ''electrical decantation'' and concentrated so as to contain up to six grams of gold per liter (a fifth of an ounce per quart).

Professor Wolfgang Pauli, of the Colloid Institute of the University of Vienna, who devised the method, has been able, by analyzing the concentrated pure sols, to identify the gold compounds which are present in small quantities in the usual gold sols and are needed to maintain the gold particles suspended in pseudo-solution in water.

These gold particles are extremely small—visible only with the aid of the ultra-microscope—and are maintained in constant ''Brownian'' motion by the bombardment of the surrounding water molecules. This alone would not be sufficient to prevent the particles of gold from coalescing. They are kept separate by the electric charge which causes them to repel one another.

The origin of this electric charge has been much discussed by colloid chemists during the last decades. Zsigmondy, one of the pioneers in this field of knowledge, maintained that the particles consist of pure gold, charged by adsorbed ions, that is, electrically charged atoms or groups of atoms attached to the surface of the gold particle. Pauli, on the other hand, brought forward the view that the surface of the gold is covered with a chemical compound of gold which breaks up or dissociates, giving positive ions to the surrounding water, while the complex iron ion with a negative charge remains attached to the gold particle. The compound in question, in the special case when the gold sol is prepared by passing electric sparks through electrodes immersed in water acidified with hydrochloric acid, has been shown to be the insoluble gold (''auro'') hydrochloride which gives up its hydrogen ion to the water.

When the gold particles are coagulated by freezing, this auro-chloride passes into solution in the form of auri-chloride, with liberation of hydrochloric acid.

The new facts discovered by Professor Pauli are of value both theoretically and practically because they will enable chemists to foretell the behavior of many metallic colloids, which have already been used in therapy.

Colloid gold itself has been employed against alcoholism, a fact rendered common knowledge by the shortest ''story of three generations'' ever told.

''Gold mine, gold spoon, gold cure.''

## HEAVY WATER

PROFESSOR GILBERT N. LEWIS, of the University of California, has obtained by experiment pure water that is heavier than ordinary water and even denser than sea water. This extraordinary water has a specific gravity of 1.035, whereas normal water is the liquid upon which specific gravity measurements are based and therefore has a value of one.

More than one third of the hydrogen in the heavy water consists of the hydrogen isotope, of atomic weight approximately two, that was discovered in 1931. This variety of hydrogen is the same chemically, but is twice as heavy as the more usual hydrogen atom. The heavy water, like ordinary water, consists of two hydrogen atoms combined with one oxygen atom, as expressed by the familiar formula, $H_2O$.

Heavy water was first produced at the U. S. Bureau of Standards in Washington last year, but Professor Lewis by using similar methods of manufacture has obtained a larger concentration of the heavy hydrogen isotope in the water and his heavy water is therefore heavier. The heavy water obtained at the University of California is 35,000 parts per million heavier than ordinary water, whereas the U. S. Bureau of Standards water is 1,400 parts per million heavier than normal.

Experiments showed that the University of California heavy water has a refractive index one tenth per cent. below that of ordinary water.

Professor Lewis used the method devised by Dr. E. W. Washburn, of the U. S. Bureau of Standards, and Professor Harold C. Urey, of Columbia University, of obtaining a concentration of the heavy hydrogen isotope. This depends upon the fact that the light weight hydrogen is given off in electrolysis of water before the double weight hydrogen, resulting in a concentration of heavier water.

## CLIMATE CHANGES AND THE LAST GLACIAL PERIOD

EVEN those portions of the earth not covered by ice during glacial periods are indirectly influenced by the ice sheet. One of the rare instances where these influences could be detected was described by Professor William Morris Davis, visiting professor of geology from Harvard University, in a recent address at the California Institute of Technology.

The unusual locality was the Santa Monica mountains which rise out of the ocean immediately west of Los Angeles. There the effects of three successive glacial periods are visible. During these the sea receded and the steep cliffs which it wore from the mountains were left to be softened and filled in by land deposits. Meanwhile the land was rising, so that after the glacier withdrew the sea could not reach its old shore-line and consequently made new sharp cliffs at the lower level. This process was repeated twice.

It is estimated that during a glacial period the sea-level may sink thirty feet or more. Since the water removed from the sea forms ice on the continents and since these cover only about one fifth of the earth's surface, the ice layer must attain an average thickness of several hundred feet, even if it is spread over half the earth. The present sheet over Greenland is several thousand feet thick.

It is well known about how fast the land is rising in California; so from the difference in level between successive cliffs estimates can be made of the elapsed time between glaciers and since the last one. It turns out that the last one was quite recent in comparison with the interval between glacial periods. Professor Davis suggested that this may indicate that the earth will get warmer before it starts to cool again prior to the next glacier. The ice caps in the polar regions may disappear entirely and the poles may become useful and inhabited places.

Even though the average temperature of the earth need drop only about five degrees below the present average to bring on a glacial period, the consequent change in climate may be enormous. If the earth warms up enough to melt all glaciers now existing a remarkable change in climate all over the world would probably result. The advantage to science would be incalculable if we could take observations and make explorations in comfort in the polar regions.

## CATCHING COLD AND BODY TEMPERATURE

WHETHER your body has a good heating system or not decides how easily you will take cold this spring, Dr. P. Schmidt, of Berlin, told a correspondent of the American Medical Association.

Dr. Schmidt had noticed for many years, that under the same circumstances, some people take cold much more easily than others. Now, using human beings as guinea-pigs, he has found out why.

Under his guidance a large number of persons exposed themselves to cold until they were thoroughly chilled. Then he measured their skin-temperature at several intervals until they had all returned to normal. He discovered that most of them regained normal skin temperature in a very short time. Some, however, were much slower to warm up to normal, and these, he discovered, were the ones who took cold from exposure.

The reason for this, says Dr. Schmidt, is the contraction of the blood-vessels and tissues at a low temperature. When contracted they are much less able to fight off germs and bacteria, just as an army of men when cramped into close quarters are unable to fight efficiently. So the persons whose temperature remained low over a long period of time gave the germs a chance to get the upper hand.

Only one tenth of all those tested had slow temperature reactions, which should mean that only one tenth of all people are naturally subject to colds. When you catch a cold, if you belong to the other nine tenths, it means that your heating system is temporarily out of order because of nervous or psychological conditions or because a prolonged unperceived draft has cooled off your bodily radiators. That last is why people have learned to think they catch cold from drafts. They do indeed, though indirectly.

Persons whose heating systems are ordinarily slow, says Dr. Schmidt, can speed them up by spending a great deal of time out of doors.

## CHILDREN'S INVENTIONS

EVEN in this day of machine-made toys, children contrive tools and playthings strikingly like those made by primitive man in the Stone Age, Dr. Rosa Katz, of the psychological laboratory of the University of Rostock, Germany, found in a study of inventive genius as it appeared in her son Julius. She has reported her study to the *Journal of Genetic Psychology*.

Julius had read "Robinson Crusoe," and probably

got from that book the inspiration to be primitive and devise tools from available materials. He did not, however, get suggestions for the particular tools constructed; those developed from his needs of the moment.

While a goose was being dressed in the kitchen, Julius found that the "wind pipe" of the bird could be used as a water hose, and caused water to flow through it into a water basin. Later he blew through it and produced a hissing sound. He then stripped off the outer tissue, bored a hole through the side of the tube, and there was a primitive flute. It was possible to produce a flute from the wind-pipe only because it had first been used for water and thus made moist. Julius noticed this relationship.

From the same goose, Julius also made a primitive type of ornament. He noticed that the breast bone resembled somewhat a face, and immediately made of it a mask.

A suggestion of how primitive man may have bound up wounds in the absence of surgical gauze or muslin bandages is found in another invention of the boy. Julius was gathering up some wood shavings left in the house by a carpenter. In so doing he injured a finger. He sought out the thinnest of the shavings, moistened them, and with them bound up the wound.

Among the boy's other inventions were a milling stone in which he ground the kernels of hazelnuts, a flint scraper for removing bark, a tomahawk which during peaceful times served also as a hammer, a spear and a snail shell pendant for a feather garland. Snail-shells were used as pendants during the Stone Age.

But Julius's best achievement was probably his ax. He split the end of a stick previously made free from bark. He clamped a stone in the cleft and wound the shaft with a cord.

"There is no doubt that this was the essential appearance of the first ax swung by the human hand," according to Dr. Katz.

## ITEMS

AS the scattered members of Dr. Sven Hedin's Asiatic expedition gather in Peiping, to report their discoveries, alarm is beginning to be felt because Dr. Nils Ambolt, astronomer, has not arrived. Dr. Ambolt was expected in November, according to advices received in Berlin. He has been in northern Tibet, mapping unknown territory. It is feared that robbers may have attacked the party as it journeyed toward Peiping.

BLINDED completely in one eye, with his other eye weakened, and with his hearing affected, Professor Gustave Aartovaara, of the Helsingfors Technical University, is a martyr to his search for a missing chemical element. In 1931, while engaged in the chemical concentration of the missing chemical element, 87, he was the victim of a laboratory explosion, the effects of which have prevented his continuance of research. To Professor Fred Allison, of the Alabama Polytechnic Institute, Professor Aartovaara sent specimens that he believed contained element 87 and Professor Allison detected this element by his magneto-optical method of analysis.

THE most significant progress in the search for the cause of cancer is being made in laboratories where these glands are being studied, Dr. James Ewing, himself an eminent cancer authority and director of cancer research at Memorial Hospital, New York City, told members of the American Society for the Control of Cancer. Cancers of certain glands secrete the powerful hormones of these glands. A specific test for one group of cancers, those of the sex glands, has been devised as a result of discovering a hormone substance in all these cancers.

TWO new isotopes of the element mercury have been discovered by Professor F. W. Aston, of the Cavendish Laboratory of the University of Cambridge. They have atomic weights 197 and 203. The detection was made through the obtaining of mass-spectra of mercury on new, very sensitive photographic plates. Isotopes 197 and 203 are estimated to be present only to the extent of one hundredth of one per cent. and six thousandths of one per cent., respectively. The mean atomic weight used by chemists is therefore affected only negligibly.

X-RAYS as intense as all the radium in the world could produce, and of a penetration and frequency equal to that of radium's gamma rays, have been produced from a new porcelain insulated, grounded anode x-ray tube of new design described to the American Physical Society by Cyrus A. Poole, of the Kelley-Koett-Manufacturing Co., Covington, Kentucky. Its design is an outgrowth of the work done by Professor C. C. Lauritsen at Pasadena, but embodies a transmission anode and is to be operated on direct current. The new tube operates on 800,000 volts furnished by a system of cascade electrical transformers and it is the first x-ray tube to operate on constant potential direct current at this high voltage.

AUTHORITIES in London are apprehensive of an outbreak of yellow fever in the Orient. At a meeting of the Ross Institute Advisory Board, Sir Malcolm Watson and others pointed out the grave danger now existing of this disease being spread from its focus in West Africa to East and South Africa by airplanes. Air travel has brought various parts of the vast African continent so close together that a person might become infected in West Africa with yellow fever and reach the eastern or southern part of the continent before the three- or four-day period necessary for the disease to appear in him. Airplanes may also convey mosquitoes, which may spread this disease. From East Africa it is a short jump to the Orient with its teeming millions who have never been exposed to yellow fever and consequently have probably no resistance to the disease. Quarantine regulations of air travel between South America, where the disease also has a focus, and the United States have been instituted by the U. S. Public Health Service. Similar regulations may be considered for air travel in Africa and between various African, Oriental and Australian points.

# SCIENCE NEWS

*Science Service, Washington, D. C.*

## THE SOUTHERN CALIFORNIA EARTHQUAKE

The earthquake which shook southern California on the night of March 10 was not much larger than the one that eight years ago (June 29, 1925) damaged Santa Barbara, and the great 1906 San Francisco earthquake was much larger. It will rank, however, as one of California's major earthquakes. The probable origin of the quake, as determined from records at the Seismological Laboratory, Pasadena, was in the San Pedro Channel within the triangle formed by Point Firmin, Avalon on Catalina Island and Laguna Beach on the mainland.

Drs. H. O. Wood and Charles O. Richter, seismologists in charge of the cooperatively maintained earthquake laboratory which is set in solid rock back of Pasadena, explained to *Science Service:* "At just twenty seconds past 5:54 P. M. Friday our instruments began recording a moderately strong local shock which was sharply felt in the laboratory and which was evidently sufficient to cause damage near its source. The source appears to be sixty to seventy miles southeast of this laboratory, but because of peculiarities in the geological structure a precise distance can not yet be given. A large number of aftershocks have been recorded with very brief interruptions. Three or four of these have been stronger than the rest and have been barely felt at the laboratory. One or two hundred shocks have been recorded on the less sensitive instruments and it is probable that the more sensitive instruments will record a great many more." Six auxiliary seismologic stations placed at strategic points in California recorded the earth movements, and Drs. Wood and Richter explained that the precise location will not be possible before the receipt of these records.

This earthquake had been expected by seismologists for over a decade, although few definite public predictions had been issued in consideration of public fears. Geologists studying the crust of the earth and earthquake specialists operating sensitive recording instruments and listing the past history of southern California earth movements felt that conditions were ripe for a serious earth disturbance in that region. While residents of southern California had not in general recognized the existing earthquake danger, leading citizens and investigators cooperated to study the conditions.

Not for 78 years has the Los Angeles region suffered a large earthquake, although on July 8, 1929, a moderately severe shock was felt in the region surrounding Los Angeles and centering at Whittier. On June 21, 1920, the Inglewood earthquake occurred near Los Angeles and partially destroyed some weakly constructed buildings.

But the great earthquakes of Los Angeles recorded in history occurred in 1769, 1852 and 1855. Four violent shocks, on July 28, 1769, with strong aftershocks on five days following, are listed in the records of the California missions. This earthquake was probably strongest along San Pedro Bay near the present harbor of Los Angeles. This is the location of the present earthquake center. October and November, 1852, brought many earth shocks to the southern California of gold-rush days. October 26 saw eleven severe shocks at Los Angeles. On July 10, 1855, a quite severe earthquake did considerable damage in Los Angeles.

The ocean region off the San Pedro-Long Beach coast near Los Angeles lying between the coast and Catalina Island is known as San Pedro Channel. Geologists describe it as the San Pedro submarine fault zone and they know that this is an area where the mountains are growing. It is probable that the present earthquake was caused by an earth crustal adjustment in this area under the sea.

Professor Albert Einstein walked through the earthquake and did not notice it. He had just emerged from a California Institute of Technology building after attending his last seminar with local scientists before leaving for New York. Walking with Dr. Beno Gutenberg, the eminent authority on earthquakes, both he and Dr. Gutenberg were so absorbed that they said later they had not noticed the earthquake.

Buildings of the California Institute of Technology at Pasadena creaked and swayed greatly, but no damage was done to these structures especially designed to withstand earthquakes.

## A NEW STRAIN OF BARLEY

"Out of rough and black get smooth and white." This problem, reminiscent of one of the ancient riddles of the Sphinx, confronted Professor B. D. Leith, of the University of Wisconsin, at one stage of his endeavor to produce a new strain of barley that could be grown with profit by farmers in Wisconsin and other Grain Belt states.

It was not so impossible a task as it might sound, for he had already put the smooth and the white qualities into the genetic mixture where they were covered over by the rough and the black. All he had to do was plant his cross-bred grain and let the old reliable Mendelian mode of segregation do the work.

To go back to the beginning: Wisconsin farmers used to raise a strain of barley known as Oderbrucker. It was good barley, good for stock feed and good for the once-great Milwaukee brewing industry. But it had one fatal drawback: the beard on its heads was armed with innumerable little back-pointing barbs that would cause these bristly hairs to work their way through the threshermen's overalls, and made life so miserable for them that they finally rebelled at working with it at all. Also, it was subject to a destructive fungus disease known as stripe.

Professor Leith set to work to produce a hybrid barley that would have a smooth beard, and, if possible, be stripe-resistant, yet preserve the virtues of Oderbrucker barley—good white grain, high yield and stiff straw.

His first crosses, with other strains of domestic barley, were not very successful. But in 1917 a new smooth-bearded barley from Southeast Russia was brought in. It was black-grained, but that did not bother Professor Leith, for he was sure he could juggle the undesired color character out of the hybrid strains.

When he crossed Oderbrucker with the new Russian barley the first generation offspring were as undesirable as could be imagined, for the beard was as rough as in Oderbrucker and the grain was black as in the Russian barley. Here, then, was his Sphinx-riddle: out of black and rough to get smooth and white.

Professor Leith, like all good students of Mendelian behavior in heredity, knew that the blackness and roughness were "dominant" characters in any mixed strain, hiding but not destroying their "recessive" opposites, whiteness and smoothness. He knew also that such recessive characters segregate out when the hybrid first generation is inbred.

This he did, and the second generation barleys came out in approximately the following ratio: 9 rough and black, 3 rough and white, 3 smooth and black, 1 smooth and white. The last, a hybrid containing only recessives in its pairs of characters, was what he was hunting for; and he knew also that so long as it was inbred neither roughness nor blackness could reappear.

This smooth-white strain forms the basis of the barley strain now known as Wisconsin Barbless, Pedigree 38. In several years of practical crop growing by a large number of farmers, some of them outside the state, it has out-yielded Oderbrucker, resisted drought, and proved highly resistant to stripe, though not to other diseases. Most important of all, its smooth beard makes it possible to harvest and thresh the new barley without making life a burden for the farmer or the threshermen.

With an eye to the eventual return of beer, the owner of one of the most famous of the old-time Milwaukee breweries has made large-scale tests of the malting qualities of the new barley at his own expense, and reports that so far as its chemical make-up is concerned it is at least the equal of the best of the old barleys.

## PETRIFICATION IN THE YELLOWSTONE NATIONAL PARK

TREE stumps now undergoing the process of petrification are an interesting sight in the Upper Geyser Basin, in Yellowstone National Park. Upper Geyser Basin is the general name for that portion of the park containing Old Faithful and other famous geysers.

On the north side of Old Faithful there are at least six or eight stumps in which the wood-fibers have been found to contain a large amount of silica. Evidently this silica is being deposited at intervals from the geyser water, according to the park naturalist, C. Max Bauer. The petrification of the stumps is a very slow process.

The Yellowstone already has an interesting display of fossil forests located over extensive areas in the northern part of the park. These, however, are the result of successive outbreaks of volcanic activity in the past. What happened in these cases apparently was that a standing forest was engulfed in great clouds of volcanic dust until the trees were completely buried. Water seeped through this dust and into the buried trees, carrying with it silica from the volcanic ash. The woody structure of the trees was dissolved and the silica deposited in its place. The trees thus became fossilized.

Long afterwards, when the volcanic activity had quieted and sufficient soil had accumulated on top of the buried trees, another forest grew, only to meet the same fate. This happened again and again.

To-day, at Specimen Ridge in the northeast portion of the park, trained observers can distinguish in some places a succession of these forests, twelve in number, one above the other.

## JANUARY MORTALITY RECORDS

THE good health records for the United States and Canada maintained during the last few years will probably not be continued in 1933. Judging from the January death reports, the health outlook for the coming year is anything but promising, officials of the Metropolitan Life Insurance Company point out in their most recent report.

The January, 1933, death-rate of 10.8 per thousand is the highest recorded for the first month of any year since 1929 and with the exception of 1929, it is the highest for more than a decade.

Influenza and pneumonia were responsible for nearly one fifth of all the deaths during January, 1933. In addition, deaths from cancer, diabetes, cerebral hemorrhage, heart disease and suicide increased sharply over the deaths from these causes a year ago.

The death rate for diabetes reached a new high figure in January, 1933, which has never been even closely approached in any month of any preceding year. This is thought to be the result of the influenza epidemic. Diabetics who become victims of influenza are frequently without sufficient resistance to withstand both diseases, and their deaths occur during the influenza outbreaks instead of later.

A number of years have made excellent health records despite bad beginnings. The year 1929, which started with a bad influenza outbreak, is given as a conspicuous example. "Nevertheless health conditions from now on will need to be exceptionally good to counterbalance the January setback and to establish a record for the year at or near the remarkably low mortality figure for 1932."

## MEDIEVAL CONSERVATION

CONSERVATION of natural resources in Germany is no new thing. It has its roots in the Middle Ages, a recent examination of old records has disclosed.

Long before pearls appeared in any numbers from distant India and Ceylon, ladies in Central European castles wore excellent fresh-water pearls that came from the tributaries of the Danube in the Bavarian and Bohemian mountains. In Passau, where the River Inn flows into the Danube, a long line of Bishops of the Church held sway also as temporal princes, their reigns lasting from 739 to 1803 in uninterrupted succession. These bishops gave thorough protection to the pearl-producing river mussels and clams, and decreed severe punishment to poachers. This protection ended when the temporal rule of the bishops was broken and the secular authorities sought wealth in the timber of the mountains. The logging operations kept the streams so constantly roiled that not only were the pearl mussels vastly reduced in numbers but the salmon, beaver and otter were practically wiped out. Not until 1929 did this destruction cease.

The churchmen-princes protected other forms of native animal life besides the wealth-bringing pearl mussels. They protected meadows where wild swans, herons and storks bred, and maintained regular beaver preserves. They even sent their retainers out to fight when neighboring noblemen attempted to raid these game sanctuaries. Not even the Peasants' War of Reformation times, with its attendant hardships and anarchy, was able to wipe out the beaver. They held out until the wars of the eighteenth century, and a few were seen alive even into the nineteenth.

The pearl mussels have survived, though in much reduced numbers. At a recent fisheries exhibition held in Passau, native pearls were displayed which compared favorably with pearls in Ceylon.

## ITEMS

A HEAVENLY object that may be a new comet or a minor planet has been found on the photographic plates of the Harvard College Observatory by Dr. F. L. Whipple. It is faint and visible only through large telescopes.

SPRING of 1933 will commence at 8: 43 P. M., Eastern Standard Time, on Monday, March 20, according to computations made at the Nautical Almanac Office, in the U. S. Naval Observatory. At that moment, the sun, which has been traveling northwards through the sky since last December, will cross the equator, and enter the zodiacal sign of Aries. This is called the vernal equinox and at this time of year the sun is below the horizon just as long as it is above, so that days and nights are of equal length. Also, on this date, the sun rises directly east and sets due west. Spring will continue until June 21, when the sun ceases its northward journey, and will start south again.

PUBLIC health need not suffer when budgets are reduced. Evidence of this is found in Chicago, the American Medical Association has pointed out. In this city during 1932 the infant death rate and the general death rate were reduced below the records of any other year, although the health department budget was reduced $500,000 in this one year. For a cosmopolitan as well as metropolitan center like Chicago, the American Medical Association considers this an achievement of the first magnitude.

YELLOWSTONE PARK beavers are not slaves of one material in their engineering efforts. Park Ranger F. Sheldon Dart has found a beaver dam built of stones on a small stream in the Thorofare district. The dam is approximately six feet long and varies from one to two feet in width. It is two and a half feet high at the highest point. Only a few willow twigs appear in its construction, almost all of its material being stone. The rocks range in size from pieces as large as a man's fist to some ten inches in diameter and twelve to fourteen inches in length.

GERMANY'S moose herds, relatives of the great antlered animals of the American and Canadian woods, are facing the danger that comes to them annually in the early spring flooding of the rivers that flow through the flat woods of East Prussia where they live. Burdened with ice, the streams sweep down the strongest swimmers among them. Another menace that the floods bring to the moose is that of starvation. The inundations force the moose to abandon their usual habitats and take to higher lands or to refuge islands which have been especially constructed for them. As long as the food supply holds out all is well, but the amount of browse available on these limited areas will not suffice the crowded herds long, especially if the waters rise high. Losses through starvation are especially large among the young animals, which can not reach the higher branches of the shrubs on which they feed. In a really bad flood year all the calves may starve.

THE nation-wide government inventory, or census, of Sweden's forest supply has now been completed after eight years of incessant work and at a total cost of about $280,000. The census was made by means of examining all trees within many parallel forest belts ten meters (30 feet) wide and drawn at certain fixed intervals. The combined length of the lines thus covered by the tree checkers is about 52,000 kilometers (31,200 miles) or more than one and a quarter times around the world, and the number of tree trunks marked and examined amount to more than 12,000,000. The result of the inventory as a whole was most gratifying, in so far as it showed not only the forest wealth of the country, but also indicated that the regrowth was considerably greater than what had generally been anticipated. Sweden's total forest area is about 58,000,000 acres. The present value of the wood is estimated to be about $240,000,000. The investigators found that the regrowth is improving considerably. Another fact is the high age of the trees. Thus in Lapland 32 per cent. of the trees were found to be over 160 years and 45 per cent. over 120 years old.

EVIDENCE that moving storm areas of low barometric pressure affect radio signals of wave-lengths longer than 100 meters by varying the strength of the lower ionized layer of the earth's atmosphere was presented by Professor R. C. Colwell and I. O. Myers, of the West Virginia University, speaking at the meeting of the American Physical Society. Two ionized layers that reflect radio waves are now known to exist. One of these, the lower, Kennelly-Heaviside or E layer, has been shown by Dr. E. V. Appleton, British physicist, and others, to reflect the long waves, while a higher, or F layer, sends back to earth the short waves. This indicates to Professor Colwell that the lower, or E layer, is in the region affected by varying pressure. He finds that the E layer is concentrated in the regions of low pressure and is most active in the eastern half of the storm cyclone or whirl of winds.

# SCIENCE NEWS

*Science Service, Washington, D. C.*

## POSITRONS

THE positron is formally introduced to the world of physics in a communication by its discoverer, Dr. Carl D. Anderson, of the California Institute of Technology, to *The Physical Review.*

August 2, 1932, is given as the date of the first photograph of the positive electron, christened positron for short, which has the mass of the older negative electron but a positive electric charge like the proton, which is nearly 2,000 times more massive.

A search for a negative particle of the mass of the proton was urged by Dr. Anderson, who predicted the possibility of its existence.

To date, Dr. Anderson has obtained 15 photographs of positron tracks in a group of 1,300 photographs of cosmic ray tracks. Positrons are let loose from atoms bombarded with cosmic rays. Dr. Anderson offers the following suggestion as to what happens:

"From the fact that positrons occur in groups associated with other tracks it is concluded that they must be secondary particles ejected from an atomic nucleus. If we retain the view that a nucleus consists of protons and neutrons (and alpha particles) and that a neutron represents a close combination of a proton and electron, then from the electromagnetic theory as to the origin of mass the simplest assumption would seem to be that an encounter between the incoming primary ray and a proton may take place in such a way as to expand the diameter of the proton to the same value as that possessed by the negatron. This process would release an energy of a billion electron-volts appearing as a secondary photon. As a second possibility the primary ray may disintegrate a neutron (or more than one) in the nucleus by the ejection either of a negatron or a positron with the result that a positive or a negative proton, as the case may be, remains in the nucleus in place of the neutron, the event occurring in this instance without the emission of a photon. This alternative, however, postulates the existence in the nucleus of a proton of negative charge, no evidence for which exists. The greater symmetry, however, between the positive and negative charges revealed by the discovery of the positron should prove a stimulus to search for evidence of the existence of negative protons. If the neutron should prove to be a fundamental particle of a new kind rather than a proton and negatron in close combination, the above hypotheses will have to be abandoned, for the proton will then in all probability be represented as a complex particle consisting of a neutron and positron."

## BERYLLIUM ATOMS PROVED RADIOACTIVE

A NEW and striking case of radioactivity, the spontaneous explosion of beryllium atoms, is the discovery announced at the California Institute of Technology by Dr. R. M. Langer and his associate, Russell Raitt, a graduate student.

This is probably the first successful prediction of radioactivity and it promises to lead to many others. Dr. Langer and Mr. Raitt first predicted the radioactive disintegration of the metallic atoms of beryllium and then systematically searched for the expected effect until they found it.

The effect of the explosion is so weak that the physicists know that the average beryllium atom will live a hundred trillion years (100,000,000,000,000 or 10 to the fourteenth power) before exploding. Extended researches show that none of the known radioactive elements can be responsible for the effects that the experimenters attribute to the beryllium atoms.

Beryllium is almost as unlike the ordinary radioactive elements as it is possible to be. It has a mass only nine times that of hydrogen whereas the most active radioactive elements have masses ten or more times larger.

Data gathered from studying the spontaneous explosions of beryllium atoms into fragments are expected to provide powerful tools in unraveling the mysteries of the atomic nucleus.

The radioctivity of beryllium accounts for the puzzling fact that beryl minerals often contain much more helium than could be explained on other hypotheses. Helium is set free when beryllium explodes.

Of great interest to physicists also is the prediction by Dr. Langer and Mr. Raitt that a new form of helium atom will be found in the future. This has a mass of five instead of the usual mass of four, and it is predicted that this heavy helium will explode spontaneously and thus prove to be the lightest radioactive element.

## MOSQUITO MAY CARRY HORSE PLAGUE

A SERIOUS epidemic disease of horses and mules, popularly known as Kansas-Nebraska horse plague, may be spread by the yellow fever mosquito, *Aedes aegypti.*

Whether the mosquito actually is the villain that spread an epidemic of the disease which affected 6,000 and killed 3,000 head of horses and mules in one season in California has not yet been proved. So far neither the mosquito nor any other insect has been caught in the act of spreading the disease from horse to horse.

But strong evidence of the mosquito's possible guilt has been obtained at the Army Medical School. Major R. A. Kelser, of the Veterinary Laboratory Division, has reported the fact that the yellow fever mosquitoes can spread the disease among guinea-pigs.

Mosquitoes infected with the causative virus of the disease have so far failed to give it to a horse. This may be explained by the fact that the horse on which the infected mosquitoes were allowed to feed is an old army horse and may have been exposed to the disease and consequently developed resistance to it earlier in its career. Major Kelser plans to feed the infected mosquitoes on a young horse whose history of infection and exposure to disease is known. He is also planning investigations with monkeys as to the rôle of mosquitoes in this disease.

Known to scientists as equine encephalomyelitis, this horse plague has been known under various names in both America and Europe for half a century or more. In Europe its most common name is Borna disease, taken from a region where a disastrous epidemic raged, just as the popular name in this country, Kansas-Nebraska horse plague, comes from the wide-spread outbreak in those two states some years ago.

The disease has been confused with many other diseases, among them forage poisoning, but in 1930, 1931 and 1932, Professor K. F. Meyer, of the Hooper Foundation, and associates of the University of California and California Agricultural Experiment Station definitely proved that the disease is caused by a germ of the filtrable virus type. The virus attacks the brain and spinal cord of the animals. Two types of the disease are said to occur: the sleepy type in which the animals may drowse until disturbed, when they may have convulsions, and the walking type in which the animals pace around and around the field.

The disease attacks only horses and mules under farm conditions and is not apparently a serious menace to humans, although two cases in California were reported in which men apparently acquired the disease from handling infected animals.

In a discussion of Major Kelser's report, investigators of the U. S. Department of Agriculture brought out the fact that while yellow fever mosquitoes were not found in California, Kansas or Nebraska, where the chief epidemics of this disease have occurred, many other kinds of mosquitoes and biting insects were found. It is possible that some of these other species may have spread the disease in those localities. Studies at the Bureau of Animal Industry seemed to show that contact between healthy and infected horses is not an important factor in the spread of the disease. This supports the theory of insect transmission.

## CHEMICAL ANTIDOTES FOR BACTERIAL POISONS

WE may not have to depend forever on painfully, often uncertainly elaborated antitoxins, serums and vaccines for the combating of our bacterial foes. Eventually antidotes for germ poisons may come off the chemist's shelf instead of out of a horse's veins. But before that day, as yet far off, a great deal of fundamental research will have to be done, involving cooperation by scientists in a number of fields.

Thus Dr. Stanhope Bayne-Jones informed the Yale chapter of the Sigma Xi in a recent lecture. Dr. Bayne-Jones is professor of bacteriology at Yale University and chairman of the medical division of the National Research Council at Washington, D. C.

But before we can undertake to make synthetic antidotes for bacterial poisons we must find out what these poisons are, and that is no easy task, Dr. Bayne-Jones reminded his hearers. They are exceedingly complex in their chemical make-up, and at the same time exceedingly easy to break down, so that efforts at study often end in destroying them without finding anything about them.

However, enough has been found out about some of them to constitute at least a fair chemical "lead," and something may be accomplished without waiting for the complete solution of these chemical and pharmacological problems.

Dr. Bayne-Jones stated that "it is probable from the ability of formaldehyde to deprive bacterial poisons of toxicity that the amino nitrogen group in the molecule has a good deal to do with the poisonous effect and that this group may be vulnerable to a chemical antidote. Oxidases destroy toxins and have some protective value. Acids remove toxicity, possibly according to the benzoyl serin intramolecular rearrangements described by Bergmann. Copper and iron appear to be essential to the production of some bacterial toxins. There are evidently enough 'chemical leads' to justify a more extended investigation of the possibilities of chemical antidotes for these poisons.

"Although the search for chemical methods of neutralizing bacterial poisons in the body might have a frankly practical objective, the end could not be reached satisfactorily without extensive bacteriological, immunological, biochemical and clinical research. The problem, like that of the chemistry of tuberculosis, needs for its solution the joint endeavors of investigators in several fields."

## MORE EARTHQUAKES EXPECTED IN SOUTHERN CALIFORNIA

THE Long Beach, California, earthquake, the aftershocks of which will be felt for months, was nevertheless not a general one and probably did not relieve the strain in the earth's crust in other parts of Southern California.

This is the opinion of Professor Bailey Willis, the eminent authority on geology and seismology who is professor emeritus at Stanford University.

There is, therefore, continued danger of severe earthquakes in southern California. When these will come, whether to-morrow or a decade or more from now, neither Professor Willis nor other geologists can attempt to predict.

"The Long Beach earthquake appears to be a shock of moderate intensity on one of the several faults of the San Pedro fault zone," Professor Willis said in response to a Science Service inquiry. "This fault zone was recognized by H. O. Wood, who described it in the *Bulletin* of the Seismological Society, 1916, in his account of the 1812 quake.

"Among the effects of movements on that zone we may recognize the elevation of the San Pedro point which is terraced by marine benches up to more than 1,000 feet above sea and demonstrates activities extending back more than a million years. The zone has the earthquake habit and may be expected to behave accordingly from time to time as in the past. Aftershocks are likely to continue for several months and some of them may be strong. Measures of safety should be rigidly enforced. Although locally disastrous, this Long Beach shock is not a general one and probably does not relieve the strain in the San Jacinto or San Andreas faults. The disaster emphasizes the need of earthquake-resistant buildings under a reasonable building code recognizing earthquake hazards.''

The San Andreas fault is the long cleavage in the earth's crust which runs from north of San Francisco along the coast to northwest of the Los Angeles region inland. Along this fault the great 1906 San Francisco earthquake occurred. The San Jacinto fault is to a certain extent an extension of the San Andreas fault southward of it.

## INCREASE IN NUMBERS OF THE PRONGHORN ANTELOPE

THE pronghorn, slender and beautiful antelope-like animal of the American West, is believed to be on the increase. Thought to be even nearer extinction than the American buffalo or bison was a generation ago, they are shown by a census conducted by the New York Zoological Society to be approximately 68,000 in number in the United States, with 2,400 additional in Canada. A similar census by the U. S. Biological Survey ten years ago indicated less than 27,000 in this country and 1,327 in Canada. Figures for the present zoological society census were supplied by federal, state and dominion authorities.

Wyoming leads the list, with 25,000 animals, as estimated by that state's fish and game commission. An unofficial estimate disagrees with this, setting the number considerably lower. Other states show pronghorn populations ranging from as high as 9,000 in Oregon down to a mere baker's dozen in Nebraska.

When white men first came to the plains, pronghorn were even more numerous than the bison, but the spread of agriculture and grazing, and the relentless guns of the hunters reduced them to an even lower estate than that of their shaggy-maned companions. Only by rigid protection in most states, together with an extensive propaganda campaign urging hunters to spare the beautiful little animals, have they been given a chance to begin their hopeful comeback.

There is a small herd of a few hundred pronghorn in Yellowstone National Park, on the buffalo range in the Lamar Valley. It is here that the average citizen perhaps has the easiest chance to see them, for the Yellowstone pronghorn are even less timid than their brethren elsewhere. Confident in their remarkable running speed, they will race automobiles, being able to keep up a speed of 35 miles an hour for considerable distances.

Zoologically the pronghorn is not related to the true antelopes of the Old World, and it has no other near relatives. It is remarkable among horned creatures in that it is the only hollow-horned animal that sheds its horns every year. Deer shed their antlers, but these are solid. Cattle and sheep have hollow horns, but never shed them. It is because of this unique scientific position as well as because of its rarity that zoologists have been anxious to see the pronghorn saved.

## ITEMS

DOUBLE weight hydrogen, the newly discovered mass two isotope of this lightest of the elements, will be ''so different from common hydrogen that it will be regarded almost as a new element,'' Professor Gilbert N. Lewis, of the University of California, expressed as his belief in a communication to the *Journal* of the American Chemical Society. He recently obtained the heaviest water on record as a result of separating electrolytically hydrogen gas consisting largely of the heavier kind of hydrogen. If the heavy hydrogen proves to be as different as he expects, Professor Lewis predicts that the organic chemistry of compounds containing the heavy isotope of hydrogen will be a fascinating study.

MOTION-PICTURES of life at its lowest possible denomination were shown at the Atlantic City meeting by Dr. Frank L. Howard. Dr. Howard exhibited two films showing the activities of myxomycetes, or slime molds, which are creatures so far down the evolutionary ladder that it has never been decided definitely whether they are plants or animals. They have some of the characteristics of either. The films showed the streaming, creeping motion of the masses of naked protoplasm of which the slime molds' bodies are composed during certain stages of their lives. They showed their ripening into the reproductive stage, the production of the spores and the ingenious mechanisms by which these reproductive bodies are scattered to the wind to drift away and germinate in a new place.

SYNTHETIC vitamins manufactured by organic chemists from cheap and plentiful raw materials were predicted by Dr. George Oliver Curme, Jr., in the annual Chandler lecture which he delivered upon the occasion of his receiving the 1933 Chandler Medal for research in chemistry. Dr. Curme directs the research of the Carbide and Carbon Chemicals Corporation. Vitamins A, B and C have been found to be closely related to substances of complex molecular structure, so that synthesis ''seems entirely possible,'' he explained. In the case of other vitamins less is known, although it would be surprising from the information now available if they were beyond the range of synthetic chemistry. He predicted that adequate supplies of vitamins will soon be available from relatively cheap and abundant sources and that under the guidance of physiological chemists and dietary experts synthetic chemistry will be able to add another triumph to its many past successes.

PROPAGANDA now being spread among school officials contending that individual experimentations by students of chemistry can be replaced by lecture demonstrations, slides or motion pictures, was deplored in a statement by Professor Ross A. Baker, in charge of the College of the City of New York's department of chemistry, issued as a preliminary to the Washington meeting of the American Chemical Society. Many school boards are likely to accept inconclusive data and scrap school chemical laboratories to save expense. Sales of chemical toy sets by hundreds of thousands is evidence of the desire on the part of boys and girls to experiment. He urged organized education to answer this need or the formation of chemistry clubs with the aid of chemistry teachers.

# SCIENCE NEWS

*Science Service, Washington, D. C.*

## PAPERS PRESENTED BEFORE THE WASHINGTON MEETING OF THE AMERICAN CHEMICAL SOCIETY

STRAWBERRIES, it seems, besides being a most tasty fruit, are excellent sources of scurvy-preventing vitamin C. Two grams of them, which is about one fourteenth of an ounce and not very much in terms of big, fat berries, fed daily to guinea-pigs protected the animals from scurvy and enabled them to make good weight gains. The berries do not lose their vitamin C content on freezing, so you may purchase the commercial frozen variety, if you prefer, and you may eat them in ice cream and still be getting this important vitamin. The good news was brought to the meeting by Professor Carl R. Fellers and Merrill J. Mack, of the Massachusetts Agricultural College.

COTTONSEED meal, valuable cattle feed by-product of the cotton industry, is a rich source of vitamins B and G, according to Professor May L. Whitsitt, of the Southern Methodist University. She found cottonseed meal richer in these two important factors than an equal weight of whole wheat, dried yeast or skim milk powder. Cottonseed oil shows no trace of either of these two vitamins, while the hull bran has a varying amount of the vitamins depending on the way it is extracted. Vitamin B is necessary to prevent the development of beriberi in man or a condition known as polyneuritis in birds. Vitamin G, also known as vitamin $B_2$, is said to be the factor in certain foods, notably yeast, that prevents pellagra in man and a similar condition, black-tongue, in dogs.

HOW much vitamin A there is in milk, and in the butter made from cream, depends to a considerable extent on the kind of hay the cow gets, as reported by Dr. E. B. Meigs, A. M. Hartman and H. T. Converse, of the U. S. Bureau of Dairy Industry. Dr. Meigs and his associates found that milk and butter produced on a basis of good alfalfa hay to be definitely richer in this essential vitamin than similar products based on a poor grade of timothy hay. High-grade alfalfa fed to dairy cows is reflected later in a rich natural yellow in their butter, indicative of a high vitamin A content.

VITAMIN $B_1$, preventive of the Oriental disease beriberi and other nerve disorders, has been obtained in crystals by Dr. Atherton Seidell and Dr. M. I. Smith, of the U. S. National Institute of Health. This achievement is considered important because it makes the vitamin available in pure form for chemical study. Dr. Seidell and Dr. Smith obtained a concentrate of vitamin $B_1$ from brewers' yeast by processes already known. This they treated with picrolonic acid, precipitating out substances of no vitamin value. The liquid left over, when evaporated, yielded a partially crystalline deposit, which after further purification gave them a quantity of prismatic crystals. These crystals appear to be the vitamin in pure form. Rats suffering from a deficiency of vitamin $B_1$ were cured with as little as fifteen thousandths of a milligram—about as much as you could pick up on the point of a pin.

FARMERS of the far future may keep pans of Penicillium instead of pens of pigs. For experimenters of the U. S. Bureau of Chemistry and Soils have found a species of mold, known botanically as *Penicillium javanicum,* that beats the hogs at the job of turning carbohydrates into fat. At the meeting of the American Chemical Society, G. E. Ward and L. B. Lockwood told of their researches on this and other fat-making molds. They found several species of Penicillium that contained a good deal of fat when well fed on glucose, but the one called javanicum was the champion of the lot. Its matted mass of white threads, when dried, contained from 20 to 43 per cent. of fat, depending on culture conditions. It takes only twelve days for the mold to produce the maximum quantity of fat out of the glucose solution. When they extracted the fatty material it came out as a reddish-orange oil, with a nut-like odor. A preliminary chemical examination showed it to be built up of the same constituents as many of the fats and oils that are now familiar articles of commerce. The new "mold-oil" is still in the experimental stage, and no definite commercial use for it has been suggested, but there is no doubt that industrial uses may some day be found for it if large-scale production makes it cheap enough.

DILUTE solutions of hydrochloric acid, alkalis and mixtures of hydrochloric acid and kerosene, are being used successfully in removing poisonous sprays from fruits before they are marketed. These measures have not solved all the problems of making fruit safe for consumption while at the same time protecting it from insect pests, but gratifying progress is made each year, according to Professor R. H. Robinson, of the Oregon Agricultural College. Professor Robinson addressed a special symposium of the society on insecticides. "The most important insect enemy of apples and pears, the codling-moth, can be held in check only by lead arsenate," he explained. Previous experience has shown that the maximum amount of arsenic that can be safely left on food is one hundredth of a grain of arsenic per pound of food, W. B. White, of the U. S. Food and Drug Administration, stated. Lead is also used in insect sprays of fruits and vegetables. Mr. White reported that as little as one tenth of a milligram of lead per day will produce serious symptoms if taken over a period of seven or eight years. Fluorine, another substance used in insect sprays, produced a condition known as mottled enamel in the teeth of children when the fluorine was present in drinking water to the amount of two to three parts per million.

E. F. KOHMAN and N. H. Sanborn, of the National Canners' Association, reported that the prune may find new favor, together with fresh flavor, when it appears on the breakfast table fresh from the can. Lemon juice or possibly other fruit juices, being added to canned prunes in order to prevent corrosion of the can, improve the flavor. It is the citric acid of the fruit juices that prevents corrosion. The French or Santa Clara variety of prune must be dried in the first place in order to produce the most desirable flavor. But preparing a dried product for a meal is more of a chore than the modern housewife may care to undertake, so the industry is trying to simplify this culinary task by canning the prunes. Drying, however, increases the tendency of the prunes canned in syrup to attack the can. Citric acid, or lemon juice, takes care of this.

CALCIUM, claimed by some investigators to have a checking effect on cancer, failed in this respect in a large number of experiments on mice performed by Dr. M. J. Shear, of the U. S. Public Health Service. He transplanted cultured cancers of two types on to the bodies of some 1,200 mice, and administered three different chemical salts of calcium either in the drinking water, in the food or by injection into the body. But the results were all negative. Treatment produced no reduction in the number of takes. Slightly smaller tumors were sometimes obtained in the treated mice, but a definite, regular reduction in the size or in the rate of growth of the tumors was not obtained.

THE amount of pepsin in the stomach juice of patients suffering from stomach ulcer may give physicians a good index as to the progress and outcome of the disease. Drs. Arnold E. Osterberg and Francis R. Vanzant, of the Mayo Clinic, studied the pepsin concentration in the stomach juice of some 400 patients after an Ewald type of test meal. They found a correlation between the pepsin concentration and the severity of symptoms which indicated that the pepsin concentration is a valuable prognostic sign.

PROGRESS in the search for pain-relieving, sleep-producing drugs that are without habit-forming properties and may therefore be substituted for the dangerous morphine was reported by Dr. Lyndon F. Small, of the University of Virginia, and Dr. Nathan B. Eddy, of the University of Michigan. The researches described by Drs. Small and Eddy are being carried out under the direction of a special committee of the National Research Council. One phase of the research has consisted in changing the arrangement of the morphine molecule and then observing the pharmacological effects of the altered drug. Certain changes in the chemistry of morphine always produce certain changes in its effect.

THE thyroid gland, important in the regulation of bodily functions, varies in size according to age, and also fluctuates in size according to the season of the year. These observations were reported by Harry von Kolnitz and Dr. Roe E. Remington, of the South Carolina Food Research Commission. Messrs. von Kolnitz and Remington examined the thyroids of 150 human bodies in Charleston. They found that up to the age of forty, human thyroids increased in size; after that they declined steadily. Women's thyroids averaged larger than men's, but contained a lower percentage of iodine. Thyroids varied seasonally, increasing in weight from April to a peak in July and then decreasing to a constant level from October on through the winter. This latter result disagrees with findings of earlier investigators.

HOW the hemoglobin-producing factors of human liver are affected by various diseases was reported by Dr. G. H. Whipple, of the University of Rochester School of Medicine. Dr. Whipple was one of the pioneers whose investigations led to the liver treatment for pernicious anemia, in which disease the hemoglobin content of the blood is somewhat reduced. Acute infections reduce the store of these potent hemoglobin-producing factors in the human liver somewhat. On the other hand, chronic intoxication had very little effect. In cirrhosis or inflammation of the liver there was a marked reduction in the amount of the hemoglobin-producing factors. Pernicious anemia showed very high values for these factors. Secondary anemia due to loss of blood showed low normal values, but even long standing severe anemia will not seriously deplete this store of hemoglobin-producing factors in the liver. In anemia due to loss of blood there may be complete dissociation between the iron content and the concentration of hemoglobin-producing factors.

MOLDS are usually thought of as fungous growths that spoil things; but they can be chosen to turn their "spoiling" activities in useful directions. Research scientists of the U. S. Bureau of Chemistry and Soils described recent progress in the taming of the aspergilli and the penicillia. Two tasks at which molds have proved themselves efficient workers have been the production from glucose solutions of citric and gluconic acids. The former is the familiar acid of lemons; the latter is a rarer acid, of possible use in medicine and industry, which, thanks to the work of the government investigators, now costs dimes a pound where it used to cost dollars.

COLORED fabrics that fade on exposure to light are not fading in the same way that they do when their colors are "washed out" in the laundry. The latter process is merely a reversal of dyeing—the dyestuff merely becomes "unstuck" and diffuses out into the water. Sun-faded fabrics have their dyestuffs actually changed over into other substances, which may have colors of their own. This accounts for the fact that a sun-faded fabric may not merely be paler than it was when new, but may have a quite different hue. These facts about sun-fading were brought out by William D. Appel, of the U. S. Bureau of Standards, and William C. Smith, of the Lowell Textile Institute.

SYNTHETIC stone, made from plentiful shale deposits

or waste limestone, marble, granite and slate quarries, will rival present building materials and compete for the job of entering into the construction of skyscrapers and homes of the future. This was predicted by Professor R. Norris Shreve, of Purdue University, in presenting details of rostone developed in Purdue laboratories by R. L. Harrison and Professor H. C. Peffer. Pulverized limestone and shale, after being properly mixed and moistened to earth dampness, is pressed in a polished steel mold, under a pressure of 2,500 pounds per square inch. The mold is then permitted to dry for a time, later going into an "indurator" which is heated by steam. There the chemical reaction takes place, working as a binder in bonding the particles of limestone together. The pressed block or slab of limestone and "matrix" is then ready for immediate use or it may be polished the same as granite, or marble. The entire process of grinding, mixing, pressing, "steaming" and finishing takes barely a half day, thus giving in a few hours this man-made stone, which nature requires decades or centuries to produce.

Gas stoves and other gas-burning appliances that are safe and suitable for use in low altitudes need to have their "settings" for gas and air flow set differently for safety in high-altitude cities like Denver. J. H. Eisemann, Dr. F. A. Smith and C. J. Merritt, of the U. S. Bureau of Standards, reported on their experiments on the changes needed in gas appliances for safe operation at high altitudes. In general, they found that the maximum safe rate for the supply of gas at sea-level, measured in heat units consumed per hour, is reduced by approximately three to four per cent. for each thousand feet of altitude; but the number of cubic feet per hour of gas of given composition which can be burned completely is practically independent of altitude. The area of flue opening which will permit the flow of enough air to insure complete combustion increases somewhat more rapidly than in proportion to the altitude at each gas rate, and this effect is the greater the higher the gas rate.

When a man falls victim to a fire, if he is not burned outright he is frequently said to be "suffocated by the smoke." But in many cases he is killed by something much more deadly than smoke. Many common household things give off some of the most toxic of poisonous gases, Professor John C. Olsen, of Brooklyn Polytechnic Institute, reported. Professor Olsen has as collaborators in his investigations George E. Ferguson and Leopold Scheflan. The gases from all types of fires investigated contain toxic constituents in sufficient amount to make breathing the gases dangerous or even fatal in a relatively short period. They vary greatly in toxicity. Those most toxic come from substances containing nitrogen or sulphur or both of these elements. Textiles such as clothing, draperies, etc., cotton and rayon produce the least toxic gases, while silk and especially woolens give off hydrogen sulphide, hydrocyanic acid, sulphur dioxide and ammonia, as well as carbon monoxide.

Motion-pictures showing how ultra-violet light of certain wave-lengths kills cells were shown by Dr. Ellice McDonald, Alexander J. Allen and Rachel Franklin, of the University of Pennsylvania. They used cells from the spleen for their experimental material, and the wave-lengths turned on them ranged between 4,350 and 2,253 Ångström units. The wave-lengths that were fatal to the cells killed in from fifteen to twenty seconds. The living protoplasm of the cells became greatly agitated, bubbles appeared on the membrane and as a rule the cells finally burst. The killing effect of the shorter ultra-violet light can not be equaled by fifteen hours of exposure to strong radiation from radium, nor is the lethal effect of ultra-violet light equaled by twelve to twenty-four hours of exposure to high-voltage x-rays.

Chemistry, which has contributed so essentially to America's economic progress, is in this depression helping to camouflage inferior quality merchandise. This danger was pointed out by H. L. Derby, president of the American Cyanamid and Chemical Corporation. "One of the notable incidents of the present depression is the demand for low-priced merchandise, quality being one of the lesser considerations—quite the reverse of the prosperity type of demand," said Mr. Derby. "In past generations the distinctions between good and cheap merchandise were readily discernible by the most inexperienced observer. However, modern chemistry has largely eliminated the superficial differences by neatly and attractively covering up the inferior quality." Chemistry's large contribution to America's industry and independence from foreign sources of essential materials were cited by Mr. Derby, who also predicted the future course of this science applied to industry.

Not all the ancients who labored mysteriously with beakers and alembics were mere alchemists, either muddle-headed themselves or deliberately out to fool their neighbors. There were real chemists among them, who knew that the "gold" they were making out of base metals was not real gold. So Professor Tenney L. Davis, of the Massachusetts Institute of Technology, reported. The chemists of ancient Alexandria knew the difference, he said, and so did the medieval genius Albertus Magnus, the earliest scientist to be canonized as a saint. Albertus, said Professor Davis, wrote in his "De Alchimia" that the gold of alchemy is identical with real gold "in every test and hammering"; but he also wrote in another part of the same book that "the gold of alchemy does not gladden the heart of man, nor cure leprosy, and wounds fester which are made by it." This indicates that Albertus knew that "the gold of alchemy" was brass. Apparently independently of the West, the Chinese invented a system of alchemy about the third century B. C. The Chinese alchemists hoped to produce actual immortality by chemical means, and to become "hsien" or supernaturally endowed, benevolent immortals. Professor Davis also set forth the reasons for believing that Arabic alchemy was derived from that of the Chinese.

# SCIENCE NEWS

*Science Service, Washington, D. C.*

## CANCER FOLLOWING GERM INJECTION

Development of cancer following the injection of a germ or micro-organism is announced by the U. S. Public Health Service's National Institute of Health. The discovery was made by Drs. T. J. Glover and J. L. Engle, who have been working at the institute, although they are not attached to the regular government staff nor to the U. S. Public Health Service. They have succeeded in producing typical, unmistakable cancer in a guinea-pig. This cancer followed the injection of a culture of a micro-organism or germ isolated from the tissues of a proved case of cancer of the human breast. This traverses the prevalent opinion that cancer is not a germ disease. It is only after years of work that the announcement has been made.

Application of the new discovery to the treatment of human cancer is far in the future, but the experiments of Drs. Glover and Engle promise to blaze a new line of cancer research that appears very hopeful. "It promises to open a valuable field for further research," commented Dr. George W. McCoy, director of the institute.

Drs. Glover and Engle have found that cancer in rats follows injection of their culture of germs from human cancerous tissue. But rats develop cancer so very easily that this was not considered convincing evidence that the germ culture actually could cause cancer. The production of cancer in guinea-pigs, which, so far as any one knows or can find out, do not readily develop it, is considered much more of a feat and more convincing that the germ culture of Drs. Glover and Engle is cancer-producing.

The cancer produced in the guinea-pig has all the characteristic appearance of cancer when examined by the unaided eye and under the microscope. Furthermore it spread, producing cancer in other parts of the body, thus fulfilling another of the criteria for the diagnosis of the growth as cancer. The germ itself is what scientists call a spore-bearer. It was isolated on special media from the tissues of the human cancer.

In the report only one case of cancer in the guinea-pig is described. The diagnosis of cancer in this case was confirmed by a pathologist of the National Institute of Health, and the foremost staff bacteriologist is now checking the bacteriological side of the work.

Dr. Glover started his investigations several years ago in New York. For the last three years, the work has been carried on by him and by Dr. Engle at the National Institute of Health where the director and staff scientists could follow and check various steps of the research.

In their report they do not claim specifically to have discovered the cause of cancer, but state with characteristic scientific reserve: "It is the purpose of this report to place on record the production of metastatic malignancy in one of a group of guinea-pigs inoculated with a culture containing a spore-bearing micro-organism which was isolated on special media from the tissue of a microscopically proven carcinoma of the human breast."

Further points to be determined are whether the micro-organism they have described causes the cancer, or whether it is caused by some virus or other germ present in the culture or by some toxin or other substance produced by the bacteria of the culture. It is possible that this culture is not the cause of all types of cancer, but of one group of them. Efforts to develop a serum, either curative or protective, will be a logical outcome of this research. Investigation of the infectiousness of a type of cancer produced by bacteria as this one was in the guinea-pig will also have to be developed.

One of the two physicians making the discovery is from New York, while the second is from Philadelphia. They had worked under private research grants for about ten years before bringing their experiments to the National Institute of Health for critical testing.

## COSMIC RAYS

Cosmic rays are streams of particles or corpuscles, not electro-magnetic waves like light, x-rays or radium's gamma rays, Professor Bruno Rossi, leading Italian physicist, has concluded from experiments at the University of Padova's Institute of Physics. He finds that cosmic radiation observed at sea-level is exclusively a corpuscular radiation. From his experiments he also concludes that the primary cosmic radiation which reaches us from outer space is, in all probability, also a corpuscular radiation. In this conclusion Professor Rossi agrees closely with Dr. Arthur H. Compton and other experimenters in America who have found evidence that cosmic rays are particles, perhaps electrons.

Professor Rossi is now organizing a cosmic radiation expedition to Africa. Experiments will be made in the neighborhood of the magnetic equator with the purpose of testing his theories of how the magnetic field of the earth affects the cosmic corpuscles. On this expedition he will make tests similar to those that were a part of the world-wide surveys under the direction of Dr. Arthur H. Compton, of the University of Chicago.

"I have approached the problem of the nature of the primary cosmic radiation from the theoretical as well as from the experimental point of view," Professor Rossi said in an exclusive statement to Science Service. He is investigating the theoretical as well as the experimental evidence of the influence of the earth's magnetic field upon cosmic rays if they are corpuscles. He has already solved this problem theoretically in its general outlines.

"Since 1930 I have been devoting myself to an accurate study of certain corpuscles of very high energy, the ultra-penetrating corpuscles, which Drs. Bothe and Kolhörster, the German physicists, demonstrated as present in the atmosphere," Professor Rossi said. "The scope of this research is to study the properties of such corpuscles and their effect upon matter as well as to determine their relation to cosmic radiation—to determine whether they are generated in the atmosphere by a primary cosmic radiation of the type of gamma rays or whether they consist of the primary cosmic radiation itself.

"To this end I have carried out an accurate and extensive comparison of the absorption of complex cosmic radiation with the absorption of corpuscular radiation, following the trajectory of the corpuscles through layers of lead up to a thickness of one meter by means of a recording device which notes each corpuscle as it enters and leaves the absorbing medium. I have not found any difference between the two absorptions.

"So far as concerns the effects produced by the corpuscles of the radiation when they penetrate matter, I have been able to demonstrate by means of a system of coincidental impulses of three recording instruments that the trajectories of these corpuscles fork at certain distances. This indicates that the divisions originate in the material traversed by secondary corpuscles. I have studied the properties of the secondary corpuscles in relation to the means by which they are generated and I have shown that to them are due all those anomalies in the absorption curve which have previously been designated as the 'transition effects.'"

## ENERGY TURNED INTO MASS FOR FIRST TIME IN HISTORY

For the first time, physicists seem to have discovered a case of energy turning into mass, that is, non-material "push and shove" being converted into something material that can be weighed, as it were. Dr. Kenneth T. Bainbridge, fellow of the Franklin Institute's Bartol Research Foundation and authority on the masses of atoms, has concluded that when lithium is bombarded with the heart of a helium atom, energy may be converted into mass.

The experiments were first made by Mme. Irene Curie-Joliot, daughter of the discoverers of radium, and her husband, Dr. F. Joliot, at the Institut de Radium in Paris last year. Dr. Bainbridge examined the experiments in detail and finds that when a lithium atom of mass seven is hit by and captures an alpha particle, or helium atom heart, there is strong indication of the transfer of kinetic energy of the impinging alpha particle into what the physicists call "inertial mass." This creates an atom of boron of mass ten. This isotope of boron is found as one of the experimental products of lithium's disintegration.

"Change of energy into inertial mass must be viewed with caution," Dr. Bainbridge said in a Franklin Institute lecture, "but available experimental data make the suggestion the most plausible of four possible explanations."

While this is the first apparent case of energy being converted into mass, many cases of the changing of mass into energy are known. The transforming of mass of atoms into heat and light is a favorite mechanism for explaining how the sun and stars keep shining for billions upon billions of years.

The scientific value of disintegration and other nuclear experiments far surpasses the highly speculative economic values of release of energy from the atom, in Dr. Bainbridge's opinion. Following in the footsteps of Dr. F. W. Aston, the British physicist, who developed the mass-spectrograph to separate chemically identical isotopes and deal with them individually, Dr. Bainbridge has carried on mass-spectrograph studies at the Bartol Research Foundation.

"The spectrograph permits the investigator to determine what nuclear types exist," Dr. Bainbridge explained. "It is possible to determine the relative abundance of the isotopes of specific elements and so indirectly the chemical atomic weights and finally to make measurements of the masses of atoms to an accuracy of one part in 30,000. These measurements are important in connection with studies of the disintegration of atomic nuclei.

"The results of atomic mass measurements in cooperation with disintegration experiments furnish an experimental proof of the equivalence of mass and energy deduced theoretically by Einstein. The best example of this is given by the experiments of Cockcroft and Walton on the disintegration of the lithium seven nucleus by the capture of an incident proton resulting in the release of two helium nuclei with a combined energy of about 17,000,000 electron volts, which energy must be the result of a transformation of mass into energy."

## ITEMS

Reiteration that cosmic rays are probably electrons or other electric particles coming to earth from outer space and being deflected by the earth's magnetic field in such a way that the intensity is greater for high latitudes than near the equator is contained in a detailed report by Dr. Arthur H. Compton, of the University of Chicago, which appears in the *Physical Review*. Summarizing the researches of more than sixty physicists in a geographical study of cosmic rays throughout the world, Dr. Compton finds that at sea level the cosmic ray intensity at high latitudes is 14 per cent. greater than at the equator, at 2,000 meters (a little over a mile) it is 22 per cent. greater, and at 4,360 meters (over two miles high) it is 33 per cent. greater. Dr. Compton writes: "Consideration of the conditions necessary for deflection of high-speed electrified particles by the earth's magnetic field indicates that if the cosmic rays are electrons, they must originate not less than several hundred kilometers above the earth." He finds that his data can be quantitatively explained on the basis of the Lemaitre-Vallarta theory of electrons approaching the earth from remote space.

Testing the hearing of chimpanzees was the rather novel task of a psychologist described by J. H. Elder, of Yale University, to the recent meeting of the New York Branch of the American Psychological Association. Chimpanzees are no harder to test accurately than are human children, Mr. Elder reported. His method was to train the apes to press a key when the signal was given and not to press it when they heard nothing. Standard earphones were used and the apes were then allowed to listen to sounds of known frequency from an audiometer. The frequencies heard by the chimpanzees are within the range audible to human beings, although several of the apes could hear frequencies lower than those heard by the average human being.

# SCIENCE NEWS

*Science Service, Washington, D. C.*

## THE MOST PROFITABLE INVESTMENT OF THE FEDERAL GOVERNMENT

By Watson Davis

*Managing Editor, Science Service*



Scientific research conducted by the Federal Government is its most profitable investment. Among the millions and the billions for wars, past, present and future, for post offices, for Congress, for prohibition enforcement, for Indians, for interest on the public debt, for RFC and other dollar transfusions to the financial structure, for relief, for reforestation, there are items of a few thousands and hundreds of thousands of dollars for scientific research.

The U. S. Department of Agriculture scientists are finding new uses for familiar farm products, fighting soil erosion, improving livestock, protecting plants and crops, and safeguarding the ordinary consumer against bad food and drugs. In far off China or the tropics, explorers of the department roam to bring back strange plants that help our farmers. Within our country's borders, entomologists are combating the insect menace. U. S. Geological Survey geologists are mapping and surveying the mineral domain that the machine age may not die of starvation. U. S. Coast and Survey ships and engineers are surveying our coasts to safeguard commerce and shipping.

Out in that group of Washington laboratories, not near the oratory of Congress, there are men and women of the U. S. Bureau of Standards staff studying the rainbow of chemical elements, developing new facts about heat, stressing steel and newer metals, perfecting standards, methods and processes of incalculable value to industry and pursuing a thousand other useful scientific tasks.

Astronomers at the U. S. Naval Observatory observe the stars in order that our watches and clocks may have the correct time. Meteorologists of the U. S. Weather Bureau observe and forecast the weather for farmers, aviators and city folks. U. S. Bureau of Mines engineers by experiments, practical and theoretical, safeguard and develop the mines of the nation.

The appropriations for such scientific research functions of the federal government are the best investments made by the government. The returns to the public in terms of percentage run to figures like 50,000 per cent. instead of the conventional 6 per cent. that bankers have popularized.

True, the profits do not flow back into the U. S. Treasury directly as dollars. The profits are made not by Uncle Sam but by the American public. That is fitting for the business of the government is not to make money, but to undertake functions that benefit the whole people.

Scientific research is often a long-time investment, with the benefits going to our children and their children. It is a safe investment. Unlike bonds of maturity in the year 2000 or later, issued to pay for rails that even now are rusting away, the money spent for fundamental scientific research is a secure investment that will continue to pay public service dividends down through the ages.

If you think of the budget of the U. S. Government as a gigantic pie, the slice that is eaten to provide scientific research and service, which is perhaps the most profitable of its many activities, is so small that it can barely be seen. Of the federal dollar, less than $\frac{7}{8}$ths of a cent is expended for the constructive scientific research and service conducted to the profit of the whole nation.

This 85 hundredths of one per cent. (based on the 1931–32 expenditures) includes all the administrative, clerical and other routine expenses in connection with the government's scientific work. If the salaries of the scientists themselves and the money expended for apparatus, etc., were considered alone, the item would be much smaller, so minute that it would be difficult to find it among the millions upon millions of dollars that pass through Uncle Sam's pocketbook. Obviously the federal budget can never be balanced by eliminating any or all of the scientific work of the Federal Government.

The crippling of an essential scientific investigation or service here and another there may give a feeling of righteousness and go through the motions of cutting down government expenditures, but it will not balance the budget or materially lift the tax burden. The effect will be hardship on the farmer, the manufacturer or the consumer in later years when the much greater direct tax of undone scientific research will be felt.

Not only will the ultimate consumer and future generations lose, but Uncle Sam himself will find his day-to-day routine governmental activities made more expensive if the scientists are fired. In addition to fundamental and applied scientific research, the federal scientific bureaus perform tests that assure that the government gets its money's worth in purchasing supplies, erecting buildings, etc.

If a total is obtained of all the money spent by the government for all kinds of research, education and developmental work, not just scientific research and service, it is found that only 2.7 per cent. of the U. S. expenditures is accounted for. Who then eats Uncle Sam's budget pie?

Wars, past and future, gobble 75.2 per cent. of the federal budget. Warships, soldiers, veterans, interest and retirement of debts from past wars, and their incidentals consumed $3,758,000,000 of the United States 1931–32 expenditures. Compare this cost of warfare and national defense with $42,000,000 for scientific work, both research and service, in 1931–32. Of the 1934 budget presented to Congress last fall, less than $35,000,000 is devoted to scientific research and service.

The legislative, executive and judicial functions of the Federal Government consumed 12.6 per cent. of the 1932 expenditures, and public works in 1931–32 were responsible for 9.5 per cent. of the expenditures.

Meeting the annual bill for profitable scientific research in the United States budget is a relatively small matter from a financial standpoint. The complete elimination of the annual federal investment in scientific research, which is unthinkable, would not help materially in "balancing the budget." The annual *per capita* cost is only about 30 cents. The *per capita* cost of all federal government activities runs from $30 to $40 per year, depending upon what year is taken.

You, as one of 122,000,000 Americans, make your profitable investment in federal scientific research when you smoke five packages of cigarettes (federal tax six cents a package) use thirty gallons of gasoline in your auto (federal tax one cent a gallon); drink two gallons of beer (federal tax $5 a barrel of 31 gallons).

The total cost of scientific research and service in the many government departments is estimated at $34,768,000 in the 1934 budget submitted to Congress last fall. Since then this budget has been deeply cut, of course. The actual federal science expenditures in the peak year 1931–32 were only about $40,000,000.

This bill for some $40,000,000, which will pay immense profits both now and to future generations, could be met by: The cost of a single modern trans-ocean express steamer; the money needed to build four cruisers; one tenth of the annual U. S. tobacco tax; one third of the "pay of the army," which does not include supplies or civilian hire expenditures of the U. S. Army. Less than a tenth of the savings made by President Roosevelt in the veterans economy measures now being put into effect.

For Uncle Sam's annual investment in scientific research and service, for the 30 cents you as a citizen contribute indirectly each year, you and your children will get many dollars of real profit in every-day living, now and in the future. Figures show that typical research projects return profits of some 50,000 per cent., that is $150 for your 30 cents. And the most beneficial returns are those that can not be computed in mere dollars and cents.

Science has revolutionized the modern world. All about us are essentials and luxuries that are newly arisen from the minds of scientists and their laboratories. Millions upon millions of dollars have been created by science for industry.

Important in the progress of science have been the labors of scientists, working day after day for modest salaries in the federal departments of agriculture, commerce, interior, etc., without avaricious thought of personal gain.

As the nation waxed rich, both in money and comfort and health, did it invest an increasing amount of its wealth in scientific research? Did it plow into its science fields, like a good farmer, adequate fertilizer for future years?

Industry has to a large extent been convinced by bountiful returns that applied scientific research pays and pays well. As income to industry rose after the World War, allotments for research increased, but not perhaps as rapidly as the increase in national income. And as the depression began to take its toll upon business, the research staffs were not fired but in most cases they were preserved and even strengthened.

There has been a new rush in research to create new products and materials to replace those affected by the depression, to develop new and cheaper methods of utilizing old materials and making staple articles. Costs have been held within limited budgets through the science and ingenuity of the research staff. Surveys made by the National Research Council show that industry is continuing to a large extent its scientific research activities.

In the reorganization of the federal government now in progress, the same spirit should rule. The cost of all scientific research and its auxiliary services in the federal government is only about $35,000,000 (based on 1934 budget) and this is a mere fraction, seven eighths of one per cent., of the total budget.

In fact, all the educational, research and developmental work of the government consumes only about three per cent. of the federal cost. A smaller percentage is devoted to constructive education, research and development work now than before the World War. In 1910, 5.1 per cent. was spent for "education, research and development." In 1915 it was 5.4 per cent. In 1920 it dropped to 1.3 per cent. due to war costs. Since 1925 it has hovered between 2.5 and 3.2 per cent.

Compare this with the national income of the whole nation, not government expenditures. Figures by the National Bureau of Economic Research show that the national income in 1910 and 1915 was $31,000,000,000 to $37,000,000,000 in round billions, whereas from 1925 to 1930 it varied from about $80,000,000,000 to $90,000,000,000.

## FUNCTIONS OF THE ADRENAL GLAND

Important new functions of the vital adrenal glands, concerned with vitamin utilization and milk production, were reported by Drs. Frank A. Hartman, J. E. Lockwood and K. A. Brownell, of the University of Buffalo, at the meeting in Cincinnati of the Federation of American Societies for Experimental Biology.

At previous meetings, members of the federation have heard the Buffalo investigators describe the life-saving cortin which they extracted from the cortex part of the two small glands that lie just above the kidneys. Cortin has saved the lives of sufferers from Addison's disease, an ailment in which the adrenal glands are diseased and fail to produce enough cortin themselves for the body's needs. Animals deprived of their adrenal glands quickly die, but their lives may be prolonged indefinitely by administration of cortin.

Experiments were reported suggesting that adrenal cortical extract, possibly cortin itself, helps the body to utilize vitamins C and $B_1$. A substance that is necessary for the production of milk has been separated from cortical extract. They call this new hormone cortilactin.

The discovery of the relation of cortin to vitamin utilization came about when microscopic changes were found in adrenal gland cortex of animals getting too little of certain vitamins in their diets. This suggested that extra demands were being made on the glands to make up for the vitamin deficiency.

When an extract containing cortin was given to guinea-pigs on vitamin C deficient diets, the onset of scurvy was delayed. The extract was prepared in such a way that none of the vitamin, which itself prevents scurvy, could have been present. Injection of this extract also delayed the onset of nerve symptoms due to deficiency of vitamin $B_1$ in the diet.

Apparently this function of the adrenal gland cortex is so important that provision is made for one gland to produce more of the substance concerned in vitamin utilization in case of injury to the other gland. This extra production on the part of the remaining, healthy gland is continued for about five weeks after disease or injury has put the other out of action.

Discussing the milk-producing hormone, cortilactin, Dr. Hartman and associates explained that cortin alone does not have this action. Mother rats that have no adrenal glands can not raise litters of young, even with enough cortin to keep the mothers themselves healthy and fat. Cortilactin must be added.

## INHERITANCE AND GLANDS IN THE CONTROL OF GROWTH

CONSTITUTIONAL, inherited factors have more to do with type of body build than secretions of the body's powerful, growth-controlling glands, it appears from breeding experiments with dogs reported by Dr. Charles R. Stockard, of Cornell University Medical College, at the meeting in Cincinnati of the American Association of Anatomists.

Secretions of certain glands, notably pituitary and thyroid, are known to affect growth because when too much or too little of the powerful hormones are secreted the results may be seen in dwarfs, giants and other abnormal bodily forms.

While admitting the power of the glands over growth, Dr. Stockard believes his experiments show that the gland secretions are quite unable to regulate growth in opposition to the inherited constitution of the individual.

"For illustration," he said, "ordinary persons may not respond in their growth reactions to pituitary modification in the same manner as do those inheriting acromegaly."

Acromegaly is a disease in which the bones and the soft parts of the hands, feet and face are enlarged. The disease is associated with over-function of the pituitary gland.

According to Dr. Stockard's theory, over-functioning of the pituitary would not produce the enlarged bones typical of acromegaly in the ordinary person, but only in persons inheriting acromegaly.

Dr. Stockard has for many years engaged in breeding experiments with dogs and has learned much of how various traits are inherited. By crossing various breeds, he has found which characteristics are dominant characters that will appear in every generation, and which are due to glandular conditions.

## ITEMS

A SPECIAL balloon now under construction in Leningrad will be used by Soviet investigators in an attempt to set a new altitude record by penetrating into the stratosphere, in order to study electric and magnetic phenomena, cosmic rays and solar energy in the upper reaches of the atmosphere. The closed passenger car, which will be attached to the balloon, will have walls 10 mm (two fifths of an inch) thick. It is being constructed of a specially strong non-magnetic alloy which has been perfected by a group of specialists working under the guidance of Engineer Vasionko.

DEFINITE evidence of an anti-growth factor in the parathyroid gland has recently been found by Drs. C. J. Eastland, N. Evers and J. H. Thompson, working at Kings College, University of London, and the Royal College of Surgeons. These investigators treated fresh parathyroid gland in a special way and obtained an extract which had a harmful effect on the growth of rats, according to a report in *The Biochemical Journal*. Six rats were used as controls, and six were given daily injections of a small measured amount of the extract, other conditions being the same for both groups of rats. The factor which retarded the growth was destroyed by treatment with hydrogen peroxide.

BITTER rubberweed, a plant belonging to the aster family, has been growing into a serious problem to sheep raisers in a part of western Texas, according to A. B. Clawson, physiologist of the Bureau of Animal Industry. Due apparently to over-use of the grazing land and to climatic factors, the weed has been increasing in abundance while good forage plants have been growing scarcer, with the result that the poor sheep have been driven to this poisonous food. It is estimated that 75,000 of them died in an area of 6,000 square miles during the winters of 1929–30 and 1930–31. The cause of the sheep losses was not at first known, but because of the abundance of the bitter rubberweed in the affected area it was placed under suspicion, and an investigation by scientists of the U. S. Department of Agriculture resulted in its conviction. The plant is known to botanists as *Actinea odorata*.

SEVERAL of the larger German cities are solving part of their depression problems by a hook-up of garbage-burning plants and greenhouses. Unemployed men are given jobs building greenhouses and running the incinerators. Ashes from the burned garbage are used as fertilizer, and heat from the incinerators keeps the greenhouses warm. Plants that thrive on high-potash fertilizers, like tomatoes, cucumbers and cut flowers, are grown in the greenhouses. H. A. Kirsch, a Berlin engineer who describes the projects in *Die Umschau,* states that employment in building will be given to about 25,000 men, and that for running the finished establishment two or three thousand families can be crossed off the rolls of those receiving public aid. The projects are expected to be self-liquidating, in that they will supply large quantities of high-grade fresh vegetables that have hitherto had to be imported.

# SCIENCE NEWS

*Science Service, Washington, D. C.*

## THE REPRODUCTION OF MUSIC BY NEW METHODS

THREE loud-speakers on an empty stage, three telephone lines running to three microphones in a sound-proof room containing the Philadelphia Symphony Orchestra, Leopold Stokowski turning electrical control knobs instead of wielding a baton, telephone engineers operating the electrical circuits, was the most advanced development of musical reproduction that will be introduced to the public in a Philadelphia-Washington concert for the National Academy of Sciences on April 27.

In a private preview for scientists and music critics held at the Academy of Music in Philadelphia, the American Telephone and Telegraph Company engineers demonstrated the results of two years of scientific research conducted with the collaboration of Director Stokowski. Wagnerian music was played with whispering pianissimos and thunderous crescendos hitherto unheard by human ears. Stokowski by the turn of a control knob could subdue his orchestra, isolated in another part of the theater, to a mere trickle of sound or he could build up their music to the sound of two thousand musicians at a peak of output. Brünhilde, sung by Miss Agnes Davis, became an electrical supervocalist, rising above the orchestral accompaniment of Götterdämmerung. Wagner's music was rendered as probably he never dared to dream it might be played.

This merging of music and telephone science has introduced jointly three factors in the electrical reproduction of orchestral music: (1) auditory perspective; (2) tone and overtone control; (3) volume control. Three loud-speakers at left, right and center of the empty stage, each connected with a similarly placed microphone on the remote stage of the actual performers, give perspective to the music and sounds. Musicians could tell just where the violins or horns were placed. In one demonstration, stage hands moved across the distant stage and the audience of the empty stage "followed" them about the empty stage by using their ears. Engineers had previously felt that this illusion of auditory perspective might be obtained only with many loud-speakers on the empty stage, but three were found to give perfect results when the electrical transmission had high quality.

A wide range of nine musical octaves, from three below middle C to nearly six above, was utilized for the first time in electrical transmission of music. This corresponds to all frequencies from about 35 cycles per second to about 16,000 cycles per second. Radio by federal regulation is limited to a band of 5,000 cycles per second. When experimentally the high and low frequencies are chopped off by electrical filters the damage to the tone and overtone qualities was readily apparent. Each of the three telephone wires carried the full range of frequencies, and the frequency channels utilized therefore were roughly nine times those of the most perfect radio transmission. In loudness range, the orchestra or other sound being transmitted can be varied from an output equivalent to a millionth of a watt to a sustained hundred watts and even a kilowatt at momentary peaks without distortion. The sound in the demonstration was raised from the rustle of leaves to beyond that of a roaring airplane engine.

Practical applications are foreseen by the telephone engineers and Director Stokowski. A symphony orchestra in one place may render its concerts with perfect tonal quality and with improved volume in a hundred or a thousand different halls in distant cities. Music may be spread from high towers so that 100,000 may enjoy it in large parks. The musician and composer can add electrical amplification and control to his material out of which beautiful sound compositions are wrought.

## PAPERS AT THE CINCINNATI MEETING OF THE FEDERATION OF AMERICAN SOCIETIES FOR EXPERIMENTAL BIOLOGY

PROGRESS toward isolation and laboratory preparation of the life-saving hormone of the adrenal gland cortex and a tentative chemical name for it were reported from two research centers. This hormone has proved valuable because its use prolongs lives of patients suffering from the hitherto incurable Addison's disease. From the gland itself, Drs. Arthur Grollman and W. M. Firor, of the Johns Hopkins University, have extracted a crystalline substance that is so very powerful that it is probably the pure hormone. However, Dr. Grollman stated that several more years of investigation will be needed to make sure of this point. The chemical composition of this substance has been investigated at the Mayo Clinic by Dr. E. C. Kendall, H. L. Mason, B. F. McKenzie and C. S. Myers. Dr. Frank Hartman, of the University of Buffalo, a pioneer investigator of this hormone, had suggested the name cortin, spelled without the final e, and Dr. Kendall's research into its chemical nature shows this to be a suitable name with the addition of the final e, which indicates the presence of nitrogen. Dr. Kendall and associates are trying now to produce the hormone from the chemicals in their laboratories, and while they have not yet synthesized the entire compound, they have succeeded in obtaining a preliminary compound.

A NEW hormone of the pituitary gland that exercises control over the thyroid and seems to "double" for the secretion of that gland causing exophthalmic goiter was a leading topic of discussion among medical investigators. As one doctor expressed it: "The pituitary gland is in the driver's seat." It is small but important, located at the base of the brain. It produces many powerful hormones or chemical regulators of the body's activities. Some of these hormones have an important stimulating effect on the sex glands. Another hormone promotes growth. The latest discovery is a new hormone that influences the secretion of the thyroid gland. Exophthalmic goiter, characterized by extreme nervousness and protruding eyes, results from over-secretion of the thyroid gland. Now scientists have found the newly discovered pituitary hormone can produce the same effect. For the first time scientists have been able to produce this type of goiter in animals, which will greatly aid further research on this serious and wide-spread disease for which the only relief at present is surgical operation.

THE "chemical dissection" of a gland has been accomplished by Drs. J. B. Collip, D. L. Thomson, H. Selye and E. M. Anderson, of McGill University. The gland is the pituitary, located at the base of the brain, and apparently possessed of far greater powers than hitherto supposed. This gland secretes a number of hormones, powerful chemical regulators of body activity. One investigator estimated that twenty-two pituitary hormones had been reported by various investigators. Dr. Collip and his associates are working to get clean hormone extracts from this gland, each separate from the other, and to determine the exact effect of each on the human body. In his pocket, Dr. Collip carried a tiny bottle containing a clear, colorless fluid. One cubic centimeter, or about four drops, of this particular pituitary hormone is sufficiently powerful to produce exophthalmic goiter in two hundred guinea-pigs.

THE parathyroid glands, located next to the thyroid gland in the neck, probably play an important rôle in the mechanism which sets free the rickets-preventing vitamin D from the skin and the tissues just under the skin, according to Dr. F. L. Kozelka, of the University of Wisconsin. Investigators have believed for some time that the ultra-violet rays of sunshine change a fatty substance, ergosterol, found in the skin and subskin tissues, into the vitamin. The parathyroid glands apparently make the next move by liberating the vitamin from the tissues so that it in turn can play its part in the body chemistry.

CAUTION against too large doses of viosterol, artificial vitamin D which is widely used as a preventive of rickets in babies, was urged by Dr. Agnes Fay Morgan, of the University of California. Dr. Morgan and associates reported a new method of studying bones to find out how they were affected by vitamin D. Dr. Morgan's studies with rats have convinced her that the largest safe dose of viosterol is very much less than previously supposed. Overdoses of this substance seem to produce kidney injury, which Dr. Morgan believes is the cause of death of animals receiving too much viosterol. She emphasized that it is unwise and unsafe for mothers to buy this potent substance and give it to their children without a physician's directions as to the amount of the dose.

THE dye, methylene blue, which has been widely heralded as an antidote for deadly cyanides and carbon monoxide gas, may kill people instead of saving their lives when used to treat victims of carbon monoxide, Professor Yandell Henderson, of Yale University, reported. In his laboratories at Yale, Professor Henderson said, Dr. Howard W. Haggard has been using the dye to treat dogs that were near death from the effects of the invisible carbon monoxide gas which is found, among other places, in the exhaust gas of automobiles. The dogs would have recovered with the usual treatment for carbon monoxide poisoning. They had been exposed to the gas in amounts just short of that which causes death. When given methylene blue treatment, instead of recovering, they died. This investigation has brought out plainly that what the dye really does, Professor Henderson commented, is to convert the oxygen-carrying hemoglobin of the blood to methemoglobin. This compound is powerless to supply oxygen to the tissues and the victim then dies of asphyxia. Carbon monoxide kills in the same way, the gas forming a strong chemical union with the hemoglobin and thus preventing it from carrying oxygen to the tissues.

A FUNDAMENTAL difference between the sexes in the way the body takes care of the sugars and starches of the diet was reported by Dr. H. J. Deuel, Jr., of the University of Southern California. Fasting adult male rats had more sugar stored in their livers than did the females, Dr. Deuel and associates found, while the females had more fat stored in the liver than the males. There was no difference in immature rats. Dr. Deuel was trying to find why women develop a condition of much greater acidosis during fasting than men do. Apparently it is because of their smaller store of sugar and larger store of fat. The problem is important in connection with diabetes in which this kind of acidosis develops when the patient is on a sugar-free diet. It indicates that diabetic women might need a slightly different diet from diabetic men. When the ovaries were removed, female rats had as much sugar stored in their livers as did normal males, Dr. Deuel found. When these rats were given doses of theelin, a female sex hormone, the sugar stored in their livers was the same amount as that of normal females.

SCIENTISTS whose knowledge of nutrition taught us how to feed our fighting men during the World War are now turning their knowledge to the problem of feeding the soldiers of the depression. The fight to-day is against the "undisclosed signs of deterioration" in health resulting from malnutrition, Professor Lafayette B. Mendel, of Yale University, pointed out at the meeting. Disease due to lack of proper foods grows slowly. Scientists are trying now to recognize these diseases in their very earliest stages, just as bankers are trying to find ways of detecting unsoundness in banks early enough to prevent disaster. Early signs of the beginning of these diseases could be seen last year in the bread lines, Professor Mendel said, and on the hands of patients admitted to the wards of Bellevue Hospital in New York, doctors saw the faintest marks on the skin which meant the beginning of pellagra. In this fight we need the help of the family physician who knows his patients well enought to see the development of what Professor Mendel called "subvisible disorders."

LOOKING through a window in a rabbit's ear, University of Pennsylvania physiologists have gained a better understanding of how the body disposes of débris cast out of the blood vessels. This has been one of the important problems still unsolved by physiologists. Drs. E. R. Clark and E. L. Clark reported their observations at Cincinnati. Lymphatic tissue, which has been credited with doing this scavenging job, appears to be much less important in this relation than previouly thought, the Clarks' study showed. Enzymes which digest protein substances may play a rôle in the scavenging process, it was suggested. The window in the rabbit's ear was devised several years ago at the University of Pennsylvania laboratories. It is a sort of double window composed of two thin sheets of transparent substance, with the space between thin enough so that light can pass through the tissues that grow into it. A microscope was used to look through this window and watch what goes on in blood-vessels, the blood itself, the connective tissue and other kinds of living material.

EVIDENCE that stomach ulcers may result from diets lacking in vitamin A was presented by Dr. Ira A. Manville, of the University of Oregon Medical School. Dr. Manville reported that white rats fed a diet deficient in vitamin A developed stomach ulcers and erosions. Nearly two thirds of all the animals fed on diets that were deficient to various degrees in the vitamin showed these sores. As the vitamin deficiency became more severe, the number of animals affected became greater until nearly 100 per cent. were found to have ulcers. Vitamin A, found in liver, butter, egg yolk, cheese, cod-liver oil, spinach and the leaves of plants, is necessary to promote normal growth. In its absence growth is stunted and a severe eye disease develops. This vitamin is also considered necessary for normal functioning of the mucous membrane of nose, throat and breathing apparatus, and urinary and gastro-intestinal tracts. In this connection it has been claimed that vitamin A will prevent colds.

THE warfare and strategy that goes on in the human body when the blue dye, methylene blue, is called in to fight poisonous cyanides was revealed in a report by Dr. William B. Wendel, of Washington University School of Medicine. Dr. Wendel's study showed that methylene blue can only win the fight for life against the poison when the dose of cyanide is not great. Successful use of the dye as antidote in a case of cyanide poisoning was reported last fall by Dr. J. C. Geiger, San Francisco director of public health. The antagonistic action of the dye for cyanides has been observed by a number of scientists. Mrs. Matilda M. Brooks, of the University of California, claims to have first suggested its use as an antidote in poisoning and suicide cases. Cyanides cause death by suffocation, since they interfere with the supply of oxygen to the tissues. Methylene blue fights cyanides by converting some of the oxygen-carrying hemoglobin of the blood into a new chemical compound, methemoglobin. This new compound is able to force the cyanide out of combat by uniting with it to form the chemical union, cyan-methemoglobin, which is harmless itself, and which keeps the cyanide from interfering with the vital, oxygen-carrying activity of the rest of the blood hemoglobin.

PROGRESS in the search for a new, safe morphine was reported by Dr. Nathan B. Eddy, of the University of Michigan. Dr. Eddy is engaged in research sponsored by the drug addiction committee of the National Research Council. The object of the research is to produce, if possible, a substitute for morphine which will have that drug's valuable pain-relieving and sleep-inducing qualities, but none of its dangerous habit-forming propensity. The morphine molecule consists of a number of chemical units arranged to form a series of rings. Among these two units, known as hydroxyl groups because they are made up of hydrogen and oxygen, are appended to the rings. At present, Dr. Eddy is trying to find which of the units is responsible for relieving pain, which for quieting nerves and inducing sleep, and which for the sense of well-being that leads to habit-formation. He reported that the two hydroxyl groups have opposite effects in the action of morphine in the body. One of them increases the pain-relieving and other useful properties of morphine, while the other hydroxyl group decreases the same properties.

## ITEMS

FINAL proof that the yellow fever mosquito, *Aedes aegypti*, can transmit a serious epidemic disease of horses and mules, popularly known as Kansas-Nebraska horse plague, has been obtained by Major R. A. Kelser, of the Veterinary Laboratory Division of the Army Medical School. The proof was obtained when a horse, on which infected mosquitoes had been feeding, developed symptoms of the disease and became seriously ill. A short time ago Major Kelser reported that the yellow fever mosquitoes had spread the disease among guinea-pigs, which implicated them as possible carriers of the disease among larger animals. At that time, however, the horse on which he had fed the infected mosquitoes had not yet developed the disease. Major Kelser's investigations also showed that the mosquito is not a mechanical carrier of the disease, but that the virus of the disease undergoes a change in the mosquito's body.

FEWER children are being killed by automobiles now than any time in the last ten years, according to statistics published by the Metropolitan Life Insurance Company. The decrease in the number of child automobile deaths began in 1930. "The year 1932 was the third successive year in which there had been a considerable drop in the death-rate of children from this cause." This gratifying reduction in automobile accident deaths of children is attributed to the safety campaigns that have been waged by schools, police departments, insurance companies and women's organizations. Along with the marked reduction in the number of child victims, there has been a decline in the total number of automobile deaths during 1932.

# SCIENCE NEWS

*Science Service, Washington, D. C.*

## THE PREVALENCE OF LEPROSY

"LEPROSY is increasing in many parts of the world by leaps and bounds." This startling declaration, made by Dr. O. E. Denny, director of the U. S. Marine Hospital at Carville, Louisiana, national leper home, needs some qualifying, Dr. Denny explained in a Science Service interview.

Dr. Denny discussed the leprosy problem at the meeting of the medical board and the advisory committee on research of the Leonard Wood Memorial, a fund supported by the American public and devoted to the study of the nature and treatment of leprosy.

The number of known cases of leprosy is increasing in many countries, according to Dr. Denny. In the United States, for example, each year more cases are discovered and segregated. But there are probably no more cases of the disease now than there were twenty-five years ago. The apparent increase, that is, the increase in reported cases, is due to the fact that doctors are learning more and more to recognize cases of leprosy and to diagnose it correctly.

In India, for instance, there were about 300,000 recognized lepers about fifty years ago. Now there are between one and three million recognized lepers in that country. Whether this enormous increase is real or is apparent and due to better diagnosis and reporting is not known. Probably the increase is only apparent.

In one or two countries there is an actual increase in leprosy. In South America, authorities are concerned over the situation. In Argentina, where there was no leprosy to speak of twenty-five years ago, it seems to be increasing in actual fact. A possible explanation may be that more and more remote mountain villages and their Indian inhabitants are coming into contact with the larger towns and with civilization. Leprosy is to some extent a disease of civilization, and it is being spread as commerce grows between the remote villages and the larger towns where a few cases of the disease exist and where the Indians may come in contact with it for the first time.

In the South Pacific, in one or two of the very small islands, leprosy also is increasing and here, too, Dr. Denny believes that the increase is a real one. The largest of these islands is Naru. The population of each is only about 100 or 200. Here, with a very small increase in population, there has been a very sharp increase in leprosy during the last ten years. Twenty-five years ago, there was no leprosy on these islands. Now physicians making medical inspections are finding it and reporting it in the medical journals. The situation is, however, not alarming.

## FUTURE RESEARCH ON FOOD AND DIGESTION

NEW goals for investigators to reach in their studies of food and its digestion were set by Professor Lafayette B. Mendel, of Yale University, at the closing session in Cincinnati of the Federation of American Societies for Experimental Biology.

Ten major problems in nutrition are awaiting solution, it appeared from Professor Mendel's remarks. These are:

1. The fate of the fats in the body. This foodstuff commonly constitutes one third of our daily food fuel intake, but no satisfactory or adequate balance sheet has ever been made to account for it all. Some is used for fuel, some is stored, some is excreted, but there is a missing fraction not yet accounted for.

2. The fate of the nitrogen-containing foods. The state of knowledge concerning these important foods, more familiarly known as proteins, is nearly as unsatisfactory as in the case of the fats.

3. An appraisal is needed of the relation of the minerals in the diet to such factors as vitamins and internal secretions.

4. The possible value of a number of pigmentary substances, such as chlorophyll, the green coloring matter of plants, needs to be investigated, now that another such substance, carotene, has been found important in connection with vitamin A.

5. Glandular foods, like liver, kidney and thymus, have a new significance in the diet since the discovery of their value in pernicious anemia, and they should be investigated further.

6. Further study of vitamins is required to complete our knowledge of these important factors.

7. The problem of alcohol as a food will probably be revived for further study.

8. Dropsy as a result of faulty diet presents a relatively new problem for investigation.

9. The rôle played by the organic acids of vegetables, such as citric, malic, tartaric and oxalic acids, which must be taken in considerable quantities in the ordinary diet, needs to be discovered. Vegetables themselves are claimed to have unique advantages in the diet. "Our knowledge of what actually happens to them chemically in the long reaches of the alimentary tract is woefully limited," according to Professor Mendel.

10. The way in which products of digestion are transported to other parts of the body deserves further scientific consideration.

In the future, scientific students of nutrition will solve problems such as these, which relate not so much to the composition of the foods we eat or to their effect on the body as to their actual fate in the chemical factories of the digestive tract.

## "UNSALTING" THE GREAT SALT LAKE

THE Great Salt Lake of Utah, remnant of the prehistoric Lake Bonneville, is at last to be put to some practical use.

Scientists and engineers have perfected a method for "unsalting" a great part of it, and then harnessing it for the production of electrical power. In its present state—seven times as salty as the sea—the lake is a dead loss in a very live world.

"Unsalting" the Great Salt Lake is not so impractical as it at first seems; the idea was, in fact, long ago advanced by the French engineer, Ferdinand de Lesseps, and it has been accepted as feasible after a series of detailed surveys and laboratory tests. The diking project involves these basic elements:

1. Diking off an initial area of 146 acres.
2. Providing sluiceways to insure continuous flow of water over the dikes.
3. Allowing sufficient time for displacement of brine by fresh water.

This last point is the problematical one. R. A. Hart, engineering expert of the Salt Lake Chamber of Commerce, has demonstrated to his own satisfaction that the initial area will be fresh in two years. Some investigators in Utah disagree with him.

The most difficult feature of the project is the erection of dikes sufficiently strong to stand the battering of the heavy water. The plan is for dikes of the earth-fill type, with a very gentle slope—about 15 to 1—and a maximum distance through the base of 500 feet.

Nature has already laid the main link in the dike system. This is Antelope Island, which lies in a north and south position just west of the eastern shore. From the extremities of this island will be built the dikes, one five and a half miles long, the other two and a half. Thus the embayed area will be fed by two or three streams which will—in time—displace the brine which to-day is unusable for steam power plants.

A million dollar loan for the project is being sought from the Reconstruction Finance Corporation.

## THE FLOOD SITUATION

FLOOD stages in rivers of East and South, following recent rainy weather over most of the country east of the Rockies, were reported in a summary of the flood situation given to Science Service by M. W. Hayes, of the U. S. Weather Bureau.

In New England, the Connecticut and the Merrimac were characterized as in "rather high flood"; the highest in several years.

The Ohio and some of its tributaries are up, though not so high as they were a short time ago. The Ohio itself is rising slightly, though still well below bank-full above the mouth of the Kentucky River; from there to Paducah, Kentucky, it is due to rise again to flood stage, though not so high as it did a month ago. The Wabash is at flood stage.

The Mississippi is falling slightly above the mouth of the Ohio; below that point it is still swollen with the recent flood, although the state of the lower river is not at all serious. An upper tributary, the Illinois River, is out of its banks. A lower tributary, the Yazoo, in the State of Mississippi, is quite high; it has established a record for this late in the season.

The James, in Virginia, and the Neuse, in North Carolina, are high, but their waters are receding.

The Missouri and other rivers of the Northwest are making no trouble at all just now. The Missouri, in fact, is at a relatively low stage.

## CELLOPHANE AND THREE-COLOR PHOTOGRAPHY

THREE-COLOR photography is making rapid strides toward perfection with the aid of that versatile material Cellophane.

In the photographic laboratory on the top floor of the Army Medical Museum, R. M. Reeve has been working quietly for almost a year on a color process using Cellophane sheets. The latest products of his experiment are pictures of flowers, people, scenery, diseased body tissues, all so natural in their colors that the photographs seem like fine and extraordinarily accurate water colors. The new photographic process may in some cases replace the work of water-color artists who copy scientific material.

The process is being perfected with a view to obtaining a government-owned patent. The cost of the process is reasonable.

To take the pictures panchromatic plates or films are exposed in the camera. One records the yellow color in the subject before the lens. Another film records greenish-blue. A third records red, which is really almost purple. At present, it is necessary to expose the three-colored films in succession. Mr. Reeve hopes eventually to perfect a tri-pack film which will "shoot" the three colors at once. Three prints are then made on correspondingly dyed Cellophane sheets. Each sheet has been impregnated with a different solution. While still wet, they are placed one over the other so that the picture coincides. The whole three-layered Cellophane picture is then fastened with adhesive to a paper backing and dried.

With all due care, Mr. Reeve says, film negatives taken separately sometimes turn out to be slightly different in size. In former three-color processes, this produced blurry outlines when the colors were assembled to make the picture. Cellophane, when wet, however, is flexible and can be stretched until the outlines coincide exactly.

The Cellophane films record very exactly the fine shadings of color in diseased tissue and other medical subjects. Photographs turned out by the new process are now being used at the Army Medical School in the form of colored lantern slides. Others have been placed on exhibit in the Army Medical Museum.

The Department of Agriculture is looking into the possibilities of the color picture for use in its exhibits and publications.

## FUEL CONSUMPTION

INCREASES in the efficiency of using coal and oil may prevent increases in the annual consumption of these fuels in the United States during the next twenty years, is pointed out by Professor W. T. Thom, Jr., of Princeton University, in commenting on a recent estimate of fuel consumption for the future, which postulated an approximate doubling of fuel consumption in the United States by 1950.

Pointing to the relatively small increases in the amount of fuel used to produce power and useful energy during the boom period culminating in 1929, Professor Thom stated that it seems entirely possible that, even if our national energy requirements increase, we may, nevertheless, be able to supply a growing demand for energy, without a corresponding increase in amount of fuel used, and possibly without any increase.

Commenting upon recent estimates of fuel consumption made by Professor W. Spencer Hutchinson, of the Massachusetts Institute of Technology, and August J. Breitenstein, Ashland, Pennsylvania, engineer, Professor Thom calls attention to the fact that really to be able to predict future fuel consumption, one must first be able to predict both the degree of prosperity which our domestic industry will enjoy, and how long the present business depression will last. As he explains, a period of acute trade depression fosters the introduction of radical departures in fuel saving economy as a means of cost-cutting. Such measures of fuel economy continue in use thenceforth, possibly causing a progressive reduction in the amount of fuel used, even while power output may be increasing.

In commenting on the use of population statistics as a basis for estimating our future national energy requirements, Dr. Thom further explains in a communication to the American Institute of Mining Engineers, that one may go astray by considering the population of the United States alone. With the free outflow of manufactured exports, our consuming population is to all intents and purposes greater than our national population, whereas, if prohibitive tariffs are in force against American goods seeking to enter other countries, then this foreign addition to our domestic energy-consuming population is unavailable and our fuel consumption is correspondingly lessened.

## ITEMS

AN increase in the number of meningitis cases throughout the country has been reported to the U. S. Public Health Service. Health officials see in the situation a possible problem for the forestry camps where large numbers of young men will be concentrated. In all mobilizations of young men heretofore there has always been an increase in meningitis. The only known precaution that can be taken to prevent an outbreak of the disease in these camps is to avoid crowding in the sleeping quarters. Reports from state health officers for the week ending April 8, gave a total of 92 cases of meningitis. The total was 69 for the corresponding week of 1932. Since the first of March the number of cases reported in 1933 has been greater than in the corresponding period of 1932. This may indicate the beginning of another outbreak of the disease or it may be due to the fact that the year 1932 was unusually healthy. The 1933 figures may be nearer to the usual ones for the prevalence of this disease.

THAT oxygen in three to four and one half times the usual percentage in the air mixture breathed during muscular work seems to offer no advantages is shown by experiments by Dr. Francis G. Benedict and Robert C. Lee, of the Nutrition Laboratory of the Carnegie Institution of Washington, reported before the meeting of the American Philosophical Society. Volunteers were used who breathed ordinary air containing 21 per cent. of oxygen during part of the tests, while the rest of the time they were supplied with air mixtures containing from 60 to 90 per cent. No significant alteration was found in the total oxygen consumption per minute for the same amount of work. Neither was there any change in the ratio of oxygen used to carbon dioxide exhaled, thus indicating no change in the character of the material burned in the body. Finally, the oxygen absorbed during the recovery periods after work remained unchanged.

FAINT radiations from the night sky, not perceptible to human eyes but detected and analyzed by the spectrograph, were termed "cosmic radiations of the sky" by Dr. V. M. Slipher, director of the Lowell Observatory at Flagstaff, Arizona, speaking before the society. The radiations extend throughout the spectrum from ultraviolet to deep infra-red, generally stronger in the longer wave-lengths. Other illuminations from the night sky intercepted by Dr. Slipher's instruments have included light from auroral displays and the brief morning and evening twilight solar stimulation in the high atmosphere.

WHY plants growing in bogs, where there is always plenty of water, should have thick, tough, leathery leaves protected against evaporation, resembling desert plants in this respect has long been a puzzle to botanists. Dr. Kurt Mothes, of the University of Halle, believes he has found a possible key in the lack of nitrogen in bog water and soil, rather than anything to do with the water relationship itself. He was struck by the fact that of all bog plants the sundews, which capture insects with the sticky fingers on their leaves and thereby get plenty of nitrogen, are the least desert-like in their appearance and structure. The same might be said of two groups of American insectivorous plants, the Venus flytrap and the pitcher plants. To test the possibilities of his hypothesis, Dr. Mothes grew tobacco plants, which normally are anything but desert-like, in culture solutions containing plenty of other mineral nutrients but lacking in nitrogen. They responded by developing thick, tough, leathery leaves, with small stomata or "breathing pores" and other characteristic structures of desert plants. The full technical discussion of Dr. Mothes' experiments is published in the *Biologisches Zentralblatt*.

MALARIA has been completely routed from the Italian province of Istria, at the head of the Adriatic, by a million and a quarter little American fishes, in a campaign that has lasted for seven years. Dr. Massimo Sella, Italian director of the Italo-German Institute of Marine Biology at Rovigno d'Istria, tells how. When the work was started seven years ago, he says, the prospects were downright dismal. In the region around Rovigno there were over 800 mosquito-breeding ponds, and 94 per cent. of the population showed symptoms of malaria. But every year some 200,000 of the American top-feeding minnow, species Gambusia, were dumped into some of the ponds, while the others were treated with Paris green. The "wigglers" were eaten by the little fish or killed by the poison. In 1927 there were still 147 ponds harboring mosquito larvae; in 1931 only 7; in 1932 none whatever. For the past two years no one in the region has shown clinical symptoms of malaria. The little American fish have scored another victory.

# SCIENCE NEWS

*Science Service, Washington, D. C.*

## THE ENERGY CONTAINED IN COSMIC RAYS

By Watson Davis, *Managing Editor*

Cosmic rays, totally unknown a few decades ago, are now recognized to comprise the greater portion of the radiant energy of the universe, Dr. Robert A. Millikan, of the California Institute of Technology, told the National Academy of Sciences at its annual meeting in Washington.

As the result of new researches with sounding balloons and airplanes this past year, Dr. Millikan and his associates have determined with great accuracy the way in which cosmic rays vary downward from nearly the top of the earth's atmosphere. The recent experimental results, combined with the findings of Dr. Millikan and other experimenters in past years, allow Dr. Millikan to conclude that the total radiant energy in our galaxy in the form of cosmic rays is nearly the same as that in all the other forms of radiation, such as light and heat emitted by stars.

In the immense spaces between the galaxies of stars the starlight and heat must diminish to a small amount of that found in our own Milky Way galaxy, but the cosmic radiation coming to the earth from far beyond our neighbor stars, from the depths of the universe, must be even greater in intensity in intergalactic space. In this way Dr. Millikan concludes that cosmic radiation forms the greater part of the radiant energy of the universe.

One of the sounding balloons launched by Dr. Millikan and Dr. I. S. Bowen reached a height at which only a half of one per cent. of the atmosphere's weight remained above it, equivalent to about 20 miles altitude (16 millimeters of mercury pressure). The cosmic ray electroscope record obtained was reliable up to nearly that height, to within about 92 per cent. of the top of the atmosphere. One other balloon flight, carrying the remarkably light, automatic instruments to great heights in the stratosphere, agreed closely with the record flight and the two checked closely the results of a similar sounding balloon ascension made at the same time (last summer) by the German physicist, Regener.

With a cosmic ray electroscope, devised by Dr. H. Victor Neher, which records accurately and automatically under the strenuous conditions of rushing auto, railroad train or airplane, measurements of cosmic ray intensity have been made at altitudes up to 29,000 feet, nearly six miles. U. S. Army bombers and pursuit planes carried the instruments aloft first without screening and second screened by a shield of lead of 10 centimeters' thickness at several localities in the United States and at Panama, while commercial planes were used in experiments 17 degrees below the equator in Peru.

The results of these airplane tests bring to light the fact that cosmic rays grow rapidly softer or less penetrating as altitude increases. This softening is so marked that more than 75 per cent. of the rays existing at altitudes of 25,000 feet have insufficient energy to penetrate four inches of lead. As Dr. Carl D. Anderson in Dr. Millikan's laboratory has measured the loss of energy of cosmic rays passing through lead, Dr. Millikan can conclude that more than three fourths of the cosmic rays at 25,000-foot altitudes have energies of less than 350,000,000 volts. But particles of this voltage can not penetrate more than half of the depth of the atmosphere, and Dr. Millikan concludes that the experiments furnish convincing proof that the cosmic rays found at low altitudes are certainly secondaries which are formed in the earth's atmosphere by collision with air atoms. Photographs taken by Dr. Anderson have caught the cosmic rays, which are non-ionizing and can not be photographed themselves, in the act of smashing atomic hearts and letting loose positively and negatively charged particles.

Dr. Millikan concludes that his researches present strong evidence that all but a small fraction of the cosmic rays observed at sea-level by cosmic ray counters and other devices used by other investigators are secondary rays produced within the earth's atmosphere.

Most of the cosmic rays, then, according to his interpretation, enter the atmosphere as photons or radiation-like light, x-rays or radium's gamma-rays, not as charged particles, like electrons or positrons. The new airplane experiments also lend support to Dr. Millikan's theory that the total cosmic ray curve is to be explained by not less than three and probably four or five cosmic ray bands, corresponding to different colors of light in the visible spectrum. Those rays that reach only the upper part of the atmosphere are, he finds, with energies less than some 75,000,000 volts.

Dr. Millikan's experiments were supported by funds of the Carnegie Corporation administered by the Carnegie Institution of Washington. In the sounding balloon experiments he had the full and effective cooperation of the U. S. Weather Bureau, and in the airplane test the equally effective cooperation of the U. S. Army Air Force and the Royal Canadian Air Force.

## RADIATION OF THE NIGHT SKY

The night sky glows with a faint light that seems to come from nowhere. It certainly is not made of scattered starlight, for it is richest in wave-lengths of the red and infra-red regions of the spectrum, whereas scattered starlight is poorest in exactly these rays. This sky radiation has been called the "cosmic radiation" of the night sky by Dr. V. M. Slipher, of the Lowell Observatory, Flagstaff, Arizona, who reported on his long study of the subject at the meeting in Washington of the American Geophysical Union.

This designation, however, should not be confused with the cosmic radiation proper, which consists of extremely penetrating rays or particles studied by Hess and Kolhoerster in Germany, and by Millikan, Compton and Swann in this country. The cosmic radiation proper almost certainly comes from outer space, whereas the sky rays studied by Dr. Slipher are almost as certainly the product of the earth's atmosphere, excited into faint luminescence by radiation from the sun.

Dr. Slipher's sky rays range through the entire gamut of wave-lengths from ultra-violet to infra-red, though some of the colors are stronger than others. He spoke of a prominent yellow line that appears in his spectrographic photographs, and of a green line due to glowing nitrogen that can be caught just before dawn and just after evening twilight but not at midnight. This line seems to be identical with the most prominent band of wave-lengths in the light of the aurora.

Dr. Slipher made his studies with a specially built instrument that enabled him to obtain spectrum photographs of five parts of the sky at the same time: the four points of the compass and directly overhead. Comparing these simultaneous photographs, he discovered that the sky near the horizon gives off radiations rich in red and infra-red rays, while at the zenith these are relatively feebler, though the violet rays in the visible spectrum are as strong there as elsewhere in the sky. This effect Dr. Slipher attributed to the greater density of the atmosphere near the earth's surface, which selects out the rays of longer wave-length and partially blocks the violet and ultra-violet rays.

Dr. Slipher was called to England to receive a medal of the Royal Society just before his paper was to be read, so that the actual presentation of his paper was made by a colleague.

## EFFECTS OF EARTHQUAKES ON WATERS OF THE EARTH

STRANGE tricks that earthquakes play with rivers, lakes and subterranean waters of the earth were described to the American Geophysical Union by Captain N. H. Heck, of the U. S. Coast and Geodetic Survey.

Earthquakes often cause fountains of water or liquid mud to spurt from the ground. They sometimes change the course of subterranean streams, or the quantity of water flowing in them. In the earthquake that occurred in New York State in 1929, the Attica reservoir filled, although there had been no rain, while in a region not far distant the wells went dry.

Earthquakes often cause strange behavior by rivers and other bodies of surface water. The famous New Madrid quake in the lower Mississippi Valley over a century ago caused the great stream to flow backwards for a time, and the disturbance was followed by the formation of several entirely new lakes that are still in existence. Earthquakes may dam up streams to form lakes, or they may break down natural dams and release floods or mud flows. Some of the most disastrous effects of recent earthquakes in interior China were due to the jarring loose of masses of watersoaked fine earth, causing terrific landslides.

Water, in its turn, has effects on earthquakes. Some of the strangest, and to scientists the most puzzling, of earthquake phenomena are the so-called gravity waves of earthquakes, waves that travel visibly along the surface at express-train speeds, though they are very much slower at that than the waves that are felt but are too swift to be seen. These gravity waves are much affected in their intensity and velocity by the amount of water held by the soil through which they move. Captain Heck recommended a thorough study of the rate of wave travel through water-soaked earth as a problem promising both theoretical and practical results in the science of earthquakes.

## THE EARTH'S CORONA

THE earth, like the sun, has a corona—a luminous gaseous envelope extending far out into space. Its existence has been demonstrated by studies of the aurora borealis, or northern lights, Professor Lars Vegard, of the University of Oslo, Norway, told the American Meteorological Society at its meeting in Washington.

The earth's corona, however, shows some marked differences from the sun's. The sun's corona, so far as we know, is generated by the sun's own power; the earth's is a product of the action of the sun on gases in the earth's outer atmosphere. Furthermore, the earth's corona is decidedly eccentric, being far more extensive on the side of the earth nearest the sun than it is anywhere else.

Auroral displays have been measured at heights of from 70 to 700 or 800 kilometers (43 to 490 or 550 miles) above the surface of the earth. Spectroscopic studies of their light indicate that the glow is due mostly to electrically excited nitrogen gas, which apparently exists at considerable density even at those great heights.

"To explain this fact," the speaker continued, "we assume that in the auroral region the atmospheric matter is brought to high altitudes through the effect of electrical forces, which result from the photoelectric action of the sun's rays of short wave-length."

Singularly enough, there are no spectrographic lines indicating the presence of the light gases, helium and hydrogen, at these elevations; or at most they are exceedingly faint and feeble. This runs quite counter to the assumption often made that layers of these "balloon gases" float on the top of the earth's atmosphere. On the contrary, all the gases in the atmosphere seem to be thoroughly mixed.

Auroral light comes from rather chilly sources, though they are not so intensely cold as we are sometimes prone to think everything must be in the upper air. By comparing their spectra with those of laboratory light sources at known temperatures, Professor Vegard reached the conclusion that auroral light centers are active at temperatures about 30 degrees below zero Centigrade, or 22 degrees below zero Fahrenheit.

## HEAVY WATER

A BATTERY of electrolytic cells for the production of heavy water and hydrogen of mass 2 was announced to the American Philosophical Society by Professor Hugh S. Taylor and Henry Eyring, of Princeton University.

With this battery of 270 units each holding 200 cubic centimeters of potassium hydroxide solution it has been found possible in somewhat over seven days to concentrate by electrolysis the heavy hydrogen present in twenty-five gallons of old alkali solutions which have been used for a period of years as a source of electrolytic hydrogen and oxygen. In this way the heavy hydrogen has been concentrated to yield about three quarters of a glassful of water containing 7 per cent. of the heavy hydrogen. A weekly production on this scale can now be maintained at Princeton.

The further enrichment of this water to yield the 100 per cent. pure heavy isotope of hydrogen of mass 2, or water of mass 1.1, is being effected by a combination of further electrolysis coupled with a new process of fractionation of the hydrogen isotopes from gas absorbed on gas-mask charcoal at the temperature of liquid air. It has recently been shown by Taylor, Gould and Bleakney that this method can secure a several fold enrichment of the hydrogen in a single operation.

The hydrogen of mass 2 produced at Princeton will be employed to trace the differences in speeds of reaction of the light and heavy isotopes at surfaces and with various gases. In this way fundamental advances in our knowledge of the speed of chemical processes are expected.

The water already attained represents a two thousand-fold enrichment of the heavy water and it is calculated that 150 gallons of ordinary water must be decomposed to yield the residual ¾ glassful of water exhibited at Philadelphia.

## CANCER HOUSE DISPROVED STATISTICALLY

Do "cancer houses" exist? "No!" is the emphatic answer of two French statisticians who have recently reported their investigations to the French Academy of Medicine. Their names are Auguste Lumière and Paul Vigne, and the town whose cancer death-rate they have investigated house by house is Lyon.

Here, in the course of 20 years, there were 6,703 deaths from cancer exclusive of those occurring in hospitals and nursing homes. The number of houses in Lyon was 23,258. Were the 6,703 deaths evenly distributed throughout these houses, or was their distribution so uneven that chance alone could not explain the frequency of cancer deaths in certain houses?

It was ascertained that there were as many as 18,231 houses in which there had been no death from cancer in the 20-year period. There were 3,869 in each of which there had been one cancer death, and 953 with two cancer deaths each. At the extreme end of this list were two houses in each of which there had been as many as 7 deaths, and one in which there had been 8 deaths.

Were these latter houses really cancer houses, possessing certain sinister properties responsible for these deaths? Or was the accumulation of cancer deaths just an accident? Finding a correct answer to these questions was not only of considerable academic and scientific interest, but also of some financial importance to the owners and tenants of the suspected houses.

As the number of persons living in each house was not available for statistical study, the answer to this question had to be sought indirectly by the following means: A study was made of the numbers of births, marriages and deaths from all causes in the same period and town. All three were found to be distributed throughout the houses of Lyon in the same apparently irregular manner as were the deaths from cancer.

Now, no one has yet had the Gilbertian fantasy to suggest the existence of birth or marriage houses endowed with peculiar properties which add to the fertility of nations or their matrimonial rates. And so long as cancer deaths are distributed throughout the houses of a community with the impartial irrelevance observed in the behavior of babies and brides and bridegrooms, no one need dread renting a house because it has a reputation for being a cancer house.

## ITEMS

THE rate at which cosmic rays ionize, or electrically charge, molecules of three atmospheric gases has been determined by Dr. W. F. G. Swann, of the Bartol Research Foundation. Dr. Swann reported on his researches before the meeting of the American Philosophical Society. Dr. Swann arranged two cylinders, which could be filled with gas at a pressure of seven atmospheres, or 105 pounds per square inch. Electrical connections were arranged so that the "kick" of each molecule as it received a charge from a cosmic ray would be registered. Per centimeter (0.39 inch), the rays charged 145 molecules of oxygen, 150 of nitrogen and 200 of argon.

LIQUID helium and superconducting lead were produced at the new cryogenic laboratory of the California Institute of Technology just six months after the beginning of construction and a year after the project was started. Professor A. Goetz found that a thirty-foot coil of fine lead wire suddenly lost all trace of electrical resistance because of its immersion in liquid helium. It remained in this superconducting state for twenty minutes while he and Dr. Alfred B. Focke, research fellow, congratulated each other that the apparatus functioned perfectly as designed and needs no modification. Last December liquid hydrogen was produced as the new laboratory's first step toward liquid helium. Helium liquefies at 450 degrees Fahrenheit below zero.

SENDING up balloons and airplanes with observers and instruments to ask why the stratosphere over the equator lets out less of the earth's heat than escapes through the atmospheric envelope in the polar regions was advocated at the meeting of the American Geophysical Union in Washington, by W. J. Humphreys, of the U. S. Weather Bureau. He called attention to the anomaly that the earth loses less heat to outer space over the tropics than it does over the polar areas; less also from rainy areas than from those of prevailingly fair weather. Why this should be the case nobody knows as yet, and this gap in our scientific knowledge Professor Humphreys presented as a challenge to researchers in meteorology. He also proposed barometric measurements from high mountain tops to determine whether the temperature of the atmosphere as a whole varies with differences in solar radiation. An increase by as much as three degrees Centigrade, he said, would cause a 2.5-millimeter increase in the barometer reading.

# SCIENCE NEWS

*Science Service, Washington, D. C.*

## TOXIN TREATMENT IN THE PREVENTION OF PNEUMONIA

Pneumonia attacks may be warded off by hypodermic injections of the poison produced by the pneumonia germ, it appears from studies by Dr. Arthur F. Coca, professor of immunology at the Cornell University Medical College. He reported his investigations of this germ to the American Association of Immunologists meeting this week in Washington.

"The pneumococcus produces a substance which is highly poisonous for human beings but much less so for lower animals," he explained. Apparently this toxin may be the important injurious agent of the pneumococcus, in which case Dr. Coca's experiments indicate that it will be easy to give people resistance or immunity to pneumonia as is now done for smallpox, typhoid fever and diphtheria. When this poison or toxin is injected into human beings, an antitoxin is formed in the blood which enables the individual to resist the toxin, giving him what physicians call immunity to it. Two injections of toxin produced immunity in two thirds of the susceptible children within three weeks. Skin tests of patients who were recovering from pneumonia showed that their blood serum has been found to neutralize the toxin.

## NEW DISEASE CAUSED BY A YEAST-LIKE ORGANISM

A case of a new and unique disease, caused by a yeast-like organism, was reported by Drs. G. H. Hansmann and J. R. Schenken, of Iowa City, at the opening session on May 9 of the Washington meeting of the American Association of Pathologists and Bacteriologists. The patient was a white man, forty-three years old at the time of his death, according to the doctor's records. For the last sixteen years of his life he had suffered from a refractory skin ailment. This first appeared on the skin back of his knees in 1916. By 1929 the entire skin was involved. The ailment consisted of a scaly inflammation, underneath which the skin was somewhat thickened and reddened. During 1929 the skin became more reddened and thickened and cracked easily. In June of 1932 hard elevated spots, something like pimples, appeared. Late in July the patient developed a high fever with signs of pleurisy, and died on August 7.

Examination of one of the elevated spots from the skin and one of the lymph nodes, which had become enlarged, showed that both contained a small organism which appeared as a small yeast. This same organism was also found in the lungs and adrenal glands. Guinea-pigs, rabbits, rats and dogs develop the same sort of skin disease when infected with this organism. The yeast-like organism causing the disease is smaller than any heretofore described and probably belongs in the Oidium group. The character and distribution of the lesions in man are unlike any other disease.

## THE CAUSE OF ARTHRITIS

A certain type of arthritis, known to physicians as hypertrophic or degenerative arthritis, results from the "wear and tear" of increasing age and from repeated injury to the joints, Drs. Granville A. Bennett and Walter Bauer, of Harvard Medical School, reported at the medical meetings held this week in Washington.

These investigators do not agree that the condition is the result of some inflammatory process. They even found marked changes in the joints, indistinguishable from those of hypertrophic arthritis, in individuals who do not have important symptoms of joint disease. The word arthritis, they pointed out, is probably not the correct one to use for this particular condition, if, as their investigations show, it is nothing more than the degenerative joint changes due to the wear and tear of increasing age. Earlier studies had shown quite clearly that the cartilage of joints has a very feeble, limited ability to regenerate or renew itself. Repeated injury to displaced knee joints did result in certain animals in very marked changes like those seen in human hypertrophic arthritis.

Because of these findings, it was decided to see what changes might take place in human joints subjected to unusual use or repeated injury. For the first part of the problem they studied a single joint which had been subjected to repeated injury or constant use, comparing it with the opposite joint which had not had such use or injury. They found that such injury or constant use was in itself enough cause for marked degenerative changes of the joint.

In a second investigation, they collected and examined, with x-ray and microscope, human knee joints representing various ages from the first to the ninth decade of life. The owners of these joints had never, so far as could be determined, had symptoms of joint disease. With each succeeding decade in life beyond the second, that is, after age twenty, increasing degenerative changes in the joint were seen. The changes were identical to those commonly considered characteristic of degenerative or hypertrophic arthritis.

Finally, the studies showed that arteriosclerosis, popularly known as hardening of the arteries, was not an important factor as the cause of this disease.

## CHRONIC ARTHRITIS

A cheerful, optimistic temperament is a great asset for the patient fighting rheumatoid arthritis, Dr. Russell L. Cecil, of New York City, said in a discussion of the prognosis in chronic arthritis at the Washington meeting of the American Clinical and Climatological Association. The prospects of recovery from chronic arthritis, sometimes popularly known as rheumatism, depend primarily on the type of arthritis from which the patient is suffering.

In the case of osteo-arthritis, the characteristic degenerative changes are permanent and tend to progress slowly. The symptoms resulting from these changes, however, can usually be ameliorated or entirely cleared up by proper treatment. The chances for recovery from rheumatoid arthritis are hard to determine since there are no adequate statistics as to the percentage of permanent recoveries. "The disease never menaces life," Dr. Cecil stated, "but the danger of serious deformity and crippling always exists, especially in neglected cases."

It is in this type of arthritis that the cheerful, optimistic temperament was said to be a great asset. Young people respond to treatment better than elderly patients. Those who have an acute onset seem to have a better chance than those whose symptoms come on insidiously. Much depends on the joints involved, the knees, hips and back offering the greatest difficulty. Finally, the ability and the disposition of the patient to devote himself zealously to the régime and treatment prescribed by his physician is of the greatest importance in forecasting the chances of recovery.

## CANCER CELLS

THE size of the cell nucleolus is the distinguishing feature by which a cancer cell may be told from normal cells, according to a report by Drs. William Carpenter MacCarty and Eva Haumeder, of the Mayo Clinic, before the American Association for Cancer Research. A method of distinguishing between normal and cancer cells has long been sought. It is not always possible to tell from its gross appearance whether or not a tumor is malignant.

Surgeons about to remove a tumor generally send a small piece of it down to the hospital laboratory for diagnosis. The pathologist must, within two or three minutes, cut a paper-thin sliver from the piece of tumor tissue, fix it on a glass slide, stain it, examine it under the microscope, and report to the surgical team waiting in the operating room whether or not the tissue is cancerous. But even when examined in this way, cancer cells sometimes look so much like certain types of normal, non-malignant cells that it is extremely difficult to make an accurate diagnosis.

Drs. MacCarty and Haumeder have found that the area of the nucleolus in the cancer cell is much greater than the area of normal cell nucleoli. They conclude that the cancer cell has at least one differential characteristic and that this must be used by those who expect to reduce the mortality from cancer. The nucleolus is a very small but important part of a cell. For their investigations, a special method of measuring this small area was devised.

## THE PIGMENTED HAIRY MOLE

THE pigmented, hairy mole appears to be a link in the evolutionary chain between the hairy touch organs of man and other mammals and the colored touch organs of the amphibian-reptilian type of animal, such as the water-snake. In other words, the mole on your neck is closely related to the dark-colored bumps on snake skin. This evolutionary theory was presented by Drs. George F. Laidlaw and Margaret R. Murray, of Columbia University, at the Washington meeting of the American Association of Pathologists and Bacteriologists.

The pattern and structure of these moles does not resemble anything known in normal skin of mammals and it is a faithful reproduction of the colored, elevated and innervated spots of the amphibia and reptiles. In the course of evolution, these colored tactile spots of the snakes and amphibia were replaced in mammals by hair follicles and by mammalian touch cells. In its hair follicle, the mole is mammalian, but in its coloring, elevation and the arrangement of cells and nerves, it is reptilian.

The evolutionary theory explains many obscure points about moles, Dr. Laidlaw said. For instance, it explains why pigmented moles are rare in hairy mammals, such as cats and dogs. Their skin has specialized far beyond human skin in the production of hair. In its relative absence of hair, human skin is closer to the ancestral snake skin, and consequently, as in its pigmented moles, it bears more vestiges of former reptilian life spent half in water and half in air. "Port wine" marks may be explained as vestiges of the tangle of veins of an amphibian skin, dating from the stage when man's ancestors breathed through their skins.

## INHERITED RESISTANCE TO INFECTIOUS DISEASES

STUDIES with mice at the Rockefeller Institute, New York, show that resistance to disease is a hereditary trait like color of eyes, hair or skin. Strains of mice highly susceptible to or highly resistant to a given disease may be segregated by selective breeding, Dr. Leslie T. Webster reported at the Washington meeting of the American Association of Pathologists and Bacteriologists.

Starting with a strain of mice 37 per cent. susceptible to mouse typhoid, he selected lines 85 per cent. and 15 per cent. susceptible, respectively. The 85 per cent. susceptible lines were descendants of mice highly susceptible to mouse typhoid, while the 15 per cent. susceptible descended from relatively resistant mice. Resistance factors are dominant, and not sex-linked, Dr. Webster found.

Mice from strains resistant to disease were heavier but not more fertile than the susceptible mice. The tissues throughout the bodies of these resistant mice seemed less sensitive to the organism causing mice typhoid than did the body tissues of susceptible mice. This suggested to Dr. Webster that the hereditary factors giving resistance to disease exercise general rather than local influence in the animal body. These hereditary factors concerned with resistance or susceptibility to disease can operate against a number of but not necessarily all harmful agents. So that an animal, possibly a man or woman, may be born with ability to resist attacks of a number of diseases, but still may be susceptible to a few infectious diseases.

## THE INVASION OF THE BODY BY DISEASE GERMS

THE extent to which disease germs can invade the body depends on the amount of inflammation they cause at the site of their entry, it appears from investigations reported by Dr. Valy Menkin, of Harvard University Medical School, to the American Association of Pathologists and Bacteriologists. By injecting a dye into the body at a place where bacteria had previously been injected, Dr. Menkin found that staphylococci, the organisms that are found in boils, limit the extent of their invasion to a very small area. They do this by causing a rapid inflammation which results in mechanical obstruction of the draining lymphatics, the avenues by which the disease germs, or other foreign matter, might continue their invasion of the body.

The pneumococcus and the fearsome streptococcus, on the other hand, do not cause such rapid obstruction of these avenues. In the case of the streptococcus, Dr. Menkin found the avenues are open for as long as two days. This gives the disease germs a chance to get far in their invasion of the body and probably accounts for the serious effects on the whole system of infection with these organisms. Dr. Menkin was able to determine the speed with which the germs could invade the body by watching the rate of progress of the dye which invaded the body just after the organisms had been introduced. When the dye could not proceed any farther, he concluded that sufficient inflammation had occurred to obstruct the path for the organisms also.

## ITEMS

DISCOVERY of bacteria belonging to the Brucella group, which cause undulant fever, in diseased vertebrae of swine was reported by Drs. William H. Feldman and Carl Olson, Jr., of the Mayo Clinic, at the Washington meeting of the American Association of Pathologists and Bacteriologists. The animals did not show any signs of disease at the time of slaughter and the organs were healthy-looking. This discovery gives further evidence that swine are a dangerous source of undulant fever infection for farmers, packing house employees, retail butchers, housewives and others who handle uncooked pork.

WHEN the moon partly entered the earth's shadow last September, as seen from Europe, the shaded part reflected less than a thousandth as much violet light as the ordinary full moon, but it sent back to us about one six hundredth as much infra-red light as the uneclipsed portion. This was determined by photographs taken by Dr. R. L. Waterfield, and just announced to the British Astronomical Association. The earth's atmosphere bends some of the sun's light around into its shadow, and for that reason the shadow, when it falls on the moon and produces a lunar eclipse, is not entirely dark. Because the longer waves of the red and infra-red light pass through the earth's atmosphere more readily than the shorter blue and violet waves, the eclipsed moon usually has a ruddy color. Dr. Waterfield's data show how much of this light is so refracted into the shadow.

AN ingenious robot detective that will "frisk" a man for concealed weapons, register the fact that it has found him and takes his photograph, all without his knowledge, was recently described in an address by O. H. Caldwell, editor of *Electronics*. The device is built around an electron tube. It can be so delicately adjusted that while it will react to a mass of metal as large as a revolver, it will ignore smaller metallic objects which law-abiding men usually have about them, such as watches, coins and bunches of keys. Another device described by Mr. Caldwell counts persons passing through an entrance, no matter how fast they come or how much massed in groups. It does not overlook odd sizes and shapes: when Mr. Caldwell tried to fool it by hiding behind an umbrella as he passed it, he got counted anyway.

THE cyanide bath now widely used for copper plating of steel can be replaced by a new non-poisonous electroplating solution developed by Dr. Colin G. Fink and Chaak Y. Wong, of Columbia University, and reported to the Electrochemical Society meeting in Montreal. A complex copper salt, chemically known as disodium diaquodioxalatocupriate, is used in the new bath, along with sodium sulphate and boric acid. The new method will be available for use in large automatic plating installations where strip steel, standard steel parts, etc., are coated with copper as the first step to other coating. A satisfactory copper deposit is obtained in only one minute with a low electrical current density with the new "oxalato" bath.

MORE progress has been made in the manufacture of lubricating oils during the past few years than in the preceding thirty, Dr. Gustav Egloff, petroleum chemist, stated in an address before the Society of Chemical Industry in New York on May 12. This progress has been brought about by the requirements of the high-pressure motors needed by high-speed airplanes, automobiles and motor boats. New extreme-pressure lubricants have been developed, made up of blends of petroleum oils, vegetable or animal oils and sulphur. Crude oils for lubricants are carefully selected and improvements in the refining process have been made for this particular demand.

A KATYDID'S knees, which are that creature's own peculiar "ears," have given men the novel experience of listening in on that insect's world of sound. The story of how scientists have tapped the hearing circuit of katydids and crickets by placing electrodes against the knees of the insects, amplifying the responses picked up, and listening in on these in an ordinary telephone receiver, was related to the meeting of the New York Branch of the American Psychological Association by Drs. E. G. Wever and C. W. Bray, of Princeton University. The resulting sound was always a sort of "shushing" noise, regardless of the source of the sound. Human speech lost all characteristic qualities except the rhythm, which was preserved. But the katydid is apparently deaf to the ordinary sounds of our world and hears principally those that are beyond the reach of human ears. Sounds of frequency below 800 cycles produced no response even when very loud. But the higher frequencies, even up to 45,000 cycles per second, were picked up. The limit of man's hearing is usually about 20,000 cycles—the shrillest note of the peanut whistle.

# SCIENCE NEWS

*Science Service, Washington, D. C.*

## NEW HORMONES FROM THE PITUITARY GLAND

NEW hormones from the pituitary gland, some just discovered and others not yet found but predicted, were described at the Congress of American Physicians and Surgeons at the recent Washington meeting.

One of these new hormones is an entirely new substance, different from any other obtained from the pituitary gland, according to an announcement made by Dr. Herbert M. Evans, who is working at the Rockefeller Institute, New York City. This substance greatly increases the effect of one of the female sex hormones and apparently has a sex-stimulating effect of its own. But it is so new that Dr. Evans was not yet ready to discuss its significance. Another new pituitary hormone apparently presides over the vitally important cortex of the adrenal glands.

When the pituitary, by a very delicate operation, is removed from its protected location in the center of the head, the cortex of the adrenal gland wastes away. Without this part of the adrenal gland, or the hormone it produces, cortin, life can not go on. A certain extract of the pituitary gland, however, restores to normal the adrenal cortex that had wasted away upon removal of the pituitary gland.

Dr. Evans stated that if the research of the next few months shows this pituitary extract to be distinct from all the other pituitary hormones, it will be the new adrenalotropic hormone of the pituitary. The relation of this pituitary-adrenal situation to the adrenal cortical hormone essential for life is not yet clear.

Another dramatic development of the anterior pituitary story is the relation between this gland and the body's use of sugar. Dr. B. A. Houssay, of Buenos Aires, showed that the death which usually occurs soon after the pancreas is removed either can be prevented or averted for a long time if the pituitary gland is removed at the same time as the pancreas. The latter organ is the one that contains the insulin-producing islands of Langerhans. When this organ does not produce enough insulin, diabetes follows.

Now Dr. Evans and his associates at the University of California have found that a true diabetes can be produced in dogs merely by giving them a certain extract of the pituitary gland. This together with the work of Houssay and other investigators seems to establish the fact that there is a relation between the pituitary gland and the body's use of sugar. Dr. Evans and associates are now at work on the task of distinguishing this possible new hormone, the diabetogenic hormone, from the others of the pituitary gland.

The tendency toward the coinage of new pituitary hormones is being vigorously resisted by Dr. Evans and by other scientific workers. It would have been preferable, he said, to have considered many of the effects he described as shared by the two or three hormones now so well established as coming from this portion of the pituitary gland. At the present time four substances can be considered as separate hormones endowed with specific effects. These are the growth hormone, the gonadotropic or sex hormone, the lactogenic hormone and the thyreotropic hormone which has recently been shown to have a profound influence on the thyroid gland.

The chemistry of these pituitary hormones was discussed by Dr. J. B. Collip, of McGill University. Their application in the treatment of disease in women was discussed by Dr. Emil Novak, of the Johns Hopkins Medical School.

## ONE-CELLED ANIMALS GROWN ON AN INORGANIC DIET

ANIMALS feeding and growing new generations of themselves, on a wholly inorganic diet of a type hitherto considered suitable only for plants equipped with the green synthesizing pigment chlorophyll, have been reared in the zoological laboratory of the Johns Hopkins University by Professor S. O. Mast and Dr. D. M. Pace.

The animals were the one-celled primitive species known as *Chilomonas paramecium.* They were "planted" in a sterile culture medium containing sodium acetate, ammonium chloride, magnesium sulphate and potassium phosphate. Under normal conditions the animals reproduce rapidly by division into two parts, and they usually contain relatively large quantities of starch and fat. In the culture solution they gave rise to 3.4 new generations a day. When sodium silicate was added their reproduction rate went up to 3.9 generations a day.

When the solution was made up minus the organic salt, sodium acetate, the reproduction rate went on at the same level for three or four days, but then the animals died. But in the same totally inorganic solution with a heavy increase in carbon dioxide in the air over it—20 per cent. instead of the normal .3 per cent.—growth and reproduction went on indefinitely and specimens produced were well filled with starch and fat.

A hint of the cause of death when both the acetate and the carbon dioxide were low is contained in the fact that under these conditions the individual animals are very small, containing little starch and fat. Death under these conditions is therefore probably due to starvation.

For some unknown reason, the silicate salt seems to be necessary in the all-inorganic culture solution. If it is omitted, the animal divides a few times and then dies. Silicon is not usually an indispensable element to either plants or animals. The Johns Hopkins investigators suggest that in this case it probably acts as a catalyst, that is, as an agent for producing chemical transformations without itself taking part in them.

The results obtained, they state in conclusion, indicate that only eight chemical elements are necessary: nitrogen, carbon, hydrogen, oxygen, potassium, magnesium, phosphorus and sulphur. But they hold that traces of a number of other elements are probably also necessary.

## THE PRODUCTION OF HELIUM

Chemical evidence of the production of helium gas from paraffin and similar carbon-hydrogen compounds, by bombardment with the mixed radiation from thorium is adduced by Professor Fritz Paneth and his associate, Dr. P. L. Günther, of the University of Königsberg, and reported in a letter to *Nature*. The rays given off by thorium B and thorium C themselves contain some helium in the form of alpha particles, but after passing through paraffin, there is a surplus of helium amounting sometimes to 1000 per cent.

Helium is one of the "rare" gases, although it is now used to fill airships. It is at present obtained mostly from natural gas in America, which country has practically a monopoly on its production.

A practical method for the manufacture of helium would be of great commercial value, but the method described by Professor Paneth and his associate can not as yet be used for this purpose. The amounts they obtained were very small and were detected only by improved methods of analysis.

Nevertheless, their experiments are extremely important because this is the first indication that the transmutation of elements may be effected in amounts large enough to be chemically detectable. Until now, proofs of artificial transmutation depended upon the physical detection of single atomic destructions, observed as scintillations, or by electrical methods. Only when the new atoms formed were expelled with a large amount of energy could the transmutation be detected by these physical methods.

## SOUND WAVES AND MOLECULES

Recent investigations carried out in the University of California at Los Angeles suggest that the excessive absorption of sound in air of certain humidities is due to collisions between oxygen and water molecules. Professor Vern O. Knudsen described, at the recent meeting of the Acoustical Society of America, the Los Angeles experiments, in which Dr. H. O. Kneser, visiting physicist from the University of Marburg, cooperated.

Sound travels freely through chemically dried air, particularly at low temperatures, according to the electrical recording instruments of the California laboratory. Perhaps this accounts for the common opinion that audibility is keen on a clear, cold night. The introduction of small quantities of moisture promptly damps off the sound, especially tones of high pitch. Peculiarly, this phenomenon does not occur when pure nitrogen is substituted for the air, in spite of the fact that air is nearly 80 per cent. nitrogen. A shift to pure oxygen in the experiment reveals this latter gas as the guilty party. But oxygen alone is rather ineffective. Water vapor must also be present to affect the sound waves.

Drs. Knudsen and Kneser find their experimental records in agreement with the theory that the water molecules catalyze, or inspire oxygen molecules to pick up sound waves, convert them into heat or other motion, and thus destroy the sound. The extent to which all this occurs varies greatly with the frequency or pitch of the sound. Peculiar results may thus turn up. For example, the consonants in spoken words, which in general are of high frequency, are damped off more than the vowels of low pitch. Or in the symphony orchestra concert, if the humidity is at a certain value—not too high or too low—the message from the piccolo gets lost before it gets to the rear of the hall. Thus arises one more good argument for the new art of air-conditioning in public buildings.

More important, possibly, than the acoustic applications lies the possibility of interpreting molecular chemical reactions from the behavior of sound waves. Heretofore the vibrational responses of atoms have been supposed to require the enormous frequency values of light—whence the modern science of spectroscopy. Now it appears that even sound waves, counting but a few score or a few hundred per second, have a definite relation to intra-molecular forces. Preliminary experiments by Dr. Knudsen on ammonia, hydrogen sulfide and other gases show decided variations in behavior of the different chemical species. Thus we have a new mode of attack on the age-old mystery of molecular composition and the behavior of objects too small to be seen individually.

## THE WINTER WHEAT CROP

Winter wheat in the United States will be a short crop this year, according to the U. S. Crop Report for May. The estimated yield will be 337,485,000 bushels, as compared with 464,151,000 bushels in 1932, and a yearly average of 539,436,000 for the five-year period 1926–1930. This represents a decrease of 27 per cent. from the 1932 figure, and of 43 per cent. from the five-year average.

This is due partly to a decrease in total acreage and partly to a decline in yield per acre. This year's crop will come from 27,096,000 acres, as compared with 33,656,000 acres in 1932 and 28,560,000 acres for the 1926–1930 period. The yield per acre is expected to be 12.5 bushels, as against 13.7 for 1932 and 14.7 for the five-year average.

Figures for spring wheat are still fragmentary, because the wet spring has interfered with sowing. The spring wheat crop may also be below average in both acreage and per-acre yield. Foreign winter wheat acreage in 24 northern hemisphere countries is reported as slightly below last year's sowings, though a little above the 1931 figures. However, inasmuch as Russian wheat plantings are still largely an uncertain quantity, nothing very definite can be forecast about foreign wheat production.

The Food Research Institute at Stanford University has been conducting a survey of the wheat situation, and has a report in preparation which will be issued within a few days.

## GORILLA WITH AN EXCEPTIONAL BRAIN

What appears to be in many respects the "best" animal brain ever studied has recently been given an exhaustive examination by Dr. C. J. Connolly, of the department of psychology of the Catholic University of

America. His report was made to the Smithsonian Institution.

The brain studied by Dr. Connolly is that of a three-year-old mountain gorilla, which died in the National Zoological Park a few months ago. It was turned over to Dr. Connolly because he has made a specialty of comparative cerebral anatomy.

The brain of this little gorilla, which weighed only forty pounds at his prime, was larger than the brains of many adult gorillas which have been studied, and indeed is one of the largest great-ape brains on record, in spite of its late owner's extreme youth. It is the first brain of a mountain gorilla studied in detail; all other gorilla brains which have been examined were those of the coast gorilla subspecies.

The brain weighed 466.6 grams, a little over a pound. The average weight of the brains of six adult female coast gorillas reported by Dr. Connolly was 379.3 grams, about three quarters of a pound. The average brain weight of three young male coast gorillas, comparable in age, was only 318.3 grams.

If the gorilla's brain grows at the same rate as that of a human being, this baby mountain gorilla, had he lived, would eventually have had a brain weighing more than 600 grams. The lightest normal human brain weighs about 1,100 grams. If the assumption of an eventual 600-gram adult brain-weight for the male mountain gorilla is correct, this represents substantially more than half the human brain-weight; and hitherto apes have been allowed less than half. The mountain gorilla may therefore set a new record for animal brains.

However, Dr. Connolly points out that this estimate may be upset by other factors; it is even possible, he says, that the little three-year-old gorilla may have had as heavy a brain as he would ever have possessed had he lived to full growth.

The brain is described as "typically anthropoid." The cerebellum, which is concerned with balance and muscular coordination in general, is relatively massive, as in all ape brains. The cerebrum, where the higher sense organs have their centers, and which seems to be the seat of consciousness and thinking, has a relatively high development, distinctly in advance of the coast gorilla brains examined. Dr. Connolly found a rich pattern of convolutions, especially in the frontal lobe, which some authorities believe most closely associated with intelligence.

In spite of his seemingly exceptional brain, however, the gorilla was in life no ape genius. His movements were deliberate, and even clumsy. He always seemed, said Director William Mann, of the National Zoological Park, "just a normal gorilla."

## ITEMS

If we could see the earth from a distance out in the heavens it would appear as a bluish planet, Professor V. M. Slipher, of Lowell Observatory, Flagstaff, Arizona, stated in the George Darwin lecture delivered in London before the Royal Astronomical Society. The gold medal of this leading astronomical organization was presented to Professor Slipher in the presence of a distinguished scientific audience that included Dr. Willem de Sitter, Sir Arthur Eddington and Sir James Jeans. Professor F. J. M. Stratton, president, made the presentation. The blueness of the earth was determined by Professor Slipher from spectrograms made photographically of the earthshine on the moon. Light from the earth was reflected by the moon back to Professor Slipher's delicate instruments. Pluto, the most recent of the planets to be discovered, which was found at Lowell Observatory, is a reddish planet which is brighter to the eye than it is on a photographic plate.

Cosmic rays smash into the atmosphere of Mexico City with more intensity from the west than from the east, Dr. Thomas H. Johnson, of the Bartol Research Foundation, has found in the course of an expedition arranged with the cooperation of the Carnegie Institution of Washington. His experimental results presented to the American Physical Society on Dr. Johnson's behalf by Dr. W. F. G. Swann, director of the Bartol Research Foundation, uphold the idea that cosmic rays are composed principally of positively charged corpuscles or particles. With three cosmic ray counters arranged in line so that a record was made only when all three were coincidentally discharged by cosmic radiation, Dr. Johnson pointed his instrument at various elevations. Comparing the intensities of cosmic radiation on the east and west sides of the magnetic meridian of Mexico City, percentage differences were found between east and west ranging from 1 per cent. at 25 degrees distance from the zenith to 25 per cent. at 65 degrees distance to the zenith. "These results are just those to be expected on the basis of the theory of the latitude variations of Lemaitre and Vallarta," Dr. Swann explained, "and they show that the principal corpuscular component of the primary cosmic radiation is positively charged."

Coal is now being mined with a saw instead of being broken loose with explosives. The development of the coal saw to its present highly practical state has improved quality and value of coal, according to C. D. McLaughlin, superintendent of the Pioneer Coal Company, speaking before the American Mining Congress. It has also improved working conditions and safety in mines without any change in organization and supervision, and without displacement of labor. Large lump coal that stands handling and transportation well results from saw mining.

Pigmy chimpanzees, constituting an animal race entirely new to science, were described before the meeting of the American Society of Mammalogists by Harold J. Coolidge, Jr., of the Museum of Comparative Anatomy, Harvard University. The species, known zoologically as *Pan paniscus*, is found south of the Congo River in Africa. It is the smallest chimpanzee in the world, and is characterized by small teeth, close-set eyes, small, almost covered ears and narrow back and shoulders. The only specimen thus far brought to this country is in the American Museum of Natural History, New York City.

# SCIENCE NEWS

*Science Service, Washington, D. C.*

## PROFESSOR BOHR AT PASADENA

By Dr. R. M. Langer
*California Institute of Technology*

Pairs of electrons, one positive and one negative, are sometimes produced when gamma rays from the element thorium pass through matter. This was reported by Dr. Carl D. Anderson, of the California Institute of Technology, in a conference, as a support of Dr. R. A. Millikan's contention that cosmic rays are originally mostly photons, or "bits of light," like gamma rays. Dr. Anderson has observed that among the energetic cosmic ray electrons there are about as many positive as negative electrons, as if they were produced in pairs.

Dr. Niels Bohr, the great Danish physicist now in Pasadena, said that after listening to the evidence it was scarcely possible to doubt the reality of the positron. He is the particular authority for modern theoretical physicists, yet he gave them something of a shock when he said that although theory had predicted the positron few theoretical physicists would have dared emphasize that before experiment had brought it out. The basis for our belief in the positron is therefore almost entirely an experimental one.

Dr. Bohr, on May 18, began a series of lectures on the foundations of atomic mechanics. He began with a careful discussion of the famous uncertainty principle, which has in recent years received unhappy treatment. He explained how the act of observation disturbs an electron or atom so that we must remain uncertain as to what its behavior would have been had we not observed it. If we give up the idea of trying to find what it would have done we save ourselves a great deal of worry and see the problem more rationally. Paradoxes then all disappear and atomic mechanics can describe all phenomena, provided we do not inquire about the atomic constitution of our measuring apparatus. When, however, we examine too closely we get into trouble with relativity. Physicists are stumped at this point and need further experiments to help them out.

If you are in a hurry you can't be too particular about energy. This is a version of the so-called uncertainty principle, which Professor Niels Bohr, of the University of Copenhagen, is driving home to physicists at Pasadena. When one body shoots by another and transfers energy to it, one can not inquire too closely as to whether the principle of conservation of energy has been violated, because it takes time to measure energy exactly. This fact helps clarify certain difficulties which old-fashioned physicists worried about.

Professor Bohr's main purpose is to get investigators to stop worrying about questions which have no possible solution. In return for this sacrifice of vain curiosity, he points out that paradoxes which have been proposed by Einstein and others dissolve themselves.

The Danish scientist is a master of simplification, and presents in brief and elementary form proofs which others achieve only after complicated mathematical developments. He showed in a few lines how material particles scatter each other according to the same law as that deduced for light by Lord Rayleigh when he explained why the sky is blue. In the optical case the blue light is more easily scattered than the red. Blue photons are heavier, so that here is a case where heavier bodies are pushed aside more easily than light ones. The same curious fact is shown when neutrons scatter protons a million times more frequently than the much lighter electrons.

## A STRATOSPHERE BALLOON ASCENT

With the goal of floating eleven or more miles above the earth, higher than man has ever gone before, a stratosphere balloon with airtight man-carrying gondola of special design will rise from Soldiers Field, Chicago, in late June or early July as a part of the science program of the Century of Progress international exhibition.

Within the seven-foot diameter ball hung from the 600,000 cubic foot balloon will be two men, one a pilot and the other a scientist.

Lieutenant-Commander T. G. W. Settle, Navy expert who is licensed and qualified to pilot every type of aircraft known, will be in charge of navigating the balloon to its great height and back to earth.

Professor Auguste Piccard, the Belgian physicist, whose ten-mile-high balloon ascensions in Europe now are world records will probably be the scientist. If Professor Piccard can not make the flight, Professor A. H. Compton, of the University of Chicago, will designate one of his colleagues in cosmic ray research to take the stratosphere ride in the interest of science. Measurements of cosmic rays will be one of the main scientific objectives of the ascension.

A magnesium metal alloy, known as dowmetal, will be used in constructing the spherical gondola in which the men and scientific instruments will be housed during the flight. Dowmetal is a third lighter than aluminum. It is the metallurgical creation of the Dow Chemical Company of Michigan, who are now constructing the gondola. This saving in weight, coupled with a balloon that is a fifth larger than the one used by Professor Piccard on his previous flight, makes the exploration of the eleventh and even the twelfth miles above the earth extremely likely. The Piccard flights reached a little over ten miles altitude.

Tentative plans have been made to broadcast the flight, minute by minute, from the stratosphere to a ground radio station from which it would be relayed over one of the national radio chains.

The National Aeronautic Association has given its approval of the ascension and it will provide altitude instruments which will make the height records official for world record acceptance.

Near the top of the atmosphere in the stratosphere the balloon will hold 500,000 cubic feet of gas, which is

100,000 cubic feet more than the previous Piccard balloon. But at the start only about 125,000 cubic feet of very pure hydrogen gas will inflate the giant gas bag, which will have a pear shape due to its inflation to only about one fifth capacity. As the balloon rises, and most of the atmosphere and its pressure is left behind, the gas will expand tremendously and at the greatest height the balloon will be fully filled.

To obtain the greatest possible lift the Union Carbide and Chemical Company will furnish hydrogen gas of a purity of 99½ per cent. or better. Oxygen carried in tanks and released as needed within the gondola will allow the crew of two to live safely at stratosphere altitudes where there is practically no air. The balloon is being made by builders of the Navy's giant airships, the Goodyear Zeppelin Corporation at Akron, where Commander Settle is at present serving as airship inspector for the Navy.

The take-off will occur at ten or eleven o'clock in the evening, to take advantage of the cool night temperature during the early hours of the flight. As the sun rises the balloon will rise with it, ascending into thinner and thinner air as the heat of the sun expands the gas.

The greatest height above the earth should be reached about mid-afternoon when the sun is hottest. Then the descent will be made and the landing should be made in the evening about dark.

The great crowd of spectators which will throng famous Soldiers Field to watch the beginning of the flight will get a thrill as the balloon rises. A few hundred yards to the southeast of the starting point there are the 628-foot towers and cables of the Century of Progress skyride and the balloon will be shot up at about twenty miles per hour in order to clear this hazard with safety.

The exact day of the start will depend upon weather conditions. Where the balloon will land will depend on wind directions and other meteorological factors. Even if the magnesium metal sphere drops into one of the Great Lakes, it and its human and scientific freight will be rescued safely because the air-tight ball will float for hours.

## HOW FILMS HOLD FAST TO METALS

Better protection for metal surfaces against rust and corrosion may be one of the practical results of an important discovery in pure science just reported to the Royal Society by two British physicists, Professor G. Finch and Dr. Quarrell, of the Imperial College, London.

Their discovery has to do with the way thin films of atoms or molecules arrange themselves when they are deposited on the surfaces of other metals by the special electrical method known as "sputtering." They found that the atoms in such films arranged themselves in the shapes of the metallic crystals underlying them, and not in the crystal shapes proper to their own natural makeup. Thus aluminum deposited on platinum assumed the dimensions of the platinum crystals so far as length and breadth were concerned, though the aggregations of atoms kept the greater height characteristic of aluminum. In this case the aluminum actually became denser than normal, because in two of its dimensions it had patterned itself upon the denser metal, platinum.

A deposit of zinc oxide upon zinc again crowded its crystals to fit them to the dimensions of the smaller zinc crystals. However, in this case the zinc oxide crystals grew taller than normal, so that their total volume remained unchanged.

The significance of the shaping of the deposited substance's crystals to fit the shapes of the underlying metal lies in the fact that there must exist between the crystals of the deposit and those of the substratum a special union or bond that will hold very firmly against any disruptive force. The deposited film is no mere loose layer laid over the surface, but is gripped hard by every atom in it.

The influence of the underlying metal extends for some little distance upwards. The crystal shapes of the underlying metal were preserved through a deposited layer as much as fifty atoms thick, their x-ray photographs showed. These studies of the physical properties of the films they have already deposited are being continued and new films are being made for further research.

## ROBOT CLOCK ANNOUNCES TIME FROM THE PARIS OBSERVATORY

Call an Odéon exchange telephone number in Paris at any hour of day or night. In clear, human tones the exact time, correct to a small fraction of a second, will be heard. Not a living operator but an automatic machine speaks. This speaking clock is set up at the Paris Observatory where time is determined by astronomical observations for the French nation.

At a recent meeting of the Société Astronomique de France, Dr. Ernest Esclangon, director of the Paris Observatory, described the device. The idea was first conceived, and preliminary experiments made, by M. Edouard Belin, pioneer inventor in the transmission of pictures by wire and radio. The final apparatus as now installed was made by the Maison Brillié, scientific instrument makers of Paris, under the supervision of their director, M. Mayer, and engineer, M. Nimier.

The speaking clock uses essentially the same methods that have made possible talking motion pictures, and the machine is driven by a synchronous electric motor, which is controlled by an accurate pendulum clock. In ordinary sound film a narrow strip along one edge carries the sound record, either in the form of a black line of varying width, or a series of cross lines of varying density. In both types, the light from an electric bulb shines through the sound track on to a photoelectric cell, which converts the variations in brightness, caused by the passing film, into a varying electric current. This current is amplified and operates the loud speakers.

In the Brillié machine, time speaking sound record is recorded on strips of paper, wound around an aluminum drum. Instead of having the light pass through the film, it is reflected from a small strip on its surface, into the photoelectric cell. As light or dark parts of the strip pass under the light, the reflected illumination varies, and the cell produces the necessary varying current. There are 90 strips of paper, 24 for the hours, 60 for the minutes and 6 for the seconds. The drum, which is about a foot in diameter and two feet long, turns continually on a horizontal axis at the speed of one revolution in two seconds.

There are three reproducers, each consisting of the necessary electric lamp, lenses and photocell, which are carried along the drum. Each hour the one for announcing the hours shifts from one strip to the next; each minute the minute reproducer steps ahead and every ten seconds the reproducer for seconds makes progress. At midnight the first one goes back to start over again, at the end of each hour the minute reproducer returns, while the seconds one starts over at the beginning of each minute. Connections are automatically made so that the reproducers speak in the proper order, giving first the hour, then the minute and then the second, which is followed by a click marking the exact moment that has been announced. Announcements are given every ten seconds.

At the end of each minute, however, the announcement is different. Then it says "At the third click it will be exactly . . . such an hour . . . such a minute," then, at seconds 58, 59 and 60, there are clicks.

Though the machine is kept in motion continually, the exciting lamps, and the requisite amplifier tubes, are ordinarily turned off. When a telephone connection is put through to the clock at the observatory, relays operate to turn them on for an announcement. Thirty telephone lines to the clock allow that number of subscribers to call simultaneously.

The clock's announcement is also broadcast every morning at 8:30. Dr. Esclangon suggested that it might be well to devote a radio station especially to it, and let announcements of the time be given continually through the day and night.

## THE ORIGIN OF PETROLEUM

PETROLEUM, now one of the principal wealths of the world, was originally garbage—offal from the endless complex banquet of the sea, that not even the bacteria in the bottom slime would eat.

This un-pretty picture of the origin of "black gold" comes from a report presented at the meeting of the American Petroleum Institute held at Tulsa, Oklahoma, by Dr. Parker D. Trask, of the U. S. Geological Survey. Dr. Trask and his associates have for a number of years been conducting an exhaustive study of both modern and ancient sea-bottom deposits, seeking for further knowledge of how petroleum was formed in the first place, so that seekers after oil may have a better idea of what kinds of geological formations are likely to yield paying results to their expensive drillings.

They found that fine-grained beds contain more organic matter than coarse-grained—clay more than silt, silt more than sand. They learned, as was to be expected, that where the sea bottom is rolling and irregular, richer deposits are to be found in the hollows than on the submarine hilltops or slopes. They found, above all, that the dead bodies of the myriad sea plants that escaped eating by fish and other marine animals were not left as raw materials for oil-making until even the bacteria of the bottom slime had taken from them such materials as they wanted for themselves.

This bottom bacterial action seems to be of the highest importance in the formation of the stuffs that eventually become petroleum. Crude plant materials, and such fishes and other animal carcasses as settle to the bottom, have relatively high nitrogenous and carbohydrate contents, which are unsuitable for working over into oil. The food requirements of the bacteria seem to be especially aimed at these non-oil-producing food materials, thereby leaving the organic débris in better condition for the oil-making processes themselves.

Oil-making seems to be an exceedingly slow job. It is not going on in the sediments now forming on the ocean bottom, but it is in progress in sediments laid down on the sea bottoms of geological yesterdays. The steps are not known with anything like satisfactory certainty, but there seems to be no doubt that great increase in sedimentary thickness, with resulting pressure and heat, squeeze and fry out the material that eventually becomes petroleum. It then seeps along migration paths through sandy strata, and collects in pools where impervious rock layers bar its further wanderings.

## ITEMS

AFTER several months in which they have kept fairly far apart, Jupiter and Mars, the two bright planets that shine high in the evening southern sky, are approaching close together. Jupiter is the brightest object in the evening sky at present, with the exception of the moon, and Mars, reddish in color, is a short distance to the right. Now about five degrees apart, at the end of the month they will only be a degree from each other, and on June 4 they will be separated by a quarter of a degree, about half the moon's diameter. Mars will then be to the south of its larger neighbor. A few days previously, on June 1, the moon will pass close to both of the planets, making an interesting spectacle.

CORN planting has been so much delayed by the long period of wet weather over almost the entire eastern half of the country that the situation is now described as "critical" by the U. S. Weather Bureau. In the central Mississippi and Ohio valleys, much of the land has not even been plowed, let alone planted, and a great deal that has been prepared will have to be reworked because of its packed condition, the result of long-continued heavy rains. In Iowa, planting during the week continued slow or at a standstill. Other crops, especially spring wheat and oats, are also being held back in the soggy corn belt states. But more cheerful reports come from the drier lands to the northwest; offset again by stories of drought in the southwestern grain areas.

HIGH blood-pressure, known to physicians as hypertension, runs in families, it appears from a study of statistics reported by Dr. William Allan, of Charlotte, North Carolina, at the Congress of American Physicians and Surgeons meeting in Washington. In one series of cases, both parents of patients having high blood-pressure also suffered from the condition. In 349 out of 480 cases, one of the patient's parents suffered from the same condition. In 121 families with both parents having high blood-pressure more than three fourths of the children suffered from it also. In 216 families with one parent having this condition, over two thirds of the children also had it. In 349 families, three fifths of the brothers and sisters of high blood-pressure patients were found also to have the condition.

DR. L. THATCHER has reported to the *Edinburgh Medical Journal* that a child of eighteen months was admitted to a hospital in Edinburgh, much under weight and unable to walk alone because of weakness. Doctors at the hospital diagnosed the ailment as a kidney inflammation. The child died. Then it was found that the child had received a daily dose of irradiated ergosterol equal to twice the recommended dose and that this severe dose was continued during the summer despite the fact that he was living an outdoor life at the seashore. The double dose of vitamin D resulted in calcium being deposited not only in the bones but in the kidneys. Death in this case was caused by too much vitamin D.

A GELATIN diet has given physicians new knowledge about a certain type of Bright's disease. Results of feeding gelatin to patients suffering from this condition were reported by Dr. G. Philip Grabfield, of Boston, to the American Society for Clinical Investigation. The gelatin diet was used because gelatin is one of the protein foods that does not contain sulfur. Dr. Grabfield was investigating the fact that patients suffering from this particular form of kidney disease tend to hold on to the sulfur in the diet even more than to the nitrogen. Patients who get swollen ankles and legs, known as edema, fail to excrete sulfur as well as nitrogen, while patients suffering from the same disease but without the swelling or edema fail to excrete nitrogen alone.

TEN minutes instead of ten days is the time required by a jeweler to regulate a watch to maximum time-keeping efficiency with the use of a new electric watch timer demonstrated to the Horological Institute. Accurate time intervals are given by a special electrical current of 100 cycles per second accurate to one part in ten million furnished by telephone companies from a constant frequency generator in New York. This current drives a synchronous motor similar to those that have come into such wide use in electric clocks. Within the new timer developed by the Bell Telephone Laboratories an image of the watch balance wheel is reflected on a mirror and a flashing lamp controlled by the precise synchronous motor flashes. This makes the watch's balance wheel seem to stand still when the watch and motor have exactly the same speed. The stroboscopic effect allows the jewelers to inspect and diagnose any trouble in a watch as well as regulate its rate of time-keeping quickly and accurately.

# SCIENCE NEWS

*Science Service, Washington, D. C.*

## SCIENCE AT THE CENTURY OF PROGRESS EXPOSITION



SCIENCE that has remade the world in the last hundred years is glorified at Chicago's Century of Progress exposition.

First of all, the very ground upon which the miles of buildings rest was created out of the shallow water of Lake Michigan by an engineering operation.

Then for the past three years engineers have been at work designing and rearing the buildings which are to serve for the next six months and then be demolished, much like the settings of a movie city. Yet while it lasts, the Century of Progress city will entertain millions of visitors and exhibit millions of dollars worth of displays and treasures. It will serve millions of meals. Adequate fire protection must be provided and hundreds of police, guides and other personnel will inhabit the exhibition city during the exhibition hours.

Some of the buildings strike new notes in modern architecture. The bright hues of many-colored paints are spread over the pylons, towers and walls, and unusual lighting effects blaze their contributions to the fair's decorative scheme at night.

Within the exhibition buildings and in outdoor exhibits, the imprint of science upon our everyday life is exemplified.

From the hemispherical planetarium at the northern corner to the gigantic transportation hall near the southern end of the exposition's expanse, there awaits the visitor a liberal education in science and its effects on human life.

The Hall of Science, to which the cross-bannered court of honor of the principal entrance leads directly, contains an array of mechanized, self-operating demonstrations and exhibits in chemistry, biology, physics, medicine and the earth sciences.

For nearly three years a corps of scientists has been at work designing, planning and building these exhibits, which are arranged in gaily painted booths upon wide aisles. In some cases the visitor or attendant pushes a button and the machine goes through its cycle of demonstrating a basic science principle. In other cases the exhibit methodically carries out its demonstration every few minutes without the prodding of button pushing.

Some of the machines talk their message by means of sound film or phonograph attachments, while others use more prosaic labels in ordinary or transparent lettering. Lantern slides automatically projected are parts of many demonstrations.

Giant electric machines, automatic telephones and switchboards and the thousands of devices developed by science and used in communication or the electrical arts are displayed in the great halls of communication and electricity. Here the large electrical manufacturers, the telephone and telegraph companies have their exhibits.

In the gold-domed Federal Building and the Hall of States with its emblematic façades, the federal and state governments show their public service and governmental activities, particularly along scientific lines.

The Adler Planetarium, as yet America's only mechanical show of the stars, is a part of the exhibition. In this richly somber dome the astronomical exhibits are contained.

America's agricultural interests are represented by a low, long building decorated in black, red and blue-green.

On Northerly Island, across the lagoon from the Hall of Science, is also the Hall of the Social Sciences, in which exhibits will recall the social consequences of the century of progress and suggest how the problems can be met.

Southward along the lake front, beyond concession buildings designed to amuse or convince the throngs commercially, is an area devoted to America's aborigines.

Rising to a commanding position is a reproduction of one of America's earliest and most striking architectural developments, a Maya temple. With strange carvings of huge mask heads, great serpents and other elaborate designs, painted brilliant yellow and green, there is duplicated a portion of the Munjas or Nunnery at Uxmal in Yucatan, built by the Maya Indians many years before Columbus discovered America. Within it can be seen some of the most valuable of the Maya treasures loaned by American museums.

In the shadow of the Maya temple five groups of American Indians will live primitive existences as their ancestors did before them. This will be their contribution to the Century of Progress. Nootka Indians from the American Northwest will raise their totem poles. Winnebagoes in wigwams will represent the woodland tribes. The plains Indians whose existence depended upon the buffalo will be represented by a group of Sioux Indians living in tipis, while the Pueblos will dwell in reproductions of their terraced villages, which were America's earliest apartment houses. Navahos, too, will show the part they played in the old Southwest. For the visitors these Indians will dance their ceremonials and sing their chants.

Close by the Indian villages and the Maya temple are the exhibition buildings of leading automobile manufacturers. Here may be seen the operating assembly line where complete cars are built from piles of parts.

The pageant of a century of transportation will be shown under the gigantic sky-hung dome of the travel and transport building, so large that railroad cars and transport airplanes seem lost beneath it. Antique vehicles used years ago will be contrasted with the most modern in transport. Along the lake front will be found famous ships of to-day and yesterday.

Enter the great central portion of the Hall of Science and a great globe will be slowly spinning before your eyes, while below there are samples and information on the ninety-three building blocks of the earth, arranged in the form of the chemist's periodic table.

These ninety-three chemical elements are the stuff from which all the rest of the fair's exhibits are made. They are the basic materials of the world and the universe. They have therefore been given a central position in the Century of Progress. Those who learned in school that there are 92 elements are informed that neuton is the one added to the periodic table in the last year.

Some of the samples in the display are rare specimens of chemical elements that were totally unknown a few years ago. Upon the model of the world above, there are shown the locations on the earth's surface where the elements are found most abundantly.

Man's highest into the stratosphere and lowest into the ocean's depths are represented by two historic spheres. One of these is the light aluminum gondola that Professor Auguste Piccard used in his world record balloon flights over Europe, while the other is the heavy steel ball in which Dr. William Beebe descended into the sea off the Bermuda coast for a world's record.

Atom smashing is symbolized by the original operating high voltage generator designed by Dr. Robert J. Van de Graaff, then of Princeton, and now of Massachusetts Institute of Technology. It is producing millions of volts for the enlightenment of the visitors.

A year's growth of a quarter-inch tree twig is visualized in 75 seconds by a $7\frac{1}{4}$ foot model in another corner of the hall. In a most realistic manner, the ingenious mechanical linden twig model adds wood on the inside of the growing zone and bark on its outside just as it does invisibly in the actual miniature twig.

A complete miniature oil refinery, all constructed in glass and actually making gasoline and lubricating oil, is seen in full operation in the central alcove.

From this main exhibition hall, the visitor can set out on exciting excursions into three floors of booths and displays dynamically telling the stories of physics, chemistry, biology, medicine and mathematics. To race through the exhibits would take three or four solid hours. If the visitor wishes to see each one operate and is determined to study each one quickly but understandingly, two or three days should be spent in the Hall of Science.

Nineteen of the world's greatest scientific men have their names emblazoned on the wall of the exhibition foyer of the Hall of Science.

The two Americans on this list of scientific immortals are Rowland and Michelson, both physicists. Professor H. A. Rowland was the famous physicist of the Johns Hopkins University who determined the mechanical equivalent of heat and made diffraction gratings for spectrum analysis known the world over. Professor Albert A. Michelson, of the University of Chicago, made the most accurate determinations of the velocity of light. He died in 1931.

Aristotle heads the list. Dr. Henry Crew, chief of division of basic sciences of the Century of Progress, who directed the extensive science displays and selected the list, explained that it was not intended to pick a science honor roll with which all would agree. He will agree with any who comment that there are famous names omitted.

The list of scientists and the fields of their researches is as follows: Aristotle—Biology, Archimedes—Mathematics, Euclid—Mathematics, Hipparchus—Astronomy, Leonardo—Anatomy, Galileo—Physics, Huygens—Astronomy, Harvey—Physiology, Newton—Mathematics, Lavoisier—Chemistry, Dalton—Chemistry, Darwin—Biology, Pasteur—Medicine, Faraday—Physics, Helmholtz—Physics, Maxwell—Physics, Mendelejeff—Chemistry, Rowland—Physics, Michelson—Physics.

The history of science has been written in 151 words of lyric prose and lettered upon the wall of the principal exhibition room.

The text, written by Dr. Henry Crew, formerly professor of physics at Northwestern University and now head of the division of basic sciences of the Century of Progress, is as follows:

Pythagoras named the cosmos; Euclid shaped geometry . . . Archimedes physics.

Xenophanes gazing upon the Heavens saw them to be one. Copernicus placed central in that one, our shining sun.

In the motions of physical bodies Galileo beheld law; thence Newton and the principle of universal gravitation.

Democritus glimpsed the atomic theory of the structure of matter; Dalton established it.

When in the nineteenth century Lamarck and Darwin formulated the great principle of organic evolution, the science of life was first seen as a cosmic progression of nature.

For the saving of life through inoculation men give honor to Jenner and Pasteur.

The century of progress saw Oersted and Faraday set forth, and Maxwell and Hertz advance the theory of electromagnetism.

Through the labors of Becquerel, of the Curies and of Thomson, to our own day are revealed fragile atoms and electrons.

Planck's quantum and Einstein's relativity theory open new epochs to science.

From the vast literature of science fourteen quotations have been selected and written upon a wall of the Hall of Science as a concise summary of scientific philosophy. Poets and public men as well as scientists are among those who wrote the collected sentences. The quotations are as follows:

Science and peace will triumph over ignorance and war.—Pasteur

Man is the interpreter of nature. . . . Science the right interpretation.—Whewell

Nature never proclaims her secrets aloud, but always whispers them.—John Owen

Science has but one fashion. . . . To lose nothing once gained.—Stedman

There is nothing so powerful as truth, often nothing so strange.—Daniel Webster

Scientific education is an essential condition of industrial progress.—Huxley

If there is one way better than another, it is the way of nature.—Aristotle

The first and the last thing required of genius is the love of truth.—Goethe

Nature is not to be governed except through obeying her.—Bacon

More important than particular truths is the love of truth.—C. J. Little

The common experiences of normal people are the matter of science.—H. Dingle

Reason's voice and God's, Nature's and duty's, never are at odds.—Whittier

The essence of science is to discover identity in difference.—F. S. Marvin

Scientific law is a description, not a prescription. —Karl Pearson

Mechanical men reveal to the visitors of the exposition the physiology and chemistry of the human body.

The famous transparent man, manufactured in Germany, as a life-sized display of the vital organs of human anatomy is a central exhibit in the medical section of the Hall of Science.

An American robot, ten feet high, who speaks and gestures and explains an illuminated interior view of himself, is a part of the chemical exhibit.

The life-size model transparent man, obtained from the famous Hygiene Museum at Dresden, has his exterior made of a synthetic transparent material. Heart, lungs, the stomach, liver and other interior organs are lighted in rotation to show vividly to the visitor their relation to the surface of the skin.

"Now, ladies and gentlemen, I shall swallow," the chemical robot tells his audience many times each day in exhibiting the mechanical movements of his stomach and intestines by illuminated dynamic pictures of his interior. "You will see the mouthful of food passing down my esophagus. The food is forced down by the contractions of the esophagus. Now you see the swallow entering the top door of my stomach. Watch my stomach contract to churn up the food."

The robot, who is a handsome well-dressed young man, except for the fact that his upper garments are pulled aside to show his digestive area, can point to the various happenings within him. He gives practical advice to the audience upon nutrition and the kinds of food that should be eaten.

A talking motion picture provides both the speech and the interior views of the robot, while ingenious mechanisms allow him to wave his arms when he orates.

Automatically and continuously, one of the many chemical exhibits is making gunpowder by mixing carbon, sulfur and niter and then exploding it before the eyes of the visitors by dropping it on a hot plate.

In other Century of Progress exhibits which show the principles and processes of chemistry that underlie our modern civilization, fire and sparks flash as there are repeated by the self-operating exhibits some of the famous and fundamental experiments that have made history.

Once a minute for ten hours each day, a dynamic display heats mercuric oxide in a test-tube and shows that metallic mercury, such as is contained in thermometers, and oxygen gas are given off. This repeats the experiment that resulted in the discovery of oxygen.

A ribbon of iron is burned in oxygen with a brilliant display of fire and another element, phosphorus, is allowed to burn simply by exposing it to the air.

Every two minutes in another booth the famous thermite reaction used in one kind of welding is performed to show the principle of chemical exchange or double decomposition. Iron oxide is mixed with aluminum dust and when the mixture is ignited there results molten iron and aluminum oxide.

That water can start fire is proved by an experiment in which the metal potassium is dropped into water with the result that it burns.

The breaking up of water into hydrogen and oxygen gas by an electric current is shown in another experiment and then these two gases are recombined into water by allowing them to burn.

Some materials cause a chemical change to take place without themselves participating in it. Such a catalytic action is illustrated by an operating experiment which shows ammonia being turned into powerful nitric acid. Before the catalytic change, the ammonia gas is basic and therefore turns a litmus solution blue when it is bubbled through it. After it is made into an acid a litmus solution is turned pink by the nitric acid gas bubbling through it.

Because sulfuric acid is one of the basic chemicals of modern industry, its manufacture is explained. The mining of the sulfur from the ground, its conversion into sulfur dioxide by burning, and its transformation into sulfuric acid by the catalytic contact process is carried out before the eyes of the visitors. Ninety-nine per cent. pure sulfuric acid is produced and the Cottrell electrical precipitator is seen changing the fog of sulfuric acid into a heavy liquid.

In another booth a dazzling color display of actual crystals being produced from a liquid and projected on a screen is to be seen.

Cherry red gold, the precious metal in finely divided solid suspension in a liquid, may also be seen. This is colloidal gold. A little acid added automatically to the solution turns the red gold to blue and then when more acid is added the gold is completely thrown down out of solution.

How gold mined from the earth is extracted from the rock is demonstrated in a complete ore flotation unit, where the gold ore is crushed, pulverized and then put through the flotation process to separate it from the lead and zinc sulfide with which it is associated.

A rubber tree with its latex sap flowing out of a gash in its bark is another exhibit which is the starting point for a complete story of the utilization of rubber in industry. Electroplating with rubber and vulcanization processes used in making automobile tires are shown in actual operation.

An automatic chromium plating plant built especially for the exposition will demonstrate this new process of electroplating as it produces appropriate souvenir letter openers which have impressed upon them a representation of chemistry's fundamental periodic table.

# SCIENCE NEWS

*Science Service, Washington, D. C.*

## MATTER CREATED FROM LIGHT AND COSMIC RAYS

Tangible matter is being created out of light and cosmic rays which come to earth from outer space. Radiation produced here on earth is also manufacturing in some proved instances matter out of intangible waves.

Conversion of mass of the stars to produce light and heat has been the favorite method of explaining their long life. That has been the classic example of the interchange of matter and radiation.

Now evidence is accumulating for the reverse process, the creation of matter out of radiation, not in the far-distant stars, but here on earth.

The idea that matter is created by light or photons was put forth by Dr. P. M. S. Blackett and G. Occhialini, of the Cavendish Laboratory of the University of Cambridge. The light prefers to perform this miracle only in the neighborhood of an atomic nucleus. The matter is created in the form of a pair of electrons, one positive and one negative. The theory is formulated on the basis of Dr. Carl D. Anderson's discovery of the positive electron and the subsequent confirming researches at Cambridge.

Experimental evidence for the creation of matter is contained in the bursts of electrons due to cosmic rays observed by Dr. Anderson in his apparatus at the California Institute of Technology. And Dr. Anderson recently found pairs of electrons formed by the gamma rays given off by thorium. The positrons or positive electrons so formed do not live long, however, since they unite with negatives to form photons or light again.

The latest development is that Dr. J. R. Oppenheimer, of the California Institute of Technology, and Dr. Milton Plesset, a National Research fellow, have found that the theoretical equation of Dr. P. A. M. Dirac is quite in accord with the facts. This has led to important predictions bearing on cosmic rays.

Photons of high energy much prefer to produce the pair of electrons than to transfer their energy to a single ordinary electron. All of the photons or cosmic rays are equally effective in producing new pairs.

After discussing these new developments at Pasadena, Dr. Niels Bohr, the Danish physicist who is spending some weeks at the California Institute of Technology, commented that the calculations by Drs. Oppenheimer and Plesset have convinced him that the Dirac equation instead of being false is the greatest acquisition to human knowledge in the past few years.

## MUSCULAR WEAKNESS IN GRAVES' DISEASE

The extreme muscular weakness that marks Graves' disease has a chemical basis and is not just due to the nervousness which also features the ailment, Drs. E. Shorr, H. B. Richardson and H. G. Wolff, of the Cornell Medical School and New York Hospital, reported at the Washington meeting of the American Society for Clinical Investigation.

This is a disease involving the thyroid gland. Some patients suffering from it have marked goiters and bulging eyes, as well as the nervousness, muscular weakness and increased metabolism. The disease is also marked by the excretion from the body of large amounts of a chemical substance called creatine.

Creatine is present in the muscles as part of the compound phosphocreatine. When muscles contract, this compound breaks down into creatine and phosphoric acid. In the recovery of the muscle the two substances are recombined into phosphocreatine. If the latter substance is not adequately rebuilt in the muscles, they will fail to function properly. In Graves' disease, one of the parts, creatine, of the essential phosphocreatine is excreted from the body in abnormal amounts instead of being completely recombined with phosphoric acid.

This abnormal excretion of creatine also occurs in another condition known as progressive muscular dystrophy, characterized by marked muscular weakness associated with degenerative changes in the muscles.

These investigators found many points in common between the two conditions. Most of the chemical reactions formerly considered characteristic of the creatinuria of muscular dystrophy were consistently found by them in patients with Graves' disease. An additional point of resemblance between the two conditions is that actual muscle degeneration, especially of the eye muscles, has also been observed in Graves' disease.

These observations do not imply that these diseases have a common origin, but suggest that a similar damage to the important phosphocreatine mechanism is sustained in both, and is responsible for the muscular weakness.

For these reasons, the creatine excretion in thyroid disease is regarded as potentially dangerous to the functional and anatomical integrity of the muscles. It can be abolished by giving iodine, which has long been established as an important therapeutic agent in Graves' disease.

## CHEMICAL WARFARE BY INSECTS

Chemical warfare with special weapons is waged by certain species of insects in India, according to Dr. Thomas E. Snyder, of the Bureau of Entomology, U. S. Department of Agriculture. Dr. Snyder has recently completed a study of a large collection of these insects in the U. S. National Museum.

The insects are termites, often incorrectly called "white ants." Termites are not ants, and are related to them only insofar as both termites and ants are insects. Ants, indeed, are among their worst enemies, and it is against ants that the chemical weapons studied by Dr. Snyder are most effectively employed.

The termites bearing these weapons belong to a special "caste" within the termite nest; they are developed for defending the colony just as others of their nestmates are specialized into a worker "caste." In these particular species the soldier termites have as chief weapon a long protrusion from the front of the head. Originally it developed from a third eye, but now its function is to secrete and discharge a powerful corrosive acid. Some of them can squirt it almost an inch, but such cases are exceptional.

When enemy ants invade the termite nests guarded by these chemically armed warriors, the latter rush to the combat. They know the weak spot in their opponents' armor, and go straight for it. Shoving their long snout-like weapons against the ant's "waist" or pedicle, they smear it with the corrosive secretion. The ant quickly becomes helpless.

Termites, whose depredations in wooden structures in New York have recently caused something of a stir, are primarily animals of the tropics, although a few destructive species have become widely distributed over the southern and eastern parts of our own country. They feed primarily on wood and other cellulose substances, and can cause immense damage if not guarded against. In the tropics they can hollow out a house and all the wooden furniture in it, besides eating up all books, stored clothing, and almost any other vegetable fiber they can fasten their jaws into.

## THE CAUSE OF FATAL DISEASE IN YOUNG LAMBS

DURING the California lambing season, a disease hitherto of unknown origin has inflicted heavy losses upon newly-born lambs on farms that are widely separated.

Dr. Hilda Hempl Heller, while at Hooper Foundation for Medical Research of the University of California, fastened the apparent guilt of causing this disease upon one kind of the very common colon bacilli, the sort of germs widely found in the intestinal tract of animals.

An unusual circumstance of this disease is that, though it is an infection, the mechanism of its action resembles that of a food poisoning. The little lamb, just after being born, drinks its mother's milk, which is not poisonous. When in some way it is infected with the colon bacillus at a virulent stage, the germs form a poison in the milk within the lamb's alimentary tract. The lamb dies from absorbed poison rather than from the direct attack of the germs.

The germs charged by Dr. Heller with causing the disease are extremely variable and they have been found to change their deadliness rapidly.

Dr. Heller, who is an authority on botulinus poisoning, began work on the disease because it was thought that it was a disease caused by an anaerobe, or air-hating germ. She found that a powerful poison was present in the lamb intestines, of which five drops would kill a mouse in two and a half hours. The blame for forming this poison could not be fastened upon any anaerobic germ.

The poison-producing power of the colon bacilli found in the lambs was then demonstrated by Dr. Heller. When grown in test-tubes the isolated germs produced a poison identical in effect with that obtained from the lambs. Dr. Heller, who worked on this problem with the cooperation of the University of California's Division of Veterinary Science, located at Davis, California, did not have the opportunity to clinch the proof by infecting lambs, because when the presumably guilty organism was isolated and proved to be rapidly fatal for guinea-pigs, the lambing season was over.

Dr. Heller hopes to be able to continue research upon this lamb disease. It seems probable that it is widespread in the sheep-raising areas of this and other countries, and must cause a loss amounting to many thousands of dollars annually. It may also be related to a similar disease of calves which is responsible for even larger financial losses.

## THE WHEAT CROP

WINTER wheat in the United States promises the shortest crop since 1904, the May issue of *Wheat Studies* of the Food Research Institute estimates. The official forecast as of May 1 indicated a crop of only 337 million bushels, 125 million below the standing estimate of last year's crop. Acreage abandonment was unprecedentedly high, over 32 per cent., leaving the smallest area for harvest since 1912.

Reports of farmers' intention to plant spring wheat indicated that the acreage sown this spring in North America may be four or five per cent. smaller than the area planted in 1932. Since the publication of the institute's report, unfavorable weather has held back spring wheat planting, along with practically all other crops, so that some shortage in spring wheat may be expected also, though whether it will be as great as that in winter wheat can not now be predicted.

One major wheat harvest of the world, that in India, has already been reaped. It is officially estimated at 340 million bushels, a trifle larger than the 1932 crop. It is not expected that the Indian crop will have much influence on world wheat prices during the May–July period.

European wheat-importing countries are still striving for as much self-sufficiency as possible in wheat. They are expected to harvest as large an area as last year's, if not a little larger, but the crop is expected to be smaller by 100 to 150 million bushels. This will be at least partly balanced, however, by a larger crop anticipated from the great wheat-exporting regions on the Danube, where last year's crop was a virtual failure in Rumania and Jugo-Slavia.

In Russia the area sown to winter wheat was more than four million acres smaller this year than last, and spring wheat plantings will probably be no larger. But even if the crop increases, as is fairly likely, much of the early surplus normally exported will have to go for the relief of the domestic food shortage.

Prices on wheat are expected to advance, but more from currency and general economic causes than because of crop conditions.

The current report of the Food Research Institute was written by M. K. Bennett and Helen C. Farnsworth, with the advice of Joseph S. Davis and Holbrook Working.

## THE PURE FOOD AND DRUG BILL TO CONGRESS

AT the direction of President Roosevelt, Secretary of Agriculture Wallace has sent a bill for a new national pure food and drug law to Congress.

The new bill has been carefully planned to remedy the deficiencies of the present food and drug law, which was enacted nearly 27 years ago after a strenuous campaign by the late Dr. Harvey W. Wiley.

The limitations of the present law make it impossible to carry out its intention of protecting the public from impure or harmful foods and drugs, Secretary Wallace pointed out in submitting the new bill.

Under the new bill, the secretary is authorized to set definitions and standards of purity for foods, just as there are now legal standards for official drugs. Under the present law such standards may be set for canned foods only.

False advertising is to be prevented under the new bill. At present there is no way, under the Food and Drugs Act, to control the serious abuses in this field.

The present law prohibits false or misleading statements on the labels of foods and drugs, but under the new bill, labels must tell enough about the product so that the consumer will know what he is getting and can buy intelligently and discriminatingly.

Cosmetics are to be brought under federal control so as to prevent the serious injuries that have occurred through the sale and use of harmful cosmetic products.

Another important feature of the bill is the provision directed at the sale of drugs labeled as treatments for various diseases. The Food and Drug Administration under the new bill will be able to prevent the sale of such drug products if the claims for them are contrary to general agreement of medical opinion. At present an influenza cure, for example, which physicians agree will not remedy influenza, can not be kept off the market unless the Food and Drug Administration can prove that the claims for the remedy are not only false but made with the intention of deceiving the public.

## ITEMS

DIFFICULTY in measuring the energy of cosmic rays presents the greatest problem to the physicists studying them, Dr. R. A. Millikan stated in a discussion following a summary of recent experiments presented by his colleague, Dr. H. Victor Neher, at the California Institute of Technology. Dr. Paul S. Epstein presented a very successful theory which pictured the cosmic rays as a stream of photons accompanied by several weaker groups of electrons. But the experimenters were warned against accepting theories until energy measurements of the rays became more complete. Meanwhile, all investigations indicate that photons predominate in cosmic rays, but that some electrons also enter the earth's atmosphere. A strong support for the photon idea was presented by Dr. Carl D. Anderson, who announced that he had produced positive electrons or positrons with photons from thorium. If photons are known to produce positrons and if no other method is known then the positrons which are found with cosmic rays were probably produced by photons too.

INTRODUCING "deuton" as a new name for the double-weight hydrogen atom only known to science for a little over a year, Professor Ernest O. Lawrence, of the University of California, reported to physicists meeting at Pasadena what happens when the heavy isotope of hydrogen is used as a projectile in smashing various elements. Only about a month ago, Dr. Gilbert N. Lewis supplied Professor Lawrence and his associates, Drs. Henderson and M. Stanley Livingston, with some deutons. The atom-smashing was done with the aid of potential up to 1,500,000 volts imparted to the deutons with Professor Lawrence's magnetic method of creating high voltages. Lithium, beryllium, boron, nitrogen, fluorine, aluminum and sodium gave good results. Transmutations occurred, alpha rays were formed, and probably other processes yet to be examined followed.

SPECTRA lying between the x-rays and the ultra-violet rays of 1,200 Ångstrom units, in which absorption spectra have hitherto been unknown, have been found by Dr. H. Beutler, Berlin physicist. The elements giving the newly discovered spectra are rubidium, caesium, cadmium and mercury. Helium was exposed to a condensed discharge to produce light from 900 to 600 Ångstrom units. The light source and the test vapor could not be separated from the vacuum spectrograph used by a window or other device because no material known allows these rays to pass through. The new lines can not be observed in emission but only in absorption. They are interpreted as arising from a change in the quantum numbers of an inner electron while the valence electrons remain unexcited and they thus represent a transition from optical to Roentgen spectra.

DR. JAMES CHADWICK, of Cambridge, discoverer of the neutron, delivering the Bakerian lecture of the Royal Society, awarded a tentative decision against the neutron as the cause of formation of the positron, another newly discovered particle of matter, when radiations from radioactive beryllium pass through a lead plate. The radiation from beryllium consists of neutrons and gamma rays. The neutron can be thought of as a corpuscle, but gamma rays are like light, x-rays and radio waves in being electromagnetic waves. Positrons or free positive electrons are produced by atom smashing when the mixed beryllium radiation is allowed to attack lead. The neutrons were accused at first, but now Dr. Chadwick believes that the gamma rays, not the neutrons, may be responsible. Out of 300 electron tracks produced in his experiments, 200 were made by the familiar, long-known negative electrons, while 70 were positive. Dr. Chadwick's work at Cavendish Laboratory agrees generally with researches by Dr. Carl D. Anderson, of California Institute of Technology, who last fall discovered the positron.

BEAUTIFUL phosphorescent light given off by certain sponges living in shallow waters is really due to small worms that inhabit them, according to Professor Emanuel Trojan, of Prague. The little light-producing worm is scarcely a quarter of an inch long, but can send branches an inch and a half in all directions. Professor Trojan tells *Nature* how he coaxed the little animal out of its hiding place by attaching the sponge to the edge of an inclined bowl, allowing the water to drip slowly out of the sponge into the bowl. As the sponge became too dry for comfort, the water-loving worms came out of their hiding-place.

# SCIENCE NEWS

*Science Service, Washington, D. C.*

## THE FIFTH PACIFIC SCIENCE CONGRESS

Fish are commonly reputed to be voiceless, yet some species can make sounds that apparently serve as calls to their mates. So stated Dr. Shinkishi Hatai, marine biologist of the Tohoku Imperial University, Japan, before the meeting of the congress at Vancouver on June 5. Several species of fish produce distinct sounds, he said, either by friction of the fins, grinding their teeth, emitting air through a narrow passage or through special developed sound-producing organs. These sounds may serve as warnings as well as for mate-calls. Dr. Hatai developed this point during a discussion of the sensitiveness of fish and other marine organisms to vibrations in general. A very little movement of a boat's oars served to attract to his boat numerous specimens of the handsome red Japanese fish called ''tai'' at a distance of forty yards. This sensitiveness of fish to changes in their environment, imperceptible to human organs or man-made instruments, may have considerable importance, both scientific and economic, in connection with the almost incessant earthquakes with which Japan is visited. Before two recent rather severe earthquakes the uneasiness of the sea fish in certain regions was noted. On both occasions they consistently refused baited hooks. The consequences of an earthquake that changes the level of the sea-bottom may be revolutionary to the animal societies living on it or in the water above it. Most bottom communities are adjusted to a given depth of water, as it affects quality and intensity of light, oxygen concentration, and other factors. In turn, these anchored animals and plants are related to the swimming animal population in the rôles of food, shelter, enemies, etc. An earthquake that revolutionizes the life balance on a given stretch of sea-bottom may very well ruin a whole fishing community, though it does not wreck a house or a boat, simply through the changes it brings to pass in the animal communities that constitute the support of the people.

The ups and downs of the isthmus that at various times in the past connected the continents of North America and Asia where now the Bering Strait separates them were described by Dean Edward W. Berry, of the Johns Hopkins University. This land bridge, over which the two continents exchanged plant and animal populations, has been above water some five separate times during the Age of Reptiles and the succeeding Age of Mammals. Its most recent emergence was during the Pleistocene or great Ice Age, when woolly mammoths and giant bison tramped back and forth across it.

The rocks underlying the Pacific Ocean are different from those of the other ocean basins of the world as well as from those of the land areas, according to Dr. B. Gutenberg, of the California Institute of Technology. The granites and sedimentary rocks that make up the bulk of the continental masses are absent, as are also the basic rocks that underlie them and form the floors of the other oceans. Instead, the Pacific bottom appears to consist of even more strongly basic rocks, that may continue downward without any sudden change to a depth as great as 1,200 kilometers (about 725 miles). Dr. Gutenberg has been led to these conclusions by a study of the rates of earthquake-wave travel through various regions of the earth.

Sea-level is not strictly on the level. It is higher in some places than it is in others, according to H. G. Avers, chief mathematician of the division of geodesy, U. S. Coast and Geodetic Survey. At Prince Rupert, B. C., mean sea-level is 1.64 feet higher than it is at Halifax, N. S.; at Seattle it is 1.18 feet higher than at Portland, Maine, and at San Diego, California, it is 1.74 feet higher than it is at Fernandino, Florida.

Botanists at the congress heard from Dr. W. L. Waterhouse, of the University of Sydney, Australia, of the quandary into which the wheat breeders of his country have been thrust by the mysterious behavior of a parasitic fungus, the rust disease of grains. They had been used to fighting several well-known, almost standardized forms of this disease. Suddenly there appeared an entirely new form of grain rust, which has quite displaced the enemies they had become used to and could deal with fairly effectually. This new foe is the more troublesome since all Australian grain varieties are extremely susceptible to it. Nobody knows where it came from or how it got to Australia.

The great unpopulated spaces of the North, ranged by wild animals good for food and fur, can become a permanent reservoir of these supplies if properly administered, Dr. R. M. Anderson, biologist of the Canadian Department of Mines, reported. Furthermore, the fauna of the Canadian and Alaskan North are of high scientific interest, because of the many suggestions on the origin and migration routes of large mammals which they offer.

Glamorous ideas, bred largely in Hollywood studios, about the simple idyllic life of ''primitive'' South Sea tribes received a jolt at the hands of Professor R. Thurnwald, of Yale University, who spoke before the congress. Their lives are anything but paradisiacal and their culture anything but simple, he said. To that extent at least they can not be said to be primitive. Neither is it possible to assume a common origin of two groups because one finds a few traits in common between them, like similar language or a similar way of building houses or hunting heads. A group in its history and migrations may borrow customs from many of its neighbors. Professor Thurnwald told of finding a people on the northern coast of New Guinea who used a Papual vocabulary with a Melanesian grammar. It reminded him, he said, of a community of Negroes in one part of Texas, whose language is a Bavarian dialect. Their one-time German masters have long since moved away and blended with the general American population, but these Afro-Americans keep the old speech.

## THE MEDICAL MEETINGS IN MILWAUKEE

PHYSICIANS of the future apparently are going to know their economics and the business side of medicine. No longer will the saying be true that physicians, along with other professional men, are not socially minded and have no knowledge of economics. An outline of medical economics to be used in medical schools is being prepared by the American Medical Association, as announced at the opening session of the annual meeting on June 6. This is to meet the increasing need for persons starting to practise medicine to have some information concerning economics, ethics and organization.

CONTROL of narcotic drugs should be a function of state rather than of the federal government, according to the legal department of the American Medical Association. A uniform narcotic law, such as has been recently adopted by Indiana, Nevada and New York, was urged by this committee. Efficient state control will be better able than federal control to prevent the abuse of these drugs. "Unless the individual states strengthen their efforts in this direction, the federal government may attempt to take over the production, manufacture, distribution and use of narcotic drugs under its treaty-making power. This would result in the loss by the states of their right to authorize physicians to prescribe narcotics and thus there is partial control of the practise of medicine by a Washington bureau. The people of a state pay for enforcement of federal narcotic laws when they might more economically enforce a state law."

THE physician of the future may become an "immunisator" or even something of a regulator of body and even of mind, according to Dr. Clyde Brooks, of New Orleans, at the meeting of the American Medical Association. Dr. Brooks discussed the present status of treating diseases by injecting foreign substances into the body. One example is use of specific vaccines made from killed or weakened germs of the disease, such as antityphoid inoculations. Another example of this type of treatment is the use of substances such as egg white or milk which have no connection with the disease. These are used on the theory that introducing any foreign material into the body will call out all its defensive forces against the invading disease. When the treatment uses a specific vaccine, as in typhoid fever, the process is said to be one of producing immunity to the disease. From this Dr. Brooks suggests the title "immunisator" for the future physician who, he believes, may treat diseases of the body and even of the mind largely by immunologic methods. The present status of this field, however, is like a jigsaw puzzle, he said. There are many isolated areas of information, some of which fit together to give a glimpse of some of the figures in the final picture, but no one yet knows what the picture will be. But enough is known to convince workers that the physician of the future will treat the sick largely by immunization.

THE vital cortex of the adrenal glands may have an influence on the regulation of salt and water in the body similar to that of insulin on sugar, the parathyroid glands on calcium and the thyroid gland on iodine. Evidence indicating that this may be the case was presented by Dr. R. L. Zwemer, of the College of Physicians and Surgeons, Columbia University, and his associate, Dr. Ruth Sullivan, at the meeting on June 8 of the Association for the Study of Internal Secretions. The salt in this case is sodium. According to Dr. Zwemer it is a loss of sodium from the body rather than any great increase in acid that produces the lower carbon dioxide combining power of the blood which is an early indicator of insufficient functioning of the adrenal glands. In cats that have lost their adrenal glands, extract of the adrenal cortex increases the amount of sodium and chloride in the blood. Drs. Zwemer and Sullivan working with animals, and Drs. Robert Loeb and Dana Atchley treating patients, found that giving common salt by mouth is helpful in conditions like Addison's disease in which the cortex of the adrenal gland is not producing enough of the necessary hormone. Cats that were given salt after removal of the adrenal glands survived twice as long as similar animals that got no salt. While salt is helpful in these conditions of adrenal insufficiency, some of the adrenal cortex hormone or extract must also be given.

A NEW, hitherto unrecognized glandular disorder was reported by Dr. Leonard G. Rowntree, of Philadelphia, and Dr. Louis A. Brunsting, of the Mayo Clinic, to the Association for the Study of Internal Secretions. The disorder was seen in two young women, twenty years old, who were brought to the Mayo Clinic because they had suddenly become very fat. They could not get rid of the excess weight by any of the measures for reducing. "Both patients were superlatively feminine in appearance with luxuriant hair and exaggerated feminine configuration," the physicians found on examination. Both patients had matured at a younger age than the normal. With the idea that the obesity was due to derangement in the body's handling of water, the patients were given treatment to remove the water from their bodies. This was done by the use of ammonium salts and the newer mercury compounds. As a result, the weights of the two patients were reduced to practically normal. After their return home, one patient regained the weight she had lost. The other patient was able to keep her weight down by continuing the ammonium and mercurial compounds and by restricting the amount of water she took. Drs. Rowntree and Brunsting suggested that the condition might be the result of an early excess of one of the hormones of the pituitary gland, known as Prolan A.

CHILDREN are more flexible than adults in their bodies' readjustment of sugar utilization in various conditions, according to studies of Dr. Henry J. John, of the Cleveland Clinic, reported at the meeting of the Association for the Study of Internal Secretions. He studied the sugar tolerance of groups of children from 4 to 20 years old who were suffering from various conditions that might affect the sugar utilization and compared this with the tolerance of adults suffering from the same ailments. These were obesity, hyperthyroidism, rheumatic disease and pituitary disease. The part played by infections in upsetting the sugar utilization may be temporary or permanent diabetes. "Diabetes is looked upon mainly as a degenerative disease, rising rapidly after the fourth decade and reaching its maximum in the seventh decades."

BOTH the birth rate and the health of new-born babies are affected by the season of the year, Dr. Lee Bivings, of Atlanta, Georgia, found from a study of Negro infants in his city. The diet of the prospective mother and the amount of sunshine also apparently influence the birth rate and infant health. The birth rate for 1930, 1931 and 1932 was consistently higher in the winter quarter. This fact suggests that the mothers who had the benefit of spring and summer sunshine in the period before the babies were born were more likely to give birth to healthy children. The average weight of babies born in 1931 was higher than that of babies born in 1932. While many factors were involved, Dr. Bivings believes the greater amount of sunshine in 1931 had some influence. This opinion was borne out by the fact that babies born in Los Angeles, St. Petersburg and Atlanta, Georgia, weighed more than those born in Iowa City and New Haven, Connecticut. The studies showed that the health of the babies was not as good when their prenatal life began in the winter. Dr. Bivings explained this on the ground that it is during the winter months that the prospective mother's diet lacks sufficient vitamin B which is believed to have an important effect on the prenatal development of a child. These are likewise the months of least sunshine.

AS a result of careful control by the Department of Agriculture of the spraying of vegetables and fruits to check insect pests few products with a dangerous arsenic content reach the consumer, it was stated at the meeting of the American Medical Association on June 15. The statement was made in the course of a discussion by W. V. Evans and H. H. Rowley, chemists of Northwestern University, on the dangers of poisoning from these sprays. Successful use of the spray method of fighting the boll weevil in cotton led to enormous increase in this method of fighting insect pests. Sprays began to be used in wholesale quantities in every kind of crop. The growth of truck farming has also had an influence in the increased use of sprays, because the greater concentration of foodstuffs in this type of farming led to an increase in insects. The sprays most often used contain chiefly arsenic and lead, both deadly poisons to human beings. The danger of acute poisoning is not so great as that of cumulative poisoning, which may result from consumption of these substances over long periods through the residue left on fruits and vegetables. Chemical solvents to remove the arsenical residues have been found effective. A solution of hydrochloric acid is recommended for fruits. Stripping the outer tainted leaves of such products as celery and cabbage removes the poison residue. Government workers are actively engaged in seeking non-poisonous sprays that will be as effective in protecting the crops.

## ITEMS

LONDON'S new Museum of Practical Geology had a strange début for a museum on June 12. Its construction was hastened to completion so that the fifteen hundred delegates to the world economic conference might move in. Exhibit halls have been turned into conference rooms, reception rooms and lounges for the delegates. The great central hall was the formal meeting place for the sessions, with rows of desks installed and a dais where the King of England stood on the opening day to greet the conferees. The institution which will take over the new building when the conference departs was established in 1837, through efforts of the founder of England's Geological Survey, to preserve specimens of ores and metals and gem stones collected by the survey. Its new home is a dignified structure of white stone located between the Science Museum and the Natural History Museum in South Kensington.

SUDDEN hot weather and a cessation of rains, coming on the heels of a most persistently wet, cold spring, has already undone much of the mischief wrought by the earlier unfavorable conditions, a survey by the U. S. Weather Bureau has disclosed. Over most of the grain belt states, where spring planting was held back until farmers had begun to be alarmed, the bulk of the crop is in. Farmers have put in extra long hours at the planting, in many cases working late at night. The high temperatures, ranging from 10 to 13 degrees above normal, have favored the quick germination and growth of the crops. On the basis of past records, the weather during May and to date in June should be favorable for a good yield of spring wheat.

SCIENTIFIC study of birds, which has been conducted by the Commonwealth of Massachusetts for many years, has been brought to an abrupt end by act of the Legislature, as interpreted by the Commissioner of Agriculture. The state ornithologist has been dismissed and all files containing data on birds have been placed in storage. All inquiries concerning birds, whether purely scientific or bearing on such economic aspects as game-bird distribution and habits, oil pollution and the relation of birds to special crops, will be answered only by a brief statement that the commonwealth has no information available.

WITH seven leaflets to each leaf instead of the usual three, and big in all its parts, a new giant clover species has been discovered in the state of Washington by J. W. Thompson, of Seattle. It was growing on dry sagebrush slopes near the mouth of Swakane Creek, Chelan County, Washington. Mr. Thompson sent a specimen to the U. S. National Herbarium, where it was examined by C. V. Morton. Mr. Morton found it to be a plant hitherto entirely unknown, and therefore gave it a technical description in the *Journal* of the Washington Academy of Sciences. He named it *Trifolium thompsoni*, in honor of its discoverer.

# SCIENCE NEWS

*Science Service, Washington, D. C.*

A METHOD for detecting a strange disease, argyria, in its earliest stages, was reported to the American Medical Association, meeting in Milwaukee, by Dr. Irving S. Wright, of the New York Post Graduate Medical School of Columbia University.

Argyria is a condition in which the patient turns a greyish-blue color. In the final stages the color is very pronounced, and if the patient is exposed to sunlight, his skin turns a very dark mahogany brown. The condition is becoming more common all the time. There is no way of treating it. Argyria results from taking medicines containing silver salts for a long period of time. Such medicines are often given in the treatment of nose and throat ailments. Frequently patients who have used these medicines under a physician's directions will use them again on their own initiative when suffering a repetition of the nose and throat ailment.

Formerly it was thought that the blue discoloration, which makes its first appearance around the base of the nails, was due to stoppage of the blood flow through the tiny blood vessels, the capillaries. But Dr. Wright and his associates have recently developed a microscope for observing the capillaries and watching the blood flow through them. When they used this apparatus to examine the capillaries of the nail cuticle in cases of argyria, they found that there was no stoppage of the blood flow and no evidence of congestion. This led to discovery that continued administration of silver-containing medicines results in the precipitation of silver albuminate in the tissues, which produces the blue color.

Once the color is established, there is no satisfactory remedy for the condition. But if the first appearance of it around the nails is noted and the dosage of silver-containing medicines stopped, it is believed the condition will not go farther. While the condition does not impair the health, it is most disfiguring.

Dr. Wright used the capillary microscope to examine another group of patients. These are a class in whom several observers had found that the surface of the fingers was actually colder after smoking one or several cigarettes. Dr. Wright and associates observed that in a few of these patients they could detect with the new apparatus a slowing down and occasionally a stoppage for several seconds of the blood flow in the capillaries of the nail cuticle. This accounts for the drop in temperature, but the constituent in tobacco which produces this effect is not known at present.

This and other methods of examining the blood vessels and for determining surface temperature of the hands and feet were shown in an exhibit sponsored by the association and contributed to by the New York Post Graduate Medical School, the Mayo Clinic, Northwestern University, the University of Pennsylvania, the University of California and the Presbyterian Hospital of New York. These new methods have enabled physicians to make early diagnosis of a number of diseases of the extremities formerly considered hopeless. As a result the conditions may be greatly relieved by surgical and medical treatment.

SKULL change is a new key to the past function of the gland which influences growth, sexual development and possible mentality. Studies showing this were reported by Dr. Hector Mortimer, of Boston, to the Association for the Study of Internal Secretions. It appeared from his report that the history of the functioning of an individual's pituitary gland throughout his life with all that tells of the individual's health and physical and mental development, can be read in changes in his skull that may be seen in x-ray photographs.

Four basic types of skull changes were found by Dr. Mortimer and Drs. George Levene and Allan Winter Rowe, of Boston, after a review of a collection of documented acromegalic crania in museums in America, England and Scotland. The first type is characterized by expansion of the face and sinuses, especially the frontal sinuses. This expansion changed, affecting all bones and mechanically producing the well-known deformities of acromegaly, including the large jaws. The second type is characterized by a small head, small face and very dense skull. This chiefly affects women who are usually fat, and is a sign of failure of the gland, not of over-activity as in the first type. The third type begins as a type one, with over-active gland; the gland subsequently fails and the bones become dense like old bones, even in young people of eighteen. Failure of the gland is, in other words, premature aging of the individual. The skull becoming dense, which means not that it is thick, but that it is so compact as to be almost like ivory, is an indication of failure of the gland. This is a feature of both groups two and three. In these groups there are ten times more women than men. The mechanism behind all this accounts for the fact that women age more quickly than men and are more liable to become stout. The fourth type of skull change is found in dwarfs and other persons whose pituitary gland has never been fully active. This type can be recognized by failure of the frontal and other sinuses to develop completely. In many of these persons the frontal sinuses never develop at all. This gland failure also means that the sexual development is much below par or even absent.

BONE development is now being used as a guide in treating certain children who are mentally retarded or emotionally unstable. Dr. E. Kost Shelton, of Santa Barbara, California, has found the stage of bone development, or bone age, a good index to the speed with which certain vital transformations are going on in the body. These transformations are the processes by which energy for the body's activities is obtained from the burning of food and oxygen. When these processes, called metabolism, proceed at either too fast or too slow a rate, the health is seriously affected.

Dr. Shelton found that the bone age, which can be determined by x-ray examination, is correlated with the metabolic rate, and can be used as a guide in treatment of certain types of disordered metabolism. "Any metabolic disorder in childhood, when sufficiently severe to produce mental or emotional symptoms, will be reflected in bone development." He believes that the rate of bone development is determined by the metabolic speed and therefore is the best guide to the latter. Dr. Shelton described a number of patients suffering from retarded growth and defective mental development, in whom he also found very much retarded bone growth. Treatment with extract from the thyroid gland, which speeds up the rate of metabolism, improved markedly the condition of the patients. Additions of vitamins A and D and feeding an otherwise adequate diet had no effect on metabolic speed or the developmental age.

THE death rate from one type of pneumonia can be cut in half when serum is used in treatment during the first four days of the disease, according to a report presented by Drs. Gaylord Anderson and Roderick Heffron, of Boston. They gave details of a study made by the Massachusetts State Department of Health. Pneumonia takes a terrific toll at the economic prime of life. It is practically impossible to prevent pneumonia through such measures as quarantine or vaccination. In two of the types, however, it is possible to modify the course of the disease by injection of serum during the first few days. Poor economic status with unhealthful living conditions does not influence the occurrence of pneumonia or the mortality, evidence from another phase of the study showed. Seasons, however, play an important part, according to Dr. Wilson G. Smillie, of the Harvard University School of Public Health. All types of the disease were less prevalent in the summer and early fall than in winter and spring.

IF scarlet fever antitoxin is given within the first day or two after a person has become sick with scarlet fever, the disease is much less severe and complications are less likely to develop, according to Dr. Luke W. Hunt, of Chicago. His report was based on a study of more than 2,000 cases, in nearly 900 of which the antitoxin was given. If enough antitoxin was given early, the rash faded within twenty-four hours and the fever fell several degrees. An important discovery was that the subsiding of these symptoms made it possible to find the complications which are more to be feared than the disease itself.

INFECTION of the esophagus, the canal which connects the throat with the stomach, leads to thickening of the layers of tissue in the organ. As a result, the tube may become so narrow that food can pass only with difficulty, if at all. This condition was described by Dr. Harris P. Mosher, of Boston. He demonstrated a method of determining where the thickening is and of stretching the tissues to widen the opening so that the patient may swallow comfortably. The infection may arise in the esophagus itself, or infection in other parts of the body may harm the canal. Dr. Mosher found some narrowing of the canal in persons who had pneumonia, ulcers of the stomach, infections of gallbladder, kidneys and other organs and in other conditions.

IF your shoulder has been gradually getting painful and stiff, for no apparent reason, it may be that you have torn the tendon which helps to support the shoulder joint. This tendon may be torn by a sudden jerk or by repeated strain without your knowing it at the time. Dr. E. B. Fowler, of Chicago, found 56 such ruptures in a study of 340 shoulders. Because there is little or no pain at the time of the tear, the injured shoulder is generally not seen by the physician until the patient is severely disabled. Immediate rest would probably result in complete repair of the tissue without other treatment. If rest does not relieve the condition, Dr. Fowler recommends an operation to determine whether the tendon actually is ruptured.

HOW surgeons can reattach the lining of the eye that has become separated by disease or accidental injury was told by Dr. Peter C. Kronfeld, of Chicago. In the condition known as "detached retina" the inner coat of the eye, the retina, which receives the optical image, may be partly or completely detached, with disturbance or loss of vision. The eye can be restored to nearly normal function so that the patient's vision is nearly normal, if the operation is done within a reasonably short time. The age of the patient also has a bearing on recovery, older patients being less fortunate in this respect. The condition affects color vision as well as vision in general. In the cases in which a color blindness for blue and green was noted, this defect was corrected.

A QUEER condition of sensitiveness to heat, cold or effort was demonstrated by Dr. W. W. Duke, of Kansas City, Missouri. He calls the condition physical allergy. The patients have many of the symptoms of sufferers from allergy due to pollens and food proteins. One patient became much depressed and was reduced to tears by warmth and exertion. With cold applications she got immediate relief from her depression and was seized with uncontrollable laughter. Another patient raised his arm three times and had convulsions. Relaxation and relief followed cold applications. Headache, asthma, partial blindness and skin eruptions were also caused by slight effort and relieved by cold applications. Temporary relief may be obtained by applying the opposite of what caused the attack. Permanent relief in many cases, amounting to cure, was obtained after six months of treatment.

HAY fever sufferers who have neglected to go for treatments until their pollen season has arrived and have found themselves sneezing and sniffing can still obtain relief by treatments during the season. While physicians specializing in the treatment of these disorders have for some years recommended desensitizing treatment before the hay-fever season started, the association endorsed both methods of treatment. It finds that treatment during the season gives satisfactory results with the use of air-conditioned rooms in which temperature and ventilation are regulated, as in many theaters and some trains, and gives promise of being as useful in treating hay fever and asthma as the desensitization treatments. However, this new method is still in the investigative stage. Its chief disadvantage is the high cost of installation. Patients are not advised to install such rooms in their homes for the present, until further study has established their value.

A THREE-HOUR bath in tannic acid as a feature of the modern treatment of extensive burns was described by Dr. Donald B. Wells, of Hartford, Connecticut. The use of tannic acid relieves the pain sufficiently so that the burned areas can be thoroughly cleaned. In this way infection can be prevented. Infection alone was the cause of the exhausting illness, many of the complications and a majority of the deaths from burns in the old days. The person with extensive burns is placed in a large tub of tannic acid solution, according to Dr. Wells' plan of treatment. "He receives quantities of liquids to drink, in order to balance the loss of water. As soon as his pain is somewhat relieved, several attendants begin to work. For three hours they remove burned tissue as the solution loosens it and clean unburned areas with soap and water. By the time the patient is ready to be placed in bed a tan has formed over the burned portions. Then for seventy-two hours warm air is blown on him from an ordinary hair drier, while he is more or less constantly sprayed with tannic acid solution. After this the blower is used alone until the tissue has become perfectly firm, for only a little perspiration may break it and invite invasion by germs." The method is especially successful in burns from gasoline explosions, ignited clothing and extensive scalds. It can be used in any well-equipped hospital.

BURNED faces are more numerous now as a result of the machine age than they were in war time, according to Dr. Howard L. Updegraff, of Hollywood, California. Dr. Updegraff described the methods by which burned faces are restored and reconstructed. Surgery plays an important part, but chemistry and gland treatment are helpful and the final procedure is instruction in the use of make-up. For this purpose a professional make-up artist is employed in Dr. Updegraff's hospital. The instruction in the use of make-up has brought about a great improvement in the mental attitude of the patients, many of whom naturally feel that their fate is hopeless. Before the make-up artist starts instructions, however, the surgeon has done his work, which begins by study of old and new photographs of the face. Plaster models are also used. The actual operative work is usually delayed until the burns have healed. Eyelids are made from skin from another portion of the body. The membranous lining of the lid is supplied by taking a graft from the mucous membrane lining of the mouth. Eyebrows and even lashes are made from pieces of scalp. Noses, lips and ears are also reconstructed.

THREE means of controlling and preventing outbreaks of food poisoning were suggested by Dr. J. C. Geiger, San Francisco director of public health. First of the three measures is regulation and supervision of all persons who handle food. Second is thorough inspection of plants where food is prepared. Third, and most essential to real control of the situation, is education of the public. Food poisoning is as definitely preventable as smallpox or diphtheria. Yet, like those two diseases, it continues to occur because preventive measures are neglected. While outbreaks of food poisonings are so frequent as to constitute a challenge to students of public health and preventive medicine, Dr. Geiger believes that only a small proportion of the cases that actually occur are reported.

DR. PHILIP B. MATZ, of the U. S. Veterans' Administration, Washington, stated that gas warfare is the most humane of the methods of warfare. He pointed out that of 70,752 casualties as a result of gas in the American forces during the war, only 200 died immediately. The results of a careful investigation of the clinical records of nearly 500 men gassed by various gases were presented. Most serious after affects appeared in cases of gassing with phosgene. In this group a number of cases of nervous and mental ailments as well as lung diseases developed. The gas was not directly responsible for the mental ailments, but its severe effect on the individual man, particularly the swelling of the lungs which interfered with breathing, provided the exciting factor in persons with a constitutional defect of brain and nervous system.

ALTHOUGH the American Medical Association is opposed to state medicine, it was pointed out at one of its sessions that during the present economic situation we are actually having a modified form of state medicine. Fifteen per cent., almost one sixth, of the families in New York State, exclusive of New York City, are receiving medical care through state aid, according to a statement made by Dr. Thomas Parran, Jr., N. Y. State health officer. In addition to comprehensive health laws for the prevention of disease, the types of care now given by government agencies include treatment of mental disease through a system of hospitals; child guidance clinics and clinics for after-care; treatment of tuberculosis; care and treatment of crippled children; the construction and operation of public general hospitals; physical examination and corrective treatment of school children; treatment of venereal disease; state and local diagnostic laboratory service, and the state-wide program for furnishing general medical care as a necessity of life as part of emergency unemployment relief.

# SCIENCE NEWS

*Science Service, Washington, D. C.*

## PAPERS READ BEFORE THE CHICAGO MEETINGS OF THE AMERICAN ASSOCIATION FOR THE ADVANCEMENT OF SCIENCE

MAN'S superior brain makes it possible for him to live in a world of extreme kinds of weather and other varying conditions, according to Professor James Barcroft, the British physiologist, a Century of Progress guest. The highly evolved brain of the human being holds unconscious control of his blood's chemistry and physics. The resulting constancy of his blood conditions make him relatively independent of heat, cold and other changes in the outside world that hamper the lives of his less fortunate lower animal kin. In the evolution of life, as pictured by Professor Barcroft, efforts of the lowest organisms to make themselves more at home in the world were at first aimed merely at so arranging their own lives that outside conditions would be less hard on them. They did not make much progress at changing and controlling their own internal conditions. Higher in the evolutionary scale, Professor Barcroft believes that the first steps toward internal regulation were chemical. Then control by the nervous system began to assert itself until finally the brain became dominant in maintaining the continuing uniformity of the blood.

PROFESSOR C. U. ARIENS KAPPERS, of the Central Dutch Institute for Brain Research, Amsterdam, told of researches that upset the old idea that the shape of the skull is always determined by the growth of the brain in its earlier stages. He has found that the skull often determines the shape and size of the brain. The small brain of a fish has plenty of room, even in the small space allowed it in the fish's skull. On the other hand, the bird's skull compels the brain it contains to fold and pack itself closely to make use of relatively limited space. Similarly among human races the various skull types—long, medium and broad—have been shown to influence the arrangement of the parts of the brain. There is, however, as yet no evidence that this influence of skull on brain makes any one race superior to another.

POTENTIAL food substances equivalent to twenty thousand times the wheat harvest of the world are dissolved in the waters of the Atlantic Ocean, according to Dr. August Krogh, the Danish zoologist. This immense amount of organic material is wasted unless it is found that, as some investigators have suggested, bacteria and microorganisms, as yet unrecognized but possibly existing in the depths of the sea, are turning it into food that larger units of sea life can eat and thus utilize.

HEREDITY is not a matter of chromosomes and genes alone. The jelly or protoplasm of the cell that surrounds these specialized living bits within the cell has much to do with whether people are tall or short, blonde or brunette. Professor Richard Goldschmidt, of Berlin's Kaiser Wilhelm Institute for Biology, reported that experiments on lower animals show that the cytoplasm, or bulk of the cell, has a distinctly modifying action on the genes, or chromosome units, that American research in the past three decades has shown to be the bearers of heredity. Genes give orders, but Dr. Goldschmidt's conception is that the surrounding cytoplasm does not always stick to the ordered plan, but acts like craftsmen who sometimes insert their own innovations.

WHEN motion stops, the organism is dead. This is the thesis of the French biologist, Dr. Jean Dufrénoy, of Bordeaux, who explained that within the living plants and animals that we consider the most stationary and motionless there is a ceaseless and intense motion of the protoplasmic jelly that makes up their cells. The more alive a cell is, the more furious is its motion, presenting a large surface to the nourishing sap or liquid. When death comes, three things happen: The protoplasm stops moving, its surface decreases markedly, its smooth unmarked granules break up into granules that can be seen only with the powerful ultramicroscope.

DR. EMILIO MIRA, of the University of Barcelona, Spain, speaking before the psychologists, stated that fear, rage and affection are the three basic human emotions that form the foundation of human moral behavior types. Fear gives rise to moral systems that express themselves in prohibitions and compulsions. Among children and people of low evolutionary level such systems are most fully developed. Rage induces the morals of anarchy and focuses upon material pleasures. True and human morality, in Dr. Mira's definition, is based on the third emotional state of affection.

THE Tropics would be hotter than they are and the Polar regions would be colder, were it not for the fact that there is an immense aerial interchange of heat in the winds, according to Professor J. Bjerknes, Norwegian meteorologist, also a guest of the Century of Progress. The most heat from the sun arrives upon earth in the equatorial zones and the least at the poles. The equatorial zone receives more heat than it radiates away and the polar caps receive less than they lose. The air transport system used by the Tropics in sending their surplus heat to the Arctic and Antarctic is the winds. Professor Bjerknes computed that it would take 303 millions of tons of air traveling across latitude thirty degrees to do this. Large as this sounds, the wind need travel only about six feet a second. Professor Bjerknes visualizes the atmosphere dividing itself into sections that can be called compartments and each maintaining its own circulation, with the usual trade winds nearer the surface and in some cases an anti-trade wind rushing along much higher. To get more information on just how and when the winds blow to equalize the heat on the earth, Professor Bjerknes urged investigators to send up sounding balloons with radio reporting weather instruments to signal what is happening in the regions above the Tropics.

FOR the first time in history "H" has been knocked out of matter by artificial means. The "H" in this case stands for hydrogen. The ejection of a proton, or hydrogen heart, from a collision between a heavy-weight hydrogen atomic heart and a carbon atom, reported by Professor E. O. Lawrence, of the University of California, is considered an important step forward in our knowledge of the constitution of matter and its relation to energy. Professor Lawrence, with his unique "merry-go-round" magnetic device for accelerating atomic projectiles, hurled some of the newly discovered double-weight hydrogen atoms at carbon of mass twelve. The carbon gained one unit of mass, or weight, and a hydrogen atom of ordinary weight was expelled in the form of a proton. One and a half million volts was fed into this synthesis and seven and a half million volts were emitted, which is a large release of energy. About two decades ago Lord Rutherford, in England, was the first to perform an atomic synthesis and knock "H" out of matter. He used the streams of helium atomic hearts, or alpha particles, that are released in the radioactivity of radium and other elements. Professor Lawrence's success in performing synthetic transmutation of a heavier element out of a lighter one with significant release of energy is an important new development.

NEW successes in a new method of element transmutation were announced by Dr. J. D. Cockcroft, from the Cavendish Laboratory, at Cambridge. The idea that atomic particles have wave-like properties and can force themselves into the hearts of atoms led to atom smashing that released very large amounts of energy. Lord Rutherford's first transmutations two decades ago were atom building without energy release. Dr. Cockcroft first turned lithium and a projected hydrogen heart into two helium atoms. Now he announced the disintegration of boron into three helium atoms, the breaking up of fluorine into oxygen and helium and the change of beryllium into lithium and helium when bombarded with hydrogen.

DR. THEODOR SVEDBERG, of Sweden, a recipient of a Nobel prize in chemistry, told how he had used the ultra-centrifuge, which is a scientific spinning top, to discover how many weights of proteins there are in blood serum. A few drops of blood and other complex substances, such as dyes, carbohydrates and hydrocarbons, whirled with 300,000 times the force of gravity, are separated, although the kinds of materials in them are extremely close to being the same weight. Dr. Svedberg photographs the substances while they revolve at high speeds. Living organisms can survive the terrific pull upon them in an ultra-whirling top, a force nearly three million times that to which our bodies are subjected by the ordinary force of gravity, as shown by experiments made at Stanford University.

EXPLANATION for the long-known but little understood tendency of wild plants to "sport" new varieties freely when introduced into cultivation, which they rarely or never do so long as they are in the natural state, was advanced before the botanists by Sir Daniel Hall, director of the John Innes Horticultural Institution. An earlier theory, accepted by Charles Darwin, held that plants were somehow encouraged to produce these new varieties by the better nourishment and care they got under cultivation. This theory made environment dominant over heredity. Sir Daniel held that the true explanation is to be sought elsewhere. Many, perhaps all, wild species bear within their germ-cells some of these varying traits, but they are "recessive" characters and are masked by their corresponding "dominants," also present. Whenever, by any thousand-to-one chance, a seed is formed that might produce a variant plant if it grew, the chances are still heavily against its reaching full growth; for in nature hundreds or even thousands of seeds are scattered for every one that grows. Furthermore, the chances are always that a new departure will have less "survival value" in the evolutionary struggle than the old, conservative original pattern, which has proved its worth against stern competition. So in the natural plant population the recessives stay buried. But when a gardener brings a wild species into his breeding ground, he first eliminates the chances against the seeds. Instead of only one in a thousand being allowed to reach maturity, something like nine hundred in a thousand are encouraged to grow. Thus the chance recessive combinations have an opportunity to come out and be seen. If they happen to be something that the gardener thinks is valuable—new color in the petals, new flavor in the fruit—he will single them out and inbreed them, preventing the re-masking by dominant characters that would be their fate in the cross-breeding of the wild state. Moreover, the gardener is not concerned at all with the natural "survival value" of an emerging character. He will shield the most ill-adapted plant, against all competition and enemies, if it has something he wants. If he happens to be a scientist rather than a commercial gardener, he will help even the most crippled and misfit plants to breed, should they promise biological information. In this combination of the encouragement of all seeds to develop to full growth, and the discouragement of re-immersion in the type and the checking of the ruthless course of natural selection, human choice gives the "recessives" repressed in nature their opportunity to express themselves. This does not preclude the arising of wholly new "mutations" in the cultivated stock, which were not present in the germ-plasm of the wild plants. These brand-new variations also occur, especially when encouraged to do so by such modern artificial means as x-raying or radium treatment. But these new mutations are much rarer than the segregation of the recessive characters that were always there but never had a chance.

DEATH is a great parting, not only between him who dies and his friends, but between the most intimately united parts of the microscopic cells of the body. When death comes, the constituents of the protoplasm part company. How this is seen in the dying cells of plants was described by Dr. Jean Dufrénoy, of the Plant Pathology Station at Brive, France. Living protoplasm, Dr. Dufrénoy said, is smooth, uniform, without even ultramicroscopically visible markings. As it streams around the cell, the only way its progress can be marked is by watching certain foreign bodies included in it, such as crystals and oil droplets. These show its movements as chips on the surface and loose pebbles on the bottom show the current of a crystal-clear brook. But when death comes, all is changed. The flow of the protoplasm slows down and stops, and the highest powers of the microscope disclose the appearance of numberless granules—the sure sign that the once uniformly assimilated substance has broken down and separated into distinct and unlike parts. While a cell is living, Dr. Dufrénoy continued, all its vital activities are carried on at the various surfaces of its protoplasm, where they front on its sap cavity, oil droplets, etc. Its chemistry is all surface chemistry. An outstanding exchange, indispensable to the continued life of the cell, is the taking up of oxygen and the voiding of carbon dioxide. The more active the cell, the more surface it exposes for this and other chemical exchanges, by throwing out extra folds and filaments of its protoplasm. But there can be too much of a good thing, in plants as well as in human beings and animals. Dr. Dufrénoy described a condition seen in the cells of plants afflicted with certain diseases, where there is an excessive development of these oxygen-exchanging protoplasmic surfaces. An examination of the respiration of such plants shows it to be much in excess of that of healthy plants: the sick plants are suffering from a real fever.

TWENTY thousand pairs of photographs were taken at the University of Chicago to show what occurs when an atomic nucleus is disintegrated when it is struck by a neutron—an atom of zero atomic number and zero electrical charge. So Professor William D. Harkins told the American Physical Society. Among the results of this long research, Professor Harkins enumerated the following: The slowest neutron which disintegrated an atomic nucleus had a velocity of 11,000 miles per second. The highest velocity for any neutron was found to be 35,000 miles per second, or about one fifth the velocity of light. This is an extremely great velocity for a particle of the mass of an atom. The energy of this neutron was extremely high, 16,000,000 electron volts, or very much higher than could be obtained by any artificial means now known. The mean velocity of the neutrons which disintegrated nitrogen nuclei was found to correspond to a temperature of 46 billion degrees. Such a temperature is not attained except possibly in the interior of a star. Since nothing is known by astronomers about the temperature of the interior of a star, except that it is very high, anything may be assumed. The nuclei of nitrogen atoms were found to disintegrate relatively often, while those of carbon and neon are very much more difficult to disintegrate. Evidence was obtained that the neutron, when it causes the disintegration of an atom is itself captured by the nucleus of the atom, but no good evidence was obtained to show that any disintegration can occur if the neutron is not captured. It was found that when an atom is disintegrated by the impact of a neutron, energy disappears, and gamma-rays, a very penetrating form of radiation, much more penetrating than x-rays, are given off. A new apparatus has been built for the photography of atomic disintegrations or syntheses. During the last day of operation this apparatus gave 6,400 pairs of photographs of excellent quality. Two motion picture machines are used to take the photographs, and to aid in the mathematical analysis of the photographs. Professor Harkins has suggested the name Neuton for this new element made up of all of the free neutrons in the universe. This is in many ways the most remarkable of all of the elements, since it is as different from all the others as the number zero is different from all positive whole numbers.

BRIGHT light "cures" nerve tissue poisoned with carbon monoxide in much the same manner that oxygen revives nerve tissue asphyxiated by oxygen starvation. This was announced by Professor Herbert Gasser, of Cornell University Medical College. When a nerve is stimulated it develops a sudden high charge or potential of electricity which comes and passes in a few thousandths of a second. This is followed by a longer period of milder electrification called the "after-potential." This potential can be diminished by various types of poisoning including carbon monoxide and asphyxiation. The after-potential is not only restored to normal but is raised above the usual level by the light or oxygen "cures."